Heparin-Induced Thrombocytopenia
Fifth Edition

Edited by

Theodore E. Warkentin

*Michael G. DeGroote School of Medicine, McMaster University,
and Hamilton Regional Laboratory Medicine Program,
Hamilton, Ontario, Canada*

Andreas Greinacher

*Universitätsmedizin, Ernst-Moritz-Arndt-Universität Greifswald,
Greifswald, Germany*

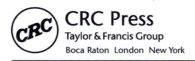

CRC Press
Taylor & Francis Group
Boca Raton London New York

CRC Press is an imprint of the
Taylor & Francis Group, an **informa** business

CRC Press
Taylor & Francis Group
6000 Broken Sound Parkway NW, Suite 300
Boca Raton, FL 33487-2742

© 2013 by Taylor & Francis Group, LLC
CRC Press is an imprint of Taylor & Francis Group, an Informa business

No claim to original U.S. Government works

Typeset by Exeter Premedia Services Pvt Ltd, Chennai, India
Printed in the United Kingdom on acid-free paper
Version Date: 20121015

ISBN: 978-1-84184-860-0 (Hardback); 978-1-84184-861-7 (eBook)

Visit the Taylor & Francis Web site at
http://www.taylorandfrancis.com

and the CRC Press Web site at
http://www.crcpress.com

To the late Professor Michael F. X. Glynn, for initiating my hemostasis interests; to Dr. John G. Kelton, for amplifying these through boundless opportunities; and to Erica, Andrew, Erin, and Nathan, for downregulating my passion, as a caring family must.

—T.E.W.

To my co-workers and students for their contributions and efforts; to Sabine, Sebastian, Anja, and Jan.

—A.G.

Contents

Contributors

Jean Amiral Hyphen Biomed Research, Zac Neuville-Université, Neuville-Sur-Oise, France

Susanne Alban Christian-Albrechts-University of Kiel, Kiel, Germany

Gowthami M. Arepally Duke University Medical Center, Durham, North Carolina, USA

John R. Bartholomew Cleveland Clinic, Cleveland, Ohio, USA

Martin Beiderlinden Marienhospital, Osnabrück, Germany

Beng Hock Chong St. George Hospital and University of New South Wales, Kogarah, New South Wales, Australia

Douglas B. Cines Perelman School of Medicine at the University of Pennsylvania, Philadelphia, Pennsylvania, USA

Adam Cuker Perelman School of Medicine at the University of Pennsylvania, Philadelphia, Pennsylvania, USA

Gregory A. Denomme BloodCenter of Wisconsin, Milwaukee, Wisconsin, USA

John W. Eikelboom Michael G. DeGroote School of Medicine, McMaster University, Hamilton, Ontario, Canada

Andreas Greinacher Universitätsmedizin, Ernst-Moritz-Arndt-Universität Greifswald, Greifswald, Germany

McDonald K. Horne III Retired, formerly of Warren G. Magnuson Clinical Center, National Institutes of Health, Bethesda, Maryland, USA

Marcie J. Hursting Clinical Science Consulting, Austin, Texas, USA

Anne F. Klenner Universitätsmedizin, Ernst-Moritz-Arndt-Universität Greifswald, Greifswald, Germany

Andreas Koster Ruhr Universität Bochum, Bad Oeynhausen, Germany

Krystin Krauel Universitätsmedizin, Ernst-Moritz-Arndt-Universität Greifswald, Greifswald, Germany

David H. Lee Queen's University, Kingston, Ontario, Canada

Lori-Ann Linkins Michael G. DeGroote School of Medicine, McMaster University, Hamilton, Ontario, Canada

Harry N. Magnani Medical Consultant, Oss, The Netherlands

Steven E. McKenzie Thomas Jefferson University, Philadelphia, Pennsylvania, USA

Mortimer Poncz The Children's Hospital of Philadelphia, and Perelman School of Medicine at the University of Pennsylvania, Philadelphia, Pennsylvania, USA

Jayne Prats The Medicines Company, Parsippany, New Jersey, USA

Lubica Rauova The Children's Hospital of Philadelphia and Perelman School of Medicine at the University of Pennsylvania, Philadelphia, Pennsylvania, USA

Lawrence Rice The Methodist Hospital, Houston, Texas, USA

Bruce S. Sachais Perelman School of Medicine at the University of Pennsylvania, Philadelphia, Pennsylvania, USA

Sixten Selleng Ernst-Moritz-Arndt-Universität Greifswald, Greifswald, Germany

Anne Marie Vissac Hyphen Biomed Research, Zac Neuville-Université, Neuville-Sur-Oise, France

Theodore E. Warkentin Michael G. DeGroote School of Medicine, McMaster University and Hamilton Regional Laboratory Medicine Program, Hamilton, Ontario, Canada

Preface

The first edition of *Heparin-Induced Thrombocytopenia* appeared 13 years ago. Even then we were asked: *Why write a book about HIT?* After all, heparin use will progressively diminish, and so correspondingly will incidents of HIT. Yet, both of us continue to see patients with HIT regularly in our own practices, and every week our reference laboratories confirm the presence of platelet-activating anti-platelet factor 4 (PF4)/heparin antibodies in several new patients referred from other hospitals.

We continue to learn new aspects of HIT treatment. For example, "PTT confounding" describes the situation where systematic interruption and underdosing of partial thromboplastin time (PTT)-adjusted direct thrombin inhibitor (DTI) therapy occurs in a patient with HIT who has concomitant coagulopathy, potentially resulting in treatment failure; avoiding this problem with (non-PTT-adjusted) danaparoid (and possibly also fondaparinux) therapy illustrates one of the new treatment concepts that first appears in this fifth edition.

Patients with ventricular assist devices—including "bridge to transplant" candidates—are at highest risk for HIT. If this reaction occurs, the concept of using heparin for subsequent cardiac transplantation—as long as the functional assay is negative, and even if the antigen assay is still positive—is another important result of recent HIT research.

New ideas regarding pathogenesis have emerged: HIT plausibly represents a misdirected antimicrobial immune response, as the key immunogen (PF4) binds not only to heparin but also to bacteria, thereby triggering a "presensitizing" anti-PF4/heparin immune response. Indeed, the rare occurrences of HIT in unusual clinical settings—such as post-infection or after orthopedic surgery performed without heparin use (so-called "spontaneous" HIT)—or perhaps even as a consequence of heparin adulterated with oversulfated chondroitin sulfate—illustrate new aspects of HIT immunopathogenesis.

The growing recognition of heparin-*in*dependent platelet-activating properties of some HIT antibodies—and their transience—helps explain certain unusual presentations such as "delayed-onset" HIT. This phenomenon also accounts for misattribution of heparin-bonded vascular grafts as a cause of HIT post-vascular surgery; in this situation, the more likely explanation is the unusual "autoimmune-like" nature of the HIT antibodies themselves.

Newer, rapid immunoassays to detect HIT antibodies are being developed, but to avoid HIT "overdiagnosis", the importance of quantitative interpretation of immunoassays and of testing for platelet-activating antibodies remains central for correct diagnosis.

Since the fourth edition, fondaparinux has emerged as a rational—and simple—therapy for HIT that might presage future success with the *new* oral anticoagulants (e.g., rivaroxaban, apixaban, dabigatran). This is in marked contrast to the *old* oral anticoagulants—warfarin and other vitamin K antagonists—which are *contraindicated* for managing acute HIT because of their propensity to precipitate microthrombosis and limb gangrene. Partially desulfated heparin, which binds to PF4 despite having minimal anticoagulant activity, has the potential to reduce risk of HIT when given together with heparin.

These and numerous other paradoxes and myths concerning HIT are of importance to clinicians who encounter thrombocytopenic patients in diverse clinical settings.

SPECIAL THANKS

A multi-author book depends on many contributors. For us, as editors, it was a delight to produce this fifth edition with many of our colleagues throughout the world. We want to acknowledge the publishing team (Manoj Arun, Oscar Heini, and Claire Bonnett), and also Erin Warkentin for the cover art. In Hamilton, we would like to thank Maria Adamek, Jo-Ann Sheppard, James Smith, Jane Moore, Carol Smith, Diana Moffatt, Aurelio Santos, Rumi Clare, Ishac Nazi, Donnie Arnold, Menaka Pai, Peter Horsewood, and John Kelton; in Greifswald, gratitude is owed to Uta Alpen, Sixten and Kathleen Selleng, Tamam Bakchoul, Thomas Thiele, Gregor Hron, Ariane Sümnig, Birgitt Fürll, Ulrike Strobel, Ricarda Raschke, and Carmen Blumentritt, for their invaluable technical and administrative support, for ideas and discussions, and especially for being part of the team dedicated to research in HIT.

Theodore E. Warkentin
Andreas Greinacher

1 History of heparin-induced thrombocytopenia

Theodore E. Warkentin

THE DISCOVERY OF HEPARIN AND ITS FIRST CLINICAL USE

The following account of the discovery and first clinical development of heparin was recorded by the physiologist Best (1959), a codiscoverer of insulin as well as a pioneer in the studies of heparin. Incidentally, in 1916, while working at Johns Hopkins University to characterize procoagulant substances, McLean (1916) identified a natural anticoagulant substance. Further studies of this material were performed by his supervisor, Dr. Howell, who coined the term, "heparin" to indicate its first extraction from animal hepatic tissues (Gr. ἥπαρ [hepar], liver) (Howell and Holt, 1918). Despite its *in vitro* anticoagulant action, the inability of heparin to prevent platelet-mediated thrombosis (Shionoya, 1927) made it uncertain whether it had antithrombotic potential. However, animal (Mason, 1924) and human studies (Crafoord, 1937) showed that heparin could prevent thrombosis. By the 1950s, heparin was established as an important therapeutic agent in the treatment of venous and arterial thrombosis.

THE PARADOX OF HEPARIN AS A POSSIBLE CAUSE OF THROMBOSIS
Weismann and Tobin

On June 1, 1957, at the Fifth Scientific Meeting of the International Society of Angiology (North American Chapter) in New York, two physicians suggested that heparin might cause arterial embolism in some patients. Rodger E. Weismann, a 43-year-old Assistant Professor of Clinical Surgery at the Dartmouth Medical School (Fig. 1.1), and his Resident in Surgery, Dr. Richard W. Tobin, presented their 3-year experience with 10 patients who developed unexpected peripheral arterial embolism during systemic heparin therapy at the Mary Hitchcock Memorial Hospital, in Hanover, New Hampshire. Their first patient with this complication was reported in detail, and to this day represents a classic description of the syndrome:

> This 62-yr-old white woman was admitted to the Hitchcock Hospital Feb 8, 1955, with left retinal detachment, complicating longstanding myopia ... Left scleral buckling was carried out on Feb 10, and strict bed rest was required during the ensuing 3 wk. On her beginning ambulation, on March 6, signs and symptoms of left iliofemoral thrombophlebitis were noted, for which systemic heparinization was begun (... heparin sodium in divided subcutaneous doses, totaling 150–300 mg per day...). On March 16, after 10 days of anticoagulation therapy, sudden signs of right common femoral arterial occlusion led to the diagnosis of common femoral arterial embolism. Successful femoral embolectomy was carried out. She was kept on adequate heparinization and made a satisfactory initial recovery until March 19, ... when signs of sudden occlusion of the distal aorta appeared.

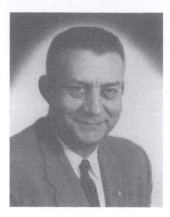

FIGURE 1.1   Photograph of Dr. Rodger Elmer Weismann, taken *circa* 1958.

... [P]rompt transperitoneal distal aortic and bilateral iliac embolectomies were performed. In the ensuing 24 h, because unsatisfactory distal circulation persisted, the patient underwent left femoral exploration, with negative findings, and right popliteal exploration, revealing an embolus. She subsequently pursued a favorable course, ... never showing more serious ischemic changes than a small area of superficial gangrene of the right great toe and several small areas of skin infarction of the right leg (Weismann and Tobin, 1958).

The report included a photograph of the emboli removed from the distal aorta and both iliac arteries, with the authors noting their "unusual length and cylindrical shape, suggesting origin in [the] proximal aorta," as well as a corresponding photomicrograph of the embolus. The thromboemboli were described by the authors as "pale, soft, salmon-colored clots" that "histologically ... were comprised mostly of fibrin, platelets and leukocytes; red cells were rare." This appearance was distinguishable from the typical appearance of thrombi originating in the heart (i.e., mulberry-colored thrombi tending to contain cellular elements of the blood in approximately normal proportions), leading the authors to propose "the source for the emboli ... to be aortic mural platelet-fibrin thrombi."

A summary of the 10 reported patients noted that the onset of arterial embolism began between 7 and 15 days, inclusive, of commencing heparin treatment (mean, day 10). Multiple thromboemboli occurred in nine patients; six of the patients died as a direct result of these complications; two survived with extensive amputations, and two were discharged with their extremities intact. The temporal time frame was consistent with the later realization by others that this syndrome represented an immune-mediated reaction initiated by the heparin.

The authors noted that further embolization stopped when the heparin was discontinued, leading to their recommendation that "heparin should be promptly reduced in dosage, and, if possible, discontinued if the presence of fibrin-platelet thrombi adherent to the intima of the aorta is suspected." Aggressive surgical management of emboli was also recommended, as some limbs were salvageable in this way. The authors summarized well the clinical dilemma: "In each instance there was a feeling of futility in the management of the problem, due to anticipation of further emboli from the same or similar sources. Heparin was badly needed to retard distal thrombosis; yet the agent was probably seriously altering the integrity and attachment of the thrombotic source" (Weismann and Tobin, 1958).

Roberts and Colleagues

The communication of Weismann and Tobin was met with considerable skepticism. When a show of hands was elicited to indicate those surgeons who had also observed similar events, none was raised (Weismann, personal communication, July 1998). However, a few years later, Roberts and colleagues from the University of Pennsylvania in Philadelphia described a series of patients who were remarkably similar to those reported by Weismann and Tobin (Roberts et al., 1964; Barker et al., 1966; Kaupp and Roberts, 1972). The key features were summarized as follows:

> To witness a series of apparently paradoxical events is disconcerting as well as challenging. When such paradoxes involve totally unexpected results following the use of a major therapeutic agent, it is at first difficult to know whether the relationship is causal or merely coincidental. When, however, the same series of events has been seen repeatedly it is difficult to escape the conclusion that there is some causal relationship, even though the mechanism by which it is accomplished may be unknown ... . During the last 9 yr at the Hospital of the University of Pennsylvania, we have seen a group of 11 patients who suffered unexplained arterial embolization for the first time while being treated with heparin for some condition that could not of itself reasonably be expected to cause arterial emboli ... . All patients had been receiving heparin for 10 days or more when the initial embolus occurred ... . All emboli removed were of a light color, seemingly made up primarily of fibrin and platelets, and microscopically appeared to be relatively free of red cells. All patients in this group had multiple emboli ... . Of the four deaths, three were attributed to cerebral vascular accidents presumably embolic in origin and one was thought to have resulted from a perforation of the small bowel 2 wk after the removal of a mesenteric embolus (Roberts et al., 1964).

Roberts' group also viewed the likely pathogenesis as that of embolization of platelet–fibrin-rich material originating within the aorta, rather than the heart. Furthermore, they believed that the thrombi were initially formed on aortic ulcerations that acted as a nidus for thrombus formation. This pathogenesis was suggested by the observation that such adherent thrombi could be removed from the proximal aorta in a few of the patients (Roberts et al., 1964; Kaupp and Roberts, 1972).

An Immune Basis for Heparin-Induced Thrombosis?

The delay between initiation of heparin therapy and onset of embolization caused Roberts and colleagues (1964) to speculate that the etiology could represent an "antiheparin factor," resulting perhaps from "an antigen–antibody mechanism." Furthermore, the observation that the first 21 patients reported with this syndrome from both Hanover and Philadelphia had received heparin exclusively by subcutaneous or intramuscular, rather than intravenous, injection also was offered by Roberts' group as support for immune sensitization. Apparent heparin-induced thrombosis did not seem rare to these investigators: at least 13 of 110 (12%) patients with peripheral arterial emboli managed by the Philadelphia group over a decade were believed to have been caused by preceding heparin treatment (Barker et al., 1966).

HEPARIN-INDUCED THROMBOCYTOPENIA AND PARADOXICAL THROMBOSIS

Heparin-Induced Thrombocytopenia

Routine platelet count measurements were not a feature of hospital laboratory practice until the 1970s, and neither the Hanover nor Philadelphia surgeons reported thrombocytopenia in their patients with heparin-induced arterial thrombosis. Ironically, the first report of severe heparin-induced thrombocytopenia (HIT) involved a patient who did not develop paradoxical thrombosis. Natelson and coworkers (1969) reported on a 78-year-old man with prostate carcinoma and pulmonary embolism (PE), who on day 10 of treatment with therapeutic-dose heparin developed severe thrombocytopenia. Three days after discontinuing the heparin therapy, the patient's fibrinogen level dropped to 1 g/L, attributed to carcinoma-associated disseminated intravascular coagulation (DIC). Heparin treatment was restarted, and although fibrinogen levels normalized, the platelet count reduced to 5×10^9/L, rising to 115×10^9/L six days after stopping heparin administration. Simultaneously, however, the fibrinogen value fell to less than 0.5 g/L. When heparin was given for the third time, the platelet count fell over two days to 10×10^9/L, although the fibrinogen values again normalized. *In vitro* studies showed that heparin added to the patient's citrated platelet-rich plasma produced platelet count reductions. This early report of severe HIT is interesting, as it illustrates the dichotomy of heparin reproducibly producing severe thrombocytopenia while maintaining anticoagulant activity (correction of DIC). However, it remained for later workers to link thrombocytopenia and thrombosis to heparin therapy.

Rhodes, Dixon, and Silver: "HIT with Thrombotic and Hemorrhagic Manifestations"

Laboratory evidence implicating an immune basis for HIT was first provided by studies performed by a vascular surgeon (Donald Silver; Fig. 1.2), together with a hematology resident (R. H. Dixon) and a medical student (Glen R. Rhodes),

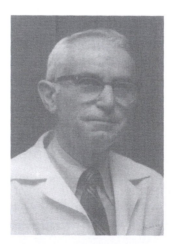

FIGURE 1.2 Photograph of Dr. Donald Silver, taken *circa* 1975.

who subsequently became a vascular surgeon. The first two patients described by Silver's group (Rhodes et al., 1973) developed severe thrombocytopenia (platelet count nadirs, 8 and 10×10^9/L), myocardial infarction, petechiae, and heparin resistance, with complete platelet count recovery on discontinuing heparin treatment.

Both patients developed rapid recurrence of thrombocytopenia when heparin rechallenges were given within 1 week of platelet count recovery.

The immune basis of this syndrome was suggested by several laboratory observations. First, increased platelet consumption was suggested by increased numbers of marrow megakaryocytes, as well as immediate recurrence of thrombocytopenia on reexposure to heparin. Second, a circulating platelet-activating substance was found in both the patients' blood: patient, but not control, serum resulted in aggregation of normal donor platelets in the presence of heparin (Fig. 1.3). Third, the possible identity of the aggregating agent as an immunoglobulin G (IgG) was shown by fractionation of one patient's serum to show the presence of heparin-dependent, complement-fixing activities within the IgG fraction.

A second report from this group (Rhodes et al., 1977) represented the landmark study in establishing HIT as a distinct syndrome. Eight patients were reported with thrombocytopenia that occurred during intravenous therapeutic-dose or subcutaneous prophylactic-dose heparin. The mean platelet count nadir was 25 (range, $5–54 \times 10^9$/L). The predominance of thrombotic, rather than hemorrhagic, complications was demonstrated: seven patients had new or recurrent thromboembolic events, and the remaining patient had a stroke leading to evacuation of a temporal lobe hematoma. Complement-fixing, heparin-dependent antibodies were identified in five of the patients. The authors also cited the previous works by Weismann and Tobin (1958) and Roberts and colleagues (1964) as likely representing the identical syndrome. Thus, for the first time, the concept of an immune-mediated hypercoagulable state, with a predisposition to arterial thromboembolism that occurred in association with thrombocytopenia, was proposed.

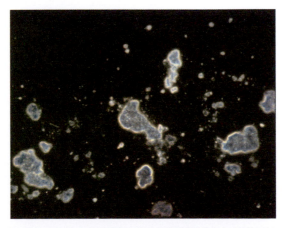

FIGURE 1.3 Heparin-induced thrombocytopenia antibody–induced platelet aggregates from an experiment in the early 1970s. Magnification approximately 250–500x. Photomicrograph provided by Dr. Glen R. Rhodes, Palmyra, VA. *Source*: From Warkentin (2011a).

Platelet-Activating Antibodies in the Pathogenesis of HIT

Although some limited studies of heparin-dependent platelet aggregation by patient serum were performed in the classic paper by Rhodes and colleagues (1973), the next few years saw increasing emphasis on this characteristic feature of HIT antibodies. In 1975, National Institutes of Health investigators Fratantoni et al. described a patient who developed severe thrombocytopenia ($4 \times 10^9/L$) and PE while receiving therapeutic-dose unfractionated heparin (UFH) to treat deep vein thrombosis (DVT). Recurrent thrombocytopenia resulted following heparin rechallenge. The patient's serum produced both aggregation and serotonin release from normal platelets in the presence of heparin. The platelet-activating factor was presumed, but not proved, to be caused by an antibody.

During the next 5 years, at least eight groups of investigators reported similar patients, confirming the presence of heparin-dependent, platelet-activating antibodies (Babcock et al., 1976; Green et al., 1978; Nelson et al., 1978; Trowbridge et al., 1978; Wahl et al., 1978; Cimo et al., 1979; Hussey et al., 1979; Cines et al., 1980). Babcock and colleagues (1976) described five patients who developed thrombocytopenia (mean platelet count nadir, $28 \times 10^9/L$) during heparin treatment; heparin-dependent antibodies were detected that produced platelet factor 3 activity (i.e., patient globulin fractions incubated with heparin, platelet-rich plasma, and celite-activated contact product shortened the clotting time following recalcification). Three patients developed thrombotic complications, and none developed hemorrhage. The five patients were observed within a 6-week time span, leading the authors to suggest that "this syndrome may occur more often than has previously been suspected."

A consistent theme was evident from these various reports. Patients developed arterial or venous thrombotic complications, in association with thrombocytopenia, that generally began after five or more days of heparin treatment. A platelet-activating antibody that aggregated platelets suspended in citrated plasma was usually detected. The platelet count nadirs seen in some of the larger series (e.g., 33 and $48 \times 10^9/L$, respectively) observed by Cimo et al. (1979) and Hussey et al. (1979), were higher than in previous reports, indicating that as recognition of the syndrome grew, less severely thrombocytopenic patients were recognized.

The "White Clot Syndrome"

Jonathan Towne, a vascular surgeon in Milwaukee, reported with his colleagues that the pale thrombi characteristic of this syndrome consisted of fibrin–platelet aggregates (electron microscopy). These workers coined the term "white clot syndrome" to describe the characteristic appearance of these arterial thromboemboli (Towne et al., 1979). Ironically, their report was also the first to note the occurrence of phlegmasia cerulea dolens (severe venous limb ischemia) that progressed to venous limb gangrene in two of their patients (i.e., a syndrome of limb loss due to extensive venous thrombosis without arterial white clots). Nonetheless, the designation of white clot syndrome has become virtually synonymous with HIT in both North America and Europe (Benhamou et al., 1985; Stanton et al., 1988), despite the lack of specificity of these thrombi for HIT (see chap. 2).

NONIMMUNE HEPARIN-ASSOCIATED THROMBOCYTOPENIA
Nonimmune Mechanisms in Heparin-Associated Thrombocytopenia

Klein and Bell (1974) reported on two patients who developed severe thrombocytopenia, thrombotic complications, and DIC, with hypofibrinogenemia and microangiopathic red cell abnormalities; that is, these patients probably had severe HIT. This experience prompted Bell to perform the first prospective study investigating the frequency of thrombocytopenia complicating therapeutic-dose UFH (Bell et al., 1976). Sixteen of 52 patients (31%) developed a platelet count fall to less than $100 \times 10^9/L$, and some of these patients developed hypofibrinogenemia and elevated fibrin(ogen) degradation products. The authors speculated that a "thromboplastic contaminant" extracted along with heparin from beef lung could explain the thrombocytopenia. A subsequent randomized controlled trial by Bell and Royall (1980) found the frequency of thrombocytopenia to be higher in patients who received bovine heparin (26%) compared with heparin of porcine intestinal origin (8%).

These investigators found no platelet-activating antibodies in plasma from the patients who developed thrombocytopenia (Alving et al., 1977), leading Bell (1988) to challenge the view that an immune pathogenesis explained HIT. However, as the Johns Hopkins group did not report thrombotic complications in any of their 37 patients who developed thrombocytopenia in their prospective studies, and given the apparent early onset of thrombocytopenia in many of their patients, it is likely that most of their patients did not have immune-mediated HIT.

Nonimmune (Type I) *vs* Immune (Type II) HIT
A confusing situation arose. The terms "heparin-induced thrombocytopenia" or "heparin-associated thrombocytopenia" were often applied to any patient who developed thrombocytopenia during heparin therapy, whether presumed or proved to be caused by heparin-dependent antibodies or otherwise. Investigators in Australia, led by Chong (1981), also observed patients with thrombocytopenia in whom heparin-dependent, platelet-activating IgG antibodies could be identified. In a subsequent report that appeared in the *Lancet*, two distinct syndromes of "HIT" were described by Chong and colleagues (1982). The first, called "group 1," developed severe, delayed-onset thrombocytopenia with thrombotic complications in association with IgG antibodies that caused platelet activation. In contrast, "group 2" patients had mild asymptomatic thrombocytopenia of early onset.

In 1989, at a Platelet Immunobiology Workshop in Milwaukee, it was suggested to Chong that terminology describing these two types of HIT be formalized. Accordingly, Chong recommended the terms in a review article that appeared in Blut (Chong and Berndt, 1989), although (in reverse of the *Lancet* article nomenclature) the early, nonimmune disorder was named "HIT type I" and the later-onset, immune disorder was referred to as "HIT type II." These terms subsequently became popular.

LABORATORY TESTING TO CHARACTERIZE THE HIT SYNDROME
A Sensitive and Specific Platelet Activation Assay for HIT
The development and application of sensitive and specific laboratory tests for detecting HIT antibodies resulted in a new era in HIT research. Historical accounts of these developments can be found elsewhere (Kelton and Warkentin, 2008; Warkentin, 2012).

Many clinical laboratories began to use platelet aggregation assays (Fratantoni et al., 1975; Babcock et al., 1976) to diagnose HIT. Problems with this type of assay, however, included low sensitivity (Kelton et al., 1984) as well as technical limitations in simultaneous evaluation of multiple patient and control samples. In 1983–1984, while working as a research fellow in the McMaster University laboratory of John Kelton, Dave Sheridan overcame problems of low test sensitivity by showing that washed platelets, resuspended in a buffer containing physiologic concentrations of divalent cations, were very sensitive to platelet activation by HIT sera (Sheridan et al., 1986). The assay, known as the "platelet serotonin release assay (SRA)," was adapted from a method of platelet washing developed at McMaster University by the laboratory of Dr. Fraser Mustard. In particular, the emphasis on using physiologic calcium concentrations was based on observations that "artifacts" of agonist-induced platelet activation were caused by the use of citrate anticoagulation resulting in low plasma calcium concentrations. One example of an artifact induced by citrate is that of two-phase aggregation triggered by adenosine diphosphate (ADP). At physiologic calcium concentrations, only weak single-phase aggregation without thromboxane generation is triggered by ADP (Kinlough-Rathbone et al., 1983). Fortuitously, the washed platelet technique previously developed at McMaster University by Mustard and colleagues that Sheridan evaluated for its HIT serum-sparing properties rendered platelets far more sensitive to the platelet-activating properties of HIT antibodies than assays based on citrated platelet-rich plasma. Modified washed platelet assays have subsequently been developed by other investigators (see chap. 11).

Sheridan and colleagues also made the observation that heparin concentrations strongly influenced platelet activation by HIT sera: therapeutic (0.05–1 U/mL), but not high (10–100 U/mL), heparin concentrations resulted in platelet activation, that is, the characteristic "two-point" serotonin release activation profile of HIT. Later, Greinacher and colleagues (1994) showed that high heparin concentrations in solution release platelet factor 4 (PF4) from PF4/heparin (PF4/H) complexes bound covalently to a solid phase, with a corresponding decrease in binding of HIT antibodies to the surface. Thus, the inhibition of platelet activation by high heparin concentrations probably results from a similar disruption of the multimolecular antigen complex on the platelet surface.

The high sensitivity of washed platelets to activation by HIT antibodies led to new insights into the pathogenesis of platelet activation. For example, 2 years after describing their washed platelet assay for HIT, Kelton and coworkers (1988) reported that the platelet activation process was critically dependent on the platelet Fc receptor. This represented a fundamental new pathobiologic mechanism in a drug-induced thrombocytopenic disorder.

Prospective Studies of Serologically Defined HIT

Although several prospective studies of the frequency of HIT were performed (see chap. 4), until the 1990s, none had systematically evaluated serum or plasma from study participants for HIT antibodies. Often the distinction between "early" and "late" thrombocytopenia was blurred. Thus, the relative frequency and clinical importance of immune versus nonimmune HIT were unclear. This is illustrated by a prospective study reported by Powers and colleagues (1979) that found HIT to be "uncommon" during treatment with porcine mucosal heparin, as "only" four of 120 (3%) patients developed thrombocytopenia, in contrast to the 26–31% frequency of thrombocytopenia reported for bovine lung heparin. However, two of these 120 patients probably died as a result of HIT-associated thrombosis (Warkentin and Kelton, 1990), underscoring the need for a specific laboratory marker for this immune-mediated syndrome.

In a prospective study of HIT that performed systematic testing for HIT antibodies (Warkentin et al., 1995), the authors showed the dramatic clinical effects of

HIT. Of 665 patients participating in a clinical trial of UFH versus low molecular weight heparin (LMWH) after orthopedic surgery, nine patients developed "late" thrombocytopenia serologically confirmed to represent HIT. These patients had a thrombotic event rate far greater than controls. Moreover, the spectrum of thrombosis in HIT patients included venous thromboembolism, rather than only the classic problem of arterial thrombosis. This study also showed that early postoperative thrombocytopenia occurred frequently, but was not explained by HIT antibodies (see chap. 3).

However, even this study did not initially capture the complete clinical profile of HIT. This is because it defined the platelet count fall indicating possible HIT using the "standard" definition of thrombocytopenia, that is, a platelet count fall to less than 150×10^9/L (Warkentin et al., 1995). Subsequent review of the database, together with correlative analysis of the results of systematic serologic testing for HIT antibodies (performed in most study subjects), showed that this standard definition underestimated the number of patients who had HIT (Warkentin et al., 2003). Rather, a proportional fall in platelet count (50% or greater)—in relation to the postoperative peak platelet count—provided a more accurate definition of thrombocytopenia (applicable at least to this postoperative patient population). This improved definition identified twice as many patients as having had HIT in this clinical trial, without compromising diagnostic specificity. Indeed, the study suggested that the risk of immune HIT is about 5% (16/332 = 4.8%) in postoperative orthopedic surgery patients receiving UFH for a week or more (see chap. 4).

THE TARGET ANTIGEN OF HIT: PF4/HEPARIN

In 1992, Jean Amiral, working in the laboratory of Dominique Meyer, reported that the antigen recognized by HIT antibodies was a complex between heparin and PF4, an endogenous platelet α-granule protein (Amiral et al., 1992). This important discovery created an explosion of basic studies in numerous laboratories that led to further characterization of the basic pathogenesis of HIT (see chaps. 5–10). Amiral's discovery also fostered the development of new assays for HIT antibodies based on enzyme immunoassay techniques (see chap. 11).

The antigen site(s) recognized by HIT antibodies were identified as being on PF4, rather than on heparin itself or a compound antigen (Li et al., 2002) (see chaps. 6 and 7). This observation highlights intriguing parallels between HIT and the antiphospholipid syndrome. This latter disorder is also characterized by pathogenic antibodies directed against one or more proteins that express neoepitopes when bound to certain negatively charged phospholipid surfaces (see chap. 3). The presence of neoepitopes on the "self" protein, PF4, suggests that HIT can be conceptualized as a transient, drug-induced, platelet- and coagulation-activating autoimmune disorder. Indeed, high-titer HIT antibodies that are able to activate platelets *in vitro* even in the absence of pharmacologic heparin have been associated with the onset of thrombocytopenia and thrombosis beginning several days after heparin has been discontinued, so-called delayed-onset HIT (Warkentin and Kelton, 2001) (see chap. 2).

CENTRAL PARADIGM OF HIT

The "central paradigm" of HIT is that of a clinicopathologic syndrome in which laboratory detectability of heparin-dependent IgG antibodies is central (Warkentin et al., 1998, 2011b; Warkentin, 2011a,b), as the pathologic antibodies activate platelets via their FcγIIa receptors (i.e., the platelet IgG receptors). This concept of HIT was also supported by a murine double transgenic model expressing both human PF4 and FcγIIa receptors (Reilly et al., 2001) (see chap. 10).

HIT as a Clinicopathologic Syndrome
The term "clinicopathologic" (or "clinical-pathological") syndrome, as applied to HIT, indicates that a patient must have one or more clinically evident events—almost always prominent thrombocytopenia and oftentimes associated new or progressive thrombotic events—as well as detectability of heparin-dependent platelet-activating antibodies. (The term "detectability" is used to indicate that antibodies are expected to be present if the appropriate assay is performed using a blood sample obtained during—or soon after—the period of thrombocytopenia. However, in practice, the presence of such antibodies is often inferred when high levels of anti-PF4/H antibodies are detected by a PF4-dependent immunoassay.) Thus, a patient without discernable clinical events does not have HIT, and a patient in whom these antibodies cannot be detected—no matter how persuasive the clinical picture—also does not have HIT (see chaps. 3 and 11).

Iceberg Model of HIT
Serosurveillance studies of heparin-treated patients led to the recognition that platelet-activating HIT antibodies comprise a subset of patients with anti-PF4/H antibodies of IgG class, and that patients with IgG class antibodies represent a subset of those who form antibodies of any of the three major immunoglobulin classes, IgG, IgA, and IgM. Crucially, clinical HIT is found only within the patients who form platelet-activating antibodies. Figure 1.4 depicts these interrelationships as an "iceberg model," in which clinically evident HIT is represented by the portion of the iceberg that protrudes above the waterline (Warkentin, 2011b). Just as only 10% of an iceberg juts out of the water, similarly only approximately 10% of immunoassay-positive patients in one clinical trial developed HIT (Warkentin et al., 2005b) (however, in certain other patient populations, such as postcardiac surgery patients, less than 2% of immunoassay-positive patients evince HIT) (Warkentin et al., 2000). More recently, the striking relationship between strength of immunoassay test result [expressed in optical density (OD) values], and the probability of platelet-activating antibodies being detected, has been recognized (Fig. 1.4).

Overdiagnosis of HIT
Because thrombocytopenia occurs very often for non-HIT reasons among heparin-treated patients, and because many immunoassay-positive patients do not have HIT, a growing problem has been the "overdiagnosis" of HIT. Overall, approximately 50% of immunoassay-positive patients recognized through clinically driven test requests will not have HIT (Greinacher et al., 2007; Lo et al., 2007; Warkentin et al., 2008b), and this proportion increases to 80–85% when critically ill patients are considered (Levine et al., 2010).

TREATMENT OF THROMBOSIS COMPLICATING HIT
Thrombosis is a remarkably common complication of HIT. The greatly increased relative risk for thrombosis in HIT (~10 to 15) exceeds that of virtually all other prothrombotic risk factors (see chap. 2). And, unlike most other risk factors, HIT

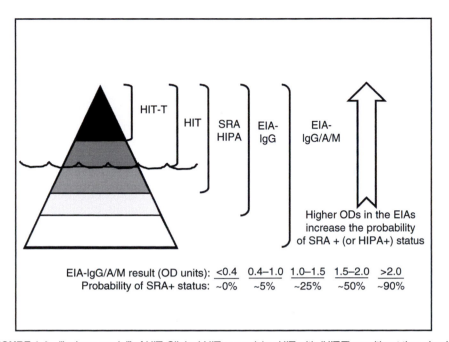

FIGURE 1.4 "Iceberg model" of HIT. Clinical HIT, comprising HIT with (HIT-T) or without thrombosis, is represented by the portion of the iceberg above the waterline; the portion below the waterline represents subclinical anti-PF4/H seroconversion. Three types of assays are highly sensitive for the diagnosis of HIT: the washed platelet activation assays, SRA, and HIPA test, the IgG-specific PF4-dependent EIAs (EIA-IgG), and the polyspecific EIAs that detect anti-PF4/H antibodies of the three major immunoglobulin classes (EIA-IgG/A/M). In contrast, diagnostic specificity varies greatly among these assays, being the highest for the platelet activation assays (SRA and HIPA) and lowest for the EIA-IgG/A/M. This is because the EIA-IgG/A/M is most likely to detect clinically irrelevant, non–platelet-activating anti-PF4/H antibodies. The approximate probability of SRA+ status in relation to a given EIA result, expressed in OD units, was obtained from the literature (Warkentin et al., 2008b). *Abbreviations*: EIA, enzyme immunoassay; HIPA, heparin-induced platelet activation (test); HIT, heparin-induced thrombocytopenia; OD, optical density; PF4/H, PF4/heparin; SRA, serotonin release assay. *Source*: From Warkentin (2011b).

exerts its prothrombotic effects only over a few weeks. The treatment of HIT is discussed in chapters 12–17. Here, we discuss only a few vignettes relating to the initial use of selected treatments for HIT.

Danaparoid Sodium

In 1982, a 48-year-old vacationing American developed DVT and PE following a transatlantic flight to Germany. Heparin treatment was complicated by thrombocytopenia and progression of venous thrombosis. Professor Job Harenberg of Heidelberg University, who had performed phase I evaluations of the experimental glycosaminoglycan anticoagulant, danaparoid, requested this agent from the manufacturer (NV Organon, The Netherlands). The platelet count recovered and the venous thrombosis resolved (Harenberg et al., 1983, 1997). Over the next 6 years, this patient developed recurrent thromboembolic events, and was successfully treated each time with danaparoid. This favorable experience led to a named-patient, compassionate-release program ending in March 1997, during which time, more than 750 patients were treated with this agent. Additionally, Chong and colleagues (2001) performed a randomized, controlled clinical trial evaluating danaparoid for treatment of HIT (see chap. 16)—this remains the only successfully completed randomized trial evaluating a therapy for HIT.

Recombinant Hirudins (Lepirudin, Desirudin)

The medicinal leech, *Hirudo medicinalis*, has been used for medical purposes for many centuries. Given the observation that the medicinal leech can prevent clotting of blood it has ingested, crude preparations derived from this animal were given experimentally at the beginning of the twentieth century. However, because this treatment's daily cost (75 Reichsmark) in 1908 was equivalent to the monthly salary of a factory worker, it was judged to be infeasible. After World War I, Haas, at Justus-Liebig University in Giessen, began his experiments using crude extracts of leech heads for hemodialysis. The major complication in these animal experiments was severe bleeding. The first human hemodialysis patients were treated by him with hirudin during dialysis when a more purified, but still crude protein extract of leech heads became available (Haas, 1925).

In 1956, Dr. F. Markwardt began his work to extract the active component of the leech at the Ernst-Moritz-Arndt University, in Greifswald. Still today, elderly peasants in the small villages around Greifswald tell stories of how they earned their pocket money by collecting leeches for the researchers at the nearby medical school.

The production of large amounts of hirudin by recombinant technology allowed the assessment of this direct thrombin inhibitor in clinical trials. Dr. Andreas Greinacher, at that time working at the Justus-Liebig University in Giessen, first used a recombinant hirudin, or r-hirudin (lepirudin [Refludan]) to anticoagulate a patient who developed acute HIT following heart transplantation. After Greinacher's move to Greifswald, he further assessed the use of r-hirudin in patients with HIT in two clinical studies that led to the first approval of a drug for parenteral anticoagulation of patients with HIT in both the European Union (March 1997) and the United States (March 1998) (Greinacher et al., 1999) (Table 1.1).

Fifteen years after its first approval, the manufacturer (Bayer) announced that they would discontinue marketing lepirudin on a worldwide basis effective March 31, 2012; however, it may continue to be available in some jurisdictions through another manufacturer (Cellgene, U.K.)/distributor (Pharmore, Germany). In addition, another r-hirudin, desirudin (Revasc [E.U.], Iprivask [U.S.A.])—first approved in the E.U. (1997) and subsequently in the United States (2003)—is now available in both Europe and the United States, albeit for an indication other than HIT (Table 1.1). In the Middle East, r-hirudin rb variant (Thrombexx, Rhein-Minapharm, 10th of Ramadan City, Egypt) is another therapeutic option (see chap. 14).

Warfarin-Induced Venous Limb Gangrene

A theme of this book is the central importance of increased thrombin generation in the pathogenesis of thrombosis complicating HIT. The recognition that warfarin therapy can be deleterious in some patients with HIT illustrates the importance of uncontrolled thrombin generation in this disorder.

In December 1992, in Hamilton, Canada, while receiving ancrod and warfarin treatment for DVT complicating HIT, a 35-year-old woman developed progressive venous ischemia, culminating in venous limb gangrene. This occurred despite a

TABLE 1.1 U.S. Approvals for Four Direct Thrombin Inhibitors

Use	Date of U.S. approval			
	Lepirudin	**Desirudin**	**Argatroban**	**Bivalirudin**
HIT indications				
For patients with HIT and associated thromboembolic disease to prevent further thromboembolic complications	March 6, 1998			
For prophylaxis or treatment of thrombosis in patients with HIT[a]			June 30, 2000	
Anticoagulation in patients with or at risk for HIT undergoing PCI			April 3, 2002	
For patients with or at risk of HIT/HITTS undergoing PCI				November 30, 2005
Non-HIT indications				
Use as an anticoagulant in patients with unstable angina undergoing PTCA				December 15, 2000
Use (with provisional use of GP IIb/IIIa inhibitor) as an anticoagulant in patients undergoing PCI				June 13, 2005
Prophylaxis of DVT in patients undergoing elective hip replacement surgery[b]		April 4, 2003[c]		

[a]Dosing guidance from U.S. Food and Drug Administration for seriously ill pediatric patients, May 3, 2008.
[b]Approval in EU is for hip and knee replacement surgery.
[c]Approval in the EU received November 11, 1997.
Abbreviations: DVT, deep vein thrombosis; GP, glycoprotein; HIT, heparin-induced thrombocytopenia; HITTS, heparin-induced thrombocytopenia/thrombosis syndrome; PCI, percutaneous coronary intervention; PTCA, percutaneous transluminal coronary angioplasty.

supratherapeutic international normalized ratio (INR). The following day, Kelton observed an area of skin necrosis on the abdomen of this patient, suggesting the diagnosis of warfarin-induced skin necrosis. The author questioned whether the warfarin had also contributed to the pathogenesis of the venous limb gangrene. This hypothesis was directly tested just 2 months later when a second young woman developed severe phlegmasia cerulea dolens of an upper limb during treatment of DVT complicating HIT with ancrod and warfarin. Treatment with vitamin K and plasma given by pheresis reversed the phlegmasia. Further laboratory studies supported this hypothesis of a disturbance in procoagulant–anticoagulant balance during treatment of HIT with warfarin (Warkentin et al., 1997) (see chaps. 2, 3, and 12).

Increasingly, HIT became viewed as a syndrome characterized by multiple prothrombotic events, including not only platelet and endothelial cell activation, but also profound activation of coagulation pathways. This conceptual framework provides a rationale for antithrombotic therapy that reduces thrombin generation in patients with HIT (Warkentin et al., 1998).

TREATMENT OF ISOLATED HIT

Isolated HIT refers to HIT diagnosed on the basis of thrombocytopenia alone, rather than because of HIT-associated thrombosis. Often, the initial reason for administering heparin includes routine postoperative prophylaxis or a medical indication, such as acute stroke or myocardial infarction. Until the early 2000s, the standard approach upon suspecting HIT in such patients was discontinuation of heparin, sometimes with substitution of oral anticoagulants.

Natural History of Isolated HIT

During the mid-1990s, new data indicated a high risk for venous thrombosis in postoperative orthopedic patients who developed HIT, particularly for PE (Warkentin et al., 1995) (see chap. 2). Thus, HIT came to be viewed as a dramatic, albeit transient, prothrombotic state, even when the original indication for heparin was routine antithrombotic prophylaxis.

In July 1992, the author became aware of a 68-year-old patient whose platelet count fell from 151 to 51×10^9/L between days 5 and 8 after coronary artery bypass surgery, during routine postoperative heparin antithrombotic prophylaxis. The heparin was stopped, and laboratory testing confirmed HIT. The platelet count recovered, and the patient was discharged to home on postoperative day 12. Three days later, the patient complained of dyspnea, and then died suddenly. Postmortem examination showed massive PE (Warkentin, 2005). This tragic outcome prompted the question: Is mere cessation of heparin sufficient for a patient with isolated HIT?

To address this problem, the author studied the natural history of HIT (Warkentin and Kelton, 1996). From a database of patients with serologically proven HIT, a 62-patient cohort with isolated HIT was identified: the cumulative 30-day thrombotic event rate was 52.8% (see Fig. 4.5 in chap. 4). The rate of thrombosis was similarly high whether heparin was simply stopped or substituted with warfarin.

Similar findings were reported later by Wallis and colleagues (1999) from Loyola University. These investigators also found a high frequency of subsequent thrombosis (43 of 113, or 38%) in patients with isolated HIT managed by discontinuation of heparin. Surprisingly, a trend was observed for the highest risk of thrombosis in those patients in whom heparin was stopped most promptly (see Table 4.7).

Further evidence supporting an unfavorable natural history of untreated HIT was provided by a prospective cohort study (Greinacher et al., 2000). These investigators found that the thrombotic event rate was 6.1% per day during the mean 1.7-day interval between diagnosis of HIT (and cessation of heparin) and initiation of lepirudin therapy. This event rate corresponded closely to the 10% rate of thrombosis observed in the Hamilton study in the first 48 hours after diagnosis of isolated HIT (Warkentin and Kelton, 1996).

Argatroban

A synthetic small-molecule thrombin inhibitor derived from L-arginine, now known as argatroban, was used in Japan during the 1980s as a treatment for chronic arterial occlusion (Tanabe, 1986). During this time, argatroban also underwent investigation as treatment for HIT in Japan, particularly in the setting of hemodialysis (Matsuo et al., 1988). In 1993, exclusive rights to the compound for the United States and Canada were acquired from Mitsubishi-Tokyo Pharmaceuticals, Inc. (now Mitsubishi Tanabe Pharma Corporation) by Texas Biotechnology Corporation (TBC; Houston, Texas, U.S.A.). In 1995, clinical evaluation of this agent for HIT began in the United States, using a prospective, multicenter, open-label design with historical controls, the ARG-911 study (Lewis et al., 2001) (see chap. 13). Two groups of patients were studied: HIT without thrombosis (i.e., isolated HIT) and HIT complicated by thrombosis (HIT/thrombosis syndrome [HITTS]). Eligibility was based on clinical suspicion of HIT, and serologic confirmation of the diagnosis, therefore, was not required. Both patient groups received the identical therapeutic-dose regimen of argatroban (initially, $2\,\mu g/kg/min$, then adjusted by activated partial thromboplastin time [aPTT]). The favorable results of the ARG-911 and subsequent studies (ARG-915, ARG-915X) led to the approval of argatroban on June 30, 2000, by the U.S. Food and Drug Administration (FDA) as "anticoagulant for prophylaxis or treatment of thrombosis in patients with HIT" (Table 1.1). Thus, for the first time in the United States, a drug was approved for the novel indication of prevention of thrombosis in isolated HIT. A marketing partnership between TBC (subsequently, Encysive; later acquired by Pfizer) and Smith-Kline Beecham [now, GlaxoSmithKline (GSK)] commenced in August 1997. Marketing of argatroban began on November 13, 2000. In April 2002, argatroban received approval for anticoagulation in patients with or at risk for HIT undergoing percutaneous coronary intervention (PCI).

In the United States, marketing exclusivity of GSK for argatroban ended in May 2011. Currently (February 2012), there are ready-to-use "alternative formulations" of this compound available from Sandoz (125 mL vial [1 mg/mL]) and from the Medicines Company (50 mL vial [1 mg/mL]), as well as the GSK product (2.5 mL vial [100 mg/mL], to be reconstituted into 250 mL). GSK continues to hold patent rights covering the formulation of argatroban until June 2014.

In Canada, market authorization for argatroban began on June 4, 2001. Table 1.2 provides information for approval status and date of market authorization for argatroban use in HIT in Asia and Europe.

Therapeutic-Dose Anticoagulation for Isolated HIT

The approval by the FDA of identical therapeutic-dose regimens of argatroban for both prophylaxis and treatment of HIT highlighted the emerging view that HIT is a high-risk prothrombotic state. This contrasted with the earlier concept that HIT was

TABLE 1.2   Availability of Argatroban For Use in HIT Outside of North America

Country	Trade name	Date of market authorization	Use[a]
Japan	Novastan and Slonnon	July 16, 2008	HIT
		May 20, 2011	Hemodialysis in HIT
			PCI in HIT
Sweden	Novastan	October 15, 2004	HIT
Netherlands	Arganova	May 25, 2005	HIT
Germany	Argatra	June 1, 2005	HIT
Austria	Argatra	September 22, 2005	HIT
Iceland	Novastan	October 31, 2005	HIT
Denmark	Novastan	January 3, 2006	HIT
Norway	Novastan	January 20, 2006	HIT
Italy	Novastan	March 13, 2008	HIT
Finland	Novastan	April 12, 2011	HIT
France	Arganova	June 21, 2011	HIT
Spain	Pending	November 2011	HIT

[a]Indication wording may vary by country.
Abbreviations: HIT, heparin-induced thrombocytopenia; PCI, percutaneous coronary intervention.

generally benign, provided that thrombocytopenia was promptly recognized and heparin discontinued. Further support for the new view included studies showing HIT to be a profound hypercoagulable state (markedly elevated molecular markers of *in vivo* thrombin generation) (Warkentin et al., 1997; Greinacher et al., 2000) and recognition that many patients already have subclinical DVT at the time that isolated HIT is first recognized (Tardy et al., 1999).

Indeed, therapeutic doses of an alternative anticoagulant might be generally applicable for treatment of most patients with isolated HIT (Farner et al., 2001) (see chaps. 12–17). For example, although the prophylactic-dose regimen of lepirudin for HIT is initially lower than the therapeutic-dose regimen (0.10 mg/kg/hr, rather than 0.15 mg/kg/hr, and without an initial lepirudin bolus), subsequent dose adjustments are made using the aPTT; thus, the eventual infusion rate approaches the one given using the therapeutic regimen. A high success rate (91.4%) was observed using such "prophylactic" doses of lepirudin for isolated HIT (Farner et al., 2001).

In contrast, the prophylactic-dose regimen using danaparoid (750 U bid or tid) may be somewhat less effective than therapeutic-dose danaparoid (usually, 150–200 U/hr after an initial bolus) for preventing new thromboembolic complications in acute HIT: 81.4% versus 91.6% (Farner et al., 2001) (see chap. 16). If this difference is real, it could be explained by greater efficacy of the therapeutic-dose regimen, in which at least twice as much danaparoid is usually given (3600–4800 *vs* 1500–2250 U/24 hr). The implication of Farner's study is that the approved prophylactic-dose regimen of danaparoid may not be optimal, either when used for its approved indication in Europe (i.e., prevention of HIT-associated thrombosis) or for the corresponding "off-label" use for HIT elsewhere (Warkentin, 2001) (see chap. 16).

Bivalirudin

The 20-amino acid hirudin analog, bivalirudin (Angiomax, formerly, Hirulog), was first used over 10 years ago in the United States on a compassionate use basis for the treatment of four patients with HIT (Nand, 1993; Reid and Alving, 1994; Chamberlin et al., 1995). Since then, it has undergone limited off-label use for the treatment of HIT (Francis et al., 2003), often in patients with both renal and hepatic compromise (see chap. 15). In contrast to its limited use in managing HIT, bivalirudin is widely used for anticoagulation in the setting of percutaneous transluminal coronary angioplasty as well as other types of PCI (Warkentin et al., 2008a). Indeed, bivalirudin is the only direct thrombin inhibitor that is approved for an indication beyond that involving HIT (Table 1.1). In November 2005, approval was also granted for use of bivalirudin for anticoagulation of patients with (or at risk of) HIT (or HIT-associated thrombosis) undergoing PCI (Table 1.1).

REDUCING THE RISK OF HIT
Low Molecular Weight Heparin

For over 50 years, UFH has been used in numerous clinical situations. However, UFH has several limitations, and efforts to develop potentially superior LMWH preparations began during the 1980s. Advantages of LMWH included better pharmacokinetics (e.g., improved bioavailability, predictable and stable dose response obviating the need for monitoring, lower risk of resistance to anticoagulation, longer plasma half-life) and favorable benefit–risk ratios in experimental animals (Hirsh, 1994; Hirsh et al., 2001). Advantages of UFH include its low cost, widely available laboratory monitoring, and potential for neutralization using protamine. But the question remained: Was the risk of HIT lower with LMWH? This was an important and relevant question, particularly as differences in risk of HIT exist even among UFH preparations derived from different animal sources (see chap. 4). As discussed earlier ("Prospective Studies of Serologically Defined HIT"), there is indeed evidence that LMWH has both a lower risk of HIT antibody formation and (more importantly) a lower risk of HIT and HIT-associated thrombosis. Table 1.3 provides a historical timeline of the introduction of the LMWH enoxaparin in the United States in various clinical situations.

Fondaparinux

Fondaparinux (Arixtra) is a synthetic pentasaccharide anticoagulant modeled after the antithrombin-binding site of heparin. It selectively binds to antithrombin, causing rapid and specific inhibition of factor Xa. In contrast to LMWH, HIT antibodies usually fail to recognize PF4 mixed with fondaparinux, both in platelet activation and PF4-dependent antigen assays (Warkentin et al., 2005a).

Interestingly, evidence suggests that although HIT antibody formation occasionally occurs in association with fondaparinux use, such antibodies fail to react in HIT assays in which fondaparinux replaces UFH or LMWH *in vitro* (Pouplard et al., 2005; Warkentin et al., 2005a). These *in vitro* observations underwent direct *in vivo* confirmation when a serologic substudy of the "Matisse trials" of venous thromboembolism therapy proved that fondaparinux was substantially less likely than heparin (unfractionated or LMWH) to precipitate rapid-onset HIT among patients who had unrecognized heparin-dependent platelet-activating antibodies [0/10 (0%) *vs* 4/4 (100%); $P < 0.001$] (Warkentin et al., 2011a). Although HIT has rarely been observed in association with fondaparinux thromboprophylaxis

TABLE 1.3   U.S. Approvals for Enoxaparin and Fondaparinux

Use[a]	Date of U.S. approval (if applicable)	
	Enoxaparin[b]	Fondaparinux
Prophylaxis after hip replacement surgery	March 29, 1993	December 7, 2001
Prophylaxis after knee replacement surgery	March 9, 1995	December 7, 2001
Prophylaxis after hip fracture surgery		December 7, 2001
Extended prophylaxis after hip replacement surgery	January 30, 1998	
Extended prophylaxis after hip fracture surgery		June 17, 2003
Prophylaxis after general (abdominal) surgery	May 6, 1997	May 26, 2005
Prophylaxis for unstable angina and non-Q wave myocardial infarction (given together with aspirin)[c]	March 27, 1998	
Acute DVT, with or without PE, together with warfarin[d,e]	December 31, 1998	May 28, 2004
Prophylaxis in medical patients at risk for DVT or PE	November 17, 2000	

[a]Use described may not necessarily conform precisely to the wording of the approved indications.
[b]Other LMWH preparations (dalteparin, tinzaparin) have been approved (at later times) for various indications (not shown).
[c]Fondaparinux has been studied for treatment of patients with acute coronary syndrome, and is approved in Canada (although not in the United States) for this indication.
[d]Wording of approved indication for enoxaparin includes "inpatient" treatment of acute DVT with or without PE and "outpatient" treatment of acute DVT without PE.
[e]Wording of approved indication for fondaparinux: "for the treatment of acute DVT when administered in conjunction with warfarin sodium; and the treatment of acute PE when administered in conjunction with warfarin sodium when initial therapy is administered in the hospital."
Abbreviations: DVT, deep vein thrombosis; LMWH, low molecular weight heparin; PE, pulmonary embolism.

following orthopedic surgery (Warkentin et al., 2007; Salem et al., 2010; Burch and Cooper, 2012), the frequency appears to be less than that of LMWH; further, for theoretical reasons, even this putative association between fondaparinux and HIT does not mean that fondaparinux might not itself be a highly effective therapy for HIT (discussed subsequently; see also chaps. 12 and 17).

Fondaparinux is approved in the United States, Canada, and the European Union for antithrombotic prophylaxis in orthopedic surgery as well as other clinical situations (Table 1.3). Data exclusivity for fondaparinux in the United States expired in 2008, and in July 2011, a generic formulation of fondaparinux entered the U.S. marketplace (produced by Dr. Reddy's Laboratories); in September 2011, an "authorized generic" supplied by GSK and marketed by Apotex became available. Data exclusivity for fondaparinux expired in the EU in spring 2012.

RECENT DEVELOPMENTS
HIT as a Misdirected Ancient Immune Response
Recently, Greinacher and coworkers provided evidence that bacterial infection can be associated with anti-PF4/H antibody formation in mice (Krauel et al., 2011). The pathophysiologic basis was the observation that bacterial surfaces bind PF4, thereby creating the HIT antigens. A human correlate was identified by this same group

(Greinacher et al., 2011), when it was reported that periodontitis—a common bacterial infection that is increasingly prevalent in the older population—is associated with natural levels of anti-PF4/H antibodies. The concept has emerged that HIT could represent a misdirected ancient immune response, as PF4-dependent antibodies triggered by bacterial infection would automatically be able to recognize numerous different bacterial species (as many species bind PF4), but that would have the adverse effect of predisposing to HIT if the powerful polyanion, heparin, is administered. Indeed, there is evidence that antiphospholipid antibodies might also have connections with antibacterial effects—in this case, β_2-glycoprotein I (which is highly conserved in the animal kingdom) plays a role in scavenging of lipopolysaccharide (Agar et al., 2011a,b). Thus, PF4 and β_2-glycoprotein I could play key roles in innate immunity, and both HIT and antiphospholipid syndrome could be examples of a misdirected host defense.

HIT Treatment: From Niche to Mainstream?
To date, treatment of HIT has focused on "niche" agents—danaparoid, argatroban, r-hirudin—that have few or no indications beyond that of HIT and associated thrombosis. However, in recent years, several new oral anticoagulants (e.g., dabigatran, rivaroxaban, apixaban, edoxaban; see chap. 17) have entered the marketplace in one or more jurisdictions. It seems likely that as these nonheparin agents become increasingly used for treating patients of diverse clinical scenarios, that some of these will include HIT and HIT-associated thrombosis. Just as fondaparinux has numerous (non-HIT) indications, and has gradually gained traction as a reasonable option for management of suspected HIT (see chaps. 12 and 17), perhaps too these newer agents will undergo a similar evolution to plausible HIT treatment options (Krauel et al., 2012). If this proves to be the case, management of HIT could eventually become as simple as taking a pill once or twice a day!

REFERENCES
Agar C, de Groot PG, Marquart JA, Meijers JC. Evolutionary conservation of the lipopolysaccharide binding site of β_2-glycoprotein I. Thromb Haemost 106: 1069–1075, 2011a.

Agar C, de Groot PG, Mörgelin M, Monk SD, van Os G, Levels JH, de Laat B, Urbanus RT, Herwald H, van der Poll T, Meijers JC. β_2-glycoprotein I: a novel component of innate immunity. Blood 117: 6939–6947, 2011b.

Alving BM, Shulman NR, Bell WR, Evatt BL, Tack KM. In vitro studies of heparin associated thrombocytopenia. Thromb Res 11: 827–834, 1977.

Amiral J, Bridey F, Dreyfus M, Vissac AM, Fressinaud E, Wolf M, Meyer D. Platelet factor 4 complexed to heparin is the target for antibodies generated in heparin induced thrombocytopenia. Thromb Haemost 68: 95–96, 1992.

Babcock RB, Dumper CW, Scharfman WB. Heparin-induced thrombocytopenia. N Engl J Med 295: 237–241, 1976.

Barker CF, Rosato FE, Roberts B. Peripheral arterial embolism. Surg Gynecol Obstet 123: 22–26, 1966.

Bell WR. Heparin-associated thrombocytopenia and thrombosis. J Lab Clin Med 111: 600–605, 1988.

Bell WR, Royall RM. Heparin-associated thrombocytopenia: a comparison of three heparin preparations. N Engl J Med 303: 902–907, 1980.

Bell WR, Tomasulo PA, Alving BM, Duffy TP. Thrombocytopenia occurring during the administration of heparin. A prospective study in 52 patients. Ann Intern Med 85: 155–160, 1976.

Benhamou AC, Gruel Y, Barsotti J, Castellani L, Marchand M, Guerois C, Leclerc MH, Delahousse B, Griguer P, Leroy J. The white clot syndrome or heparin associated thrombocytopenia and thrombosis (WCS or HATT). Int Angiol 4: 303–310, 1985.

Best CH. Preparation of heparin, and its use in the first clinical cases. Circulation 19: 79–86, 1959.

Burch M, Cooper B. Fondaparinux-associated heparin-induced thrombocytopenia. Proc (Baylor Univ Med Cent) 25: 13–15, 2012.

Chamberlin JR, Lewis B, Wallis D, Messmore H, Hoppensteadt D, Walenga JM, Moran S, Fareed J, McKiernan T. Successful treatment of heparin-associated thrombocytopenia and thrombosis using Hirulog. Can J Cardiol 11: 511–514, 1995.

Chong BH, Berndt MC. Heparin-induced thrombocytopenia. Blut 58: 53–57, 1989.

Chong BH, Grace CS, Rozenberg MC. Heparin-induced thrombocytopenia: effect of heparin platelet antibody on platelets. Br J Haematol 49: 531–540, 1981.

Chong BH, Pitney WR, Castaldi PA. Heparin-induced thrombocytopenia: association of thrombotic complications with heparin-dependent IgG antibody that induces thromboxane synthesis and platelet aggregation. Lancet 2: 1246–1249, 1982.

Chong BH, Gallus AS, Cade JF, Magnani H, Manoharan A, Oldmeadow M, Arthur C, Rickard K, Gallo J, Lloyd J, Seshadri P, Chesterman CN. Prospective randomised open-label comparison of danaparoid with dextran 70 in the treatment of heparin-induced thrombocytopenia with thrombosis: a clinical outcome study. Thromb Haemost 86: 1170–1175, 2001.

Cimo PL, Moake JL, Weinger RS, Ben-Menachem Y, Khalil KG. Heparin-induced thrombocytopenia: association with a platelet aggregating factor and arterial thromboses. Am J Hematol 6: 125–133, 1979.

Cines DB, Kaywin P, Bina M, Tomaski A, Schreiber AD. Heparin-associated thrombocytopenia. N Engl J Med 303: 788–795, 1980.

Crafoord C. Preliminary report on postoperative treatment with heparin as a preventive of thrombosis. Acta Chir Scand 79: 407–426, 1937.

Farner B, Eichler P, Kroll H, Greinacher A. A comparison of danaparoid and lepirudin in heparin-induced thrombocytopenia. Thromb Haemost 85: 950–957, 2001.

Francis JL, Drexler A, Gwyn G, Moroose R. Bivalirudin, a direct thrombin inhibitor, in the treatment of heparin-induced thrombocytopenia. J Thromb Haemost 1(Suppl 1): 1909, 2003.

Fratantoni JC, Pollet R, Gralnick HR. Heparin-induced thrombocytopenia: confirmation of diagnosis with in vitro methods. Blood 45: 395–401, 1975.

Green D, Harris K, Reynolds N, Roberts M, Patterson R. Heparin immune thrombocytopenia: evidence for a heparin-platelet complex as the antigenic determinant. J Lab Clin Med 91: 167–175, 1978.

Greinacher A, Pötzsch B, Amiral J, Dummel V, Eichner A, Mueller-Eckhardt C. Heparin-associated thrombocytopenia: isolation of the antibody and characterization of a multimolecular PF4–heparin complex as the major antigen. Thromb Haemost 71: 247–251, 1994.

Greinacher A, Völpel H, Janssens U, Hach-Wunderle V, Kemkes-Matthes B, Eichler P, Mueller-Velten HG, Pötzsch B. For the HIT Investigators Group. Recombinant hirudin (lepirudin) provides safe and effective anticoagulation in patients with heparin-induced thrombocytopenia. Circulation 99: 73–80, 1999.

Greinacher A, Eichler P, Lubenow N, Kwasny H, Luz M. Heparin-induced thrombocytopenia with thromboembolic complications: metaanalysis of two prospective trials to assess the value of parenteral treatment with lepirudin and its therapeutic aPTT range. Blood 96: 846–851, 2000.

Greinacher A, Juhl D, Strobel U, Wessel A, Lubenow N, Selleng K, Eichler P, Warkentin TE. Heparin-induced thrombocytopenia: a prospective study on the incidence, platelet-activating capacity and clinical significance of anti-PF4/heparin antibodies of the IgG, IgM, and IgA classes. J Thromb Haemost 5: 1666–1673, 2007.

Greinacher A, Holtfreter B, Krauel K, Gätke D, Weber C, Ittermann T, Hammerschmidt S, Kocher T. Association of natural anti-platelet factor 4/heparin antibodies with periodontal disease. Blood 118: 1395–1401, 2011.

Haas G. Versuche der Blutauswaschung am Lebenden mit Hilfe der Dialyse. Klin Wochenschr 4: 13–14, 1925.

Harenberg J, Zimmermann R, Schwarz F, Kubler W. Treatment of heparin-induced thrombocytopenia with thrombosis by new heparinoid. Lancet 1: 986–987, 1983.

Harenberg J, Huhle G, Piazolo L, Wang LU, Heene DL. Anticoagulation in patients with heparin-induced thrombocytopenia type II. Semin Thromb Hemost 23: 189–196, 1997.

Hirsh J. From bench to bedside: history of development of LMWHs. Orthop Rev 23(Suppl l): 40–46, 1994.

Hirsh J, Warkentin TE, Shaughnessy SG, Anand SS, Halperin JL, Raschke R, Granger C, Ohman EM, Dalen JE. Heparin and low molecular weight heparin: mechanisms of action, pharmacokinetics, dosing, monitoring, efficacy, and safety. Chest 119(Suppl): 64S–94S, 2001.

Howell WH, Holt E. Two new factors in blood coagulation—heparin and pro-antithrombin. Am J Physiol 47: 328–341, 1918.

Hussey CV, Bernhard VM, McLean MR, Fobian JE. Heparin induced platelet aggregation: in vitro confirmation of thrombotic complications associated with heparin therapy. Ann Clin Lab Sci 9: 487–493, 1979.

Kaupp HA, Roberts B. Arterial embolization during subcutaneous heparin therapy. Case report. J Cardiovasc Surg 13: 210–212, 1972.

Kelton JG, Warkentin TE. Heparin-induced thrombocytopenia: a historical perspective. Blood 112: 2607–2616, 2008.

Kelton JG, Sheridan D, Brain H, Powers PJ, Turpie AG, Carter CJ. Clinical usefulness of testing for a heparin-dependent platelet-aggregating factor in patients with suspected heparin-associated thrombocytopenia. J Lab Clin Med 103: 606–612, 1984.

Kelton JG, Sheridan D, Santos A, Smith J, Steeves K, Smith C, Brown C, Murphy WG. Heparin-induced thrombocytopenia: laboratory studies. Blood 72: 925–930, 1988.

Kinlough-Rathbone RL, Packham MA, Mustard JF. Platelet aggregation. In: Harker LA, Zimmerman TS, eds. Methods in Hematology. Measurements of Platelet Function. Edinburgh: Churchill Livingstone, 64–91, 1983.

Klein HG, Bell WR. Disseminated intravascular coagulation during heparin therapy. Ann Intern Med 80: 477–481, 1974.

Krauel K, Pötschke C, Weber C, Kessler W, Fürll B, Ittermann T, Maier S, Hammerschmidt S, Bröker BM, Greinacher A. Platelet factor 4 binds to bacteria [corrected], inducing antibodies cross-reacting with the major antigen in heparin-induced thrombocytopenia. Blood 117: 1370–1378, 2011.

Krauel K, Hackbarth C, Fürll B, Greinacher A. Heparin-induced thrombocytopenia: in vitro studies on the interaction of dabigatran, rivaroxaban, and low-sulfated heparin, with platelet factor 4 and anti-PF4/heparin antibodies. Blood 119: 1248–1255, 2012.

Levine RL, Hergenroeder GW, Francis JL, Miller CC, Hursting MJ. Heparin–platelet factor 4 antibodies in intensive care patients: an observational seroprevalence study. J Thromb Thrombolysis 30: 142–148, 2010.

Lewis BE, Wallis DE, Berkowitz SD, Matthai WH, Fareed J, Walenga JM, Bartholomew J, Sham R, Lerner RG, Zeigler ZR, Rustagi PK, Jang IK, Rifkin SD, Moran J, Hursting MJ, Kelton JG, for the ARG-911 Study Investigators. Circulation 103: 1838–1843, 2001.

Li ZQ, Liu W, Park KS, Sachais BS, Arepally GM, Cines AB, Poncz M. Defining a second epitope for heparin-induced thrombocytopenia/thrombosis antibodies using KKO, a murine HIT-like monoclonal antibody. Blood 99: 1230–1236, 2002.

Lo GK, Sigouin CS, Warkentin TE. What is the potential for overdiagnosis of heparin-induced thrombocytopenia? Am J Hematol 82: 1037–1043, 2007.

Mason EC. Blood coagulation. The production and prevention of experimental thrombosis and pulmonary embolism. Surg Gynecol Obstet 39: 421–428, 1924.

Matsuo T, Chikahira Y, Yamada T, Nakao K, Ueshima S, Matsuo O. Effect of synthetic thrombin inhibitor (MD805) as an alternative drug on heparin induced thrombocytopenia during hemodialysis. Thromb Res 52: 165–171, 1988.

McLean J. The thromboplastic action of cephalin. Am J Physiol 41: 250–257, 1916.

Nand S. Hirudin therapy for heparin-associated thrombocytopenia and deep venous thrombosis. Am J Hematol 43: 310–311, 1993.

Natelson EA, Lynch EC, Alfrey CP Jr, Gross JB. Heparin-induced thrombocytopenia. An unexpected response to treatment of consumption coagulopathy. Ann Intern Med 71: 1121–1125, 1969.

Nelson JC, Lerner RG, Goldstein R, Cagin NA. Heparin-induced thrombocytopenia. Arch Intern Med 138: 548–552, 1978.

Pouplard C, Couvret C, Regina S, Gruel Y. Development of antibodies specific to polyanion-modified platelet factor 4 during treatment with fondaparinux. J Thromb Haemost 3: 2813–2815, 2005.

Powers PJ, Cuthbert D, Hirsh J. Thrombocytopenia found uncommonly during heparin therapy. JAMA 241: 2396–2397, 1979.

Reid T III, Alving BM. Hirulog® therapy for heparin-associated thrombocytopenia and deep venous thrombosis. Am J Hematol 43: 352–353, 1994.

Reilly MP, Taylor SM, Hartman NK, Arepally GM, Sachais BS, Cines DB, Poncz M, McKenzie SE. Heparin-induced thrombocytopenia/thrombosis in a transgenic mouse model requires human platelet factor 4 and platelet activation through FcγRIIA. Blood 98: 2442–2447, 2001.

Rhodes GR, Dixon RH, Silver D. Heparin induced thrombocytopenia with thrombotic and hemorrhagic manifestations. Surg Gynecol Obstet 136: 409–416, 1973.

Rhodes GR, Dixon RH, Silver D. Heparin induced thrombocytopenia: eight cases with thrombotic-hemorrhagic complications. Ann Surg 186: 752–758, 1977.

Roberts B, Rosato FE, Rosato EF. Heparin—a cause of arterial emboli? Surgery 55: 803–808, 1964.

Salem M, Elrefai S, Shrit MA, Warkentin TE. Fondaparinux thromboprophylaxis-associated heparin-induced thrombocytopenia syndrome complicated by arterial thrombotic stroke. Thromb Haemost 104: 1071–1072, 2010.

Sheridan D, Carter C, Kelton JG. A diagnostic test for heparin-induced thrombocytopenia. Blood 67: 27–30, 1986.

Shionoya T. Studies on experimental extracorporeal thrombosis. III. Effects of certain anticoagulants (heparin and hirudin) on extracorporeal thrombosis and on the mechanism of thrombus formation. J Exp Med 46: 19–26, 1927.

Stanton PE Jr, Evans JR, Lefemine AA, Vo RN, Rannick GA, Morgan CV Jr, Hinton JP, Read M. White clot syndrome. South Med J 81: 616–620, 1988.

Tanabe T. Clinical results of MD-805, antithrombin agent, on chronic arterial occlusion. J Clin Ther Med 2: 1645, 1986.

Tardy B, Tardy-Poncet B, Fournel P, Venet C, Jospe R, Dacosta A. Lower limb veins should be systematically explored in patients with isolated heparin-induced thrombocytopenia. Thromb Haemost 82: 1199–1200, 1999.

Towne JB, Bernhard VM, Hussey C, Garancis JC. White clot syndrome. Peripheral vascular complications of heparin therapy. Arch Surg 114: 372–377, 1979.

Trowbridge AA, Caraveo J, Green JB III, Amaral B, Stone MJ. Heparin-related immune thrombocytopenia. Studies of antibody-heparin specificity. Am J Med 65: 277–283, 1978.

Wahl TO, Lipschitz DA, Stechschulte DJ. Thrombocytopenia associated with antiheparin antibody. JAMA 240: 2560–2562, 1978.

Wallis DE, Workman DL, Lewis BE, Steen L, Pifarre R, Moran JF. Failure of early heparin cessation as treatment for heparin-induced thrombocytopenia. Am J Med 106: 629–635, 1999.

Warkentin TE. Heparin-induced thrombocytopenia: yet another treatment paradox? Thromb Haemost 85: 947–949, 2001.

Warkentin TE. Heparin-induced thrombocytopenia, part 2. Clinical course and treatment. J Crit Illn 20: 36–43, 2005.

Warkentin TE. HIT paradigms and paradoxes. J Thromb Haemost 9(Suppl 1): 105–117, 2011a.

Warkentin TE. How I diagnose and manage HIT. Hematol Am Soc Hematol Educ Program 2011: 143–149, 2011b.

Warkentin TE. HITlights: a career perspective on heparin-induced thrombocytopenia. Am J Hematol 87(Suppl 1): S92–S99, 2012.

Warkentin TE, Kelton JG. Heparin and platelets. Hematol Oncol Clin North Am 4: 243–264, 1990.

Warkentin TE, Kelton JG. A 14-year study of heparin-induced thrombocytopenia. Am J Med 101: 502–507, 1996.
Warkentin TE, Kelton JG. Delayed-onset heparin-induced thrombocytopenia and thrombosis. Ann Intern Med 135: 502–506, 2001.
Warkentin TE, Levine MN, Hirsh J, Horsewood P, Roberts RS, Gent M, Kelton JG. Heparin-induced thrombocytopenia in patients treated with low molecular weight heparin or unfractionated heparin. N Engl J Med 332: 1330–1335, 1995.
Warkentin TE, Elavathil LJ, Hayward CPM, Johnston MA, Russett JI, Kelton JG. The pathogenesis of venous limb gangrene associated with heparin-induced thrombocytopenia. Ann Intern Med 127: 804–812, 1997.
Warkentin TE, Chong BH, Greinacher A. Heparin-induced thrombocytopenia: towards consensus. Thromb Haemost 79: 1–7, 1998.
Warkentin TE, Sheppard JI, Horsewood P, Simpson PJ, Moore JC, Kelton JG. Impact of the patient population on the risk for heparin-induced thrombocytopenia. Blood 96: 1703–1708, 2000.
Warkentin TE, Roberts RS, Hirsh J, Kelton JG. An improved definition of immune heparin-induced thrombocytopenia in postoperative orthopedic patients. Arch Intern Med 163: 2518–2524, 2003.
Warkentin TE, Cook RJ, Marder VJ, Sheppard JI, Moore JC, Eriksson BI, Greinacher A, Kelton JG. Anti-platelet factor 4 antibodies in orthopedic surgery patients receiving antithrombotic prophylaxis with fondaparinux or enoxaparin. Blood 106: 3791–3796, 2005a.
Warkentin TE, Sheppard JI, Moore JC, Moore KM, Sigouin CS, Kelton JG. Laboratory testing for the antibodies that cause heparin-induced thrombocytopenia: how much class do we need? J Lab Clin Med 146: 341–346, 2005b.
Warkentin TE, Maurer BT, Aster RH. Heparin-induced thrombocytopenia associated with fondaparinux. N Engl J Med 356: 2653–2654, 2007.
Warkentin TE, Greinacher A, Koster A. Bivalirudin. Thromb Haemost 99: 830–839, 2008a.
Warkentin TE, Sheppard JI, Moore JC, Sigouin CS, Kelton JG. Quantitative interpretation of optical density measurements using PF4-dependent enzyme-immunoassays. J Thromb Haemost 6: 1304–1312, 2008b.
Warkentin TE, Davidson BL, Büller HR, Gallus A, Gent M, Lensing AWA, Piovella F, Prins MH, Segers AEM, Kelton JG. Prevalence and risk of preexisting heparin-induced thrombocytopenia antibodies in patients with acute VTE. Chest 140: 366–373, 2011a.
Warkentin TE, Greinacher A, Gruel Y, Aster RH, Chong BH, on behalf of the Scientific and Standardization Committee of the International Society on Thrombosis and Haemostasis. Laboratory testing for heparin-induced thrombocytopenia: a conceptual framework and implications for diagnosis. J Thromb Haemost 9: 2498–2500, 2011b.
Weismann RE, Tobin RW. Arterial embolism occurring during systemic heparin therapy. Arch Surg 76: 219–227, 1958.

2 Clinical picture of heparin-induced thrombocytopenia

Theodore E. Warkentin

INTRODUCTION

Heparin-induced thrombocytopenia (HIT) is a distinct clinicopathologic syndrome caused by platelet-activating antibodies that recognize complexes of platelet factor 4/heparin (PF4/H). Its strong association with venous and arterial thrombosis represents a striking paradox. However, thrombocytopenia itself is common in clinical medicine. Furthermore, heparin is usually given to patients who either have thrombosis, or who are judged to be at a high risk for thrombosis. Thus, thrombocytopenia with or without thrombosis during heparin treatment does not necessarily indicate a diagnosis of HIT. Indeed, several disorders can closely resemble HIT (see chap. 3).

HIT is also associated with a wide spectrum of unusual thrombotic and other complications (Table 2.1). Unrecognized HIT may have been an important contributing factor in otherwise bizarre clinical events that have occurred in certain heparin-treated patients (Anderson et al., 1981; Solomon et al., 1988; Pfueller et al., 1990; Muntean et al., 1992). Laboratory documentation of HIT antibodies has been crucial in determining the clinical scope of the HIT syndrome. Accordingly, this chapter emphasizes clinical data obtained from prospective and retrospective studies that have used diagnostic testing for HIT antibodies.

Estimated frequencies of the various complications of HIT are taken from reports with serologic confirmation of the diagnosis (Warkentin et al., 1995, 1997; Warkentin and Kelton, 1996). "Rare" indicates an estimated frequency <3% of HIT patients.

THROMBOCYTOPENIA

Thrombocytopenia, using the standard definition of a platelet count of less than $150 \times 10^9/L$, is the most common clinical effect of HIT, occurring in 85–90% of patients (Warkentin, 1998a). An even higher proportion develops "thrombocytopenia" if a definition appropriate for the clinical situation is used.

Timing

The characteristic delay of five or more days between initiation of heparin and onset of thrombocytopenia was the major clue that led early investigators to recognize the immune pathogenesis of HIT (Roberts et al., 1964; Rhodes et al., 1973). King and Kelton (1984) noted that thrombocytopenia occurred between days 6 and 15 for more than 90% of patients in whom HIT occurred during their first exposure to heparin. In contrast, for patients who developed HIT during a repeat course of heparin, the onset of thrombocytopenia was often more rapid, occurring within two

TABLE 2.1   Thrombotic and Other Sequelae of HIT

Venous thrombosis	Arterial thrombosis	Miscellaneous
DVT (50%): new, progressive, recurrent; lower limb (often bilateral); upper limb (at site of venous catheter); phlegmasia cerulea dolens	Aortic or iliofemoral thrombosis resulting in acute limb ischemia/infarction (5–10%) or spinal cord infarction (rare)	Heparin-induced skin lesions at heparin injection sites (10–20%):
		Erythematous plaques
		Necrotizing skin lesions
	Acute thrombotic stroke (3–5%)	Coumarin-induced skin necrosis complicating HIT
Coumarin-induced venous limb gangrene (~5–10% of DVT treated with warfarin)	Myocardial infarction (3–5%)	involving "central" sites (breast, abdomen, thigh, leg, and so on) (rare)
	Cardiac intraventricular or intra-atrial thrombosis, *in situ* or via embolization of DVT (rare)	
Pulmonary embolism (25%): with or without right-sided cardiac intra-atrial or intraventricular thrombi	Thrombosis involving miscellaneous arteries (rare): upper limb, renal, mesenteric, spinal, and other arteries	Acute systemic reactions postintravenous heparin bolus (~25% of sensitized patients who receive an iv UFH bolus or sc LMWH injection):
Cerebral dural sinus thrombosis (rare)		Inflammatory: e.g., fever, chills, flushing
Splanchnic vein thrombosis: adrenal hemorrhagic infarction (rare)—bilateral (acute or chronic adrenal failure) or unilateral; mesenteric or portal vein thrombosis	Embolization of thrombus from heart or proximal aorta can also contribute to microvascular ischemic syndromes	Cardiorespiratory: e.g., tachycardia, hypertension, dyspnea; cardiopulmonary arrest (rare)
DIC, with (relative) hypofibrinogenemia and acquired natural anticoagulant deficiency, causing multiple venous and arterial thromboses, including microvascular thrombosis (rare)		Gastrointestinal: nausea, vomiting, diarrhea
		Neurologic: transient global amnesia, headache

Abbreviations: DIC, disseminated intravascular coagulation; DVT, deep vein thrombosis; HIT, heparin-induced thrombocytopenia; iv, intravenous; LMWH, low molecular weight heparin; UFH, unfractionated heparin; sc, subcutaneous.

days. These data have been interpreted as indicating an "anamnestic" (Gr., memory) or "secondary" immune response in HIT; that is, the immune system produces HIT antibodies more quickly on reencountering an antigen "remembered" within its memory cell repertoire. It is now known that this concept is incorrect, and that "typical" and "rapid" onset of thrombocytopenia in HIT reflects only a single type of immune response (discussed subsequently).

Typical Onset of HIT

A prospective study of serologically confirmed HIT showed that the platelet count typically begins to fall between days 5 and 10 (inclusive) of postoperative subcutaneous (sc) heparin prophylaxis (Warkentin et al., 1995, 2003) (Fig. 2.1). (Note that the data refer to the day the platelet count *begins* to fall, and not the later day on which an arbitrary threshold defining thrombocytopenia is crossed.) This study also showed that most patients who developed thrombocytopenia beginning after

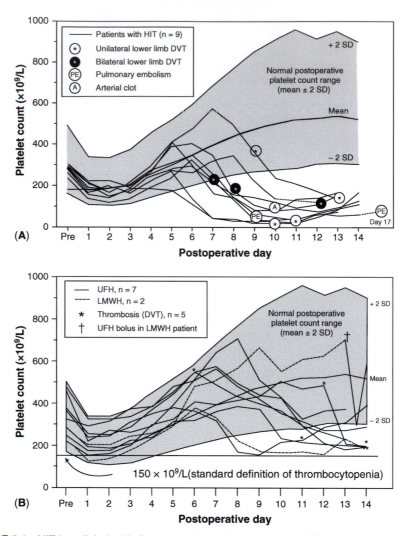

FIGURE 2.1   HIT in a clinical trial of postoperative orthopedic patients. (**A**) Serial platelet counts of nine patients with HIT (platelet count nadir < 150 × 10⁹/L). The bold line and shaded area indicate the mean (±2 SD) platelet count in the reference population (367 patients who tested negative for HIT antibodies). The reference population indicates the occurrence of postoperative thrombocytopenia (days 1–3), followed by postoperative thrombocytosis (maximal, days 11–14). Nine patients developed serologically confirmed HIT, with a platelet count fall to <150 × 10⁹/L; eight of the nine patients developed HIT-associated thrombosis (see insert for description of the types of thrombi observed; all thrombi were venous, except for a mesenteric artery thrombosis). (**B**) Serial platelet counts of nine patients with HIT (platelet nadir > 150 × 10⁹/L, but platelet count fall > 50%). Five patients developed DVT. (For one of the patients, the platelet count began to fall on day 5 after UFH "flushes" were received through an intra-arterial catheter placed at the time of surgery.) HIT developed in seven patients receiving UFH and two receiving LMWH (The platelet count fell abruptly on day 12 (postoperative day 13), together with symptoms and signs of an acute systemic (anaphylactoid) reaction, following administration of a 5000 U iv UFH bolus. However, the first clinical manifestation of HIT was on day 9 (erythematous skin lesions at LMWH injection sites). The platelet count fell abruptly on postoperative day 13 when 5000 U of iv UFH was given. (*Continued*)

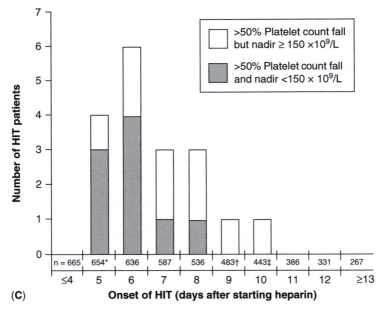

FIGURE 2.1 (*Continued*) (**C**) Day of onset of HIT for 18 patients observed in a clinical trial. HIT began between days 5 and 10, inclusive, in all 18 patients. Length of heparin treatment was variable; thus, the remaining number of patients at risk for HIT for each day of followup is shown (*n*). *For one of the patients, the platelet count began to fall on day 5 after heparin "flushes" were given through an intraoperative arterial line. †The platelet count fell abruptly on day 13 after giving a 5000 U bolus of UFH (see † on Fig 2.1B); however, heparin-induced skin lesions were evident on day 9. ‡The platelet count fell abruptly on day 10 after administration of a 5000 U iv UFH bolus, followed by therapeutic-dose UFH infusion. *Abbreviations*: DVT, deep vein thrombosis; HIT, heparin-induced thrombocytopenia; iv, intravenous; LMWH, low molecular weight heparin; UFH, unfractionated heparin. *Source*: (**A, C**) From Warkentin et al. (1995), and Warkentin (2000); (**B**) from Warkentin et al. (1995, 2003).

day 5 had HIT rather than another explanation for the thrombocytopenia. The data suggest the following clinical rule:

Rule 1

A thrombocytopenic patient whose platelet count fall began between days 5 and 10 of heparin treatment (inclusive) should be considered to have HIT unless proved otherwise (first day of heparin use is considered "day 0").

HIT-IgG antibodies generally are not detectable before day 4 or 5 of heparin treatment, but are readily detectable using sensitive assays when the platelet count first begins to fall due to HIT (Warkentin et al., 2009).

Warkentin and Kelton (2001b), analyzing temporal aspects of the platelet count fall in 243 patients with serologically confirmed HIT in relation to heparin use (both past and present), found that the onset of the platelet count fall typically occurs between days 5 and 10 (Fig. 2.2). Interestingly, among these patients with typical onset of HIT, there was no significant difference in the time to onset of HIT, irrespective of whether or not the patients had been exposed to heparin in the past. For most patients with typical onset of HIT, previous heparin exposure had occurred in the "remote" past, arbitrarily defined as more than 100 days earlier (Fig. 2.2).

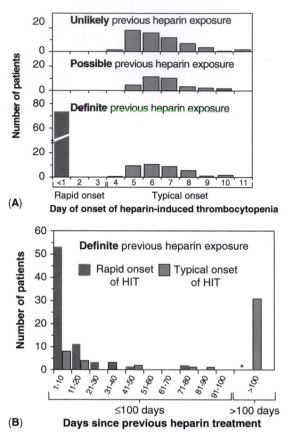

FIGURE 2.2 Temporal patterns of HIT in 243 patients in relation to previous treatment with heparin. (**A**) Data are shown for the patients in whom the day of onset of HIT could be determined to within a 3-day period. Among 170 patients with typical onset of HIT, there was no significant difference in the onset of HIT (median day), irrespective of whether previous heparin exposure had been definite (6.5, $n = 47$), possible (7.0, $n = 49$), or unlikely (6.0, $n = 74$) ($P = 0.88$, definite *vs* unlikely). Among 120 patients who had definite previous exposure to heparin, 73 had rapid onset of HIT. (**B**) For the subgroup of patients with definite previous exposure to heparin, the 73 patients with rapid onset of HIT invariably had been exposed to heparin within the past 100 days (i.e., no patients shown at the asterisk [*]); in contrast, only 16/47 patients with typical onset of HIT had been exposed to heparin within the past 100 days ($P < 0.001$). *Abbreviation*: HIT, heparin-induced thrombocytopenia. *Source*: From Warkentin and Kelton (2001b).

Gruel and colleagues (2003) have reported that the onset of the platelet count fall may occur on average several days later in patients who develop HIT during low molecular weight heparin (LMWH) therapy. More time may be required to generate clinically important levels of HIT-IgG so as to activate platelets in the presence of PF4/LMWH, rather than PF4/H, complexes.

Diminishing Risk of HIT After Day 10
The risk of HIT decreases after the day 5–10 "window" passes (Fig. 2.1C). In my experience, a platelet count fall after day 10 is usually caused by another

pathologic process, such as septicemia. As a notable exception, sometimes an invasive procedure "resets the clock"; that is, a platelet count fall that begins on day 12 of a course of heparin that consists of two 6-day treatments with heparin (before and after intervening surgery) is likely HIT (see Fig. 3.10 in chap. 3). Perhaps the surgery causes circumstances that favor seroconversion (e.g., release of PF4). Tholl and colleagues (1997) reported on a patient who for 9 years uneventfully received unfractionated heparin (UFH) for hemodialysis; nevertheless, HIT complicating hemodialysis began shortly after the patient underwent parathyroidectomy.

Rapid Onset of HIT
Sometimes patients develop *rapid-onset HIT*. This is defined as an unexpected fall in the platelet count that begins soon after heparin is started. Indeed, it is generally evident on the first postheparin platelet count, whether obtained minutes, hours, or a day later. Patients who develop such a rapid fall in the platelet count and who are confirmed serologically to have HIT antibodies almost invariably have received heparin in the past (Warkentin and Kelton, 2001b; Lubenow et al., 2002). A characteristic feature of this prior heparin exposure is that it usually has occurred in the *recent* past, usually within the past 2–3 weeks, and almost always within the past 100 days (Figs. 2.2 and 2.3).

This temporal profile of onset of HIT can be explained as follows: the rapid fall in platelet count represents abrupt onset of platelet activation caused by residual circulating HIT antibodies that resulted from the recent heparin treatment, rather than antibodies newly generated by the subsequent course of heparin.

This explanation is supported by other observations. First, for patients with typical onset of HIT, there was no difference in its median day of onset, irrespective of whether or not patients had previously been exposed to heparin (Warkentin and Kelton, 2001b; Warkentin et al., 2009). Second, patients did not generally develop thrombocytopenia that began between days 2 and 4. Had there truly been an anamnestic immune response more rapid than the usual 5- to 10-day period, one might have expected to identify such a group of patients. Third, patients reexposed to heparin following disappearance of HIT antibodies do not necessarily form HIT antibodies again; those who do appear to form antibodies after day 5 (Gruel et al., 1990; Warkentin and Kelton, 2001b). Indeed, several patients with well-documented previous HIT have received full treatment courses of heparin several months or years later without incident (Warkentin and Kelton, 2001b; Lindhoff-Last et al., 2002).

HIT Antibodies are Transient
There is a plausible biologic basis to explain why patients who develop rapid-onset HIT have received heparin in the recent, rather than in the remote, past: HIT antibodies are transient and become undetectable at a median of 50 days [95% confidence interval (CI), 32–64 days] after first testing positive, using the platelet serotonin release assay (SRA), an "activation assay". The median time to a negative test is somewhat longer (85 days; 95% CI, 64–124 days) using an enzyme immunoassay (EIA), or "antigen assay" (Fig. 2.4). At 100-day follow-up, the probability of the activation and antigen assays being negative is approximately 90% and 60%, respectively (Warkentin and Kelton, 2001b).

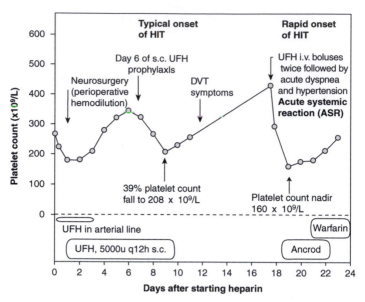

FIGURE 2.3 A 49-yr-old patient exhibiting both typical- and rapid-onset HIT: The platelet count began to fall on day 6 of sc UFH injections given for antithrombotic prophylaxis after neurosurgery (typical HIT). An abrupt fall in platelet count occurred twice on day 18, each after a 5000 U iv UFH bolus (rapid HIT). Symptoms and signs of acute systemic reaction occurred 10 min after each bolus (dyspnea, tachypnea, hypertension, chest tightness, restlessness). Note that the patient's platelet count never fell below 150×10^9/L, although her serum tested strongly positive for HIT antibodies by serotonin release assay. She developed proximal DVT shortly after developing HIT. *Abbreviations*: ASR, acute systemic reaction; DVT, deep vein thrombosis; HIT, heparin-induced thrombocytopenia; iv, intravenous; sc, subcutaneous; UFH, unfractionated heparin.

Rule 2

A rapid fall in the platelet count that began soon after starting heparin therapy is unlikely to represent HIT unless the patient has received heparin in the recent past, usually within the past 30, and latest, 100 days.

To summarize, the rapid fall in platelet count appears to be caused by the repeat administration of heparin to a patient with residual circulating HIT antibodies, rather than resulting from a rapid regeneration of HIT antibodies.

HIT Represents an Atypical Immune Response

Evaluation of serial plasma samples from clinical trials of heparin thromboprophylaxis have shown the relationship between anti-PF4/H antibody seroconversion and the development of HIT (Warkentin et al., 2009). These studies have revealed a characteristic "timeline" of the HIT immune response (Fig. 2.5), as follows:

1. HIT antibodies are generated rapidly (detectability, median day 4) and without IgM class precedence, suggesting that HIT is an atypical, perhaps secondary, immune response.
2. There is a specific sequence of events: antibody detectability (median, day 4) followed by the onset of the HIT-associated platelet count fall (median, day 6)

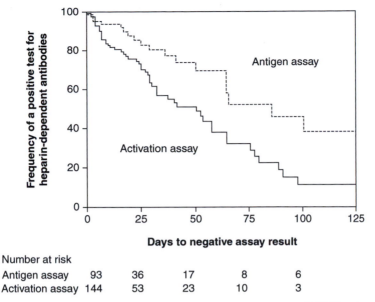

Number at risk

Antigen assay	93	36	17	8	6
Activation assay	144	53	23	10	3

FIGURE 2.4 Proportion of patients with HIT antibodies after an episode of HIT. The time (in days) to a negative test by the activation assay ($n = 144$) or the antigen assay ($n = 93$) is shown. The antigen test tended to become negative more slowly than did the activation assay ($P = 0.007$). *Abbreviation*: HIT, heparin-induced thrombocytopenia. *Source*: From Warkentin and Kelton (2001b).

that increases substantially (>50% fall at median day 8) followed by thrombosis (median, day 10).

3. Per this timeline, HIT antibodies are readily detectable in patient serum or plasma at the onset of the platelet count fall attributable to HIT.

These observations are consistent with a "point immunization" phenomenon, whereby the triggering of the immune response occurs during a narrow time window (see Fig. 7.10 in chap. 7). In these postoperative thromboprophylaxis studies, the immunization likely is triggered by the first postoperative injection of heparin, that is, when PF4 levels from activated platelets likely are highest.

The explanation for these atypical features are unknown. Prior sensitization to PF4-related antigens, for example, through infection (because PF4 binds to negatively charged bacterial surfaces), could explain the relatively rapid IgG response and lack of IgM precedence (Krauel et al., 2011; Greinacher et al., 2011), but does not explain the transience of the immune response. However, given that the HIT antigens are comprised of two autologous substances (PF4 and heparin), HIT can be viewed as an *autoimmune* disorder. Sometimes, transient IgG-mediated autoimmune responses can occur, particularly when the responsible antibodies have a relatively low affinity for the neoepitope (thus having avoided prior clonal deletion as occurs with lymphocytes that have high-affinity binding to autoantigens). In this situation, the antibodies are generated only as long as the autoantigen is present, thus explaining why there is a rapid fall in anti-PF4/H antibodies soon after discontinuation of heparin—or even in spite of continuation of heparin

(Greinacher et al., 2009). The affinity of the HIT antibodies may be substantially enhanced when both Fab "arms" of the IgG molecule can bind to linked epitopes, potentially even two PF4 molecules bound to a single heparin molecule (Newman and Chong, 1999).

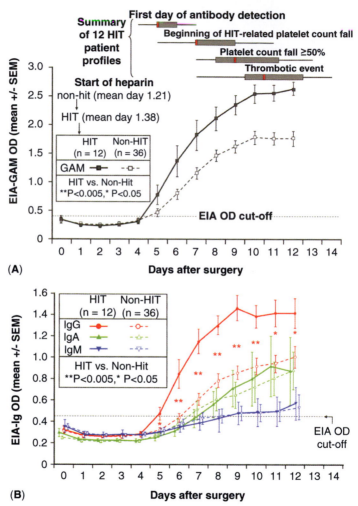

(A)

(B)

FIGURE 2.5 Characteristic timeline of HIT: anti-PF4/H antibodies (by EIA) per postoperative day in 12 patients with HIT and 36 seropositive non-HIT patients. **(A)** Mean (± SEM) OD of anti-PF4/H antibodies detected using commercial EIA from Gen-Probe GTI Diagnostics (Waukesha, WI, U.S.A.) that detects antibodies of all three major immunoglobulin classes, IgG, IgA, and IgM (EIA-GAM). HIT patients are indicated by solid squares and seropositive non-HIT controls by open squares. On each day beginning on postoperative day 6, there was a significant difference in the mean of the OD levels between the patients with HIT and the seropositive non-HIT controls (*P* < 0.05 by nonpaired *t* test). At the top of the figure, summary data for the 12 HIT patient profiles are shown for four key events (first day of antibody detection, beginning of HIT-related platelet count fall, platelet count fall >50%, and thrombotic event), summarized as median (small red squares within rectangles), IQR (rectangles), and range (ends of thin black lines). (*Continued*)

FIGURE 2.5 (*Continued*) (**B**) Mean (± SEM) OD values of anti-PF4/H antibodies detected using an in-house EIA (EIA-Ig) of the McMaster Platelet Immunology Laboratory that detect antibodies of the individual immunoglobulin classes, IgG (red circles), IgA (green triangles), and IgM (blue inverted triangles) for HIT (solid symbols) and non-HIT (open symbols). On each postoperative day beginning on day 5, there is a significant difference in the mean of the OD units for the EIA-IgG between the patients with HIT and the seropositive non-HIT controls (**$P < 0.005$ for days 6–10; *$P < 0.05$ for days 5, 11, and 12). In addition, among the 34 non-HIT controls who tested positive for IgG antibodies, mean (± SEM) maximum OD values for the EIA-IgG were significantly greater in the eight patients who tested positive in the SRA compared with the 26 patients who tested negative in the SRA ($1.30 ± 0.15$ vs $0.96 ± 0.07$; $P = 0.025$). Among the 20 patients who tested positive in the SRA, mean (± SEM) maximum OD values for the EIA-IgG showed a trend to higher levels in the 12 patients with clinical HIT, compared with the eight seropositive non-HIT controls ($1.63 ± 0.09$ vs $1.30 ± 0.15$ units; $P = 0.059$). *Abbreviations*: EIA, enzyme immunoassay; HIT, heparin-induced thrombocytopenia; IQR, interquartile range; OD, optical density; PF4/H, platelet factor 4/heparin; SEM, standard error of mean; SRA, serotonin release assay. *Source*: From Warkentin et al. (2009).

This hypothesis could explain several unusual aspects of the timing of HIT, such as (*i*) why HIT tends to occur fairly rapidly, beginning as soon as five days after starting heparin even in a patient who has never been exposed previously to heparin (autoreactive T-cell or B-cell clones might already be present in small numbers prior to starting heparin); (*ii*) why HIT occurs more often in certain patient populations, such as postoperative patients (cytokine-driven immune responses); and (*iii*) why HIT does not necessarily recur in patients with a previous history of HIT who are subsequently treated with heparin: there is a rapid loss of HIT antibodies after resolution of HIT—with paucity of specific memory B-cells (Selleng et al., 2010b)—and the specific circumstances that favored immune stimulation the first time—for example, large, stoichiometric concentrations of PF4 and heparin, occurring in an inflammatory milieu—may not be recapitulated during the subsequent heparin exposure.

Implications for Repeat Use of Heparin in a Patient with a History of HIT

The (*i*) transient nature of the HIT antibody, the (*ii*) apparent minimum of five days to regenerate clinically significant HIT antibodies even in a patient who once had HIT, and (*iii*) the observation that HIT antibodies do not necessarily recur, despite heparin rechallenge in a patient with definite prior HIT, all suggest that it may be safe to readminister heparin to such patients. Indeed, following disappearance of HIT antibodies, successful resumption of UFH or LMWH anticoagulation for hemodialysis has been reported in patients with previous HIT (Hartman et al., 2006; Wanaka et al., 2010).

Besides hemodialysis, UFH is also the unparalleled drug of choice for heart surgery and vascular surgery. Consequently, for patients with a previous history of HIT (especially since >100 days) who require cardiac or vascular surgery, a rational approach is to prove serologically that HIT antibodies are no longer present, and then to give heparin for a brief time to permit the surgery (Olinger et al., 1984; Pötzsch et al., 2000; Warkentin and Kelton, 2001b; Warkentin et al., 2008a; Linkins et al., 2012) (see chap. 19). We have even used this approach successfully in patients who required heparin for cardiac or vascular surgery as early as one month following an episode of HIT, when the HIT antibodies had just become undetectable (by SRA). After surgery, it seems prudent to avoid postoperative heparin completely and to administer an alternative anticoagulant. The actual risk of recurrent HIT beginning 5–10 days later, either following a transient intraoperative heparin exposure or even during prolonged postoperative heparin use, is unknown, but appears to be low.

For planning a brief reexposure to heparin in a patient who had HIT in the past few weeks or months, a dilemma would arise if the follow-up patient serum now tested negative using a sensitive activation assay (e.g., SRA), but positive by EIA. Platelet activation assays are better at detecting clinically significant levels of HIT antibodies (Warkentin, 2011b) (see chap. 11). Thus, use of heparin in this situation is recommended (Selleng et al., 2008a; Warkentin et al., 2008a). Continued watchful waiting is another option, given the transience of HIT antibodies.

Sensitization by Incidental Heparin Exposure

Sensitizing exposures to heparin can be relatively obscure. For example, incidental use of intraoperative line "flushes" that were not even documented in the medical records has led to HIT antibody formation or acute onset of HIT, with tragic consequences (Brushwood, 1992; Ling and Warkentin, 1998). Greinacher and colleagues (1992) reported a patient who developed recurrent HIT when reexposed to heparin present in prothrombin complex concentrates. Physicians should suspect possible heparin exposure in a patient whose clinical course suggests HIT, especially if the patient was recently hospitalized or has undergone procedures in which heparin exposure may have occurred.

Delayed Onset of HIT

Rarely, HIT begins several days after discontinuing heparin therapy or persists for several weeks, although heparin administration has been stopped (Castaman et al., 1992; Tahata et al., 1992; Warkentin and Kelton, 2001a; Rice et al., 2002; Shah and Spencer, 2003; Warkentin and Bernstein, 2003; Levine et al., 2004; Smythe et al., 2005; Arepally and Ortel, 2006; Jackson et al., 2006; Refaai et al., 2007; Alsaleh et al., 2008; Linkins and Warkentin, 2011) (Fig. 2.6). A dramatic case encountered by the author was a 68-year-old female outpatient who presented with transient global amnesia and a platelet count of $40 \times 10^9/L$ seven days after receiving two doses of UFH; despite the diagnosis and serologic confirmation of HIT and avoidance of all heparin, this patient's platelet count fell over the next four days to $14 \times 10^9/L$, along with laboratory evidence for disseminated intravascular coagulation (DIC) (low fibrinogen and elevated fibrin D-dimer levels). This patient's platelet counts gradually recovered to normal over several months, during which time recurrent thrombotic events were managed successfully with an alternative anticoagulant. (This clinical course was reported as patient 1 in Warkentin and Kelton, 2001a; the platelet activation profile induced by this patient's serum is shown in Fig. 20.4C of chap. 20.)

The term "delayed onset" HIT is not ideal because the onset of the platelet count fall usually occurs during the same day 5–10 window of "typical onset" HIT. Moreover, there are patients who develop typical-onset HIT while receiving heparin (ranging from "flushes" to therapeutic-dose heparin) where the thrombocytopenia subsequently continues to worsen—together with progressive consumptive coagulopathy—despite stopping all heparin (Warkentin, 2010, 2011a). These cases also are consistent with the concept of delayed onset (or "autoimmune-like") HIT.

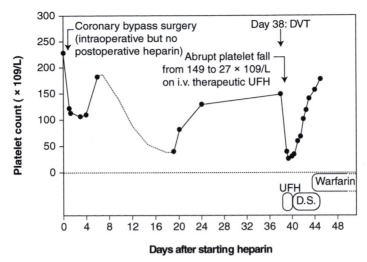

FIGURE 2.6 Delayed onset of HIT: a 68-yr-old woman who received UFH for heart surgery was noted to have a platelet count of 40 × 10⁹/L on postoperative day 19 and a "rash" of her lower extremities. She presented on day 38 with symptomatic DVT and developed rapid-onset recurrent thrombocytopenia after receiving iv UFH. The patient was successfully treated with D.S. and warfarin. In retrospect, the thrombocytopenia first observed on postoperative day 19 almost certainly was caused by delayed onset of HIT. *Abbreviations*: D.S., danaparoid sodium; DVT, deep venous thrombosis; iv, intravenous; UFH, unfractionated heparin.

Since such patients usually reach their maximum degree of HIT intensity (judged by platelet count nadir and degree of consumptive coagulopathy) approximately 14 days after the immunizing heparin exposure, this means that irrespective of whether the preceding period of heparin exposure is 1 or 7 days, the HIT episode can intensify for at least 1 week after all heparin has been stopped (see Fig. 12.4 in chap. 12).

The unusual clinical course of these patients presumably is related to very high titers of platelet-activating IgG antibodies; moreover, substantial platelet activation *in vitro* is caused by these patients' sera even in the absence of added heparin (Warkentin and Kelton, 2001a). This finding of substantial heparin-independent platelet activation is not an uncommon feature of HIT sera (Linkins and Warkentin, 2011), although patients with clinical features consistent with "delayed-onset HIT" (including progressive or persisting thrombocytopenia despite stopping heparin and/or HIT-associated consumptive coagulopathy) occurs in approximately 10–20% of patients with HIT. Also, with trends toward earlier patient discharge from hospital and a higher index of suspicion for this syndrome means that delayed onset of HIT is becoming a relatively more common presentation of HIT.

Delayed onset of HIT, however, should not be confused with delayed clinical manifestation of HIT-associated thrombosis. For example, Figure 2.3 shows a patient who developed typical onset of HIT while receiving postoperative heparin prophylaxis. However, isolated HIT was not clinically recognized, and the patient presented subsequently with a deep vein thrombosis (DVT) and a normal platelet count; when heparin boluses were given, rapid onset of thrombocytopenia occurred. Presumably, subclinical HIT-associated DVT that began during the episode of isolated HIT progressed to symptomatic thrombosis in the absence of anticoagulation. In contrast, patients with delayed onset of HIT develop thrombocytopenia that begins or worsens after the use of heparin and thus are usually thrombocytopenic when they present with thrombosis. Exacerbation of thrombocytopenia occurs if further heparin is given.

The existence of delayed onset of HIT presents a diagnostic dilemma in patients who are no longer receiving heparin but who develop thrombocytopenia five or more days after placement of a heparin-coated device, for example, certain intravascular grafts or stents (see chap. 20). In my view, either delayed onset or a protracted course of thrombocytopenia could reflect the generation and persistence of unusual "autoimmune" HIT antibodies without the need to invoke any effects of continuing exposure to heparin within the device.

Spontaneous HIT

Rarely, patients present with a clinical disorder that strongly resembles HIT on both clinical and serologic grounds but without any history of proximate heparin exposure (Warkentin et al., 2008b; Olah et al., 2012; Perrin et al., 2012). The clinical features include thrombocytopenia, thrombosis and—if UFH or LMWH is administered for treatment of suspected thrombosis—postheparin anaphylactoid reactions. The serologic features include strong positive tests for HIT antibodies—both PF4-dependent EIAs and platelet activation assays. In most cases, the sera exhibit the additional property of heparin-independent platelet activation (as observed in sera of patients with delayed onset of HIT). Interestingly, reported patients often have had preceding infections (Warkentin et al., 2008b; Olah et al., 2012): perhaps, PF4 binding to bacterial cell walls has triggered an anti-PF4/polyanion immune response (Krauel et al., 2011).

The so-called "spontaneous HIT" has also been observed in patients who have undergone preceding orthopedic surgery with warfarin (rather than heparin) thromboprophylaxis (Jay and Warkentin, 2008; Pruthi et al., 2009; Mallik et al., 2011). Interestingly, most such patients have undergone knee (rather than hip) replacement surgery. The reason that on rare occasions a patient who undergoes surgery can develop the HIT syndrome in the absence of any perioperative heparin exposure remains unknown. The existence of postoperative HIT in the absence of heparin exposure also creates an issue of attribution of causation with respect to fondaparinus-associated HIT: after all, given that there are several reports of the HIT syndrome after warfarin thromboprophylaxis, how can one be sure that the occasional case of HIT complicating fondaparinux thromboprophylaxis is really caused by the pentasaccharide anticoagulant? (see also chap. 17).

Severity of Thrombocytopenia

Figure 2.7 shows the platelet count nadirs of patients with SRA-positive HIT: the median platelet count nadir was approximately 60×10^9/L (Warkentin, 1998a, 2007). This contrasts with "typical" drug-induced immune thrombocytopenic purpura (e.g., caused by quinine/quinidine, sulfa antibiotics, or vancomycin), for which the median platelet count nadir is 20×10^9/L or less, and patients usually develop bleeding (Pedersen-Bjergaard et al., 1997). The platelet count is 20×10^9/L or fewer in only about 5–10% of patients with HIT (Warkentin, 2003, 2007). But even in this minority of HIT patients with very severe thrombocytopenia, thrombosis, rather than bleeding, predominates (see Fig. 12.5 in chap. 12).

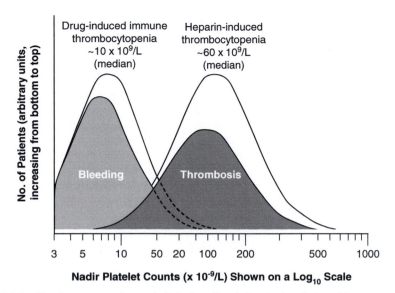

Nadir Platelet Counts (x 10⁻⁹/L) Shown on a Log₁₀ Scale

FIGURE 2.7 Platelet count nadirs and clinical profile of classic drug-induced immune-mediated thrombocytopenia *versus* serologically confirmed HIT. "Classic" drug-induced immune-mediated thrombocytopenia (e.g., caused by quinine, vancomycin, or glycoprotein IIb/IIIa antagonists, among other drugs) typically produces severe thrombocytopenia (median platelet count nadir, approximately 10×10^9/L) and associated mucocutaneous bleeding. In contrast, HIT typically results in mild-to-moderate thrombocytopenia (median platelet count nadir, about 60×10^9/L) and associated venous or arterial thrombosis. Note that the relative heights of the two peaks are not drawn to scale, as HIT is much more common than all other causes of drug-induced immune-mediated thrombocytopenia combined. *Abbreviation*: HIT, heparin-induced thrombocytopenia. *Source*: From Warkentin (2007).

Definition of Thrombocytopenia

Figure 2.7 illustrates that HIT is associated with thrombosis even when the platelet count nadir is more than 150×10^9/L. This suggests that the standard definition of thrombocytopenia ($<150 \times 10^9$/L) may be inadequate for many patients with HIT. Particularly in postoperative patients, a major fall in the platelet count can occur without the nadir falling to less than 150×10^9/L (Figs. 2.1B and 2.3). Indeed, studies indicate that a 50% or greater fall in the platelet count from the postoperative peak is strongly associated with HIT antibodies, even when the platelet count nadir remains higher than 150×10^9/L (Ganzer et al., 1997; Warkentin et al., 2003). Moreover, this patient subgroup is at increased risk for thrombosis.

Rule 3

A platelet count fall of more than 50% from the postoperative peak between days 5 and 14 after surgery associated with heparin treatment can indicate HIT even if the platelet count remains higher than 150×10^9/L.

It is possible that a greater than 50% platelet count fall definition is also appropriate for medical patients (Girolami et al., 2003). Regardless of the patient population, a clinician should have a high index of suspicion when unexpected large-percentage declines in the platelet count occur during heparin treatment, irrespective of whether an arbitrary absolute threshold for "thrombocytopenia" is crossed. Indeed, some investigators have used other thresholds to define thrombo-cytopenia, such as platelet count declines of 40% (Pouplard et al., 2005) or even 30% (Greinacher et al., 2005a; Lo et al., 2006).

Platelet Count Monitoring in Patients Receiving Heparin
In postoperative patients, the onset of HIT coincides with rising platelet counts (postoperative thrombocytosis); thus, the platelet count profile of HIT resembles an "inverted V" (Λ; Fig. 2.1 A,B). The postoperative peak platelet count preceding HIT is often higher than the preoperative platelet count. Therefore, the postopera-tive peak platelet count is the appropriate baseline for calculating the magnitude of a subsequent platelet count fall (Warkentin et al., 2003; Pouplard et al., 2005) (Table 2.2).

HIT-Associated Thrombosis Without Thrombocytopenia
Anecdotal reports indicate that HIT-associated thrombosis can occur in the absence of thrombocytopenia, as conventionally defined (Phelan, 1983; Hach-Wunderle et al., 1994; Warkentin, 1996a, 1997; Houston, 2000). However, most of these patients do have an associated fall in the platelet count, although the nadir remains higher than $150 \times 10^9/L$. Perhaps the most dramatic example of this phenomenon—reported as "ET gets HIT"—was a patient with essential thrombocythemia (ET) who developed serologically confirmed HIT: the platelet count fell by 49% from 1235 to 633, that is, concomitant "thrombocytopenia" and thrombocytosis (Risch et al., 2000).

A study suggested that HIT antibody formation without thrombocytopenia is not associated with a thrombosis rate greater than control patients (Warkentin et al., 1995, 2003). However, the subset of patients who formed HIT antibodies and whose platelet count fell by 50% or more—but remained above $150 \times 10^9/L$—did have an increased risk for thrombosis (odds ratio, 6.0). Figure 2.8 illustrates this concept of the central importance of thrombocytopenia (defined broadly as a large relative fall in the platelet count) in determining risk for thrombosis. These observations pro-vide indirect evidence suggesting that *in vivo* platelet activation by HIT antibodies probably contributes to the pathogenesis of HIT-associated thrombosis.

As shown in Figure 2.7, thrombosis commonly complicates HIT irrespective of the severity of the thrombocytopenia. Nevertheless, there is evidence that both the frequency and the severity of thrombotic complications increase somewhat in relation to the magnitude of the platelet count decline, whether quantitated in relative or absolute terms (Warkentin et al., 2003; Greinacher et al., 2005b; Lewis et al., 2006).

Platelet Count Recovery Following Discontinuation of Heparin, Including Persisting HIT
The median time to platelet count recovery to more than $150 \times 10^9/L$ after stopping heparin administration is about four days, although several more days may be required for the platelet count to reach a stable plateau. For 90% of patients with HIT, platelet count recovery occurs within one week. In approximately 1% of patients, it can take four weeks or more for the platelet count to recover (Warkentin and Kelton, 2001a). It seems likely that in such patients with "persisting HIT," there

TABLE 2.2 Determining the Day of Onset of Thrombocytopenia: A 35-Year-Old Woman Who Developed HIT After Heart Surgery

	Postoperative day												
	−1	0 (surgery)	1	2	3	4	5	6	7	8	9	10	11
Heparin used	UFH during CPB	Line flushes		Nil	Nil	UFH 5000 b.i.d. sc	UFH 5000 b.i.d. sc	UFH 5000 b.i.d. sc	UFH 5000 b.i.d. sc	D.S	D.S	D.S	D.S
Platelet count	227	98	137	209	255	300	374	378	310	224 (PE[a])	166	171	161 (nadir)
Percent platelet count fall							Rising platelet count	Peak platelet count	18% (378→ 310)	41% (378→ 224)	56% (378→ 166)	No further fall	57% (378→ 161)

(Shaded annotation, days 0–4: Platelet fall during day 0–4 is unlikely to be HIT unless there was recent heparin use (past 100 days) and the magnitude of the platelet fall is greater than expected)

[a]PE occurred on postoperative day 8, in association with a platelet count fall of 41%, from 378 (postoperative peak) to 224 × 10^9/L. The platelet count began to fall on day 7. The case illustrates why it is wrong to use the preoperative platelet count value as the "baseline," as the fall in platelet count from 227 [preoperative (day −1)] to 224 (day 7) would be considered trivial, although HIT-associated pulmonary embolism occurred. The preoperative (day −1) and first three postoperative days should be censored in the interpretation of platelet counts in HIT. In this patient, the abrupt fall in platelet count from 227 to 98 (day 0) is expected (heart surgery). This patient was treated successfully with D.S, with longer-term anticoagulation with warfarin.

Abbreviations: b.i.d., twice daily; D.S., danaparoid sodium; HIT, heparin-induced thrombocytopenia; PE, pulmonary embolism; UFH, unfractionated heparin.

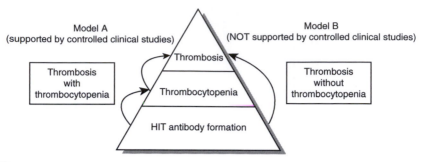

FIGURE 2.8 "Iceberg" model of HIT: Model A indicates that thrombosis occurs in patients who develop HIT antibody formation and thrombocytopenia. This model is supported by clinical data. In contrast, model B indicates the possibility of HIT antibody formation contributing to thrombosis without the intermediary process of thrombocytopenia. Although anecdotal experience suggests occasional patients consistent with model B, controlled studies indicate that HIT antibody formation without thrombocytopenia does not have an increased frequency of thrombosis, compared with controls (Warkentin et al., 1995, 2003). Note that thrombocytopenia is broadly defined and includes patients with large relative falls in the platelet count, even if the platelet nadir is >150 × 10^9/L. *Abbreviation*: HIT, heparin-induced thrombocytopenia. *Source*: From Warkentin (1999).

is somewhat longer detectability than usual of HIT antibodies with heparin-independent platelet-activating properties. Given the wide spectrum of platelet count recovery profiles in HIT, ranging from recovery despite continued heparin (Greinacher et al., 2009) to persistence of thrombocytopenia for several months (Warkentin and Kelton, 2001a), it points to the limitations of using platelet count recovery as a diagnostic feature of HIT.

THROMBOSIS
The HIT Paradox: Thrombosis but not Hemorrhage
Table 2.1 summarizes the clinical spectrum and approximate frequency of clinical sequelae associated with HIT. Spontaneous hemorrhage is not characteristic of HIT, and petechiae are not typically observed, even in those occasional patients whose platelet count is less than 10 × 10^9/L. Bleeding complications were not increased over controls in two prospective studies of HIT (Cipolle et al., 1983; Warkentin et al., 1995).

> *Rule 4*
>
> Petechiae, mucosal hemorrhages, and other signs of spontaneous bleeding are not clinical features of HIT, even in patients with very severe thrombocytopenia.

The explanation for this clinical feature is unknown, but could be related to unique pathophysiologic aspects of HIT, such as *in vivo* platelet activation, generation of procoagulant, platelet-derived microparticles, and procoagulant alterations of endothelium and monocytes (see chaps. 8 and 9).

HIT Is a Hypercoagulable State
A large controlled study (Warkentin et al., 1995, 2003) concluded that HIT is independently associated with thrombosis, even in a patient population at a high

TABLE 2.3   The Prothrombotic Nature of HIT: Comparison with Other Hypercoagulable States

Hypercoagulable state	Odds ratio for thrombosis
Heparin-induced thrombocytopenia:	–
Platelet count <150 × 10⁹/L	36.9
Platelet fall >50% beginning ≥5 days of heparin	12.4
Platelet fall >50%, but platelet count remains > 150 × 10⁹/L	6.0
Factor V Leiden	6.6
Congenital protein C deficiency	14.4
Congenital protein S deficiency	10.9
Congenital antithrombin deficiency	24.1
Dysfibrinogenemia	11.3
Lupus anticoagulant	5.4

Source: From Warkentin (1995); Warkentin et al. (1995, 2003).

baseline risk for thrombosis (postoperative orthopedic patients). Moreover, both venous and arterial thrombosis was seen. Thus, HIT can be considered a *hypercoagulable state* (Table 2.3), a designation consistent with increased *in vivo* thrombin generation seen in almost all patients with HIT (Warkentin et al., 1997; Greinacher et al., 2000).

The overall risk of thrombosis in HIT—expressed as a relative risk (RR)—is approximately 12.0 (95% CI, 7.0–20.6) (Warkentin, 2012), based on the analysis of a postorthopedic surgery thromboprophylaxis trial (Warkentin et al., 1995, 2003) with a high frequency of HIT. The calculation is based on the frequency of proximal DVT, PE, and/or arterial thrombosis of 10/18 (55.6%) in patients with HIT compared with a control rate of 30/647 (4.6%) among non-HIT patients. Given that postoperative heparin prophylaxis confers a risk reduction of 0.68 for postoperative DVT (i.e., an RR of 0.32 *vs* placebo control) (Collins et al., 1988), this suggests that the overall risk of thrombosis in a patient with HIT is almost fourfold greater than if the patient had never received any postoperative heparin at all, that is, $0.32 \times 12.0 = 3.84$. Moreover, the types of thrombi that occur in some patients with HIT—limb-threatening arterial thrombosis, DIC with venous limb gangrene, adrenal infarction—are unusually severe and not characteristic of usual postoperative complications.

Timing of Thrombotic Complications

Thrombosis occurs in association with HIT in at least four ways. Only the last three situations are conventionally considered as HIT-associated thrombosis. First, thrombosis can precede heparin treatment, for which it usually represents the initial indication for heparin therapy. Second, HIT can be the presenting clinical manifestation of HIT, sometimes even occurring prior to the platelet count fall (Greinacher et al., 2005b) (Fig. 2.9). Indeed, new thrombosis is the initial clinical manifestation in about 40–50% of all HIT patients (Warkentin and Kelton, 1996; Greinacher et al., 1999, 2005b).

Third, thrombosis can occur during the period of thrombocytopenia or early platelet count recovery despite discontinuation of the heparin (discussed subsequently). Finally, thrombosis can occur following platelet count recovery (Gallus et al., 1987; Warkentin and Kelton, 1996). In these patients, it is possible that subclinical thrombosis occurred during the thrombocytopenia, but became clinically

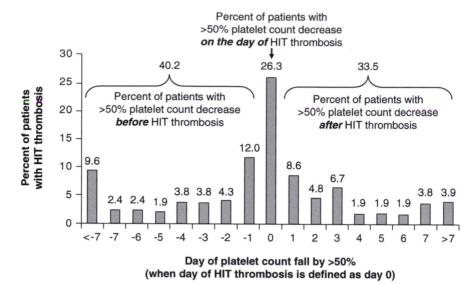

FIGURE 2.9 Relationship between onset of platelet count decrease and onset of HIT-associated thrombosis. The data summarize 209 patients with HIT-associated thrombosis. About one quarter (26.3%) of patients develop thrombosis on the same day that the thrombocytopenia occurs (defined arbitrarily as the day the platelet count has fallen by more than 50%), and in 33.5% the platelet count reached thrombocytopenia levels only *after* the occurrence of thrombosis. *Abbreviation*: HIT, heparin-induced thrombocytopenia. *Source*: From Greinacher et al. (2005b).

evident only later. The term *heparin-induced thrombocytopenia-thrombosis (syndrome)*, also known as HITT or HITTS, is sometimes used to describe patients with HIT-associated thrombosis.

Natural History of "Isolated HIT"

There is a high probability of subsequent thrombosis even when heparin administration is stopped because of thrombocytopenia caused by HIT. A retrospective cohort study (Warkentin and Kelton, 1996) identified 62 patients with serologically confirmed HIT in whom the diagnosis was clinically suspected because of thrombocytopenia alone, and not because of signs and symptoms indicative of possible new thrombosis. Thus, this cohort was identified without an apparent recognition bias caused by symptomatic thrombosis. Nevertheless, the 30-day thrombosis event rate was about 50% (Fig. 4.5 in chap. 4). This high frequency of thrombosis occurred whether the heparin administration was simply stopped or substituted by warfarin.

Subsequently, Wallis and colleagues (2009) provided further support for this concept that isolated HIT had an unfavorable natural history. In their retrospective cohort study of 113 patients with serologically confirmed HIT, these workers also found a relatively high risk of thrombosis (23–38% at 30-day follow-up, depending on whether patients who developed thrombosis at the time heparin was stopped are included) in patients with isolated HIT managed by cessation of heparin. Furthermore, early cessation of heparin (within 48 hours after a 50% or greater fall in platelet count) did not appear to reduce the risk of thrombosis, compared with patients in whom heparin was discontinued later.

More recently, Zwicker and coworkers (2004) performed a retrospective study that evaluated the risk of symptomatic thrombosis among patients with isolated HIT, based on the magnitude of a positive EIA for anti-PF4/H antibodies. Thrombosis was seen in five (36%) of 14 patients with a strong positive EIA (>1.0 optical density units), but only three (9%) of 34 patients with a weak positive test ($P = 0.07$). Baroletti and colleagues (2012) recently reported a strong relationship between OD levels and risk of thrombosis. These studies are consistent with data indicating that the greater the magnitude of a positive EIA, the greater the likelihood that the patient has heparin-dependent platelet-activating antibodies and, hence, "true" HIT (Warkentin et al., 2005c, 2008c).

Meta-analyses of two prospective cohort studies also found a high initial thrombotic event rate (5.1% per day after stopping heparin therapy and before beginning alternative anticoagulant therapy with lepirudin) (Greinacher et al., 1999, 2000) (Fig. 14.5 in chap. 14). Taken together, these large retrospective and prospective cohort studies suggest the following rule:

Rule 5

HIT is associated with a high frequency of thrombosis despite discontinuation of heparin therapy with or without substitution by coumarin: the initial rate of thrombosis is about 5–10% per day over the first 1–2 days; the 30-day cumulative risk is about 50%.

About 5% of patients (3 of 62) in the largest study died suddenly, two with proved or probable pulmonary embolism (Warkentin and Kelton, 1996). This experience supports the recommendation that further anticoagulation be considered for patients in whom isolated HIT has been diagnosed (Hirsh et al., 1998, 2001; Warkentin and Greinacher, 2004; Warkentin et al., 2008a; Linkins et al., 2012) (see chaps. 1 and 12–17).

Clinical Factors in the Pathogenesis of HIT-Associated Thrombosis

Clinical factors help determine the location of thrombosis in HIT. For example, Makhoul and colleagues (1986) observed prior vessel injury (e.g., recent angiography) in 19 of 25 patients with lower-limb HIT-associated thrombosis. Similarly, central venous catheters are crucial for the occurrence of an upper-limb DVT in patients with HIT (Hong et al., 2003).

Prospective studies of HIT in medical patients show that venous and arterial thrombotic events occur in approximately equal numbers; in contrast, there is a marked predominance of venous thrombosis when HIT occurs in surgical patients (Table 4.6 in chap. 4). In a retrospective study, Boshkov and colleagues (1993) found that HIT patients with cardiovascular disease were more likely to develop arterial thrombosis, whereas venous thrombosis was strongly associated with the postoperative state.

Rule 6

Localization of thrombosis in patients with HIT is strongly influenced by independent acute and chronic clinical factors, such as the postoperative state, arteriosclerosis, or the location of intravascular catheters in central veins or arteries.

Venous Thrombosis

Large case series suggest that venous thrombotic complications predominate in HIT (Warkentin and Kelton, 1996; Nand et al., 1997; Greinacher et al., 2005b) (Tables 4.6 and 4.7 in chap. 4). Indeed, pulmonary embolism occurs more often than all arterial thrombotic events combined. Furthermore, the strength of association between HIT and venous thromboembolism (VTE) increases in relation to the severity of thrombosis (Table 2.4). Other unusual venous thrombotic events complicating HIT include cerebral vein (dural sinus) thrombosis, adrenal vein thrombosis, hepatic vein thrombosis (Theuerkauf et al., 2000), mesenteric vein thrombosis (Muslimani et al., 2007), and perhaps retinal vein thrombosis (Nguyen et al., 2003). Thus:

Rule 7

In patients receiving heparin, the more unusual or severe a subsequent thrombotic event, the more likely the thrombosis is caused by HIT.

Regardless of the severity of thrombosis, in any patient who develops a symptomatic venous or arterial thrombosis while receiving heparin, the platelet count should be measured to evaluate whether HIT could be present.

Levine and colleagues (2006) estimated from published data that HIT could be present in about one in eight patients who develop VTE subsequent to UFH treatment or prophylaxis. However, the risk could be substantially higher (~45–75%) among patients who develop *symptomatic* VTE following postoperative UFH thromboprophylaxis (Warkentin, 2006c; Greinacher et al., 2005a).

Lower-Limb DVT

Lower-limb DVT is the most frequent thrombotic manifestation of HIT. Many venous thrombi are extensive and are often bilateral (Table 2.4).

Sometimes the DVT is sufficiently severe on clinical grounds as to merit use of the term "phlegmasia cerulea dolens" (i.e., an inflamed, blue, painful limb). However, progression of phlegmasia to venous limb gangrene is rare in the absence of coumarin anticoagulation (discussed subsequently).

There is slight left-sided predominance involving lower-limb DVT: we found that 76/137 (56%) of lower-limb DVT complicating HIT involved the left lower limb (Hong et al., 2003), a similar proportion as in control patients (57%). A slight left-sided predominance (~55 *vs* ~45%) for lower-limb DVT has also been noted in non-HIT populations (Kerr et al., 1990; Markel et al., 1992). This is attributed to the left iliac vein crossing the left iliac artery, causing an increase in left-sided lower-limb venous pressures. Pregnancy amplifies further this phenomenon, thus explaining the marked predominance (~90%) of left lower-limb DVT in pregnancy (Ginsberg et al., 1992; Chan et al., 2010).

Upper-Limb DVT

Upper-limb DVT is relatively common in HIT, occurring in about 5% of patients with HIT (Hong et al., 2003). Notably, in these patients the upper-limb DVT occurred at the site of a current or recent central venous catheter. Most (86%) of the patients therefore had right upper-limb DVT complicating HIT, reflecting strong physician preference to using the right neck veins for insertion of central lines. This study suggests that a systemic hypercoagulable state (HIT) interacts with a local factor (location of central lines) to result in clinical events (upper-limb DVT).

TABLE 2.4 Association of HIT and Thrombosis

Patient population (Ref.)	Thrombosis	Thrombosis rate		OR (95% CI)	P value
		HIT	Controls		
Postorthopedic surgery[a] (Warkentin et al., 1995, 2003)	Proximal DVT	8/18 (44.4%)	26/647 (4.0%)	19.1 (5.9–58.3)	<0.001
	Bilateral proximal DVT	2/18 (11.1%)	4/647 (0.6%)	20.1 (1.7–150)	0.01
	Pulmonary embolism	2/18 (11.1%)	2/647 (0.3%)	40.3 (2.7–572)	0.004
	Any thrombosis	13/18 (72.2%)	112/647 (17.3%)	12.4 (4.0–45.2)	<0.001
Patients with central line[b] (Hong et al., 2003)	Upper-limb DVT	14/145 (9.7%)	3/484 (0.6%)	17.1 (4.9–60.5)	<0.001
Medical[a] (Girolami et al., 2003)	Any thrombosis	3/5 (60%)	21/593 (3.5%)	40.8 (5.2–163)	<0.001

[a]HIT defined as >50% platelet count fall.
[b]HIT defined as any abnormal platelet count fall with positive HIT serology (platelet fall was >50% in 93% of study patients).
Abbreviations: CI, confidence interval; DVT, deep vein thrombosis; HIT, heparin-induced thrombocytopenia; OR, odds ratio.

Recurrence of VTE

Gallus and colleagues (1987) identified HIT as a significant risk factor for recurrence of VTE in a prospective treatment study: three of the nine patients with HIT developed recurrent VTE, compared with 12 of the 223 patients in whom HIT was not diagnosed (odds ratio, 8.8; $P < 0.01$).

Warfarin-Induced Venous Limb Gangrene

Venous limb gangrene is one of two clinical syndromes associated with HIT in which coumarin anticoagulation paradoxically plays an important pathogenic role (Fig. 2.10). Venous limb gangrene is defined as acral (distal extremity) necrosis that occurs in a limb affected by DVT. Additional features include (*i*) absence of large artery occlusion (i.e., there are palpable or Doppler identifiable pulses); (*ii*) extensive thrombotic occlusion of large and small veins, as well as venules; and (*iii*) the characteristic hallmark of a *supra*therapeutic international normalized ratio (INR), generally >4.0 (Fig. 2.11).

Anticoagulation with warfarin, phenprocoumon, or other coumarins is a crucial factor to explain the progression of DVT to venous limb gangrene (Warkentin, 1996b; Warkentin et al., 1997). A case–control study of eight patients with HIT-associated venous limb gangrene found a higher median INR, compared with 58 control HIT patients treated with warfarin for DVT who did not develop venous gangrene (5.8 *vs* 3.1; $P < 0.001$). Laboratory studies showed a characteristic hemostatic profile for patients with venous gangrene: persisting *in vivo* thrombin generation (elevated thrombin–antithrombin complex levels), together with reduced protein C activity (Fig. 2.12). The high INR is a surrogate marker for severely reduced protein C (through parallel coumarin-induced reduction in factor VII). Thus, venous limb gangrene appears to result from a profound disturbance in procoagulant–anticoagulant balance.

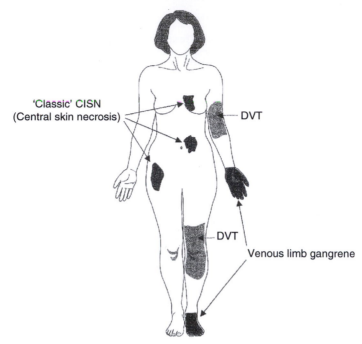

FIGURE 2.10 Coumarin-induced necrosis: HIT is associated with two forms of necrosis: (*i*) venous limb gangrene, affecting extremities with active DVT, and (*ii*) "classic" CISN, which involves central (nonacral) tissues, such as breast, abdomen, thigh, flank, and leg, among other tissue sites. Coumarin-induced necrosis complicating HIT typically manifests as venous limb gangrene (~90%) (Warkentin et al., 1997, 1999), whereas CISN in other clinical settings most commonly affects central tissues (~90%) (Cole et al., 1988). *Abbreviations*: DVT, deep vein thrombosis; CISN, coumarin-induced skin necrosis; HIT, heparin-induced thrombocytopenia. *Source*: From Warkentin (1996b).

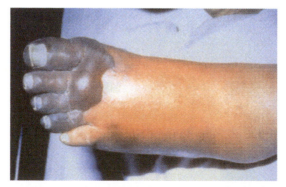

FIGURE 2.11 Warfarin-associated venous limb gangrene. Progression of DVT to acral necrosis (leading to below-the-knee amputation) occurred despite the presence of palpable arterial foot pulses in this 49-yr-old woman with HIT treated with warfarin (INR = 7.2 at the onset of limb gangrene). *Abbreviations*: DVT, deep vein thrombosis; HIT, heparin-induced thrombocytopenia; INR, international normalized ratio. *Source*: From Warkentin et al. (1997).

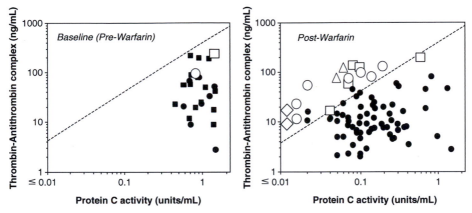

FIGURE 2.12 TAT complexes compared with protein C activity in patients with HIT: each data point represents TAT complexes and protein C activity per single treatment day per patient. In both panels the open symbols represent three patients with warfarin-induced venous limb gangrene and one patient with phlegmasia cerulea dolens (*open squares*). The diagonal line represents an arbitrary ratio of TAT complex to protein C of 400. (*Left*) Results when HIT was first diagnosed and before warfarin therapy. Control samples included eight patients (*closed circles*) who subsequently received warfarin for DVT without developing venous limb gangrene and 14 patients (*closed squares*) without DVT who did not later receive warfarin. (*Right*) Results in 16 patients who were receiving warfarin for HIT, including four patients (*open symbols*) who developed venous limb gangrene/phlegmasia and 12 patients (*closed circles*) who received warfarin without developing venous limb gangrene. The data suggest that patients who develop venous limb gangrene or phlegmasia have a higher ratio of TAT to protein C, consistent with a disturbance in procoagulant–anticoagulant balance during warfarin treatment of HIT. *Abbreviations*: DVT, deep vein thrombosis; HIT, heparin-induced thrombocytopenia; TAT, thrombin–antithrombin. *Source*: From Warkentin et al. (1997).

The association between venous limb gangrene and HIT was first reported by Towne and colleagues (1979). They noted a prodrome of phlegmasia cerulea dolens before progression to distal gangrene (information on possible coumarin treatment was not given). Other reports of venous limb gangrene complicating HIT, however, do suggest that warfarin had been used during the evolution to necrosis (Thomas and Block, 1992; Hunter et al., 1993; Kaufman et al., 1998).

Patients have also developed venous limb gangrene during combined treatment with both ancrod and warfarin (Warkentin et al., 1997; Gupta et al., 1998); because thrombin generation *increases* during treatment of HIT with ancrod (Warkentin, 1998b; Fig. 12.2 in chap. 12), ancrod could predispose to a greater risk for venous gangrene during warfarin treatment.

Several patients have been reported who developed venous limb gangrene during the transition to coumarin from parenteral anticoagulation with a direct thrombin inhibitor (DTI, lepirudin or argatroban) (Smythe et al., 2002; Srinivasan et al., 2004; Warkentin, 2006a). Typically, patients had symptomatic DVT in the affected limb and had their DTI started and stopped while they remained thrombocytopenic. Additionally, the INR was supratherapeutic at the time that limb ischemia or gangrene occurred *after stopping* the DTI. This experience indicates that the transition from parenteral anticoagulation to coumarin therapy should proceed cautiously, as suggested by the following "rule" (see chap. 12):

Rule 8

Venous limb gangrene is characterized by (*i*) *in vivo* thrombin generation associated with acute HIT; (2) active DVT in the limb(s) affected by venous gangrene; and (3) a supratherapeutic INR during coumarin anticoagulation. This syndrome can be prevented by (*i*) delaying initiation of coumarin anticoagulation during acute HIT until there has been substantial recovery of the platelet count (to at least 150×10^9/L) while receiving an alternative parenteral anticoagulant (e.g., lepirudin, argatroban, danaparoid, fondaparinux), and only if the thrombosis has clinically improved; (*ii*) initiating coumarin in low, maintenance doses (e.g., 2–5 mg warfarin); (*iii*) ensuring that both parenteral and oral anticoagulant overlap for at least five days, with at least the last two days in the target therapeutic range; and (*iv*) if applicable, physicians should reverse coumarin anticoagulation with intravenous (iv) vitamin K in a patient recognized with acute HIT after coumarin therapy has been commenced.

The frequency of venous limb gangrene in HIT patients with DVT who receive warfarin is unknown. This complication happened in 8 of 66 (12.1%; 95% CI, 5.4–22.5%) patients with HIT-associated DVT treated with warfarin (with or without ancrod) in Hamilton; venous limb gangrene was a more frequent cause of limb loss in HIT patients than was arterial occlusion in this medical community. Venous gangrene also occurred in 1 of 21 (4.8%; 95% CI, 0.12–23.8%) patients treated with phenprocoumon in Germany (Greinacher et al., 2000). In contrast, this complication was not observed by Wallis and colleagues in any of the 51 patients who received warfarin with a diagnosis of HIT, although only 16 patients received warfarin to manage HIT-associated thrombosis (95% CI, for 0/16, 0–20.6%). Besides cotherapy with ancrod, factors that could influence the risk for venous gangrene include the dosing of coumarin, the rate of coagulation factor turnover/consumption related to HIT severity and/or DIC, and vitamin K deficiency.

Rarely, coumarin therapy contributes to microvascular thrombosis and acral limb ischemia in the absence of DVT. Figure 2.13 shows multiple digital necrosis of the right hand complicating the initiation of warfarin therapy (maximal INR = 4.3) in a patient with Raynaud's phenomenon who developed HIT after aortic valve

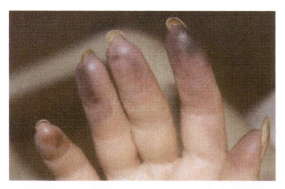

FIGURE 2.13   Warfarin-associated multiple digital necrosis of the right hand in a 61-yr-old woman with paraneoplastic Raynaud's phenomenon and adenocarcinoma-associated thrombotic endocarditis who developed HIT after aortic valve replacement surgery (see text for additional clinical details). *Abbreviation*: HIT, heparin-induced thrombocytopenia. *Source*: From Warkentin et al. (2004).

replacement for adenocarcinoma-associated noninfective thrombotic endocarditis (Warkentin et al., 2004). Although digital necrosis occurred in all four limbs in this patient, only the right foot (which exhibited the greatest amount of ischemic necrosis) was found to have DVT by duplex ultrasonography. It was hypothesized that microcirculatory disturbances secondary to paraneoplastic Raynaud's phenomenon interacted with altered procoagulant–anticoagulant balance (secondary to HIT and warfarin therapy) to cause this dramatic clinical syndrome.

Cerebral Venous (Dural Sinus) Thrombosis

Thrombosis of the dural venous sinuses is an unusual cause of stroke in HIT patients (Stevenson, 1976; Fesler et al., 2011). Often, there is a second hypercoagulable state, such as pregnancy (Van der Weyden et al., 1983; Calhoun and Hesser, 1987) or myeloproliferative disease (Kyritsis et al., 1990) that may have interacted with HIT to cause this complication. Platelet-rich "white clots" were identified in the superior sagittal venous sinus in one necropsy study (Meyer-Lindenberg et al., 1997). Clinicians should have a high index of suspicion for dural sinus thrombosis when a patient develops progressive focal neurologic signs, decreased level of consciousness, seizures, or headache during or soon after stopping heparin treatment (Beland et al., 1997; Pohl et al., 1999, 2000; Warkentin and Bernstein, 2003). Treatment includes discontinuation of heparin, use of an alternative anticoagulant, and possibly, iv gammaglobulin (see chap. 12).

Adrenal Hemorrhagic Infarction (Adrenal Vein Thrombosis)

Clinicians should suspect bilateral adrenal hemorrhagic infarction when thrombocytopenic patients develop abdominal pain and/or hypotension in association with heparin treatment (Arthur et al., 1985; Dahlberg et al., 1990; Ernest and Fisher, 1991; Bleasel et al., 1992; Delhumeau and Granry, 1992; Kovacs et al., 2001; Warkentin, 2002a, 2006b; Rosenberger et al., 2011; Thota et al., 2012). Fever and hyponatremia occur in some patients. These patients require corticosteroid replacement to prevent death from acute or chronic adrenal failure (Rowland et al., 1999). Unilateral adrenal hemorrhagic infarction typically presents with ipsilateral flank pain without signs of adrenal failure (Warkentin, 1996a). HIT explained at least 5% of patients with adrenal hemorrhage at one institution (Vella et al., 2001).

This hemorrhagic manifestation of HIT is caused by thrombosis of adrenal veins leading to hemorrhagic necrosis of the glands (Warkentin 2002a, 2006b). Other hypercoagulable states associated with adrenal necrosis include DIC complicating meningococcemia (Waterhouse–Friderichsen syndrome) and the antiphospholipid antibody syndrome (McKay, 1965; Carette and Jobin, 1989).

DIC, Acquired Anticoagulant Deficiency, and PTT Confounding

Although increased thrombin generation occurs in virtually all patients with HIT, overt *decompensated DIC*, defined as reduced fibrinogen levels or an otherwise unexplained increase in the INR, is relatively uncommon, occurring in about 5–10% of patients (Natelson et al., 1969; Klein and Bell, 1974; Zalcberg et al., 1983; Castaman et al., 1992; Betrosian et al., 2003). Protein C consumption is also well compensated, as protein C levels are usually within the normal range when HIT is diagnosed (Warkentin et al., 1997).

Nevertheless, acquired natural anticoagulant failure from DIC could contribute to thrombosis in some patients with HIT. Markedly reduced antithrombin levels were found in a young woman with three-limb DVT and bilateral adrenal infarction complicating HIT; after recovery, antithrombin levels were normal (unpublished observations of the author). This hypothesis implies that plasmapheresis could benefit patients by correcting acquired anticoagulant deficiency; if so, the replacement fluid must be plasma, rather than albumin, to correct antithrombin and other natural anticoagulant deficiencies.

Other patients with HIT-associated DIC evince clinical signs of microvascular thrombosis. For example, Figure 2.14 shows livedo reticularis and patchy foot necrosis (despite palpable foot pulses) in a postoperative cardiac surgery patient with HIT (platelet count nadir, 39×10^9/L) complicated by hypofibrinogenemic DIC. Evidence for acquired natural anticoagulant failure included mildly reduced antithrombin levels (0.76 U/mL; normal, 0.77–1.30 U/mL) and moderately reduced protein C activity (0.50 U/mL; normal, 0.70–1.80 U/mL) that subsequently resolved. Free protein S levels were normal (1.12 U/mL; normal, 0.62–1.38 U/mL). Evidence

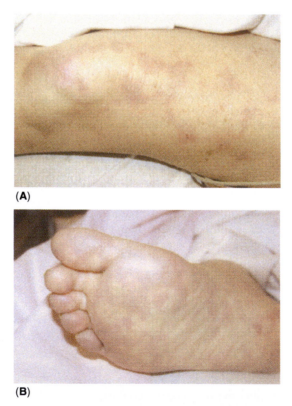

(A)

(B)

FIGURE 2.14   Clinical manifestations of DIC. **(A)** Livedo reticularis. **(B)** Patchy ischemic necrosis of right foot. This 70-yr-old woman developed HIT-associated DIC with hypofibrinogenemia, elevated INR, and reduced antithrombin and protein C activity levels nine days after emergency cardiac surgery for cardiac catheterization-associated dissection of the left main coronary artery (see text for additional clinical information). *Abbreviations*: DIC, disseminated intravascular coagulation; HIT, heparin-induced thrombocytopenia; INR, international normalized ratio.

for DIC included a fibrinogen of 1.2 g/L (normal, 1.5–4.0 g/L) that rose to 4.7 g/L 1 week later during therapeutic-dose danaparoid therapy, a strongly positive prot-amine sulfate paracoagulation assay (4+ reactivity at 15 minutes; normal, no reac-tivity), a fibrin D-dimer level that was greater than 2000 µg/L (normal, <500 µg/L), and the presence of red cell fragments. Additionally, the INR was elevated at 1.6 (normal, 0.9–1.2), although coagulation factors VII, V, X, and II all measured between 0.73 and 0.83 U/mL (normal, 0.50–1.50 U/mL). The anticoagulant treatment was successful in avoiding limb amputation. In my experience, limb ischemia, and necrosis associated with DIC that occurs in the absence of large artery thrombotic occlusion or warfarin therapy is an uncommon explanation for limb loss in HIT.

Livedo reticularis is also discussed on p. 56.

More recently, HIT-associated DIC has been recognized as a factor that can explain DTI treatment failure via "partial thromboplastin time (PTT) confounding"; here, supratherapeutic PTT values attained after initiating DTI therapy prompt repeated dose interruptions/reductions, with associated progression in micro- and macrovascu-lar thrombosis (Greinacher and Warkentin, 2008; Warkentin, 2010; see chap. 12). The key concept is that the supratherapeutic PTT does *not* accurately reflect supratherapeu-tic drug levels, but rather the combined effects of DTI and consumptive coagulopathy in raising the PTT; thus, the patient is not adequately anticoagulated. Figure 2.15 pro-vides an example of "PTT confounding" contributing to multiple limb loss.

Congenital Hypercoagulability and HIT-Associated Thrombosis

Gardyn and associates (1995) reported a patient with fatal HIT and widespread microvascular thrombosis. The investigators identified heterozygous factor V Leiden (G1691A mutation) in this patient, and they speculated that this contributed to the severe clinical course. However, the complications may also have been related to the treatment with LMWH and warfarin.

The interaction between factor V Leiden and thrombotic sequelae of HIT was formally investigated in a study of 165 patients with HIT, 16 (9.7%) of whom had factor V Leiden (Lee et al., 1998). No increase in the number or severity of venous or arterial thrombosis was seen. This result is not surprising, as thrombosis occurs in about 50–75% of patients with HIT (Warkentin and Kelton, 1996). Thus, even if the most common congenital hypercoagulable disorders, factor V Leiden and the pro-thrombin G20210A mutation (each occurring in about 5% of the population), were strongly associated with increased risk for thrombosis in HIT, only a few HIT-associated thromboses could thereby be explained.

Carlsson and colleagues (2003) studied 142 patients with HIT (79 with throm-bosis) to determine whether any of the 10 established or putative platelet receptor or clotting factor polymorphisms (including factor V Leiden and prothrombin G20210A mutation) was associated with thrombosis. None was found.

Lindhoff-Last et al. (2002) also found no association between factor V Leiden or prothrombin G20210A mutation and thrombosis in a smaller study of 21 patients. However, they found that more HIT patients had elevated factor VIII levels (at mean 29 months follow-up) than matched normal controls (16/21 *vs* 4/21). The significance of this finding is unclear.

Arterial Thrombosis

Lower-limb artery thrombosis was the first recognized complication of HIT (Weismann and Tobin, 1958; Roberts et al., 1964; Rhodes et al., 1973, 1977). Arterial thrombosis most commonly involves the distal aorta (e.g., saddle embolism) or the

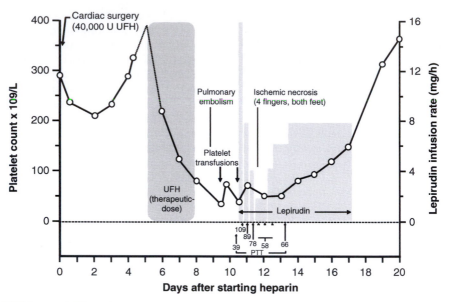

FIGURE 2.15 PTT confounding as a factor explaining multiple limb necrosis during lepirudin anti-coagulation of HIT complicated by overt (decompensated) DIC. A 56-yr-old 107-kg male underwent coronary artery bypass surgery. On postoperative day 6 he received iv therapeutic-dose UFH because of atrial fibrillation and dyspnea. In addition, over the next 3 days, intermittent acrocyanosis of the fingers and toes was observed. On postoperative day 9, pulmonary embolism was diagnosed (confirmed by high-probability ventilation–perfusion lung scan). At this time, the platelet count was 40×10^9/L, the INR was 2.1 (normal range, 0.9–1.2), the PTT was 39 sec (normal range, 22–33 sec); the fibrinogen was 3.6 g/L (normal range, 1.5–4.5 g/L), and the fibrin split products were increased (>80 μg/L; normal range, <10 μg/L). The serum creatinine was normal (1.2 mg/dL; normal range, 0.8–1.5 mg/dL). Lepirudin therapy was commenced at the approved dosing regimen, namely, an initial 43 mg bolus (~0.4 mg/kg, given iv over 20 min) plus infusion at 16 mg/hr (~0.15 mg/kg/hr). As shown, three subsequent dose interruptions (2 hr each) plus three dose reductions were made (each by 50%) until the patient was receiving only 2 mg/hr (~0.019 mg/kg/hr). After the third dose reduction, progression to severe multiple limb ischemic necrosis occurred, ultimately necessitating amputations of four digits (left hand), the left midfoot, and the right forefoot. The patient case questions the appropriateness—at least in some patients—of monitoring by PTT in the setting of HIT-associated DIC, and also raises the issue of "rebound" hypercoagulability, i.e., abrupt worsening of thrombosis soon after dose interruption. *Abbreviations*: DIC, disseminated intravascular coagulation; HIT, heparin-induced thrombocytopenia; INR, international normalized ratio; PTT, partial thromboplastin time; UFH, unfractionated heparin. *Source*: From Greinacher and Warkentin (2008).

large arteries of the lower limbs, leading to acute limb ischemia with absent pulses. Sometimes, platelet-rich thromboemboli from the left heart or proximal aorta explain acute lower-limb arterial ischemia (Vignon et al., 1996). Other arterial thrombotic complications that are relatively common in HIT include acute throm-botic stroke and myocardial infarction. The relative frequency of arterial thrombosis in HIT by location, namely, lower-limb artery occlusion >> stroke syndrome > myocardial infarction (Benhamou et al., 1985; Kappa et al., 1987; Warkentin and Kelton, 1996; Nand et al., 1997), is reversed from that observed in the non-HIT population (myocardial infarction > stroke syndrome > lower-limb artery occlusion).

Uncommon but well-described arterial thrombotic events in HIT include mesenteric artery thrombosis (bowel infarction), brachial artery thrombosis (upper-limb gangrene), and renal artery thrombosis (renal infarction). Multiple arterial thrombotic events have been reported. Occasionally, microembolization of thrombus originating from the heart or aorta causes foot or toe necrosis with palpable arterial pulses.

Angiographic Appearance

Lindsey and colleagues (1979) reported a distinct angiographic appearance of heparin-induced thromboembolic lesions, described as "broad-based, isolated, gently lobulated excrescences, which produced 30–95% narrowing of the arterial lumen. The abrupt appearance of such prominent luminal contour deformities in arterial segments that were otherwise smooth and undistorted was unexpected and impressive .... In each case, the lesions were located proximal to sites of arterial occlusion." The radiologic and surgical experience described suggests that distal embolization of "white" clots composed of "platelet-fibrin aggregates" accounted for the limb ischemia.

Graft, Prosthetic Device, and Extracorporeal Circuit Thrombosis

HIT predisposes to thrombosis of blood in contact with native or prosthetic grafts or vascular fistulae, valve or other intravascular prostheses, as well as extracorporeal circuits (Towne et al., 1979; Silver et al., 1983; Bernasconi et al., 1988; AbuRahma et al., 1991; Hall et al., 1992; Lipton and Gould, 1992). This presents serious management problems in certain situations, such as renal hemodialysis (see chap. 18). Clinicians should check for unexpected platelet count declines, and test for HIT antibodies, in patients who develop thrombosis of grafts, prostheses, or other devices during heparin treatment. Whether heparin bound covalently to intravascular grafts could explain postoperative HIT seems unlikely, given the rarity of these cases, their inevitable confounding with intra-/postoperative heparin, and a plausible alternative explanation through delayed-onset HIT–related mechanisms (see chap. 20).

MISCELLANEOUS COMPLICATIONS OF HIT
Heparin-Induced Skin Lesions at sc Injection Sites

Skin lesions that occur at the site(s) of sc heparin injection are a manifestation of the HIT syndrome. For unknown reasons, only 10–20% of patients who form HIT antibodies during sc UFH or LMWH treatment develop these lesions (Warkentin et al., 2005b). Furthermore, about 50–75% of patients who develop heparin-induced skin lesions do not develop thrombocytopenia, although heparin-dependent, platelet-activating HIT antibodies are readily detectable (Warkentin, 1996a, 1997; Handschin et al., 2005).

The skin abnormalities range in appearance from indurated, erythematous nodules or plaques (Fig. 2.16A) to frank necrotizing lesions (Fig. 2.16B) that start five or more days (median, day 8) after beginning heparin injections (Hasegawa, 1984; MacLean et al., 1990; Wütschert et al., 1999). The lesions can occur earlier if there was recent treatment with heparin given by another route that resulted in the formation of HIT antibodies. Some erythematous plaques have an eczematous appearance. Necrotic lesions typically consist of a central black eschar surrounded

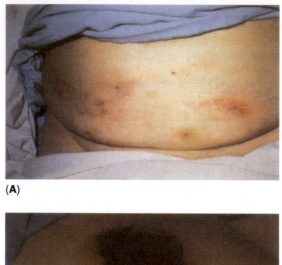

(A)

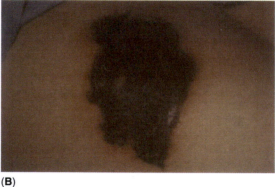

(B)

FIGURE 2.16 Heparin-induced skin lesions. (**A**) Heparin-induced erythematous plaques: UFH injections into the lower abdomen resulted in painful erythematous plaques beginning on day 7 of sc UFH treatment; at this time, the platelet count fell only by 9% from 340 to 311×10^9/L. HIT antibody seroconversion from a negative baseline was shown using the serotonin release assay (from 0 to 84% serotonin release). (**B**) Heparin-induced skin necrosis: UFH injections into the right anterior thigh led to skin necrosis: a large black eschar with irregular borders is surrounded by a narrow band of erythema. The platelet count fell to 32×10^9/L; despite stopping heparin, the patient developed symptomatic proximal deep vein thrombosis 10 days later. *Abbreviations*: HIT, heparin-induced thrombocytopenia; UFH, unfractionated heparin. *Source*: (**B**) From Warkentin (1996a).

by a cuff of induration and erythema (Fig. 2.16B). Complex skin lesions can result—for example, several discrete areas of necrosis (each lesion corresponding to a different heparin injection site), each with a surrounding violaceous halo, with all circumscribed by a diffuse erythema. Even the least severe forms of heparin-induced skin lesions usually cause pain or pruritus.

Both UFH and LMWH can cause these reactions (Handschin et al., 2005). Patients who develop UFH-induced skin lesions generally will develop further lesions if LMWH is substituted for the UFH (Bircher et al., 1990). In contrast, it is uncommon for danaparoid or fondaparinux to cause these reactions de novo (Schindewolf et al., 2010b), or to cross-react when substituted for patients with UFH- or LMWH-induced delayed hypersensitivity reaction (DHR) (Weberschock et al., 2011).

Schindewolf and coworkers (2010a) found that non-necrotizing skin lesions at heparin (primarily LMWH) injection sites are usually a manifestation of DHR, rather than of HIT. This suggests that when using the 4Ts scoring system—in which non-necrotizing skin lesions at sc heparin injection sites are scored as 1 point (for category "Thrombosis")—that a score of 0 points be assigned for the category "oTher", given that DHR is a definite alternative explanation for these lesions (Warkentin and Linkins, 2010).

In my experience, both necrotizing and (HIT-related) nonnecrotizing skin lesions are much less common than in the 1980s and early 1990s, perhaps because their most common clinical setting—postorthopedic surgery thromboprophylaxis with UFH (Warkentin, 1996a, Warkentin et al., 2005b)—is rarely encountered nowadays.

Histopathology
Lymphocyte infiltration of the upper and middermis that can extend into the epidermis characterizes the erythematous plaque (Bircher et al., 1990). Dermal and epidermal edema (spongiosis) is observed in lesions that appear eczematous. The T lymphocytes of helper–suppressor (CD4+) phenotype predominate, together with CD1+/DR+ dendritic (Langerhans) cells, and are consistent with a (type IV) DHR. Cytokine synthesis by activated CD4 cells could explain the peripheral blood eosinophilia that has been reported in a few patients (Bircher et al., 1994). In contrast, histopathology of lesions associated with cutaneous necrosis usually shows intravascular thrombosis of dermal vessels, with or without perivascular inflammation and red cell extravasation of variable degree (Hall et al., 1980; Kearsley et al., 1982; Cohen et al., 1988; MacLean et al., 1990; Balestra et al., 1994).

Management
Heparin-induced skin lesions should be considered a possible marker for the HIT syndrome (Warkentin et al., 2005b). Platelet count monitoring, if not already being performed, should be initiated and continued for several days, even after stopping heparin administration. The reason is that some patients develop a fall in platelet count, together with thrombosis (often affecting limb arteries), that begins several days after stopping the heparin (Warkentin, 1996a, 1997). An alternative anticoagulant, such as danaparoid, lepirudin, or argatroban, should be given, particularly in patients whose original indication for anticoagulation still exists or who develop progressive thrombocytopenia. The skin lesions themselves should be managed conservatively whenever possible, although some patients require debridement of necrotic tissues followed by skin grafting (Hall et al., 1980).

> *Rule 9*
>
> Erythematous or (especially) necrotizing skin lesions at heparin injection sites should be considered dermal manifestations of the HIT syndrome, irrespective of the platelet count, unless proved otherwise. Patients who develop thrombocytopenia in association with heparin-induced skin lesions are at an increased risk for venous and, especially, arterial thrombosis.

Classic Coumarin-Induced Skin Necrosis
Classic coumarin-induced skin necrosis (CISN) is a very rare complication of oral anticoagulant therapy (Cole et al., 1988). In its classic form, it is characterized by dermal necrosis, usually in a central (nonacral) location, such as breast, abdomen, thigh, or leg, that begins 3–6 days after starting therapy with warfarin or other coumarin anticoagulants (Fig. 2.10). Initially, there is localized pain, induration,

and erythema that progresses over hours to central purplish-black skin discoloration and blistering, ultimately evolving to well-demarcated, full-thickness necrosis involving skin and subdermal tissues. Some patients require surgical debridement. Case reports suggest that congenital deficiency of natural anticoagulant proteins, especially protein C, is sometimes a pathogenic factor (Broekmans et al., 1983; Comp, 1993).

There is evidence that HIT also predisposes to classic CISN (Celoria et al., 1988; Cohen et al., 1989; Warkentin et al., 1999; Srinivasan et al., 2004). Theoretically, this could result from increased consumption of anticoagulant factors, thereby leading to greater reduction in protein C in the setting of increased thrombin generation in HIT (Tans et al., 1991; Warkentin et al., 1997). However, central lesions of CISN seem less likely to complicate HIT than the related syndrome of coumarin-induced venous limb gangrene (Warkentin et al., 1997, 1999). Perhaps active DVT in HIT localizes the progressive microvascular thrombosis to acral tissues already affected by extensive venous thrombosis.

Other Heparin-Associated Skin Lesions
Skin Necrosis in the Absence of Coumarin Therapy
Other patients have developed skin lesions during iv heparin therapy, or at locations otherwise distant from sc injection sites, in the absence of coumarin therapy. Hartman and colleagues (1988) reported a man who received iv heparin for saphenous vein thrombosis: the platelet count fell from 864 to $44 \times 10^9/L$ (day 10). On day 7, when the platelet count had fallen by 33% to $575 \times 10^9/L$, progressive necrosis of skin in the thigh at the region of the thrombosed vein occurred, necessitating surgical excision. Thrombosis of veins and capillaries, with arterial sparing, was noted. Balestra et al. (1994) reported a patient who developed thrombocytopenia ($75 \times 10^9/L$) and skin necrosis of the thigh on day 9 of sc injections of LMWH given into the lower abdominal wall. A skin biopsy showed small vessel thrombosis with a mild inflammatory reaction.

Other clinicians have reported patients with HIT antibodies who developed skin lesions that occurred at locations distant from subcutaneous LMWH injection sites, even in the absence of thrombocytopenia (Tietge et al., 1998).

Other Skin Lesions Associated with Heparin Treatment
Livedo Reticularis. The bluish, reticulated (network-like), mottled appearance of livedo reticularis was reported in a patient with HIT complicating iv UFH given for atrial fibrillation after heart surgery (Gross et al., 1993). This patient also had DIC, microangiopathic peripheral blood abnormalities, and fibrin thrombi noted within small dermal vessels. The livedo appearance results from microvascular thrombosis, with slowing of blood flow and dilation of the horizontally oriented dermal venous drainage channels (Copeman, 1975). Fig. 2.14A (see p. 50) shows livedo reticularis associated with HIT and DIC.

Urticaria and Other Miscellaneous Lesions. Other dermatologic consequences of heparin treatment do not appear to be related to HIT. These range from common lesions (ecchymosis) to rare effects of iv heparin, such as vasculitis (Jones and Epstein, 1987) and cutaneous necrosis with hemorrhagic bullae (Kelly et al., 1981). Some patients have developed widespread urticarial lesions, sometimes accompanied by angioedema, during treatment with sc or iv heparin (Odeh and Oliven, 1992; Patriarca et al., 1994). In one patient skin testing suggested a generalized reaction against the preservative chlorbutol (Dux et al., 1981). Although LMWH injections were claimed to have caused distal extremity dermal lesions in a patient with HIT (Payne and Kovacs, 2003), it is possible these were related to concomitant warfarin therapy.

Cutaneous (Type IV) Delayed Hypersensitivity Reactions. Not all cutaneous lesions that develop at UFH or LMWH injection sites represent HIT. The so-called type IV delayed hypersensitivity reactions, which are characterized by pruritic infiltrations or blistering erythematous reactions of variable size at heparin injection sites, are usually not associated with the presence of anti-PF4/H antibodies (Schindewolf et al., 2010b). More than 90% of affected patients are females, with high body mass index, and many are pregnant (Ludwig et al., 2006; Schindewolf et al., 2009). The histopathology consists of epidermal spongiosis, dermal edema, and lymphocytic infiltrates accompanied by numerous eosinophils in the papillary dermis (Grasseger et al., 2001). Cutaneous allergy testing usually shows variable cross-reactivity with other heparin(oids), with frequency of cross-reactivity reportedly related to molecular weight, as follows (UFH > LMWH > danaparoid > fondaparinux) (Ludwig et al., 2005, 2006). However, some investigators have observed patients with cutaneous cross-reactivity against various LMWH preparations but not with UFH (Grasseger et al., 2001).

The distinction between non-HIT and HIT-associated skin lesions is not trivial: whereas iv heparin administration is appropriate for managing patients who cannot tolerate sc injections because of DHR (Koch et al., 1991; Gaigl et al., 2005; Ludwig et al., 2006), iv bolus heparin administration to a patient with HIT-associated skin lesions can lead to rapid-onset HIT and an associated acute systemic reaction (ASR) (Platell and Tan, 1986).

Acute Systemic (Anaphylactoid) Reactions Following IV Bolus Heparin

ASR refers to a variety of symptoms and signs that characteristically begin 5–30 minutes after an iv heparin bolus is given to a patient with circulating HIT antibodies (Nelson et al., 1978; Warkentin et al., 1992, 1994; Popov et al., 1997; Ling and Warkentin, 1998; Warkentin, 2002b; Mims et al., 2004; Warkentin and Greinacher, 2009) (Table 2.5; Fig. 2.3). Only about one quarter of at-risk patients who receive a heparin bolus develop such a reaction. Less commonly, patients develop similar reactions within 1 hour after sc injection of LMWH (Srinivasan et al., 2004; Warkentin et al., 2008b; Hillis et al., 2011). The most common signs and

---

TABLE 2.5 Clinical Features of Postheparin Acute Systemic Reactions

Timing: onset 5–30 min after iv heparin bolus, or within 60 min of sc LMWH injection
Clinical context: recent use of heparin (past 5–100 days)
Laboratory features: abrupt, reversible fall in the platelet count
Signs and symptoms
    Inflammatory: chills, rigors, fever, flushing
    Cardiorespiratory: tachycardia, hypertension, tachypnea, dyspnea, chest pain or tightness, cardiopulmonary arrest (rare)
    Gastrointestinal: nausea, vomiting, diarrhea
    Neurological: headache, transient global amnesia (rare)

Abbreviations: iv, intravenous; LMWH, low molecular weight heparin; sc, subcutaneous.

symptoms are fever and chills, hypertension, and tachycardia. Less common are flushing, headache, chest pain, dyspnea, tachypnea, and large-volume diarrhea. In some patients, severe dyspnea is the predominant sign, termed "pseudopulmonary embolism" (Popov et al., 1997; Hartman et al., 2006); multiple small perfusion defects on radionuclide lung scans can be shown (Nelson et al., 1978; Ling and Warkentin, 1998). Fatal cardiac and respiratory arrest has been reported (Ansell et al., 1986; Platell and Tan, 1986; Hewitt et al., 1998; Warkentin and Greinacher, 2009).

An abrupt fall in the platelet count invariably accompanies these reactions. However, the platelet count drop is often transient (Warkentin et al., 2005b). Thus, physicians should determine the platelet count immediately on suspecting the diagnosis and test for HIT antibodies. Heparin must be discontinued, as further use can lead to fatal complications (Ling and Warkentin, 1998).

Rule 10

Any inflammatory, cardiopulmonary, or other unexpected acute event that begins 5–30 min after an iv heparin bolus, or within 60 min of a sc LMWH injection, should be considered acute HIT unless proved otherwise. The postreaction platelet count should be measured promptly and compared with prereaction levels, because the platelet count fall is abrupt and often transient.

The clinical features of ASR are not typical of IgE-mediated anaphylaxis (i.e., urticaria, angioedema, and hypotension are *not* seen). Rather, the syndrome resembles febrile transfusion reactions commonly observed after platelet transfusions, suggesting a common pathogenesis of proinflammatory cytokines associated with cellular activation (Heddle et al., 1994). Moreover, there are similarities between ASR and the administration of ADP in humans, including acute dyspnea, tachycardia, and transient thrombocytopenia (Davey and Lander, 1964).

A few patients have developed acute, transient impairment of anterograde memory (i.e., the ability to form new memories) following an iv heparin bolus in association with acute HIT (Warkentin et al., 1994; Pohl et al., 2000). This syndrome resembles that of transient global amnesia, a well-characterized neurologic syndrome of uncertain pathogenesis.

Heparin Resistance

Difficulty in maintaining therapeutic anticoagulation despite increasing heparin dosage, or heparin resistance, is a common finding in patients with HIT-associated thrombosis (Rhodes et al., 1977; Silver et al., 1983). Possible explanations include neutralization of heparin by PF4 released from activated platelets (Padilla et al., 1992) or pathophysiologic consequences of platelet-derived microparticles (Bode et al., 1991). Heparin resistance is not specific for HIT, however, and occurs in many patients with extensive thrombosis of various etiologies (e.g., cancer).

SPECIAL CLINICAL SITUATIONS
Cardiac and Neurologic Complications of HIT

Although HIT can affect almost any organ system, some clinical specialties observe a wider spectrum of thrombotic and other sequelae of HIT. Table 2.6 lists complications encountered in cardiology and neurology. Several studies of HIT in postcardiac

TABLE 2.6 Cardiologic and Neurologic Complications of HIT

Cardiologic Complications
    Myocardial infarction (Rhodes et al., 1973; Van der Weyden et al., 1983)
    Occlusion of saphenous vein grafts postcoronary artery bypass surgery[a]
    Intra-atrial thrombus (left and right[b] heart chambers) (Scheffold et al., 1995; Olbricht et al., 1998)
    Intraventricular thrombus (left and right[b] heart chambers) (Commeau et al., 1986; Dion et al.,
        1989; Vignon et al., 1996)
    Prosthetic valve thrombosis (Bernasconi et al., 1988; Vazquez-Jimenez et al., 1999)
    Right heart failure secondary to massive pulmonary embolism
    Cardiac arrest post-iv heparin bolus (Ansell et al., 1986; Platell and Tan, 1986; Hewitt et al., 1998)
Neurologic complications
    Stroke syndrome
        In situ thrombosis
        Progressive stroke in patients receiving heparin for treatment of stroke
            (Ramirez-Lassepas et al., 1984)
        Cardiac embolization (Scheffold et al., 1995)
        Cerebral vein (dural venous sinus) thrombosis (Van der Weyden et al., 1983; Kyritsis et al.,
            1990; Meyer-Lindenberg et al., 1997; Warkentin and Bernstein, 2003); complicating
            pregnancy (Calhoun and Hesser, 1987)
        Amaurosis fugax (Theuerkauf et al., 2000)
        Ischemic lumbosacral plexopathy (Jain, 1986)
        Paraplegia, transient (Maurin et al., 1991) or permanent (Feng et al., 1993), associated with
            distal aortic thrombosis
        Transient global amnesia (Warkentin et al., 1994; Teh et al., 2010)
        Headache[c]

[a]Thrombosis preferentially affects saphenous vein grafts rather than internal mammary artery grafts (Liu et al., 2002; Ayala et al., 2004).
[b]Although adherent thrombi that likely developed *in situ* have been reported (Dion et al., 1989), emboli originating from limb veins can explain right-sided intra-atrial or intraventricular clots.
[c]Headache as a feature of HIT is suggested by *(i)* its occurrence in patients with acute systemic reactions postheparin bolus; and *(ii)* its concurrence with onset of thrombocytopenia in several patients who developed HIT in a clinical trial (unpublished observations of the author).
Abbreviation: HIT, heparin-induced thrombocytopenia.

surgery patients have been reported (Wan et al., 2006; Kerendi et al., 2007; Thielmann et al., 2010). Mortality rates appeared high, but this was likely due to non-HIT factors since one study found uniformly high mortality among EIA-positive patients irrespective of whether the platelet activation assay was positive or negative (Thielmann et al., 2010).

HIT in Pregnancy

HIT has complicated UFH treatment given for VTE complicating pregnancy (Van der Weyden et al., 1983; Meytes et al., 1986; Copplestone and Oscier, 1987; Greinacher et al., 1992) or the postpartum period (Calhoun and Hesser, 1987). HIT seems to be rare in this patient population; no pregnant patients have been diagnosed with HIT over a 25-year period in Hamilton. Plasma glycosaminoglycans are increased during pregnancy (Andrew et al., 1992), which could contribute to lower frequency or pathogenicity of HIT antibodies. HIT antibodies cross the placenta (Greinacher et al., 1993), so it is at least theoretically possible that a heparin-treated newborn delivered from a mother with acute HIT could develop this drug reaction.

Pregnant patients with HIT have developed unusual events, such as cerebral dural sinus thrombosis (Van der Weyden et al., 1983; Calhoun and Hesser, 1987). Treatment options for pregnant patients with life-threatening thrombosis include danaparoid or fondaparinux as these drugs do not cross the placenta (see chaps. 12, 16, and 17). The more benign syndrome of heparin-induced skin lesions without thrombocytopenia has also been reported in pregnant patients (Drouet et al., 1992). Danaparoid was reported to be effective in a patient who developed LMWH-induced skin lesions (de Saint-Blanquat et al., 2000).

HIT in Children and Neonates

There are anecdotal reports of HIT occurring in children, some as young as three months of age (Laster et al., 1987; Oriot et al., 1990; Potter et al., 1992; Murdoch et al., 1993; Klement et al., 1996; Butler et al., 1997; Ranze et al., 1999, 2001; Klenner et al., 2004;) (see chap. 21). However, not all of these patients underwent confirmatory testing with specific diagnostic assays. HIT in children has a similar, often dramatic clinical course, as is seen in adults. The frequency of HIT in the pediatric population is unknown.

The frequency and clinical import of HIT in neonates receiving heparin in intensive care settings is controversial. Spadone and colleagues (1992) investigated 34 newborn infants (average gestational age, 29 weeks) who developed thrombocytopenia or thrombosis, beginning an average of 22 days after starting heparin therapy. Platelet aggregation studies suggested the presence of HIT antibodies in 41% of these neonates. Aortic thrombosis complicating umbilical artery catheter use was the most common complication. Another group (Butler et al., 1997), also using platelet aggregation studies, reported a neonate who may have developed fatal HIT shortly after birth. More specific activation or antigen assays were not performed in either study, however. A recent study of 108 neonates who received UFH flushes found no HIT antibodies using a sensitive antigen assay (Klenner et al., 2003).

HIT in Bone Marrow and Solid Organ Transplantation

Given the widespread use of heparin to maintain patency of indwelling catheters, it is surprising that there are few reports of HIT in patients undergoing intensive anti-cancer chemotherapy. Two reports describe patients with apparent HIT complicating allogeneic or autologous marrow or stem cell transplantation (Tezcan et al., 1994; Sauer et al., 1999). Subclavian vein thrombosis occurred in one patient. It is possible that the combination of intensive chemotherapy and treatment-induced thrombocytopenia reduces the likelihood of HIT antibody formation or clinical expression of HIT.

There is an intriguing report of a man recently recovered from HIT who was about to receive autologous marrow transplantation. When his marrow was collected into heparin anticoagulant, substantial *ex vivo* thrombus formation occurred, preventing adequate cell collection (Bowers and Jones, 2002).

Solid organ or tissue transplantation is rarely complicated by postoperative HIT (Hourigan et al., 2002; Anderegg et al., 2005; Rastellini et al., 2006). Whether postoperative immunosuppression reduces the risk of HIT compared with other postoperative patient populations is unknown.

RISK FACTORS FOR HIT: IMPLICATIONS FOR CLINICAL PRESENTATION AND PLATELET COUNT MONITORING

Risk Factors for HIT

Besides duration of heparin administration, other risk factors for HIT include the following: (*i*) type of heparin (UFH >> LMWH >> fondaparinux); (*ii*) type of patient (postsurgical > medical > obstetric/pediatric); (*iii*) patient sex (female > male) (Warkentin et al., 1995, 2005a, 2006) (see chap. 4). Ironically, despite the greater risk of HIT in females (odds ratio, 1.5–2.0) (Warkentin et al., 2006), HIT is rare in pregnancy (Fausett et al., 2001), and has not been reported with LMWH administered during pregnancy (Greer and Nelson-Piercy, 2005). In addition, major (*vs* minor) trauma is a risk factor for HIT (Lubenow et al., 2010), as may be proinflammatory conditions, such as malignancy (Opatrny and Warner, 2004; Prandoni et al., 2007; Linkins and Warkentin, 2011; Sandset, 2012).

HIT in Surgical Patients

These aforementioned risk factors—particularly surgery—help to explain the various clinical scenarios in which HIT is usually encountered. For example, the high seroconversion risk associated with heparin given intra- or postoperatively helps to explain why typical- (or delayed-) onset HIT usually occurs in postoperative patients. This results in a characteristic platelet count profile: the patient first evinces an early, transient postoperative thrombocytopenia that partially or completely recovers, followed by an unexpected *secondary* platelet count fall indicative of typical- (or delayed-) onset HIT that begins between postoperative days 5 and 10 (inclusive) (Fig. 2.17A, red solid line). It is rare for early postoperative thrombocytopenia to be explained by HIT (although we have occasionally encountered such patients) (Warkentin and Sheppard, 2007; Warkentin et al., 2012b). Sometimes, a postoperative patient will develop rapid-onset HIT (Fig. 2.17A, red dotted line), for example, if a patient who received intra- or postoperative heparin subsequently receives therapeutic-dose heparin to treat thrombosis.

HIT in Medical Patients

In contrast, a "medical" patient who presents with VTE and whose platelet count abruptly falls within hours of receiving heparin may have rapid-onset HIT (Fig. 2.17B, red solid line). Indeed, such a patient might be better classified as a "surgical" patient if the presence of HIT antibodies can be explained by recent surgery (past three months) and associated heparin exposure. Indeed, in the Matisse VTE trials, there were 14 patients who presented with VTE and who had heparin-dependent, platelet-activating antibodies at the time of study enrolment: four of these patients received heparin (UFH or LMWH), and all four developed rapid onset of thrombocytopenia (none of the remaining 10 patients who received fondaparinux developed thrombocytopenia; see Fig. 17.4 in chap. 17) (Warkentin et al., 2011). In contrast, there were only 6 patients in the Matisse trials who developed seroconversion to a positive SRA as a result of treatment with study drug exposure (to UFH, LMWH, or fondaparinux) in the clinical trials themselves (unpublished observations). Given the relatively low frequency of de novo HIT in a medical patient (Fig. 2.17B, red dotted line), it may well be that HIT in "medical" patients is more often the result of recent "surgical" status and associated heparin-induced immunization.

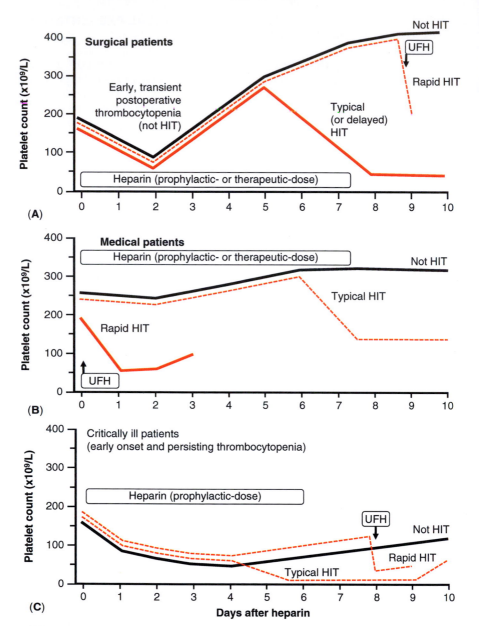

FIGURE 2.17 Characteristic profiles of HIT in relation to clinical setting. (**A**) HIT in surgical patients. The most common presentation is typical- (or delayed-) onset HIT (solid red line). Less often, patients develop rapid-onset HIT in the postoperative period when heparin is restarted (or the dose increased), often because of thrombosis (red dashed line). (**B**) HIT in medical patients. Most often, patients develop rapid-onset HIT when they receive UFH (or LMWH) to treat VTE (solid red line). Although classified as "medical" patients, these are often postsurgical patients (when the reason for HIT antibodies is because of recent perioperative heparin exposure). Less often, medical patients develop typical-onset HIT (red dashed line). (*Continued*)

FIGURE 2.17 (*Continued*) (**C**) HIT in critically ill patients. Only a small minority of thrombocytopenic critically ill patients have HIT; clinical clues include a superimposed "typical" onset of thrombocytopenia or an abrupt (rapid-onset) exacerbation of thrombocytopenia if heparin dose is restarted or increased (two red dashed lines).

HIT in Critically Ill Patients versus (Non-HIT) Early-Onset and Persisting Thrombocytopenia

In a critically ill medical or surgical patient, early-onset and persisting thrombocytopenia most likely represents a non–HIT-related illness, such as septicemia or multiorgan dysfunction syndrome, even if tests for anti-PF4/H antibodies subsequently become positive (Selleng et al., 2010a). The risk of such a patient additionally developing HIT appears to be low (<2%), and would be suggested by a *superimposed* drop in platelet count with temporal features consistent with HIT, particularly if accompanied by thrombosis (Selleng et al., 2008b; Warkentin, 2010; Warkentin et al., 2012a) (Fig. 2.17C). Functional (platelet activation) tests are diagnostically useful, given the high frequency of subclinical anti-PF4/H seroconversion.

Platelet Count Monitoring for HIT

Platelet count monitoring for HIT is controversial. Several years ago, regular platelet count monitoring for HIT—ranging from every three to four days (Hyers et al., 1989) to daily monitoring (Hirsh et al., 1992, 1995; Hyers et al., 1995)—was mentioned in guidelines for VTE treatment with UFH (a situation in which daily blood testing for anticoagulant monitoring by PTT is standard). In contrast, contemporaneous thromboprophylaxis recommendations did not discuss platelet count monitoring (e.g., Clagett et al., 1995). However, the recognition that HIT could occur at a frequency of at least 1% in the setting of postoperative thromboprophylaxis with UFH suggested that platelet count monitoring might be appropriate in these patients as well (Hirsh et al., 1998). Moreover, in postoperative patients, regular platelet counts are needed to identify the appropriate "baseline" platelet count—which could be a markedly elevated platelet count on day 7 or 8—that precedes the subsequent HIT-associated platelet count decline (Warkentin et al., 2003).

The differing risks of HIT, depending on the clinical situation, resulted in the concept of stratifying the intensity of platelet count monitoring depending on the patient's risk of developing HIT (Warkentin, 2002c; Warkentin and Greinacher, 2004; Warkentin et al., 2008a) (Table 2.7). For a high-risk situation (frequency >1%), daily or every-other-day platelet monitoring (from day 4 to 10, while receiving heparin) might be appropriate, whereas no monitoring would be reasonable when HIT was rare (<0.1%). Recently, the 2012 American College of Chest Physicians Antithrombotic Guidelines recommended less intensive monitoring (every two or three days) for high-risk patients, and no monitoring for patients with risk <1% (Linkins et al., 2012).

Arguments exist both for and against platelet count monitoring for HIT.

FOR

1. There is consensus that strongly suspected (or confirmed) isolated HIT warrants nonheparin anticoagulant therapy; however, by definition, isolated HIT can only be identified by measuring the platelet count (assumes absence of signs of symptoms of thrombosis).

TABLE 2.7 American College of Chest Physicians Recommendations for Platelet Count Monitoring for HIT

	Risk of HIT and platelet count monitoring (Day 4 to 14, while on heparin[a])		
Year	High risk (>1%)[b]	Intermediate risk (0.1–1.0%)[c]	Low risk (<0.1%)[d]
2004	At least EOD	Every 2–3 days (when practical[e])	Not recommended
2008	At least EOD	Every 2–3 days (when practical[e])	Not recommended
2012	Every 2–3 days	Not recommended	Not recommended

[a]The crucial time period for monitoring "typical onset" HIT is between days 4 to 14 (first day of heparin = day 0), where the highest platelet count from day 4 (inclusive) onward represents the "baseline." Platelet count monitoring can cease before day 14 when heparin is stopped.
[b]High risk: patients receiving prophylactic- or therapeutic-dose UFH after major surgery.
[c]Intermediate risk: medical/obstetrical patients receiving prophylactic- or therapeutic-dose UFH, or receiving LMWH after first receiving UFH; postsurgery patients receiving prophylactic-dose LMWH or UFH "flushes."
[d]Low risk: medical/obstetric patients receiving LMWH, or only UFH "flushes"; any patient receiving UFH or LMWH ≤4 days; any patient receiving prophylactic- or therapeutic-dose fondaparinux.
[e]Platelet count monitoring may not be practical when UFH or LMWH is given to outpatients.
Abbreviations: EOD, every other day; HIT, heparin-induced thrombocytopenia; LMWH, low molecular weight heparin; UFH, unfractionated heparin.

2. The frequency and clinical severity of HIT-associated thrombosis is most common in the setting of antithrombotic prophylaxis. Since the goal of prophylaxis is to prevent thrombosis, this would seem to justify attempts to identify an adverse drug effect that paradoxically increases the risk of thrombosis far beyond that of thromboprophylaxis not being applied (see section "HIT Is a Hypercoagulable State").

3. Regular platelet counts are required to identify postoperative platelet count changes—including postoperative thrombocytosis—which identifies the "baseline" platelet count needed to assess the magnitude of the subsequent HIT-associated platelet count decline (which otherwise would be underestimated).

AGAINST

1. Platelet count monitoring may lead to HIT "overdiagnosis," with inappropriate discontinuation of heparin or substitution with alternative anticoagulants.
2. Risks and benefits of platelet count monitoring have not been proven.
3. Cost and burden.

REFERENCES
AbuRahma AF, Boland JP, Witsberger T. Diagnostic and therapeutic strategies of white clot syndrome. Am J Surg 162: 175–179, 1991.
Alsaleh KA, Al-Nasser SM, Bates SM, Patel A, Warkentin TE, Arnold DM. Delayed-onset heparin-induced thrombocytopenia caused by low molecular weight heparin manifesting during fondaparinux prophylaxis. Am J Hematol 83: 876–878, 2008.
Anderegg BA, Baillie GM, Lin A, Lazarchick J. Heparin-induced thrombocytopenia in a renal transplant recipient. Am J Transplant 5: 1537–1540, 2005.
Anderson KC, Kihajda FP, Bell WR. Diagnosis and treatment of anticoagulant-related adrenal hemorrhage. Am J Hematol 11: 379–385, 1981.
Andrew M, Mitchell L, Berry L, Paes B, Delorme M, Ofosu F, Burrows R, Khambalia B. An anticoagulant dermatan sulfate proteoglycan circulates in the pregnant woman and her fetus. J Clin Invest 89: 321–326, 1992.

Ansell JE, Clark WP Jr, Compton CC. Fatal reactions associated with intravenous heparin. Drug Intell Clin Pharm 20: 74–75, 1986.

Arepally GM, Ortel TL. Clinical practice. Heparin-induced thrombocytopenia. N Engl J Med 355: 809–817, 2006.

Arthur CK, Grant SJB, Murray WK, Isbister JP, Stiel JN, Lauer CS. Heparin-associated acute adrenal insufficiency. Aust NZ J Med 15: 454–455, 1985.

Ayala E, Rosado MF, Morgensztern D, Kharfan-Dabaja MA, Byrnes JJ. Heparin-induced thrombocytopenia presenting with thrombosis of multiple saphenous vein grafts and myocardial infarction. Am J Hematol 76: 383–385, 2004.

Balestra B, Quadri P, Demarmels Biasiutti F, Furlan M, Lämmle B. Low molecular weight heparin-induced thrombocytopenia and skin necrosis distant from injection sites. Eur J Haematol 53: 61–63, 1994.

Baroletti S, Hurwitz S, Conti NA, Fanikos J, Piazza G, Goldhaber SZ. Thrombosis in suspected heparin-induced thrombocytopenia occurs more often with high antibody levels. Am J Med 125: 44–49, 2012.

Beland B, Busse H, Loick HM, Ostermann H, van Aken H. Phlegmasia cerulea dolens, cerebral venous thrombosis, and fatal pulmonary embolism due to heparin-induced thrombocytopenic thrombosis syndrome. Anesth Analg 85: 1272–1274, 1997.

Benhamou AC, Gruel Y, Barsotti J, Castellani L, Marchand M, Guerois C, Leclerc MH, Delahousse B, Griguer P, Leroy J. The white clot syndrome or heparin-associated thrombocytopenia and thrombosis (WCS or HATT). Int Angiol 4: 303–310, 1985.

Bernasconi F, Metivet F, Estrade G, Garnier D, Donatien Y. Thrombose d'une prothèse valvulaire mitrale au cours d'une thrombopénie induite par l'héparine. Traitement fibrinolytique. Presse Med 17: 1366, 1988. [in French]

Betrosian AP, Theodossiades G, Lambroulis G, Kostantonis D, Balla M, Papanikolaou M, Georgiades G. Heparin-induced thrombocytopenia with pulmonary embolism and disseminated intravascular coagulation associated with low molecular weight heparin. Am J Med Sci 325: 45–47, 2003.

Bircher AJ, Fluckiger R, Buchner SA. Eczematous infiltrated plaques to subcutaneous heparin: a type IV allergic reaction. Br J Dermatol 123: 507–514, 1990.

Bircher AJ, Itin PH, Buchner SA. Skin lesions, hypereosinophilia, and subcutaneous heparin. Lancet 343: 861, 1994.

Bleasel JF, Rasko JEJ, Rickard KA, Richards G. Acute adrenal insufficiency secondary to heparin-induced thrombocytopenia-thrombosis syndrome. Med J Aust 157: 192–193, 1992.

Bode AP, Castellani WJ, Hodges ED, Yelverton S. The effect of lysed platelets on neutralization of heparin in vitro with protamine as measured by the activated coagulation time (ACT). Thromb Haemost 66: 213–217, 1991.

Boshkov LK, Warkentin TE, Hayward CPM, Andrew M, Kelton JG. Heparin-induced thrombocytopenia and thrombosis: clinical and laboratory studies. Br J Haematol 84: 322–328, 1993.

Bowers MJ, Jones FGC. Thrombus in harvested marrow from a patient with recent heparin-induced thrombocytopenia. Br J Haematol 119: 294, 2002.

Broekmans AW, Bertina RM, Loeliger EA, Hofmann V, Klingemann HG. Protein C and the development of skin necrosis during anticoagulant. therapy. Thromb Haemost 49: 251, 1983.

Brushwood DB. Hospital liable for allergic reaction to heparin used in injection flush. Am J Hosp Pharm 49: 1491–1492, 1992.

Butler TJ, Sodoma LJ, Doski JJ, Cheu HW, Berg ST, Stokes GN, Lancaster KJ. Heparin-associated thrombocytopenia and thrombosis as the cause of a fatal thrombus on extracorporeal membrane oxygenation. J Pediatr Surg 32: 768–771, 1997.

Calhoun BC, Hesser JW. Heparin-associated antibody with pregnancy: discussion of two cases. Am J Obstet Gynecol 156: 964–966, 1987.

Carette S, Jobin F. Acute adrenal insufficiency as a manifestation of the anticardiolipin syndrome? Ann Rheum Dis 48: 430–431, 1989.

Carlsson LE, Lubenow N, Blumentritt C, Kempf R, Papenberg S, Schröder W, Eichler P, Herrmann FH, Santoso S, Greinacher A. Platelet receptor and clotting factor polymorphisms as genetic risk factors for thromboembolic complications in heparin-induced thrombocytopenia. Pharmacogenetics 13: 253–258, 2003.

Castaman G, Ruggeri M, Girardello R, Rodeghiero F. An unusually prolonged case of heparin-induced thrombocytopenia and disseminated intravascular coagulation. Haematologica 77: 174–176, 1992.

Celoria GM, Steingart RH, Banson B, Friedmann P, Rhee SW, Berman JA. Coumarin skin necrosis in a patient with heparin-induced thrombocytopenia—a case report. Angiology 39: 915–920, 1988.

Chan WS, Spencer FA, Ginsberg JS. Anatomical distribution of deep vein thrombosis in pregnancy. CMAJ 182: 657–660, 2010.

Cipolle RJ, Rodvoid KA, Seifert R, Clarens R, Ramirez-Lassepas M. Heparin-associated thrombocytopenia: a prospective evaluation of 211 patients. Ther Drug Monit 5: 205–211, 1983.

Clagett GP, Anderson FA Jr, Heit J, Levine MN, Wheeler HB. Prevention of venous thromboembolism. Chest 108(4 Suppl): 312S–334S, 1995.

Cohen GR, Hall JC, Yeast JD, Field-Kriese D. Heparin-induced cutaneous necrosis in a postpartum patient. Obstet Gynecol 72: 498–499, 1988.

Cohen DJ, Briggs R, Head HD, Acher CW. Phlegmasia cerulea dolens and its association with hypercoagulable states: case reports. Angiology 40: 498–500, 1989.

Cole MS, Minifee PK, Wolma FJ. Coumarin necrosis—a review of the literature. Surgery 103: 271–277, 1988.

Collins R, Scrimgeour A, Yusuf S, Peto R. Reduction in fatal pulmonary embolism and venous thrombosis by perioperative administration of subcutaneous heparin. Overview of results of randomized trials in general, orthopaedic, and urologic surgery. N Engl J Med 318: 1162–1173, 1988.

Commeau P, Grollier G, Charbonneau P, Troussard X, Lequerrec A, Bazin C, Potier JC. Thrombopenie immunoallergique induite par l'heparine responsable d'une thrombose intraventriculaire gauche. Therapie 41: 345–347, 1986. [in French]

Comp PC. Coumarin-induced skin necrosis. Incidence, mechanisms, management and avoidance. Drug Safety 8: 128–135, 1993.

Copeman PWM. Livedo reticularis. Signs in the skin of disturbance of blood viscosity and of blood flow. Br J Dermatol 93: 519–522, 1975.

Copplestone A, Oscier DG. Heparin-induced thrombocytopenia in pregnancy. Br J Haematol 65: 248, 1987.

Dahlberg PJ, Goellner MH, Pehling GB. Adrenal insufficiency secondary to adrenal hemorrhage. Two case reports and a review of cases confirmed by computed tomography. Arch Intern Med 150: 905–909, 1990.

Davey MG, Lander H. Effect of adenosine diphosphate on circulating platelets in man. Nature 201: 1037–1039, 1964.

Delhumeau A, Granry JC. Heparin-associated thrombocytopenia. Crit Care Med 20: 1192, 1992.

de Saint-Blanquat L, Simon L, Toubas MF, Hamza J. Traitement par le danaparoi'de de de sodium au cours de la grossesse chez une patiente presentant une allergie cutanee aux heparines de bas poids moleculaire. Ann Fr Anesth Reanim 19: 751–754, 2000. [in French]

Dion D, Dumesnil JG, LeBlanc P. In situ right ventricular thrombus secondary to heparin induced thrombocytopenia. Can J Cardiol 5: 308–310, 1989.

Drouet M, Le Pabic F, Le Sellin J, Bonneau JC, Sabbah A. Allergy to heparin. Special problems set by pregnant women. Allergol Immunopathol 20: 225–229, 1992.

Dux S, Pitlik S, Perry G, Rosenfeld JB. Hypersensitivity reaction to chlorbutol-preserved heparin. Lancet 1: 149, 1981.

Ernest D, Fisher MM. Heparin-induced thrombocytopenia complicated by bilateral adrenal haemorrhage. Intensive Care Med 17: 238–240, 1991.

Fausett MB, Vogtlander M, Lee RM, Esplin MS, Branch DW, Rodgers GM, Silver RM. Heparin-induced thrombocytopenia is rare in pregnancy. Am J Obstet Gynecol 185: 148–152, 2001.

Feng WC, Singh AK, Bert AA, Sanofsky SJ, Crowley JP. Perioperative paraplegia and multiorgan failure from heparin-induced thrombocytopenia. Ann Thorac Surg 55: 1555–1557, 1993.

Fesler MJ, Creer MH, Richart JM, Edgell R, Havlioglu N, Norfleet G, Cruz-Flores S. Heparin-induced thrombocytopenia and cerebral venous thrombosis: case report and literature review. Neurocrit Care 15: 161–165, 2011.

Gaigl Z, Pfeuffer P, Raith P, Brocker EB, Trautmann A. Tolerance to intravenous heparin in patients with delayed-type hypersensitivity to heparins: a prospective study. Br J Haematol 128: 389–392, 2005.

Gallus AS, Goodall KT, Tillett J, Jackaman J, Wycherley A. The relative contributions of anti-thrombin III during heparin treatment, and of clinically recognisable risk factors, to early recurrence of venous thromboembolism. Thromb Res 46: 539–553, 1987.

Ganzer D, Gutezeit A, Mayer G, Greinacher A, Eichler P. Thromboembolieprophylaxe als Ausloser thrombembolischer Komplikationen. Eine Untersuchung zur Inzidenz der Heparin-induzierten Thrombozytopenie (HIT) Typ II. Z Orthop Ihre Grenzgeb 135: 543–549, 1997. [in German]

Gardyn J, Sorkin P, Kluger Y, Kabili S, Klausner JM, Zivelin A, Eldor A. Heparin-induced thrombocytopenia and fatal thrombosis in a patient with activated protein C resistance. Am J Hematol 50: 292–295, 1995.

Ginsberg JS, Brill-Edwards P, Burrows RF, Bona R, Prandoni P, Büller HR, Lensing A. Venous thrombosis during pregnancy: leg and trimester of presentation. Thromb Haemost 67: 519–520, 1992.

Girolami B, Prandoni P, Stefani PM, Tanduo C, Sabbion P, Eichler P, Ramon R, Baggio G, Fabris F, Girolami A. The incidence of heparin-induced thrombocytopenia in hospitalized medical patients treated with subcutaneous unfractionated heparin: a prospective cohort study. Blood 101: 2955–2959, 2003.

Grasseger A, Fritsch P, Reider N. Delayed-type hypersensitivity and cross-reactivity to heparin and danaparoid: a prospective study. Dermatol Surg 27: 47–52, 2001.

Greer IA, Nelson-Piercy C. Low molecular weight heparins for thromboprophylaxis and treatment of venous thromboembolism in pregnancy: a systematic review of safety and efficacy. Blood 106: 401–407, 2005.

Greinacher A, Warkentin TE. The direct thrombin inhibitor hirudin. Thromb Haemost 99: 819–829, 2008.

Greinacher A, Michels I, Mueller-Eckhardt C. Heparin-associated thrombocytopenia: the antibody is not heparin specific. Thromb Haemost 67: 545–549, 1992.

Greinacher A, Eckhardt T, Mussmann J, Mueller-Eckhardt C. Pregnancy complicated by heparin associated thrombocytopenia: management by a prospectively in vitro selected heparinoid (Org 10172). Thromb Res 71: 123–126, 1993.

Greinacher A, Völpel H, Janssens U, Hach-Wunderle V, Kemkes-Matthes B, Eichler P, Mueller-Velten HG, Pötzsch B; For the HIT Investigators Group. Recombinant hirudin (lepirudin) provides safe and effective anticoagulation in patients with heparin-induced thrombocytopenia: a prospective study. Circulation 99: 73–80, 1999.

Greinacher A, Eichler P, Lubenow N, Kwasny H, Luz M. Heparin-induced thrombocytopenia with thromboembolic complications: meta-analysis of 2 prospective trials to assess the value of parenteral treatment with lepirudin and its therapeutic aPTT range. Blood 96: 846–851, 2000.

Greinacher A, Eichler P, Lietz T, Warkentin TE. Replacement of unfractionated heparin by low molecular weight heparin for postorthopedic surgery antithrombotic prophylaxis lowers the overall risk of symptomatic thrombosis because of a lower frequency of heparin-induced thrombocytopenia. Blood 106: 2921–2922, 2005a.

Greinacher A, Farner B, Kroll H, Kohlmann T, Warkentin TE, Eichler P. Clinical features of heparin-induced thrombocytopenia including risk factors for thrombosis. A retrospective analysis of 408 patients. Thromb Haemost 94: 132–135, 2005b.

Greinacher A, Kohlmann T, Strobel U, Sheppard JI, Warkentin TE. The temporal profile of the anti-PF4/heparin immune response. Blood 113: 4970–4976, 2009.

Greinacher A, Holtfreter B, Krauel K, Gätke D, Weber C, Ittermann T, Hammerschmidt S, Kocher T. Association of natural anti-platelet factor 4/heparin antibodies with periodontal disease. Blood 118: 1395–1401, 2011.

Gross AS, Thompson FL, Arzubiaga MC, Graber SE, Hammer RD, Schulman G, Ellis DL, King LE Jr. Heparin-associated thrombocytopenia and thrombosis (HATT) presenting with livedo reticularis. Int J Dermatol 32: 276–279, 1993.

Gruel Y, Lang M, Darnige L, Pacouret G, Dreyfus X, Leroy J, Charbonnier B. Fatal effect of reexposure to heparin after previous heparin-associated thrombocytopenia and thrombosis. Lancet 336: 1077–1078, 1990.

Gruel Y, Pouplard C, Nguyen P, Borg JY, Derlon A, Juhan-Vague I, Regnault V, Samama M. Biological and clinical features of low molecular weight heparin-induced thrombocytopenia. Br J Haematol 121: 786–792, 2003.

Gupta AK, Kovacs MJ, Sauder DN. Heparin-induced thrombocytopenia. Ann Pharmacother 32: 55–59, 1998.

Hach-Wunderle V, Kainer K, Krug B, Müller-Berghaus G, Pötzsch B. Heparin-associated thrombosis despite normal platelet counts. Lancet 344: 469–470, 1994.

Hall JC, McConahay D, Gibson D. Heparin necrosis. An anticoagulation syndrome. JAMA 244: 1831–1832, 1980.

Hall AV, Clark WF, Parbtani A. Heparin-induced thrombocytopenia in renal failure. Clin Nephrol 38: 86–89, 1992.

Handschin AE, Trentz O, Kock HJ, Wanner GA. Low molecular weight heparin-induced skin necrosis—a systematic review. Langenbecks Arch Surg 390: 249–254, 2005.

Hartman AR, Hood RM, Anagnostopoulos CE. Phenomenon of heparin-induced thrombocytopenia associated with skin necrosis. J Vasc Surg 7: 781–784, 1988.

Hartman V, Malbrain M, Daelemans R, Meersman P, Zachée P. Pseudo-pulmonary embolism as a sign of acute heparin-induced thrombocytopenia in hemodialysis patients: safety of resuming heparin after disappearance of HIT antibodies. Nephron Clin Pract 104: c143–c148, 2006.

Hasegawa GR. Heparin-induced skin lesions. Drug Intell Clin Pharm 18: 313–314, 1984.

Heddle NM, Klama L, Singer J, Richards C, Fedak P, Walker I, Kelton JG. The role of the plasma from platelet concentrates in transfusion reactions. N Engl J Med 331: 625–628, 1994.

Hewitt RL, Akers DL, Leissinger CA, Gill JI, Aster RH. Concurrence of anaphylaxis and acute heparin-induced thrombocytopenia in a patients with heparin-induced antibodies. J Vasc Surg 28: 561–565, 1998.

Hillis C, Warkentin TE, Taha K, Eikelboom JW. Chills and limb pain following administration of low molecular weight heparin for treatment of acute venous thromboembolism. Am J Hematol 86: 603–606, 2011.

Hirsh J, Dalen JE, Deykin D, Poller L. Heparin: mechanism of action, pharmacokinetics, dosing considerations, monitoring, efficacy, and safety. Chest 102(4 Suppl): 337S–351S, 1992.

Hirsh J, Raschke R, Warkentin TE, Dalen JE, Deykin D, Poller L. Heparin: mechanism of action, pharmacokinetics, dosing considerations, monitoring, efficacy, and safety. Chest 108(4 Suppl): 258S–275S, 1995.

Hirsh J, Warkentin TE, Raschke R, Granger C, Ohman EM, Dalen JE. Heparin and low molecular weight heparin. Mechanisms of action, pharmacokinetics, dosing considerations, monitoring, efficacy, and safety. Chest 114(1 Suppl): 489S–510S, 1998.

Hirsh J, Warkentin TE, Shaughnessy SG, Anand SS, Halperin JL, Raschke R, Granger C, Ohman EM, Dalen JE. Heparin and low molecular weight heparin: mechanisms of action, pharmacokinetics, dosing, monitoring, efficacy, and safety. Chest 119(1 Suppl): 64S–94S, 2001.

Hong AP, Cook DJ, Sigouin CS, Warkentin TE. Central venous catheters and upper-extremity deep-vein thrombosis complicating immune heparin-induced thrombocytopenia. Blood 101: 3049–3051, 2003.

Hourigan LA, Walters DL, Keck SADec GW. Heparin-induced thrombocytopenia: a common complication in cardiac transplant recipients. J Heart Lung Transplant 21: 1283–1289, 2002.

Houston DS. Heparin-induced thrombocytopenia without thrombocytopenia in a patient with essential thrombocythemia. Am J Hematol 65: 331–332, 2000.

Hunter JB, Lonsdale RJ, Wenham PW, Frostick SP. Heparin-induced thrombosis: an important complication of heparin prophylaxis for thromboembolic disease in surgery. Br Med J 307: 53–55, 1993.

Hyers TM, Hull RD, Weg JG. Antithrombotic therapy for venous thromboembolic disease. Chest 95(2 Suppl): 37S–51S, 1989.

Hyers TM, Hull RD, Weg JG. Antithrombotic therapy for venous thromboembolic disease. Chest 108(4 Suppl): 335S–351S, 1995.

Jackson MR, Neilson JW, Lary M, Baay P, Web K, Clagett GP. Delayed-onset heparin-induced thrombocytopenia and thrombosis after intraoperative heparin anticoagulation—four case reports. Vasc Endovasc Surg 40: 67–70, 2006.

Jain A. Ischemic lumbosacral plexus neuropathy secondary to possible heparin-induced thrombosis following aortoiliac bypass [abstr]. Arch Phys Med Rehabil 67: 680, 1986.

Jay RM, Warkentin TE. Fatal heparin-induced thrombocytopenia (HIT) during warfarin thromboprophylaxis following orthopedic surgery: another example of 'spontaneous' HIT? J Thromb Haemost 6: 1598–1600, 2008.

Jones BF, Epstein MT. Cutaneous heparin necrosis associated with glomerulonephritis. Australas J Dermatol 28: 117–118, 1987.

Kappa JR, Fisher CA, Berkowitz HD, Cottrell ED, Addonizio VP Jr. Heparin-induced platelet activation in sixteen surgical patients: diagnosis and management. J Vasc Surg 5: 101–109, 1987.

Kaufman BR, Zoldos J, Bentz M, Nystrom NA. Venous gangrene of the upper extremity. Ann Plast Surg 40: 370–377, 1998.

Kearsley JH, Jeremy RW, Coates AS. Leukocytoclastic vasculitis and skin necrosis following subcutaneous heparin calcium. Aust NZ J Med 12: 288–289, 1982.

Kelly RA, Gelfand JA, Pincus SH. Cutaneous necrosis caused by systemically administered heparin. JAMA 246: 1582–1583, 1981.

Kerendi F, Thourani VH, Puskas JD, Kilgo PD, Osgood M, Guyton RA, Lattouf OM. Impact of heparin-induced thrombocytopenia on postoperative outcomes after cardiac surgery. Ann Thorac Surg 84: 1548–1555, 2007.

Kerr TM, Cranley JJ, Johnson JR, Lutter KS, Riechmann GC, Cranley RD, True MA, Sampson M. Analysis of 1084 consecutive lower extremities involved with acute venous thrombosis diagnosed by duplex scanning. Surgery 108: 520–527, 1990.

King DJ, Kelton JG. Heparin-associated thrombocytopenia. Ann Intern Med 100: 535–540, 1984.

Klein HG, Bell WR. Disseminated intravascular coagulation during heparin therapy. Ann Intern Med 80: 477–481, 1974.

Klement D, Rammos S, von Kries R, Kirschke W, Kniemeyer HW, Greinacher A. Heparin as a cause of thrombus progression. Heparin-associated thrombocytopenia is an important differential diagnosis in paediatric patients even with normal platelet counts. Eur J Pediatr 155: 11–14, 1996.

Klenner AF, Fusch C, Rakow A, Kadow I, Beyersdorff E, Eichler P, Wander K, Lietz T, Greinacher A. Benefit and risk for maintaining peripheral venous catheters in neonates: a placebo-controlled trial. J Pediatr 143: 741–745, 2003.

Klenner AF, Lubenow N, Raschke R, Greinacher A. Heparin-induced thrombocytopenia in children: 12 new cases and review of the literature. Thromb Haemost 91: 719–724, 2004.

Koch P, Bahmer FA, Schafer H. Tolerance of intravenous low molecular weight heparin after eczematous reaction to subcutaneous heparin. Contact Dermatitis 25: 205–206, 1991.

Kovacs KA, Lam YM, Pater JL. Bilateral massive adrenal hemorrhage. Assessment of putative risk factors by the case-control method. Medicine (Balt) 80: 45–53, 2001.

Krauel K, Pötschke C, Weber C, Kessler W, Fürll B, Ittermann T, Maier S, Hammerschmidt S, Bröker BM, Greinacher A. Platelet factor 4 binds to bacteria, [corrected] inducing antibodies cross-reacting with the major antigen in heparin-induced thrombocytopenia. Blood 117: 1370–1378, 2011.

Kyritsis AP, Williams EC, Schutta HS. Cerebral venous thrombosis due to heparin-induced thrombocytopenia. Stroke 21: 1503–1505, 1990.

Laster J, Cikrit D, Waler N, Silver D. The heparin-induced thrombocytopenia syndrome: an update. Surgery 102: 763–770, 1987.

Lee DH, Warkentin TE, Denomme GA, Lagrotteria DD, Kelton JG. Factor V Leiden and thrombotic complications in heparin-induced thrombocytopenia. Thromb Haemost 79: 50–53, 1998.

Levine RL, Hursting MJ, Drexler A, Lewis BE, Francis JL. Heparin-induced thrombocytopenia in the emergency department. Ann Emerg Med 44: 511–515, 2004.

Levine RL, McCollum D, Hursting MJ. How frequently is venous thromboembolism in heparin-treated patients associated with heparin-induced thrombocytopenia? Chest 130: 681–687, 2006.

Lewis BE, Wallis DE, Hursting MJ, Levine RL, Leya F. Effects of argatroban therapy, demographic variables, and platelet count on thrombotic risks in heparin-induced thrombocytopenia. Chest 129: 1407–1416, 2006.

Lindhoff-Last E, Wenning B, Stein M, Gerdsen F, Bauersachs R, Wagner R. Risk factors and long-term follow-up of patients with the immune type of heparin-induced thrombocytopenia. Clin Appl Thrombosis/Hemostasis 8: 347–352, 2002.

Lindsey SM, Maddison FE, Towne JB. Heparin-induced thromboembolism: angiographic features. Radiology 131: 771–774, 1979.

Ling E, Warkentin TE. Intraoperative heparin flushes and acute heparin-induced thrombocytopenia. Anesthesiology 89: 1567–1569, 1998.

Linkins LA, Warkentin TE. Heparin-induced thrombocytopenia: real world issues. Semin Thromb Hemost 37: 653–663, 2011.

Linkins LA, Dans AL, Moores LK, Bona R, Davidson BL, Schulman S, Crowther M. Treatment and prevention of heparin-induced thrombocytopenia. Antithrombotic Therapy and Prevention of Thrombosis, 9th ed: American College of Chest Physicians Evidence-Based Clinical Practice Guidelines. Chest 141(Suppl): e495S–e530S, 2012.

Lipton ME, Gould D. Case report: heparin-induced thrombocytopenia—a complication presenting to the vascular radiologist. Clin Radiol 45: 137–138, 1992.

Liu JC, Lewis BE, Steen LH, Grassman ED, Bakhos M, Blakeman B, Wrona L, Leya F. Patency of coronary artery bypass grafts in patients with heparin-induced thrombocytopenia. Am J Cardiol 89: 979–981, 2002.

Lo GK, Juhl D, Warkentin TE, Sigouin CS, Eichler P, Greinacher A. Evaluation of pretest clinical score (4 T's) for the diagnosis of heparin-induced thrombocytopenia in two clinical settings. J Thromb Haemost 4: 759–765, 2006.

Lubenow N, Kempf R, Eichner A, Eichler P, Carlsson LE, Greinacher A. Heparin-induced thrombocytopenia: temporal pattern of thrombocytopenia in relation to initial use or reexposure to heparin. Chest 122: 37–42, 2002.

Lubenow N, Hinz P, Thomaschewski S, Lietz T, Vogler M, Ladwig A, Jünger M, Nauck M, Schellong S, Wander K, Engel G, Ekkernkamp A, Greinacher A. The severity of trauma determines the immune response to PF4/heparin and the frequency of heparin-induced thrombocytopenia. Blood 115: 1797–1803, 2010.

Ludwig RJ, Schindewolf M, Alban S, Kaufmann R, Lindhoff-Last E, Wolf-Henning B. Molecular weight determines the frequency of delayed type hypersensitivity reactions to heparin and synthetic oligosaccharides. Thromb Haemost 94: 1265–1269, 2005.

Ludwig RJ, Schindewolf M, Utikal J, Lindhoff-Last E, Boehnke WH. Management of cutaneous type IV hypersensitivity reactions induced by heparin. Thromb Haemost 96: 611–617, 2006.

MacLean JA, Moscicki R, Bloch KJ. Adverse reactions to heparin. Ann Allerg 65: 254–259, 1990.

Makhoul RG, Greenberg CS, McCann RL. Heparin-associated thrombocytopenia and thrombosis: a serious clinical problem and potential solution. J Vasc Surg 4: 522–528, 1986.

Mallik A, Carlson KB, DeSancho MT. A patient with 'spontaneous' heparin-induced thrombocytopenia and thrombosis after undergoing knee replacement. Blood Coagul Fibrinolysis 22: 73–75, 2011.

Markel A, Manzo RA, Bergelin RO, Strandness DE Jr. Pattern and distribution of thrombi in acute venous thrombosis. Arch Surg 127: 305–309, 1992.

Maurin N, Biniek R, Heintz B, Kierdorf H. Heparin-induced thrombocytopenia and thrombosis with spinal ischaemia—recovery of platelet count following a change to a low molecular weight heparin. Intensive Care Med 17: 185–186, 1991.

McKay DG. Late manifestations of intravascular coagulation—tissue necrosis. In: McKay DG, ed. Disseminated Intravascular Coagulation. An Intermediary Mechanism of Disease. New York: Harper & Row, 392–471, 1965.

Meyer-Lindenberg A, Quenzel EM, Bierhoff E, Wolff H, Schindler E, Biniek R. Fatal cerebral venous sinus thrombosis in heparin-induced thrombotic thrombocytopenia. Eur Neurol 37: 191–192, 1997.

Meytes D, Ayalon H, Virag I, Weisbort Y, Zakut H. Heparin-induced thrombocytopenia and recurrent thrombosis in pregnancy. A case report. J Reprod Med 31: 993–996, 1986.

Mims MP, Manian P, Rice L. Acute cardiorespiratory collapse from heparin: a consequence of heparin-induced thrombocytopenia. Eur J Haematol 72: 366–369, 2004.

Muntean W, Finding K, Gamillscheg A, Zenz W. Multiple thromboses and coumarin induced skin necrosis in a young child with antiphospholipid antibodies. Thromb Haemorrh Disord 5: 43–45, 1992.

Murdoch IA, Beattie RM, Silver DM. Heparin-induced thrombocytopenia in children. Acta Paediatr 82: 495–497, 1993.

Muslimani AA, Ricaurte B, Daw HA. Immune heparin-induced thrombocytopenia resulting from preceding exposure to heparin catheter flushes. Am J Hematol 82: 652–655, 2007.

Nand S, Wong W, Yuen B, Yetter A, Schmulbach E, Gross Fisher S. Heparin induced thrombocytopenia with thrombosis: incidence, analysis of risk factors, and clinical outcomes in 108 consecutive patients treated at a single institution. Am J Hematol 56: 12–16, 1997.

Natelson EA, Lynch EC, Alfrey CP Jr, Gross JB. Heparin-induced thrombocytopenia. An unexpected response to treatment of consumption coagulopathy. Ann Intern Med 71: 1121–1125, 1969.

Nelson JC, Lerner RG, Goldstein R, Cagin NA. Heparin-induced thrombocytopenia. Arch Intern Med 138: 548–552, 1978.

Newman PM, Chong BH. Further characterization of antibody and antigen in heparin-induced thrombocytopenia. Br J Haematol 107: 303–309, 1999.

Nguyen QD, Do DV, Feke GT, Demirjian ZN, Lashkari K. Heparin induced anti-heparin platelet antibody associated with retinal venous thrombosis. Ophthalmology 110: 600–603, 2003.

Odeh M, Oliven A. Urticaria and angioedema induced by low molecular weight heparin. Lancet 340: 972–973, 1992.

Olah Z, Kerenyi A, Kappelmayer J, Schlammadinger A, Razso K, Boda Z. Rapid-onset heparin-induced thrombocytopenia without previous heparin exposure. Platelets 23: 495–498, 2012.

Olbricht K, Wiersbitzky M, Wacke W, Eichler P, Zinke H, Schwock M, Mox B, Kraatz G, Motz W, Greinacher A. Atypical heparin-induced thrombocytopenia complicated by intracardiac thrombus, effectively treated with ultra-low-dose rt-PA lysis and recombinant hirudin (Lepirudin). Blood Coagul Fibrinolysis 9: 273–277, 1998.

Olinger GN, Hussey CV, Olive JA, Malik MI. Cardiopulmonary bypass for patients with previously documented heparin-induced platelet aggregation. J Thorac Cardiovasc Surg 87: 673–677, 1984.

Opatrny L, Warner MN. Risk of thrombosis in patients with malignancy and heparin-induced thrombocytopenia. Am J Hematol 76: 240–244, 2004.

Oriot D, Wolf M, Wood C, Brun P, Sidi D, Devictor D, Tchernia G, Huault G. Thrombopenie severe induite par l'heparine chez un nourrisson porteur d'une myocardite aigue. Arch Fr Pediatr 47: 357–359, 1990. [in French]

Padilla A, Gray E, Pepper DS, Barrowcliffe TW. Inhibition of thrombin generation by heparin and low molecular weight (LMW) heparins in the absence and presence of platelet factor 4 (PF4). Br J Haematol 82: 406–413, 1992.

Patriarca G, Rossi M, Schiavino D, Schinco G, Fais G, Varano C, Schiavello R. Rush desensitization in heparin hypersensitivity: a case report. Allergy 49: 292–294, 1994.

Payne SM, Kovacs MJ. Cutaneous dalteparin reactions associated with antibodies of heparin-induced thrombocytopenia. Ann Pharmacother 37: 655–658, 2003.

Pedersen-Bjergaard U, Andersen M, Hansen PB. Drug-induced thrombocytopenia: clinical data on 309 cases and the effect of corticosteroid therapy. Eur J Clin Pharmacol 52: 183–189, 1997.

Perrin J, Barraud D, Toussaint-Hacquard M, Bollaert PE, Lecompte T. Rapid onset heparin-induced thrombocytopenia (HIT) without history of heparin exposure: a new case of so-called 'spontaneous' HIT. Thromb Haemost 107: 795–797, 2012.

Pfueller SL, David R, Firkin BG, Bilston RA, Cortizo F. Platelet aggregating IgG antibody to platelet surface glycoproteins associated with thrombosis and thrombocytopenia. Br J Haematol 74: 336–341, 1990.

Phelan BK. Heparin-associated thrombosis without thrombocytopenia. Ann Intern Med 99: 637–638, 1983.

Platell CFE, Tan EGC. Hypersensitivity reactions to heparin: delayed onset thrombocytopenia and necrotizing skin lesions. Aust NZ J Surg 56: 621–623, 1986.

Pohl C, Klockgether T, Greinacher A, Hanfland P, Harbrecht U. Neurological complications in heparin-induced thrombocytopenia. Lancet 353: 1678–1679, 1999.

Pohl C, Harbrecht U, Greinacher A, Theuerkauf I, Binick R, Hanfland P, Klockgether T. Neurologic complications in immune-mediated heparin-induced thrombocytopenia. Neurology 54: 1240–1245, 2000.

Popov D, Zarrabi MH, Foda H, Graber M. Pseudopulmonary embolism: acute respiratory distress in the syndrome of heparin-induced thrombocytopenia. Ann J Kidney Dis 29: 449–452, 1997.

Potter C, Gill JC, Scott JP, McFarland JG. Heparin-induced thrombocytopenia in a child. J Pediatr 121: 135–138, 1992.

Pötzsch B, Klovekorn WP, Madlener K. Use of heparin during cardiopulmonary bypass in patients with a history of heparin-induced thrombocytopenia. N Engl J Med 343: 515, 2000.

Pouplard C, May MA, Regina S, Marchand M, Fusciardi J, Gruel Y. Changes in platelet count after cardiac surgery can effectively predict the development of pathogenic heparin-dependent antibodies. Br J Haematol 128: 837–841, 2005.

Prandoni P, Falanga A, Piccioli A. Cancer, thrombosis and heparin-induced thrombocytopenia. Thromb Res 120(Suppl 2): S137–S140, 2007.

Pruthi RK, Daniels PR, NambudirGS, Warkentin TE. Heparin-induced thrombocytopenia (HIT) during postoperative warfarin thromboprophylaxis: a second example of postorthopedic surgery 'spontaneous' HIT? J Thromb Haemost 7: 499–501, 2009.

Ramirez-Lassepas M, Cipolle RJ, Rodvold KA, Seifert RD, Strand L, Taddeini L, Cusulos M. Heparin-induced thrombocytopenia in patients with cerebrovascular disease. Neurology 34: 736–740, 1984.

Ranze O, Ranze P, Magnani HN, Greinacher A. Heparin-induced thrombocytopenia in paediatric patients—a review of the literature and a new case treated with danaparoid sodium. Eur J Pediatr 158(Suppl 3): S130–S133, 1999.

Ranze O, Rakow A, Ranze P, Eichler P, Greinacher A, Fusch C. Low dose danaparoid sodium catheter flushes in an intensive care infant suffering from heparin-induced thrombocytopenia. Pediatr Crit Care Med 2: 175–177, 2001.

Rastellini C, Brown ML, Cicalese L. Heparin-induced thrombocytopenia following pancreatectomy and islet autotransplantation. Clin Transplant 20: 156–158, 2006.

Refaai MA, Warkentin TE, Axelson M, Matevosyan K, Sarode R. Delayed-onset heparin-induced thrombocytopenia, venous thromboembolism, and cerebral venous thrombosis: a consequence of heparin "flushes". Thromb Haemost 98: 1139–1140, 2007.

Rhodes GR, Dixon RH, Silver D. Heparin-induced thrombocytopenia with thrombotic and hemorrhagic manifestations. Surg Gynecol Obstet 136: 409–416, 1973.

Rhodes GR, Dixon RH, Silver D. Heparin-induced thrombocytopenia: eight cases with thrombotic-hemorrhagic complications. Ann Surg 186: 752–758, 1977.

Rice L, Attisha WK, Drexler A, Francis JL. Delayed-onset heparin-induced thrombocytopenia. Ann Intern Med 136: 210–215, 2002.

Risch L, Pihan H, Zeller C, Huber AR. ET gets HIT-thrombocytotic heparin-induced thrombocytopenia (HIT) in a patient with essential thrombocythemia (ET). Blood Coagul Fibrinolysis 11: 663–667, 2000.

Roberts B, Rosato FE, Rosato EF. Heparin—a cause of arterial emboli? Surgery 55: 803–808, 1964.

Rosenberger LH, Smith PW, Sawyer RG, Hanks JB, Adams RB, Hedrick TL. Bilateral adrenal hemorrhage: the unrecognized cause of hemodynamic collapse associated with heparin-induced thrombocytopenia. Crit Care Med 39: 833–838, 2011.

Rowland CH, Woodford PA, De Lisle-Hammond J, Nair B. Heparin-induced thrombocytopenia: thrombosis syndrome and bilateral adrenal hemorrhage after prophylactic heparin use. Aust NZJ Med 29: 741–742, 1999.

Sandset PM. CXCL4-platelet factor 4, heparin-induced thrombocytopenia and cancer. Thromb Res 129(Suppl 1): S97–S100, 2012.

Sauer M, Gruhn B, Fuchs D, Altermann WW, Greinacher A, Völpel H, Zintl F. Anticoagulation with recombinant hirudin following bone marrow transplantation in a patient with activated protein C resistance and heparin-induced antibodies showing cross-reactivity to the heparinoid danaparoid. Med Pediatr Oncol 32: 457–458, 1999.

Scheffold N, Greinacher A, Cyran J. Intrakardiale Thrombenbildung bei Heparin-assoziierter Thrombozytopenie Typ II. Dtsch Med Wochenschr 120: 519–522, 1995. [in German]

Schindewolf M, Schwaner S, Wolter M, Kroll H, Recke A, Kaufmann R, Boehnke WH, Lindhoff-Last E, Ludwig RJ. Incidence and causes of heparin-induced skin lesions. CMAJ 181: 477–481, 2009.

Schindewolf M, Kroll H, Ackermann H, Garbaraviciene J, Kaufmann R, Boehncke WH, Ludwig RJ, Lindhoff-Last E. Heparin-induced non-necrotizing skin lesions: rarely associated with heparin-induced thrombocytopenia. J Thromb Haemost 8: 1486–1491, 2010a.

Schindewolf M, Scheuermann J, Kroll H, Garbaraviciene J, Hecking C, Marzi I, Wolter M, Kaufmann R, Boehnke WH, Lindhoff-Last E, Ludwig RJ. Low allergenic potential with fondaparinux: results of a prospective investigation. Mayo Clin Proc 85: 913–919, 2010b.

Selleng S, Haneya A, Hirt S, Selleng K, Schmid C, Greinacher A. Management of anticoagulation in patients with subacute heparin-induced thrombocytopenia scheduled for heart transplantation. Blood 112: 4024–4027, 2008a.

Selleng S, Selleng K, Wollert HG, Muellejans B, Lietz T, Warkentin TE, Greinacher A. Heparin-induced thrombocytopenia in patients requiring prolonged intensive care unit treatment after cardiopulmonary bypass. J Thromb Haemost 6: 428–435, 2008b.

Selleng S, Malowsky B, Strobel U, Wessel A, Ittermann T, Wollert HG, Warkentin TE, Greinacher A. Early-onset and persisting thrombocytopenia in post-cardiac surgery patients is rarely due to heparin-induced thrombocytopenia even when antibody tests are positive. J Thromb Haemost 8: 30–36, 2010a.

Selleng K, Schütt A, Selleng S, Warkentin TE, Greinacher A. Studies of the anti-platelet factor 4/heparin immune response: adapting the enzyme-linked immunosorbent spot assay for detection of memory B cells against complex antigens. Transfusion 2010: 50: 32–39, 2010b.

Shah MR, Spencer JP. Heparin-induced thrombocytopenia occurring after discontinuation of heparin. J Am Board Fam Pract 16: 148–150, 2003.

Silver D, Kapsch DN, Tsoi EKM. Heparin-induced thrombocytopenia, thrombosis, and hemorrhage. Ann Surg 198: 301–306, 1983.

Smythe MA, Warkentin TE, Stephens JL, Zakalik D, Mattson JC. Venous limb gangrene during overlapping therapy with warfarin and a direct thrombin inhibitor for immune heparin-induced thrombocytopenia. Am J Hematol 71: 50–52, 2002.

Smythe MA, Stephens JL, Mattson JC. Delayed-onset heparin-induced thrombocytopenia. Ann Emerg Med 45: 417–419, 2005.

Solomon SA, Cotton DWK, Preston FE, Ramsay LE. Severe disseminated intravascular coagulation associated with massive ventricular mural thrombus following acute myocardial infarction. Postgrad Med J 64: 791–795, 1988.

Spadone D, Clark F, James E, Laster J, Hoch J, Silver D. Heparin-induced thrombocytopenia in the newborn. J Vasc Surg 15: 306–312, 1992.

Srinivasan AF, Rice L, Bartholomew JR, Rangaswamy C, La Perna L, Thompson JE, Murphy S, Baker KR. Warfarin-induced skin necrosis and venous limb gangrene in the setting of heparin-induced thrombocytopenia. Arch Intern Med 164: 66–70, 2004.

Stevenson MM. Thrombocytopenia during heparin therapy. N Engl J Med 295: 1200–1201, 1976.

Tahata T, Miki S, Kusuhara K, Ueda Y, Okita Y, Matsuo S. [Delayed onset of heparin induced thrombocytopenia: a case report]. Nippon Kyobu Geka Gakkai Zasshi 40: 456–458, 1992. [in Japanese]

Tans G, Rosing J, Thomassen MC, Heeb MJ, Zwaal RF, Griffin JH. Comparison of anticoagulant and procoagulant activities of stimulated platelets and platelet-derived microparticles. Blood 77: 2641–2648, 1991.

Teh CH, Robertson MN, Warkentin TE, Henriksen PA, Brackenbury ET, Anderson JAM. Transient global amnesia as the presenting feature of heparin-induced thrombocytopenia. J Card Surg 25: 300–302, 2010.

Tezcan AZ, Tezcan H, Gastineau DA, Armitage JO, Haire WD. Heparin-induced thrombocytopenia after bone marrow transplantation: report of two cases. Bone Marrow Transplant 14: 487–490, 1994.

Theuerkauf I, Lickfett L, Harbrecht U, Pohl C, Fischer HP, Pfeifer U. Segmental hepatic vein thrombosis associated with heparin-induced thrombocytopenia II. Virchows Arch 436: 88–91, 2000.

Thielmann M, Bunschkowski M, Tossios P, Selleng S, Marggraf G, Greinacher A, Jakob H, Massoudy P. Perioperative thrombocytopenia in cardiac surgical patients--incidence of heparin-induced thrombocytopenia, morbidities and mortality. Eur J Cardiothorac Surg 37: 1391–1395, 2010.

Tholl U, Greinacher A, Overdick K, Anlauf M. Life-threatening anaphylactic reaction following parathyroidectomy in a dialysis patient with heparin-induced thrombocytopenia. Nephrol Dial Transplant 12: 2750–2755, 1997.

Thomas D, Block AJ. Thrombocytopenia, cutaneous necrosis, and gangrene of the upper and lower extremities in a 35–year-old man. Chest 102: 1578–1580, 1992.

Thota R, Porter J, Ganti AK, Peters E. Hemodynamic collapse following bilateral knee arthoplasty: a mysterious case. J Thromb Thrombolysis 33: 3–5, 2012.

Tietge UJF, Schmidt HH, Jackel C, Trautwein C, Manns MP. LMWH-induced skin necrosis occurring distant from injection sites and without thrombocytopenia. J Intern Med 243: 313–315, 1998.

Towne JB, Bernhard VM, Hussey C, Garancis JC. White clot syndrome. Peripheral vascular complications of heparin therapy. Arch Surg 114: 372–377, 1979.

Van der Weyden MB, Hunt H, McGrath K, Fawcett T, Fitzmaurice A, Sawers RJ, Rosengarten DS. Delayed-onset heparin-induced thrombocytopenia. A potentially malignant syndrome. Med J Aust 2: 132–135, 1983.

Vazquez-Jimenez JF, Janssens U, Sellhaus B, Hermanns B, Huegel W, Hanrath P, Messmer BJ. Thrombosis of a mitral valve prosthesis in a patient with heparin-induced thrombocytopenia type II. J Thorac Cardiovasc Surg 118: 751–753, 1999.

Vella A, Nippoldt TB, Morris JC III. Adrenal hemorrhage: a 25–year experience at the Mayo Clinic. Mayo Clin Proc 76: 161–168, 2001.

Vignon P, Guéret P, Francois B, Serhal C, Fermeaux V, Bensaid J. Acute limb ischemia and heparin-induced thrombocytopenia: the value of echocardiography in eliminating a cardiac source of arterial emboli. J Am Soc Echocardiogr 9: 344–347, 1996.

Wallis DE, Workman DL, Lewis BE, Steen L, Pifarre R, Moran JF. Failure of early heparin cessation as treatment for heparin-induced thrombocytopenia. Am J Med 106: 629–635, 1999.

Wan C, Warner M, DeVarennes B, Ergina P, Cecere R, Lachapelle K. Clinical presentation, temporal relationship, and outcome in thirty-three patients with type 2 heparin-induced thrombocytopenia after cardiotomy. Ann Thorac Surg 82: 21–27, 2006.

Wanaka K, Matsuo T, Matsuo M, Kaneko C, Miyashita K, Asada R, Matsushima H, Nakajima Y. Re-exposure to heparin in uremic patients requiring hemodialysis with heparin-induced thrombocytopenia. J Thromb Hemost 8, 616–618, 2010.

Warkentin TE. Hemostasis and arteriosclerosis. Can J Cardiol 11(Suppl C): 29C–34C, 1995.

Warkentin TE. Heparin-induced skin lesions. Br J Haematol 92: 494–497, 1996a.

Warkentin TE. Heparin-induced thrombocytopenia: IgG-mediated platelet activation, platelet microparticle generation, and altered procoagulant/anticoagulant balance in the pathogenesis of thrombosis and venous limb gangrene complicating heparin induced thrombocytopenia. Transfusion Med Rev 10: 249–258, 1996b.

Warkentin TE. Heparin-induced thrombocytopenia, heparin-induced skin lesions, and arterial thrombosis. Thromb Haemost 77(Suppl): 562, 1997.

Warkentin TE. Clinical presentation of heparin-induced thrombocytopenia. Semin Hematol 35(Suppl 5): 9–16, 1998a.

Warkentin TE. Limitations of conventional treatment options for heparin-induced thrombocytopenia. Semin Hematol 35(Suppl 5): 17–25, 1998b.

Warkentin TE. Heparin-induced thrombocytopenia: a clinicopathologic syndrome. Thromb Haemost 82(Suppl): 439–447, 1999.

Warkentin TE. Venous thromboembolism in heparin-induced thrombocytopenia. Curr Opin Pulm Med 6: 343–351, 2000.

Warkentin TE. Heparin-induced thrombocytopenia. Curr Hematol Rep 1: 63–72, 2002a.

Warkentin TE. Heparin-induced thrombocytopenia and the anesthesiologist. Can J Anesth 49(Suppl): S36–S49, 2002b.

Warkentin TE. Platelet count monitoring and laboratory testing for heparin-induced thrombocytopenia. Arch Pathol Lab Med 126: 1415–1423, 2002c.

Warkentin TE. Heparin-induced thrombocytopenia: pathogenesis and management. Br J Haematol 121: 535–555, 2003.

Warkentin TE. Should vitamin K be administered when HIT is diagnosed after administration of coumarin? J Thromb Haemost 4: 894–896, 2006a.

Warkentin TE. Think of HIT. Hematology Am Soc Hematol Educ Program 408–414, 2006b.

Warkentin TE. Think of HIT when thrombosis follows heparin. Chest 130: 631–632, 2006c.

Warkentin TE. Drug-induced immune-mediated thrombocytopenia: from purpura to thrombosis. N Engl J Med 356: 891–893, 2007.

Warkentin TE. Agents for the treatment of heparin-induced thrombocytopenia. Hematol/ Oncol Clin N Am 24: 755–775, 2010.

Warkentin TE. HIT paradigms and paradoxes. J Thromb Haemost 9(Suppl 1): 105–117, 2011a.

Warkentin TE. How I diagnose and manage HIT. Hematology Am Soc Hematol Educ Program 2011: 143–149, 2011b.

Warkentin TE. HITlights: a career perspective on heparin-induced thrombocytopenia. Am J Hematol 87(Suppl 1): S92–S99, 2012.

Warkentin TE, Bernstein RA. Delayed-onset heparin-induced thrombocytopenia and cerebral thrombosis after a single administration of unfractionated heparin. N Engl J Med 348: 1067–1069, 2003.

Warkentin TE, Greinacher A. Heparin-induced thrombocytopenia: recognition, treatment, and prevention: the Seventh ACCP Conference on Antithrombotic and Thrombolytic Therapy. 126(3 Suppl): 311S–337S, 2004.

Warkentin TE, Greinacher A. Heparin-induced anaphylactic and anaphylactoid reactions: two distinct but overlapping syndromes. Expert Opin Drug Saf 8: 129–144, 2009.

Warkentin TE, Kelton JG. A 14–year study of heparin-induced thrombocytopenia. Am J Med 101: 502–507, 1996.

Warkentin TE, Kelton JG. Delayed-onset heparin-induced thrombocytopenia and thrombosis. Ann Intern Med 135: 502–506, 2001a.

Warkentin TE, Kelton JG. Temporal aspects of heparin-induced thrombocytopenia. N Engl J Med 344: 1286–1292, 2001b.

Warkentin TE, Linkins LA. Non-necrotizing heparin-induced skin lesions and the 4T's score. J Thromb Haemost 8: 1483–1485, 2010.

Warkentin TE, Sheppard JI. Clinical sample investigation (CSI) hematology: pinpointing the precise onset of heparin-induced thrombocytopenia (HIT). J Thromb Haemost 5: 636–637, 2007.

Warkentin TE, Soutar RL, Panju A, Ginsberg JS. Acute systemic reactions to intravenous bolus heparin therapy: characterization and relationship to heparin-induced thrombocytopenia [abstr]. Blood 80(Suppl 1): 160a, 1992.

Warkentin TE, Hirte HW, Anderson DR, Wilson WEC, O'Connell GJ, Lo RC. Transient global amnesia associated with acute heparin-induced thrombocytopenia. Am J Med 97: 489–491, 1994.

Warkentin TE, Levine MN, Hirsh J, Horsewood P, Roberts RS, Gent M, Kelton JG. Heparin-induced thrombocytopenia in patients treated with low molecular weight heparin or unfractionated heparin. N Engl J Med 332: 1330–1335, 1995.

Warkentin TE, Elavathil LJ, Hayward CPM, Johnston MA, Russett JI, Kelton JG. The pathogenesis of venous limb gangrene associated with heparin-induced thrombocytopenia. Ann Intern Med 127: 804–812, 1997.

Warkentin TE, Sikov WM, Lillicrap DP. Multicentric warfarin-induced skin necrosis complicating heparin-induced thrombocytopenia. Am J Med 62: 44–48, 1999.

Warkentin TE, Roberts RS, Hirsh J, Kelton JG. An improved definition of immune heparin-induced thrombocytopenia in postoperative orthopedic patients. Arch Intern Med 163: 2518–2524, 2003.

Warkentin TE, Whitlock RP, Teoh KHT. Warfarin-associated multiple digital necrosis complicating heparin-induced thrombocytopenia and Raynaud's phenomenon after aortic valve replacement for adenocarcinoma-associated thrombotic endocarditis. Am J Hematol 75: 56–62, 2004.

Warkentin TE, Cook RJ, Marder VJ, Sheppard JI, Moore JC, Eriksson BI, Greinacher A, Kelton JG. Anti-platelet factor 4/heparin antibodies in orthopedic surgery patients receiving antithrombotic prophylaxis with fondaparinux or enoxaparin. Blood 106: 3791–3796, 2005a.

Warkentin TE, Roberts RS, Hirsh J, Kelton JG. Heparin-induced skin lesions and other unusual sequelae of the heparin-induced thrombocytopenia syndrome. A nested cohort study. Chest 127: 1857–1861, 2005b.

Warkentin TE, Sheppard JI, Moore JC, Moore KM, Sigouin CS, Kelton JG. Laboratory testing for the antibodies that cause heparin-induced thrombocytopenia: how much class do we need? J Lab Clin Med 146: 341–346, 2005c.

Warkentin TE, Sheppard JI, Sigouin CS, Kohlmann T, Eichler P, Greinacher A. Gender imbalance and risk factor interactions in heparin-induced thrombocytopenia. Blood 108: 2937–2941, 2006.

Warkentin TE, Greinacher A, Koster A, Lincoff AM. Treatment and prevention of heparin-induced thrombocytopenia. American College of Chest Physicians evidence-based clinical practice guidelines (8th edition). Chest 133(6 Suppl): 340S–380S, 2008a.

Warkentin TE, Makris M, Jay RM, Kelton JG. A spontaneous prothrombotic disorder resembling heparin-induced thrombocytopenia. Am J Med 121: 632–636, 2008b.

Warkentin TE, Sheppard JI, Moore JC, Sigouin CS, Kelton JG. Quantitative interpretation of optical density measurements using PF4-dependent enzyme-immunoassays. J Thromb Haemost 6: 1304–1312, 2008c.

Warkentin TE, Sheppard JI, Moore JC, Cook RJ, Kelton JG. Studies of the immune response in heparin-induced thrombocytopenia. Blood 113: 4963–4969, 2009.

Warkentin TE, Davidson BL, Büller HR, Gallus A, Gent M, Lensing AWA, Piovella F, Prins MH, Segers AEM, Kelton JG. Prevalence and risk of preexisting heparin-induced thrombocytopenia antibodies in patients with acute VTE. Chest 140: 366–373, 2011.

Warkentin TE, Moore JC, Vogel S, Sheppard JI, Warkentin NI, Eikelboom JW. The serological profile of early-onset and persisting post-cardiac surgery thrombocytopenia complicated by "true" heparin-induced thrombocytopenia. Thromb Haemost 107: 998–1000, 2012a.

Warkentin TE, Pai M, Cook RJ. Intraoperative anticoagulation and limb amputations in patients with immune heparin-induced thrombocytopenia who require vascular surgery. J Thromb Haemost 10: 148–150, 2012b.

Weberschock T, Meister AC, Bohrt K, Schmitt J, Boehncke WH, Ludwig RJ. The risk for cross-reactions after a cutaneous delayed-type hypersensitivity reaction to heparin preparations is independent of their molecular weight: a systematic review. Contact Dermatitis 65: 187–194, 2011.

Weismann RE, Tobin RW. Arterial embolism occurring during systemic heparin therapy. Arch Surg 76: 219–227, 1958.

Wütschert R, Piletta P, Bounameaux H. Adverse skin reactions to low molecular weight heparins: frequency, management and prevention. Drug Safety 20: 515–525, 1999.

Zalcberg JR, McGrath K, Dauer R, Wiley SJ. Heparin-induced thrombocytopenia with associated disseminated intravascular coagulation. Br J Haematol 54: 655–660, 1983.

Zwicker JI, Uhl L, Huang WY, Shaz BH, Bauer KA. Thrombosis and ELISA optical density in hospitalized patients with heparin-induced thrombocytopenia. J Thromb Haemost 2: 2133–2137, 2004.

Differential diagnosis of heparin-induced thrombocytopenia and scoring systems

Theodore E. Warkentin and Adam Cuker

INTRODUCTION

Differential Diagnosis of Heparin-Induced Thrombocytopenia

Heparin exposure and thrombocytopenia are common events in hospitalized patients; indeed, their combination does not usually indicate the occurrence of heparin-induced thrombocytopenia (HIT). Early postoperative platelet count declines in patients receiving heparin thromboprophylaxis virtually never represent HIT, but rather the expected pattern of transient postsurgical platelet count declines. However, among such patients, a *second* platelet count fall that begins 5 to 10 days after the preceding intra- or early postoperative heparin exposure has a high likelihood of representing HIT, that is, "typical-onset" HIT; if such a platelet count fall occurs (or worsens) after heparin has been stopped, the term "delayed-onset" HIT would be appropriate.

In this chapter, we discuss some of the non-HIT conditions—both common and rare—that can explain thrombocytopenia in heparin-treated patients. Sometimes the condition resembles HIT sufficiently closely that the term "pseudo-HIT" (v.i.) may be appropriate. First, however, we discuss a common clinical scenario—early postoperative thrombocytopenia—that precedes most episodes of "true" HIT, but which on its own may be confused with HIT.

Perioperative Thrombocytopenia

Early postoperative thrombocytopenia is due to a combination of hemodilution (from intra-/early postoperative administration of fluid/blood products) and increased platelet consumption (Greinacher and Warkentin, 2012). The platelet count declines can be substantial, for example, 30–70% postcardiac surgery (Warkentin and Greinacher, 2003), and are approximately proportional to the amount of crystalloid, colloid, or blood products given. There is concomitant dilutional coagulopathy, for example, transient increases in the prothrombin time and (activated) partial thromboplastin time (aPTT).

Immediate perioperative hemodilution is also accompanied by increased platelet consumption, which helps to explain progressive platelet count declines over the first one to three postoperative days; indeed, the normal postoperative platelet count nadir ranges from postoperative days 1 to 4 (median, day 2) (Warkentin et al., 1995; Greinacher and Selleng, 2010) (Fig. 3.1). Subsequently, there is a rise in the platelet count that usually peaks at approximately day 14, at levels that are two to three times the patient's preoperative baseline (*postoperative thrombocytosis*), before it returns to baseline over the next one to two weeks.

The aforementioned normal platelet count profile of initial decline, followed by a subsequent rise to transient postoperative thrombocytosis, is explained by

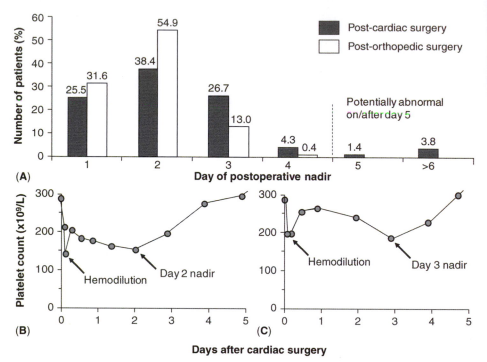

FIGURE 3.1   Profile of early postoperative platelet count declines. **(A)** Distribution of early postoperative count nadirs. For both orthopedic and cardiac surgery patients, day 2 represents the most common day for the postoperative platelet count nadir to occur (data exclude day 0 = day of surgery); beyond postoperative day 4, it is likely that a superimposed thrombocytopenic disorder is occurring. Orthopedic surgery data obtained from Warkentin et al. (1995) and cardiac surgery data obtained from Greinacher and Selleng (2010). **(B)** and **(C)** Representative postcardiac surgery platelet count declines. Both patients illustrate early hemodilution effects (day 0) and subsequent additional early platelet count declines with nadirs of **(B)** day 2 and **(C)** day 3. Neither patient received platelet transfusions. *Source*: From Greinacher and Warkentin (2012).

thrombopoietin (TPO) physiology (Greinacher and Warkentin, 2012). TPO is constitutively produced by the liver, and because TPO binds to platelet receptors (c-mpl), TPO levels are inversely proportional to the platelet mass. Consequently, TPO levels rise when the postsurgery platelet count declines occur. However, there is a lag between megakaryocyte stimulation by TPO and subsequent release of new platelets. This is illustrated by the observation that platelet count increase begins three to five days after the application of a TPO analogue, romiplostim (Wang et al., 2004). This early platelet count fall that is characteristic of perioperative thrombocytopenia must be distinguished from a postsurgery HIT-related platelet count fall, which begins at least five days after surgery in which intraoperative or early postoperative heparin is given.

Perioperative platelet transfusions can alter this platelet count profile somewhat: platelet transfusion produces an abrupt increase in the platelet count, but the subsequent clearance of the transfused platelets can shift the postoperative platelet count nadir one or two days later.

The Concept of Pseudo-Heparin-Induced Thrombocytopenia

HIT is strongly associated with life- and limb-threatening venous and arterial thrombosis, including pulmonary embolism, venous limb gangrene, and large vessel arterial occlusion. However, HIT is by no means a unique explanation for the combination of thrombocytopenia and thrombosis (Table 3.1). In these "pseudo-HIT" disorders—so named because they strongly mimic HIT on clinical grounds—thrombocytopenia usually occurs early during the course of heparin treatment. This could reflect the prothrombotic process associated with the patient's primary diagnosis. Alternatively, heparin could exacerbate the platelet count fall by nonimmune proaggregatory effects on platelets (see chap. 5). If the patient previously received heparin, physicians might consider HIT in the differential diagnosis of the platelet count fall.

However, one pseudo-HIT syndrome in particular closely resembles even the typical day 5–10 timing of thrombocytopenia characteristic of HIT: adenocarcinoma-associated disseminated intravascular coagulation (DIC). In these patients, the fall in platelet count begins soon after stopping heparin treatment. Because the patients usually will have received heparin for 5–10 days to treat adenocarcinoma-associated thrombosis, the timing of the onset of thrombocytopenia closely resembles immune HIT. Furthermore, the frequent occurrence of new or progressive thrombosis in this setting also suggests HIT.

The crucial concept in defining the notion of pseudo-HIT is the presumption that no matter how closely the thrombocytopenic disorder resembles HIT on clinical grounds, pathologic HIT antibodies, that is, those characterized by strong heparin-dependent, platelet-activating properties, are *not* detectable in the patient's blood. This concept is credible given the high sensitivity of certain assays for detecting such antibodies (Warkentin et al., 2011) (see chap. 11).

This chapter draws attention to those clinical disorders that can mimic and, thereby, be confused with HIT. This is not a trivial distinction: whereas heparin is contraindicated in patients with HIT, it often is the optimal treatment of patients with pseudo-HIT. Second, the close clinical parallels between HIT and certain pseudo-HIT disorders can provide insights into the pathogenesis of thrombosis. For example, the recognition that venous limb gangrene can complicate metastatic adenocarcinoma, and the clinical parallels with a similar syndrome in HIT patients, suggests that a common factor (coumarin anticoagulation) may play a crucial pathogenic role in both disorders (Warkentin, 2001). Likewise, similarities between HIT and the antiphospholipid syndrome (APS) suggest that they could also share common pathogenic mechanisms (Arnout, 1996, 2000; Gruel, 2000).

PSEUDO-HIT SYNDROMES
Adenocarcinoma

Mucin-producing adenocarcinoma is an important cause of venous and arterial thrombosis that occurs in association with thrombocytopenia. In these patients, DIC is often the predominant explanation for thrombocytopenia. The diagnosis is suggested by reduced fibrinogen levels, elevated prothrombin time, and elevated cross-linked (D-dimer) fibrin degradation products (or a positive protamine sulfate "paracoagulation" test).

Adenocarcinoma-associated DIC can strongly resemble HIT (Fig. 3.2). Typically, a patient presents with idiopathic deep vein thrombosis (DVT), sometimes

TABLE 3.1 Pseudo-HIT Disorders

Pseudo-HIT disorders	Pathogenesis of thrombocytopenia and thrombosis	Timing
Prothrombotic disorders		
Adenocarcinoma	DIC secondary to procoagulant material(s) produced by neoplastic cells	Late[a]
Pulmonary embolism	Platelet activation by clot-bound thrombin	Early[b] or late
Diabetic ketoacidosis	Hyperaggregable platelets in ketoacidosis (?)	Early[c]
Antiphospholipid syndrome	Multiple mechanisms described, including platelet activation by antiphospholipid antibodies (?)	Early
Thrombolytic therapy	Platelet activation by thrombin bound to fibrin degradation products (?)	Early[d]
Septicemia-associated purpura fulminans	Symmetrical peripheral gangrene secondary to DIC with depletion of protein C and antithrombin	Early
Hepatic necrosis/limb necrosis syndrome	Hypotension-associated ischemic hepatitis ("shock liver") and DIC with depletion of natural anticoagulants (e.g., protein C, antithrombin)	Early[e]
Infective endocarditis	Infection-associated thrombocytopenia; ischemic events secondary to septic emboli	Early
Paroxysmal nocturnal hemoglobinuria	Platelets susceptible to complement-mediated damage; platelet hypoproduction	Early
Postsurgical TTP	Anti-ADAMTS13 autoantibodies modulated by the postoperative state (?)	Early or late
Prohemorrhagic disorders		
GPIIb/IIIa antagonist-induced thrombocytopenia	Usually secondary to natural anti-GPIIb/IIIa antibodies; bleeding more common than thrombosis	Early
PTP	"Pseudospecific" alloantibody-mediated platelet destruction (exception: bleeding, not thrombosis)	Late

Note: These pseudo-HIT disorders can mimic HIT by causing thrombocytopenia and thrombosis in association with heparin treatment. An exception is PTP, which causes bleeding, but not thrombosis; however, PTP can resemble HIT because both disorders usually occur about a week after major surgery requiring blood and postoperative heparin. The pseudo-HIT disorders can be categorized based on whether the onset of thrombocytopenia is typically "early" (<5 days) or "late" (>5 days) in relation to the heparin. (?) indicates that the proposed pathogenesis remains uncertain.

[a]See Figure 3.2 for an example of pseudo-HIT caused by adenocarcinoma-associated DIC.
[b]See Figure 3.4 for early thrombocytopenia associated with pulmonary embolism.
[c]See Figure 3.5 for early thrombocytopenia associated with diabetic ketoacidosis.
[d]See Figure 3.6 for early thrombocytopenia caused by thrombolytic therapy.
[e]See Figures 3.7 and 3.8 for early thrombocytopenia in the setting of hepatic necrosis.

Abbreviations: ADAMTS, **a** **d**isintegrin **a**nd **m**etalloprotease with **t**hrombospondin-1-like domains; DIC, disseminated intravascular coagulation; GP, glycoprotein; HIT, heparin-induced thrombocytopenia; PTP, posttransfusion purpura; TTP, thrombotic thrombocytopenic purpura.

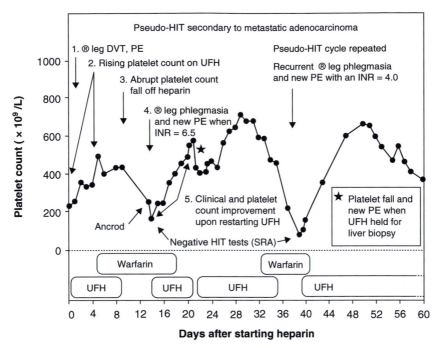

FIGURE 3.2 Pseudo-HIT: adenocarcinoma with thrombocytopenia and phlegmasia cerulea dolens after stopping administration of UFH. The late presentation of thrombocytopenia suggested HIT, prompting use of an alternative anticoagulant (ancrod). Heparin was restarted when HIT antibodies were not detected by SRA. Subsequently, discontinuation of heparin led to the recurrence of thrombocytopenia and warfarin-associated phlegmasia cerulea dolens (repeat of pseudo-HIT cycle). *Abbreviations*: DVT, deep vein thrombosis; HIT, heparin-induced thrombocytopenia; INR, international normalized ratio; PE, pulmonary embolism; SRA, serotonin release assay; UFH, unfractionated heparin.

with mild-to-moderate thrombocytopenia. During treatment with therapeutic-dose unfractionated or low molecular weight heparin (LMWH), the platelet count rises, probably because of improved control of DIC by the heparin. In our experience, this often dramatic rise in the platelet count during heparin treatment of "idiopathic" DVT is a clinically useful marker for adenocarcinoma-associated DIC. During the 5- to 10-day period of heparin treatment with overlapping warfarin anticoagulation, no problems are encountered. However, there is rapid recurrence of thrombocytopenia within hours or days of discontinuing the heparin, despite apparent therapeutic anticoagulation with warfarin, during which time the patient develops new or progressive venous, or even arterial, thrombosis. Thus, the onset of thrombocytopenia and thrombosis may occur within the characteristic 5- to 10-day "window" that suggests HIT.

Venous Limb Gangrene Complicating Adenocarcinoma

The venous thrombotic events complicating adenocarcinoma include DVT, phlegmasia cerulea dolens, and even venous limb gangrene (Everett and Jones, 1986; Adamson and Currie, 1993). Clinical and laboratory parallels between HIT and

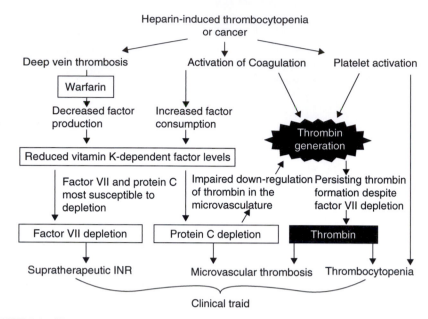

FIGURE 3.3 The pathogenesis of warfarin-associated venous limb gangrene is shown in relation to its typical clinical triad—supratherapeutic INR, microvascular thrombosis, and thrombocytopenia. The central paradox is the persisting formation of thrombin despite markedly depleted plasma factor VII level, which is paralleled by severely depleted protein C activity, leading to impaired downregulation of thrombin generation in the microvasculature and, consequently, microvascular thrombosis. *Abbreviation*: INR, international normalized ratio. *Source*: From Warkentin (2001).

adenocarcinoma suggest that, paradoxically, coumarin treatment could contribute to the pathogenesis of venous gangrene in these patients through a disturbance in procoagulant–anticoagulant balance (Warkentin, 1996, 2001; Klein et al., 2004; Ng and Crowther, 2006; White et al., 2006; Gunn et al., 2009; Chang et al., 2010; Warkentin et al., 2012). Figure 3.3 summarizes the proposed pathogenesis of this syndrome from the perspective of the characteristic clinical triad of venous limb gangrene: (*i*) thrombocytopenia caused by HIT or adenocarcinoma-associated DIC; (*ii*) acute DVT with acral (distal) microvascular thrombosis; and (*iii*) a supratherapeutic international normalized ratio (INR) associated with coumarin therapy.

Venous limb gangrene appears to result from failure of the protein C anticoagulant pathway to downregulate thrombin generation within the microvasculature (Warkentin 1996; Warkentin et al., 1997, 2012; see chap. 2). Here, the elevated INR represents a surrogate marker for marked reduction in functional protein C levels (by a parallel reduction in factor VII); the thrombocytopenia is a surrogate marker for uncontrolled thrombin generation associated either with HIT or adenocarcinoma (Fig. 3.3). As venous limb gangrene occurs in a limb with preceding active DVT, this suggests that local factors, such as direct extension of thrombosis, as well as exacerbation of distal thrombosis by venous stasis, contribute to large- and small-vessel thrombosis characteristic of this syndrome.

Venous thrombosis complicating adenocarcinoma, especially when associated with DIC or severe venous ischemia/necrosis, should be treated with heparin, rather than warfarin or other coumarin anticoagulants. Reversal of warfarin anticoagulation (intravenous vitamin K, with or without plasma infusion) and prompt control of DIC with heparin could salvage a limb with severe phlegmasia, or limit damage in a patient with venous gangrene. An effective agent often is LMWH (Prandoni, 1997; Lee et al., 2003). We recommend monitoring using anti-factor Xa levels, because some patients have heparin "resistance" and require high doses of heparin to achieve therapeutic anticoagulation.

Ironically, one of the problems of heparin in these patients is its efficacy: thus, if heparin is discontinued for any reason, rapid recurrence of thrombocytopenia and thrombosis results. Figure 3.2 shows an example in which thrombocytopenia and pulmonary embolism occurred (day 21) when heparin was briefly held to permit a liver biopsy to diagnose metastatic carcinoma. One of us (TEW) observed a patient with lung adenocarcinoma in whom heparin was held to permit limb amputation; postanesthesia, the patient was aphasic (intraoperative stroke).

Pulmonary Embolism

Mild thrombocytopenia is common in patients with pulmonary embolism. Sometimes the thrombocytopenia is severe and associated with laboratory markers of DIC (Stahl et al., 1984; Mustafa et al., 1989; Leitner et al., 2010) (Fig. 3.4). The thrombocytopenia presumably results from thrombin-induced platelet activation and/or platelet accretion within the thromboemboli (Welch, 1887; Kitchens, 2004). Studies of experimental venous thromboembolism in dogs show abrupt increase in plasma fibrinopeptide levels upon embolization, consistent with intensification of the thrombotic process (Morris et al., 2004). Large thromboemboli within the high-flow pulmonary vessels may act as a reservoir for clot-bound thrombin that is relatively protected from inhibition by antithrombin-dependent inhibitors (Weitz et al., 1990). This view is indirectly supported by the observation that thrombocytopenia commonly occurs in patients with pulmonary embolism, but not in patients with DVT alone (Monreal et al., 1991; Warkentin et al., 2003b). Furthermore, increased heparin clearance has been demonstrated in experimental pulmonary embolism (Chiu et al., 1977), which could also contribute to increased thrombin generation.

Because HIT is also strongly associated with pulmonary embolism (Warkentin et al., 1995, 2003b), a diagnostic and therapeutic dilemma results when a patient presents with pulmonary embolism and thrombocytopenia five or more days after surgery managed with postoperative heparin prophylaxis. Initiating therapeutic heparin could have catastrophic consequences for the patient who has circulating HIT antibodies, although in sufficient doses it is effective for a patient with pulmonary embolism and DIC without HIT. Because these two possibilities cannot be readily distinguished on clinical grounds alone, one should manage such a patient with an alternative anticoagulant until the results of HIT antibody testing become available (Warkentin, 2000).

Diabetic Ketoacidosis

Diabetic ketoacidosis (DKA) can be associated with acute thromboembolic complications. *In vitro* studies indicate that high glucose levels enhance platelet activation by adenosine diphosphate (ADP) and other platelet agonists (Sudic et al., 2006). Evidence for *in vivo* platelet activation was observed in one study of 10 patients who had elevated plasma levels of platelet factor 4 (PF4) and β-thromboglobulin during DKA that resolved following recovery (Campbell et al., 1985). Evidence for activation

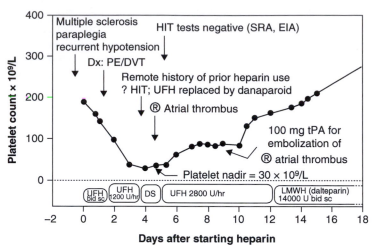

FIGURE 3.4 Pseudo-HIT secondary to PE and DIC: An obese, 50-year-old man with paraplegia was admitted for recurrent hypotension. He initially received bid sc UFH for antithrombotic prophylaxis, as the initial diagnosis was septicemia. DVT and PE were then diagnosed (Dx), and therapy changed to intravenous UFH, 1200 U/hr. The platelet count fell over four days to a nadir of 30 × 10⁹/L; DS was given because of concern over possible HIT (there was a remote history of previous heparin use). An echocardiogram showed large right atrial thrombus (likely representing a leg vein embolus), and the patient was transferred to a cardiac surgical center. The platelet count fall was judged too rapid to be HIT (see chap. 2), a viewpoint supported by negative testing for HIT antibodies by SRA and PF4/heparin EIA. UFH administration was restarted in higher doses with antifactor Xa monitoring to overcome heparin resistance. Recurrent hypotension occurred when the right atrial thrombus embolized; full hemodynamic and platelet count recovery occurred following t-PA administration, followed by UFH, then LMWH, and (later) warfarin treatment. The patient was well at 3-yr follow-up, without evidence of carcinoma. *Abbreviations*: bid, twice-daily; DIC, disseminated intravascular coagulation; DVT, deep vein thrombosis; DS, danaparoid sodium; EIA, enzyme immunoassay; HIT, heparin-induced thrombocytopenia; LMWH, low molecular weight heparin; PE, pulmonary embolism; SRA, serotonin release assay; sc, subcutaneous; t-PA, tissue plasminogen activator; UFH, unfractionated heparin.

of coagulation includes elevated fibrin degradation products and reduced antithrombin (Paton, 1981). Figure 3.5 illustrates a patient with "white clots" in the femoral artery, leading to amputation, who was initially thought to have HIT. However, HIT antibody testing and subsequent clinical events proved that the patient did not have HIT as the initial explanation for this dramatic clinical presentation of thrombocytopenia and thrombosis complicating DKA (although HIT occurred later in the clinical course). We are also aware of a patient with essential thrombocythemia who developed postoperative DKA, thrombocytopenia, and bilateral lower-limb artery thrombosis that occurred too early (days 2–3) during thromboprophylaxis with unfractionated heparin (UFH) to have been caused by immune HIT. A similar example of early-onset severe thrombocytopenia and arterial thrombosis resulting in amputation of an arm was reported in a patient with DKA and adult respiratory distress syndrome (ARDS) (Phillips et al., 1994). Although the authors suggested HIT secondary to heparin "flushes" as the diagnosis, pseudo-HIT seems more likely based on the temporal features of the case, as well as the negative laboratory testing

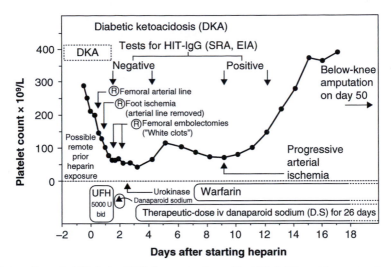

FIGURE 3.5 Pseudo-HIT during DKA, later complicated by HIT: A 27-yr-old man developed rapid onset of thrombocytopenia and white clots in the left femoral artery (at a femoral artery catheter site) during management of DKA that included prophylactic-dose UFH. HIT was suspected errone-ously on the basis of a possible previous remote heparin exposure (gastric surgery 10 yr earlier). The patient underwent two embolectomies as well as treatment with urokinase and iv danaparoid. The patient developed a second platelet count fall during danaparoid treatment that began on day 6 in relation to the initial course of UFH. Tests for HIT antibodies changed from negative (SRA: days 1 and 4, serotonin release <5%) to positive (days 9 and 12, serotonin release 92% and 80%, respectively). By PF4/heparin–EIA (set up to detect IgG antibodies), the day 1 sample also was negative (OD, 0.262; negative, <0.450), the day 4 sample was weakly positive (0.804), and the day 9 and l2 samples were strongly positive (1.863 and 1.002, respectively). Although the possibility of *in vivo* cross-reactivity of danaparoid with the HIT antibodies is suggested by the thrombocytopenia and progression of limb ischemia, the platelet count subsequently rose during danaparoid treat-ment, and no additional thromboembolic events occurred. *In vitro* cross-reactivity was detected on day 9, but not on day 12, blood sample. *Abbreviations*: HIT, heparin-induced thrombocytopenia; DKA, diabetic ketoacidosis; UFH, unfractionated heparin; iv, intravenous; OD, optical density; SRA, serotonin release assay; EIA, enzyme immunoassay.

for HIT antibodies. Casteels et al. (2003) observed the combination of rhabdomyolysis, thrombocytopenia, and anemia in a child presenting with DKA.

Antiphospholipid Syndrome or Lupus Anticoagulant Syndrome
Clinical Features
Antiphospholipid antibodies can be detected either as "lupus anticoagulants" (nonspecific inhibitors) or as anticardiolipin or anti-β_2-glycoprotein I antibodies (Asherson et al., 1989; Ginsberg et al., 1995).

APS is characterized by increased risk for thrombosis and recurrent fetal loss, limb or intra-abdominal vein thrombosis, cerebral venous (dural sinus) thrombo-sis, nonatheromatous arterial thrombosis, cardiac valvulitis, and microvascular thrombosis (e.g., acrocyanosis, "blue toe syndrome," digital ulceration or gan-grene, livedo reticularis) (Hojnik et al., 1996; Gibson et al., 1997). Many patients have thrombocytopenia (Morgan et al., 1993; Galli et al., 1996), which is typically mild and intermittent. The explanation for thrombocytopenia is uncertain: Some patients have platelet-reactive autoantibodies (Galli et al., 1994; Lipp et al., 1998), but platelet-activating effects of IgG are also suspected (Vermylen et al., 1997).

The explanation for the prothrombotic tendency of APS is also elusive. A multifactorial pathogenesis is likely, because the antibodies recognize complexes of negatively charged phospholipids with many different protein cofactors, such as β_2-glycoprotein I (β_2GPI), prothrombin, protein C, protein S, and annexin V (Galli, 1996; Triplett, 1996). Indeed, interference with endothelial cell function, impaired fibrinolysis, disturbances in protein C anticoagulant pathway activities, and antibody-mediated platelet activation have all been described (for review see Petri, 1997; Gruel, 2000; Arnout and Vermylen, 2003).

Parallels Between APS and HIT

Table 3.2 lists some common features of APS and HIT. Both clinicopathologic disorders are characterized by thrombocytopenia, a paradoxical risk for venous and arterial thrombosis, and associated antibodies that can be detected by either functional or antigen assays (see chap. 11). Moreover, for both APS and HIT, positive functional assays are more strongly associated with thrombosis than positive antigen assays (Ginsberg et al., 1995; Warkentin et al., 2000; Galli et al., 2003). The parallels between these disorders led Arnout (1996) to hypothesize that IgG-mediated platelet activation could explain thrombosis in APS. Supportive experimental data include the observations that antiphospholipid antibodies enhance platelet activation induced by other agonists (Martinuzzo et al., 1993). Furthermore, Arvieux et al. (1993) observed murine monoclonal antibodies reactive against β_2GPI induced

TABLE 3.2   Clinical Parallels Between HIT and APS

	HIT	APS
Thrombotic paradox	Thrombosis despite thrombocytopenia	Thrombosis despite prolonged coagulation tests (± thrombocytopenia)
Spectrum of thrombotic events	Venous > arterial thrombosis; adrenal infarction, dural sinus thrombosis	Venous > arterial thrombosis; adrenal infarction, dural sinus thrombosis
Severity of thrombocytopenia	Mild to moderate thrombocytopenia	Mild to moderate thrombocytopenia
Laboratory diagnosis by (*i*) functional or (*ii*) antigen assays	(*i*) Platelet activation assays (e.g., serotonin release assay, heparin-induced platelet activation test); (*ii*) platelet factor 4/heparin–EIA	(*i*) Lupus anticoagulant (i.e., prolonged phospholipid-dependent coagulation assay in presence of patient plasma); (*ii*) β_2GPI-dependent anticardiolipin-EIA
Pathogenesis	Platelet activation by platelet Fc receptors; endothelial activation by immune injury	Uncertain pathogenesis: immune platelet activation and endothelial injury are possible factors

Note: Further laboratory parallels between HIT and APS are discussed in chapter 11.
Abbreviations: β_2GPI, β_2-glycoprotein I; EIA, enzyme immunoassay; HIT, heparin-induced thrombocytopenia; APS, antiphospholipid syndrome.

platelet activation in the presence of subthreshold concentrations of ADP and epinephrine, an effect dependent on binding to platelet FcγIIa receptors. However, other workers were unable to demonstrate enhanced platelet activation in the presence of IgG antiphospholipid antibodies (Shi et al., 1993; Ford et al., 1998) or showed no role for platelet FcγIIa receptors (Lutters et al., 2001; Jankowski et al., 2003).

Thrombocytopenia in Patients with APS Receiving Heparin

In retrospective studies, Auger and colleagues (1995) reported that platelet counts typically fell by about 50% in patients with chronic thromboembolic disease and the lupus anticoagulant who were treated with heparin. Neither timing of the onset of thrombocytopenia nor results of specific antigen or activation assays for HIT antibodies were reported, so it remains uncertain whether these patients had (immune) HIT. Perunicic et al. (2008) reported a patient with APS whose thrombocytopenia worsened with heparin: although these authors initially considered the patient to have pseudo-HIT, their final conclusion was "HIT" despite the negative functional and antigen assays (we would have retained the designation of "pseudo-HIT").

It is possible that nonidiosyncratic platelet activation caused by heparin could increase the thrombocytopenic potential of antiphospholipid antibodies in the absence of HIT antibodies. Alternatively, some patients with APS may have low levels of circulating HIT antibodies even in the absence of previous heparin exposure (Lasne et al., 1997; Martinuzzo et al., 1999). We observed a young woman with ischemic stroke who developed thrombocytopenia and lower-limb thrombosis when therapeutic-dose heparin was given; pretreatment blood samples contained both antiphospholipid antibodies and platelet-activating anti-PF4/heparin (PF4/H) IgG (Lo et al., 2006); subsequently, this patient was included in a case-series of "spontaneous" HIT (Warkentin et al., 2008).

Bourhim and colleagues (2003) showed that affinity-purified IgM anti-β_2GPI from a patient with APS gave a positive reaction in PF4-dependent enzyme immunoassays (EIAs). Furthermore, mice actively immunized with the purified IgM anti-β_2GPI generated anti-β_2GPI antibodies (via an idiotype–anti-idiotype mechanism) that also cross-reacted with PF4/H. More recently, Pauzner and coworkers (2009) reported that patients with APS and systemic lupus erythematosus could have false-positive tests for anti-PF4/H antibodies by EIA because of the presence of anti-PF4 (*not* anti-PF4/H) antibodies.

Thrombolytic Therapy

Early-onset thrombocytopenia occurs in about 1% of patients with acute coronary syndrome whether treated by heparin or nonheparin anticoagulants (Eikelboom et al., 2001). The frequency of thrombocytopenia is even higher in patients treated with streptokinase, especially when this thrombolytic agent is combined with heparin (Balduini et al., 1993) (Fig. 3.6). This could represent a direct, activating stimulus of heparin on platelets that perhaps is exacerbated by procoagulant effects of thrombolytic therapy. For example, fibrin degradation products generated by thrombolytic agents bind and protect thrombin from inhibition by heparin (Weitz et al., 1998). Such a mechanism could explain thrombocytopenia after the use of any thrombolytic drug. However, some investigators have reported that plasma containing antistreptokinase antibodies can activate platelets through their Fcγ receptors in the presence of streptokinase (Vaughan et al., 1988; Lebrazi et al., 1995;

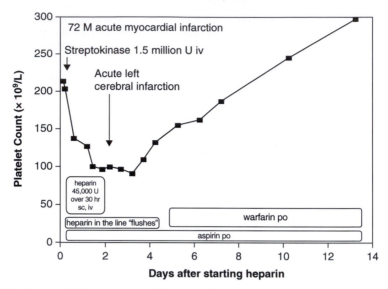

FIGURE 3.6 Pseudo-HIT associated with thrombolytic therapy. A 72-yr-old man developed moderate thrombocytopenia shortly after receiving streptokinase and heparin, which resolved following discontinuation of heparin. The early onset of thrombocytopenia, as well as the negative testing for HIT-IgG using the platelet serotonin release assay, was consistent with pseudo-HIT. *Abbreviations*: HIT, heparin-induced thrombocytopenia; iv, intravenous; po, per os; sc, subcutaneous. *Source*: From Warkentin and Kelton (1994).

Regnault et al., 2003). Thus, high-titer antistreptokinase antibodies found in some normal individuals could explain the occasional occurrence of thrombocytopenia and thrombosis following treatment with streptokinase.

Septicemia-Associated Purpura Fulminans
Septicemia complicated by DIC occasionally results in progressive ischemia and necrosis of fingers or hands and toes or feet, producing a syndrome of symmetrical peripheral gangrene also known as purpura fulminans (Knight et al., 2000). The association with DIC suggests that increased thrombin generation *in vivo*, together with severe consumption and depletion of natural anticoagulant factors (e.g., protein C, protein S, antithrombin), leads to dysregulated fibrin deposition in the microvasculature. Other contributing factors can include hypotension or shock, pharmacologic vasoconstriction (e.g., dopamine, epinephrine, norepinephrine) (Winkler and Trunkey, 1981; Hayes et al., 1992), vessel injury from invasive catheters, impaired hepatic synthesis of natural anticoagulants (e.g., vitamin K deficiency, postoperative hepatic dysfunction or failure), postsplenectomy status, or congenital deficiency of natural anticoagulants. Rarely, purpura fulminans occurs several weeks after varicella infection, usually because of autoantibodies reactive against protein S (Smith and White, 1999).

Meningococcemia in particular is often complicated by peripheral tissue necrosis that seems to parallel the severity of protein C depletion (Fijnvandraat et al., 1995). Clinical studies suggest that protein C replacement therapy improves the natural history of this infection (Smith and White, 1999; White et al., 2000).

Other infections that sometimes are complicated by symmetrical peripheral gangrene include septicemia secondary to pneumococcus (Johansen and Hansen Jr., 1993), *Escherichia coli* (Rinaldo and Perez, 1982), *Haemophilus influenzae* type b (Hayes et al., 1992), and *Capnocytophaga canimorsus* (Kullberg et al., 1991), among others. Sometimes severe systemic inflammatory response syndromes, such as ARDS, in the absence of demonstrable infection, can be complicated by limb necrosis (Bone et al., 1976). Acquired antithrombin deficiency in such patients with ARDS could be associated with thrombosis (Owings et al., 1996).

The development of acral tissue ischemia or necrosis in a thrombocytopenic, septic patient receiving heparin may suggest HIT. Although a common therapeutic response to such a diagnostic dilemma might be to stop heparin pending results of diagnostic testing for HIT antibodies, this could result in further ischemic injury, because anticoagulants might help prevent microvascular thrombosis (White et al., 2000). Furthermore, alternative nonheparin anticoagulants could be relatively contraindicated in a patient with significant renal or hepatic dysfunction. Thus, a reasonable treatment approach might well include continued heparin if clinical judgment posited a higher likelihood of septicemia, rather than HIT, as the cause of the microvascular thrombosis.

Only a small minority of septic patients develop acral limb ischemia or necrosis. Many, however, develop thrombocytopenia, with or without laboratory evidence for DIC. The predominant explanation for increased platelet destruction in sepsis is uncertain, but appears to involve the underlying inflammatory host response (Aird, 2003a,b). Since hospitalized septic patients frequently are exposed to heparin, diagnostic confusion with HIT can result. Low protein C levels correlate with poor outcomes in sepsis (Yan et al., 2001), and recombinant human activated protein C (drotrecogin, Xigris) has been shown to reduce mortality in septic patients (Bernard et al., 2001). It is possible that this therapy might reduce the risk of limb ischemia from microvascular thrombosis in this patient population. A potential dilemma is that septic patients with severe thrombocytopenia ($<30 \times 10^9$/L) were excluded in the clinical trials because of the bleeding potential of drotrecogin; however, as relative and absolute efficacy was greatest in the patients with the most severe sepsis, it has been suggested that otherwise eligible patients with such severe thrombocytopenia be considered as candidates for drotrecogin following platelet transfusion (Warkentin et al., 2003a).

Hepatic Necrosis-Limb Necrosis

Acute ischemic necrosis—as can occur in hypotensive, critically ill patients following surgery—can be complicated by progressive acral ischemic limb necrosis despite palpable arterial pulses (Figs. 3.7 and 3.8). Concomitant factors include DIC and vasopressor therapy. The contributory role of liver failure to microvascular thrombosis includes depletion of natural anticoagulants, such as protein C and antithrombin as well as confounding of aPTT-monitored anticoagulant therapy through associated coagulopathy (Warkentin, 2011; Siegal et al., 2012).

Infective Endocarditis

Infective endocarditis is frequently complicated by thrombocytopenia. These patients are also at risk for septic emboli manifesting as thrombotic or hemorrhagic stroke, myocardial infarction, renal infarction, or even acute limb ischemia (de Gennes et al., 1990). Thus, the profile of macrovascular thrombosis and thrombocytopenia characteristic of HIT can be mimicked, especially as heparin is often used to anticoagulate

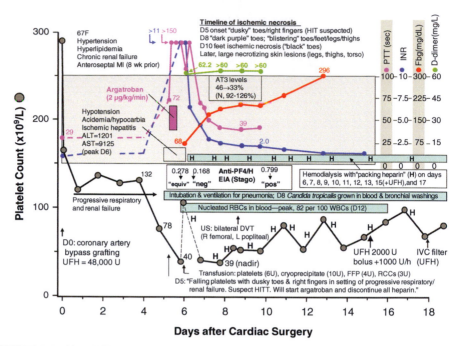

FIGURE 3.7 Non–HIT-associated thrombocytopenia and coagulopathy treated as HIT: PTT confounding in the setting of acute ischemic hepatitis. A 67-yr-old woman with recent myocardial infarction underwent coronary artery bypass grafting. The early postoperative course (day [D] 1–4) was characterized by progressive respiratory failure with pulmonary infiltrates (treated with bilevel positive airway pressure, antibiotics, corticosteroids, and high-dose intravenous gammaglobulin) and progressive renal failure [rise in serum creatinine from 1.9 to 3.1 mg/dL (normal, 0.6–1.3 mg/dL)]; no postoperative heparin prophylaxis was given. On D5 the patient developed hypotension (treated with albumin, dopamine, and neosynephrine), acidemia/hypocarbia, and ischemic hepatitis (marked increase in ALT and AST); the platelet count fell from 132 (D4) to 78 (D5) × 10^9/L. Several hours later the toes and right fingers appeared "dusky" and HIT-associated thrombosis (HITT) was suspected (despite the patient not having received heparin since surgery). Argatroban (Arg) was started, but was stopped approximately 4 hr later when the PTT measured >150 sec (target PTT range, 60–90 sec). The next morning (D6), the platelet count had fallen further to 40; the PTT remained >150, the INR was >11 (normal, 0.9–1.1), and the fibrinogen measured only 68 mg/dL (normal, 200–450 mg/dL). The patient received platelets, cryoprecipitate, FFP, and RCCs. The PF4-dependent EIA from Diagnostica Stago (Asnieres-sur-Seine, France) was reported as "equivocal" ("equiv") and a repeat test performed the next day was reported as "negative" ("neg"). Despite "therapeutic" (or greater) PTT and INR values, by D8, progression to ischemic necrosis of the toes was evident (despite Doppler-identifiable pulses), as well as blistering of numerous sites on the lower extremities; in addition, bilateral lower-limb DVT was documented by US, but anticoagulation was not restarted because of (minor) gastrointestinal bleeding. A repeat EIA measured "positive" ("pos") on D10. Ultimately, the patient developed numerous large, full-thickness, burn-like necrotic skin lesions involving feet, legs, thighs, buttocks, and torso. This patient case illustrates failure to prevent extensive acral limb and multiple central necrotizing skin lesions despite prompt institution of alternative nonheparin anticoagulation for clinically suspected HIT. Despite the positive PF4-dependent EIA on D10, the patient did not have HIT, based on (*i*) equivocal/negative EIAs (D5, D6) despite established thrombocytopenia; (*ii*) a clear alternative explanation for thrombocytopenia (fungemia); and (*Continued*)

FIGURE 3.7 (*Continued*) (*iii*) lack of platelet count fall when the patient inadvertently received UFH on D15 (during hemodialysis) and D18 (during insertion of IVC filter); it is unlikely that "packing heparin" administered into the tubing immediately after dialysis (H) played any deleterious role. The dramatic multicentric skin necrosis probably resulted from a profound disturbance in procoagulant–anticoagulant balance, resulting from (*i*) DIC and (*ii*) natural anticoagulant failure [marked antithrombin (AT3) depletion (note: protein C and protein S levels were not measured, but likely were also profoundly reduced)]. On D7 and D8, the patient had the combination of high fibrin D-dimer levels [>60 mg/L (normal, <2.8 mg/L)] and profoundly low AT3 levels (D8 nadir, 33% of normal). The case also illustrates the issue of coagulopathy-associated confounding of PTT-adjusted argatroban therapy. The high baseline PTT (72 sec immediately before argatroban)—likely reflecting both DIC and hepatic dysfunction—meant that subsequent (supra)therapeutic PTTs did not indicate therapeutic or supratherapeutic concentrations of argatroban. *Abbreviations*: ALT, alanine transaminase; AST, aspartate transaminase; DIC, disseminated intravascular coagulation; DVT, deep vein thrombosis; EIA, enzyme immunoassay; Fbg, fibrinogen; FPP, fresh-frozen plasma; HIT, heparin-induced thrombocytopenia; HITT, HIT-associated thrombosis; INR, international normalized ratio; IVC, inferior vena cava; PTT, partial thromboplastin time; RCCs, red cell concentrates; PF4, platelet factor 4; US, ultrasound; UFH, unfractionated heparin. *Source*: From Warkentin et al. (2011).

patients with septic endocarditis (Delahaye et al., 1990). Microembolization leading to multiple small infarcts or microabscesses, in such organs as muscles, adrenal glands, and spleen, is an additional feature of endocarditis (Ting et al., 1990) that is not seen in HIT. When endocarditis-associated thrombocytopenia is unusually severe, potential explanations include platelet-reactive autoantibodies (Arnold et al., 2004) or procoagulant monocyte-stimulating factors secreted by microorganisms from within large vegetations (Selleng et al., 2007). One reported case of bilateral venous limb gangrene complicating presumptive infective endocarditis (Awad et al., 1998) seems more likely to represent warfarin-induced microthrombosis in the setting of cancer-associated DIC and marantic endocarditis, as blood cultures were negative, limb necrosis coincided with postcardiac surgery warfarin administration, and autopsy showed extensive lower-limb DVT and metastatic adenocarcinoma.

Paroxysmal Nocturnal Hemoglobinuria
Paroxysmal nocturnal hemoglobinuria (PNH) is a clonal myeloid disorder characterized by an acquired defect in the X-linked phosphatidylinositol glycan class A (PIG-A) gene, leading to loss of cell surface glycosylphosphatidylinositol-anchored proteins (for review see Pu and Brodsky, 2011). Loss of the complement-regulating glycosylphosphatidylinositol-linked surface proteins, decay-accelerating factor, and membrane attack complex inhibitory factor, causes the red cells to be exquisitely sensitive to complement-mediated hemolysis. Some patients have thrombocytopenia, and unusual, life-threatening venous thrombotic events, such as hepatic vein thrombosis, occur in some patients. Thus, the clinical profile of HIT potentially can be mimicked. The thrombocytopenia could be related either to decreased platelet production or to complement-mediated formation of procoagulant platelet-derived microparticles (Wiedmer et al., 1993).

Postsurgical Thrombocytopenic Thrombocytopenia Purpura
Thrombotic thrombocytopenic purpura (TTP) is a life-threatening disorder characterized by thrombocytopenia and microangiopathic hemolytic anemia (Coombs-negative hemolysis with prominent red cell fragmentation). Ischemic necrosis of

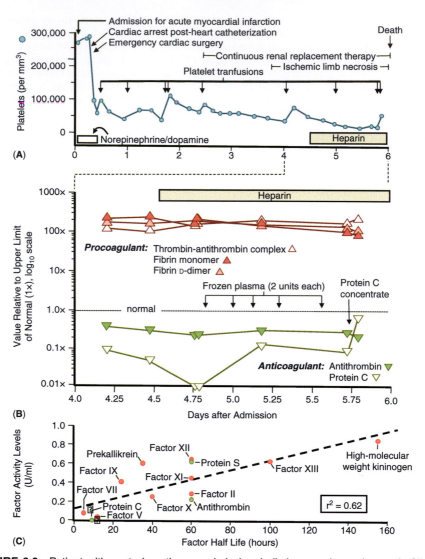

FIGURE 3.8 Patient with acute hepatic necrosis-ischemic limb necrosis syndrome. A. Clinical course and platelet counts. Ischemic limb necrosis began approximately 4 days post-cardiac arrest, and progressed despite heparin therapy. B. Disturbed procoagulant-anticoagulant balance. Soon after onset of ischemic limb necrosis, procoagulant markers (fibrin D-dimer, fibrin monomer, thrombin-antithrombin complexes) were elevated by approximately 100- to 200-times the upper limit of normal, whereas the natural anticoagulants, protein C and antithrombin, attained nadir levels that were only approximately 1% (0.01 U/ml [reference range, 0.70 to 1.80]) and 20% (0.20 U/ml [reference range, 0.77 to 1.25]) of normal (at day 4.75), respectively, with subsequent increases in protein C following transfusion of frozen plasma and protein C concentrate. C. Coagulation factor activity levels (analyzing mean values of two plasma samples obtained approximately 4.75 days post-admission, and prior to plasma administration) versus factor half-lives. Factor VIII coagulant levels measured approximately four-times elevated (not shown), consistent with its role as an acute phase reactant. *Source*: From Ref. Siegal et al. 2012. With permission of Massachusetts Medical Society.

brain, kidneys, heart, pancreas, and other tissues can result from disseminated arteriolar occlusions by platelet-von Willebrand factor (vWF) microthrombi. In many patients, there is evidence for autoantibodies that inhibit or clear the enzyme, *a* disintegrin *a*nd *m*etalloprotease with *t*hrombospondin-1–like domains (ADAMTS13), which is responsible for cleaving ultralarge vWF multimers released from endothelium. Thus, the pathogenesis of idiopathic (primary) TTP likely reflects the formation of arteriolar-occluding complexes of ultralarge vWF multimers and platelets, thereby explaining both the thrombocytopenia and the tissue ischemia. "Secondary" TTP has been reported to occur in association with pregnancy, certain drugs (e.g., ticlopidine, clopidogrel, quinine, cyclosporine, mitomycin), autoimmune disorders (systemic lupus erythematosus), organ transplantation, and infections (human immunodeficiency virus, bacterial endocarditis). TTP clinically resembles a nephrotropic microangiopathic hemolytic anemia known as hemolytic uremic syndrome (HUS); however, there are certain unique triggers of HUS (especially preceding infection with *E. coli* O157:H7 and O104:H4) and anti-ADAMTS13 autoantibodies are not detected in HUS. Recently, an autoimmune humoral pathogenesis of postinfectious HUS was suggested based on clinical response to IgG depletion through immunoadsorption (Greinacher et al., 2011).

In recent years, an entity known as postoperative TTP has been recognized (Naqvi et al., 2004). The most common clinical setting is postcardiac surgery, with cases seen beginning 2–19 days (median, day 5–6) after surgery (Chang et al., 1996; Pavlovsky and Weinstein, 1997; Almehmi et al., 2004; Chang and Ikhlaque, 2004). Other preceding events have included vascular surgery (Chang et al., 1996; Lee et al., 2011), abdominal surgery (Robson and Abbs, 1997; Chang et al., 2000; Lee et al., 2011), and orthopedic surgery (Iosifidis et al., 2006). The authors advocate plasmapheresis (the therapeutic mainstay of primary TTP) when postoperative TTP is diagnosed. Given the frequent formation of anti-PF4/H antibodies after surgery in heparin-treated patients, it is possible that coincidental formation of nonpathogenic anti-PF4/H antibodies could cause a false diagnosis of HIT in a patient with this rare entity of postoperative TTP. On the other hand, peripheral digit ischemic syndrome leading to amputations has been reported in postcardiac surgery TTP (Chang and Ikhlaque, 2004), further blurring the distinctions between HIT and TTP. One patient has been reported in whom the authors believed the patient had concomitant TTP and HIT (Benke and Moltzan, 2005); an alternative explanation is that HIT-associated DIC produced thrombi in the renal microvasculature (thus, HIT may have mimicked TTP).

Glycoprotein IIb/IIIa Antagonist-Induced Thrombocytopenia

Glycoprotein (GP) IIb/IIIa antagonists (abciximab, tirofiban, eptifibatide) are used during coronary angioplasty to reduce platelet-mediated thrombosis. However, in a few patients, acute thrombocytopenia begins within hours of GPIIb/IIIa antagonist use (Aster et al., 2006; Warkentin, 2007). The thrombocytopenia is typically severe (usually $<20 \times 10^9$/L) and life-threatening bleeding can sometimes occur. Interestingly, most reported cases have occurred after *first* exposure to one of these drugs, although the frequency may be higher with repeat exposures (especially with abciximab) (Curtis et al., 2002). Platelet counts usually recover in 2–5 days after discontinuing the drug. Thrombocytopenia occurring after first exposure to a GPIIb/IIIa antagonist is explained by naturally occurring antibodies that recognize GPIIb/IIIa in the presence of the provoking drug (Bougie et al., 2002). Delayed onset of thrombocytopenia is explained by persistence of platelet-bound drug for several weeks after treatment, rendering platelets susceptible to destruction by newly formed antibodies (Curtis et al., 2004). A serologic problem is the distinction of "pathologic" from "benign" antibodies found commonly among normal individuals. The blood film should always be examined when "thrombocytopenia" appears after abciximab use: this is because in some patients this GPIIb/IIIa antagonist can induce platelet clumping *ex vivo* (when the blood is drawn into a calcium-chelating anticoagulant), resulting in a "pseudothrombocytopenia" that is clinically benign (unless inappropriate platelet transfusions are initiated) (Sane et al., 2000).

In some patients with acute thrombocytopenia triggered by tirofiban or eptifibatide, platelet-activating effects of the antibodies—mediated through platelet FcγIIa receptors—may contribute to prothrombotic consequences (Dunkley et al., 2003; Gao et al., 2009), potentially explaining the increased mortality of patients who develop thrombocytopenia when treated with GPIIb/IIIa antagonists (Abrams and Cines, 2002). Here, the parallels with immune HIT are striking.

What should the clinician suspect when a patient develops abrupt onset of severe thrombocytopenia immediately after cardiac angioplasty in which both heparin and a GPIIb/IIIa antagonist have been used? (Assume also that heparin has been given previously, but not a GPIIb/IIIa antagonist.) The surprising answer is that this clinical scenario almost always is caused by the GPIIb/IIIa antagonist. Thus, it would be wrong to treat such a patient presumptively as rapid-onset HIT, particularly because further anticoagulation with therapeutic doses of a nonheparin anticoagulant could lead to dangerous bleeding, especially considering the patient's severe thrombocytopenia and GPIIb/IIIa-antagonized platelets.

Posttransfusion Purpura

Posttransfusion purpura (PTP) is a rare syndrome characterized by severe thrombocytopenia and mucocutaneous bleeding that begins 5–10 days after blood transfusion, usually red cell concentrates. More than 95% of affected patients are older women, in keeping with its pathogenesis of an anamnestic recurrence of platelet-specific alloantibodies in women previously sensitized by pregnancy. Destruction of autologous platelets is believed to result from the pseudospecificity of the alloimmune response, for example, the high-titer antihuman platelet antigen-la (anti-HPA-la) alloantibodies (the most frequent cause of the syndrome) probably somewhat recognize the autologous HPA-lb alloantigen.

Because both PTP and HIT typically occur about a week after surgery managed with perioperative blood transfusions and postoperative heparin prophylaxis, a diagnostic dilemma can arise (Lubenow et al., 2000). Indeed, in a review of PTP Mueller-Eckhardt (1986) stated: "A frequent misdiagnosis was HIT supposedly because these patients had received heparin prophylactically after operations." Several reports have commented on the diagnostic confusion between PTP and HIT (Araújo et al., 2000; Shtalrid et al., 2006; Woelke et al., 2006). For distinguishing these conditions, a useful clinical clue is the presence or absence of petechiae: PTP almost invariably is characterized by this hallmark of severe thrombocytopenia, whereas patients with HIT generally do not develop petechiae, even if they have very severe thrombocytopenia. In the differential diagnosis,

Lubenow and coworkers pointed out that a platelet count less than $15 \times 10^9/L$ points to PTP, whereas a platelet count above this threshold indicates likely HIT. To prove the diagnosis of PTP, high titers of platelet-reactive alloantibodies must be demonstrated in patient blood.

RECOGNITION AND TREATMENT OF PSEUDO-HIT

Many patients with pseudo-HIT can be distinguished from HIT because of the early onset of thrombocytopenia (Table 3.1). Unless the patient received heparin within the past 30, and at most 100, days, the early platelet count fall is strong evidence against HIT (Warkentin and Kelton, 2001; Lubenow et al., 2002) (see chap. 2).

However, for patients with adenocarcinoma-associated DIC, or postoperative pulmonary embolism, in whom the platelet count fall can occur after five days of heparin treatment, the diagnosis initially could be uncertain. As alternative anticoagulants (danaparoid, fondaparinux, bivalirudin, or argatroban) are available in most countries, treatment with one of these agents before obtaining results of HIT antibody testing may be appropriate. For patients with adenocarcinoma without HIT antibodies, management is more successful with LMWH or UFH than with warfarin (Prandoni, 1997; Lee et al., 2003).

Pseudo-HIT Complicated by HIT

HIT is a relatively common complication of heparin therapy. It may be even more common in patients who have baseline platelet activation and PF4 release, as occurs in adenocarcinoma-associated DIC or DKA. Therefore, a patient with early thrombocytopenia attributable to a pseudo-HIT disorder may subsequently develop clinically significant HIT antibodies (Greinacher, 1995) (Fig. 3.5). Another example is that of a patient with lung cancer and DVT who developed a platelet count rise during intravenous heparin therapy, followed by recurrent thrombocytopenia and, ultimately, venous limb gangrene during anticoagulation with warfarin and ancrod (Fig. 3.9). In this situation, one might have expected platelet count recovery during a second course of heparin. However, an intravenous heparin challenge resulted in worsening of thrombocytopenia, and the patient had a strong positive assay for HIT antibodies, indicating the concurrence of cancer-associated DIC and HIT.

Opatrny and Warner (2004) observed 11 patients with cancer who also developed evidence for HIT, three of whom required amputations for venous limb gangrene (one case attributable to warfarin treatment). The authors suggested that the risk of thrombotic sequelae—particularly limb ischemia—is especially high when HIT complicates anticoagulation for cancer. The wider availability of assays to detect HIT antibodies should help clinicians better elucidate when HIT plays a pathogenic role in explaining such unusual thrombotic events.

SCORING SYSTEMS FOR HIT
The 4T's
Several scoring systems have been developed to assist clinicians in estimating the pre-test probability of HIT. The most extensively studied of these systems, the 4T's, incorporates four clinical features: magnitude of Thrombocytopenia, Timing of the onset of thrombocytopenia or thrombosis with respect to heparin

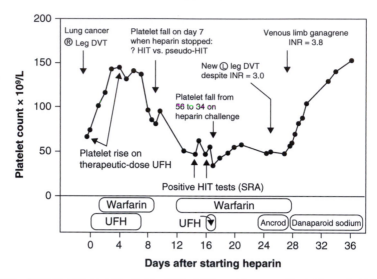

FIGURE 3.9 Pseudo-HIT complicated by HIT: A 78-yr-old man, with right proximal lower-limb DVT and thrombocytopenia, developed progressive platelet count increase during therapeutic-dose UFH treatment. Recurrent thrombocytopenia developed after UFH was stopped and when the patient was anticoagulated with warfarin. A liver biopsy on day 9 showed metastatic adeno-carcinoma (primary lung neoplasm), and adenocarcinoma-associated DIC was diagnosed. However, a heparin challenge produced a further platelet count fall; HIT antibody testing was strongly positive (SRA: 88% serotonin release at 0.1 U/mL heparin; <15% release at 0 and 100 U/mL heparin). Subsequently, the patient developed new left-sided DVT, as well as venous gangrene of the left foot during treatment with warfarin and ancrod (peak INR = 3.8). Although the clinical course was initially identical with pseudo-HIT (rising platelet count on heparin therapy; abrupt platelet count fall after heparin administration was stopped), the subsequent heparin-induced fall in the platelet count, and strong positive HIT test results, indicate the patient also had HIT. *Abbreviations*: DIC, disseminated intravascular coagulation; DVT, deep vein thrombosis; HIT, heparin-induced thrombocytopenia; INR, international normalized ratio; SRA, serotonin release assay; UFH, unfractionated heparin.

exposure, the presence of Thrombosis or other clinical sequelae, and the likelihood of oTher potential causes of thrombocytopenia. Each feature is assigned a score of 0, 1, or 2, yielding a maximum possible summative score of 8. Total scores of 0–3, 4–5, and 6–8 correspond to low, intermediate, and high pre-test probabilities, respectively.

Since its initial description in 2003 (Warkentin and Heddle, 2003), the 4T's has undergone a number of modifications. The latest iteration (Figure 3.10) is currently under prospective study (Warkentin and Linkins, 2010). The performance of a previous version (Lo et al., 2006) has been evaluated in a variety of clinical settings. Table 3.3 shows all published studies of 40 or more patients with suspected HIT in which the 4T's system was compared with a gold standard. Altogether, these studies enrolled almost 3000 patients from eight countries. Although the validity of a pooled analysis is limited by differences in patient population and gold standard, it is informative in several respects. First, the negative predictive value (NPV) of a low probability 4T's score is 0.99 (95% CI, 0.99–1.00), affirming that HIT is essentially

	Score = 2	Score = 1	Score = 0
Thrombocytopenia Compare the highest platelet count within the sequence of declining platelet counts with the lowest count to determine the % of platelet fall. **(Select only 1 option)**	○ >50% Platelet fall AND a nadir of 20 AND no surgery within preceding 3 days	○ >50% Platelet fall BUT surgery within preceding 3 days OR ○ Any combination of platelet fall and nadir that does not fit criteria for Score 2 or Score 0 (e.g., 30–50% platelet fall or nadir 10–19)	○ <30% Platelet fall ○ Any platelet fall with nadir <10
Timing (of platelet count fall or thrombosis)[a] Day 0 = first day of most recent heparin exposure[b] **(Select only 1 option)**	○ Platelet fall day 5–10 after start of heparin ○ Platelet fall within 1 day of start of heparin AND exposure to heparin within past 5–30 days	○ Consistent with platelet fall day 5–10 but not clear (e.g., missing counts) ○ Platelet fall within 1 day of start of heparin AND exposure to heparin in past 31–100 days ○ Platelet fall after day 10	○ Platelet fall ≤ day 4 without exposure to heparin in past 100 days
Thrombosis (or other clinical sequelae) **(Select only 1 option)**	○ Confirmed new thrombosis (venous or arterial) ○ Skin necrosis at injection site(s) ○ Anaphylactoid reaction to iv UFH bolus/sc LMWH ○ Adrenal hemorrhage	○ Recurrent venous thrombosis in a patient receiving therapeutic anticoagulants ○ Suspected thrombosis (awaiting confirmation with imaging) ○ Erythematous skin lesions at heparin injection site(s)	○ Thrombosis not suspected

		Possible other cause is evident:	Probable other cause present:
oTher cause for cthrombocytopenia[c] **(Select only 1 option)**	○ No alternative explanation for platelet fall is evident	○ Sepsis without proven microbial source ○ Thrombocytopenia associated with initiation of ventilator ○ Other:	○ Within 72 hours of surgery ○ Confirmed bacteremia/fungemia ○ Chemotherapy or radiation within past 20 days ○ DIC Due to non-HIT cause ○ Posttransfusion purpura (PTP) ○ Thrombotic thrombocytopenic purpura (TTP) ○ Platelet count < 20 AND given a drug implicated in causing D-ITP (see list) ○ Non-necrotizing skin lesions at LMWH injection sites (presumed DHR) ○ Other:

Drugs implicated in drug-induced immune thrombocytopenic purpura (D-ITP)
Relatively Common: glycoprotein IIb/IIIa antagonists (abciximab, eptifibatide, tirofiban); quinine, quinidine, sulfa antibiotics, carbamazepine, vancomycin
Less Common: actinomycin, amitriptyline, amoxicillin/piperacillin/nafcillin, cephalosporins (cefazolin, ceftazidime, ceftriaxone), celecoxib, ciprofloxacin, esomeprazole, fexofenadine, fentanyl, fucidic acid furosemide, gold salts, levofloxacin, metronidazole, naproxen, oxaliplatin, phenytoin, propranolol, propoxyphene, ranitidine, rifampin, suramin, trimethoprim. Note: this is a partial list.

FIGURE 3.10   4T's scoring system.

[a]In some circumstances, it may be appropriate to judge "Timing" based upon clinical sequelae, such as timing of onset of thrombosis or skin lesions.

[b]The day the platelet count begins to fall is considered the day of onset of thrombocytopenia (it generally takes 1–3 more days until an arbitrary threshold that defines thrombocytopenia is passed). In general, giving heparin during or soon after surgery is most likely to induce immunization.

[c]Usually, "oTher" scores "0 points" if thrombocytopenia is not present. However, it may be appropriate to judge "oTher" based upon clinical sequelae, such as whether heparin-induced skin lesions are necrotizing (2 points, i.e., a non-HIT explanation is unlikely) or non-necrotizing (0 points, i.e., a non-HIT explanation is likely. DIC, disseminated intravascular coagulation; DHR, delayed-type hypersensitivity reaction, iv, intravenous; LMWH, low molecular weight heparin; sc, subcutaneous.

TABLE 3.3 Pooled analysis of studies evaluating the 4T's

Study setting (n)	Study population[a]	Reference	Definition of HIT	High probability (4T's score 6–8) HIT+	HIT-	Intermediate probability (4T's score 4–5) HIT+	HIT-	Low probability (4T's score 0–3) HIT+	HIT-
Canada (100)	Unselected	Lo et al., 2006	Positive SRA	8	0	8	20	1	63
Germany (236)	Unselected	Lo et al., 2006	Positive HIP	9	33	11	128	0	55
France (213)	Unselected	Pouplard et al., 2007	Positive SRA	8	2	14	115	0	74
Australia (246)	Unselected	Bryant et al., 2008	Positive SRA	4	8	5	87	0	142
Belgium (102)	Unselected	Denys et al., 2008	Positive flow cytometric assay	6	3	4	58	0	31
Germany (500)	Unselected	Bakchoul et al., 2009	Positive HIPA	26	28	9	121	0	316
US (104)	Surgical ICU patients	Berry et al., 2011	Positive SRA	6	8	9	23	5	53
Canada (49)	ICU patients	Crowther et al., 2010	Positive SRA	1	0	1	8	0	39
US (50)	Unselected	Cuker et al., 2010	Consensus diagnosis of expert adjudicator panel	2	3	5	21	0	19
Switzerland (1291)	Unselected	Nellen et al., 2011	Positive PAT	39	35	50	308	7	852
Egypt (50)	Unselected	Tawfik et al., 2011	Positive SRA	3	5	2	24	0	16
US (43)	Cardiothoracic surgical patients	Demma et al., 2011	Positive SRA	5	0	6	13	0	19
Total (2984)				117	125	124	926	13	1679

[a]All studies included only patients with suspected HIT.

Abbreviations: SRA, serotonin release assay; HIPA, heparin-induced platelet activation assay; PAT, heparin-induced platelet aggregation test.

excluded by a score ≤3. Second, approximately half of patients with a high probability score have true HIT [positive predictive value (PPV) 0.48, 95% CI 0.42–0.55], whereas most patients with an intermediate probability 4T's score do not (PPV 0.12, 95% CI 0.10–0.14).

The HEP Score

The HIT Expert Probability (HEP) Score is an alternative scoring system for HIT based on the opinions of 26 clinical HIT experts from North America (Cuker et al., 2010). It is comprised of eight clinical features, including magnitude of platelet count fall, timing of platelet count fall, nadir platelet count, thrombosis, skin necrosis, acute systemic reaction, bleeding, and other causes of thrombocytopenia (Table 3.4). Integral weights, ranging from −3 (feature argues strongly against HIT) to +3 (feature argues strongly in favor of HIT), are assigned to each feature and correspond to the median opinions of the 26 experts on which the model is based. In a retrospective single center study, the HEP Score showed good agreement with the serotonin release assay and the consensus diagnosis of an independent panel of expert adjudicators. A cutoff score of ≥5 was associated with a PPV of 0.55 (95% CI 0.25–0.82) and a NPV of 0.97 (95% CI 0.85–1.00), operating characteristics similar to those observed with the 4T's. A retrospective comparison of the HEP Score and 4T's in 47 Thai patients with suspected HIT did not demonstrate a significant difference in performance between the two models (Uaprasert et al., 2011).

Other Scoring Systems

Several other pre-test scoring systems for HIT have been developed, but have not been prospectively evaluated or compared with other models (Lillo-Le Louët et al., 2004; Messmore et al., 2011). One of the systems, the Lillo-Le Louët model, is designed for estimation of the probability of HIT in patients following cardiopulmonary bypass (CPB). The model, which incorporates three variables that were predictive of HIT in a derivation set (a biphasic platelet count profile from CPB to the first day of suspected HIT, an interval of ≥5 days from CPB to the first day of suspected HIT, and a CPB duration of ≤118 minutes), has not been evaluated in an independent validation set (Lillo-Le Louët et al., 2004). In addition to the aforementioned pre-test probability models, several authors have proposed scoring systems that include platelet count recovery after heparin cessation and/or platelet response to heparin rechallenge (Greinacher et al., 1994; Lecompte et al., 1995; Pouplard et al., 1999; Alberio et al., 2003). Because these variables are generally not available to clinicians at the time HIT is initially suspected, these "post-test" models have limited applicability to clinical practice. They have, however, been used as research tools, for instance, in studies evaluating novel laboratory assays or biomarkers for HIT.

Applying Scoring Systems to Individual Patients

Although scoring systems for HIT are intended to standardize clinical diagnosis, the interpretation and scoring of various clinical features may nonetheless prove challenging in the context of an individual patient. For example, both the 4T's and HEP Score require an assessment of the percent fall in platelet count from peak to nadir, but how to define the peak platelet count is not always apparent to providers. We define the peak platelet count as the highest platelet count after initial heparin

TABLE 3.4 HIT Expert Probability Score

Clinical features	Score
1. Magnitude of fall in platelet count	
(Measured from peak platelet count to nadir platelet count since heparin exposure.)	
a. <30%	−1
b. 30–50%	1
c. >50%	3
2. Timing of fall in platelet count	
For patients in whom typical onset HIT is suspected:	
a. Fall begins <4 days after heparin exposure	−2
b. Fall begins 4 days after heparin exposure	2
c. Fall begins 5–10 days after heparin exposure	3
d. Fall begins 11–14 days after heparin exposure	2
e. Fall begins >14 days after heparin exposure	−1
For patients with previous heparin exposure in last 100 days in whom rapid onset HIT is suspected:	
f. Fall begins <48 hr after heparin re-exposure	2
g. Fall begins >48 hr after heparin re-exposure	−1
3. Nadir platelet count	
a. ≤20 × 10⁹/L	−2
b. >20 × 10⁹/L	2
4. Thrombosis (Select no more than one.)	
For patients without a previous heparin exposure in last 100 days:	
a. New VTE or ATE ≥4 days after heparin exposure	3
b. Progression of pre-existing VTE or ATE while receiving heparin	2
For patients with a previous heparin exposure in last 100 days:	
c. New VTE or ATE after heparin exposure	3
d. Progression of pre-existing VTE or ATE while receiving heparin	2
5. Skin necrosis	
a. Skin necrosis at subcutaneous heparin injection sites	3
6. Acute systemic reaction	
a. Acute systemic reaction following intravenous heparin bolus	2
7. Bleeding	
a. Presence of bleeding, petechiae, or extensive bruising	−1
8. Other causes of thrombocytopenia (Select all that apply.)	
a. Presence of a chronic thrombocytopenic disorder	−1
b. Newly initiated nonheparin medication known to cause thrombocytopenia	−2
c. Severe infection	−2
d. Severe DIC (defined as fibrinogen <100 mg/dL and D-dimer >5.0 μg/mL)	−2
e. Indwelling intra-arterial device (e.g. IABP, VAD, ECMO)	−2
f. Cardiopulmonary bypass within previous 96 hr	−1
g. No other apparent cause	3

Abbreviations: ATE, arterial thromboembolism; DIC, disseminated intravascular coagulation; ECMO, extracorporeal membrane oxygenation; IABP, intra-aortic balloon pump; VAD, ventricular assist device; VTE, venous thromboembolism.

exposure rather than the platelet count at the time heparin is initiated. This distinction is particularly important in surgical patients, who commonly experience a postoperative thrombocytosis (Warkentin et al., 2003b). As Figure 3.11 illustrates, use of the platelet count at the time of initiation of heparin, rather than the highest platelet count after heparin exposure, as the peak platelet count may lead to an

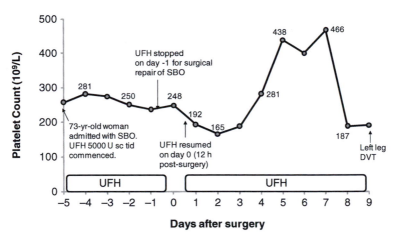

FIGURE 3.11 Typical-onset HIT presenting in the postoperative setting. A 73-yr-old woman was admitted on day −5 with an SBO. She received UFH 5000 U by sc route tid from admission through day −1. Her bowel obstruction did not respond to conservative management and she underwent surgical repair on day 0. UFH was resumed on the evening of day 0, approximately 12 hr after surgery. Her postoperative platelet count initially declined to approximately 33% of the preoperative platelet count, reaching a nadir of 165×10^9/L on day 2. Typical postoperative thrombocytosis followed with the platelet count rising to 466×10^9/L by day 7. On day 8, the platelet count fell abruptly to 187×10^9/L. The following day, the patient developed symptomatic left common femoral vein DVT confirmed by compression ultrasonography. The patient's blood tested strongly positive for HIT antibodies by enzyme immunoassay and SRA. This case illustrates two important points about presentation of HIT in the postoperative setting. First, heparin exposure during or after surgery is more likely to induce HIT antibody formation than preoperative heparin administration. In this example, resumption of UFH on the evening of surgery (day 0) should be considered the most likely immunizing exposure with a characteristic fall in platelet count 8 days later (day 8). Second, in assessing the likelihood of HIT, the percent fall in platelet count should be measured from the peak platelet count after initiation of heparin (466×10^9/L) to the nadir platelet count (187×10^9/L), corresponding to a 60% fall in this case. If fall in platelet count is calculated from the platelet count at the time of initiation of heparin after surgery (248×10^9/L) rather than from the peak platelet count, the magnitude of platelet count fall will be underestimated at 25% and mistakenly interpreted to be inconsistent with HIT, which is typically associated with a platelet count fall > 50%. *Abbreviations*: DVT, deep vein thrombosis; HIT, heparin-induced thrombocytopenia; INR, international normalized ratio; PE, pulmonary embolism; SBO, small bowel obstruction; sc, subcutaneous; SRA, serotonin release assay; tid, three times a day; UFH, unfractionated heparin.

underestimation of the percent fall in platelet count and, more importantly, an underestimation of the pre-test probability of HIT.

Similarly, evaluation of the timing of onset of thrombocytopenia relative to heparin exposure requires careful consideration of the date of the initial *immunizing* heparin exposure (i.e., day 0), a determination that is often challenging in patients with a previous recent heparin exposure. For example, many patients undergoing cardiac surgery have received heparin for coronary angiography within the previous 100 days. Are these patients therefore at risk for rapid-onset HIT immediately after surgery, or are they more susceptible to the development of typical-onset HIT 5–10 days after their operation? In our experience, preoperative heparin exposure during catheterization is rarely of clinical importance and typical-onset HIT in this population is more likely. We therefore perform our initial score with the heparin exposure we judge most likely to induce antibody formation as day 0 (generally the intraoperative heparin exposure for cardiac and vascular surgery, and the first post-operative dose of thromboprophylaxis for noncardiovascular surgeries) (Fig. 3.11), and calculate secondary scores with other heparin exposures as warranted by the clinical scenario.

A third component of scoring models, which appears to be highly subject to personal interpretation, is the likelihood of other causes of thrombocytopenia. Alternative causes of hospital-acquired thrombocytopenia, such as infection, medications other than heparin, hemodilution, and intravascular appliances (e.g., intra-aortic balloon pumps, ventricular assist devices, extracorporeal circuits) are common in patients with suspected HIT. Clinicians differ substantially in their estimation of the contribution of these etiologies to thrombocytopenia in individual patients (Cuker et al., 2010; Strutt et al., 2011).

In view of the challenges and subjectivity inherent in applying scoring systems to individual patients, it is not surprising that existing models exhibit substantial interobserver variability (Strutt et al., 2011; Nagler et al., 2012). Newer models include more detailed and explicit itemization of clinical features in an attempt to clarify their meaning and enhance reproducibility among raters (Cuker et al., 2010; Warkentin and Linkins, 2010).

Scoring Systems as Clinical Decision Rules
A clinical decision rule (CDR) is a clinical tool that quantifies the individual contributions that various components of the history, physical examination, and basic laboratory and imaging results make toward the diagnosis of an individual patient. According to McGinn et al. in their contribution to the seminal *User's Guides to the Medical Literature*, CDRs are most likely to be useful in situations where decision making is complex, the clinical stakes are high, and there are opportunities to achieve cost savings without compromising patient care (McGinn et al., 2000). This description would seem to fit the evaluation of patients with suspected HIT to a tee: clinical diagnosis is complex and requires synthesis of a number of clinical features (Fig. 3.10 and Table 3.4), the consequences of missing a case of HIT may be catastrophic, and the costs of unnecessarily exposing thrombocytopenic patients without HIT to expensive alternative anticogulants and their attendant bleeding risk are substantial. Not surprisingly then, current work is focused on evaluating the utility of pre-test scoring systems for HIT as CDRs. Indeed, one series suggested that management guided by the HEP Score was associated with the potential to safely reduce the number of patients receiving a direct thrombin inhibitor by 41% (Cuker et al., 2010). Proper validation will require prospective comparison of scoring systems with standard gestalt-driven clinical diagnosis and formal analysis of the impact of model-guided diagnosis and management on clinical behavior and outcomes (McGinn et al., 2000).

REFERENCES
Abrams CS, Cines DB. Platelet glycoprotein IIb/IIIa inhibitors and thrombocytopenia: possible link between platelet activation, autoimmunity and thrombosis. Thromb Haemost 88: 888–889, 2002.

Adamson DJA, Currie JM. Occult malignancy is associated with venous thrombosis unresponsive to adequate anticoagulation. Br J Clin Pract 47: 190–191, 1993.

Aird WC. The role of the endothelium in severe sepsis and the multiple organ dysfunction syndrome. Blood 101: 3765–3777, 2003a.

Aird WC. The hematologic system as a marker of organ dysfunction in sepsis. Mayo Clin Proc 78: 869–881, 2003b.

Alberio L, Limmerle S, Baumann A, Taleghani BM, Biasiutti FD, Lämmle B. Rapid determination of anti-heparin/platelet factor 4 antibody titers in the diagnosis of heparin-induced thrombocytopenia. Am J Med 114: 528–536, 2003.

Almehmi A, Malas A, Juhelirer SJ. Thrombotic thrombocytopenic purpura following cardiovascular surgery: a case report. W V Med J 69: 84–86, 2004.

Araújo F, Sá JJ, Araújo V, Lopes M, Cunha-Ribeiro LM. Post-transfusion purpura vs. heparin-induced thrombocytopenia: differential diagnosis in clinical practice. Transfus Med 10: 323–324, 2000.

Arnold DM, Smaill F, Warkentin TE, Christjanson L, Walker I. Cardiobacterium hominis endocarditis associated with very severe thrombocytopenia and platelet autoantibodies. Am J Hematol 76: 373–377, 2004.

Arnout J. The pathogenesis of the antiphospholipid antibody syndrome: a hypothesis based on parallelisms with heparin-induced thrombocytopenia. Thromb Haemost 75: 536–541, 1996.

Arnout J. The role of β_2–glycoprotein I-dependent lupus anticoagulants in the pathogenesis of the antiphospholipid syndrome. Verh K Acad Geneeskd Belg 62: 353–372, 2000.

Arnout J, Vermylen J. Current status and implications of autoimmune antiphospholipid antibodies in relation to thrombotic disease. J Thromb Haemost 1: 931–942, 2003.

Arvieux J, Roussel B, Pouzol P, Colomb MG. Platelet activating properties of murine monoclonal antibodies to β_2–glycoprotein I. Thromb Haemost 70: 336–341, 1993.

Asherson RA, Khamashta MA, Ordi-Ros J, Derksen RH, Machin SJ, Barquinero J, Outt HH, Harris EN, Vilardell-Torres M, Hughes GR. The "primary" antiphospholipid syndrome: major clinical and serological features. Medicine 68: 366–374, 1989.

Aster RH, Curtis BR, Bougie DW, Dunkley S, Greinacher A, Warkentin TE, Chong BH. Thrombocytopenia associated with the use of GPIIb/IIIa inhibitors: position paper of the ISTH working group on thrombocytopenia and GPIIb/IIIa inhibitors. J Thromb Haemost 4: 678–679, 2006.

Auger WR, Permpikul P, Moser KM. Lupus anticoagulant, heparin use, and thrombocytopenia in patients with chronic thromboembolic pulmonary hypertension: a preliminary report. Am J Med 99: 392–396, 1995.

Awad WI, Coumbe A, Walesby RK. Venous gangrene of the lower limbs following aortic valve replacement for native valve endocarditis. Eur J Cardiothorac Surg 14: 440–442, 1998.

Bakchoul T, Giptner A, Najaoui A, Bein G, Santoso S, Sachs UJH. Prospective evaluation of PF4/heparin immunoassays for the diagnosis of heparin-induced thrombocytopenia. J Thromb Haemost 7: 1260–1265, 2009.

Balduini CL, Noris P, Bertolino G, Previtali M. Heparin modifies platelet count and function in patients who have undergone thrombolytic therapy for acute myocardial infarction. Thromb Haemost 69: 522–532, 1993.

Benke S, Moltzan C. Co-existence of heparin-induced thrombocytopenia and thrombotic thrombocytopenic purpura in a postoperative cardiac surgery patient. Am J Hematol 80: 288–291, 2005.

Bernard GR, Vincent JL, Laterre PF, LaRosa SP, Dhainaut JF, Lopez-Rodriguez A, Steingrub JS, Garber GE, Helterbrand JD, Ely EW, Fisher JC Jr. Efficacy and safety of recombinant human activated protein C for severe sepsis. N Engl J Med 344: 699–709, 2001.

Berry C, Tcherniantchouk O, Ley EJ, Salim A, Mirocha J, Martin-Stone S, Stolpner D, Margulies DR. Overdiagnosis of heparin-induced thrombocytopenia in surgical ICU patients. J Am Coll Surg 213: 10–18, 2011.

Bone RC, Francis PB, Pierce AK. Intravascular coagulation associated with the adult respiratory distress syndrome. Am J Med 61: 585–589, 1976.

Bougie DW, Wilker PR, Wuitschick ED, Curtis BR, Malik M, Levine S, Lind RN, Pereira J, Aster RH. Acute thrombocytopenia after treatment with tirofiban or eptifibatide is associated with antibodies specific for ligand-occupied GPIIb/IIIa. Blood 100: 2071–2076, 2002.

Bourhim M, Darnige L, Legallais C, Arvieux J, Cevallos R, Pouplard C, Vigayalakshmi MA. Anti-β_2-glycoprotein I antibodies recognizing platelet factor 4-heparin complex in antiphospholipid syndrome in patient substantiated with mouse model. J Mol Recognit 16: 125–130, 2003.

Bryant A, Low J, Austin S, Joseph JE. Timely diagnosis and management of heparin-induced thrombocytopenia in a frequent request, low incidence single centre using clinical 4T's score and particle gel immunoassay. Br J Haematol 143: 721–726, 2008.

Campbell RR, Foster KJ, Stirling C, Mundy D, Reckless JPD. Paradoxical platelet behaviour in diabetic ketoacidosis. Diabet Med 3: 161–164, 1985.

Casteels K, Beckers D, Wouters C, Van Geet C. Rhabdomyolysis in diabetic ketoacidosis. Pediatr Diabetes 4: 29–31, 2003.

Chang JC, Ikhlaque N. Peripheral digit ischemic syndrome can be a manifestation of postoperative thrombotic thrombocytopenic purpura. Ther Apher Dial 8: 413–418, 2004.

Chang JC, Shipstone A, Llenado MA. Postoperative thrombotic thrombocytopenic purpura following cardiovascular surgeries. Am J Hematol 53: 11–17, 1996.

Chang JC, El-Tarabily M, Gupta S. Acute thrombotic thrombocytopenic purpura following abdominal surgeries: a report of three cases. J Clin Apher 15: 176–179, 2000.

Chang IH, Ha MS, Chi BH, Kown YW, Lee SJ. Warfarin-induced penile necrosis in a patient with heparin-induced thrombocytopenia. J Korean Med Sci 25: 1390–1393, 2010.

Chiu HM, van Aken WG, Hirsh J, Regoeczi E, Horner AA. Increased heparin clearance in experimental pulmonary embolism. J Lab Clin Med 90: 204–215, 1977.

Crowther MA, Cook DJ, Albert M, Williamson D, Meade M, Granton J, Skrobik Y, Langevin S, Mehta S, Hebert P, Guyatt GH, Geerts W, Rabbat C, Douketis J, Zytaruk N, Sheppard J, Greinacher A, Warkentin TE. For the Canadian Critical Care Trials Group. the 4Ts scoring system for heparin-induced thrombocytopenia in medical-surgical intensive care unit patients. J Crit Care 25: 287–293, 2010.

Cuker A, Arepally G, Crowther MA, Rice L, Datko F, Hook K, Propert KJ, Kuter DJ, Ortel TL, Konkle BA, Cines DB. The HIT Expert Probability (HEP) Score: a novel pre-test probability model for heparin-induced thrombocytopenia based on broad expert opinion. J Thromb Haemost 8: 2642–2650, 2010.

Curtis BR, Swyers J, Divgi A, McFarland JG, Aster RH. Thrombocytopenia after second exposure to abciximab is caused by antibodies that recognize abciximab-coated platelets. Blood 99: 2054–2059, 2002.

Curtis BR, Divgi A, Garritty M, Aster RH. Delayed thrombocytopenia after treatment with abciximab: a distinct clinical entity associated with the immune response to the drug. J Thromb Haemost 2: 985–992, 2004.

De Gennes C, Souilhem J, Du LTH, Chapelon C, Raguin G, Wechsler B, Bletry O, Godeau P. Embolie arterielle des membres au cours des endocardites infectieuses sur valves natives. Presse Med 19: 1177–1181, 1990.

Delahaye JP, Poncet P, Malquarti V, Beaune J, Gare JP, Mann JM. Cerebrovascular accidents in infective endocarditis: role of anticoagulation. Eur Heart J 1: 1074–1078, 1990.

Demma LJ, Winkler AM, Levy JH. A diagnosis of heparin-induced thrombocytopenia with combined clinical and laboratory methods in cardiothoracic surgical intensive care unit patients. Anesth Analg 113: 697–702, 2011.

Denys B, Stove V, Philippé J, Devreese K. A clinical-laboratory approach contributing to a rapid and reliable diagnosis of heparin-induced thrombocytopenia. Thromb Res 123: 137–145, 2008.

Dunkley S, Lindeman R, Evans S, Casten R, Jepson N. Evidence of platelet activation due to tirofiban-dependent platelet antibodies: double trouble. J Thromb Haemost 1: 2248–2250, 2003.

Eikelboom JW, Anand SS, Mehta SR, Weitz JI, Yi C, Yusuf S. Prognostic significance of thrombocytopenia during hirudin and heparin therapy in acute coronary syndrome without ST elevation. organization to assess strategies for ischemic syndromes (OASIS-2) study. Circulation 103: 643–650, 2001.

Everett RN, Jones FL Jr. Warfarin-induced skin necrosis. A cutaneous sign of malignancy? Postgrad Med 79: 97–103, 1986.

Fijnvandraat K, Derkx B, Peters M, Bijlmer R, Sturk A, Prins MH, van Deventer SJH, ten Cate JW. Coagulation activation and tissue necrosis in meningococcal septic shock: severely reduced protein C levels predict a high mortality. Thromb Haemost 73: 15–20, 1995.

Ford I, Urbaniak S, Greaves M. IgG from patients with antiphospholipid syndrome binds to platelets without induction of platelet activation. Br J Haematol 102: 841–849, 1998.

Galli M. Non β_2–glycoprotein I cofactors for antiphospholipid antibodies. Lupus 5: 388–392, 1996.

Galli M, Daldossi M, Barbui T. Anti-glycoprotein Ib/IX and IIb/IIIa antibodies in patients with antiphospholipid antibodies. Thromb Haemost 71: 571–575, 1994.

Galli M, Finazzi G, Barbui T. Thrombocytopenia in the antiphospholipid syndrome. Br J Haematol 93: 1–5, 1996.

Galli M, Luciani D, Bertolini G, Barbui T. Lupus anticoagulants are stronger risk factors for thrombosis than anticardiolipin antibodies in the antiphospholipid syndrome: a systematic review of the literature. Blood 101: 1827–1832, 2003.

Gao C, Boylan B, Bougie D, Gill JC, Birenbaum J, Newman DK, Aster RH, Newman PJ. Eptifibatide-induced thrombocytopenia and thrombosis in humans require $Fc\gamma RIIa$ and the integrin $\beta 3$ cytoplasmic domain. J Clin Invest 119: 504–511, 2009.

Gibson GE, Su WP, Pittelkow MR. Antiphospholipid syndrome and the skin. J Am Acad Dermatol 36:970–982, 1997.

Ginsberg JS, Wells PS, Brill-Edwards P, Donovan D, Moffatt K, Johnston M, Stevens P, Hirsh J. Antiphospholipid antibodies and venous thromboembolism. Blood 86: 3685–3691, 1995.

Greinacher A. Antigen generation in heparin-associated thrombocytopenia: the non-immunologic type and the immunologic type are closely linked in their pathogenesis. Semin Thromb Hemost 21: 106–116, 1995.

Greinacher A, Selleng K. Thrombocytopenia in the intensive care unit patient. Hematology Am Soc Hematol Educ Program 2010: 135–143, 2010.

Greinacher A, Warkentin TE. Acquired non-immune thrombocytopenia. In: Marder VJ, Aird WC, Bennett JS, Schulman S, White GC, eds. Hemostasis and Thrombosis: Basic Principles and Clinical Practice, 6th edn. Philadelphia: Lippincott Williams & Wilkins, 2013; in press.

Greinacher A, Amiral J, Dummel V, Vissac A, Kiefel V, Mueller-Eckhardt C. Laboratory diagnosis of heparin-associated thrombocytopenia and comparison of platelet aggregation test, heparin-induced platelet activation test, and platelet factor 4/heparin enzyme-linked immunosorbent assay. Transfusion 34: 381–385, 1994.

Greinacher A, Friesecke S, Abel P, Dressel A, Stracke S, Fiene M, Ernst F, Selleng K, Weissenborn K, Schmidt BM, Schiffer M, Felix SB, Lerch MM, Kielstein JT, Mayerle J. Treatment of severe neurological deficits with IgG depletion through immunoadsorption in patients with Escherichia coli O104:H4-associated haemolytic uremic syndrome: a prospective trial. Lancet 378: 1166–1173, 2011.

Gruel Y. Antiphospholipid syndrome and heparin-induced thrombocytopenia: update on similarities and differences. J Autoimmun 15: 265–268, 2000.

Gunn SK, Farolino D, McDonald AA. A case of warfarin-associated venous limb gangrene: implications of anticoagulation in a palliative care setting. J Palliat Med 12: 269–272, 2009.

Hayes MA, Yau EH, Hinds CJ, Watson JD. Symmetrical peripheral gangrene: association with noradrenaline administration. Intensive Care Med 18: 433–436, 1992.

Hojnik M, George J, Ziporen L, Shoenfeld Y. Heart valve involvement (Libman-Sacks endocarditis) in the antiphospholipid syndrome. Circulation 93: 1579–1587, 1996.

Iosifidis MI, Ntavlis M, Giannoulis I, Malioufas L, Ioannou A, Giantsis G. Acute thrombotic thrombocytopenic purpura following orthopedic surgery: a case report. Arch Orthop Trauma Surg 126: 335–338, 2006.

Jankowski M, Vreys I, Wittevrongel C, Boon D, Vermylen J, Hoylaerts MF, Arnout J. Thrombogenicity of β_2–glycoprotein I dependent antiphospholipid antibodies in a photochemically induced thrombosis model in the hamster. Blood 101: 157–162, 2003.

Johansen K, Hansen ST Jr. Symmetrical peripheral gangrene (purpura fulminans) complicating pneumococcal sepsis. Am J Surg 165: 642–655, 1993.

Kitchens CS. Thrombocytopenia due to acute venous thromboembolism and its role in expanding the differential diagnosis of heparin-induced thrombocytopenia. Am J Hematol 76: 69–73, 2004.

Klein L, Galvez A, Klein O, Chediak J. Warfarin-induced limb gangrene in the setting of lung adenocarcinoma. Am J Hematol 76: 176–179, 2004.

Knight TT Jr, Gordon SV, Canady J, Rush DS, Browder W. Symmetrical peripheral gangrene: a new presentation of an old disease. Am Surg 66: 196–199, 2000.

Kullberg BJ, Westendorp RGJ, van't Wout JW, Meinders AE. Purpura fulminans and symmetrical peripheral gangrene caused by capnocytophaga canimorsus (formerly DF-2) septicemia—a complication of dog bite. Medicine (Balt) 70: 287–292, 1991.

Lasne D, Saffroy R, Bachelot C, Vincenot A, Rendu F, Papo T, Aiach M, Piette JC. Tests for heparin-induced thrombocytopenia in primary antiphospholipid syndrome. Br J Haematol 97. 939, 1997.

Lebrazi J, Helft G, Abdelouahed M, Elalamy I, Mirshahi M, Samama MM, Lecompte T. Human anti-streptokinase antibodies induce platelet aggregation in an Fc receptor (CD32) dependent manner. Thromb Haemost 74: 938–942, 1995.

Lecompte T, Stieltjes N, Shao-Kai L, Morel MC, Kaplan C, Samama MM. Heparin- and streptokinase-dependent platelet-activating immunoglobulin G : mechanism and diagnosis. Semin Thromb Hemost 21: 95–105, 1995.

Lee AY, Levine MN, Baker RI, Bowden C, Kakkar AK, Prins M, Rickle FR, Julian JA, Haley S, Kovacs MJ, Gent M. Low molecular weight heparin versus a coumarin for the prevention of recurrent venous thromboembolism in patients with cancer. N Engl J Med 349: 109–111, 2003.

Lee DW, Seo JW, Cho HS, Kang Y, Kim HJ, Chang SH, Park DJ. Two cases of postoperative thrombotic thrombocytopenic purpura. Ther Apher Dial 15: 594–597, 2011.

Leitner JM, Jilma B, Spiel AO, Sterz F, Laggner AN, Janata KM. Massive pulmonary embolism leading to cardiac arrest is associated with consumptive coagulopathy presenting as disseminated intravascular coagulation. J Thromb Haemost 8: 1477–1482, 2010.

Lillo-Le Louët A, Boutouyrie P, Alhenc-Gelas M, Le Beller C, Gautier I, Aiach M, Lasne D. Diagnostic score for heparin-induced thrombocytopenia after cardiopulmonary bypass. J Thromb Haemost 2: 1882–1888, 2004.

Lipp E, von Felten A, Sax H, Miiller D, Berchtold P. Antibodies against platelet glycoproteins and antiphospholipid antibodies in autoimmune thrombocytopenia. Eur J Haematol 60: 283–288, 1998.

Lo GK, Juhl D, Warkentin TE, Sigouin CS, Eichler P, Greinacher A. Evaluation of pretest clinical score (4 T's) for the diagnosis of heparin-induced thrombocytopenia in two clinical settings. J Thromb Haemost 4: 759–765, 2006.

Lubenow N, Eichler P, Albrecht D, Carlsson LE, Kothmann J, Rossocha W, Hahn M, Quitmann H, Greinacher A. Very low platelet counts in post-transfusion purpura falsely diagnosed as heparin-induced thrombocytopenia. Report of four cases and review of literature. Thromb Res 100: 115–125, 2000.

Lubenow N, Kempf R, Eichner A, Eichler P, Carlsson LE, Greinacher A. Heparin-induced thrombocytopenia: temporal pattern of thrombocytopenia in relation to initial use or reexposure to heparin. Chest 122: 37–42, 2002.

Lutters BC, Meijers JC, Derksen RH, Arnout J, de Groot PG. Dimers of β_2–glycoprotein I mimic the in vitro effects of β_2–glycoprotein I-anti-β_2–glycoprotein I antibody complexes. J Biol Chem 276: 3060–3067, 2001.

Martinuzzo ME, Maclouf J, Carreras LO, Levy-Toledano S. Antiphospholipid antibodies enhance thrombin-induced platelet activation and thromboxane formation. Thromb Haemost 70: 667–671, 1993.

Martinuzzo ME, Forastiero RR, Adamczuk Y, Pombo G, Carreras LO. Antiplatelet factor 4-Heparin antibodies in patients with antiphospholipid antibodies. Thromb Res 95: 271–279, 1999.

McGinn TG, Guyatt GH, Wyer PC, Naylor CD, Stiell IG, Richardson WS. Users' guide to the medical literature: XXII: how to use articles about clinical decision rules. Evidence-Based Medicine Working Group. JAMA 284: 79–84, 2000.

Messmore HL, Fabbrini N, Bird ML, Choudhury AM, Cerejo M, Prechel M, Jeske WP, Siddiqui A, Thethi I, Wehrmacher WH, Walenga JM. Simple scoring system for early management of heparin-induced thrombocytopenia. Clin Appl Thromb Hemost 17: 197–201, 2011.

Monreal M, Lafoz E, Casals A, Ruiz J, Arias A. Platelet count and venous thromboembolism. A useful test for suspected pulmonary embolism. Chest 100: 1493–1496, 1991.

Morgan M, Downs K, Chesterman CN, Biggs JC. Clinical analysis of 125 patients with the lupus anticoagulant. Aust NZ J Med 23: 151–156, 1993.

Morris TA, Marsh JJ, Chiles PG, Pedersen CA, Konopka RG, Gamst AC, Loza O. Embolization itself stimulates thrombus propagation in pulmonary embolism. Am J Physiol Heart Circ Physiol 287: H818–H822, 2004.

Mustafa MH, Mispireta LA, Pierce LE. Occult pulmonary embolism presenting with thrombocytopenia and elevated fibrin split products. Am J Med 86: 490–491, 1989.

Mueller-Eckhardt C. Post-transfusion purpura. Br J Haematol 64: 419–424, 1986.

Nagler M, Fabbro T, Wuillemin WA. Prospective evaluation of the interobserver reliability of the 4Ts score in patients with suspected heparin-induced thrombosytopenia. J Thromb Haemost 10: 151–152, 2012.

Naqvi TA, Baumann MA, Chang JC. Post-operative thrombotic thrombocytopenic purpura: a review. Int J Clin Pract 58: 169–172, 2004.

Nellen V, Sulzer I, Barizzi G, Lämmle B, Alberio L. Rapid exclusion or confirmation of heparin-induced thrombocytopenia: a single-center experience with 1,291 patients. Haematologica 97: 89–97, 2012.

Ng HJ, Crowther MA. Malignancy-associated venous thrombosis with concurrent warfarin-induced skin necrosis, venous limb gangrene and thrombotic microangiopathy. Thromb Haemost 95: 1038–1039, 2006.

Opatrny L, Warner MN. Risk of thrombosis in patients with malignancy and heparin-induced thrombocytopenia. Am J Hematol 76: 240–244, 2004.

Owings JT, Bagley M, Gosselin R, Romac D, Disbrow E. Effect of critical injury on plasma antithrombin activity: low antithrombin levels are associated with thromboembolic complications. J Trauma 41: 396–405, 1996.

Paton RC. Haemostatic changes in diabetic coma. Diabetologia 21: 172–177, 1981.

Pauzner R, Greinacher A, Selleng K, Althaus K, Shenkman B, Seligsohn U. False-positive tests for heparin-induced thrombocytopenia in patients with antiphospholipid syndrome and systemic lupus erythematosus. J Thromb Haemost 7: 1070–1074, 2009.

Pavlovsky M, Weinstein R. Thrombotic thrombocytopenic purpura following coronary artery bypass graft surgery: prospective observations of an emerging syndrome. J Clin Apher 12: 159–164, 1997.

Perunicic J, Antonijevic NM, Miljic P, Djordjevic V, Mikovic D, Kovac M, Djokic M, Mrdovic I, Nikolic A, Vasiljevic Z. Clinical challenge: heparin-induced thrombocytopenia type II (HIT II) or pseudo-HIT in a patient with antiphospholipid syndrome. J Thromb Thrombolysis 26: 142–146, 2008.

Petri M. Pathogenesis and treatment of the antiphospholipid antibody syndrome. Adv Rheumatol 81: 151–177, 1997.

Phillips DE, Payne DK, Mills GM. Heparin-induced thrombotic thrombocytopenia. Ann Pharmacother 28: 43–46, 1994.

Pouplard C, Amiral J, Borg JY, Laporte-Simitsidis S, Delahousse B, Gruel Y. Decision analysis for use of platelet aggregation test, carbon 14-serotonin release assay, and heparin-platelet factor 4 enzyme-linked immunosorbent assay for diagnosis of heparin-induced thrombocytopenia. Am J Clin Pathol 111: 700–706, 1999.

Pouplard C, Gueret P, Fouassier M, Ternisien C, Trossaert M, Régina S, Gruel Y. Prospective evaluation of the '4Ts' score and particle gel immunoassay specific to heparin/PF4 for the diagnosis of heparin-induced thrombocytopenia. J Thromb Haemost 5: 1373–1379, 2007.

Prandoni P. Antithrombotic strategies in patients with cancer. Thromb Haemost 78: 141–144, 1997.

Pu JJ, Brodksy RA. Paroxysmal nocturnal hemoglobinuria from bench to bedside. Clin Transl Sci 4: 219–224, 2011.

Regnault V, Helft G, Wahl D, Czitrom D, Vuillemenot A, Papouin G, Roda L, Danchin N, Lecompte T. Antistreptokinase platelet-activating antibodies are common and heterogeneous. J Thromb Haemost 1: 1055–1061, 2003.

Rinaldo JE, Perez H. Ischemic necrosis of both lower extremities as a result of the microembolism syndrome complicating the adult respiratory distress syndrome caused by Escherichia coli pneumonia and septicemia. Am Rev Respir Dis 126: 932–935, 1982.

Robson MO, Abbs IC. Thrombotic thrombocytopenic purpura following hemicolectomy for colonic carcinoma. Nephrol Dial Transplant 12: 198–199, 1997.

Sane DC, Damaraju LV, Topol EJ, Cabot CF, Mascelli MA, Harrington RA, Simoons ML, Califf RM. Occurrence and clinical significance of pseudothrombocytopenia during abciximab therapy. J Am Coll Cardiol 36: 75–83, 2000.

Selleng K, Warkentin TE, Greinacher A, Morris AM, Walker IR, Heggtveit HA, Eichler P, Cybulsky IJ. Very severe thrombocytopenia and fragmentation hemolysis mimicking thrombotic thrombocytopenic purpura associated with a giant intracardiac vegetation infected with Staphylococcus epidermidis: role of monocyte procoagulant activity induced by bacterial supernatant. Am J Hematol 82: 766–771, 2007.

Shi W, Chong BH, Chesterman CN. β_2–Glycoprotein I is a requirement for anti-cardiolipin antibodies binding to activated platelets: differences with lupus anticoagulants. Blood 81: 1255–1262, 1993.

Shtalrid M, Shvidel L, Vorst E, Weinmann EE, Berrebi A, Sigler E. Post-transfusion purpura: a challenging diagnosis. IMAJ 8: 672–674, 2006.

Siegal DM, Cook RJ, Warkentin TE. Acute hepatic necrosis and ischemic limb necrosis. N Engl J Med 2012; in press.

Smith OP, White B. Infectious purpura fulminans: diagnosis and treatment. Br J Haematol 104: 202–207, 1999.

Stahl RL, Javid JP, Lackner H. Unrecognized pulmonary embolism presenting as disseminated intravascular coagulation. Am J Med 76: 772–778, 1984.

Strutt JK, Mackey JE, Johnson SM, Sylvia LM. Assessment of the 4Ts pretest clinical scoring system as a predictor of heparin-induced thrombocytopenia. Pharmacotherapy 31: 138–145, 2011.

Sudic D, Razmara M, Forslund M, Ji Q, Hjemdahl P, Li N. High glucose levels enhance platelet activation: involvement of multiple mechanisms. Br J Haematol 133: 315–322, 2006.

Tawfik NM, Hegazy MA, Hassan EA, Ramadan YK, Nasr AS. Egyptian experience of reliability of 4T's score in diagnosis of heparin induced thrombocytopenia syndrome. Blood Coagul Fibrinolysis 22: 701–705, 2011.

Ting W, Silverman NA, Arzouman DA, Levitsky S. Splenic septic emboli in endocarditis. Circulation 82(5 Suppl): IV105–IV109, 1990.

Triplett DA. Lupus anticoagulants/antiphospholipid-protein antibodies: the great imposters. Lupus 5: 431–435, 1996.

Uaprasert N, Rojnuckarin P, Akkawat B. Comparison of diagnostic performance of heparin expert probability (HEP) and 4'Ts score in screening for heparin-induced thrombocytopenia (HIT) [abstr]. J Thromb Haemost 9(2 Suppl): 81, 2011.

Vaughan DE, Kirshenbaum JM, Loscalzo J. Streptokinase-induced, antibody-mediated platelet aggregation: a potential cause of clot propagation in vivo. J Am Coll Cardiol 11: 1343–1348, 1988.

Vermylen J, Hoylaerts MF, Arnout J. Antibody-mediated thrombosis. Thromb Haemost 78: 420–426, 1997.

Wang B, Nichol JL, Sullivan JT. Pharmacodynamics and pharmacokinetics of AMG 531, a novel thrombopoietin receptor ligand. Clin Pharmacol Ther 76: 628–638, 2004.

Warkentin TE. Heparin-induced thrombocytopenia: IgG-mediated platelet activation platelet microparticle generation, and altered procoagulant/anticoagulant balance in the pathogenesis of thrombosis and venous limb gangrene complicating heparin-induced thrombocytopenia. Transfusion Med Rev 10: 249–258, 1996.

Warkentin TE. Venous thromboembolism in heparin-induced thrombocytopenia. Curr Opin Pulm Med 6: 343–351, 2000.

Warkentin TE. Venous limb gangrene during warfarin treatment of cancer-associated deep venous thrombosis. Ann Intern Med 135: 589–593, 2001.

Warkentin TE. Drug-induced, immune-mediated thrombocytopenia—from purpura to thrombosis. N Engl J Med 356: 891–893, 2007.

Warkentin TE. Heparin-induced thrombocytopenia in critically ill patients. Crit Care Clin 27: 805–823, 2011.

Warkentin TE, Greinacher A. Heparin-induced thrombocytopenia and cardiac surgery. Ann Thorac Surg 76: 2121–2131, 2003.

Warkentin TE, Heddle NM. Laboratory diagnosis of immune heparin-induced thrombocytopenia. Curr Hematol Rep 2: 148–157, 2003.

Warkentin TE, Kelton JG. Interaction of heparin with platelets, including heparin-induced thrombocytopenia. In: Bounameaux H, ed. Low Molecular Weight Heparins in Prophylaxis and Therapy of Thromboembolic Diseases. New York: Marcel Dekker, 75–127, 1994.

Warkentin TE, Kelton JG. Temporal aspects of heparin-induced thrombocytopenia. N Engl J Med 344: 1286–1992, 2001.

Warkentin TE, Linkins LA. Non-necrotizing heparin-induced skin lesions and the 4T's score. J Thromb Haemost 8: 1483–1485, 2010.

Warkentin TE, Levine MN, Hirsh J, Horsewood P, Roberts RS, Gent M, Kelton JG. Heparin-induced thrombocytopenia in patients treated with low molecular weight heparin or unfractionated heparin. N Engl J Med 332: 1330–1335, 1995.

Warkentin TE, Elavathil LJ, Hayward CPM, Johnston MA, Russett JI, Kelton JG. The pathogenesis of venous limb gangrene associated with heparin-induced thrombocytopenia. Ann Intern Med 127: 804–812, 1997.

Warkentin TE, Sheppard JI, Horsewood P, Simpson PJ, Moore JC, Kelton JG. Impact of the patient population on the risk for heparin-induced thrombocytopenia. Blood 96: 1703–1708, 2000.

Warkentin TE, Aird AC, Rand J. Platelet-endothelial interactions: sepsis, HIT, and antiphospholipid syndrome. Hematology (Am Soc Hematol Educ Program) 497–519, 2003a.

Warkentin TE, Roberts RS, Hirsh J, Kelton JG. An improved definition of immune heparin-induced thrombocytopenia in postoperative orthopedic patients. Arch Intern Med 163: 2518–2524, 2003b.

Warkentin TE, Makris M, Jay RM, Kelton JG. A spontaneous prothrombotic disorder resembling heparin-induced thrombocyctopenia. Am J Med 121: 632–636, 2008.

Warkentin TE, Greinacher A, Gruel Y, Aster RH, Chong BH. On behalf of the scientific and standardization committee of the International Society on thrombosis and haemostasis. laboratory testing for heparin-induced thrombocytopenia: a conceptual framework and implications for diagnosis. J Thromb Haemost 9: 2498–2500, 2011.

Warkentin TE, Sarode R, Johnston MA, Crowther MA. The pathogenesis of warfarin-associated venous limb ischemia and gangrene complicating cancer: clinical and laboratory parallels with heparin-induced thrombocytopenia (HIT) [abstr]. Thromb Res 129(Suppl 1): S159–S160, 2012.

Weitz JI, Hudoba M, Massel D, Maraganore J, Hirsh J. Clot-bound thrombin is protected from inhibition by heparin-antithrombin III but is susceptible to inactivation by antithrombin Ill-independent inhibitors. J Clin Invest 86: 385–391, 1990.

Weitz JI, Leslie B, Hudoba M. Thrombin binds to soluble fibrin degradation products where it is protected from inhibition by heparin-antithrombin but susceptible to inactivation by antithrombin-independent inhibitors. Circulation 97: 544–552, 1998.

Welch WH. The structure of white thrombi. Trans Pathol Soc Philadelphia 13: 25–43, 1887.

White B, Livingstone W, Murphy C, Hodgson A, Fafferty M, Smith OP. An open-label study of the role of adjuvant hemostatic support with protein C replacement therapy in purpura fulminans-associated meningococcemia. Blood 96: 3719–3724, 2000.

White CA, Chung DA, Thomas M, Marrinan MT. Warfarin-induced skin necrosis and heparin-induced thrombocytopenia following mitral valve replacement for marantic endocarditis. J Heart Valve Dis 15: 716–718, 2006.

Wiedmer T, Hall SE, Ortel TL, Kane WH, Rosse WF, Sims PJ. Complement-induced vesiculation and exposure of membrane prothrombinase sites in platelets of paroxysmal nocturnal hemoglobinuria. Blood 82: 1192—1196, 1993.

Winkler MJ, Trunkey DD. Dopamine gangrene. Am J Surg 142: 588–589, 1981.

Woelke C, Eichler P, Washington G, Flesch BK. Post-transfusion purpura in a patient with HPA-1a and GPIa/IIa antibodies. Transfus Med 16: 69–72, 2006.

Yan SB, Helterbrand JD, Hartman DL, Wright TJ, Bernard GR. Low levels of protein C are associated with poor outcome in severe sepsis. Chest 120: 915–922, 2001.

4 Frequency of heparin-induced thrombocytopenia

Lori-Ann Linkins and David H. Lee

Reviewing the literature for studies evaluating the frequency of HIT requires an understanding of the difference between the development of antiplatelet factor 4/heparin (PF4/H) antibodies (*immunization*) and the development of *clinical HIT* (platelet-activating anti-PF4/H antibodies that cause thrombocytopenia and/or thrombosis). As illustrated by the Iceberg Model (see Fig. 1.4 in chap. 1 and Fig. 11.9 in chap. 11), only anti-PF4/H antibodies of IgG class that possess platelet-activating properties are associated with risk of clinical HIT. Consequently, there are two different types of HIT frequency studies: (*i*) studies that evaluated the frequency of immunization by heparin (and related molecules) in specific patient populations, and (*ii*) studies that evaluated the frequency of clinical HIT in patients who are suspected to have this condition based on clinical features (typically, thrombocytopenia).

The frequency of HIT immunization and clinical HIT are now known to be *variable*. Drug-related factors, such as chain length and degree of sulfation, help to explain the difference in frequency of HIT seen in patients receiving unfractionated heparin (UFH) *versus* low molecular weight heparin (LMWH) *versus* fondaparinux. However, these factors are only part of the story. Over the last few years, appreciation has grown for the importance of the role of non–drug related factors, such as patient setting, severity of trauma, and gender, in determining the frequency of HIT.

Determining the frequency of clinical HIT in patients with thrombocytopenia is particularly difficult because thrombocytopenia is such a common problem in hospitalized patients. For patients receiving heparin, there are three general explanations for thrombocytopenia: (*i*) heparin-induced thrombocytopenia (HIT), (*ii*) nonimmune heparin-induced platelet activation (see chap. 5), and—more often—(*iii*) an unrelated clinical problem, either common (e.g., hemodilution, septicemia) or rare (e.g., posttransfusion purpura, drug-induced immune thrombocytopenic purpura) (see chap. 3). The availability of sensitive and specific laboratory assays [e.g., enzyme immunoassay (EIA) and serotonin release assay (SRA)] for pathogenic HIT antibodies means that patients with HIT can usually be readily distinguished from those with the other conditions (see chap. 11). However, many early studies of HIT frequency either did not perform laboratory testing or used relatively insensitive or nonspecific assays to diagnose HIT (Table 4.1 lists various biologic and technical explanations that underlie the reported variability in frequency of HIT among prospective studies). In contrast, more recent studies have used one, or even two, sensitive and complementary assays. Perhaps for this reason, the understanding of the frequency and clinical impact of HIT has shifted over the years.

TABLE 4.1 Explanations for Variable Frequency of HIT Among Prospective Studies

---

Biologic explanations
 Patient population studied (frequency of HIT antibody formation differs among patient
  populations, possibly because of differences in platelet activation and PF4 release)
 Type of heparin used: immunogenicity (bovine UFH > porcine UFH > porcine LMWH ~
  fondaparinux) and *in vivo* cross-reactivity (UFH > LMWH >> fondaparinux); also, possibility
  of lot-to-lot variability in immunogenicity/cross-reactivity among heparins
 Variable duration of heparin treatment (HIT typically begins between days 5 and 10)
 Gender: female > male (exception: HIT is rare during pregnancy)
 Dose of heparin used (dose-dependent thrombocytopenia)
Technical explanations
 Variable definition of thrombocytopenia used
 Differing baseline platelet counts permitted for study entry
 Requirement to repeat platelet count testing to confirm thrombocytopenia
 Variable intensity of platelet count surveillance
 Variable intensity of surveillance for thrombotic events
Failure to exclude nonimmune heparin-associated thrombocytopenia
 Lack of use of *in vitro* test for HIT antibodies
 Use of insensitive or nonspecific HIT antibody assays
 Inclusion of patients with "early" thrombocytopenia
 Failure to exclude patients whose platelet count recovered during continued heparin treatment
 Failure to exclude patients with other explanations for thrombocytopenia

---

Abbreviations: HIT, heparin-induced thrombocytopenia; LMWH, low molecular weight heparin; PF4, platelet factor 4; UFH, unfractionated heparin.

Clinical HIT is recognized as a *clinicopathologic syndrome* because diagnosis requires (*i*) one or more clinical events (thrombocytopenia or thrombosis); and (*ii*) laboratory evidence of heparin-dependent antibodies (Warkentin et al., 1998a, 2011b). The importance of confirmatory laboratory testing should not be underestimated: systematic studies (Greinacher et al., 2007; Lo et al., 2007; Warkentin et al., 2008c) suggest that only 6–15% of sera referred for evaluation test positive for (platelet-activating) HIT antibodies. Consequently, this chapter primarily focuses on studies that have used *in vitro* testing to confirm the presence of HIT antibodies in patients with clinical features of HIT.

FREQUENCY OF CLINICAL HIT
Drug-Related Factors
Type of Heparin
The frequency of HIT varies substantially with the type of heparin used with highest to lowest frequency as follows: UFH > LMWH > fondaparinux. Differences in the polysaccharide chain length and degree of sulfation of these drugs are believed to be responsible for this observation (Greinacher et al., 1995; Rauova et al., 2005).

Fondaparinux (Arixtra) is the heparin with the shortest chain length (i.e., one-third the length of heparin). It is a synthetic pentasaccharide modeled after the antithrombin-binding region of heparin (Turpie, 2004). However, despite its small size, fondaparinux has been shown to stimulate the production of anti-PF4/H antibodies (immunization) (Warkentin, 2010). In fact, in prospective sero-surveillance studies, anti-PF4/H antibodies were generated at approximately the

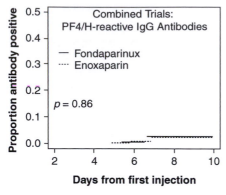 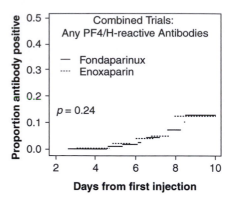

FIGURE 4.1 Anti-PF4/H antibody formation in patients receiving fondaparinux or enoxaparin after orthopedic surgery (current status analysis). Data are combined for patients undergoing knee and hip replacement. (*Left*) Anti-PF4/H antibodies of IgG class. There is no significant difference between the study drug groups (P = 0.86). (*Right*) All anti-PF4/H antibodies. There is no significant difference between the study drug groups (P = 0.24). *Abbreviation*: PF4/H, platelet factor 4/heparin. *Source*: From Warkentin et al. (2005a).

same frequency in patients who received fondaparinux as patients who received LMWH (enoxaparin) for thromboprophylaxis following elective orthopedic surgery (Warkentin et al., 2005a, 2010; Pouplard et al., 2005) (Fig. 4.1). No cases of clinical HIT were reported in either treatment group.

HIT immunization is frequent with fondaparinux, whereas cross-reactivity (i.e., ability to promote HIT antibody binding to PF4 *in vitro* and to promote platelet activation by HIT antibodies) is not. In the MATISSE clinical trials that compared fondaparinux with a heparin (either enoxaparin or UFH) for treatment of patients with venous thromboembolism, treatment with fondaparinux significantly reduced the risk of precipitating rapid-onset HIT among the small subset of patients who had platelet-activating HIT antibodies at the time of study enrolment (Warkentin et al., 2011a). Furthermore, it has been shown *in vitro* that anti–PF4/H antibodies (whether obtained from fondaparinux-treated patients or from patients with HIT) rarely cross-react with PF4/fondaparinux, although they react strongly with PF4/ UFH or PF4/LMWH (Warkentin et al., 2005a). These observations suggest that there is a *dissociation* between immunization by fondaparinux (i.e., ability to generate anti-PF4/H antibodies) and the cross-reactivity of fondaparinux (i.e., ability to promote HIT antibody binding to PF4 *in vitro* and to promote platelet activation by HIT antibodies). While induction of HIT by fondaparinux is biologically plausible, it is rare based on the dearth of such reports to date (Warkentin, 2010). Thus, fondaparinux offers the possibility of a negligible risk of HIT, a concept that can be illustrated using the iceberg model (Fig. 4.2) (Warkentin, 2006).

Origin of Heparin (Bovine vs Porcine)
Heparin derived from bovine lung is no longer available on the market (possibly due to concern about bovine spongiform encephalopathy); therefore, it is not discussed in detail in this chapter. Earlier studies showed a higher frequency of HIT with bovine heparin than with heparin derived from porcine sources (see Table 2 in

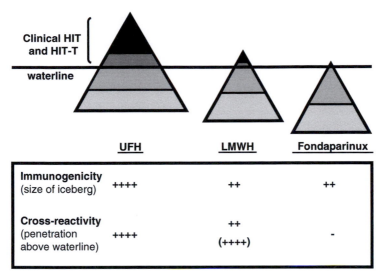

FIGURE 4.2 Dissociation in immunogenicity and cross-reactivity: comparison of UFH, LMWH, and fondaparinux. Of the three sulfated polysaccharide anticoagulants, UFH is most immunogenic (largest iceberg), whereas LMWH and fondaparinux exhibit similar immunogenicity. However, in contrast to UFH and LMWH, which can form well the antigens recognized by HIT antibodies, fondaparinux only poorly forms antigens with PF4 *in vitro* that are recognized by HIT antibodies. (Note: LMWH is indicated by ++ and ++++ to indicate that its cross-reactivity appears to differ *in vivo* [++] and *in vitro* [++++].). *Abbreviations*: HIT, heparin-induced thrombocytopenia; HIT-T, HIT-associated thrombosis; LMWH, low molecular weight heparin; UFH, unfractionated heparin. *Source*: From Warkentin (2006).

Lee and Warkentin, 2007). This is biologically plausible given that bovine heparin has a higher sulfate:disaccharide ratio than does porcine heparin (Casu et al., 1983), and it is better able to activate platelets *in vitro* (Barradas et al., 1987). These properties could lead to greater platelet activation *in vivo* and, consequently, greater potential for PF4 release. Moreover, the bovine heparin chains would be expected to better form the large multimolecular complexes that compose the target antigen for HIT antibodies.

Duration of Heparin Treatment
As HIT typically begins 5–10 days after starting therapy with heparin, it follows that the length of heparin treatment can influence the risk for HIT, for example, a 10- to 14-day course of UFH is far more likely to result in clinical HIT than a one-day treatment period (>2% *vs* 0.02%, i.e., an OR of ~100). Of note, there is evidence that the risk of HIT begins to decline after 10 days of uninterrupted heparin use (see Fig. 2.1, chap. 2). In a large study of postoperative orthopedic surgical patients receiving postoperative heparin prophylaxis, no patient developed HIT antibodies after day 10, although many patients received heparin for up to 14 days (Warkentin et al., 1995). These data are consistent with a "point immunization" model for risk of HIT (Warkentin, 2012) in which there is a brief time shortly after surgery when high circulating PF4 levels coincide with the first few subcutaneous heparin injections

resulting in favorable conditions for the development of anti-PF4/H antibodies (discussed further in Patient-Related Factors). However, it is important to note that even if HIT antibody formation occurs during the day 5–10 window period, thrombocytopenia itself can occur somewhat later, particularly if a larger dose of heparin is given, or UFH is substituted for LMWH.

Patient-Related Factors
Stoichiometry Model for HIT
The HIT antigen is a cryptic autoantigen, or neoantigen, on PF4 that is formed when PF4 binds to heparin (see chaps. 6 and 7). Only stoichiometric concentrations of heparin and PF4 will form the antigen (Greinacher et al., 2008). Thus, it can be hypothesized that the frequency of anti-PF4/H antibody formation will be influenced not only by heparin dose and composition, but also by circulating PF4 levels.

Greinacher and colleagues (2008) used photon correlation spectroscopy to determine at which concentrations UFH, LMWH, and fondaparinux form complexes with PF4. Using this technique, they found the optimal ratio at which the largest complexes were formed, as well as the PF4/polysaccharide ratios at which complexes reached 50% of maximum size. They then used these ratios to model the concentration ranges at which PF4/polysaccharide complexes form optimally at different PF4 concentrations.

These *in vitro* experiments led to the following conclusions: (*i*) at therapeutic doses, UFH will form complexes with PF4 primarily in situations of major platelet activation (resulting in very high concentrations of PF4); (*ii*) UFH is more likely to form complexes with PF4 at prophylactic doses than at therapeutic doses, but complex formation will still primarily occur in situations with moderate to major platelet activation; (*iii*) at therapeutic doses, LMWH concentrations are too high for optimal complex formation with PF4; (*iv*) at prophylactic doses, LMWH will form complexes with PF4 in situations of major platelet activation; and (*v*) at prophylactic doses, fondaparinux concentrations are too low for optimal complex formation with PF4. Consequently, in most clinical settings with little platelet activation, UFH or LMWH are present in considerably higher concentrations than required to form PF4/H complexes and the concentration of fondaparinux is too low. This stoichiometric model has been used to explain how the frequency of HIT may be influenced by the patient-related factors discussed in the following section (Warkentin et al., 2010).

Patient Setting
The frequency of clinical HIT according to patient setting in prospective studies is given in Tables 4.2 and 4.3. Overall, the highest to lowest frequency of HIT is as follows: surgical patients (particularly, orthopedic and cardiovascular surgery patients) > medical patients > obstetric patients. These patient populations, along with HIT in the setting of incidental heparin flushes, heparin-coated devices, and ventricular assist devices (VADs), are reviewed in the following sections.

Frequency of HIT in Surgical Patients Receiving UFH
Orthopedic Surgery   Two large prospective studies suggest that the frequency of HIT is high in orthopedic patients receiving UFH (Warkentin et al., 1995, 2003, 2005b; Greinacher et al., 2005a). When using a proportional fall in platelet count (e.g., 50% or greater) that began on or after day 5 of heparin treatment, and that

TABLE 4.2 The Frequency of HIT: Prospective Studies of Surgical Patients Using Confirmatory *In Vitro* Laboratory Testing of Patient Serum or Plasma

Study	Major indication for heparin	*In Vitro* test	Route, dose	Frequency of (immune) HIT (%)			Timing of platelet count fall reported?	Definition of thrombocytopenia (×10⁹/L)
				UFH	LMWH	Fondaparinux		
Leyvraz et al., 1991	Orthopedic	PRP	sc proph	2/204 (1.0)	0/205 (0)		Yes	<100, >40% fall
Warkentin et al., 1995	Orthopedic	SRA	sc proph	9/332 (2.7)	0/333 (0)		Yes	<150[a]
Warkentin et al., 2003, 2005b	Orthopedic	SRA/EIA	sc proph	16/332 (4.8)	2/333 (0.6)		Yes	>50% fall[a]
Geerts et al., 1996	Trauma	EIA	sc proph	2/136	0/129		No	Not stated
Lubenow et al., 2010	Trauma	EIA, HIPA	sc proph	4/316 (1.3)	1/298 (0.3)		Yes	Not stated
Warkentin et al., 1998b	Orthopedic	SRA/EIA	sc proph		2/246 (0.8)		Yes	<150 or >50% fall
Ganzer et al., 1997, 1999b	Orthopedic	HIPA	sc proph	15/307 (4.9)	0/325 (0)		Yes	>50% fall[c]
Marx et al., 1999	Orthopedic	EIA, SRA	sc proph	5/252 (2.0)	0/586 (0)		NA	>50% fall
Mahlfeld et al., 2002	Orthopedic	HIPA	sc proph		1/252 (0.4)		Yes	>40% fall
Greinacher et al., 2005ab	Orthopedic	HIPA, EIA	sc proph	12/231 (5.2)	0/271 (0)		Yes	>30% fall[c]
Warkentin et al., 2005a	Orthopedic	EIA, SRA	sc proph		0/1349 (0)	0/1377 (0)	NA	>50% fall
Trossaert et al., 1998	Cardiac	PRP/EIA	sc proph	0/51 (0)			NA	Not stated
Warkentin et al., 2000	Cardiac	SRA	sc proph	1/100 (1.0)			Yes	>50% fall
Pouplard et al., 1999, 2002	Cardiac	SRA, EIA	sc proph	9/263 (3.4)	1/370 (0.3)		No	<100 or >40% fall
Kannan et al., 2005	Cardiac	EIA, PRP, SRA	iv ther	5/33 (15.2)			No	<100 or 35% baseline
Selleng et al., 2010	Cardiac	EIA, HIPA	sc proph iv ther	3/327 (0.9%)	0/149		Yes	>50% fall

[a]Results of same RCT reported using two different definitions of thrombocytopenia (<150 and >50% fall).

[b]There is overlap in patients reported by Ganzer et al. (1997, 1999) and Greinacher et al. (2005a).

[c]Patients underwent laboratory testing for HIT antibodies if thrombosis developed even in the absence of thrombocytopenia. An additional five patients in the Ganzer et al., 1997 study developed thrombosis and positive HIPA test in the absence of platelet count fall >50%, i.e., overall HIT frequency 20/307 = 6.5%.

Abbreviations: EIA, PF4/heparin enzyme immunoassay; HIPA, heparin-induced platelet activation test (aggregation of washed platelets); HIT, heparin-induced thrombocytopenia; iv ther, intravenous therapeutic-dose heparin; LMWH, low molecular weight heparin; NA, not applicable; PRP, HIT assay using citrated platelet-rich plasma; sc proph, subcutaneous prophylactic-dose heparin; RCT, randomized controlled trial; SRA, serotonin release assay using washed platelets; UFH, unfractionated heparin.

TABLE 4.3 The Frequency of HIT: Prospective Studies of HIT in Medical Patients Using *In Vitro* Testing of Patient Serum/Plasma for HIT Antibodies

Study	Major indication for heparin	*In Vitro* test	Route, dose	Frequency of (Immune) HIT (%)		Timing of platelet count fall reported?	Definition of thrombocytopenia (×10⁹/L)
				UFH	LMWH		
Predominant treatment for VTE or ATE							
Cipolle et al., 1983; Ramirez-Lassepas et al., 1984 [stroke subgroup]	VTE, ATE	PRP	iv ther	1/111 (0.9) [1/83] (1.2)		Yes	<100
Rao et al., 1989	Multiple indications	PRP (SR)	iv ther sc proph	0/94 (0) 0/99 (0)		NA	<100
Lindhoff-Last et al., 2002	VTE	EIA	iv ther; sc ther	1/356 (0.3)[a]	0/720[a] (0)	Yes	<100 or >50% fall
Büller et al., 2003	VTE	EIA	iv ther, sc ther	0/1110 (0)		NA[b]	<100 or >40%
Büller et al., 2004	VTE	EIA	sc ther		0/1101 (0)	NA[b]	<100 or >40%
Prandoni et al., 2005	Multiple indications	EIA, HIPA	sc proph, ther		14/1754 (0.8)[c]	Yes	>50% fall
Kawano et al., 2011	Ischemic stroke	EIA, SRA	iv ther	3/172 (1.7)[d]		Yes	4T's score ≥4
Predominant use of heparin for prophylaxis							
Girolami et al., 2003	Prophylaxis, VTE, ATE	HIPA, EIA	sc proph sc ther	5/360 (1.4)[e] 0/238 (0)		Yes	>50% fall
Harbrecht et al., 2004; Pohl et al., 2005	Prophylaxis, neurology	EIA, HIPA	sc proph, iv ther	5/200 (2.5)	0/111 (0)[f]	Yes	<120 or >50% fall
Predominant treatment for MI/ACS							
Kappers-Klunne et al., 1997	MI/ACS	HIPA, EIA	iv ther	1/358 (0.3) 2/358 (0.6)		Yes	<60 and >50% fall (<120)
Romeril et al., 1982	MI/ACS	PRP	sc proph	0/45 (0)		NA	<150
Foo et al., 2006	Cardiac catherization	EIA	iv ther	0/357 (0)		NA	Not stated
Gluckman et al., 2005	PCI	EIA, SRA	iv ther	0/94 (0)		NA	Not stated

Study						Platelet count definition
Matsuo et al., 2005	ACS	EIA	iv ther	4/252 (1.6)	No	<100 or >50% fall
Hemodialysis						
Yamamoto et al., 1996	New onset HD	EIA, PRP	iv ther	6/154 (3.9) 3/154 (1.9)	Yes	Clotting and >20% fall (>50% fall)
Pena de la Vega et al., 2005	Chronic HD	EIA, HIPA	iv ther	1/57 (1.8)	No	<150 or >50% fall
Skouri et al., 2006	Pediatric chronic HD	EIA, HIPA	iv ther	0/38 (0)	No	Not stated

Note: Where uncertainty existed as to the number of patients with probable HIT, the lower number was indicated in the table, to avoid overestimating the number of patients with HIT. Some data relating to Cipolle et al. (1983) were obtained by personal communication, as reported by Warkentin and Kelton (1991).

[a] Thrombocytopenic patients with negative EIA testing were excluded.

[b] Platelet counts performed at baseline, day 4 and end of initial treatment.

[c] Frequencies of HIT in patients with and without previous exposure to UFH or LMWH were 10/598 (1.7%) and 1/1156 (0.3%), respectively.

[d] Authors cannot exclude that two patients out of three may not have had HIT.

[e] Antibody testing could not be performed in two out of these five patients.

[f] These authors compared the frequency of HIT among a prospective cohort of LMWH-treated neurology patients with their previous UFH-treated patient cohort (*P* =0.17).

Abbreviations: ATE, arterial thromboembolism; EIA, PF4/heparin enzyme immunoassay; HD, hemodialysis; HIPA, heparin-induced platelet activation test; HIT, heparin-induced thrombocytopenia; iv ther, intravenous therapeutic-dose heparin; LMWH, low molecular weight heparin; MI/ACS, myocardial infarction/acute coronary syndromes; NA, not applicable; PCI, percutaneous coronary intervention; PRP, HIT assay using citrated platelet-rich plasma (PRP/SR, with serotonin release); sc proph, subcutaneous prophylactic-dose heparin; sc ther, subcutaneous therapeutic-dose heparin; RCT, randomized controlled trial; SRA, serotonin release assay using washed platelets; UFH, unfractionated heparin; VTE, venous thromboembolism.

was confirmed by serologic testing for HIT antibodies, both studies observed a frequency of HIT of about 5% (Table 4.2). Each study used porcine mucosal heparin, derived from a different manufacturer, given by the subcutaneous (sc) route at a dosage of 15,000 U/day. Other studies of postorthopedic UFH thromboprophylaxis (using confirmatory *in vitro* testing) have shown frequencies of HIT of about 2.0% (Leyvraz et al., 1991; Mahlfeld et al., 2002). Applying the stoichiometry model proposed by Greinacher and colleagues, it is likely that the high risk of HIT seen in this patient population is explained by the release of large amounts of PF4 by the surgical procedure, which facilitates the formation of immunogenic PF4/H complexes.

It is important to note that the high frequency of HIT reported in the orthopedic studies above was, at least in part, due to the duration of exposure (10–14 days). The frequency of HIT in modern day orthopedic patients is significantly lower due to shorter durations of exposure when heparin is administered (Smythe et al., 2007), and the availability of alternative nonheparin anticoagulants for thromboprophylaxis.

Cardiac Surgery   Three studies have been performed on postoperative cardiac surgical patients who also received postoperative UFH in addition to high doses of UFH during preceding cardiopulmonary bypass (CPB) (Trossaert et al., 1998; Pouplard et al., 1999; Warkentin et al., 2000) (Table 4.2). Pooling these three studies, about 2% of patients developed serologically confirmed HIT. This frequency is consistent with a number of retrospective studies (Glock et al., 1988; Walls et al., 1992a,b; Singer et al., 1993) that reported a frequency of HIT of up to 5%, but with an overall frequency of about 2% (Lee and Warkentin, 2007). Interestingly, the frequency of HIT in this population appears to be lower than in orthopedic patients receiving UFH, although the cardiac surgical patients appear to have a higher frequency of HIT immunization (Warkentin et al., 2000).

Trauma Surgery   Lubenow and colleagues (2010) reported an overall incidence of HIT of 2.2% (95% CI, 0.3–4.1) in a randomized trial of UFH *versus* LMWH for thromboprophylaxis following trauma. From their analysis of blood samples collected at baseline and between day 10 and 14 (or at the time of discharge), they also determined that the rate of HIT seroconversion was higher in surgical patients who experienced major trauma (fractured humerus, hip, femur, tibia, pelvis, or extended tissue trauma) compared with patients who experienced minor trauma (all other surgical interventions) [OR 7.98 (95% CI 2.06–31.00; $P = 0.003$)]. As with orthopedic surgery, it is believed that major trauma probably results in release of a larger amount of PF4, which can bind to UFH (or LMWH) to form immunogenic PF4/H complexes.

Frequency of HIT in Surgical Patients Receiving LMWH

Clinical trial data suggest that the frequency of HIT in surgery patients who receive LMWH is less than 1%. A meta-analysis of five surgical thromboprophylaxis prospective cohort studies and RCTs (four postorthopedic, one postcardiac) that defined HIT using both clinical and serologic criteria found a substantial reduction in HIT frequency (odds ratio [OR], 0.10; $P < 0.001$) with LMWH compared with UFH (Martel et al., 2005) (Fig. 4.3). The authors found the absolute risk of HIT to be 0.2% with LMWH and 2.6% with UFH. In contrast, when they examined the OR for

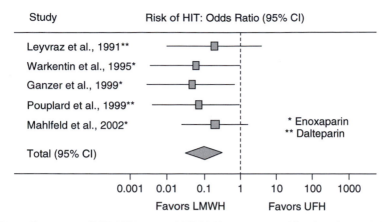

FIGURE 4.3 Frequency of HIT: UFH *versus* LMWH. Meta-analysis of five thromboprophylaxis studies comparing the frequency of serologically confirmed HIT between UFH and LMWH (enoxaparin, three studies; dalteparin, two studies). *Abbreviations*: HIT, heparin-induced thrombocytopenia; LMWH, low molecular weight heparin; UFH, unfractionated heparin. *Source*: From Martel et al. (2005).

HIT using a nonserologically defined definition of thrombocytopenia, the difference in risk of apparent HIT was less marked.

Orthopedic Surgery The strongest evidence that LMWH is associated with a lower frequency of HIT in orthopedic patients was provided by an randomized controlled trial (RCT) that directly compared the frequency of HIT between the two types of heparin (Warkentin et al., 1995, 2003, 2005b). The frequency of HIT in patients treated with the LMWH (enoxaparin) was lower than that seen in patients treated with UFH, irrespective of whether a standard definition [platelet fall to $<150 \times 10^9/L$ on or after day 5 of heparin treatment (0% *vs* 2.7%)] or a more sensitive definition [>50% platelet count fall from the postoperative peak (0.6% *vs* 4.8%)] of thrombocytopenia was used (Table 4.2). The frequency of HIT antibody formation also differed between the two patient groups, using either the SRA (Warkentin et al., 1995, 2005b) or a PF4/H (or PF4/polyanion) EIA (Warkentin et al., 2000, 2005b).

Warkentin and colleagues also analyzed the results of four large RCTs comparing LMWH (enoxaparin) with fondaparinux for thromboprophylaxis following orthopedic surgery to determine the frequency of seroconversion as a surrogate marker for the risk of HIT (Warkentin et al., 2010). In these studies, 6324 out of 7344 randomized patients were screened serologically using the GTI-PF4 EIA (prestudy and one postsample at day 5 or later). Samples with positive results were then tested with an inhouse PF4/H EIA and SRA. The proportion of patients who developed anti-PF4/H antibodies (seroconversion) was 3% (191/6324), 37 patients had a positive SRA, and one patient met the definition for clinical HIT.

From these studies, they made the following observations: (*i*) the rate of seroconversion was higher for patients who received enoxaparin following knee arthroplasty compared with hip arthroplasty [relative risk (RR) = 3.97 (95% CI 2.01–7.87)]; (*ii*) there was a trend toward lower seroconversion rates when enoxaparin was started preoperatively compared with postoperatively in hip arthroplasty patients [RR = 0.39 (95% CI 0.15–1.05)]; and (*iii*) a trend toward higher seroconversion rates for enoxaparin started preoperatively compared with postoperatively in hip fracture surgery patients [RR = 2.08 (95% CI 0.81–5.36)]. The differences in rates of seroconversion outlined above were not observed in patients who received fondaparinux [with the exception of an increased rate of seroconversion when fondaparinux was started preoperatively compared with postoperatively in hip fracture patients; RR = 2.52 (95% CI 1.15–5.55)].

Warkentin and colleagues postulated that this variability in the rate of seroconversion observed in the orthopedic RCTs could be explained by the influence of the factors described above on the concentration of PF4 available for forming immunogenic PF4/H complexes. For example, knee arthroplasty and hip fracture surgery likely release higher concentrations of PF4 (than elective hip arthroplasty), which shifts the PF4:heparin ratio in favor of forming PF4/H complexes. They also hypothesized that in elective hip arthroplasty patients, some of the PF4 that is normally bound to endothelial cell heparin sulfate becomes mobilized and then "sequestered" when the first dose of enoxaparin (or fondaparinux) is given preoperatively, which shifts the PF4:heparin ratio away from forming PF4/H complexes in the postoperative setting (Warkentin et al., 2010).

UFH appeared also to stimulate a higher frequency of anti-PF4/H antibody formation than LMWH (reviparin) in a randomized trial of post-hip surgery and -knee surgery patients (Ahmad et al., 2003b). HIT antibodies occurred somewhat more often in knee surgery patients. The same investigators also examined HIT antibody formation in orthopedic patients immobilized in a plaster cast who were randomized to receive reviparin or placebo (Ahmad et al., 2003a). A surprising finding was that the number of patients who apparently formed anti-PF4/polyanion antibodies (by EIA) was higher in the placebo group (10 cases *vs* 6). No patient in either study developed clinical HIT, but up to 18% developed a positive EIA for anti-PF4/H antibodies.

Cardiac Surgery The influence of postoperative UFH or LMWH on the frequency of HIT antibody formation and clinical HIT following cardiac surgery has been examined by two groups of investigators (Pouplard et al., 1999, 2002, 2005; Selleng et al., 2010). In their multiyear observational studies involving nonrandomized comparisons between UFH and LMWH, Pouplard and colleagues found a significant difference in risk of HIT: UFH = 11/437 (2.5%) *versus* LMWH = 8/1874 (0.4%); $P < 0.0001$. However, differences in patient composition prevent firm conclusions. Notably, the frequency of antibody formation was similar in both groups of patients using a commercial EIA that detects IgM, IgA, and IgG antibodies. This suggests that "point immunization" from intraoperative UFH use, rather than any major influence from postoperative UFH or LMWH, is responsible for the formation of anti-PF4/H antibodies in the post-cardiac surgery patient population.

Selleng and colleagues (2010) also evaluated post-cardiac surgery patients, but in their prospective cohort study, UFH was given in therapeutic doses to patients who required full anticoagulation, and LMWH was given in prophylactic doses to all other patients. The incidence of HIT in patients who received UFH was 0.9% (3/327) compared with 0% (0/149) in patients who received LMWH ($P = 0.23$) (Table 4.2).

Trauma Surgery In trauma patients, Lubenow and colleagues (2010) reported a lower incidence of HIT in patients who received LMWH thromboprophylaxis compared with patients who received UFH, although the difference did not reach statistical significance (LMWH 1.3% *vs* UFH 0.3%; $P = 0.37$).

Frequency of HIT in Medical Patients Treated with UFH

From prospective studies using confirmatory laboratory tests, the incidence of HIT in medical patients receiving prophylactic-dose UFH appears to be lower than that observed in surgical patients receiving UFH prophylaxis. Girolami et al. (2003) prospectively evaluated 598 hospitalized medical patients who received prophylactic ($n = 360$) or therapeutic ($n = 238$) dose UFH. Overall, five patients developed HIT, all of whom were receiving UFH in prophylactic doses (0.8% of combined group, or 1.4% of patients receiving prophylactic-dose UFH).

The incidence of HIT in medical patients receiving intravenous, therapeutic-dose UFH, usually for venous thromboembolism (VTE) and myocardial infarction and acute coronary syndromes (MI/ACS), appears to be slightly less than 1%. The largest modern study that systematically evaluated platelet counts at baseline, on day 4, and at the end of initial treatment for VTE, reported an incidence of HIT of 0% in 1110 patients who received therapeutic UFH for a median duration of 6.9 ± 2.2 days (Büller et al., 2003) (Table 4.3).

In contrast, HIT appears to be more frequent in chronic HD patients who receive UFH with a reported incidence of 2% (Yamamoto et al., 1996). Whether this is a real difference that reflects increased platelet activation (and PF4 release) during HD or it reflects a more sensitive definition of thrombocytopenia (any platelet count fall associated with line clotting) is unknown. Whether the incidence of elevated levels of anti-PF4/H antibodies and clinical HIT are dependent on the time since the initiation of HD is also unclear. Some have suggested that the frequency of anti-PF4/H antibody increases with time (Palomo et al., 2005), whereas others have found no association (Pena de la Vega et al., 2005). Two studies suggest that the antibodies tend to develop early after initiation of HD, and may disappear after months, despite ongoing heparin exposure (Nakamoto et al., 2005; Skouri et al., 2006). Most studies have not found an association between vascular access thrombosis and elevated levels of anti-PF4/H antibodies (Greinacher et al., 1996; Sitter et al., 1998; O'Shea et al., 2002; Palomo et al., 2005; Pena de la Vega et al., 2005; Carrier et al., 2007).

Frequency of HIT in Medical Patients Treated with LMWH

Although there have been several RCTs evaluating the efficacy of LMWH for prophylaxis in medical patients, published descriptions of secondary safety endpoints, such as HIT, are usually brief and often inadequate to judge whether the occurrences of thrombocytopenia were due to HIT or not (Samama et al., 1999; Turpie, 2000; Leizorovicz et al., 2004). One meta-analysis of randomized trials for the treatment of VTE reported no significant difference in the incidence of HIT between patients who received LMWH [0.3% (3/1058)] and UFH [0.1% (2/1426)] (Morris et al., 2007). However, the methodologic rigor with which HIT was identified in the studies included in this meta-analysis has been questioned (Warkentin and Greinacher, 2007).

In one RCT that systematically compared the incidence of HIT in patients who were treated for deep vein thrombosis (DVT), none of 720 patients who received LMWH developed (antibody-positive) HIT, whereas one of 356 (0.3%)

patients treated with UFH manifested this complication (Lindhoff-Last et al., 2002). Interestingly, if the definition of HIT in that study was expanded to include thrombosis and a positive test for anti-PF4/H antibodies (even without thrombocytopenia), then a greater event-rate was observed in the UFH-treated patients (2.2% vs 0.1%; $P = 0.00087$) (Warkentin and Greinacher, 2005). This RCT also showed a greater frequency of antibody formation in the UFH-treated arm (21.1% vs 6.2%; $P < 0.0001$).

In a prospective cohort study specifically designed to ascertain the incidence of HIT in medical patients receiving LMWH, 14/1754 (0.8%) developed HIT (Prandoni et al., 2005), a frequency similar to that reported by the same investigators in medical patients receiving UFH (Girolami et al., 2003). In "before–after" prospective cohort studies performed in neurologic patients, the frequency of HIT tended to be lower in patients treated with LMWH (nadroparin) compared with UFH (0% vs 2.5%; $P = 0.17$), with a significantly lower frequency of heparin-dependent antibody formation among the patients receiving LMWH (1.8% vs 10.5%; $P < 0.001$) (Harbrecht et al., 2004; Pohl et al., 2005) (Table 4.3).

Frequency of HIT in Critically Ill Patients

Thrombocytopenia is common in critically ill patients, occurring in 20–50% of all patients in the intensive care unit (ICU). In this population, the presence of thrombocytopenia is associated with increased mortality, and depending on severity and etiology, is associated with increased hemorrhagic risk as well. ICU patients often have several potential causes of thrombocytopenia, making evaluation challenging. Heparin exposure (in the form of line flushes, prophylaxis, or therapeutic anticoagulation) is virtually ubiquitous in the ICU, making HIT a frequent diagnostic consideration.

The PROTECT study (PROphylaxis for ThromboEmbolism in Critical Care Trial) provides the strongest data for the frequency of HIT with UFH versus LMWH prophylaxis in ICU patients (Table 4.4). In this multicenter trial, 3764 patients were randomized to receive either dalteparin (5000 IU once a day) or UFH (5000 IU twice a day) while they were in the ICU (Cook et al., 2011). The incidence of HIT, confirmed by the SRA, was a secondary study endpoint. By intention-to-treat analysis, 12 of 1873 (0.6%) patients randomized to receive UFH developed HIT, compared with 5 of 1873 (0.3%) patients randomized to receive dalteparin [hazard ratio, 0.47 (95% CI 0.16–1.35; $P = 0.16$)]. However, in a prespecified per-protocol analysis, the frequency of HIT was significantly lower in patients who received dalteparin [hazard ratio, 0.27; (95% CI 0.08–0.98; $P = 0.046$)].

Two groups of investigators have conducted prospective studies to determine the frequency of HIT, confirmed by the SRA, in critically ill patients (Verma et al., 2003; Crowther et al., 2010). Crowther and colleagues (2010) reported that 50 out of 528 patients (9.5%) admitted to medical-surgical ICUs (across three prospective studies) were investigated for HIT with an overall incidence of 0.4%. Verma and colleagues (2003) reported the same frequency of HIT in their prospective study of 267 patients who were admitted to a single-center combined coronary/ICU over a two-year period. Indeed, if the frequency of HIT is only about 0.4% in ICU patients, yet the overall risk of thrombocytopenia is about 20–50%, then a useful clinical "rule" is that the true risk of HIT is only about one in 100 among all ICU patients who develop thrombocytopenia (Napolitano et al., 2006; Warkentin, 2006; Selleng et al., 2007).

TABLE 4.4 Frequency of HIT in Critically Ill Patients

| Study | Population | HIT clinical criteria | Frequency of thrombocytopenia n/N (%) | Suspected HIT n/N (%) | HIT cases | | | Comments |
					Positive HIT serology n/N (%)	HIT with thrombosis n/N (%)	In Vitro test	
Prospective studies								
Crowther et al., 2010	528 patients[a] critically ill medical and surgical patients	Thrombocytopenia was defined as a platelet count <150 × 10⁹/L; <50% of admission platelet count; clinically suspected	Not stated	50/528 (9.5)	2/527[b] (0.4)	NA	SRA, EIA	Postop orthopedic and cardiac surgery patients not studied. Positive SRA needed to diagnose HIT (n = 66 tested)
Verma et al., 2003	748 UFH-treated patients admitted to a combined ICU and CCU over 2-yr. 267 had sufficient exposure to be considered at risk for HIT	>2 consecutive platelet counts <150 × 10⁹/L, or >33% drop, ≥5 days after UFH exposure, or sooner if previously exposed within preceding 8 wk	Not stated	40/267 (15.0)	1/259 (0.4)	0/1 (0)	EIA, SRA	Serology missing from 8/40 patients with clinically suspected HIT. Positive SRA needed to diagnose HIT (n = 32 tested)

(Continued)

TABLE 4.4 (Continued) Frequency of HIT in Critically Ill Patients

Study	Population	HIT clinical criteria	Frequency of thrombocytopenia n/N (%)	Suspected HIT n/N (%)	HIT cases			Comments
					Positive HIT serology n/N (%)	HIT with thrombosis n/N (%)	In Vitro test	
Strauss et al., 2002	145 consecutive patients admitted to a medical ICU with a normal platelet count	Thrombocytopenia was defined as a platelet count <150 × 10⁹/L; other clinical criteria for HIT not stated	64/145 (44%)	Not stated	2/145 (1.4)	Not stated	Not stated	Clinical criteria for HIT not stated. Two HIT cases reported to be confirmed by laboratory testing, but type of assay not stated
Stéphan et al., 1999	147 consecutive patients admitted to a surgical ICU over 6-mo period	Thrombocytopenia was defined as a platelet count <100 × 10⁹/L; other criteria for HIT not stated	52/147 (35%)	Not stated	No cases described	No cases described	Not stated	UFH and LMWH were not found to be independent risk factors for the development of thrombocytopenia
Bouman et al., 2002	106 critically ill patients enrolled in a clinical trial of CRRT	Not stated	Not stated	Not stated	Not stated	Not stated	Not stated	5/106 (4.7%) Patients were diagnosed with HIT, but criteria for diagnosis were not stated

ªIncluded patients from three prospective studies with similar inclusion/exclusion criteria.
ᵇOne patient with positive EIA who did not undergo SRA testing was excluded from the analysis.
Abbreviations: CRRT continuous renal replacement therapy; CCU, coronary care unit; CT, computed axial tomography; EIA, enzyme immunoassay; HIT, heparin-induced thrombocytopenia; ICU, intensive care unit; LMWH, low molecular weight heparin; NA, not applicable; PAT, platelet aggregation test; SRA, serotonin release assay; UFH, unfractionated heparin.

Other retrospective analyses using anti-PF4/polyanion EIAs (which are much less specific for clinical HIT) raise the possibility that certain patient subgroups may be at higher risk for HIT (Lee and Warkentin, 2007). However, prospective studies using platelet activation assays are required to ascertain the true frequencies of clinical HIT among these and other patient subgroups.

When HIT does occur in critically ill patients, it appears to be associated with a high risk of venous and arterial thrombotic events, similar to that observed in non–critically ill patients with HIT. Retrospective studies report a thrombosis frequency of 20–50%, or even greater (Wester et al., 2004; Hoh et al., 2005; Gettings et al., 2006, Trehel-Tursis et al., 2012). The HIT-associated mortality in these studies also appears to be high, although not necessarily higher than in non-HIT thrombocytopenic patients in the ICU (Trehel-Tursis et al., 2012).

Frequency of HIT During Pregnancy

HIT appears to be uncommon during pregnancy even with UFH treatment. Fausett and colleagues (2001) reported that none of 244 pregnant women developed HIT during UFH use, although HIT occurred in 10 of 244 (4%) nonpregnant patients who received UFH ($P = 0.0014$). In a literature review, Sanson and colleagues (1999) identified no cases of HIT among 486 women who received LMWH during pregnancy. Ellison et al (2000) studied 57 pregnancies in 50 patients and also found no episodes of HIT in pregnant women who received enoxaparin. Similarly, Lepercq and colleagues (2001) found no cases of HIT in 624 pregnancies among 604 women treated with LMWH. More recently, a systematic review of studies published up to the end of 2003 found no cases of HIT in 2777 pregnancies (Greer and Nelson-Piercy 2005).

Role of Incidental UFH Flushes in the Frequency of HIT

There are two ways that "incidental" exposure to heparin by "flushing" of intravascular catheters can affect the frequency or clinical effect of HIT. First, such minor heparin exposures can trigger the formation of HIT antibodies (Ling and Warkentin, 1998; Warkentin et al., 1998b). And second, in patients who have already formed potent HIT antibodies for any reason, any ongoing or recurrent heparin exposure—including small-dose exposure—could lead to recurrence or exacerbation of thrombocytopenia or thrombosis (Rice and Jackson, 1981) (however, a confounding issue is that such patients may also have "autoimmune"-like antibodies that are able to cause HIT irrespective of ongoing small-dose heparin exposure—see chaps. 2 and 20). Several patients have been reported in whom severe HIT occurred while only small amounts of heparin were being given as flushes to maintain the patency of intravascular catheters (Doty et al., 1986; Heeger and Backstrom, 1986; Kappa et al., 1987; Rama et al., 1991; Brushwood, 1992; Parney and Steinke, 2000).

In most of the reports of patients developing HIT during LMWH treatment, recent prior exposure to UFH was not excluded. Indeed, incidental exposure to UFH by intraoperative invasive catheters could lead to the formation of HIT antibodies that are inappropriately attributed to later postoperative LMWH prophylaxis (Shumate, 1995).

To address this issue, a randomized, double-blind clinical trial was performed to test the hypothesis that incidental exposure to UFH by intraoperative invasive lines, rather than postoperative LMWH antithrombotic prophylaxis, was the predominant explanation for postoperative HIT antibody formation (Warkentin et al., 1998b). Patients were randomized to receive either UFH or normal saline flushes during surgery. Surprisingly, the results of this study ruled against the hypothesis: the frequency of HIT antibodies was not higher in the patients who were randomized to receive UFH flushes (2.2% vs 2.7%; $P = 0.73$). Rather, the results suggested that postoperative LMWH prophylaxis administered to both groups was the predominant factor in causing HIT antibody formation. However, HIT antibody formation occurred in two patients who received UFH flushes, but who subsequently were given warfarin anticoagulation. Because intraoperative UFH flushes occasionally result in the formation of high levels of HIT antibodies that can lead to life-threatening, acute HIT if therapeutic-dose UFH is administered a few weeks later (Ling and Warkentin, 1998), and because there is no clinical benefit to flushing intravascular catheters with UFH (Warkentin et al., 1998b), it seems reasonable to recommend that normal saline flushes be considered for routine flushing of intravascular catheters used during surgery.

A double-blind placebo-controlled trial of UFH for maintaining peripheral vein catheter patency in neonates also evaluated the incidence of anti-PF4/H antibodies and clinical HIT. None of the 108 neonates who were allocated to receive heparin developed HIT or heparin-dependent antibodies (Klenner et al., 2003).

It is possible that heparin flushes for venous access devices in cancer patients can cause anti-PF4/H antibody formation. In a serosurveillance study, Mayo and colleagues (1999) found that about one-third of 49 such patients tested formed low levels of antibodies (detected by EIA) at least once. However, only one patient developed a positive SRA, and no patient developed thrombocytopenia.

In recent years, many centers have substituted saline for heparin to intermittently "flush" peripheral venous catheters. This is because saline flushing of such devices "locked" between use have similar patency rates as when heparin flushes are used (Randolph et al., 1998b). In contrast, heparin may help prolong the patency of intra-arterial, central venous, and pulmonary artery catheters (Randolph et al., 1998a), and consequently exposure to heparin by these routes remains common.

HIT and Heparin-Coated Devices

Heparin can be bonded to artificial surfaces (Larsson et al., 1987), either through ionic attachment, as used for pulmonary artery catheters (Eldh and Jacobsson, 1974; Almeida et al., 1998b), or by end-linked covalent bonding [e.g., Carmeda BioActive Surface (CBAS)] (Larm et al., 1983) (see chap. 20). CBAS has been used for CPB circuits and filters (Borowiec et al., 1992a,b, 1993), extracorporeal membrane oxygenation (ECMO) devices (Koul et al., 1992), and coronary stents (Serruys et al., 1996). During use in patients, ionically attached heparin is displaced by albumin from the catheter surface, where it could contribute to HIT (discussed subsequently). End-linked heparin is an effective and longer-lasting anticoagulant, as the immobilized, but flexible, heparin chains are able to interact with fluid-phase antithrombin and thrombin (Elgue et al., 1993). Nevertheless, the end-linked, but relatively unconstrained, heparin is capable of interacting with PF4 (Suh et al., 1998). Although it is theoretically possible that covalent heparin-bonded devices could result in the formation of HIT antibodies, this effect would seem trivial compared with the much higher doses of systemic UFH that are given when these devices are implanted. Potentially, covalently bonded heparin in implanted devices (e.g., grafts) might contribute to HIT pathogenesis, although there are several arguments against this (see chap. 20). Use of heparin-coated pulmonary catheters in contributing to HIT has been implicated by Laster and Silver (1988). These workers reported 10 patients with HIT whose platelet counts did not rise until the removal of their heparin-coated pulmonary catheters, despite discontinuing all other sources of heparin. Incubation of the heparin-coated catheters with platelets in the presence of patient sera resulted in catheter-induced platelet aggregation. Based on the identification of four such cases, during which time 1112 heparin-coated catheters had been used, they estimated the frequency of catheter-associated HIT to be 0.4%.

HIT and Ventricular Assist Devices

VADs are surgically implanted mechanical pumps that have a large foreign surface area in direct contact with flowing blood, thereby creating an inherently prothrombotic environment. In a nonrandomized study of patients who received heparin-coated and uncoated VADs, there was no difference in the development of anti-PF4/H antibodies and thromboembolism between the groups (Koster et al., 2001). In two more recent studies, 10/113 (8.8%) (Schenk et al., 2006, 2007) and 28/358 (7.8%) (Koster et al., 2007) of VAD patients developed apparent HIT. In both studies, the frequency of anti-PF4/H antibody formation (by EIA) was over 60%. While these apparent frequencies of clinical HIT (~8%) are among the highest reported in any patient population, it is unclear how to distinguish true clinical HIT from a patient with cardiogenic shock or other non-HIT explanations for thrombocytopenia who coincidentally develop heparin-dependent platelet-activating antibodies (Warkentin and Crowther, 2007).

Gender

Ironically, in view of the rarity of HIT in pregnancy, it is now recognized that female gender is a modest risk factor for HIT (OR, 1.5–2.0). Warkentin et al. (2006) found an overrepresentation of the female gender in their analysis of a national HIT database and prospective studies comparing UFH with LMWH. Interestingly, they also found that the relationship between female gender and a higher frequency of HIT was predominantly seen in patients who received UFH; it was less clear in patients treated with LMWH. Whether the increased frequency of HIT in women is related to gender differences in frequency of antibody formation, or in antibody levels, or in susceptibility of platelets to be activated by HIT antibodies, has not been reported.

Body Mass Index

Warkentin and colleagues also examined the relationship between body mass index (BMI) and the frequency of anti-PF4/H antibody formation in the orthopedic studies previously discussed in Patient-Related Factors. (Warkentin et al., 2010). Using the data from these studies, the authors showed that the effect of increasing BMI quartiles on the RR of immunization for fondaparinux *versus* enoxaparin was consistent with predictions based on their stoichiometry-based model. In brief, the RR of immunization decreased with increasing BMI due to an increase in the rate of immunization with enoxaparin (likely as a result of a decrease in enoxaparin to levels more compatible with complex formation and no appreciable change in fondaparinux levels) (Fig. 4.4).

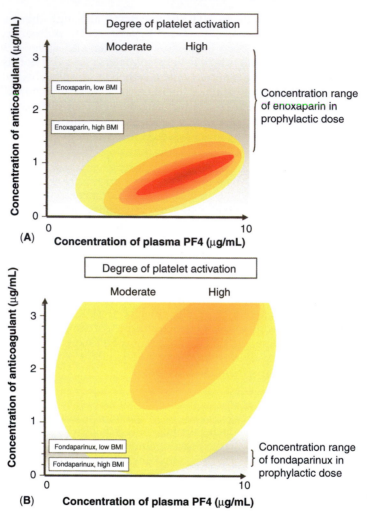

FIGURE 4.4 Implications of a stoichiometry-based schematic model of immunization against PF4-containing immunogenic complexes. The concentration ranges indicated are estimates derived from *in vitro* and *ex vivo* studies. (**A**) Enoxaparin. The colored area indicates greatest risk of forming multimolecular complexes of PF4/enoxaparin, as follows: red > red-orange > orange > yellow. In general, factors that tend to increase the degree of platelet activation, and associated PF4 release and availability, will tend to increase immunization risk. The range of concentrations of enoxaparin achieved during prophylactic dose anticoagulation tends to be higher than those required for optimal formation of immunogenic concentrations; thus, patients with a high BMI—and, consequently, a tendency to lower drug levels with a fixed dose enoxaparin regimen—would be expected to have a greater immunization risk compared with low BMI patients (see text). (**B**) Fondaparinux. The colored area indicates greatest risk of forming multimolecular complexes of PF4/fondaparinux, as follows: orange > yellow-orange > yellow. As with enoxaparin, factors that tend to increase the degree of platelet activation, and associated PF4 release and availability, will tend to increase the risk of immunization. However, in contrast to enoxaparin, the range of concentrations of fondaparinux achieved during prophylactic-dose anticoagulation tends to be lower than those that are optimal for forming immunogenic concentrations. (*Continued*)

FIGURE 4.4 (*Continued*) Thus, patients with high BMI (and, consequently, a tendency to lower drug levels with a fixed-dose fondaparinux regimen) would be expected to have a lower immunization risk compared with low BMI patients. Consequently, the RR of immunization observed with fondaparinux compared with that observed for enoxaparin, should decrease with progressively greater BMI values, a hypothesis we specifically tested. *Abbreviations*: BMI, body mass index; PF4, platelet factor 4; RR, relative risk. *Source*: From Warkentin et al. (2010).

Risk Factor Interactions
Table 4.5 summarizes the data supporting the role of three major risk factors for HIT: heparin type (UFH > LMWH), patient type (surgical > medical), and patient gender (female > male) (Warkentin et al., 2006). (A fourth major risk factor, namely, duration of heparin therapy, is not shown.) Note that the influence of heparin type is most striking in a female patient receiving postoperative thromboprophylaxis: HIT is much more likely to occur with UFH than with LMWH in such a patient [OR, 17.39 (95% CI, 4.22–71.70); $P < 0.0001$]; in contrast, the benefit of LMWH is significantly less in males receiving postsurgical thromboprophylaxis.

HIT in the Absence of Heparin
HIT Caused by Other Sulfated Polysaccharides
The cryptic HIT autoantigen comprises conformationally altered PF4 when it forms a multimolecular complex with heparin. Other negatively charged polysaccharides can interact with PF4 to produce the HIT antigen (Wolf et al., 1983; Anderson, 1992; Greinacher et al., 1992a,b,c) (see chap. 7). These considerations explain why a number of high-sulfated polysaccharides, 10 or more subunits in length, have been reported to cause a syndrome of thrombocytopenia and thrombosis that essentially mimics HIT. These drugs include the semi-synthetic five-carbon subunit-based "heparinoid" pentosan polysulfate (Gouault-Heilman et al., 1985; Vitoux et al., 1985; Follea et al., 1986; Goad et al., 1994; Tardy-Poncet et al., 1994; Rice et al., 1998), polysulfated chondroitin sulfate (Van Aken, 1980; Wolf et al., 1983; Greinacher et al., 1992c; Greinacher and Warkentin, 2008; Warkentin and Greinacher, 2009), and the antiangiogenic agent, PI-88 (Rosenthal et al., 2002). The frequency of immune-mediated thrombocytopenia, with or without thrombosis, after exposure to these compounds is unknown, but may be high. Also on very rare occasions, a syndrome resembling HIT may be triggered by the pentasaccharide anticoagulant, fondaparinux (Warkentin et al., 2007; see also chap. 17).

Danaparoid, a mixture of anticoagulant glycosaminoglycans, has not been reported to cause HIT *de novo*. However, some HIT sera "cross-react" *in vitro* with danaparoid, and cases of apparent *in vivo* cross-reactivity have been reported (see chap. 16) (Magnani and Gallus, 2006).

Spontaneous HIT
On exceptionally rare occasions, patients spontaneously develop an illness that clinically resembles HIT, that is, thrombocytopenia, thrombosis, and presence of platelet-activating anti-PF4/H (HIT) antibodies, in the absence of heparin exposure (Warkentin et al., 2008b). Typically, there is a preceding inflammatory or surgical event that promotes generation of these antibodies (Jay and Warkentin, 2008; Warkentin et al., 2008b; Pruthi et al., 2009; Mallik et al., 2011). Of the six cases of spontaneous HIT reported to date, three occurred after orthopedic surgery (Jay and

TABLE 4.5 Factors Influencing the Risk of HIT: Type of Heparin, Type of Patient Population, and Gender (Fixed-Effects Statistical Analysis)

Group (Number of studies)	Common OR for HIT	95% CI common OR		P value
		Lower	Upper	
Overall effect of heparin type: UFH vs LMWH (7)	5.29	2.84	9.86	<0.0001
Overall effect of patient type: surgical vs medical (7)[a]	3.25	1.98	5.35	<0.0001
Overall effect of gender: female vs male (7)	2.37	1.37	4.09	0.0015
Studies of *interactions* of gender (females, males), patient type (surgical, medical), or both (female/ surgical; female/medical) on risk of HIT for UFH vs LMWH[b]	Common OR for HIT: UFH vs LMWH			
Female (7)	9.22	3.87	21.97	<0.0001
Male (7)[a]	1.83	0.64	5.23	0.2907
Comparison of the treatment effect of heparin type in females vs the treatment effect in males, $P = 0.0199$				
Surgical (4)	13.93	4.33	44.76	<0.0001
Medical (3)	1.75	0.73	4.22	0.2327
Comparison of the treatment effect of heparin type in surgical vs the treatment effect in medical patients, $P = 0.0054$				
Female/surgical (4)	17.39	4.22	71.70	<0.0001
Female/medical (3)	3.75	1.16	12.17	0.0252
Comparison of the treatment effect of heparin type in female surgical patients vs the treatment effect in female medical patients, $P = 0.1028$				

[a]Studies were pooled across patient type to produce a simple 2 × 2 table; surgical (42/1999) and medical (25/3811), Fisher's exact test (two-sided) P value.
[b]Male/surgical and male/medical not considered due to lack of events.
Source: From Warkentin et al. (2006).
Abbreviations: HIT, heparin-induced thrombocytopenia; UFH, unfractionated heparin; LMWH, low molecular weight heparin.

Warkentin, 2008; Pruthi et al., 2009; Mallik et al., 2011). It is unclear whether the PF4 tetramers are rendered immunogenic by exposure to a polyanionic bacterial surface (Greinacher et al., 2011; Krauel et al., 2011) or to chondroitin sulfates released during surgery or to other unknown mechanisms.

Sometimes, patients with antiphospholipid syndrome develop thrombocytopenia rapidly upon receiving heparin treatment, consistent with pre-existing HIT antibodies associated with their autoimmune diathesis (Martinuzzo et al., 1999; Bourhim et al., 2003). Furthermore, determining the frequency of HIT in patients with antiphospholipid syndrome and/or systemic lupus erythematosus is complicated by the tendency of this patient population to demonstrate false-positive results with HIT antigen testing (Pauzner et al., 2009).

FREQUENCY OF THROMBOSIS COMPLICATING HIT

Ironically, although thrombosis was the first manifestation of the HIT syndrome, first recognized almost 50 years ago (Weismann and Tobin, 1958), widespread recognition that thrombosis was a common complication of HIT did not occur until recently. Indeed, until 1995 no study of HIT had compared the frequency of thrombosis with a matched control population (Warkentin et al., 1995). This study quantitated the strength of the association between HIT and thrombosis and further noted that the more unusual the thrombotic event (e.g., bilateral DVT, pulmonary embolism), the stronger the association with HIT (see chap. 2).

Table 4.6 summarizes the thrombotic events that have been observed during prospective studies of HIT. The major observation is that thrombosis is relatively common in HIT patients, occurring in approximately one-third of medical patients and about half of postoperative surgical patients. The data also support findings from a prior retrospective study (Boshkov et al., 1993) that found the type of thrombotic event complicating HIT was influenced by the patient population. Table 4.6 suggests that the ratio of arterial to venous thrombosis is about 1:1 in medical patients, many of whom might have had arterial disease as their basis for hospitalization. Additionally, the therapeutic dose heparin used in many of these studies may have partially protected against VTE, although it may not have prevented platelet-mediated arterial occlusion. In contrast, there appears to be a strong predisposition to VTE in postoperative orthopedic patients who have developed HIT (venous:arterial ratio at least 14:1).

The retrospective identification of patients with serologically confirmed HIT permits analysis of large groups of HIT patients (Table 4.7). This provides an alternative assessment of the spectrum of thrombotic complications in HIT. Three large studies (Warkentin and Kelton, 1996; Nand et al., 1997; Wallis et al., 1999) showed a predominance of venous thrombosis complicating HIT. Indeed, pulmonary embolism was even more frequent than all types of arterial thromboses combined.

In contrast, a different spectrum of thrombotic complications was reported by investigators at the University of Missouri-Columbia Health Sciences Center (Silver et al., 1983; Laster et al., 1987; Almeida et al., 1998a). Arterial, rather than venous, thromboembolism predominates in these patient series. Because this work is from the perspective of a vascular surgery service, it is possible that patients with arterial thrombosis are either more likely to be recognized as having HIT, or greater numbers of patients with pre-existing arteriopathy are treated with heparin, and thus at a higher risk of developing arterial thrombosis if HIT develops.

Another pattern that emerges from the Missouri series is a progressively decreasing frequency of reported thrombotic or hemorrhagic complications, from 61% in 1983, to 23% in 1987, then to 7.4% in 1998. The authors believe this to be the result of earlier recognition of HIT. However, an alternative explanation could be greater awareness of HIT over time, and thus a higher likelihood of identifying patients with less severe HIT. Indeed, a study by Wallis and colleagues (1999) suggests that earlier recognition of HIT may *not* reduce the risk of thrombosis (Table 4.7).

TABLE 4.6 Proportion of Patients with HIT Developing HIT-Associated Thrombosis in Prospective Studies of Porcine Mucosal UFH Employing *In Vitro* Laboratory Testing

Study	Major indication for heparin	*In Vitro* test	Number treated	Definition of thrombocytopenia ($\times 10^9$/L)	Patients with HIT (Using more sensitive definition of HIT)	Thrombotic complication of HIT Venous	Thrombotic complication of HIT Arterial
Medical patients (therapeutic dose heparin)							
Gallus et al., 1980	VTE	PRP	166	<100	5	1	0
Malcolm et al., 1979	Multiple	PRP	66	<100	1	1	0
Kappers-Klunne et al., 1997	Acute coronary syndromes	HIPA, EIA	358	<120, >30% fall (<60 or >50% fall)	2 (1)	1 (1)	0 (0)
Yamamoto et al., 1996	Hemodialysis	PRP, EIA	154	Clotting, platelet fall	5	0	1
Prandoni et al., 2005	Medical patients	EIA, HIPA	1754	>50% fall	14	2	2
Total medical: venous/arterial thrombosis ratio = 5/3 = 1.7			2498		27	5	3
Medical patients (prophylactic dose heparin)							
Girolami et al., 2003	Prophylaxis	EIA, HIPA	360	>50% fall	5	1	3
Harbrecht et al., 2004	Neurology patients	EIA, HIPA	200	<120 or >50% fall	5	5[a]	2[a]
Total medical: venous/arterial thrombosis ratio = 6/5 = 1.2			560		10	6	5
Orthopedic surgical patients (total joint arthroplasty)							
Warkentin et al., 1995, 2003	Hip	SRA	332	<150 (50% fall)	9 (18)	7 (12)	1 (1)
Warkentin et al., 1998b	Hip, knee	SRA	246	<150, >50%	2	0	0
Ganzer et al., 1997	Hip, knee	HIPA	307	>50% fall	15	5[b]	0
Leyvraz et al., 1991	Hip	PRP	175	<100, >40% fall	2	2	0
Total orthopedic: venous/arterial thrombosis ratio = 14/1 = 14.0			1060	(>50% fall)	28 (37)	14 (19)	1 (1)

Note: Where there was uncertainty over the numbers of patients with HIT, the higher estimated value was indicated in the table, to minimize the bias toward a high frequency of HIT-associated thrombosis (contrast analysis shown in Table 4.2).

[a]Thromboses diagnosed only at autopsy were not included; one stroke due to paradoxical embolism through patent foramen ovale classified as venous thrombosis.

[b]Another five patients developed venous thrombosis in association with a positive HIPA assay, but the platelet count did not fall by >50%.

Abbreviations: ATE, arterial thromboembolism; EIA, PF4/heparin enzyme-linked immunosorbent assay; HIPA, heparin-induced platelet activation test (aggregation of washed platelets); HIT, heparin-induced thrombocytopenia; LMWH, low molecular weight heparin; MI/ACS, myocardial infarction or acute coronary syndromes; PRP, HIT assay using citrated platelet-rich plasma; SRA, serotonin release assay using washed platelets; UFH, unfractionated heparin; VTE, venous thromboembolism.

TABLE 4.7   Frequency of Thrombosis Complicating HIT in Retrospective Studies

Study	Patients with HIT	Mean platelet count nadir ($\times 10^9$/L)	Number of patients with thrombosis No. (%)	Ratio of venous/ arterial thrombosis	Number of deaths no. (%)
Warkentin and Kelton, 1996	127	59[a]	97 (76)	4.3	26 (20)
Subgroup with "isolated" thrombocytopenia	62	57	32 (52)[b]	4	13 (21)
Nand et al., 1997	108	58	32 (29)	2.5	5 (5)[c]
Wallis et al., 1999	113	54	43 (38)	1.4	31 (27)
Subgroup with heparin cessation <48 hr	40	56	18 (45)	1.4	10 (25)
Subgroup with heparin cessation >48 hr	73	54	25 (34)	1.4	21 (29)
Silver et al., 1983	62	Range: 5–83	38 (61)	0.6	20 (32)[d]
Laster et al., 1987	169	57	30 (18)	0.5	20 (12)
Almeida et al., 1998a	94[e]	>108	7 (7)	0.6[f]	0 (0)
Sturtevant et al., 2006	22	39	14 (67)	5.5[g]	7 (32)[h]
Greinacher et al., 2005b	408	41	227 (56)	2.4	Not stated
Mureebe et al., 2004	45	Not stated	Not stated	1.5[i]	10/35 (29)[j]
Murray and Hursting, 2006	6	35	1 (17)	Not stated[k]	3/6 (50)

Note: Where there was uncertainty over the numbers of patients with HIT, the higher estimated value was indicated in the table, to minimize the bias toward a high frequency of HIT-associated thrombosis (contrast analysis shown in Table 4.2).

[a]The mean platelet count nadir for 127 patients with HIT and platelet count <150 × 10^9/L, and the median platelet count nadir for all 142 patients diagnosed with HIT (including those whose platelet count nadir was >150 × 10^9/L), were both 59 × 10^9/L (Warkentin and Kelton, 1996; Warkentin, 1998).

[b]The cumulative 30-day frequency of new thrombosis in patients with isolated thrombocytopenia following recognition of HIT was 52.8% by Kaplan-Meier analysis.

[c]Only deaths in patients who developed thrombosis were reported. Total number of deaths in the HIT cohort was not reported.

[d]Fourteen of the 20 deaths were judged to be caused by HIT-associated thrombosis.

[e]Of 100 consecutive patients with positive *in vitro* testing, six were previously known to have heparin-dependent antibodies and were not subsequently reexposed to heparin.

[f]Two thromboses of arteriovenous grafts were excluded from classification into arterial or venous thrombosis.

[g]Two thromboses on the dialysis membrane were excluded from classification into arterial or venous thrombosis.

[h]In four of the seven deaths, HIT was judged to be contributory.

[i]Thrombosis of temporary (4) or permanent (10) dialysis access excluded from classification into arterial or venous thrombosis.

[j]Complete data available on 35 patients.

[k]Type of thrombosis not stated.

Abbreviation: HIT, heparin-induced thrombocytopenia.

A progressive reduction in HIT-associated mortality over time was also observed by the Missouri group (Table 4.7). However, early discontinuation of heparin was not associated with significantly lower mortality in another study (Wallis et al., 1999). This issue is complicated by the observation that deaths apparently unrelated to thrombosis are relatively common in patients with HIT (Warkentin and Kelton, 1996; Greinacher et al., 1999).

It is possible that nonthrombotic mortality may be higher than expected by chance in patients with HIT. This speculation is based on the observation that only a minority of patients who form anti-PF4/H antibodies develop HIT; a corollary to this statement is that comorbid factors that tend to result in increased pathogenicity of heparin-dependent antibodies may also independently contribute to increased patient morbidity and mortality (i.e., patients with septicemia or multisystem organ failure may be more likely to have platelet activation in the presence of HIT antibodies than "well" patients). Alternatively, because the patients develop thrombocytopenia they are tested for heparin-dependent antibodies, and nonpathogenic antibodies are detected.

ISOLATED HIT

Isolated HIT is defined as the initial recognition of HIT because of thrombocytopenia alone, rather than because symptoms or signs of thrombosis draw attention to the possibility of underlying HIT. Retrospective studies have suggested that the subsequent frequency of new, progressive, or recurrent thrombosis is relatively high in such a patient population with serologically confirmed HIT (Warkentin and Kelton, 1996, Wallis et al., 1999).

This observation was confirmed in a meta-analysis of prospective cohort studies of patients treated for isolated HIT (Warkentin et al., 2008a), which reported a rate of new thrombosis ranging from 15–22% in the historical control arms (i.e., the majority of patients in this group were treated with discontinuation of heparin alone or substitution of heparin with a vitamin K antagonist). This rate was reduced to 4% in patients who were treated with lepirudin, and 7% in patients who were treated with argatroban.

A secondary analysis of patients enrolled in the lepirudin treatment trials mentioned above provided further evidence supporting an unfavorable natural history of untreated HIT (Greinacher et al., 2000). These investigators found that the thrombotic event rate was 6.1% per day during the mean 1.7-day interval between diagnosis of HIT (and cessation of heparin) and initiation of lepirudin therapy. This event rate ($6.1 \times 1.7 = 10.4\%$) corresponds closely to the 10% rate of thrombosis observed in a retrospective Hamilton study in the first 48 hours after diagnosis of isolated HIT with a 30-day cumulative risk of 52.8% (Warkentin and Kelton, 1996) (Fig. 4.5).

A high risk for thrombosis in HIT is also supported by a prospective study (Warkentin et al., 1995), in which five of six HIT patients developed thrombosis either on the first day that their platelet count fell below $150 \times 10^9/L$ or within the next few days despite the discontinuation of heparin.

Wallis and colleagues (1999) from Loyola University confirmed the high risk for thrombosis among patients in whom HIT is identified by platelet count monitoring, even with discontinuation of heparin (Table 4.7). Overall, the 30-day thrombotic event rate was 43/113 (38%), with a ratio of venous to arterial thrombosis of just 1.4. The relatively low predominance of venous thrombosis could be explained by the

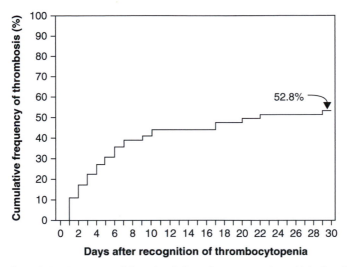

FIGURE 4.5 Cumulative frequency of thrombosis in patients presenting with isolated HIT ($n = 62$). Approximately 50% of HIT patients initially recognized with isolated HIT developed objective evidence for thrombosis during the subsequent 30-day period. The 1- and 2-day thrombotic event rates were approximately 10% and 18%, respectively. About 5% (3/62) patients developed sudden death as their presenting thrombotic event. *Abbreviation*: HIT, heparin-induced thrombocytopenia. *Source*: From Warkentin and Kelton (1996).

large number of patients (59%) in this study who developed HIT following cardiac surgery (i.e., a patient population had relatively high risk for arterial thrombosis).

An intriguing finding of the Wallis report is that early cessation of heparin did not appear to improve clinical outcomes. For 40 of the 113 patients with HIT (35%), heparin was discontinued within 48 hours of onset of thrombocytopenia (defined as a platelet count fall to less than $100 \times 10^9/L$, or a greater than 50% fall from the peak platelet count after initiating heparin). Indeed, there was a trend to a *higher* rate of thrombosis in the patients with early heparin cessation, compared with the remaining 65% of patients in whom heparin was stopped later (45% *vs* 34%; $P = 0.26$) (Table 4.7).

Taken together, these studies provide the basis for the recommendation that alternative anticoagulant therapy (in therapeutic doses) is appropriate for most patients strongly suspected (or confirmed) to have isolated HIT (Hirsh et al., 2001; Warkentin et al., 2008a; Linkins et al., 2012) (see chap. 12). Other data to support this concept include the high probability of detecting subclinical DVT by duplex ultrasonography in patients with isolated HIT (Tardy et al., 1999), as well as the persistence of marked *in vivo* thrombin generation for several days in patients with acute HIT even following discontinuation of heparin (Warkentin et al., 1997; Greinacher et al., 2000).

Key Points
1. The risk of thrombosis in patients with HIT is higher than previously recognized (up to 50%), and remains high despite the discontinuation of heparin.

Mortality in patients with HIT is significant, although it remains uncertain what proportion is related to HIT-associated thrombosis, and to what extent these can be prevented by effective treatment.

2. Most thrombotic events are venous, rather than arterial, although this predominance may not be observed in patient populations at high risk for arterial disease. Pulmonary embolism appears to be the most frequent life-threatening consequence of HIT.

POPULATION-BASED STUDIES OF HIT ANTIBODY SEROCONVERSION

Usually, serologic investigation for HIT antibodies is performed on patients who develop thrombocytopenia during heparin treatment. Since 1995, however, many studies have systematically assessed heparin-dependent antibody seroconversion using sensitive assays (EIA, SRA, or both), irrespective of whether or not thrombocytopenia occurred. Some interesting insights into the pathogenesis of HIT have emerged from these reports.

Table 4.8 shows the results of prospective studies which (*i*) systematically screened for HIT antibodies using a sensitive assay, and (*ii*) enrolled more than 100 patients. Three main types of patient population have been investigated: medical patients receiving therapeutic-dose UFH, LMWH, or fondaparinux; orthopedic patients receiving UFH or LMWH; and cardiac surgical patients receiving UFH or LMWH. There appear to be distinct frequencies of HIT antibody formation, as well as varying risks of "breakthrough" of HIT, among these different populations. Several observations emerge from these studies:

1. The prevalence of seroconversion depends on the diagnostic assay used. The PF4/H EIA is more sensitive than the SRA for the detection of anti-PF4/H antibodies (Pouplard et al., 1999; Warkentin et al., 2000, 2005b; Warkentin and Sheppard, 2006a); however, this increase in sensitivity does not necessarily translate into greater predictive value for clinical HIT (see chap. 11).

2. With use of PF4/polyanion EIA, the frequency of seroconversion after cardiac surgery ranges to as high as about 75% (Visentin et al., 1996; Warkentin et al., 2000; Warkentin and Sheppard, 2006a). A high frequency of seroconversion (13–20%) was also observed using the SRA. Despite the highest frequency of HIT seroconversion reported in this patient population, the likelihood of developing HIT appears to be less than in orthopedic patients treated with postoperative UFH.

3. Seroconversion occurs frequently without thrombocytopenia or thrombosis. Indeed, few patients who form anti-PF4/H antibodies develop HIT. The proportion who develop HIT, however, is highest among the patients who have a positive SRA. This suggests that HIT antibodies "strong" enough to activate platelets are more likely to be clinically significant. Patient-dependent factors also must be important, however, because the probability of a positive SRA indicating clinical HIT ranges from about <10% (cardiac surgery) to approximately 50% (orthopedic surgery patients receiving UFH).

4. Regardless of which diagnostic assay is used, new seroconversion occurs more frequently after exposure to UFH than LMWH (Warkentin et al., 1995, 2000, 2003, 2005b; Ahmad et al., 2003b) (Fig. 4.1).

TABLE 4.8 Studies Describing Systematic Screening for HIT Antibodies Using Sensitive Assays in Patients Receiving Heparin

Study	Trial design	Heparin	Number of patients	HIT assay used	Patients with anti-PF4/H antibodies (%)	Patients with HIT, n (%)
Medical patients						
Kappers-Klunne et al., 1997	Prospective	iv ther UFH	358	EIA-IgG	9 (2.5)	2 (0.6)
				HIPA	30 (8.4)	0 (0)
Harbrecht et al., 2004	Prospective	iv ther, sc proph UFH	200	EIA-IgG/A/M	41 (20.5)[a]	5 (2.5)
Pohl et al., 2005	Prospective	sc proph LMWH	111	EIA-IgG/A/M	2/111 (1.8)	0 (0)
Kawano et al., 2011	Prospective	iv ther, sc proph UFH	172	EIA-IgG/A/M	22/172 (12.8)	3 (1.7)
Hemodialysis patients						
Greinacher et al., 1996	Prevalence study	iv ther UFH	165	HIPA	7 (4.2)	0 (0)
Boon et al., 1996	Prevalence study	iv ther UFH	128	EIA-IgG/M	4 (3.1)	0 (0)[b]
				EIA-IgG	3 (2.3)	
		LMWH	133	EIA-IgG/M	1 (0.8)	0 (0)[c]
				EIA-IgG	1 (0.8)	
Yu et al., 2002	Prevalence study	iv ther UFH	100	EIA-IgG/A/M	6 (6.0)	0 (0)
Palomo et al., 2005	Prevalence study	iv ther UFH	207	EIA-IgG/A/M	37 (17.9)[d]	Not stated
Nakamoto et al., 2005	Prevalence study	iv ther UFH	105	EIA	2 (1.9)	Not stated
Carrier et al., 2007	Prevalence study	iv ther UFH	419	EIA-IgG/A/M	54 (12.9)	Not stated
				EIA-IgG	9 (2.1)	
				SRA	0 (0)	
Cardiac patients						
Yeh et al., 2006[e]	Prospective	iv ther UFH	311	EIA-IgG/A/M	25 (8.0)	Not stated
Foo et al., 2006[e]	Prospective	iv ther UFH	357	EIA-IgG/A/M	36 (10.1)	Not stated
Matsuo et al., 2005	Prospective	iv ther UFH	252[f]	EIA	22 (8.7)[f]	4 (1.6)

(Continued)

TABLE 4.8 (*Continued*) Studies Describing Systematic Screening for HIT Antibodies Using Sensitive Assays in Patients Receiving Heparin

Study	Trial design	Heparin	Number of patients	HIT assay used	Patients with anti-PF4/H antibodies (%)	Patients with HIT, n (%)
Orthopedic postoperative surgical patients						
Warkentin et al., 1995, 2000	Substudy of RCT	sc proph UFH	205	EIA-IgG SRA	29 (14.1) 19 (9.3)	10 (4.9)
		sc proph LMWH	182	EIA-IgG SRA	11 (6.0) 5 (2.7)[g]	2(1.1)
Marx et al., 1999	Prospective	sc proph LMWH	265	EIA	13 (4.9)[h]	0 (0)
Warkentin et al., 2000	Prospective	sc proph LMWH	257	EIA-IgG SRA	22 (8.6) 9 (3.5)[g]	2 (0.8)
Warkentin et al., 2005b	Substudy of RCT	sc proph LMWH	1349	EIA-IgG/A/M EIA-IgG SRA	30 (2.2) 6 (0.4) 1 (0.1)	0(0)
		sc proph fondaparinux	1377	EIA-IgG/A/M EIA-IgG SRA	26 (1.9) 9 (0.7) 3 (0.2)	0 (0)
Greinacher et al., 2005a	Prospective	sc proph UFH	231	EIA-IgG/A/M HIPA	46 (23.5) 25 (12.4)	12 (5.2)
		sc proph LMWH	271	EIA-IgG/A/M HIPA	19 (8.3) 13 (5.5)	0 (0)
Cardiac postoperative surgical patients (all received porcine UFH at cardiopulmonary bypass)						
Pouplard et al., 1999	Prospective	sc proph UFH	157	EIA-IgG/A/M EIA-IgG SRA	46 (29.3) 24 (15.3) 6 (3.8)	6 (3.8)
		sc proph LMWH	171	EIA-IgG/A/M EIA-IgG SRA	37 (21.6) 24 (14.0) 2 (1.2)	0 (0)
Warkentin et al., 2000	Prospective	CPB: UFH; sc proph UFH	100	EIA-IgG SRA	50 (50.0) 20 (20.0)	1 (1.0)

Koster et al., 2003	Prospective	CPB; VAD: UFH	100	EIA-IgG/A/M	63 (63)	Not stated
Francis et al., 2003	RCT	CPB: porcine UFH	108	EIA-IgG/A/M	33 (30.6)[i]	0 (0)
Screening precardiac surgery						
Bennett-Guerrero et al., 2005	Prospective	Previous UFH exposure	466	EIA-IgG/A/M	59 (12.7)	Not stated
Trauma patients						
Lubenow et al., 2010	RCT	sc proph UFH	316	EIA and HIPA	21 (6.6)	4 (1.3)
		sc proph LMWH	298		5 (1.7)	1 (0.3)

[a] HIPA positive in 3/41 (7.3%) of EIA-positive sera.

[b] Results of platelet aggregation testing are not included since there was a false-positive rate of 33% in control uremic patients not yet exposed to heparin.

[c] Two patients with HIT antibodies had mild thrombocytopenia, but a causal relation to heparin was not stated.

[d] Twelve of 22 EIA positive sera also tested positive by SRA

[e] Yeh et al. (2006) and Foo et al. (2006) describe similar inception cohorts with a baseline prevalence of HIT-Ig of 15/500 (3.0%).

[f] Of patients undergoing PCI, 20/163 (12.3%) were EIA-positive; Of the non-PCI patients, 2/89 (2.2%) were EIA-positive; 22/252 represents new seroconversions [2/254 (0.8%) EIA-positive at baseline].

[g] Twenty percent serotonin release used in the study by Warkentin et al. (2000), rather than 50% serotonin release cutoff used in the study by Warkentin et al. (1995).

[h] Ten of 265 (3.8%) were found to have HIT-Ig prior to surgery.

[i] Excludes patients testing positive for HIT antibodies at baseline.

Abbreviations: CPB, cardiopulmonary bypass; EIA, PF4/heparin enzyme-linked immunosorbent assay (–IgG/A/M, one or more of IgG, IgA, and IgM antibodies present; –IgG, IgG antibodies only present); HIPA, heparin-induced platelet activation assay; HIT, heparin-induced thrombocytopenia; iv ther, intravenous therapeutic-dose heparin; LMWH, low molecular weight heparin; MI, myocardial infarction; NPH, no postoperative heparin; PCI, percutaneous coronary intervention; PRP, HIT assay using citrated platelet-rich plasma; RCT, randomized controlled trial; sc proph, subcutaneous prophylactic dose heparin; SRA, serotonin release assay using washed platelets; UFH, unfractionated heparin; VAD, ventricular assist device; VTE, venous thromboembolism.

Adverse Prognosis of Anti-PF4/H Antibodies

A controversial issue is whether anti-PF4/H antibodies confer adverse prognosis even in the absence of clinically overt HIT. Mattioli and coworkers (2000) found a higher 1 year event-rate (death, MI, recurrent angina, revascularization, or stroke) among patients who formed anti-PF4/H antibodies after UFH treatment for unstable angina (66% vs 44%; $P < 0.01$). Williams and colleagues (2003), using blood samples obtained 48 hours after entry into a clinical trial of non–ST-segment elevation MI, found that death or MI was increased at 1 month (OR, 4.0; $P = 0.0093$) among patients with a positive anti-PF4/polyanion EIA. Finally, Carrier and colleagues (2008) found an association between anti-PF4/H antibodies and all-cause mortality in a prospective cohort study of chronic HD patients. In none of these studies did clinically evident HIT appear to explain these differences. However, a recent systematic review of patients undergoing cardiac surgery did not support an association between thromboembolic complications and death in patients documented to have preoperative anti-PF4/H antibodies (Yusuf et al., 2012).

Despite the implication that these antibodies might be pathogenic, an alternative view is that unrecognized confounders explain their apparent adverse prognosis. For example, these antibodies could represent a *surrogate marker* for another key risk factor, such as inflammation—a known risk factor for atherosclerosis-associated mortality (Ridker et al., 1997). This distinction is critical: if these antibodies are truly pathogenic ("forme fruste HIT"), avoiding heparin might be beneficial, whereas this is unlikely to be the case if the antibodies are merely a marker for other vascular risk factors (Warkentin and Sheppard, 2006b).

NONIMMUNE THROMBOCYTOPENIA

The distinction between thrombocytopenia that begins early (within four days) or late (five or more days after beginning heparin treatment) is a simple clinical feature that is useful to distinguish nonimmune heparin-associated thrombocytopenia (HAT), which begins early, from (immune) HIT, which begins late. For this assessment, the first day of heparin use is considered day 0. There is an important exception to this rule of timing for HIT: a rapid fall in platelet count on starting heparin therapy can represent acute HIT, but only if a patient already has circulating HIT antibodies, usually the result of a recent heparin exposure. HIT antibodies are transient, which could explain why the risk for rapid-onset HIT is restricted to a period of about 100 days following exposure to heparin (Warkentin and Kelton, 2001) (see chap. 2).

Typically, nonimmune HAT begins one to two days after starting heparin administration and resolves during continued heparin therapy (Johnson et al., 1984; Chong and Berndt, 1989; Warkentin and Kelton, 1994; Greinacher, 1995; Warkentin et al., 1995). The platelet count fall is usually mild, with a nadir between 75 and $150 \times 10^9/L$. This early platelet count fall may be the result of a direct activating effect of heparin on platelets (Chong and Castaldi, 1986; Chong and Ismail, 1989) or of comorbid clinical factors.

Early nonimmune HAT occurs in up to 30% of patients receiving heparin (Bell et al., 1976; Nelson et al., 1978; Warkentin et al., 1995). Systematic serologic investigation of patients with early thrombocytopenia was performed in one study comparing UFH with LMWH for postoperative antithrombotic prophylaxis in patients who underwent hip replacement surgery (Warkentin et al., 1995). With $150 \times 10^9/L$

as a platelet count threshold, early thrombocytopenia was observed in 189/665 (28%) patients; however, HIT antibodies were not detected in any of the 98 patients tested, and platelet count recovery to more than $150 \times 10^9/L$ within three days occurred despite continuing the heparin. No difference in the frequency of early thrombocytopenia was observed between patients who received UFH (28%) and those who received LMWH (29%). This suggests that unrelated clinical factors, such as perioperative hemodilution with fluid and blood products, were primarily responsible. In contrast, the onset of late thrombocytopenia (i.e., between days 5 and 10 of heparin treatment) was strongly associated with the formation of heparin-dependent platelet-activating antibodies and occurred significantly more frequently in the patients who received UFH.

ACKNOWLEDGMENTS

Studies described in this chapter were supported by grants from the Heart and Stroke Foundation of Ontario. Dr. Linkins was supported by New Investigator Career Award from the Heart and Stroke Foundation of Canada.

REFERENCES

Ahmad S, Bacher P, Lassen MR, Hoppensteadt DA, Leitz H, Misselwitz F, Walenga JM, Fareed J. Investigations of the immunoglobulin subtype transformation of anti-heparin-platelet factor 4 antibodies during treatment with a low molecular weight heparin (Clivarin) in orthopedic patients. Arch Pathol Lab Med 127: 584–588, 2003a.

Ahmad S, Haas S, Hoppensteadt DA, Lietz H, Reid U, Bender N, Messmore HL, Misselwitz F, Bacher P, Gaikwad BS, Jeske WP, Walenga JM, Fareed J. Differential effects of clivarin and heparin in patients undergoing hip and knee surgery for the generation of anti-heparin-platelet factor 4 antibodies. Thromb Res 108: 49–55, 2003b.

Almeida JI, Coats R, Liem TK, Silver D. Reduced morbidity and mortality rates of the heparin-induced thrombocytopenia syndrome. J Vasc Surg 27: 309–316, 1998a.

Almeida JI, Liem TK, Silver D. Heparin-bonded grafts induce platelet aggregation in the presence of heparin-associated antiplatelet antibodies. J Vasc Surg 27: 896–901, 1998b.

Anderson GP. Insights into heparin-induced thrombocytopenia. Br J Haematol 80: 504–508, 1992.

Barradas MA, Mikhailidis DP, Epemolu O, Jeremy JY, Fonseca V, Dandona P. Comparison of the platelet proaggregatory effect of conventional unfractionated heparins and a low molecular weight heparin fraction (CY 222). Br J Haematol 67: 451–457, 1987.

Bell WR, Tomasulo PA, Alving BM, Duffy TP. Thrombocytopenia occurring during the administration of heparin. A prospective study in 52 patients. Ann Intern Med 85: 155–160, 1976.

Bennett-Guerrero E, Slaughter TF, White WD, Welsby IJ, Greenberg CS, El-Moalem H, Ortel TL. Preoperative anti-PF4/heparin antibody level predicts adverse outcome after cardiac surgery. J Thorac Cardiovasc Surg 130: 1567–1572, 2005.

Boon DMS, van Vliet HHDM, Zietse R, Kappers-Klunne MC. The presence of antibodies against a PF4–heparin complex in patients on haemodialysis. Thromb Haemost 76: 480, 1996.

Borowiec J, Thelin S, Bagge L, Hultman J, Hansson H-E. Decreased blood loss after cardiopulmonary bypass using heparin-coated circuit and 50% reduction of heparin dose. Scand J Thorac Cardiovasc Surg 26: 177–185, 1992a.

Borowiec J, Thelin S, Bagge L, Nilsson L, Venge P, Hansson HE. Heparin-coated circuits reduce activation of granulocytes during cardiopulmonary bypass. A clinical study. J Thorac Cardiovasc Surg 104: 642–667, 1992b.

Borowiec JW, Bylock A, van der Linden J, Thelin S. Heparin coating reduces blood cell adhesion to arterial filters during coronary bypass: a clinical study. Ann Thorac Surg 55: 1540–1545, 1993.

Boshkov LK, Warkentin TE, Hayward CPM, Andrew M, Kelton JG. Heparin-induced thrombocytopenia and thrombosis: clinical and laboratory studies. Br J Haematol 84: 322–328, 1993.

Bouman CS, Oudemans-Van Straaten HM, Tijssen JG, Zandstra DF, Kesecioglu J. Effects of early high-volume continuous venovenous hemofiltration on survival and recovery of renal function in intensive care patients with acute renal failure: a prospective, randomized trial. Crit Care Med 30: 2205–2011, 2002.

Bourhim M, Darnige L, Legallais C, Arvieux J, Cevallos R, Pouplard C, Vijayalakshmi MA. Anti-β_2-glycoprotein I antibodies recognizing platelet factor 4–heparin complex in antiphospholipid syndrome in patient substantiated with mouse model. J Molec Recognit 16: 125–130, 2003.

Brushwood DB. Hospital liable for allergic reaction to heparin used in injection flush. Am J Hosp Pharm 49: 1491–1492, 1992.

Büller HR, Davidson BL, Decousus H, Gallus A, Gent M, Piovella F, Prins MH, Raskob G, van den Berg-Segers AE, Cariou R, Leeuwenkamp O, Lensing AW. Matisse investigators. subcutaneous fondaparinux versus intravenous unfractionated heparin in the initial treatment of pulmonary embolism. N Engl J Med 349: 1695–1702, 2003.

Büller HR, Davidson BL, Decousus H, Gallus A, Gent M, Piovella F, Prins MH, Raskob G, Segers AE, Cariou R, Leeuwenkamp O, Lensing AW. Matisse investigators. fondaparinux or enoxaparin for the initial treatment of symptomatic deep venous thrombosis: a randomized trial. Ann Intern Med 140: 867–873, 2004.

Carrier M, Knoll GA, Kovacs MJ, Moore JC, Fergusson D, Rodger MA. The prevalence of antibodies to the platelet factor 4–heparin complex and association with access thrombosis in patients on chronic hemodialysis. Thromb Res 120: 215–220, 2007.

Carrier M, Rodger MA, Fergusson D, Doucette S, Kovacs MJ, Moore J, Kelton JG, Knoll GA. Increased mortality in hemodialysis patients having specific antibodies to the platelet factor 4–heparin complex. Kidney Int 73: 213–219, 2008.

Casu B, Johnson EA, Mantovani M, Mulloy B, Oreste P, Pescador R, Prino G, Torri G, Zoppetti G. Correlation between structure, fat-clearing and anticoagulant properties of heparins and heparin sulphates. Arzneimittal, forschung Drug Res 33: 135–142, 1983.

Chong BH, Berndt MC. Heparin-induced thrombocytopenia. Blut 58: 53–57, 1989.

Chong BH, Castaldi PA. Platelet proaggregating effect of heparin: possible mechanism for nonimmune heparin-associated thrombocytopenia. Aust NZ J Med 16: 715–716, 1986.

Chong BH, Ismail F. The mechanism of heparin-induced platelet aggregation. Eur J Haematol 43: 245–251, 1989.

Cipolle RJ, Rodvoid KA, Seifert R, Clarens R, Ramirez-Lassepas M. Heparin-associated thrombocytopenia: a prospective evaluation of 211 patients. Ther Drug Monit 5: 205–211, 1983.

Cook D; PROTECT Investigators for the Canadian Critical Care Trials Group and the Australian and New Zealand Intensive Care Society Clinical Trials Group. Dalteparin versus unfractionated heparin in critically ill patients. N Engl J Med 364: 1305–1314, 2011.

Crowther MA, Cook DJ, Albert M, Williamson D, Meade M, Granton J, Skrobik Y, Langevin S, Mehta S, Hebert P, Guyatt GH, Geerts W, Rabbat C, Douketis J, Zytaruk N, Sheppard J, Greinacher A, Warkentin TE; Canadian Critical Care Trials Group. The 4Ts scoring system for heparin-induced thrombocytopenia in medical-surgical intensive care unit patients. J Crit Care 25: 287–293, 2010.

Doty JR, Alving BM, McDonnell DE, Ondra SL. Heparin-associated thrombocytopenia in the neurosurgical patient. Neurosurgery 19: 69–72, 1986.

Eldh P, Jacobsson B. Heparinized vascular catheters: a clinical trial. Radiology 111: 289–292, 1974.

Elgue G, Blomback M, Olsson P, Riesenfeld J. On the mechanism of coagulation inhibition on surfaces with end point immobilized heparin. Thromb Haemost 70: 289–293, 1993.

Ellison J, Walker ID, Greer IA. Antenatal use of enoxaparin for prevention and treatment of thromboembolism in pregnancy. BJOG 107: 1116–1121, 2000.

Fausett MB, Vogtlander M, Lee RM, Esplin MS, Branch DW, Rodgers GM, Silver RM. Heparin-induced thrombocytopenia is rare in pregnancy. Am J Obstet Gynecol 185: 148–152, 2001.

Follea G, Hamandijan I, Trzeciak MC, Nedey C, Streichenberger R, Dechavanne M. Pentosane polysulfate associated thrombocytopenia. Thromb Res 42: 413–418, 1986.

Foo SY, Everett BM, Yeh RW, Criss D, Laposata M, Van Cott EM, Jang IK. Prevalence of heparin-induced thrombocytopenia in patients undergoing cardiac catheterization. Am Heart J 152: 290. e1–7, 2006.

Francis JL, Palmer GJ, Moroose R, Drexler A. Comparison of bovine and porcine heparin in heparin antibody formation after cardiac surgery. Ann Thorac Surg 75: 17–22, 2003.

Gallus AS, Goodall KT, Beswick W, Chesterman CN. Heparin-associated thrombocyto-penia: case report and prospective study. Aust NZ J Med 10: 25–31, 1980.

Ganzer D, Gutezeit A, Mayer G, Greinacher A, Eichler P. Thromboembolieprophylaxe als ausloser thrombembolischer Komplicationen. Eine Untersuchung zur inzidenz der heparin-induzierten thrombozytopenie (HIT) typ II. Z Orthop 135: 543–549, 1997.

Ganzer D, Gutezeit A, Mayer G. Gefahrenpotentiale in der medikamentösen Thromboseprophylaxe-Niedermolekuläre Heparine versus Standardheparin. Z Othop Ihre Grenzget 137: 457–461, 1999.

Geerts WH, Jay RM, Code KI, Chen E, Szalai JP, Saibil EA, Hamilton PA. A comparison of low-dose heparin with low molecular weight heparin as prophylaxis against venous thromboembolism after major trauma. N Engl J Med 335: 701–707, 1996.

Gettings EM, Brush KA, Van Cott EM, Hurford WE. Outcome of postoperative critically ill patients with heparin-induced thrombocytopenia: an observational retrospective case-control study. Crit Care 10. R161, 2006.

Girolami B, Prandoni P, Stefani PM, Tanduo C, Sabbion P, Eichler P, Ramon R, Baggio G, Fabris F, Girolami A. The incidence of heparin induced thrombocytopenia in hospitalized medical patients treated with subcutaneous unfractionated heparin: a prospective cohort study. Blood 101: 2955–2959, 2003.

Glock Y, Szmil E, Boudjema B, Boccalon H, Fournial G, Cerene AL, Puel P. Cardiovascular surgery and heparin-induced thrombocytopenia. Int Angiol 7: 238–245, 1988.

Gluckman TJ, Segal JB, Fredde NL, Saland KE, Jani JT, Walenga JM, Prechel MM, Citro KM, Zidar DA, Fox E, Schulman SP, Kickler TS, Rade JJ. Incidence of antiplatelet factor 4/heparin antibody induction in patients undergoing percutaneous coronary revascularization. Am J Cardiol 95: 744–747, 2005.

Goad KE, Horne MK III, Gralnick HR. Pentosan-induced thrombocytopenia: support for an immune complex mechanism. Br J Haematol 88: 803–808, 1994.

Gouault-Heilman M, Payen D, Contant G, Intrator L, Huet Y, Schaeffer A. Thrombocytopenia related to synthetic heparin analogue therapy. Thromb Haemost 54: 557, 1985.

Greer IA, Nelson-Piercy C. Low molecular weight heparins for thromboprophylaxis and treatment of venous thromboembolism in pregnancy: a systematic review of safety and efficacy. Blood 106: 401–407, 2005.

Greinacher A. Antigen generation in heparin-associated thrombocytopenia: the non-immunologic type and the immunologic type are closely linked in their pathogenesis. Semin Thromb Hemostas 21: 106–116, 1995.

Greinacher A, Warkentin TE. Contaminated heparin. N Engl J Med 359: 1291–1292, 2008.

Greinacher A, Drost W, Michels I, Leitl J, Gottsmann M, Kohl HG, Glaser M, Mueller-Eckhardt C. Heparin-associated thrombocytopenia successfully treated with the heparinoid org 10172 in a patient showing cross-reaction to LMW heparins. Ann Haematol 64: 40–42, 1992a.

Greinacher A, Michels I, Muller-Eckardt C. Heparin-associated thrombocytopenia: the antibody is not heparin-specific. Thromb Haemost 67: 545–549, 1992b.

Greinacher A, Michels I, Schafer M, Kiefel V, Muller-Eckhardt C. Heparin-associated thrombocytopenia in a patient treated with polysulphated chondroitin sulphate: evidence for immunological crossreactivity between heparin and polysulphated glycosaminoglycan. Br J Haematol 81: 252–254, 1992c.

Greinacher A, Alban S, Dummel V, Franz G, Mueller-Eckhardt C. Characterization of the structural requirements for a carbohydrate based anticoagulant with a reduced risk of inducing the immunological type of heparin-associated thrombocytopenia. Thromb Haemost 74: 886–892, 1995.

Greinacher A, Zinn S, Wizemann Birk UW. Heparin-induced antibodies as a risk factor for thromboembolism and haemorrhage in patients undergoing chronic haemodialysis. Lancet 348: 764, 1996.

Greinacher A, Völpel H, Janssens U, Hach-Wunderle V, Kemkes-Matthes B, Eichler P, Mueller-Velten HG, Pötzsch B. Recombinant hirudin (lepirudin) provides effective and safe anticoagulation in patients with the immunologic type of heparin-induced thrombocytopenia. Circulation 99: 73–80, 1999.

Greinacher A, Eichler P, Lubenow N, Kwasny H, Luz M. Heparin-induced thrombocytopenia with thromboembolic complications: meta-analysis of 2 prospective trials to assess the value of parenteral treatment with lepirudin and its therapeutic aPTT range. Blood 96: 846–851, 2000.

Greinacher A, Eichler P, Lietz T, Warkentin TE. Replacement of unfractionated heparin by low molecular weight heparin for postorthopedic surgery antithrombotic prophylaxis lowers the overall risk of symptomatic thrombosis because of a lower frequency of heparin-induced thrombocytopenia. Blood 106: 2921–2922, 2005a.

Greinacher A, Farner B, Kroll H, Kohlmann T, Warkentin TE, Eichler P. Clinical features of heparin-induced thrombocytopenia including risk factors for thrombosis. a retrospective analysis of 408 patients. Thromb Haemost 94: 132–135, 2005b.

Greinacher A, Juhl D, Strobel U, Wessel A, Lubenow N, Selleng K, Eichler P, Warkentin TE. Heparin-induced thrombocytopenia: a prospective study on the incidence, platelet-activating capacity and clinical significance of anti-PF4/heparin antibodies of the IgG, IgM, and IgA classes. J Thromb Haemost 5: 1666–1673, 2007.

Greinacher A, Alban S, Omer-Adam MA, Weitschies W, Warkentin TE. Heparin-induced thrombocytopenia: a stoichiometry-based model to explain the differing immunogenicities of unfractionated heparin, low molecular weight heparin, and fondaparinux in different clinical settings. Thromb Res 122: 211–220, 2008.

Greinacher A, Holtfreter B, Krauel K, Gätke D, Weber C, Itterman T, Hammerschmidt S, Kocher T. Association of natural anti-platelet factor 4/heparin antibodies with periodontal disease. Blood 118: 1395–1410, 2011.

Harbrecht U, Bastians B, Kredteck A, Hanfland P, Klockgether T, Pohl C. Heparin-induced thrombocytopenia in neurologic disease treated with unfractionated heparin. Neurology 62: 657–659, 2004.

Heeger PS, Backstrom JT. Heparin flushes and thrombocytopenia. Ann Intern Med 105: 143, 1986.

Hirsh J, Warkentin TE, Shaughnessy SG, Anand SS, Halperin JL, Raschke R, Granger C, Ohman Em, Dalen JE. Heparin and low molecular weight heparin. Mechanisms of action, pharmacokinetics, dosing, monitoring, efficacy, and safety. Chest 119(Suppl): 64S–94S, 2001.

Hoh BL, Aghi M, Pryor JC, Ogilvy CS. Heparin-induced thrombocytopenia Type II in subarachnoid hemorrhage patients: incidence and complications. Neurosurgery 57: 243–248, 2005.

Jay RM, Warkentin TE. Fatal heparin-induced thrombocytopenia (HIT) during warfarin thromboprophylaxis following orthopedic surgery: another example of 'spontaneous' HIT? J Thromb Haemost 6: 1598–1600, 2008.

Johnson RA, Lazarus KH, Henry DH. Heparin-induced thrombocytopenia: a prospective study. Am J Hematol 17: 349–353, 1984.

Kannan M, Ahmad S, Ahmad F, Kale S, Hoppensteadt DA, Fareed J, Saxena R. Functional characterization of antibodies against heparin-platelet factor 4 complex in heparin-induced thrombocytopenia patients in Asian-Indians: relevance to inflammatory markers. Blood Coagul Fibrinolysis 16: 487–490, 2005.

Kappa JR, Fisher CA, Berkowitz HD, Cottrell ED, Addonizio VP Jr. Heparin-induced platelet activation in sixteen surgical patients: diagnosis and management. J Vasc Surg 5: 101–109, 1987.

Kappers-Klunne MC, Boon DMS, Hop WCJ, Michiels JJ, Stibbe J, van der Zwaan C, Koudstaal PJ, van Vliet HHDM. Heparin-induced thrombocytopenia and thrombosis: a prospective analysis of the incidence in patients with heart and cerebrovascular diseases. Br J Haematol 96: 442–446, 1997.

Kawano H, Yamamoto H, Miyata S, Izumi M, Hirano T, Toratani N, Kakutani I, Sheppard JA, Warkentin TE, Kada A, Sato S, Okamoto S, Nagatsuka K, Naritomi H, Toyoda K, Uchino M, Minematsu K. Prospective multicentre cohort study of heparin-induced thrombocytopenia in acute ischaemic stroke patients. Br J Haematol 154: 378–386, 2011.

Klenner AF, Fusch C, Rakow A, Kadow I, Beyersdorff E, Eichler P, Wander K, Lietz T, Greinacher A. Benefit and risk of heparin for maintaining peripheral venous catheters in neonates: a placebo-controlled trial. J Pediatr 143: 741–745, 2003.

Koster A, Loebe M, Sodian R, Potapov EV, Hansen R, Muller J, Mertzlufft F, Crystal GJ, Kuppe H, Hetzer R. Heparin antibodies and thromboembolism in heparin-coated and noncoated ventricular assist devices. J Thorac Cardiovasc Surg 121: 331–335, 2001.

Koster A, Huebler S, Potapov E, Meyer O, Jurmann M, Weng Y, Pasic M, Drews T, Kuppe H, Loebe M, Hetzer R. Impact of heparin-induced thrombocytopenia on outcome in patients with ventricular assist device support: single-institution experience in 358 consecutive patients. Ann Thorac Surg 83: 72–76, 2007.

Koul B, Vesterqvist O, Egberg N, Steen S. Twenty-four-hour heparin-free veno-right ventricular ECMO: an experimental study. Ann Thorac Surg 53: 1046–1051, 1992.

Krauel K, Pötschke C, Weber C, Kessler W, Fürll B, Ittermann T, Maier S, Hammerschmidt S, Bröker BM, Greinacher A. Platelet factor 4 binds to bacteria, [corrected] inducing antibodies cross-reacting with the major antigen in heparin-induced thrombocytopenia. Blood 117: 1370–1378, 2011.

Larm O, Larsson R, Olsson P. A new non-thrombogenic surface prepared by selective covalent binding of heparin via a modified reducing terminal residue. Biomater Med Devices Artif Organs 11: 161–173, 1983.

Larsson R, Larm O, Olsson P. The search for thromboresistance using immobilized heparin. Ann NY Acad Sci 516: 102–115, 1987.

Laster J, Silver D. Heparin-coated catheters and heparin-induced thrombocytopenia. J Vasc Surg 7: 667–672, 1988.

Laster J, Cikrit D, Walker N, Silver D. The heparin-induced thrombocytopenia syndrome: an update. Surgery 102: 763–770, 1987.

Lee DH, Warkentin TE. Frequency of heparin-induced thrombocytopenia. In: Warkentin TE, Greinacher A, eds. Heparin-Induced Thrombocytopenia, 4th edn. New York, NY: Informa Healthcare USA, 67–116, 2007.

Leizorovicz A, Cohen AT, Turpie AG, Olsson CG, Vaitkus PT, Goldhaber SZ; PREVENT Medical Thromboprophylaxis Study Group. Randomized, placebo-controlled trial of dalteparin for the prevention of venous thromboembolism in acutely ill medical patients. Circulation 110: 874–879, 2004.

Lepercq J, Conard J, Borel-Derlon A, Darmon JY, Boudignat O, Francoual C, Priollet P, Cohen C, Yvelin N, Schved JF, Tournaire M, Borg JY. Venous thromboembolism during pregnancy: a retrospective study of enoxaparin safety in 624 pregnancies. BJOG 108: 1134–1140, 2001.

Leyvraz PF, Bachmann F, Hoek J, Biiller HR, Postel M, Samama M, Vandenbroek MD. Prevention of deep vein thrombosis after hip replacement: randomised comparison between unfractionated heparin and low molecular weight heparin. Br Med J 303: 543–548, 1991.

Lindhoff-Last E, Nakov R, Misselwitz F, Breddin HK, Bauersachs R. Incidence and clinical relevance of heparin-induced antibodies in patients with deep vein thrombosis treated with unfractionated or low molecular weight heparin. Br J Haematol 118: 1137–1142, 2002.

Ling E, Warkentin TE. Intraoperative heparin flushes and subsequent acute heparin-induced thrombocytopenia. Anesthesiology 89: 1567–1569, 1998.

Linkins LA, Dans AL, Moores LK, Bona R, Davidson BL, Schulman S, Crowther M. Treatment and prevention of heparin-induced thrombocytopenia: antithrombotic therapy and prevention of thrombosis, 9th ed: American College of Chest Physicians Evidence-Based Clinical Practice Guidelines. Chest 141: e495S–e530S, 2012.

Lo GK, Sigouin CS, Warkentin TE. What is the potential for overdiagnosis of heparin-induced thrombocytopenia? Am J Hematol 82: 1037–1043, 2007.

Lubenow N, Hinz P, Thomaschewski S, Lietz T, Vogler M, Ladwig A, Jünger M, Nauck M, Schellong S, Wander K, Engel G, Ekkernkamp A, Greinacher A. The severity of trauma determines the immune response to PF4/heparin and the frequency of heparin-induced thrombocytopenia. Blood 115: 1797–1803, 2010.

Magnani HN, Gallus A. Heparin-induced thrombocytopenia (HIT). A report of 1,478 clinical outcomes of patients treated with danaparoid (Orgaran) from 1982 to mid-2004. Thromb Haemost 95: 967–981, 2006.

Mahlfeld K, Franke J, Schaeper O, Kayser R, Grasshoff H. Heparininduzierte Thrombozytopenie als Komplikation der postoperativen Thromboseprophylaxe mit UFH/NMH-Heparinen nach Hüft- und Knieendoprothetik. Unfallchirurg 105. 327–331, 2002; German.

Malcolm ID, Wigmore TA, Steinbrecher UP. Heparin-associated thrombocytopenia: low frequency in 104 patients treated with heparin of intestinal mucosal origin. Can Med Assoc J 120: 1086–1088, 1979.

Mallik A, Carlson KB, DeSancho MT. A patient with 'spontaneous' heparin-induced thrombocytopenia and thrombosis after undergoing knee replacement. Blood Coagul Fibrinolysis 22: 73–75, 2011.

Martel N, Lee J, Wells PS. Risk for heparin-induced thrombocytopenia with unfractionated and low molecular weight heparin thromboprophylaxis: a meta-analysis. Blood 106: 2710–2715, 2005.

Martinuzzo M, Forastiero RR, Adamczuk Y, Pombo G, Carreras LO. Antiplatelet factor 4—heparin antibodies in patients with antiphospholipid antibodies. Thromb Res 95: 271–279, 1999.

Marx A, Huhle G, Hoffmann U, Wang LC, Schule B, Jani L, Harenberg J. [Heparin-induced thrombocytopenia after elective hip joint replacement with postoperative prevention of thromboembolism with low molecular weight heparintew]. Z Orthop Ihre Grenzgeb 137: 536–539, 1999; German.

Matsuo T, Tomaru T, Kario K, Hirokawa T; HIT Research Group of Japan. Incidence of heparin-PF4 complex antibody formation and heparin-induced thrombocytopenia in acute coronary syndrome. Thromb Res 115: 475–481, 2005.

Mattioli AV, Bonetti L, Sternieri S, Mattioli G. Heparin-induced thrombocytopenia in patients treated with unfractionated heparin: prevalence of thrombosis in a 1 year follow-up. Ital Heart J 1: 39–42, 2000.

Mayo DJ, Cullinane AM, Merryman PK, Horne MK III. Serologic evidence of heparin sensitization in cancer patients receiving heparin flushes of venous access devices. Support Care Cancer 7: 425–427, 1999.

Morris TA, Castrejon S, Devendra G, Gamst AC. No difference in risk for thrombocytopenia during treatment of pulmonary embolism and deep venous thrombosis with either low molecular weight heparin or unfractionated heparin: a metaanalysis. Chest 132: 1131–1139, 2007.

Mureebe L, Coats RD, Silliman WR, Shuster TA, Nichols WK, Silver D. Heparin-associated antiplatelet antibodies increase morbidity and mortality in hemodialysis patients. Surgery 136: 848–853, 2004.

Murray PT, Hursting MJ. Heparin-induced thrombocytopenia in patients administered heparin solely for hemodialysis. Ren Fail 28: 537–539, 2006.

Nakamoto H, Shimada Y, Kanno T, Wanaka K, Matsuo T, Suzuki H. Role of platelet factor 4–heparin complex antibody (HIT antibody) in the pathogenesis of thrombotic episodes in patients on hemodialysis. Hemodial Int 9(Suppl 1): S2–S7, 2005.

Nand S, Wong W, Yuen B, Yetter A, Schmulbach E, Gross Fisher S. Heparin-induced thrombocytopenia with thrombosis: incidence, analysis of risk factors, and clinical outcomes in 108 consecutive patients treated at a single institution. Am J Hematol 56: 12–16, 1997.

Napolitano LM, Warkentin TE, Almahameed A, Nasraway SA. Heparin-induced thrombocytopenia in the critical care setting: diagnosis and management. Crit Care Med 34: 2898–2911, 2006.

Nelson JC, Lerner RG, Goldstein R, Cagin NA. Heparin-induced thrombocytopenia. Arch Intern Med 138: 548–552, 1978.

O'Shea SI, Sands JJ, Nudo SA, Ortel TL. Frequency of anti-heparin-platelet factor 4 antibodies in hemodialysis patients and correlation with recurrent vascular access thrombosis. Am J Hematol 69: 72–73, 2002.

Palomo I, Pereira J, Alarcón M, Diaz G, Hidalgo P, Pizarro I, Jara E, Rojas P, Quiroga G, Moore-Carrasco R. Prevalence of heparin-induced antibodies in patients with chronic renal failure undergoing hemodialysis. J Clin Lab Anal 19: 189–195, 2005.

Parney IF, Steinke DE. Heparin-induced thrombocytopenia and thrombosis following subarachnoid hemorrhage. Case report. J Neurosurg 93: 136–139, 2000.

Pauzner R, Greinacher A, Selleng K, Althaus K, Shenkman B, Seligsohn U. False-positive tests for heparin-induced thrombocytopenia in patients with antiphospholipid syndrome and systemic lupus erythematosus. J Thromb Haemost 7: 1070–1074, 2009.

Pena de la Vega L, Miller RS, Benda MM, Grill DE, Johnson MG, McCarthy JT, McBane RD II. Association of heparin-dependent antibodies and adverse outcomes in hemodialysis patients: a population-based study. Mayo Clin Proc 80: 995–1000, 2005.

Pohl C, Kredteck A, Bastiens B, Hanfland P, Klockgether T, Harbrecht U. Heparin-induced thrombocytopenia in neurologic patients treated with low molecular weight heparin. Neurology 64: 1285–1287, 2005.

Pouplard C, May MA, Lochmann S, Amiral J, Vissac AM, Marchand M, Gruel Y. Antibodies to platelet factor 4–heparin after cardiopulmonary bypass in patients anticoagulated with unfractionated heparin or a low molecular weight heparin: clinical implications for heparin-induced thrombocytopenia. Circulation 99: 2530–2536, 1999.

Pouplard C, May MA, Regina S, Maakaroun A, Fusciardi J, Gruel Y. Changes in the platelet count after cardiopulmonary bypass can efficiently predict the development of pathogenic heparin-dependent antibodies [abstr]. Blood 100: 16a–17a, 2002.

Pouplard C, Couvret C, Regina S, Gruel Y. Development of antibodies specific to polyanion-modified platelet factor 4 during treatment with fondaparinux. J Thromb Haemost 3: 2813–2815, 2005.

Prandoni P, Siragusa S, Girolami B, Fabris F; BELZONI Investigators Group. The incidence of heparin-induced thrombocytopenia in medical patients treated with low molecular weight heparin: a prospective cohort study. Blood 106: 3049–3054, 2005.

Pruthi RK, Daniels PR, Nambudiri GS, Warkentin TE. Heparin-induced thrombocytopenia (HIT) during postoperative warfarin thromboprophylaxis: a second example of postorthopedic surgery 'spontaneous' HIT. J Thromb Haemost 7: 499–501, 2009.

Rama BN, Haake RE, Bander SJ, Ghasem-Zadeh A, Gorla C. Heparin-flush associated thrombocytopenia-induced hemorrhage: a case report. Nebr Med J 76: 392–394, 1991.

Ramirez-Lassepas M, Cipolle RJ, Rodvold KA, Seifert RD, Strand L, Taddeini L, Cusulos M. Heparin-induced thrombocytopenia in patients with cerebrovascular ischemic disease. Neurology 34: 736–740, 1984.

Randolph AG, Cook DJ, Gonzales CA, Andrew M. Benefit of heparin in central venous and pulmonary artery catheters. A meta-analysis of randomized controlled trials. Chest 113: 165–171, 1998a.

Randolph AG, Cook DJ, Gonzales CA, Andrew M. Benefit of heparin in peripheral venous and arterial catheters: systematic review and meta-analysis of randomised controlled trials. BMJ 316: 969–975, 1998b.

Rao AK, White GC, Sherman L, Colman R, Lan G, Ball AP. Low incidence of thrombocytopenia with porcine mucosal heparin. A prospective multicentre study. Arch Intern Med 149: 1285–1288, 1989.

Rauova L, Poncz M, McKenzie SE, Reilly MP, Arepally G, Weisel JW, Nagaswami C, Cines DB, Sachais BS. Ultralarge complexes of PF4 and heparin are central to the pathogenesis of heparin-induced thrombocytopenia. Blood 105: 131–138, 2005.

Rice L, Jackson D. Can heparin cause clotting? Heart Lung 10: 331–335, 1981.

Rice L, Kennedy D, Veach A. Pentosan induced cerebral sagittal sinus thrombosis: a variant of heparin induced thrombocytopenia. J Urol 160: 2148, 1998.

Ridker PM, Cushman M, Stampfer MJ, Tracy RP, Hennekens CH. Inflammation, aspirin, and the risk of cardiovascular disease in apparently healthy men. N Engl J Med 336: 973–979, 1997.

Romeril KR, Hickton CM, Hamer JW, Heaton DC. Heparin-induced thrombocytopenia: case reports and a prospective study. NZ Med J 95: 267–269, 1982.

Rosenthal MA, Rischin D, McArthur G, Ribbons K, Chong B, Fareed J, Toner G, Green MD, Basser RL. Treatment with the novel anti-angiogenic agent PI-88 is associated with immune-mediated thrombocytopenia. Ann Oncol 13: 770–776, 2002.

Samama MM, Cohen AT, Darmon JY, Desjardins L, Eldor A, Janbon C, Leizorovicz A, Nguyen H, Olsson CG, Turpie AG, Weisslinger N. A comparison of enoxaparin with placebo for the prevention of venous thromboembolism in acutely ill medical patients. Prophylaxis in Medical Patients with Enoxaparin Study Group. N Engl J Med 341: 793–800, 1999.

Sanson BJ, Lensing AWA, Prins MH, Ginsberg JS, Barkagan ZS, Lavenne Pardonge E, Brenner B, Dulitzky M, Nielsen JD, Boda Z, Turi S, MacGillavry MR, Hamulyak K, Theunissen IM, Hunt BJ, Büller HR. Safety of low molecular weight heparin in pregnancy: a systematic review. Thromb Haemost 81: 668–672, 1999.

Schenk S, El-Banayosy A, Prohaska W, Arusoglu L, Morshuis M, Koester-Eiserfunke W, Kizner L, Murray E, Eichler P, Koerfer R, Greinacher A. Heparin-induced thrombocytopenia in patients receiving mechanical circulatory support. J Thorac Cardiovasc Surg 131: 1373–1381, 2006.

Schenk S, El-Banayosy A, Morshuis M, Arusoglu L, Eichler P, Lubenow N, Tenderich Koerfer R, Greinacher A, Prohaska W. IgG classification of anti-PF4/heparin antibodies to identify patients with heparin-induced thrombocytopenia during mechanical circulatory support. J Thromb Haemost 5: 235–241, 2007.

Selleng S, Malowsky B, Strobel U, Wessel A, Ittermann T, Wollert HG, Warkentin TE, Greinacher A. Early-onset and persisting thrombocytopenia in post-cardiac surgery patients is rarely due to heparin-induced thrombocytopenia, even when antibody tests are positive. J Thromb Haemost 8: 30–36, 2010.

Selleng K, Warkentin TE, Greinacher A. Heparin-induced thrombocytopenia in intensive care patients. Crit Care Med 35: 1165–1176, 2007.

Serruys PW, Emanuelsson H, van der Giessen W, Lunn AC, Kiemeney F, Macaya C, Rutsch W, Heyndrickx G, Suryapranata H, Legrand V, Goy JJ, Materne P, Bonnier Morice M-C, Fajadet J, Belardi J, Colombo A, Garcia E, Ruygrok P, de Jaegere P, Morel M-A; on behalf of the Benestent-II Study Group. Heparin-coated Palmaz-Schatz stents in human coronary arteries. early outcome of the Benestent-II pilot study. Circulation 93: 412–422, 1996.

Shumate MJ. Heparin-induced thrombocytopenia. N Engl J Med 333: 1006–1007, 1995.

Silver D, Kapsch DN, Tsoi EK. Heparin-induced thrombocytopenia, thrombosis, and hemorrhage. Ann Surg 198: 301–306, 1983.

Singer RL, Mannion JD, Bauer TL, Armenti FR, Edie RN. Complications from heparin-induced thrombocytopenia in patients undergoing cardiopulmonary bypass. Chest 104: 1436–1440, 1993.

Sitter T, Spannagl M, Banas B, Schiffl H. Prevalence of heparin-induced PF4–heparin antibodies in hemodialysis patients. Nephron 79: 245–246, 1998.

Skouri H, Gandouz R, Abroug S, Kraiem I, Euch H, Gargouri J, Harbi A. A prospective study of the prevalence of heparin-induced antibodies and other associated thromboembolic risk factors in pediatric patients undergoing hemodialysis. Am J Hematol 81: 328–334, 2006.

Smythe MA, Koerber JM, Mattson JC. The incidence of recognized heparin-induced thrombocytopenia in a large, tertiary care teaching hospital. Chest 131: 1644–1649, 2007.

Stéphan F, Hollande J, Richard O, Cheffi A, Maier-Redelsperger M, Flahault A. Thrombocytopenia in a surgical ICU. Chest 115: 1363–1370, 1999.

Strauss R, Wehler M, Mehler K, Kreutzer D, Koebnick C, Hahn EG. Thrombocytopenia in patients in the medical intensive care unit: bleeding prevalence, transfusion requirements, and outcome. Crit Care Med 30: 1765–1771, 2002.

Sturtevant JM, Pillans PI, Mackenzie F, Gibbs HH. Heparin-induced thrombocytopenia: recent experience in a large teaching hospital. Int Med J 36: 431–436, 2006.

Suh JS, Aster RH, Visentin GP. Antibodies from patients with heparin-induced thrombocytopenia/thrombosis recognize different epitopes on heparin: platelet factor 4. Blood 91: 916–922, 1998.

Tardy B, Tardy-Poncet B, Fournel P, Venet C, Jospe R, Dacosta A. Lower limb veins should be systematically explored in patients with isolated heparin-induced thrombocytopenia. Thromb Haemost 82: 1199–1200, 1999.

Tardy-Poncet B, Tardy B, Grelac F, Reynaud J, Mismetti P, Bertrand JC, Guyotat D. Pentosan polysulfate-induced thrombocytopenia and thrombosis. Am J Hematol 45: 252–257, 1994.

Trehel-Tursis V, Louvain-Quintard V, Zarrouki Y, Imbert A, Doubine S, Stéphan F. Clinical and biological features of patients suspected to have heparin-induced thrombocytopenia in a cardiothoracic surgical ICU. Chest 8 Mar 2012. [Epub ahead of print]

Trossaert M, Gaillard A, Commin PL, Amiral J, Vissac AM, Fressinaud E. High incidence of anti-heparin/platelet factor 4 antibodies after cardiopulmonary bypass. Br J Haematol 101: 653–655, 1998.

Turpie AG. Thrombosis prophylaxis in the acutely ill medical patient: insights from the prophylaxis in MEDical patients with ENOXaparin (MEDENOX) trial. Am J Cardiol 86: 48M–52M, 2000.

Turpie AG. Fondaparinux: a factor Xa inhibitor for antithrombotic therapy. Expert Opin Pharmacother 5: 1373–1384, 2004.

Van Aken WG. Thrombocytopenia (and consumption coagulopathy) induced by heparin. A case report. Scand J Haematol 36: 85–90, 1980.

Verma AK, Levine M, Shalansky SJ, Carter CJ, Kelton JG. Frequency of heparin-induced thrombocytopenia in critical care patients. Pharmacotherapy 23: 745–753, 2003.

Visentin GP, Malik M, Cyganiak KA, Aster RH. Patients treated with unfractionated heparin during open heart surgery are at high risk to form antibodies reactive with heparin: platelet factor 4 complexes. J Lab Clin Med 128: 376–383, 1996.

Vitoux JF, Roncato M, Hourdbhaigt P, Aiach M, Fiessinger JN. Heparin-induced thrombocytopenia and pentosan polysulfate: treatment with a low molecular weight heparin despite in vitro platelet aggregation. Thromb Hemost 55: 294–295, 1985.

Wallis DE, Workman DL, Lewis BE, Steen L, Pifarre R, Moran JF. Failure of early heparin cessation as treatment for heparin-induced thrombocytopenia. Am J Med 106: 629–635, 1999.

Walls JT, Boley TM, Curtis JJ, Silver D. Heparin-induced thrombocytopenia in patients undergoing intra-aortic balloon pumping after open heart surgery. ASAIO J 38: M574–M576, 1992a.

Walls JT, Curtis JJ, Silver D, Boley TM, Schmaltz RA, Nawarawong W. Heparin-induced thrombocytopenia in open heart surgical patients: sequelae of late recognition. Ann Thorac Surg 53: 787–791, 1992b.

Warkentin TE. Clinical presentation of heparin-induced thrombocytopenia. Semin Hematol 35(Suppl 5): 9–16, 1998.

Warkentin TE. HIT: lessons learned. Pathophysiol Haemost Thromb 35: 50–57, 2006.

Warkentin TE. Fondaparinux: does it cause HIT? Can it treat HIT? Expert Rev Hematol 3: 567, 81, 2010.

Warkentin TE. HIT treatment easier, HIT prevention harder. Blood 119: 1099–1100, 2012.

Warkentin TE, Crowther MA. When is HIT really HIT? Ann Thorac Surg 83: 21–23, 2007.

Warkentin TE, Greinacher A. Unfractionated LMWH and the risk of HIT: are medical patients different? Blood 106: 2931–2932, 2005.

Warkentin TE, Greinacher A. So, does low molecular weight heparin cause less heparin-induced thrombocytopenia than unfractionated heparin or not? Chest 132: 1131–1139, 2007.

Warkentin TE, Greinacher A. Anaphylactic and anaphylactoid reactions: two distinct but overlapping syndromes. Exp Opin Drug Safety 8: 129–144, 2009.

Warkentin TE, Kelton JG. Heparin-induced thrombocytopenia. Prog Hemost Thromb 10: 1–34, 1991.

Warkentin TE, Kelton JG. Interaction of heparin with platelets, including heparin-induced thrombocytopenia. In: Bounameaux H, ed. Low Molecular Weight Heparins in Prophylaxis and Therapy of Thromboembolic Diseases. New York: Marcel Dekker, 75–127, 1994.

Warkentin TE, Kelton JG. A 14–year study of heparin-induced thrombocytopenia. Am J Med 101: 502–507, 1996.

Warkentin TE, Kelton JG. Temporal aspects of heparin-induced thrombocytopenia. N Engl J Med 344: 1286–1292, 2001.

Warkentin TE, Sheppard JI. No significant improvement in diagnostic specificity of an anti-PF4/polyanion immunoassay with use of high heparin confirmatory procedure. J Thromb Haemost 4: 281–282, 2006a.

Warkentin TE, Sheppard JI. Testing for heparin-induced thrombocytopenia antibodies. Transfus Med Rev 20: 259–272, 2006b.

Warkentin TE, Levine MN, Hirsh J, Horsewood P, Roberts RS, Gent M, Kelton JG. Heparin-induced thrombocytopenia in patients treated with low molecular weight heparin or unfractionated heparin. N Engl J Med 332: 1330–1335, 1995.

Warkentin TE, Elavathil LJ, Hayward CPM, Johnston MA, Russett JI, Kelton JG. The pathogenesis of venous limb gangrene associated with heparin-induced thrombocytopenia. Ann Intern Med 127: 804–812, 1997.

Warkentin TE, Chong BH, Greinacher A. Heparin-induced thrombocytopenia: towards consensus. Thromb Haemost 79: 1–7, 1998a.

Warkentin TE, Ling E, Ho A, Sheppard JI. "Incidental" unfractionated heparin (UFH) vs normal saline (NS) flushes for intraoperative invasive catheters and the frequency of formation of heparin-induced thrombocytopenia IgG antibodies (HIT-IgG): a randomized, controlled trial [abstr]. Blood 92(Suppl 1): 91b, 1998b.

Warkentin TE, Sheppard JI, Horsewood P, Simpson PJ Moore JC, Kelton JG. Impact of the patient population on the risk of heparin-induced thrombocytopenia. Blood 96: 1703–1708, 2000.

Warkentin TE, Roberts RS, Hirsh J, Kelton JG. An improved definition of immune heparin-induced thrombocytopenia in postoperative orthopedic patients. Arch Intern Med 163: 2518–2524, 2003.

Warkentin TE, Cook RJ, Marder VJ, Sheppard JI, Moore JC, Eriksson BI, Greinacher A, Kelton JG. Anti-platelet factor 4/heparin antibodies in orthopedic surgery patients receiving anti-thrombotic prophylaxis with fondaparinux or enoxaparin. Blood 106: 3791–3796, 2005a.

Warkentin TE, Sheppard JI, Moore JC, Moore KM, Sigouin CS, Kelton JG. Laboratory testing for the antibodies that cause heparin-induced thrombocytopenia: how much class do we need? J Lab Clin Med 146: 341–346, 2005b.

Warkentin TE, Sheppard JI, Sigouin CS, Kohlmann T, Eichler P, Greinacher A. Gender imbalance and risk factor interactions in heparin-induced thrombocytopenia. Blood 108: 2937–2941, 2006.

Warkentin TE, Maurer BT, Aster RH. Heparin-induced thrombocytopenia associated with fondaparinux. N Engl J Med 356: 2653–2655, 2007.

Warkentin TE, Greinacher A, Koster A, Lincoff AM. American College of Chest Physicians. Treatment and prevention of heparin-induced thrombocytopenia. American College of Chest Physicians Evidence-Based Clinical Practice Guidelines, 8th Edition. Chest 133: 340S–380S, 2008a.

Warkentin TE, Makris M, Jay RM, Kelton JG. A spontaneous prothrombotic discorder resembling heparin-induced thrombocytopenia. Am J Med 121: 632–636, 2008b.

Warkentin TE, Sheppard JI, Moore JC, Sigouin CS, Kelton JG. Quantitative interpretation of optical density measurements using PF4-dependent enzyme-immunoassays. J Thromb Haemost 6: 1304–1312, 2008c.

Warkentin TE, Cook RJ, Marder VJ, Greinacher A. Anti-PF4/heparin antibody formation postorthopedic surgery thromboprophylaxis: the role of non-drug risk factors and evidence for a stoichiometry-based model of immunization. J Thromb Haemost 8: 504–512, 2010.

Warkentin TE, Davidson BL, Büller HR, Gallus A, Gent M, Lensing AW, Piovella F, Prins MH, Segers AE, Kelton JG. Prevalence and risk of preexisting heparin-induced thrombocytopenia antibodies in patients with acute VTE. Chest 140: 366–373, 2011a.

Warkentin TE, Greinacher A, Gruel Y, Aster RH, Chong BH; on behalf of the Scientific and Standardization Committee of the International Society on Thrombosis and Haemostasis. Laboratory testing for heparin-induced thrombocytopenia: a conceptual framework and implications for diagnosis. J Thromb Haemost 9: 2498–2500, 2011b.

Weismann RE, Tobin RW. Arterial embolism occurring during systemic heparin therapy. Arch Surg 76: 219–227, 1958.

Wester JP, Haas FJ, Biesma DH, Leusink JA, Veth G. Thrombosis and hemorrhage in heparin-induced thrombocytopenia in seriously ill patients. Intensive Care Med 30: 1927–1934, 2004.

Williams RT, Damaraju LV, Mascelli MA, Barnathan ES, Califf RM, Simoons ML, Deliargyris EN, Sane DC. Anti-platelet factor 4/heparin antibodies. An independent predictor of 30-day myocardial infarction after acute coronary ischemic syndromes. Circulation 107: 2307–2312, 2003.

Wolf H, Nowak H, Wick G. Detection of antibodies interacting with glycosaminoglycans polysulfate in patients treated with heparin or other polysulfated glycosaminoglycans. Int Arch Allergy Appl Immunol 70: 157–163, 1983.

Yamamoto S, Koide M, Matsuo M, Suzuki S, Ohtaka M, Saika S, Matsuo T. Heparin-induced thrombocytopenia in hemodialysis patients. Am J Kidney Dis 28: 82–85, 1996.

Yeh RW, Everett BM, Foo SY, Dorer DJ, Laposata M, Van Cott EM, Jang IK. Predictors for the development of elevated anti-heparin/platelet factor 4 antibody titers in patients undergoing cardiac catheterization. Am J Cardiol 98: 419–421, 2006.

Yu A, Jacobson SH, Bygden A, Egberg N. The presence of heparin-platelet factor 4 antibodies as a marker of hypercoagulability during hemodialysis. Clin Chem Lab Med 40: 21–26, 2002.

Yusuf AM, Warkentin TE, Arsenault KA, Whitlock R, Eikelboom JW. Prognostic importance of preoperative anti-PF4/heparin antibodies in patients undergoing cardiac surgery. A systematic review. Thromb Haemost 107: 8–14, 2012.

Nonimmune heparin–platelet interactions: Implications for the pathogenesis of heparin-induced thrombocytopenia

McDonald K. Horne III and Andreas Greinacher

INTRODUCTION

Almost as soon as heparin was introduced into clinical medicine, the new drug was reported to cause immediate small, but consistent, reductions in platelet count (Sappington, 1939). Later it was also found to produce platelet dysfunction (Heiden et al., 1977), accounting for at least some of its hemorrhagic risk (Hirsh, 1984; John et al., 1993). These effects, which most likely result from direct contact between heparin and platelets, are distinct from the role heparin plays in immune-mediated, heparin-induced thrombocytopenia (HIT). However, direct heparin-platelet binding is critical in the pathogenesis of HIT as well (Horne and Hutchison, 1998). Therefore, the various "nonimmune" heparin–platelet interactions will be reviewed.

HEPARIN BINDING TO PLATELETS

Appreciation of the functional effects of heparin on platelets led to studies of heparin binding to these cells, which was found to be specific and saturable (Horne, 1988; Sobel and Adelman, 1988; Horne and Chao, 1989). The negative charge density of the ligand (heparin) largely determines its binding specificity (Horne, 1988; Horne and Chao, 1990). Polysaccharide molecules with various primary structures can displace heparin from platelets if they are sufficiently charged (Horne, 1988; Greinacher et al., 1993) (Table 5.1). The identity of the platelet-binding site(s), which provides a complementary positive charge, is uncertain. One report indicates that glycoprotein (GP)IIb/IIIa (integrin $\alpha_{IIb}\beta_3$) contains a heparin-binding site (Sobel et al., 2001), but this is inconsistent with other studies (Horne, 1988, 1991). While there might be several binding sites on platelets, GPIIb/IIIa is important for transmitting the activation signal after heparin binding onto platelets (Gao et al., 2011).

Next to negative charge density, molecular size has the greatest effect on polysaccharide binding to platelets. Heparin molecular weight, for example, affects both its platelet-binding affinity and capacity (Horne and Chao, 1990). Because medicinal heparin is a mixture of molecules varying in mass from about 4000 to about 30,000 Da, the mass of a mole of heparin (i.e., approximately 6×10^{23} molecules) depends on the mean size of the molecules in the sample. The maximum number of molecules bound per platelet is approximately the same for heparin species with molecular weights between about 5000 and 15,000 Da (Table 5.1). However, larger molecules bring more glycosaminoglycan (GAG) mass to the platelet surface than smaller molecules (Fig. 5.1). Therefore, when heparin-binding capacity is expressed

TABLE 5.1   Platelet-Binding Parameters for Heparin Fractions of Different Molecular Mass

Heparin M_r range (Da)	Sulfate/ carboxylate (mol/mol)	Dissociation constant		Binding capacity	
		(mg/L)	(nM)	(mg/10^{15} cells)	(molecules/cell)
14,000–16,000	2.0 ± 0.29[a]	4.6 ± 1.1	310 ± 73	66 ± 2.5	2600 ± 100
9500–10,500	1.8 ± 0.26	3.9 ± 2.1	390 ± 210	56 ± 8.4	3400 ± 500
4500–5500	1.9 ± 0.15	3.2 ± 1.0	640 ± 200	23 ± 5.7	2800 ± 680
2700–3300	1.7 ± 0.25	4.0 ± 2.0	1300 ± 650	10 ± 5.4	2000 ± 1100

[a]Values are means ±1 standard deviation.
Source: Horne and Chao (1990).

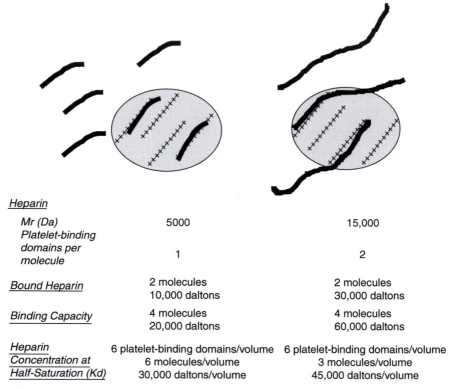

Heparin		
Mr (Da)	5000	15,000
Platelet-binding domains per molecule	1	2
Bound Heparin	2 molecules 10,000 daltons	2 molecules 30,000 daltons
Binding Capacity	4 molecules 20,000 daltons	4 molecules 60,000 daltons
Heparin Concentration at Half-Saturation (Kd)	6 platelet-binding domains/volume 6 molecules/volume 30,000 daltons/volume	6 platelet-binding domains/volume 3 molecules/volume 45,000 daltons/volume

FIGURE 5.1   Schematic binding of heparin to platelets comparing heparin of M_r 5000 Da with heparin of M_r 15,000 Da. Each "platelet-binding domain" of heparin is hypothesized to have $M_r >$ 3000 Da, whereas heparin-binding sites on the platelets (indicated by ++++) can bind 7000 Da heparin. Therefore, each binding site is not quite filled with M_r 5000 heparin but is too occupied to allow the binding of a second heparin molecule. In contrast, M_r 15,000 heparin has adequate length to occupy two binding sites on platelets, but physical constraints, such as limited heparin flexibility and the spacial distribution of binding sites, allow it to occupy only one site at a time. The scheme is consistent with the binding parameters shown in Table 5.1.

in terms of mass rather than moles or molecules, the capacity of larger heparins is greater than that of smaller heparins.

Similar distinctions apply to the parameters of binding affinity. Longer heparin molecules contain more potential platelet-binding domains than shorter molecules. Therefore, a large heparin species can half-saturate platelets at a lower molar concentration (K_d) than a smaller heparin species, although the concentration of heparin platelet-binding domains in the suspension is the same for both species at half-saturation (Horne and Chao, 1990) (Fig. 5.1).

Because of its high charge density as well as the high linear flexibility conferred by its constituent L-iduronic acid residues, heparin also binds to a variety of plasma proteins, which theoretically could compete with platelets for heparin (Casu et al., 1988; Young et al., 1994). However, heparin binding to only two plasma proteins, antithrombin and fibronectin, interferes with heparin-induced platelet activation (Salzman et al., 1980; Chong and Ismail, 1989) or with binding of heparin to platelets (Horne and Chao, 1990).

NONIDIOSYNCRATIC HEPARIN-INDUCED PLATELET ACTIVATION

The functional consequence of heparin binding to platelets is subtle cell stimulation. Antibody-independent activation of platelets by heparin *in vitro* has been reported from many laboratories. However, the results of these studies have varied, presumably because of differences in experimental conditions. In plasma, for example, heparin alone causes slight platelet aggregation, whereas platelets suspended in laboratory buffers are reported to aggregate either briskly or not at all in response to heparin (Eika, 1972; Salzman et al., 1980; Westwick et al., 1986; Chong and Ismail, 1989). In citrate-anticoagulated plasma, heparin also potentiates platelet activation by agonists, such as ADP and collagen (Holmer et al., 1980; Chen and Sylven, 1992; Xiao and Theroux, 1998; Aggarwal et al., 2002; Klein et al., 2002), and this effect is more pronounced in patients with acute illness, arterial disease, and anorexia nervosa (Mikhailidis et al., 1985; Reininger et al., 1996; Burgess and Chong, 1997).

The platelet proaggregatory effect of heparin does not appear to be an artifact of low ionized calcium concentration due to citrate anticoagulant: Chen and colleagues (1992) observed that heparin enhanced collagen-induced platelet aggregation in a dose-dependent fashion even in whole blood anticoagulated with hirudin (i.e., physiologic calcium concentrations). On the other hand, the responsiveness of washed platelets to agonists when resuspended in buffers containing physiologic calcium has been reported to be both increased and decreased by heparin (Saba et al., 1984; Westwick et al., 1986). Although the data are not always consistent, this much seems clear: direct heparin-induced platelet aggregation requires metabolic energy and is mediated by fibrinogen; therefore, it depends on platelet fibrinogen receptors (GPIIb/IIIa) and divalent cations (Chong and Ismail, 1989). There is also evidence that heparin can antagonize platelet inhibition by prostacyclin (Eldor and Weksler, 1979; Saba et al., 1979; Fortini et al., 1985; Berglund and Wallentin, 1991).

The properties of heparin that influence its platelet binding also influence its stimulating effect on platelets: heparin of a high molecular weight is more active than low molecular weight heparin (LMWH), and heparin with low affinity for antithrombin and fibronectin is more active (because it is more available) than heparin with high affinity for these plasma proteins (Holmer et al., 1980; Salzman et al., 1980;

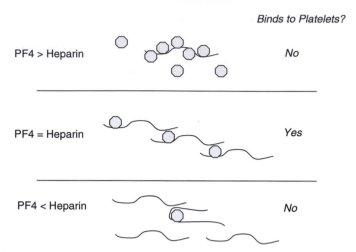

FIGURE 5.2 Schematic representation of the effect of the molar ratio of PF4 and heparin on the formation of complexes. *Abbreviation*: PF4, platelet factor 4.

Westwick et al., 1986; Chong and Ismail, 1989; Brace and Fareed, 1990; Xiao and Théroux, 1998; Aggarwal et al., 2002; Klein et al., 2002). The latter observation implies that the anticoagulant (antithrombin-dependent) activity of heparin is distinct from its platelet stimulatory effects. Furthermore, nonheparin polysaccharides can mimic the effect of heparin on platelets if they are sufficiently large and charged (Tiffany and Penner, 1981). In contrast, heparan sulfate (the predominant anticoagulant GAG in danaparoid) has negligible platelet-activating properties, as it has a relatively low degree of sulfation, despite sharing a carbohydrate backbone similar to that of heparin (Lindahl and Kjellen, 1991; Burgess and Chong, 1997).

When unfractionated heparin (UFH), LMWH, or fondaparinux bind to the GPIIb/IIIa complex (Gao et al., 2011), this causes outside-in signaling and thereby activation of phosphatidyl inositol-3 kinase (Fig. 5.2). This does not result in platelet aggregation or granule secretion, but potentiates the platelet-activating effects of low-dose ADP. In the study of Gao and coworkers, UFH and fondaparinux had similar proactivating effects, whereas in previous studies, the effects of LMWH on platelets were much less pronounced compared with UFH (Barradas et al., 1987). Platelets also bind to immobilized heparin via GPIIb/IIIa. This not only lowers the threshold for activation by other agonists, such as ADP, but also induces platelet spreading involving a slightly different pathway than binding of soluble UFH, involving phosphorylation of focal adhesion kinase (FAK). This might be of clinical relevance, as many intravascular devices are coated with heparin (however, binding properties differ from that used by Gao and colleagues). This immobilized heparin may induce mild activation of platelets on heparin-coated devices (Greinacher, 2011).

PLATELET-RELATED PROHEMORRHAGIC EFFECTS OF HEPARIN

Paradoxically, despite the *in vitro* evidence that heparin stimulates platelets, there is evidence that heparin causes bleeding partly because of its effects on platelet function (Hirsh, 1984; John et al., 1993). Heparin, for example, causes prolongation of the skin bleeding time unrelated to any effects on platelet counts. Also, the structural characteristics of heparin that enhance platelet stimulation *in vitro* (i.e., increased heparin size or sulfation; decreased affinity for antithrombin) are associated with enhanced bleeding in animal models (Hjort et al., 1960; Carter et al., 1982; Ockelford et al., 1982; Fernandez et al., 1986; Borowska et al., 1988; Van Ryn-McKenna et al., 1989).

The apparent inhibition of platelet function *in vivo* may be related to two specific actions of heparin: inhibition of thrombin-induced platelet activation and reduction of von Willebrand factor (vWf)-dependent platelet function. Thrombin is a "strong" platelet activator [i.e., it stimulates platelet secretion without intermediate platelet aggregation (Ware and Coller, 1995)]. However, in the presence of antithrombin, heparin essentially eliminates stimulation of platelets by thrombin (Westwick et al., 1986; Cofrancesco et al., 1988). This effect is likely responsible for the marked prolongation of bleeding time seen in patients receiving high doses of heparin during heart surgery (Kestin et al., 1993). Heparin also binds to vWf, preventing vWf binding to platelets (Sobel et al., 1991, 1992). This reduces vWf-mediated subendothelial adhesion of platelets flowing at high shear rates, perhaps also contributing to the heparin-related prolongation of the bleeding time.

NONIMMUNE HEPARIN-ASSOCIATED THROMBOCYTOPENIA

Nonimmune heparin-associated thrombocytopenia (HAT) describes the common clinical situation in which a patient develops a fall in platelet count within the first few days of receiving heparin. Often, there are concomitant clinical factors to explain the thrombocytopenia [e.g., hemodilution, bacteremia, or disseminated intravascular coagulation (DIC)]. In some patients, however, it is possible that a direct proaggregatory effect of heparin is responsible for the drop in platelet count (Salzman et al., 1980). The designation *associated* helps to convey the uncertain role of heparin in causing thrombocytopenia in this setting, and the term *nonimmune* distinguishes this syndrome from immune-mediated HIT (Warkentin et al., 1998).

Nonimmune HAT is typically mild, often transient, and clinically inconsequential (Gollub and Ulin, 1962; Johnson et al., 1984; Chong, 1988; Warkentin and Kelton, 1994). There is debate whether this represents a real *in vivo* phenomenon or whether the apparent thrombocytopenia is instead related to *ex vivo* platelet aggregation (Davey and Lander, 1968). Indeed, some investigators were unable to show this phenomenon at all (Heinrich et al., 1988; Xiao and Theroux, 1998). Sometimes, however, nonimmune HAT is a dramatic clinical syndrome that can be confused with HIT (Chong et al., 1982) (see chap. 3).

Balduini et al. (1993) observed that an early fall in platelet count was more frequent and of greater magnitude in patients receiving heparin following streptokinase therapy for acute myocardial infarction compared with control patients who received streptokinase alone. The heparin-treated patients also showed greater *ex vivo* spontaneous platelet aggregation, which is in line with the *in vitro* observations that heparin has a direct proaggregatory effect.

HEPARIN–PLATELET INTERACTIONS IN THE PATHOGENESIS OF HIT

Nonimmune heparin–platelet interactions are central to the pathogenesis of HIT because of the key role of platelet factor 4 (PF4). This cationic chemokine is secreted from activated platelets and binds to GAGs on the surface of platelets and endothelium (Dawes et al., 1982; Rao et al., 1983; Capitanio et al., 1985; O'Brien et al., 1985; Cines et al., 1987; Visentin et al., 1994). PF4 also binds to soluble GAGs, especially highly anionic heparin, leading to a competition between cell-bound and soluble GAGs for PF4 (Horne, 1993; Newman et al., 1998).

When complexed with GAG, PF4 exposes one or more neoantigens that stimulate the formation of HIT antibodies (Amiral et al., 1992, 1995; Kelton et al., 1994; Newman and Chong, 1999). Neoantigens are also formed by close approximation of two PF4 tetramers, which can happen when the positive charge of the PF4s is neutralized by GAGs (Greinacher et al., 2006). However, to be immunogenic, the PF4–GAG complexes presumably must be soluble and thereby accessible to the immune system. Perhaps this explains why PF4–GAG that is constitutively present on the endothelial surface is not immunogenic, but soluble PF4–heparin complexes are.

Once stimulated by exposure to PF4–heparin, HIT antibodies can bind to PF4 complexed with other GAGs (e.g., heparan sulfate and chondroitin sulfate) on cell membranes. By this mechanism, they could stimulate platelets (Rauova et al., 2006) and also (directly or indirectly) endothelial expression of tissue factor (Cines et al., 1987; Herbert et al., 1998). Such heparin-independent binding of HIT antibodies to platelets and endothelium may explain the appearance or persistence of thrombocytopenia in HIT after heparin exposure has ceased (see chap. 2). Activation of platelets in the absence of heparin, however, appears to require extensive saturation of the platelet surface with PF4, since antibody binding *in vitro* is observed only with PF4 concentrations > 300 nM, whereas the K_d for the binding of PF4 to platelets is reported to be about 30 nM (Loscalzo et al., 1985; Rauova et al., 2006). Such concentrations would be rarely, if ever, achieved *in vivo*. On the other hand, PF4 binds to endothelium even at normal plasma concentrations less than 1 nM and is readily displaced by heparin. Therefore, stimulation of endothelium by HIT antibodies seems a more probable mechanism for appearance or persistence of HIT after heparin has been discontinued.

When heparin is present, it forms soluble complexes with PF4 that it displaced from endothelium or that was secreted by activated platelets. These complexes also bind HIT antibodies, and they have the potential for docking at the platelet surface, attaching via their heparin at cationic sites rather than at the GAG (chondroitin sulfate) naturally found in the platelet cell membranes (Greinacher et al., 1993; Horne and Hutchison, 1998).

The ability of HIT–immune complexes to stimulate platelets appears to depend on the size of the PF4–heparin component (Rauova et al., 2005). The largest PF4–heparin complexes have the greatest chance of binding to platelets, and they can also carry several HIT–IgG molecules (Rauova et al., 2005). Therefore, when such a complex attaches to a platelet, it brings an especially rich trove of HIT–IgG to activate the cell through its Fcγ receptors (Horne and Alkins, 1996).

The size of PF4–heparin complexes depends on the length of the heparin chains and on the molar ratio of heparin to PF4. A heparin molecule of M_r ~11,000 Da can bind about four PF4 molecules, only partially saturating each one (Loscalzo et al., 1985). Heparin molecules about half this size (M_r 5000–7000 Da) can crosslink two or three PF4s (Bock et al., 1980). Therefore, LMWH (M_r 3000–10,000 Da) does not form ultralarge complexes as readily as UFH (M_r 4000–30,000 Da), and the pentasaccharide fondaparinux (M_r 1728 Da) does not form them at all (Rauova et al., 2005).

When UFH and PF4 are present in roughly equal molar amounts, large lattices (>670,000 Da) of heparin and PF4 can form (Bock et al., 1980; Rauova et al., 2005) (Fig. 5.2, *middle panel*). As the molar concentration of PF4 exceeds that of heparin, the size of the complexes becomes smaller and smaller until each contains only a single heparin molecule saturated with PF4 (Fig. 5.2, *upper panel*). A consequence of this is that these complexes cannot attach to platelets because the PF4 sites that might bind to platelet chondroitin sulfate are blocked by heparin, while there is no heparin free to bind to platelet cationic sites (Horne and Hutchison, 1998). If the molar ratio shifts the other way, so that heparin is in excess, the complexes will become limited to one heparin and one PF4 molecule each (Fig. 5.2, *bottom panel*). In this situation, the complexes are unlikely to bind to platelets because of competition with free heparin molecules and because the negative charge of heparin, which affects its affinity for the platelet, is partially neutralized by binding to PF4.

The critical importance of the molar ratio of heparin to PF4 probably explains why most patients who develop HIT antibodies never develop the clinical syndrome: molar ratios of PF4 and heparin favorable for platelet binding are rare or transient in most clinical situations (Amiral et al., 1996; Visentin et al., 1996; Kappers-Klunne et al., 1997; Warkentin et al., 2000; Rauova et al., 2006). While the

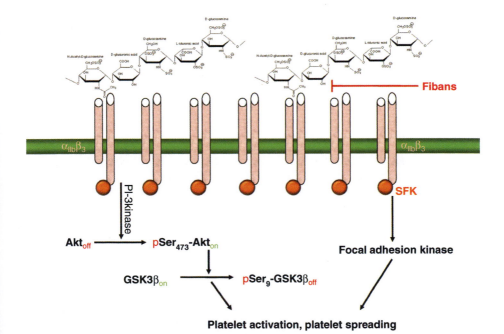

FIGURE 5.3 Schematic of the mechanism by which heparin induces outside-in, $\alpha_{IIb}\beta_3$-dependent platelet potentiation. Multivalent heparin is proposed to interact with the integrin at or near its ligand-binding site, resulting in microclustering of $\alpha_{IIb}\beta_3$ complexes on the platelet surface, transactivation of integrin-associated Src-family kinases (SFK), and subsequent activation of downstream signaling pathways that either potentiate (solution heparin) or induce (immobilized heparin) platelet activation. Fibans, such as abciximab and eptifibatide, might be effective in blocking this antibody-independent form of heparin-induced platelet activation. *Source*: From Gao et al. (2011).

plasma concentration of heparin is dose-dependent, the plasma concentration of PF4 depends on the level of platelet activation, which is affected by the degree of stimulation by HIT antibodies and on displacement of PF4 from the endothelial and platelet surfaces by heparin (O'Brien et al., 1985; Horne, 1993). Furthermore, individuals are reported to vary greatly in their platelet content of PF4 (O'Brien et al., 1984; Rauova et al., 2005).

In most clinical settings, free heparin is in considerable molar excess over PF4. Therapeutic concentrations of heparin (0.2–0.4 U/mL) correspond to about 100–200 nmol/L heparin. When heparin is given to normal individuals, plasma concentrations of PF4 from endothelial reservoirs only reach approximately 8 nM (Dawes et al., 1982). For PF4 concentrations to approach 100–200 nmol/L, marked activation of circulating platelets is necessary. Complete activation of platelets in a concentration of $250 \times 10^9/L$ will generate a plasma PF4 concentration of about 200 nM (Horne, 1993). Therefore, a molar excess of PF4 over therapeutic concentrations of heparin would be highly unlikely outside extreme clinical circumstances, although in the immediate environment of an activated platelet, the concentration of PF4 could rise much higher. On the other hand, prophylactic doses of heparin (e.g., 5000 U every 8–12 hours by subcutaneous injection) administered in a setting associated with a degree of platelet activation (e.g., after surgery) might well produce molar ratios of heparin and PF4 that would favor platelet binding of PF4-heparin complexes, and—if an immune response has occurred—platelet binding of PF4-heparin–IgG complexes. Indeed, such scenarios are the ones in which HIT is reported most frequently (Boshkov et al., 1993; Warkentin et al., 1995, 2000) (see chap. 4). As LMWH has a lower anticoagulatory activity per milligram than UFH (because some pentasaccharide sequences are disturbed during the fractionation process), LMWH is usually in large molar excess over PF4. This is likely an additional reason that HIT is much less frequent during treatment with LMWH (Greinacher et al., 2008).

IMPLICATIONS OF NONIMMUNE HEPARIN BINDING TO PLATELETS FOR THE PREVENTION OR TREATMENT OF HIT

Besides the different molar concentrations of UFH and LMWH reached during treatment, the fact that heparin's molecular size determines its platelet-binding affinity and capacity and its ability to assemble ultralarge complexes with PF4 may be one explanation why LMWH preparations are associated with a lower incidence of HIT than standard UFH and why, in some instances, LMWH has been given to patients with HIT without adverse consequences (Warkentin et al., 1995; Slocum et al., 1996). Indeed, there is increasing evidence that the smallest heparin, the synthetic pentasaccharide, fondaparinux (M_r 1728 Da), may be an effective medication for treating patients with HIT (Warkentin, 2010; Warkentin et al., 2011) (see chap. 17). Although fondaparinux apparently can bind well enough to PF4 to be immunogenic and the anti-PF4–heparin antibodies identified in patients who have received this drug can promote platelet activation *in vitro* in the presence of UFH or LMWH, they are not active in the presence of fondaparinux (Warkentin et al., 2005). In theory, this is because fondaparinux is either too small to form a stable complex with PF4 or to mediate the binding of complexes to the platelet surface (Elalamy et al., 1995; Walenga et al., 1997; Ahmad et al., 1999; Warkentin et al., 2005).

Similarly, the safety and efficacy of treating HIT patients with danaparoid, a so-called heparinoid, can be explained by the fact that its major component (approximately 84% heparan sulfate) does bind weakly to platelets (Horne, 1988; Magnani, 1993). More importantly, the specific activity of danaparoid is only 23 IU/mg, compared with 150 IU/mg UFH and ~100 IU/mg LMWH. Thus, there is a major molar excess of danaparoid, which binds PF4, detaches PF4 from the surface of platelets and other cells, and disrupts PF4/heparin complexes (Krauel et al., 2008). On the other hand, danaparoid sometimes cross-reacts with HIT antibodies in laboratory tests for HIT (see chap. 16). This is perhaps mediated by a minor component of danaparoid (about 12% dermatan sulfate) that does have weak affinity for both platelets and PF4 (Barber et al., 1972; Horne, 1988), or the 3–5% heparin sulfate with high binding affinity to AT, which has been shown to bind to PF4 and to generate the HIT antigen (Greinacher et al., 1992).

ACKNOWLEDGMENT

This work was supported by the Intramural Research Program of the NIH.

REFERENCES

Aggarwal A, Sobel BE, Schneider DJ. Decreased platelet reactivity in blood anticoagulated with bivalirudin or enoxaparin compared with unfractionated heparin: implications for coronary intervention. J Thromb Thrombolysis 13: 161–165, 2002.

Ahmad S, Jeske WP, Walenga JM, Hoppensteadt DA, Wood JJ, Herbert JM, Messmore HL, Fareed J. Synthetic pentasaccharides do not cause platelet activation by anti-heparin-platelet factor 4 antibodies. Clin Appl Thromb Hemost 5: 259–266, 1999.

Amiral J, Bridey F, Dreyfus M, Vissac AM, Fressinaud E, Wolf M, Meyer D. Platelet factor 4 complexed to heparin is the target for antibodies generated in heparin-induced thrombocytopenia. Thromb Haemost 68: 95–96, 1992.

Amiral J, Bridey F, Wolf M, Boyer-Neumann C, Fressinaud E, Vissac AM, Peynaud-Debayle E, Dreyfus M, Meyer D. Antibodies to macromolecular platelet factor 4–heparin complexes in heparin-induced thrombocytopenia: a study of 44 cases. Thromb Haemost 73: 21–28, 1995.

Amiral J, Peynaud-Debayle E, Wolf M, Bridey F, Vissac AM, Meyer D. Generation of antibodies to heparin-PF4 complexes without thrombocytopenia in patients treated with unfractionated or low molecular weight heparin. Am J Hematol 52: 90–95, 1996.

Balduini CL, Noris P, Bertolino G, Previtali M. Heparin modifies platelet count and function in patients who have undergone thrombolytic therapy for acute myocardial infarction. Thromb Haemost 69: 522–523, 1993.

Barber AF, Kaser-Glanzmann R, Jakabova M, Luscher EF. Characterization of a chondroitin 4–sulfate proteoglycan carrier for heparin neutralizing activity (platelet factor 4) released from human blood platelets. Biochim Biophys Acta 286: 312–329, 1972.

Barradas MA, Mikhailidis DP, Epemolu O, Jeremy JY, Fonseca V, Dandona P. Comparison of the platelet pro-aggregatory effect of conventional unfractionated heparins and a low molecular weight heparin fraction (CY 222). Br J Haematol 67: 451–457, 1987.

Berglund U, Wallentin L. Influence on platelet function by heparin in men with unstable coronary artery disease. Thromb Haemost 66: 648–651, 1991.

Bock PE, Luscombe M, Marshall SE, Pepper DS, Holbrook JJ. The multiple complexes formed by the interaction of platelet factor 4 with heparin. Biochem J 191: 769–776, 1980.

Borowska A, Lauri D, Maggi A, Dejana E, de Gaetano G, Donati MB, Pangrazzi J. Impairment of primary haemostasis by low molecular weight heparins in rats. Br J Haematol 68: 339–344, 1988.

Boshkov LK, Warkentin TE, Hayward CPM, Andrew M, Kelton JG. Heparin-induced thrombocytopenia and thrombosis: clinical and laboratory studies. Br J Haematol 84: 322–328, 1993.

Brace LD, Fareed J. Heparin-induced platelet aggregation. II. dose/response relationships for two low molecular weight heparin fractions (CY216 and CY222). Thromb Res 59: 1–14, 1990.

Burgess JK, Chong BH. The platelet proaggregating and potentiating effects of unfractionated heparin, low molecular weight heparin and heparinoid in intensive care patients and healthy controls. Eur J Haematol 58: 279–285, 1997.

Capitanio AM, Niewiarowski S, Rucinski B, Tuszynski GP, Cierniewski CS, Hershock D, Kornecki E. Interaction of platelet factor 4 with human platelets. Biochim Biophys Acta 839: 161–173, 1985.

Carter CJ, Kelton JG, Hirsh J, Cerskus A, Santos AV, Gent M. The relationship between the hemorrhagic and antithrombotic properties of low molecular weight heparin in rabbits. Blood 59: 1239–1245, 1982.

Casu B, Petitou M, Provasoli M, Sinay P. Conformational flexibility: a new concept for explaining binding and biological properties of iduronic acid-containing glycosaminoglycans. Trends Biochem Sci 13: 221–225, 1988.

Chen J, Sylven C. Heparin potentiation of collagen-induced platelet aggregation is related to the GPIIb/GPIIIa receptor and not to the GPIb receptor, as tested by whole blood aggregometry. Thromb Res 66: 111–120, 1992.

Chen J, Karlberg KE, Sylven C. Heparin enhances platelet aggregation irrespective of anticoagulation with citrate or with hirudin. Thromb Res 67: 253–262, 1992.

Chong BH. Heparin-induced thrombocytopenia. Blood Rev 2: 108–114, 1988.

Chong BH, Pitney WR, Castaldi PA. Heparin-induced thrombocytopenia: association of thrombotic complications with heparin-dependent IgG antibody that induces thromboxane synthesis and platelet aggregation. Lancet ii: 1246–1248, 1982.

Chong BH, Ismail F. The mechanism of heparin-induced platelet aggregation. Eur J Haematol 43: 245–251, 1989.

Cines DB, Tomaski A, Tannenbaum S. Immune endothelial-cell injury in heparin-associated thrombocytopenia. N Engl J Med 316: 581–589, 1987.

Cofrancesco E, Colombi M, Manfreda M, Pogliani EM. Effect of heparin and related glycosaminoglycans (GAGs) on thrombin-induced platelet aggregation and release. Haematologica 73: 471–475, 1988.

Davey MG, Lander H. Effect of injected heparin on platelet levels in man. J Clin Pathol 21: 55–59, 1968.

Dawes J, Pumphrey CW, McLaren KM, Prowse CV, Pepper DS. The in vivo release of human platelet factor 4 by heparin. Thromb Res 27: 65–76, 1982.

Eika C. The platelet aggregating effect of eight commercial heparins. Scand J Haematol 9: 480–482, 1972.

Elalamy I, Lecrubier C, Potevin F, Abdelouahed M, Bara L, Marie JP, Samama MM. Absence of in vitro cross-reaction of pentasaccharide with the plasma heparin-dependent factor of twenty-five patients with heparin-associated thrombocytopenia. Thromb Haemost 74: 1379–1387, 1995.

Eldor A, Weksler BB. Heparin and dextran sulfate antagonize PGI_2 inhibition of platelet aggregation. Thromb Res 16: 617–628, 1979.

Fernandez F, N'guyen P, Van Ryn J, Ofosu FA, Hirsh J, Buchanan MR. Hemorrhagic doses of heparin and other glycosaminoglycans induce a platelet defect. Thromb Res 43: 491–495, 1986.

Fortini A, Modesti PA, Abbate R, Gensini GF, Neri Serneri GG. Heparin does not interfere with prostacyclin and prostaglandin D_2 binding to platelets. Thromb Res 40: 319–328, 1985.

Gao C, Boylan B, Fang J, Wilcox DA, Newman DK, Newman PJ. Heparin promotes platelet responsiveness by potentiating αIIbβ3-mediated outside-in signaling. Blood 117: 4946–4952, 2011.

Gollub S, Ulin AW. Heparin-induced thrombocytopenia in man. J Lab Clin Med 59: 430–435, 1962.

Greinacher A. Platelet activation by heparin. Blood 117: 4686–4687, 2011.

Greinacher A, Michels I, Mueller-Eckhardt C. Heparin-associated thrombocytopenia: the antibody is not heparin specific. Thromb Haemost 67: 545–549, 1992.

Greinacher A, Michels I, Liebenhoff U, Presek P, Mueller-Eckhardt C. Heparin-associated thrombocytopenia: immune complexes are attached to the platelet membrane by the negative charge of highly sulphated oligosaccharides. Br J Haematol 84: 711–716, 1993.

Greinacher A, Gopinadhan M, Gunther J, U, Omer-Adam MA, Strobel U, Warkentin TE, Papastavrou G, Weitschies W, Helm CA. Close approximation of two platelet factor 4 tetramers by charge neutralization forms the antigens recognized by HIT antibodies. Arterioscler Thromb Vasc Biol 26: 2386–2393, 2006.

Greinacher A, Alban S, Omer-Adam MA, Weitschies W, Warkentin TE. Heparin-induced thrombocytopenia: a stoichiometry-based model to explain the differing immunogenicities of unfractionated heparin, low molecular weight heparin, and fondaparinux in different clinical settings. Thromb Res 122: 211–220, 2008.

Heiden D, Mielke CH, Rodvien R. Impairment by heparin of primary haemostasis and platelet [^{14}C]-5–hydroxytryptamine release. Br J Haematol 36: 427–436, 1977.

Heinrich D, Gorg T, Schulz M. Effects of unfractionated and fractionated heparin on platelet function. Haemostasis 18(Suppl 3): 48–54, 1988.

Herbert J-M, Savi P, Jeske WP, Walenga JM. Effect of SR121566A, a potent GP IIb–IIIa antagonist, on the HIT serum/heparin-induced platelet mediated activation of human endothelial cells. Thromb Haemost 80: 326–331, 1998.

Hirsh J. Heparin induced bleeding. Nouv Rev Fr Hematol 26: 261–266, 1984.

Hjort PF, Borchgrevink CF, Iversen OH, Stormorken H. The effect of heparin on the bleeding time. Thromb Diath Haemorrh 4: 389–399, 1960.

Holmer E, Lindahl U, Backstrom G, Thunberg L, Sandberg H, Soderstrom G, Andersson L-O. Anticoagulant activities and effects on platelets of a heparin fragment with high affinity for antithrombin. Thromb Res 18: 861–869, 1980.

Horne MK III. Heparin binding to normal and abnormal platelets. Thromb Res 51: 135–144, 1988.

Horne MK III. Heparin binds normally to platelets digested with Streptomyces griseus protease. Thromb Res 61: 155–158, 1991.

Horne MK III. The effect of secreted heparin-binding proteins on heparin binding to platelets. Thromb Res 70: 91–98, 1993.

Horne MK III, Chao ES. Heparin binding to resting and activated platelets. Blood 74: 238–243, 1989.

Horne MK III, Chao ES. The effect of molecular weight on heparin binding to platelets. Br J Haematol 74: 306–312, 1990.

Horne MK III, Alkins BR. Platelet binding of IgG from patients with heparin-induced thrombocytopenia. J Lab Clin Med 127: 435–442, 1996.

Horne MK III, Hutchison KJ. Simultaneous binding of heparin and platelet factor-4 to platelets: further insights into the mechanism of heparin-induced thrombocytopenia. Am J Hematol 58: 24–30, 1998.

John LCH, Rees GM, Kovacs IB. Inhibition of platelet function by heparin. J Thorac Cardiovasc Surg 105: 816–822, 1993.

Johnson RA, Lazarus KH, Henry DH. Heparin-induced thrombocytopenia: a prospective study. Am J Hematol 17: 349–353, 1984.

Kappers-Klunne MC, Boon DMS, Hop WCJ, Michiels JJ, Stibbe J, van der Zwaan C, Koudstaal PJ, van Vliet HHDM. Heparin-induced thrombocytopenia and thrombosis: a prospective analysis of the incidence in patients with heart and cerebrovascular diseases. Br J Haematol 96: 442–446, 1997.

Kelton JG, Smith JW, Warkentin TE, Hayward CPM, Denomme GA, Horsewood P. Immunoglobin G from patients with heparin-induced thrombocytopenia binds to a complex of heparin and platelet factor 4. Blood 83: 3232–3239, 1994.

Kestin AS, Valeri CR, Khuri SF, Loscalzo J, Ellis PA, MacGregor H, Birjiniuk V, Oimet H, Pasche B, Nelson MJ, Benoit SE, Rodino LJ, Barnard MR, Michelson AD. The platelet function defect of cardiopulmonary bypass. Blood 82: 107–117, 1993.

Klein B, Faridi A, von Tempelhoff GH, Heilmann L, Mittermayer C, Rath W. A whole blood flow cytometric determination of platelet activation by unfractionated and low molecular weight heparin in vitro. Thromb Res 108: 291–296, 2002.

Krauel K, Fürll B, Warkentin TE, Weitschies W, Kohlmann T, Sheppard JI, Greinacher A. Heparin-induced thrombocytopenia—therapeutic concentrations of danaparoid, unlike fondaparinux and direct thrombin inhibitors, inhibit formation of platelet factor 4-heparin complexes. J Thromb Haemost 6: 2160–2167, 2008.

Lindahl U, Kjellen L. Heparin or heparan sulfate—what is the difference? Thromb Haemost 66: 44–48, 1991.

Loscalzo J, Melnick B, Handin RI. The interaction of platelet factor four and glycosaminoglycans. Arch Biochem Biophys 240: 446–455, 1985.

Magnani HN. Heparin-induced thrombocytopenia (HIT): an overview of 230 patients treated with orgaran (Org 10172). Thromb Haemost 70: 554–561, 1993.

Mikhailidis DP, Barradas MA, Jeremy JY, Gracey L, Wakeling A, Dandona P. Heparin-induced platelet aggregation in anorexia nervosa and in severe peripheral vascular disease. Eur J Clin Invest 15: 313–319, 1985.

Newman PM, Chong BH. Further characterization of antibody and antigen in heparin-induced thrombocytopenia. Br J Haematol 107: 303–309, 1999.

Newman PM, Swanson RL, Chong BH. Heparin-induced thrombocytopenia: IgG binding to PF4–heparin complexes in the fluid phase and cross-reactivity with low molecular weight heparin and heparinoid. Thromb Haemost 80: 292–297, 1998.

O'Brien JR, Etherington MD, Pashley M. Intra-platelet platelet factor 4 (IP.PF4) and the heparin-mobilisable pool of PF4 in health and atherosclerosis. Thromb Haemost 51: 354–357, 1984.

O'Brien JR, Etherington MD, Pashley MA. The heparin-mobilisable pool of platelet factor 4: a comparison of intravenous and subcutaneous heparin and Kabi heparin fragment 2165. Thromb Haemost 54: 735–738, 1985.

Ockelford PA, Carter CJ, Cerskus A, Smith CA, Hirsh J. Comparison of the in vivo hemorrhagic and antithrombotic effects of a low antithrombin-III affinity heparin fraction. Thromb Res 27: 679–690, 1982.

Rao AK, Niewiarowski S, James P, Holt JC, Harris M, Elfenbein B, Bastl C. Effect of heparin on the in vivo release and clearance of human platelet factor 4. Blood 61: 1208–1214, 1983.

Rauova L, Poncz M, McKenzie SE, Reilly MP, Arepally G, Weisel JW, Nagaswami C, Cines DB, Sachais BS. Ultra large complexes of PF4 and heparin are central to the pathogenesis of heparin-induced thrombocytopenia. Blood 105: 131–138, 2005.

Rauova L, Zhai L, Kowalska MA, Arepally GM, Cines DB, Poncz M. Role of platelet surface PF4 antigenic complexes in heparin-induced thrombocytopenia pathogenesis: diagnostic and therapeutic implications. Blood 107: 2346–2353, 2006.

Reininger CB, Greinacher A, Graf J, Lasser R, Steckmeier B, Schweiberer L. Platelets of patients with peripheral arterial disease are hypersensitive to heparin. Thromb Res 81: 641–649, 1996.

Saba HI, Saba SR, Blackburn CA, Hartmann RC, Mason RG. Heparin neutralization of PGI_2: effects upon platelets. Science 205: 499–501, 1979.

Saba HI, Saba SR, Morelli GA. Effect of heparin on platelet aggregation. Am J Hematol 17: 295–306, 1984.

Salzman EW, Rosenberg RD, Smith MH, Lindon JN, Favreau L. Effect of heparin and heparin fractions on platelet aggregation. J Clin Invest 65: 64–73, 1980.

Sappington SW. The use of heparin in blood transfusions. JAMA 113: 22–25, 1939.

Slocum MM, Adams JG, Teel R, Spadone DP, Silver D. Use of enoxaparin in patients with heparin-induced thrombocytopenia syndrome. J Vasc Surg 23: 839–843, 1996.

Sobel M, Adelman B. Characterization of platelet binding of heparins and other glycosaminoglycans. Thromb Res 50: 815–826, 1988.

Sobel M, McNeil PM, Carlson PL, Kermode JC, Adelman B, Conroy R, Marques D. Heparin inhibition of von Willebrand factor-dependent platelet function in vitro and in vivo. J Clin Invest 87: 1787–1793, 1991.

Sobel M, Soler DF, Kermode JC, Harris RB. Localization and characterization of a heparin binding domain peptide of human von Willebrand factor. J Biol Chem 267: 8857–8862, 1992.

Sobel M, Fish WR, Toma N, Luo S, Bird K, Mori K, Kusumoto S, Blystone SD, Suda Y. Heparin modulates integrin function in human platelets. J Vasc Surg 33: 587–594, 2001.

Tiffany ML, Penner JA. Heparin and other sulfated polyanions: their interaction with the blood platelet. Ann NY Acad Sci 370: 662–667, 1981.

Van Ryn-McKenna J, Ofosu FA, Hirsh J, Buchanan MR. Antithrombotic and bleeding effects of glycosaminoglycans with different degrees of sulfation. Br J Haematol 71: 265–269, 1989.

Visentin GP, Ford SE, Scott JP, Aster RH. Antibodies from patients with heparin-induced thrombocytopenia/thrombosis are specific for platelet factor 4 complexed with heparin or bound to endothelial cells. J Clin Invest 93: 81–88, 1994.

Visentin GP, Malik M, Cyganiak KA, Aster RH. Patients treated with unfractionated heparin during open heart surgery are at high risk to form antibodies reactive with heparin: platelet factor 4 complexes. J Lab Clin Med 128: 376–383, 1996.

Walenga JM, Jeske WP, Bara L, Samama MM, Fareed J. Biochemical and pharmacologic rationale for the development of a synthetic heparin pentasaccharide. Thromb Res 86: 1–36, 1997.

Ware AJ, Coller BS. Platelet morphology, biochemistry, and function. In: Beutler E, Lichtman MA, Coller BS, Kipps TJ, eds. Williams Hematology, 5th edn. New York: McGraw-Hill, 1161–1201, 1995.

Warkentin TE. Fondaparinux: does it cause HIT? can it treat HIT? Exp Rev Hematol 3: 567–581, 2010.

Warkentin TE, Kelton JG. Interaction of heparin with platelets, including heparin-induced thrombocytopenia. In: Bounameaux H, ed. Low Molecular Weight Heparins in Prophylaxis and Therapy of Thromboembolic Diseases. New York: Marcel Dekker, 75–127, 1994.

Warkentin TE, Levine MN, Hirsh J, Horsewood P, Roberts RS, Gent M, Kelton JG. Heparin-induced thrombocytopenia in patients treated with low molecular weight heparin or unfractionated heparin. N Engl J Med 332: 1330–1335, 1995.

Warkentin TE, Chong BH, Greinacher A. Heparin-induced thrombocytopenia: towards consensus. Thromb Haemost 79: 1–7, 1998.

Warkentin TE, Sheppard JA, Horsewood P, Simpson PJ, Moore JC, Kelton JG. Impact of the patient population on the risk for heparin-induced thrombocytopenia. Blood 96: 1703–1708, 2000.

Warkentin TE, Cook RJ, Marder VJ, Sheppard JI, Moore JC, Eriksson BI, Greinacher A, Kelton JG. Anti-platelet factor 4/heparin antibodies in orthopedic surgery patients receiving antithrombotic prophylaxis with fondaparinux or enoxaparin. Blood 106: 3791–3796, 2005.

Warkentin TE, Pai M, Sheppard JI, Schulman S, Spyropoulos AC, Eikelboom JW. Fondaparinux treatment of acute heparin-induced thrombocytopenia confirmed by the serotonin-release assay: a 30-month, 16-patient case series. J Thromb Haemost 9: 2389–2396, 2011.

Westwick J, Scully MF, Poll C, Kakkar VV. Comparison of the effects of low molecular weight heparin and unfractionated heparin on activation of human platelets in vitro. Thromb Res 42: 435–447, 1986.

Xiao Z, Theroux P. Platelet activation with unfractionated heparin at therapeutic concentrations and comparisons with a low molecular weight heparin and with a direct thrombin inhibitor. Circulation 97: 251–256, 1998.

Young E, Wells P, Holloway S, Weitz J, Hirsh J. Ex-vivo and in-vitro evidence that low molecular weight heparins exhibit less binding to plasma proteins than unfractionated heparin. Thromb Haemost 71: 300–304, 1994.

6 Role of heparin-dependent antigens in immune heparin-induced thrombocytopenia

Jean Amiral and Anne Marie Vissac

INTRODUCTION

Immune (type II) heparin-induced thrombocytopenia (HIT) remains a major iatrogenic complication of heparin therapy. It is triggered by "heparin-dependent" antibodies targeted to protein–heparin—mainly platelet factor 4 (PF4)—complexes. Its frequency could be underestimated, if HIT is not considered as a potential cause of thrombocytopenia and new thrombosis (Francis, 2005) or overestimated, if any positive PF4-dependent antibody test is considered as confirmation of HIT, as PF4-dependent immunoassays used when HIT is clinically suspected have a low diagnostic specificity (Berry et al., 2011). HIT develops more frequently during therapy with unfractionated heparin (UFH) (Poncz, 2005; Greinacher, 2006), especially in the setting of vascular alteration, blood activation, and inflammation. PF4 complexed to heparin (PF4/H) was identified as the major target antigen for heparin-dependent antibodies involved in the pathogenesis of immune HIT 20 years ago (Amiral et al., 1992, 1995) and confirmed by various investigators (Gruel et al., 1993; Greinacher et al., 1994, 1995; Kelton et al., 1994; Visentin et al., 1994). However, today, presence of anti-PF4/H antibodies (especially when they are detected using assays that recognize all three major immunoglobulin classes, IgG, IgA, and IgM) must be understood to be just a risk factor for HIT rather than an absolute indicator of this clinical complication (see chap. 11). Conversely, when thrombocytopenia (and/or thrombosis) develops five or more days after beginning heparin therapy, presence of these anti-PF4/H antibodies—especially when they are of IgG class and found at high levels—essentially confirms the diagnosis of HIT (Lindhoff-Last et al., 2001; Warkentin, 2004, 2005; Warkentin et al., 2005; Warkentin and Sheppard, 2006; Greinacher, 2006).

Occasionally, other antigens can be involved in HIT pathogenesis, such as interleukin-8 (IL-8) or neutrophil-activating peptide-2 (NAP-2), two CXC chemokines of the PF4 superfamily that exhibit affinity for heparin (Amiral et al., 1996a; Regnault et al., 2003). More recently, antibodies to protamine sulfate complexed to heparin have been identified in patients clinically suspected to have HIT but who do not have antibodies against PF4/H complexes (Amiral and Vissac, 2009).

There is increasing evidence that the risk of HIT depends on the type of heparin used, its sulfation grade (Greinacher et al., 1995), the duration of therapy, and the patient's clinical context (Kelton, 1992; Warkentin and Kelton, 1996) (see chaps. 2 and 4). However, many questions remain unresolved: How are these antibodies generated? Why are they observed in only a subgroup of patients receiving heparin? Why do they become pathogenic in only a few of these patients? Why are antibodies formed so often, but with a (relatively) low incidence of thrombocytopenia and thrombosis, particularly in some clinical contexts, such as extracorporeal circulation (Bauer et al.,

1997) or hemodialysis? What is the explanation for "delayed-onset" HIT in some patients (Warkentin and Kelton, 2001; Rice et al., 2002; Smythe et al., 2005)? Indeed, antibodies to PF4/H develop surprisingly often in many heparin-treated patients, especially in the context of platelet activation, such as heart surgery using cardiopulmonary bypass (CPB) (Amiral et al., 1996b; Visentin et al., 1996). Clinical complications of HIT are especially associated with high-titer anti-PF4/H antibodies of the IgG isotype, usually in patients with comorbid disease who are receiving UFH. Experimentally, the presence of prothrombotic factors has been demonstrated to enhance the occurrence of HIT and thrombosis in a mouse model (Reilly et al., 2006). The frequency of HIT is less with low molecular weight heparin (LMWH) (Warkentin et al., 1995, 2006; Warkentin, 2004, 2005; Greinacher, 2006). However, some studies suggest that this complication might also develop rarely in the absence of IgG isotypes (Amiral et al., 1996c; Meyer et al., 2006). In a few patients with clinically apparent HIT and with positive testing for heparin-dependent, platelet-activating antibodies, only IgA (Meyer et al., 2006) or IgM isotypes are present, although usually at very high concentrations.

In this chapter, we highlight the role of PF4 as the major antigen for the generation of heparin-dependent antibodies, although we discuss also the contribution of other antigens, such as IL-8, and the possible implication of antibodies against protamine sulfate/heparin complexes. We also focus on the current understanding of anti-PF4/H antibody generation and its contribution to the complications of HIT. Formation of the PF4/H antigen complexes and their binding to blood and endothelial cells (ECs), which targets the immune response onto these cells (Cines et al., 1987; Visentin et al., 1994; Visentin and Aster, 1995; Horne and Hutchison, 1998; Arepally and Mayer, 2001, Pouplard et al., 2001; Blank et al., 2002), thereby inducing their activation and release of tissue factor (TF) and procoagulant microparticles, are outlined. Finally, the possibility that HIT can be caused without detectable antibodies against PF4/H is reviewed, including the hypothesis that pre-existing antibodies to other chemokines, such as IL-8, or even NAP-2, are involved. These antibodies could become pathogenic during heparin treatment (Amiral et al., 1996a; Regnault et al., 2003), thereby mimicking the clinical picture of rapid-onset HIT (see chap. 2).

HOW DOES HEPARIN TRANSFORM PF4 INTO AN ALLOANTIGEN?

PF4 is a 7.8 kDa CXC chemokine protein present in platelet α-granules as a tetramer of about 30 kDa. Upon platelet activation or lysis, PF4 is released into blood as a high molecular weight complex (350 kDa) consisting of a proteoglycan dimer carrying eight PF4 tetramers. PF4 is rapidly cleared from blood through binding to EC glycosaminoglycans (GAGs), for which it has a greater affinity than for the platelet proteoglycan dimer. During heparin therapy (UFH or LMWH), PF4 tetramers are displaced from the EC storage sites (because heparins have a higher affinity for PF4 than do other GAGs) and they are released into blood at concentrations that depend on the patient's platelet activation status (Fig. 6.1). In some cases, these PF4/H complexes induce the generation of heparin-dependent antibodies (Poncz, 2005).

Antibodies to self-antigens, including certain autologous plasma proteins, can develop as a result of immune dysfunction, triggering autoimmune disease.

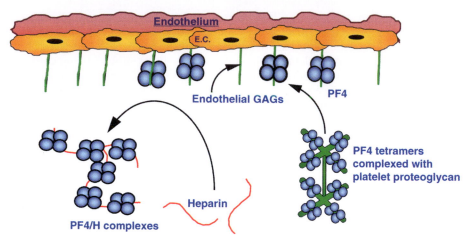

FIGURE 6.1   Release of PF4 from platelets as a high molecular weight complex of eight tetramers with a proteoglycan dimer; PF4 binds to endothelial cell GAGs, for which it has a greater affinity, but it is displaced by heparin, which exhibits a higher affinity for PF4. *Abbreviations*: E.C., endothelial cell; GAGs, glycosaminoglycans; PF4, platelet factor 4; PF4/H, PF4 complexed to heparin.

Sometimes, however, formation of complexes between an autologous protein and a foreign substance leads to new antigens on the self-protein, which can be described as *cryptic alloantigens* or *neoantigens*. Figure 6.2 shows how the PF4 tetramer can be modified by its binding to heparin, thereby exposing neoepitopes that were masked on native PF4. The immune stimulation resulting from such an altered self-epitope abates quickly once the inducing foreign substance is no longer present. Such a model explains some of the clinical events observed in HIT (see chap. 2). In HIT, PF4 constitutes the self-antigen, forming an "alloantigen" when complexed with heparin, particularly when both PF4 and heparin are present at the stoichiometric concentrations that allow the formation of multimolecular complexes and, consequently, exposure of one or more cryptic neoepitopes. Thus, the antibodies to PF4/H complexes essentially can be considered to be autoantibodies or alloantibodies (Shoenfeld, 1997). However, as a foreign substance (heparin) is involved, and as there is little evidence that complexes between PF4 and naturally occurring GAGs generate antibodies, it seems more appropriate to call those heparin-dependent antibodies, "*alloantibodies*."

As mentioned, PF4 is a positively charged tetrameric glycoprotein (GP) member of the CXC chemokine family (Brandt and Flad, 1992). The tetramer forms by sequential noncovalent association of identical PF4 monomers: two dimers are formed that self-associate into the fundamental tetrameric structure. As found within platelet α-granules, PF4 is released into blood only after platelet activation, such as seen with trauma, surgery, atherosclerosis (Dunlop et al., 1987), diabetes, CPB, inflammation, cancer, infections, and so on. *In vivo*, PF4 has many different bio-logic functions, including immunoregulation, inhibition of megakaryocytopoiesis and angiogenesis, and mediation of cell response (Nesmelova et al., 2005; Slungaard, 2005; Lambert et al., 2007). As summarized in Figure 6.1, PF4 released from platelets is in a 350 kDa complex comprising eight PF4 tetramers linked to a chondroitin-containing proteoglycan dimer (Barber et al., 1972; Luscombe et al.,

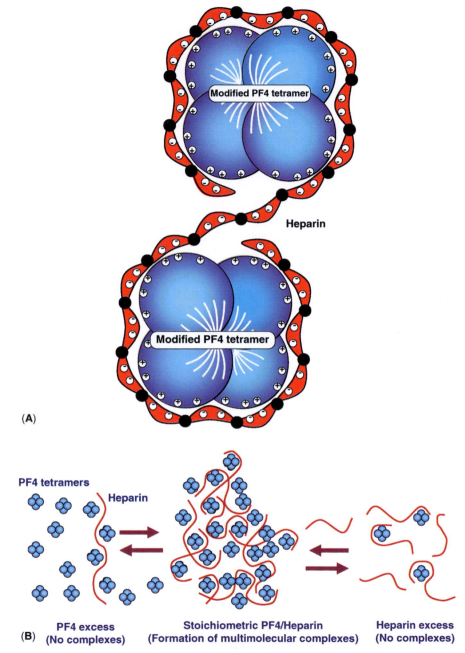

FIGURE 6.2 Schema showing the "modifications" of the PF4 tetramer after its tight binding with heparin at stoichiometry and exposure of neoepitopes **(A)** and depicting the formation of heparin and PF4 complexes at different concentrations of heparin and PF4 **(B)**. In the presence of stoichiometric concentrations of both substances, multimolecular complexes are formed. Heparin then wraps around the PF4 tetramer, altering its structure and rendering it antigenic. *Abbreviation*: PF4, platelet factor 4.

1981; Huang et al., 1982). These PF4 complexes then bind to EC proteoglycans (heparan sulfate), and heparin, when present, displaces PF4 from the EC GAGs due to its greater affinity for PF4. The resulting PF4/H complexes are released into the circulating blood.

The interaction between heparin and PF4 has been intensively studied (Bock et al., 1980; Cowan et al., 1986; Stuckey et al., 1992; Maccarana and Lindahl, 1993). In the presence of a stoichiometric concentration of heparin and PF4 (which corresponds to about 27 international units [IU], i.e., about $175 \pm 25\,\mu g$ of heparin per milligram of PF4), multimolecular PF4/H complexes are generated (Greinacher et al., 1994; Amiral et al., 1995). With stoichiometric concentrations, heparin tightly wraps around the PF4 molecule (Fig. 6.2A), altering its structure and rendering it antigenic through the exposure of neoantigens. Figure 6.2B shows the different complexes that can be formed between heparin and PF4, depending on the respective concentrations of both substances. Only multimolecular complexes, formed when well-defined ratios between PF4 and heparin exist, are believed to be antigenic. The larger PF4/H complexes formed with UFH, compared with LMWH, are believed to be more immunogenic and more pathogenic (Poncz, 2005; Rauova et al., 2005; Greinacher, 2006). Since complex formation depends strictly on the respective concentrations of heparin and PF4, if we consider the usual therapeutic range for heparin to be <0.1–$1\,IU/mL$, then the amount of PF4 required for the generation of multimolecular PF4/H complexes ranges from <3 to $40\,\mu g/mL$. In patients undergoing CPB, who receive higher heparin concentrations (up to $3\,IU/mL$), the correspondingly higher PF4 concentrations required to form immunogenic PF4/H complexes results from the intense platelet activation produced when blood is exposed to the CPB circuit. In general, the existence of favorable conditions permitting the formation of multimolecular PF4/H complexes may depend as much on the underlying disease promoting platelet activation as on the dose of heparin given (see chap. 4). Indeed, PF4 can be present at very high concentrations (exceeding the expected serum concentration of about $5\,\mu g/mL$) at pathologic sites where platelets and leukocytes are chemoattracted and then activated (Fig. 6.3), such as during major surgery (orthopedic, cardiac), acute infection or inflammation, malignancy, and so on.

The intensity of the heparin-dependent immune response thus depends on the presence and, probably, the persistence of multimolecular PF4/H complexes. In particular, the presence of high concentrations of PF4/H complexes may be important in triggering an immune response. However, heparin concentrations can vary considerably even in an individual patient during the course of heparin therapy, and so the stoichiometric concentrations allowing for PF4/H complex formation may occur frequently. But, if only low PF4 concentrations are present, formation of immunogenic complexes occurs only at corresponding low levels of heparin, for example, $0.027\,IU/mL$ of heparin for $100\,ng/mL$ of PF4, which is the approximate PF4 concentration in normal subjects receiving heparin. The chances of developing a significant immune response in this setting would be low. In contrast, PF4 concentrations are expected to be high at sites where platelets and leukocytes converge and are activated (Fig. 6.3), thus improving the chances of an immune response. The potentially important role of individual immune responsiveness to a given PF4/H antigenic stimulus is unknown. Studies have demonstrated that the immunologic response to a PF4/H immunologic stimulus is T-cell dependent (Bacsi et al., 1999; Suvarna et al., 2005).

We have reported that although antibodies to PF4/H complexes are present in most patients who develop HIT, they are absent in some patients with apparent

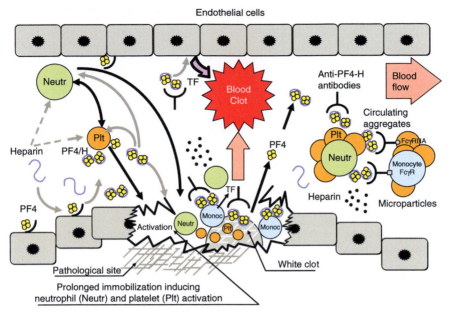

FIGURE 6.3 Cell–cell interactions in the neighborhood of blood activation or sites of inflammation: Presence of heparin-dependent antibodies increases the amount of cells available at these sites, amplifies cell–cell interactions and cellular activation, and can lead to blood clotting or release of circulating cell aggregates. The procoagulant effect is enhanced by the release of tissue factor (from endothelial cells and monocytes) and generation of microparticles. *Abbreviations*: FcγR, Fcγ receptor; IL-8, interleukin-8; Monoc, monocyte; PF4, platelet factor 4; PF4/H, platelet factor 4/heparin complex; TF, tissue factor.

HIT, including patients with positive platelet activation assays. Antibodies to IL-8 or to NAP-2 have been observed in some of these patients (Amiral et al., 1996a; Regnault et al., 2003), but in a few, no specific heparin-dependent antibodies have yet been identified. As discussed later, antibodies to IL-8 or to NAP-2 can be generated by mechanisms different from those involved in anti-PF4/H antibody formation. These antibodies can precede the heparin therapy, and could have a regulatory role for inflammation (Reitamo et al., 1993). Recently, these pre-existing antibodies have been reported also for PF4 and could already be involved in clinical thrombotic complications (Desprez et al., 2010). Administration of heparin is then the trigger for their pathologic effect, as heparin then promotes binding of these chemokines onto some blood cells (including platelets and ECs) to which they do not bind (or bind poorly) in the absence of heparin. In contrast to anti-PF4/H antibodies, these anti-IL-8 or anti-NAP-2 antibodies might be true autoantibodies (Bendtzen et al., 1995). They can be generated in many different clinical situations, and their pathologic incidence still remains unknown. Concerning pre-existing PF4-dependent antibodies, a new theory has recently been proposed: generation of these antibodies could be induced by preimmunization against bacteria coated with PF4, as PF4 binds to the bacterial surface and forms there complexes, which are recognized by anti-PF4/H antibodies (Greinacher et al., 2011; Krauel et al., 2011).

PATHOLOGIC MECHANISMS OF HEPARIN-DEPENDENT ANTIBODIES

In our experience, anti-PF4/H antibodies of the IgG isotype are present in at least 85% of patients with clinical HIT. In the remaining cases, IgA, IgM, or both isotypes—but only when present at high concentrations—could be involved. This is based on studies of HIT in which the anti-PF4/H antibodies were fully isotyped (Amiral et al., 1996c). Although the clinical picture and positive platelet aggregation tests supported the diagnosis of immune HIT, only IgM and/or IgA isotypes of anti-PF4/H antibodies were found, and no IgG was detected. This finding is nevertheless controversial, as many studies tend to demonstrate the preeminent role of the IgG isotype in the development of HIT (Lindhoff-Last et al., 2001; Warkentin, 2004, 2005; Warkentin et al., 2005; Greinacher, 2006). However, HIT cases associated with high concentrations of IgM and/or IgA isotypes (Amiral et al., 1996c; Meyer et al., 2006) could be underdiagnosed, depending on the study inclusion criteria. In any event, these intriguing observations require explanation for how IgM and IgA antibodies could trigger thrombocytopenia, with or without thrombosis.

It is well accepted that IgG antibodies to PF4/H can become pathogenic when they interact with platelets, particularly when PF4/H–IgG complexes bind to the platelet Fcγ receptors (FcγRIIa) (Kelton et al., 1988) (see chap. 8). Another group proposed that, in addition, an IgG receptor polymorphism on leukocyte FcγRIIIa, different from that of FcγRIIa, could also be involved (Gruel et al., 2004). Our observations indicate that other mechanisms for PF4/H–antibody complexes binding onto blood cells could be involved. These could result not only if the PF4/H complexes bind to the cell surfaces through their heparin-binding sites (Van Rijn et al., 1987; Horne and Alkins, 1996; Horne and Hutchison, 1998) but possibly also through PF4-binding sites (Capitanio et al., 1985; Rybak et al., 1989). Although HIT antibodies recognize PF4/H complexes in the fluid phase (Newman et al., 1998), it is uncertain whether this typically occurs *in vivo* before interaction of PF4/H–IgG complexes with the platelet surface, or whether HIT antibodies only bind after PF4/H complexes first become attached to the platelet surface. Recent reports have shown that anti-PF4/H antibodies from patients with HIT can activate ECs (especially microvascular ECs) and also monocytes, and thereby induce release of TF (Arepally and Mayer, 2001; Pouplard et al., 2001; Blank et al., 2002).

Regardless, the clinical state of the patient, determining the extent of platelet and EC activation, seems to be a key factor for determining whether clinical HIT results (Boshkov et al., 1993; Reininger et al., 1996). This contribution occurs in several ways: activated platelets release high amounts of PF4 that can complex with heparin, and activated platelets also expose a higher density of heparin-binding sites (Horne and Chao, 1989). Consequently, these platelets may be even more readily activated by heparin-dependent antibodies. This situation occurs in patients with acute or chronic platelet activation associated with CPB, atherosclerosis, inflammation, infections, cancer, diabetes, and orthopedic surgery, among others.

Another factor determining HIT antibody formation is the type of heparin that binds to PF4, which depends on its oligosaccharide composition, polysaccharide length, and grade of sulfation (Lindahl et al., 1994; Greinacher et al., 1995). Formation of PF4/H complexes requires a heparin molecule containing at least 12–14 oligosaccharide units and a high sulfation grade (more than three sulfate groups per disaccharide) (Amiral et al., 1995). Furthermore, binding of heparin to blood and ECs also increases with heparin molecule length and sulfation grade (Sobel and Adelman, 1988; Horne and Chao, 1990; Harenberg et al., 1994). Heparin structure thus has a dual effect in HIT: it is required not only to form PF4/H complexes but also to target these complexes onto cell surfaces. These factors could explain the higher frequency of anti-PF4/H antibody development and of HIT in patients receiving UFH, compared with those receiving LMWH (Poncz, 2005; Greinacher, 2006). With UFH, PF4/H complexes are larger and are more easily formed, requiring a lower heparin concentration than with LMWH. For the latter drug, only the subset of molecules containing at least 12–14 oligosaccharide units (MW > 3600 Da) can generate immunoreactive PF4/H complexes. Thus, because LMWH has a lower propensity to form PF4/H complexes and binds less readily to platelets and ECs, LMWH therapy is also less likely to result in thrombocytopenia even when pathologic HIT antibodies are already present.

PF4/H-reactive antibodies targeted at platelets induce platelet activation, resulting in thrombocytopenia and, often, thrombosis. Occasionally, heparin-induced thrombosis occurs in the absence of thrombocytopenia (Hach-Wunderle et al., 1994; Bux-Gewehr et al., 1996), or because of high platelet counts present before the occurrence of HIT (see chaps. 2 and 3). Platelet activation by the IgG isotype antibodies is mediated by interaction with platelet FcγRIIa (Kelton et al., 1988; Denomme et al., 1997). Some studies suggest an important role for an FcγRIIa polymorphism (Brandt et al., 1995; Burgess et al., 1995). However, the role of the FcγRIIa polymorphism is controversial (Arepally et al., 1997; Denomme et al., 1997; Suh et al., 1997; Bachelot-Loza et al., 1998) (see chap. 8).

Platelet activation might also occur through other mechanisms, such as direct antibody binding to exposed cell antigens (Rubinstein et al., 1995), a phenomenon that is dependent on the antigen electric charge (Schattner et al., 1993). Heparin is highly electronegative. Evidence for direct activation through antigen binding is supported by the positive platelet aggregation response produced by some patient plasma samples containing only anti-PF4/H antibodies of the IgM and/or IgA isotypes. Formation of heparin-containing immune complexes on cell surfaces can initiate blood and EC interactions, and this can enhance their activating effects. Cell–cell interactions may occur and be amplified through release products that chemoattract and activate cells or through transcellular metabolism (Nash, 1994; Marcus et al., 1995). Platelet products (e.g., PF4) and platelet-derived microparticles (Warkentin et al., 1994) can induce activation of leukocytes (Aziz et al., 1995; Jy et al., 1995; Petersen et al., 1996). Leukocyte-release products, such as cathepsin G, can directly activate platelets and cleave β-thromboglobulin to the active chemokine, NAP-2, thus establishing an amplification loop. Platelet–leukocyte aggregates can form *in vivo*, contributing to vascular occlusion, especially in limb vessels (Fig. 6.3). In a recent study, antibodies to PF4/H from patients with HIT were shown to induce synthesis of TF by monocytes in the presence of PF4 and heparin (Pouplard et al., 2001) or by microvascular ECs (Blank et al., 2002). This could be a complementary pathway for inducing thrombosis.

Variability in certain biologic characteristics of anti-PF4/H antibodies influences their potential for inducing HIT. Platelet activation caused by anti-PF4/H antibodies is usually weak and is only pathogenic when amplification mechanisms are involved. This is demonstrated by the variable lag phase observed in platelet aggregation studies performed with different plasmas or sera from HIT patients. Antibody concentration is another important factor for determining the extent of platelet activation. Antibody affinity is also crucial: the higher the affinity, the lower the concentration of antibodies required for activating platelets. A subset of antibodies to PF4/H complexes that had platelet-activating properties was isolated in three patients with HIT (Amiral et al., 2000). These platelet-activating antibodies had the highest avidity for PF4/H. In contrast, the bulk of antibodies against PF4/H in these patients had no effect on platelet activation. Also, when IgM or IgA isotypes are present, affinity for PF4/H complexes is usually lower than that of IgG isotypes and, consequently, high concentrations are necessary for pathogenicity. Lastly, HIT antibodies do not all bind to the same epitopes on PF4/H complexes, and this specificity could be an additional important factor (Horsewood et al., 1996; Pouplard et al., 1997; Suh et al., 1998). At least two neoepitopes have been identified on PF4 that are distinct from the "region of positive charge" to which heparin binds (Ziporen et al., 1998; Li et al., 2002) (see also chap. 9). Thus, anti-PF4/H antibodies are not equivalent, and those with the strongest affinity are most pathogenic.

Platelet activation in HIT involves amplification through ADP receptors (Polgár et al., 1998) and involves GPIIb/IIIa (Hérault et al., 1997; Jeske et al., 1997). These findings further emphasize the importance of platelet activation amplification loops for producing the clinical manifestations of HIT.

ROLE OF PRE-EXISTING ANTIBODIES TO CXC CHEMOKINES

Pre-existing antibodies to chemokines, such as IL-8 or NAP-2, or possibly even to PF4 itself, may be present in some patients before heparin therapy (Sylvester et al., 1992; Bendtzen et al., 1995; Warkentin et al., 2006b). These antibodies may occur naturally or be induced in pathologic states, where they might have a regulatory role in inflammation (Reitamo et al., 1993), or result from bacteria preimmunization (Greinacher et al., 2011; Krauel et al., 2011). In some diseases, they are present at high concentrations. Antibodies to IL-8 are the most common (Reitamo et al., 1993). However, in some patients, true autoantibodies to PF4 alone can also be observed. In the absence of heparin, these antibodies usually do not demonstrate any clear pathogenicity. However, during heparin therapy, PF4 and other chemokines are released into blood from their storage pools. Heparin may further localize these chemokines onto blood cells and endothelium, with deleterious consequences. The amount of chemokine/heparin complexes bound to blood cells and ECs depends on different factors: the amount of releasable chemokines (i.e., the patient's clinical state); the type and dose of heparin used; the presence of activated cells with an increased capacity to bind chemokines; and, if present, the heparin-dependent antibodies, through their binding to chemokine/heparin complexes. As with antibodies against PF4/H complexes, these natural antichemokine antibodies could initiate cell activation and cell–cell interactions as well as generate circulating cell aggregates that could lead to vessel occlusion. Figure 6.4 shows the possible mechanism for pathogenic effects of these antichemokine antibodies, as antibody localization to the target cells is enhanced by heparin therapy. In a recent observation, antibodies to PF4 alone were detected in a patient who developed thrombocytopenia and clinical symptoms of HIT soon after having received heparin for treatment of cerebral venous thrombosis (Desprez et al., 2010). In this case, pre-existing anti-PF4 antibodies could be associated with the cerebral thrombosis complication, even in the absence of preceding heparin. Finally, we can speculate that protamine sulfate, used for neutralizing heparin after CPB, could generate an immunologic stimulus for heparin-dependent immunization

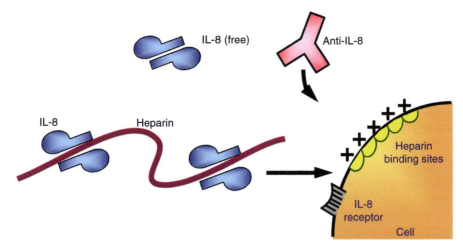

FIGURE 6.4 Possible effect of heparin for carrying pre-existing antibodies to IL-8 onto platelets (and other blood cells), through the heparin-binding sites or through the IL-8 receptors, targeting the deleterious consequences of these antibodies onto these cells. *Abbreviation*: IL-8, interleukin-8.

(Al-Mondhiry et al., 1985), especially as both protamine and heparin can induce thrombocytopenia, and protamine can induce specific antibody formation. However, in some cases, anti-protamine sulfate/heparin complex (anti-PS/H) antibodies were the only antibodies detected in patients with a high clinical suspicion of HIT, based on thrombocytopenia corresponding to proximate heparin therapy and thrombosis occurrence (Amiral and Amiral, 2009). These patients had received protamine sulfate for neutralization of heparin.

NEW ASSAYS FOR HIT BASED ON HEPARIN-DEPENDENT ANTIGENS

The present understanding of how heparin-dependent antibodies contribute to the development of HIT allowed us to develop new assays for measuring these antibodies, by mimicking closely the conditions thought to occur *in vivo*. For this approach, functionally available heparin is coated onto a solid surface, such as an enzyme immunoassay (EIA) plate or any other surface. This can be achieved by different means: coating protamine sulfate in the presence of a large excess of heparin; coating streptavidin/biotinylated heparin; or coating heparin covalently bound to a carrier protein (such as albumin) or a polymer. The patient plasma or serum is incubated with this heparinized surface. If chemokines that exhibit heparin affinity are present, they bind to the coated heparin, exposing neoepitopes, and thereby capturing heparin-dependent antibodies (Fig. 6.5). In addition, if antigenic heparin/protein complexes are present, they can also directly bind to heparin through the heparin-binding protein. Using an anti-IgG/A/M or an anti-IgG or a combination of anti-IgG, -IgA and -IgM peroxidase conjugates allows measurement of all the antibody isotypes (useful for screening for HIT) or only the IgG isotype (the preferred assay for confirming the diagnosis of HIT) or proceeding to a full isotyping of those antibodies (which remains a convenient tool for research studies). This approach is flexible, very sensitive, and highly specific for

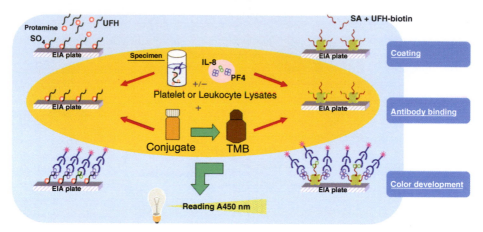

FIGURE 6.5 Assay for testing heparin-dependent antibodies, associated with HIT, by their binding to functionally available heparin through the heparin cofactor antigen (usually PF4); heparin is coated in a large excess as a complex with aprotinin or biotinylated and reacted with coated SA. *Abbreviations*: EIA, enzyme immunoassay; IL-8, interleukin-8; PF4, platelet factor 4; SA, streptavidin; TMB, tetramethyl benzidine; UFH, unfractionated heparin.

heparin-dependent antibodies. It allows identification of the antibody isotypes of clinical relevance.

An interesting improvement consists in supplementing the reaction milieu with platelet lysates or with lysates from leukocyte–platelet concentrates, or, when required, directly with PF4, IL-8, or any other high affinity heparin-binding protein. This provides PF4 or other chemokines in excess for forming the heparin-dependent antigenic target for HIT antibodies. Using platelet lysates, the assay correlates fully with the conventional EIA for measuring anti-PF4/H antibodies of IgG isotype using plasmas from patients with clinically suspected HIT ($r^2 = 0.89$), although some IgG positive patients were negative with the conventional PF4/H EIA, possibly because additional antigenic complexes are only measured with the new assay. Some of these discrepant patients, but not all of them, had anti-PS/H antibodies, which are captured onto the plate when it is coated with protamine sulfate and heparin. When comparing the assay performed with or without platelet lysates, two groups of patients with HIT are identified: those for whom the antibody binding is totally dependent on the presence of platelet lysates and those in whom antibodies in the dilute patient plasma (or serum) bind "directly" to functionally active heparin. At this time, no clinical significance has yet been identified regarding these differences.

CONCLUSIONS

PF4 complexed with heparin is the major antigen involved in HIT. Understanding the mechanisms for generating heparin-dependent antibodies, and how these antibodies become pathogenic, offers new approaches for diagnosis and management of HIT. Only a subset of antibodies to PF4/H exhibit a pathogenic effect by triggering thrombocytopenia and/or thrombosis, particularly IgG antibodies with the highest affinity for PF4/H. The conditions that permit the formation of the PF4/H target antigens involve the type of heparin used, the dose and duration of therapy, and the clinical context of the treated patient. Immunoreactive complexes between PF4 and heparin are formed only under certain conditions, with their formation in high concentrations facilitated if underlying disease favors platelet activation and release. Similar conditions enhance the pathogenicity of the HIT antibodies generated. These considerations help to unravel the seemingly random generation of HIT antibodies among heparin-treated patients as well as the apparent chance occurrence of thrombocytopenia and thrombotic events. In addition, some HIT episodes could be associated with pre-existing antibodies to chemokines, such as IL-8, NAP-2, or possibly, even PF4-dependent antigens. A possible involvement of anti-PS/H antibodies is also suspected. The use of heparin then only constitutes the abrupt trigger of pathogenicity by focusing these antibodies onto targeted blood cells and ECs. This could be the explanation for atypical presentations of HIT that can occur with pathologic states, such as malignancy, major surgery/ inflammation, or infections. Understanding how heparin-dependent antigens can induce antibody generation, how these antibodies can become pathogenic in a subset of patients, and how heparin can trigger pathologic effects for naturally occurring antichemokine antibodies, can improve recognition and management of these complications of heparin therapy. This includes the development of more appropriate diagnostic laboratory assays for this life-threatening iatrogenic complication of heparin therapy.

REFERENCES

Al-Mondhiry H, Pierce WS, Basarab RM. Protamine-induced thrombocytopenia and leukopenia. Thromb Haemost 53: 60–64, 1985.

Amiral J, Bridey F, Dreyfus M, Vissac AM, Fressinaud E, Wolf M, Meyer D. Platelet factor 4 complexed to heparin is the target for antibodies generated in heparin induced thrombocytopenia. Thromb Haemost 68: 95–96, 1992.

Amiral J, Bridey F, Wolf M, Boyer-Neumann C, Fressinaud E, Vissac AM, Peynaud-Debayle E, Dreyfus M, Meyer D. Antibodies to macromolecular platelet factor 4 heparin complexes in heparin-induced thrombocytopenia: a study of 44 cases. Thromb Haemost 73: 21–28, 1995.

Amiral J, Marfaing-Koka A, Wolf M, Alessi MC, Tardy B, Boyer-Neumann C, Vissac AM, Fressinaud E, Poncz M, Meyer D. Presence of auto-antibodies to interleukin-8 or neutrophil-activating peptide-2 in patients with heparin-associated-thrombocytopenia. Blood 88: 410–416, 1996a.

Amiral J, Peynaud-Debayle E, Wolf M, Bridey F, Vissac AM, Meyer D. Generation of antibodies to heparin-PF4 complexes without thrombocytopenia in patients treated with unfractionated or low molecular weight heparin. Am J Hematol 52: 90–95, 1996b.

Amiral J, Wolf M, Fischer AM, Boyer-Neumann C, Vissac AM, Meyer D. Pathogenicity of IgA and/or IgM antibodies to heparin-PF4 complexes in patients with heparin-induced thrombocytopenia. Br J Haematol 92: 954–959, 1996c.

Amiral J, Pouplard C, Vissac AM, Walenga JM, Jeske W, Gruel Y. Affinity purification of heparin-dependent antibodies to platelet factor 4 developed in heparin-induced thrombocytopenia: biological characteristics and effects on platelet activation. Br J Haematol 109: 336–341, 2000.

Amiral J, Vissac AM. Pseudo-HIT associated with antibodies to protamine-sulfate [Abstr PP-MO-697]. XXIIth Congress of the International Society on Thrombosis and Haemostasis, 2009 [available on-line].

Arepally GM, Mayer IM. Antibodies from patients with heparin-induced thrombocytopenia stimulate monocytic cells to express tissue factor and secrete interleukin-8. Blood 98: 1252–1254, 2001.
Arepally G, McKenzie SE, Jiang X-M, Poncz M, Cines DB. FcγRIIA H/R131 polymorphism, subclass-specific IgG anti-heparin/platelet factor 4 antibodies and clinical course in patients with heparin-induced thrombocytopenia and thrombosis. Blood 89: 370–375, 1997.
Aziz KA, Cawley JC, Zuzel M. Platelets prime PMN via released PF4: mechanism of priming and synergy with GM-CSF. Br J Haematol 91: 846–853, 1995.
Bachelot-Loza C, Saffroy R, Lasne D, Chatellier G, Aiach M, Rendu F. Importance of the FcγRIIA-Arg/His-131 polymorphism in heparin-induced thrombocytopenia diagnosis. Thromb Haemost 79: 523–528, 1998.
Bacsi S, De Palma R, Visentin GP, Gorski J, Aster RH. Complexes of heparin and platelet factor 4 specifically stimulate T cells from patients with heparin-induced thrombocytopenia/thrombosis. Blood 94: 208–215, 1999.
Bauer TL, Arepally G, Konkle BA, Mestichelli B, Shapiro SS, Cines DB, Poncz M, McNulty S, Amiral J, Hauck WW, Edie RN, Mannion JD. Prevalence of heparin-associated antibodies without thrombosis in patients undergoing cardiopulmonary bypass surgery. Circulation 95: 1242–1246, 1997.
Barber AJ, Kaser-Glanzmann R, Jakabova M, Luscher F. Characterization of a chon-droitin 4–sulfate proteoglycan carrier for heparin neutralizing activity (platelet factor 4) released from human blood platelets. Biochim Biophys Acta 286: 312–329, 1972.
Bendtzen K, Hansen MB, Ross C, Poulsen LK, Svenson M. Cytokines and autoantibodies to cytokines. Stem Cells 13: 206–222, 1995.
Berry C, Tchermiantchouk O, Ley EJ, Salim A, Mirocha J, Martin-Stone S, Stolpner D, Margulies DR. Overdiagnosis of heparin-induced thrombocytopenia in surgical ICU patients. J Am Coll Surg 213: 10–17, 2011.
Blank M, Shoenfeld Y, Tavor S, Praprotnik S, Boffa MC, Weksler B, Walenga MJ, Amiral J, Eldor A. Anti-platelet factor 4/heparin antibodies from patients with heparin-induced thrombocytopenia provoke direct activation of microvascular endothelial cells. Int Immunol 14: 121–129, 2002.
Bock PE, Luscombe M, Marshall SE, Pepper DS, Holbrook JJ. The multiple complexes formed by the interaction of platelet factor 4 with heparin. Biochem J 191: 769–776, 1980.
Boshkov LK, Warkentin TE, Hayward CPM, Andrew M, Kelton JG. Heparin-induced thrombocytopenia and thrombosis: clinical and laboratory studies. Br J Haematol 84: 322–328, 1993.
Brandt E, Flad HD. Structure and function of platelet-derived cytokines of the β-thromboglobulin/interleukin 8 family. Platelets 3: 295–305, 1992.
Brandt J, Isenhart CE, Osborne JM, Ahmed A, Anderson CL. On the role of platelet FcγRIIa phenotype in heparin-induced thrombocytopenia. Thromb Haemost 74: 1564–1572, 1995.
Burgess JK, Lindeman R, Chesterman CN, Chong BH. Single amino acid mutation of fcγ receptor is associated with the development of heparin-induced thrombocytopenia. Br J Haematol 91: 761–766, 1995.
Bux-Gewehr I, Helmling E, Sefert UT. HAT type II and platelets within a normal range. Kardiologia 85: 656–660, 1996.
Capitanio AM, Niewiarowski S, Rucinski B, Tuszynski GP, Cierniewski CS, Hershock D, Kornecki E. Interaction of platelet factor 4 with human platelets. Biochim Biophys Acta 839: 161–173, 1985.
Cines DB, Tomaski A, Tannenbaum S. Immune endothelial-cell injury in heparin-associated thrombocytopenia. N Engl J Med 316: 581–589, 1987.
Cowan SW, Bakshi EN, Machin KJ, Isaacs NW. Binding of heparin to human platelet factor 4. Biochem J 234: 485–488, 1986.
Denomme GA, Warkentin TE, Horsewood P, Sheppard JI, Warner MN, Kelton JG. Activation of platelets by sera containing IgGl heparin-dependent antibodies: an explanation for the predominance of the FcγRIIa "low responder" (his131) gene in patients with heparin-induced thrombocytopenia. J Lab Clin Med 130: 278–284, 1997.
Desprez D, Desprez P, Tardy B, Amiral J, Droulle C, Mauvieux L, Grunebaum L. Anti-PF4 antibodies and thrombophlebitis in a child with cerebral venous thrombosis. Ann Biol Clin (Paris) 68: 725–728, 2010. [in French]

Dunlop MG, Prowse CV, Dawes J. Heparin-induced platelet factor 4 release in patients with atherosclerotic peripheral vascular disease. Thromb Res 46: 409–410, 1987.

Francis JL. Detection and significance of heparin-platelet factor 4 antibodies. Semin Hematol 42(3 Suppl 3): S9–S14, 2005.

Greinacher A. Heparin-induced thrombocytopenia: frequency and pathogenesis. Pathophysiol Haemost Thromb 35: 37–45, 2006.

Greinacher A, Potzsch B, Amiral J, Dummel V, Eichner A, Mueller-Eckhardt C. Heparin-associated thrombocytopenia: isolation of the antibody and characterization of a multimolecular PF4-heparin complex as the major antigen. Thromb Haemost 71: 247–251, 1994.

Greinacher A, Alban S, Dummel V, Franz G, Mueller-Eckhardt C. Characterization of the structural requirements for a carbohydrate based anticoagulant with a reduced risk of inducing the immunological type of heparin-associated thrombocytopenia. Thromb Haemost 74: 886–892, 1995.

Greinacher A, Holtfreter B, Krauel K, Gätke D, Weber C, Ittermann T, Hammerschmidt S, Kocher T. Association of natural anti-platelet factor 4/heparin antibodies with periodontal disease. Blood 118: 1395–401, 2011.

Gruel Y, Boizard-Boval B, Wautier JL. Further evidence that α-granule components such as platelet factor 4 are involved in platelet-IgG-heparin interactions during heparin-associated thrombocytopenia. Thromb Haemost 70: 374–375, 1993.

Gruel Y, Pouplard C, Lasne D, Magdelaine-Beuzelin C, Charroing C, Wautier H. The homozygous FcγRIIIa-158V genotype is a risk factor for heparin-induced thrombocytopenia in patients with antibodies to heparin-platelet factor 4 complexes. Blood 104: 2791–2793, 2004.

Hach-Wunderle V, Kainer K, Krug B, Muller-Berghaus G, Pötzsch B. Heparin-associated thrombosis despite normal platelet counts. Lancet 344: 469–470, 1994.

Harenberg J, Malsch R, Piazolo L, Heene DL. Binding of heparin to human leukocytes. Hamostaseologie 14: 16–24, 1994.

Hérault JP, Lalé A, Savi P, Pflieger AM, Herbert JM. In vitro inhibition of heparin-induced platelet aggregation in plasma from patients with HIT by SR 121566, a newly developed Gp IIb/IIIa antagonist. Blood Coagul Fibrinolysis 8: 206–207, 1997.

Horne MK III, Alkins BR. Platelets binding of IgG from patients with heparin-induced thrombocytopenia. J Lab Clin Med 127: 435–442, 1996.

Horne MK III, Chao ES. Heparin binding to resting and activated platelets. Blood 74: 238–243, 1989.

Horne MK III, Chao ES. The effect of molecular weight on heparin binding to platelets. Br J Haematol 74: 306–312, 1990.

Horne MK III, Hutchison KJ. Simultaneous binding of heparin and platelet factor-4 to platelets: further insights into the mechanism of heparin-induced thrombocytopenia. Am J Hematol 58: 24–30, 1998.

Huang SS, Huang JS, Deul TS. Proteoglycan carrier of platelet factor 4. J Biol Chem 257: 11546–11550, 1982.

Horsewood P, Warkentin TE, Hayward CPM, Kelton JG. The epitope specificity of heparin-induced thrombocytopenia. Br J Haematol 95: 161–167, 1996.

Jeske WP, Walenga JM, Szatkowski E, Ero M, Herbert JM, Haas S, Bakhos M. Effect of glycoprotein IIb-IIIa antagonists on the HIT serum induced activation of platelets. Thromb Res 88: 271–281, 1997.

Jy W, Mao WW, Horstman LL, Tao J, Ahn YS. Platelet microparticles bind, activate and aggregate neutrophils in vitro. Blood Cells Mol Dis 21: 217–231, 1995.

Kelton J. Pathophysiology of heparin-induced thrombocytopenia. Br J Haematol 82: 778–784, 1992.

Kelton JG, Sheridan D, Santos A, Smith J, Steeves K, Smith C, Brown C, Murphy WG. Heparin-induced thrombocytopenia: laboratory studies. Blood 72: 925–930, 1988.

Kelton JG, Smith JW, Warkentin TE, Hayward CPM, Denomme GA, Horsewood P. Immunoglobulin g from patients with heparin-induced thrombocytopenia binds to a complex of heparin and platelet factor 4. Blood 83: 3232–3239, 1994.

Krauel K, Pötschke C, Weber C, Kessler W, Fürll B, Ittermann T, Maier S, Hammerschmidt S, Bröker BM, Greinacher A. Platelet factor 4 binds to bacteria, [corrected] inducing antibodies cross-reacting with the major antigen in heparin-induced thrombocytopenia. Blood 117: 1370–1378, 2011.

Lambert MP, Rauova L, Bailey M, Sola-Visner MC, Kowalska MA, Poncz M. Platelet factor 4 is an autocrine in vivo regulator of megakaryocytopoiesis: clinical and therapeutic implications. Blood 110: 1153-1160, 2007.

Li ZQ, Liu W, Park KS, Sachais BS, Arepally GM, Cines DB, Poncz M. Defining a second epitope for heparin-induced thrombocytopenia/thrombosis antibodies using KKO, a murine HIT-like monoclonal antibody. Blood 99: 1230–1236, 2002.

Lindahl U, Lidholt K, Spillmann D, Kjellen L. More to "heparin" than anticoagulant. Thromb Res 75: 1–32, 1994.

Lindhoff-Last E, Gerdsen F, Ackermann H, Bauersachs R. Determination of heparin-platelet factor 4–IgG antibodies improves diagnosis of heparin-induced thrombocytopenia. Br J Haematol 113: 886–890, 2001.

Luscombe M, Marshall SE, Pepper D, Holdbrook JJ. The transfer of platelet factor 4 from its proteoglycan carrier to natural and synthetic polymers. Biochim Biophys Acta 678: 137–142, 1981.

Maccarana M, Lindahl U. Mode of interaction between platelet factor 4 and heparin. Glycobiology 3: 271–277, 1993.

Marcus AJ, Safier LB, Broekman MJ, Islam N, Fliessbach JH, Hajjar KA, Kaminski WE, Jendraschak E, Silverstein RL, von Schacky C. Thrombosis and inflammation as multicellular processes: significance of cell-cell interactions. Thromb Haemost 74: 213–217, 1995.

Meyer O, Aslan T, Koster A, Kiesewetter H, Salama A. Report of a patient with heparin-induced thrombocytopenia type II associated with IgA antibodies only. Clin Appl Thromb Hemost 12: 373–375, 2006.

Nash GB. Adhesion between neutrophils and platelets: a modulator of thrombotic and inflammatory events? Thromb Res 74: S3–S11, 1994.

Nesmelova IV, Sham Y, Dudek AZ, van Eijk LI, Wu G, Slungaard A, Mortari F, Griffioen AW, Mayo KH. Platelet factor 4 and interleukin-8 CXC chemokine hetero-dimer formation modulates function at the quaternary structural level. J Biol Chem 280: 4948–4958, 2005.

Newman PM, Swanson RL, Chong BH. Heparin-induced thrombocytopenia: IgG binding to PF4-Heparin complexes in the fluid phase and cross-reactivity with low molecular weight heparin and heparinoid. Thromb Haemost 80: 292–297, 1998.

Petersen F, Lidwig A, Flad HD, Brandt E. TNF-a renders human neutrophils responsive to platelet factor 4. J Immunol 156: 1954–1962, 1996.

Polgar J, Eichler P, Greinacher A, Clemetson KJ. Adenosine diphosphate (ADP) and ADP receptor play a major role in platelet activation/aggregation induced by sera from heparin-induced thrombocytopenia patients. Blood 91: 549–554, 1998.

Poncz M. Mechanistic basis of heparin-induced thrombocytopenia. Semin Thorac Cardiovasc Surg 17: 73–79, 2005.

Pouplard C, Amiral J, Borg JY, Vissac AM, Delahousse B, Gruel Y. Differences in specificity of heparin-dependent antibodies developed under low molecular weight heparin therapy and higher cross-reactivity with Orgaran. Br J Haematol 99: 273–280, 1997.

Pouplard C, Iochmann I, Renard O, Hérault O, Colombat P, Amiral J, Gruel Y. Induction of monocyte tissue factor expression by antibodies to platelet factor 4 developed in heparin-induced thrombocytopenia. Blood 97: 3300–3302, 2001.

Rauova L, Poncz M, McKenzie SA, Reilly MP, Arepally G, Weisel JW, Nagaswami C, Cines DB, Sachais BS. Ultralarge complexes of PF4 and heparin are central to the pathogenesis of heparin-induced thrombocytopenia. Blood 105: 131–138, 2005.

Regnault V, de Maistre E, Carteaux JP, Gruel Y, Nguyen P, Tardy B, Lecompte T. Platelet activation induced by human antibodies to interleukin-8. Blood 101: 1419–1421, 2003.

Reilly MP, Taylor SM, Franklin C, Sachais BS, Cines DB, Williams KJ, McKenzie SE. Prothrombotic factors enhance heparin-induced thrombocytopenia and thrombosis in vivo in a mouse model. J Thromb Haemost 4: 2687–2694, 2006.

Reininger CB, Greinacher A, Graf J, Lasser R, Steckmeier B, Schweiberer L. Platelets of patients with peripheral arterial disease are hypersensitive to heparin. Thromb Res 81: 641–649, 1996.

Reitamo S, Remitz A, Varga J, Ceska M, Effenberger F, Jimenez S, Uitto J. Demonstration of interleukin 8 and autoantibodies to interleukin 8 in the serum of patients with systemic sclerosis and related disorders. Arch Dermatol 129: 189–193, 1993.

Rice L, Attisha WK, Drexler A, Francis JL. Delayed-onset heparin-induced thrombocytopenia. Ann Intern Med 136: 210–215, 2002.

Rubinstein E, Boucheix C, Worthington RE, Carroll RC. Anti-platelet antibody interactions with fcγ receptor. Semin Thromb Hemost 21: 10–22, 1995.

Rybak ME, Gimbrone MA, Davies PF, Handin RI. Interaction of platelet factor four with cultured vascular endothelial cells. Blood 73: 1534–1539, 1989.

Schattner M, Lazzari M, Trevani AS, Malchiodi E, Kempfer AC, Isturiz MA, Geffner JR. Activation of human platelets by immune complexes prepared with cationized human IgG. Blood 82: 3045–3051, 1993.

Shoenfeld Y. Heparin-induced thrombocytopenia as an autoimmune disease: idiotypic evidence for the role of anti-heparin-PF4 autoantibodies. Isr J Med Sci 33: 243–245, 1997.

Slungaard A. Platelet factor 4: a chemokines enigma. Int J Biochem Cell Biol 37: 1162–1167, 2005.

Smythe MA, Stephen JL, Mattson JC. Delayed-onset heparin-induced thrombocytopenia. Ann Emerg Med 45: 417–419, 2005.

Sobel M, Adelman B. Characterization of platelet binding of heparins and other glycosaminoglycans. Thromb Res 50: 815–826, 1988.

Stuckey JA, St Charles R, Edwards B. A model of the platelet factor 4 complex with heparin. Proteins 14: 277–287, 1992.

Suh JS, Malik MI, Aster RH, Visentin GP. Characterization of the humoral immune response in heparin-induced thrombocytopenia. Am J Hematol 54: 196–201, 1997.

Suh JS, Aster RH, Visentin GP. Antibodies from patients with heparin-induced thrombocytopenia/thrombosis recognize different epitopes on heparin: platelet factor 4. Blood 91: 916–922, 1998.

Suvarna S, Rauova L, McCracken EKE, Goss CM, Sachais BS, McKenzie SE, Reilly MP, Gunn MD, CInes DB, Poncz M, Arepally G. PF4/heparin complexes are T cell-dependent antigens. Blood 106: 929–931, 2005.

Sylvester L, Yoshimura T, Sticherling M, Schroder JM, Ceska M, Peichi P, Leonard EJ. Neutrophil attractant protein-1–immunoglobulin g immune complexes and free anti-NAP-1 antibody in normal human serum. J Clin Invest 90: 471–481, 1992.

Van Rijn JLML, Trillou M, Mardiguian J, Tobelem G, Caen J. Selective binding of heparins to human endothelial cells. implications for pharmacokinetics. Thromb Res 45: 211–222, 1987.

Visentin GP, Aster RH. Heparin induced thrombocytopenia and thrombosis. Curr Opin Hematol 2: 351–357, 1995.

Visentin GP, Ford SE, Scott JP, Aster RH. Antibodies from patients with heparin-induced thrombocytopenia/thrombosis are specific for platelet factor 4 complexed with heparin or bound to endothelial cells. J Clin Invest 93: 81–88, 1994.

Visentin GP, Malik M, Cyganiak KA, Aster RH. Patients with unfractionated heparin during open heart surgery are at high risk to form antibodies reactive with heparin: platelet factor 4 complexes. J Lab Clin Med 128: 376–383, 1996.

Warkentin TE. Heparin-induced thrombocytopenia. Diagnosis and Management. Circulation 110: 454–458, 2004.

Warkentin TE. New approaches to the diagnosis of heparin-induced thrombocytopenia. Chest 127: 35–45, 2005.

Warkentin TE, Kelton JG. A 14–year study of heparin-induced thrombocytopenia. Am J Med 101: 502–507, 1996.

Warkentin TE, Kelton JG. Delayed-onset heparin-induced thrombocytopenia and thrombosis. Ann Intern Med 135: 502–506, 2001.

Warkentin TE, Sheppard JA. Testing for heparin-induced thrombocytopenia antibodies. Transfus Med Rev 20: 259–272, 2006.

Warkentin TE, Hayward CPM, Boshkov LK, Santos AV, Sheppard JI, Bode AP, Kelton JG. Sera from patients with heparin-induced thrombocytopenia generate platelet-derived microparticles with procoagulant activity: an explanation for the thrombotic complications of heparin-induced thrombocytopenia. Blood 84: 3691–3699, 1994.

Warkentin TE, Levine MN, Hirsh J, Horsewood P, Roberts RS, Gent M, Kelton JG. Heparin-induced thrombocytopenia in patients treated with low molecular weight heparin or unfractionated heparin. N Engl J Med 332: 1330–1335, 1995.

Warkentin TE, Sheppard JI, Moore JC, Moore KM, Sigouin CS, Kelton JG. Laboratory testing for the antibodies that cause heparin-induced thrombocytopenia: how much class do we need? J Lab Clin Med 146: 341–346, 2005.

Warkentin TE, Sheppard JI, Sigouin CS, Kohlmann T, Eichler P, Greinacher A. Gender imbalance and risk factor interactions in heparin-induced thrombocytopenia. Blood 108: 2937–2941, 2006.

Warkentin TE, Makris M, Jay RM, Kelton JG. A spontaneous prothrombotic disorder resembling heparin-induced thrombocytopenia. Am J Med 121: 632–636, 2008.

Ziporen L, Li ZQ, Park KS, Sabnekar P, Liu WY, Arepally G, Shoenfeld Y, Kieber-Emmons T, Cines DB, Poncz M. Defining an antigenic epitope on platelet factor 4 associated with heparin-induced thrombocytopenia. Blood 92: 3250–3259, 1998.

Role of sulfated polysaccharides and other polyanions in the pathogenesis of heparin-induced thrombocytopenia

Susanne Alban, Krystin Krauel, and Andreas Greinacher

INTRODUCTION

Unfractionated heparin (UFH) and low molecular weight heparin (LMWH) are the anticoagulants of choice when parenteral anticoagulation is required. Both can be given by subcutaneous (sc) or intravenous (iv) routes, and both are effective in a variety of clinical settings (Hirsh and Raschke, 2004). UFH, in particular, has several limitations. These include its poor bioavailability after sc injection as well as the marked variability in the anticoagulant response to UFH treatment in patients with acute thromboembolism (Young et al., 1992; Hirsh and Raschke, 2004). Another problem is the risk of inducing heparin-induced thrombocytopenia (HIT). These limitations are closely linked (Greinacher, 1995): the underlying cause is the high density of negative charges of the heparin molecule, leading to nonspecific interactions of heparin with cells and plasma proteins other than antithrombin (AT). This results in reduced anticoagulant effects of heparin as well as in conformational changes of the proteins bound to heparin, with the potential for exposure of neoepitopes, or cryptic epitopes, which may induce an immune response.

In this chapter, the mechanism and structural requirements for complex formation between sulfated carbohydrates, especially heparin, and proteins, such as platelet factor 4 (PF4), are reviewed. The pathophysiologic consequences of these interactions in causing HIT are summarized. From these considerations, the prospects for development of carbohydrate-based heparin alternatives with a lower risk for immune thrombocytopenia are discussed. This chapter does not review the interactions of PF4 with polyanions on the surfaces of endothelial cells (ECs) and monocytes, which are reviewed in chapter 9.

INTERACTIONS OF PF4 WITH SULFATED CARBOHYDRATES
Structure of PF4

Heparin activity is neutralized by PF4, a protein released from the α-granules of activated platelets (Sear and Poller, 1973; Luscher and Kaser-Glanzman, 1975; Niewiarowski, 1976; Klener and Kubisz, 1978), which attaches to the EC surface by binding to glycosaminoglycans (GAGs) (Novotny et al., 1993). PF4 is a compact homotetrameric globular protein with a subunit molecular weight (MW) of 7780 Da (70 amino acid residues per subunit) (Kaplan and Niewiarowski, 1985; Mayo et al., 1995). With its content of 6.0% arginine, 3.2% histidine, and 12.3% lysine, PF4 is a basic (positively charged) protein (Moore et al., 1975). The NH_2 terminal residues form antiparallel β-sheet-like structures that induce noncovalent associations between dimers and also contribute to the cohesion of the tetrameric unit. Furthermore, electrostatic interactions between charged amino acid side chains and hydrogen-bonding interactions at the AB/CD dimer interface serve to stabilize the tetrameric structure. The COOH-terminal α-helices, which contain four lysine residues, are arranged as antiparallel pairs on the surface of each extended β-sheet (St. Charles et al., 1989). The lysine residues are predominantly on one side, resulting in a "ring of positive charge" that runs perpendicularly across the helices (Stuckey et al., 1992; Zhang et al., 1994) (see Fig. 9.1 in chap. 9).

Structure of Heparin

Heparin is a polydisperse mixture of GAGs with MWs ranging from 5 to 30 kDa, with an average MW of 13 kDa (Linhardt and Toida, 1997). It is composed of alternating β-D-glucosamine residues 1 → 4-linked to either α-L-iduronic acid or β-D-glucuronic acid (Casu, 1985). The occurrence of 10 distinctly substituted monosaccharides leads to considerable structural heterogeneity. The principal repeating unit in heparin is the trisulfated disaccharide [→ 4)-α-L-iduronic acid-2–O-sulfate (1 → 4)-α-D-glucosamine-2-N, 6–O-disulfate (1 →] (Fig. 7.1A), which represents 60–70% of the heparin chain (Bianchini et al., 2007). The remaining 30–40%

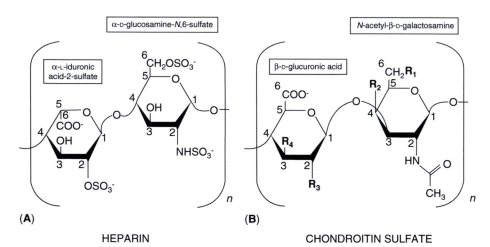

(A) HEPARIN   **(B)** CHONDROITIN SULFATE

FIGURE 7.1 Disaccharide structure of two disaccharides: **(A)** heparin and **(B)** chondroitin sulfate/OSCS. **(A)**. The major disaccharide units of heparin consist of α-1,4-linked iduronic acid (usually sulfated at the 2-position, i.e., iduronic acid-2-sulfate) and glucosamine [usually both N-sulfonated and 6-O-sulfonated (see figure), but sometimes additionally 3-O-sulfonated, a substitution crucial for AT-binding activity of the functional "pentasaccharide" moiety within heparin]. A minority of disaccharides within heparin contain glucuronic acid, rather than its epimer, iduronic acid, and/or N-acetylglucosamine and thus resemble the structure of heparan sulfate. **(B)**. The major repeat units of chondroitin sulfate consist of glucuronic acid and N-acetylgalactosamine. R_1–R_4 can be either SO_4^- or OH. Chondroitin sulfate A and C refer to disaccharides that are sulfated at position 4 (R_2) and 6 (R_1) sites, respectively, of the N-acetylgalactosamine unit. In contrast, OSCS consists of chondroitin sulfate in which R_1, R_2, R_3, and R_4 represent sulfate groups, i.e., per-O-sulfo chondroitin sulfate. *Source*: From Greinacher and Warkentin (2009). *Abbreviations*: OSCS, oversulfated chondroitin sulfate; AT, antithrombin.

of disaccharide units differ in their degree and positions of sulfation (Linhardt et al., 1988). Besides, there are disaccharides consisting of unsulfated glucuronic acid and/or N-acetylglucosamine as is rather typical for heparan sulfate. With a SO_4^-:COO^- ratio of 2.0–2.5, heparin is the GAG with the highest charge density. (For comparison, Figure 7.1B shows the disaccharide unit for chondroitin sulfate, discussed later.) By binding to domains containing positively charged amino acids, especially arginine and lysine, it interacts with many proteins, resulting in manifold biologic activities. The most prominent example is a well-defined pentasaccharide sequence with a central α-D-glucosamine-2-N, 3-O, 6-O-trisulfate unit, which binds specifically to AT (Choay, 1989) (Fig. 7.2). About 30–50% and 10–20%, respectively, of the UFH and LMWH chains contain this pentasaccharide sequence. These molecules are called high-affinity heparin in contrast to the low-affinity heparin without this AT-binding site (Casu, 1990). AT is a natural serine protease inhibitor that controls blood coagulation by forming equimolar covalent complexes with certain coagulation enzymes. The anticoagulant action of heparin is mainly based on accelerating the slow rate of factor Xa and thrombin inhibition by AT (Björk et al., 1989). The heparin pentasaccharide is sufficient for factor Xa inhibition, whereas thrombin inhibition requires a minimum heparin chain length of 18 monosaccharides (5400 Da) to permit simultaneous binding of heparin to both AT and thrombin.

PF4/Sulfated Polysaccharide Complexes

PF4 has the highest affinity to heparin among proteins stored within the platelet α-granules. Heparin molecules bind to PF4 by interactions with the positively charged residues on the surface of PF4 (see chaps. 6 and 9). Stuckey and coworkers (1992) suggested that heparin is bound to PF4 by being wrapped around the tetramer along the ring of positive charges. A heparin molecule with 16–18 monosaccharides interacts with PF4 by spanning about half of the tetramer. As a consequence, only very long molecules are able to wrap around the complete tetramer. Mayo and

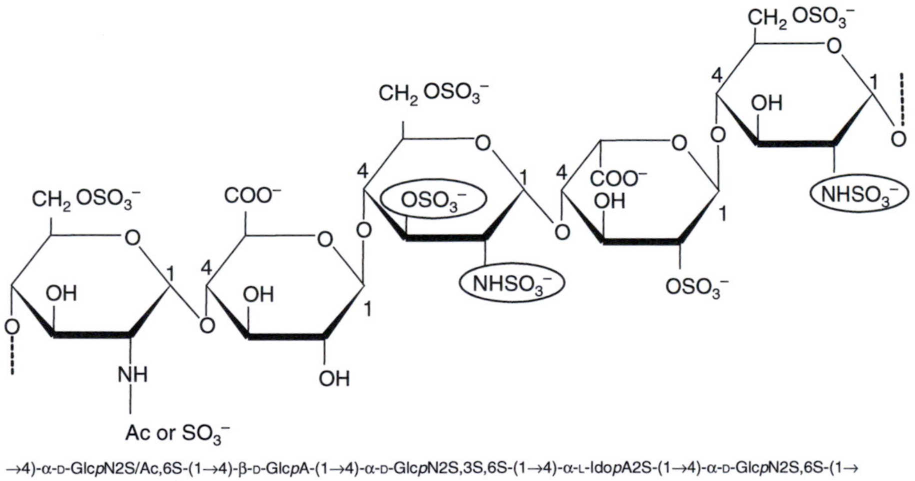

$\rightarrow$4)-α-D-Glc$p$N2S/Ac,6S-(1$\rightarrow$4)-β-D-Glc$p$A-(1$\rightarrow$4)-α-D-Glc$p$N2S,3S,6S-(1$\rightarrow$4)-α-L-Ido$p$A2S-(1$\rightarrow$4)-α-D-Glc$p$N2S,6S-(1$\rightarrow$

FIGURE 7.2   Pentasaccharide sequence of the AT-binding site of heparin. Sulfate groups essential for the AT-binding are encircled. *Abbreviation*: AT, antithrombin.

coworkers (1995) identified a loop containing Arg-20, Arg-22, His-23, and Thr-25, as well as Lys-46 and Arg-49, which are more relevant for heparin binding than the COOH-terminal lysines. For optimal interaction with PF4, a heparin molecule should consist of at least 12 monosaccharides (Mikhailov et al., 1999; Visentin, 1999). At low concentrations (0.1–1.0 IU/mL) of heparin and high concentrations of PF4, several PF4 tetramers compete for heparin binding. This permits binding of a heparin chain to more than one PF4 tetramer. Particularly, if a heparin molecule is longer than 16 monosaccharides, it is able to bind to and thereby bridge two PF4 tetramers. Thus, at certain concentrations of heparin and PF4, large, multimolecular PF4/heparin (PF4/H) complexes are formed. UFH forms larger complexes than LMWH (Rauova et al., 2005; Greinacher et al., 2006). These complexes can be dissociated in the presence of high heparin concentrations (Bock et al., 1980; Greinacher et al., 1994c, 1995).

In vitro, only heparin molecules containing 16 or more monosaccharides completely bind to immobilized PF4, resulting in total neutralization of their antifactor Xa (anti-Xa) and antithrombin (anti-IIa) activities, whereas progressively smaller oligosaccharides (without anti-IIa activity) become increasingly resistant to neutralization of their anti-Xa activity by PF4 (Denton et al., 1983; Lane et al., 1984). Also in plasma, the anti-IIa activity of LMWHs, which is mediated by molecules with MW >5400 Da, but not their anti-Xa activity, can be completely neutralized by higher PF4 concentrations (Padilla et al., 1992; Bendetowicz et al., 1994). The reduced sensitivity of LMWHs to inactivation by PF4 also explains why LMWHs are more active than UFH in platelet-rich plasma (Béguin et al., 1989).

Low- and high-affinity heparin binds to PF4 with a similar apparent K_d (Loscalzo et al., 1985). The interaction appears to be mediated by electrostatic interactions as shown by studies of heparin oligosaccharides with different charge densities (Maccarana and Lindahl, 1993). Therefore, the complexes are dissociable. Indeed, heparin can be displaced from PF4 by sulfated polysaccharides, such as other GAGs (Handin and Cohen, 1976), dextran sulfate (Loscalzo et al., 1985), or xylan sulfate (Campbell et al., 1987). The molar ratios required for complex formation increase in the order: UFH < LMWH < heparan sulfate < dermatan sulfate < chondroitin-6-O-sulfate < chondroitin-4-O-sulfate (Handin and Cohen, 1976). Besides the degree of sulfation (DS) and MW, other structural parameters, such as the type of the uronic acid and the position of the sulfate groups within the monosaccharide in the case of GAGs, influence the affinity of a polysaccharide to PF4 (Table 7.1).

In contrast to the early findings on a minimum heparin chain length (Mikhailov et al., 1999; Visentin, 1999), heparin molecules as small as the pentasaccharide were later shown to interact with PF4 as well (Greinacher et al., 2006). By atomic force microscopy and photon correlation spectroscopy, it has been demonstrated that at very high concentrations and in the absence of AT, the pentasaccharide forms clusters in which PF4 tetramers become closely apposed, although this tendency is much lower than that seen with UFH and LMWH.

In vivo, heparin and some other GAGs are able to increase plasma PF4 levels (Cella et al., 1986). Endothelial bound, rather than platelet-stored, PF4 seems to be the predominant source of the PF4 released by heparin. Most likely, heparin and other high-sulfated polysaccharides are able to displace PF4 from endothelial heparan sulfate in relation to their affinity for PF4 (O'Brien et al., 1985). Hereby, iv injection of heparin causes an increase in plasma PF4 levels, whereas sc administration does not (O'Brien et al., 1985). The maximum amount of PF4 released corresponds

TABLE 7.1 Typical Disaccharide Units of Mammalian Glycosaminoglycans, Arranged by Increasing Affinity to Platelet Factor 4

Glycosaminoglycan	Main disaccharide unit	DS[a]
Hyaluronic acid	[4]-β-D-GlcpA-(1 → 3)-β-D-GlcpNAc-(1 →]	0
Keratan sulfate	[3]-β-D-Galp-(1 → 4)-β-D-GlcpNAc6S-(1 →]	~0.6
Chondroitin sulfate A	[4]-β-D-GlcpA-(1 → 3)-β-D-GalpNAc4S-(1 →]	~0.8
Chondroitin sulfate C	[4]-β-D-GlcpA-(1 → 3)-β-D-GalpNAc6S-(1 →]	~0.8
Dermatan sulfate = ChS B	[4]-α-L-IdopA-(1 → 3)-β-D-GalpNAc4S-(1 →]	~1.4
Heparan sulfate	[4]-β-D-GlcpA-(1 → 4)-α-D-GlcpNAc6S-(1 →]	0.8–1.8
Low molecular weight heparins[b]	[4]-α-L-IdopA2S-(1 → 4)-α-D-GlcpN2S,6S-(1 →]	2.0–2.5
Unfractionated heparin	[4]-α-L-IdopA2S-(1 → 4)-α-D-GlcpN2S,6S-(1 →]	2.0–2.5

[a]DS, degree of sulfation (sulfate groups per disaccharide unit).
[b]Produced by degradation of unfractionated heparin.

to only about 5% of total platelet PF4 (Dawes et al., 1982). Thus, in situations with strong platelet activation, the amount of total PF4 can increase substantially, changing the molar ratio between PF4 and polyanions.

PF4/HEPARIN COMPLEXES AS THE MAJOR ANTIGEN RECOGNIZED BY HIT ANTIBODIES
Formation of Antigens Recognized by HIT Antibodies

The strong anionic character of heparin plays the predominant pathogenic role in the formation of the HIT antigens. Heparin adheres to both cell surface-bound and free PF4, and may additionally increase free PF4 by its platelet-activating effects (Horne and Hutchison, 1998; Newman and Chong, 2000). Heparin binding to PF4 results in clustering of PF4 (Amiral et al., 1992; Rauova et al., 2005) forming linear, ridge-like, multimolecular complexes (Greinacher et al., 2006). From experiments using the pentasaccharide, it has been shown that antigenic PF4 complexes are formed not only by bridging of two PF4 molecules, but also when charge neutralization by polyanions allows positively charged PF4 tetramers to undergo close approximation (Greinacher et al., 2006). Some patients develop antibodies (HIT antibodies) against these complexes. Most HIT antibodies recognize noncontiguous conformational epitopes on the PF4 molecule [three distinct binding sites for HIT antibodies on the PF4/H complexes have been identified (Suh et al., 1998; Li et al., 2002)] that are produced when at least two PF4 tetramers are bound together by heparin (Horsewood et al., 1996; Newman and Chong, 1999; Greinacher et al., 2006). Differences in the relative size, amount, and stability of the complexes may be responsible for the observed differences in immunogenicity (UFH > LMWH ≈fondaparinux) (Warkentin et al., 2005a) and clinically relevant cross-reactivity (UFH > LMWH >> fondaparinux) (Savi et al., 2005; Warkentin et al., 2005a) (Fig. 7.3).

Differing optimal ratios of heparin and PF4 observed to form the HIT epitopes *in vitro* are reported (Rauova et al., 2005; Greinacher et al., 2006), perhaps resulting from differences in heparin preparations used and in experimental design. The reported optimal molar ratios between PF4 and heparin are debatable because exact molar concentrations cannot be indicated for polydisperse mixtures of molecules, such as heparin.

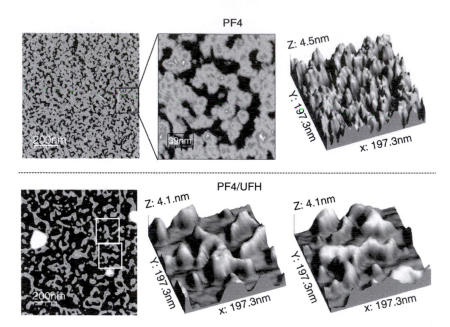

FIGURE 7.3 Atomic force microscopy of PF4 (*upper panel*) and PF4/UFH complexes (*lower panel*) shows the structural changes that PF4 undergoes when it complexes to UFH. PF4 molecules maintain a certain distance to each other due to their strong positive charges. When charges are neutralized by negatively charged heparin, PF4 molecules form linear, ridge-like clusters. *Abbreviations*: PF4, platelet factor 4; UFH, unfractionated heparin. *Source*: From Greinacher et al. (2006).

In a few cases, PF4 alone can be recognized by the HIT antibodies, as shown by the reaction of purified HIT antibodies with either PF4/H complexes or PF4 in the absence of heparin (Greinacher et al., 1994c; Newman and Chong, 1999; Amiral et al., 2000; Prechel et al., 2005). Since pretreatment of platelets with chondroitinase abolishes the platelet-activating effects of these heparin-independent antibodies (Rauova et al., 2006), endogenous platelet-associated GAGs are thought to take the role of heparin. This may also be an explanation for "delayed-onset HIT," where thrombocytopenia and thrombosis begin several days after heparin has been stopped (Warkentin and Kelton, 2001). One such patient developed high levels of antibodies against PF4/H complexes, together with thrombocytopenia and multiple thromboses, beginning about 1 week after a single 5000-unit injection of heparin (Warkentin and Bernstein, 2003). Sera from patients with delayed-onset HIT activate platelets strongly *in vitro* even in the absence of added heparin. The most likely explanation is that these patients develop autoantibodies that recognize PF4 bound to platelet surface GAGs.

Potentially, other obscure factors can induce HIT antigens. This hypothesis is strengthened by the observation that on exceptionally rare occasions, patients can be identified with a thrombocytopenic, prothrombotic disorder that serologically mimics HIT but in whom no previous heparin exposure can be identified (Warkentin et al., 2008). A related observation could be the finding that blood obtained from some patients with acute myocardial infarction contains anti-PF4/H

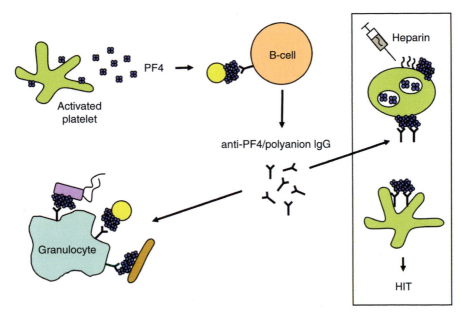

FIGURE 7.4 Schematic representation of the mechanism of how PF4 mediates antibacterial host defense and concurrently primes for HIT. Activated platelets release positively charged PF4 interacting with polyanions at the bacterial surface. This generates antigenic PF4 clusters, which initiates antibody production by B cells. Once antibodies are induced they can bind to all bacterial species, resulting in PF4/IgG clusters on bacterial surfaces, which facilitates their phagocytosis. On the other hand, these antibodies recognize PF4/H-coated platelets (which mimic PF4-coated bacteria), which leads to a misdirected host defense mechanism manifesting as HIT. *Source*: From Krauel et al. (2011).

antibodies, despite apparent absence of previous exposure to heparin (Suzuki et al., 1997).

Bacterial Surface Polyanions as the Potential Physiologic Basis for Formation of PF4/Polyanion Complexes

Bacterial surfaces consist of polyanions (Beveridge, 1999; Neuhaus and Baddiley, 2003). PF4 binds to these polyanions on bacterial surfaces, thereby inducing PF4/H-like epitopes, which are recognized by anti-PF4/H antibodies (Krauel et al., 2011). Potentially, anti-PF4/H antibodies are initially induced as a response to bacterial infections. These patients are then primed and develop a misdirected host defense mechanism in case of subsequent treatment with heparin (Fig. 7.4).

Preimmunization with PF4 bound to bacteria might be one explanation for the early occurrence of anti-PF4/H IgG without IgM precedence in patients treated with heparin for the first time (Greinacher et al., 2009; Warkentin et al., 2009). This is supported by the finding that septic mice developed anti-PF4/H antibodies (Krauel et al., 2011). To induce sepsis in mice the mouse peritoneal sepsis model colon ascendens stent peritonitis was used (Zantl et al., 1998; Maier et al., 2004). Beginning on day 3, these mice generated anti-PF4/H IgM, and from day 14 onwards, anti-PF4/H IgG, i.e., reflecting features of a primary antibody response. However, sepsis, a life-threatening disease, is relatively rare and cannot explain the occurrence of anti-PF4/H antibodies in the normal population (18.8% anti-PF4/H IgM, 6.1% anti-PF4/H IgG) (Krauel et al., 2011) and the formation of these antibodies in as many as 50–75% of patients after cardiac surgery (Warkentin and Sheppard, 2006; Selleng et al., 2010). One of the most prevalent human infections often escaping medical detection is periodontitis. In a large cross-sectional population-based study (John et al., 2001; Hensel et al., 2003) there was a highly significant association between the presence of natural anti-PF4/H antibodies and periodontitis (Greinacher et al., 2011). In accordance with this hypothesis, PF4 bound to periodontal pathogenic bacteria enabling subsequent binding of human anti-PF4/H antibodies.

Pathogenic periodontal bacteria are represented by Gram-negative species. The surface of Gram-negative bacteria is mainly composed of negatively charged lipopolysaccharide (LPS) interspersed with proteins (Fig. 7.5; Beveridge, 1999). By performing PF4 binding studies using bacterial mutants with gradually truncated LPS backbones, the lipid A moiety—which attaches LPS to the outer membrane of bacteria—was identified as the binding site for PF4 on the surface of Gram-negative bacteria (Krauel et al., 2012b). Surface exposed proteins were not involved in PF4 binding. Interaction of PF4 with lipid A was mediated by negatively charged phosphate groups. Bacterial lipid A is highly conserved, as is the heparin-binding site of PF4 (unpublished data). This further supports PF4 binding as an ancient host defense mechanism. Recently, it was described that β_2-glycoprotein I (β_2-GPI), which is the

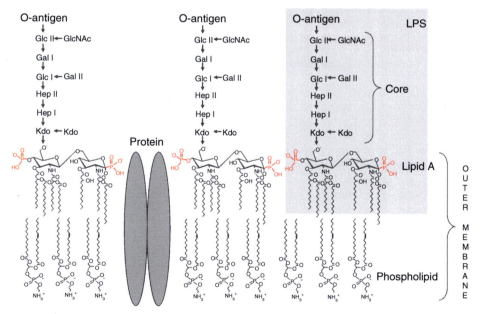

FIGURE 7.5 Exemplary structure of LPS embedded into the outer membrane of Gram-negative bacteria. LPS is a complex glycolipid composed of a highly conserved lipid A moiety (which attaches LPS to the outer membrane), the more variable core oligosaccharide, and the hypervariable antigenic O-polysaccharide (O-antigen) consisting of several copies of oligosaccharide repeating units. Phosphate groups of lipid A mediating PF4 binding are indicated in red. *Abbreviations*: Glc, glucose; Gal, galactose, GlcNAc, *N*-acetyl-D-glucosamine; Hep, heptose; Kdo: 3-deoxy-D-*manno*-oct-2-ulosonic acid.

major antigen in the antiphospholipid syndrome (APS) (de Groot and Derksen, 2005), binds to LPS inducing the antigenic open conformation (Agar et al., 2011b). Interestingly, it was further shown that the LPS binding domain of β_2-GPI is highly conserved (Agar et al., 2011a) and that β_2-GPI binds to PF4 (Sikara et al., 2010). Therefore, it is an intriguing hypothesis that PF4 and β_2-GPI act in concert to defend against bacterial infections. It currently remains unresolved which surface structures of Gram-positive bacteria are responsible for PF4 binding. Regarding APS it was already shown that the bacterial protein, protein H, induces conformational change in β_2-GPI; that mice injected with protein H of Gram-positive *Streptococcus pyogenes* develop antibodies against β_2-GPI (van Os et al., 2011); and that patients with pharyngotonsillitis caused by *S. pyogenes* also generate anti-β_2-GPI antibodies (van Os et al., 2011).

Whether such "natural" anti-PF4/polyanion antibodies have any pathogenic role is currently unresolved. A retrospective analysis of patients with acute coronary syndrome found that the presence of anti-PF4/H antibodies at hospital admission was associated with a higher risk of acute myocardial infarction and death during the follow-up period (Williams et al., 2003).

Effects of HIT Antibody-Containing Immune Complexes

HIT antibodies bind to PF4/H complexes by their F(ab')$_2$ domains (Horne and Alkins, 1996; Newman and Chong, 2000). The predominant immunoglobulin isotype in clinical HIT is IgG (Amiral et al., 1996b; Warkentin et al., 2005b; Juhl et al., 2006). Thus, divalent IgG binding to multimolecular PF4/H complexes leads to the formation of large immune complexes containing HIT-IgG on the platelet surface. The interaction of the HIT-IgG Fc with the platelet FcγIIa receptors leads to crosslinking of these receptors on the same or adjacent platelets, which triggers platelet activation (Kelton et al., 1988, 1994; Chong et al., 1989a) (see chap. 8). The HIT antibody-mediated platelet activation can be inhibited by a monoclonal antibody specific for the FcγIIa receptor, by high concentrations of Fc fragments derived from normal IgG, and by excess heparin saturating all binding sites on PF4, and thus preventing the formation of multimolecular complexes (Greinacher et al., 1994a; Visentin et al., 1994).

Besides these effects on platelets, polyclonal HIT antibodies bind to ECs (Cines et al., 1987; Visentin et al., 1994). The most convincing evidence demonstrating that these antibodies are the same ones that cause platelet activation was provided by classic adsorption-elution experiments (Greinacher et al., 1994c). Purified IgG obtained from sera of HIT patients gave positive reactions in both activation (serotonin release) and antigen (anti-PF4/H) immuno assays. This IgG fraction was then incubated with cultured ECs and, after extensive washing, the antibodies were eluted from the ECs by low pH. The eluate again tested positive in both activation and antigen assays. Thus, these experiments showed that the antibodies recognize the same epitope on platelets, ECs, and PF4/H complexes coated onto a microtiter plate. It appears most likely that the epitope on ECs comprises surface GAGs (Cines et al., 1987; Greinacher et al., 1994c; Visentin et al., 1994).

In addition to platelet and EC activation, there is concomitant activation of coagulation, as shown by marked elevations in thrombin–AT complex levels (Warkentin et al., 1997; Greinacher et al., 2000). The simultaneous activation of platelets, endothelium, and coagulation factors is in line with the development of thrombocytopenia combined with thrombosis and disseminated intravascular coagulation in some patients with HIT (see chap. 2).

Importance of HIT Antibodies in Clinical HIT

HIT antibodies occur commonly in heparin-treated patients. However, as many patients develop neither thrombocytopenia nor thrombosis (Amiral et al., 1996a; Arepally et al., 1997; Kappers-Klunne et al., 1997), it is evident that pathogenicity requires additional factors. Possible factors are number and size of the antigen complexes (Rauova et al., 2005; Greinacher et al., 2006), antibody class (Warkentin et al., 2005b; Juhl et al., 2006), and titer of the HIT antibodies (Suh et al., 1997), as well as optimal concentrations of heparin and PF4 in the blood circulation, which enable the formation of macromolecular PF4/H antigen complexes (Horne and Alkins, 1996; Horne and Hutchison, 1998). Thus, during low-dose heparin prophylaxis in a setting of minimal platelet activation, clinical HIT may occur less often than in patients with activated platelets receiving heparin (Fondu, 1995). Accordingly, HIT antibodies are most frequently induced by UFH in patients after cardiopulmonary bypass surgery (~50–75%), followed by patients undergoing major orthopedic surgery (~15–30%), and least frequently in medical patients (~3%) (see chap. 4).

Besides MW, DS, and concentration of heparin, additional factors favoring the development of clinical HIT are prethrombotic or inflammatory situations (e.g., major surgery) (Visentin et al., 1996; Lubenow et al., 2010), greater susceptibility of the platelets to activation by HIT antibodies (Salem and van der Weyden, 1983), perhaps mediated by increased PF4 binding to platelets (Capitanio et al., 1985), or expression of PF4 (Rauova et al., 2006) and FcγIIa receptors (Chong et al., 1993) on the platelet surface. Furthermore, the polymorphism of the FcγIIa receptor at position Arg-His[131] seems to be associated with a predisposition to HIT (Carlsson et al., 1998). Another poorly understood phenomenon is gender imbalance in HIT, with females having a higher risk of HIT than males, especially with UFH treatment (Warkentin et al., 2006).

OTHER PF4-BINDING SULFATED GLYCANS AND THEIR IMMUNOGENICITY AND CROSS-REACTIVITY WITH HIT ANTIBODIES

Interactions with LMWHs

Generation of the HIT antigen depends not only on the concentration, but also on the chain length of heparin. LMWH preparations (Table 7.2) have reduced affinity for platelets, ECs, and plasma proteins, such as PF4 (O'Brien et al., 1985; Horne, 1993; Turpie, 1996). Accordingly, it has been proposed that LMWHs are less likely to form multimolecular complexes with PF4 (Greinacher et al., 1993; Rauova et al., 2005), which could explain the lower frequency of HIT in patients treated with LMWH compared with UFH (Warkentin et al., 1995; Greinacher et al., 2005; Martel et al., 2005; Warkentin et al., 2006; Lubenow et al., 2010; PROTECT Investigators, 2011). Inconsistent with this hypothesis, however, is the observation that *in vitro*, LMWH shows a higher rate of inducing platelet activation in the presence of HIT antibodies (Greinacher et al., 1992). This led to an alternative concept based on the different molar concentrations reached with LMWH and UFH. As LMWH has a lower anticoagulant activity than UFH on a weight basis (Table 7.2) and a lower MW, many more LMWH molecules are required to obtain clinically relevant anti-FXa activity. When assessing complex formation between PF4 and UFH, optimal complex formation occurs at prophylactic-dose UFH and high PF4 levels. In contrast, concentrations of therapeutic-dose UFH, prophylactic-dose LMWH, and especially therapeutic-dose LMWH are generally too high for optimal complex formation, while those of both prophylactic- and therapeutic-dose fondaparinux are far below the optimal stoichiometric range

TABLE 7.2 Characteristics of Commercial Low Molecular Weight Heparins

INN (Brand name)	Degradation method	Mean MW (kDa)	Anti-Xa (IU/mg)	Anti-Xa: anti-IIa ratio[a]
Ardeparin sodium (Normiflo®)	Peroxidation at elevated temperature	4.0–6.0	120 ± 25	1.7–2.4
Bemiparin sodium[b] (Hibor®)	Basic degradation in a nonaqueous medium and fractionation	~3.6	80–90	8.1
Certoparin sodium (Mono-Embolex®)	Acid degradation with isoamylnitrite	4.2–6.2	80–120	1.5–2.5
Dalteparin sodium[c] (Fragmin®)	Acid degradation with HNO_2 and fractionation	5.6–6.4	110–210	1.9–3.2
Enoxaparin sodium[c] (Clexane®, Lovenox®)	Benzylation and alkaline β-elimination	3.8–5.0	95–125	3.3–5.3
Nadroparin calcium[c] (Fraxiparin®)	Acid degradation with HNO_2 and fractionation	3.6–5.0	95–130	2.5–4.0
Parnaparin sodium[c] (Fluxum®)	Radical-catalyzed degradation with H_2O_2 and a cupric salt	4.0–6.0	75–110	1.5–3.0
Reviparin sodium (Clivarin®)	Acid degradation with HNO_2	3.2–5.2	98–155	3.6–6.1
Semuloparin sodium[d] (Visamerin®, Mulsevo®)	Benzylation and chemoselective alkaline β-elimination	2.0–3.0	~160	~80
Tinzaparin sodium[c] (Innohep®)	Enzymatic (bacterial heparinase) β-elimination	5.6–7.5	70–120	1.5–2.5

[a]Ratio of anti-Xa activity (IU/mg) to anti-IIa activity (IU/mg).
[b]Bemiparin is the first example of second-generation LMWHs, i.e., ULMWH, which are defined to have mean MW <4.0 kDa, a proportion of fragments >6.0 kDa < 15%, and an anti-Xa:anti-IIa ratio >4:1.
[c]From Monographs in European Pharmacopoeia, 7th ed.
[d]The ULMWH semuloparin (syn. AVE-5026) (Viskov et al., 2009) is awaiting approval in the United States and the European Union for VTE prevention in cancer patients.
Abbreviations: INN, international nonproprietary name; MW, molecular weight; ULMWH, ultra-low molecular weight heparin.

(Greinacher et al., 2008). Thus, immune complex formation and immunization should occur more often in situations with major (rather than minor) platelet activation; and as prophylactic-dose UFH > therapeutic-dose UFH > prophylactic-dose LMWH, fondaparinux > therapeutic-dose LMWH. The framework provided by this model may explain the empirical observations that LMWH induces less frequently anti-PF4/H antibodies than does UFH, and that anti-PF4/H antibodies are more often found in patients undergoing major surgery than in medical patients (Greinacher et al., 2008). The findings of a secondary analysis of prospective clinical trials comparing anti-PF4/H immunization rate between LMWH (enoxaparin) and fondaparinux in patients undergoing orthopedic joint replacement surgery further corroborates this stoichiometric model of PF4/polyanion complex formation *in vivo* (Warkentin et al., 2010).

Despite their lower immunogenicity, LMWHs exhibit nearly 100% *in vitro* cross-reactivity to HIT antibodies using sensitive assays (Greinacher et al., 1994a,b; Warkentin et al., 1995; Amiral et al., 1996b; Amiral, 1997). The small variations found with different LMWH preparations *in vitro* are probably based on their individual composition of molecules with different chain length (Fareed et al., 1988). Homogenous heparin molecules consisting of 20, 18, 16, 14, and 12 monosaccharides form antigenic multimolecular complexes to which HIT antibodies bind strongly. Fragments containing 10 residues form complexes with PF4, which are recognized by the antibodies only weakly (as judged by a platelet activation assay), whereas fragments containing eight and six residues are even less reactive (Amiral et al., 1995; Greinacher et al., 1995) or nonreactive (Visentin et al., 2001). Accordingly, the ultra-LMWH semuloparin, which is mainly composed of octasaccharides (Viskov et al., 2009), may not only have a reduced risk of inducing clinical HIT, but also a low risk of cross-reacting with HIT antibodies.

Interactions with Other Sulfated Carbohydrates

The formation of platelet-activating immune complexes is not limited to heparin (Greinacher et al., 1992, 1993). Various other sulfated polysaccharides, and even polyvinylsulfonate, bind PF4 to form antigen complexes recognized by HIT antibodies. This cross-reaction depends on their structure, especially on their DS and MW (Greinacher et al., 1992, 1995; Kelton et al., 1994; Amiral et al., 1995). In vitro assays demonstrate that pentosan polysulfate, dextran sulfate, as well as a high-sulfated chondroitin sulfate, and a highly sulfated polysaccharide (PI-88) developed for antitumor treatment (Rosenthal et al., 2002) can all substitute for heparin. In contrast, neither dextran, dermatan sulfate, N-desulfated heparin, sulfated glucosamine (Weimann et al., 2001), nor the AT-binding pentasaccharide react in these assays. Accordingly, pentosan polysulfate, high-sulfated chondroitin sulfate, and PI-88 have induced thrombocytopenia and thrombosis in vivo (Greinacher et al., 1993; Tardy et al., 1994; Rosenthal et al., 2002). The corresponding antibodies can be detected by conventional anti-PF4/H enzyme immunoassay (EIA) demonstrating the cross-reactivity with heparin (Gironell et al., 1996).

Structure-Dependent Cross-Reactivity of Anticoagulant β-1,3-Glucan Sulfates with HIT-Associated Antibodies

To establish the structural requirements for the anticoagulant activity of sulfated carbohydrates, as well as for the development of platelet-activating immune complexes in the presence of HIT antibodies, we synthesized structurally well-defined sulfated polysaccharides (Greinacher et al., 1995). The resulting β-1,3-glucan sulfates (GluS) varied in their DS, MW, sulfation pattern, and chemically introduced glycosidic side chains (Fig. 7.6). Although these compounds differ structurally from heparin, they exhibit structure-dependent anticoagulant as well as antithrombotic activities (Alban et al., 1995; Franz and Alban, 1995). They also induce platelet activation in the presence of HIT antibodies (Greinacher et al., 1995). Therefore, neither uronic acids, amino groups, nor the α-1,4- or β-1,4-glycosidic linkages found in heparin are essential for these biologic properties.

An increase in the DS results in improved anticoagulant activity and, after binding to PF4, in increased formation of HIT antibody-binding sites. The MW is a second important structural parameter for anticoagulant potency of a sulfated polysaccharide, as well as its capacity to cause platelet activation in the presence of HIT antibodies. Fractions with hydrodynamic volumes between 38 and 60 kDa showed the most prominent effects (Alban and Franz, 1994a; Greinacher et al., 1995) (the hydrodynamic volumes were determined by gel filtration chromatography using neutral pullulans as MW standards; since these have lower hydrodynamic volumes owing to the missing sulfate groups, the measured hydrodynamic volumes are higher than the real MW; for example, UFH had a

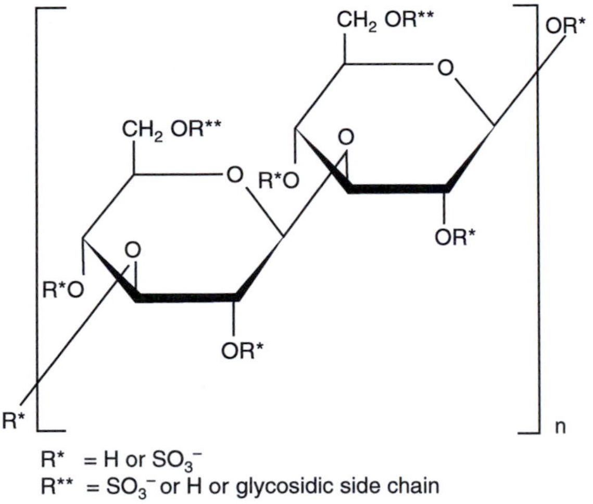

R* = H or SO_3^-
R** = SO_3^- or H or glycosidic side chain

FIGURE 7.6 Repeating unit of β-1,3-glucan sulfates: The primary OH group in position 6(**) is preferentially sulfated. Glycosidic-branched β-1,3-glucan sulfates are substituted by a glucose, rhamnose, or arabinose unit, respectively, in position 6.

mean hydrodynamic volume of 30 kDa). Therefore, this MW range, which corresponds to that of the so-called extra-large material of UFH, seems to represent the optimal chain length both for the interaction with proteins involved in the coagulation cascade as well as with PF4 to form HIT antigens. Beyond the optimal chain length, higher concentrations are required to form multimolecular PF4/GluS complexes (Greinacher et al., 1995).

Compared with linear GluS having similar DS and MW, glycosidically branched compounds generally exhibit higher anticoagulant activity than the respective linear derivatives (Alban, 1993, 1997). Glycosidic substitution changes the 3D structure of the polysaccharide chain, resulting in enhanced flexibility, and improved the interaction with proteins (Kindness et al., 1980). In addition, as the side chains are more accessible to sulfation, they represent clusters of negative charges (Alban and Franz, 1994b) facilitating binding to PF4, which results in an increased cross-reactivity with HIT antibodies.

OSCS and Oversulfated Heparin Byproducts

The world-wide "heparin scandal" in 2008 caused by counterfeit heparin manufactured in China led to about 900 reports to the U.S. Food and Drug Administration (FDA) and the Federal Institute of Drugs and Medical Devices in Germany of adverse events associated with the use of UFH (Beyer et al., 2010). The most commonly reported adverse reactions were hypotension (50%), nausea (48.7%), and shortness of breath occurring within 30 minutes after administration (37.5%), and edema, especially facial swelling (23.7%) (Blossom et al., 2008). These represent typical symptoms of anaphylactoid reactions (Greinacher and Warkentin, 2009), mediated by activation of the contact phase system with the formation of vasoactive bradykinins (Fig. 7.7). More than 240 patients died from complications associated with the use of these contaminated UFH lots in the United States

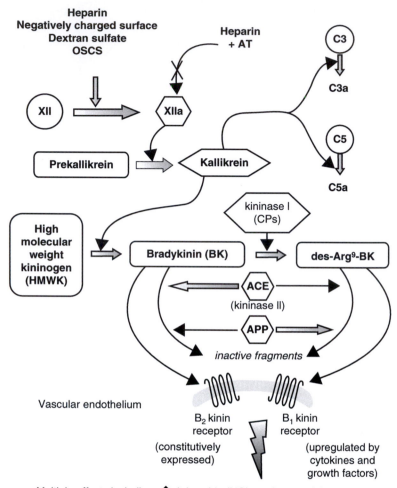

FIGURE 7.7. Consequences of activation of the contact system by polyanions including OSCS. Some polyanions, such as dextran sulfate and OSCS, and negatively charged surfaces (e.g., certain hemodialyzers, blood filters) directly facilitate autocatalysis of factor XII to the active enzyme, factor XIIa. Although heparin also facilitates this process, it additionally catalyzes the inhibition (through AT) of XIIa; therefore, pharmacologic heparin—unlike OSCS—usually does not trigger contact system activation. Factor XIIa leads to activation of the intrinsic pathway of coagulation (not shown), and also activates plasma prekallikrein to kallikrein. Kallikrein converts HMWK to bradykinin (BK), as well as the complement factors C3 and C5 to their respective anaphylatoxins, C3a and C5a. BK is converted by "kininase I" (a term that denotes various carboxypeptidases, e.g., carboxypeptidases N, M, and U) to its main metabolite, des-arg^9-BK. Both BK and des-arg^9-BK are short-lived vasoactive kinins ($t_{1/2}$, 30 sec and 8 min, respectively), which activate cells through the B_2 and B_1 kinin receptors, respectively. B_1 receptors are upregulated by cytokines and growth factors, whereas the B_2 receptors are constitutively expressed. Activation of the B_2 and B_1 receptors leads to numerous effects, including increased endothelial cell nitric oxide synthase activity, which results in increased levels of nitric oxide, a potent vasodilator. (*Continued*)

FIGURE 7.7. (*Continued*) Regulation of the kinin system includes the enzyme, peptidyl-dipeptidase A, also known as ACE and "kininase II." Although ACE is the major enzyme that degrades BK, another enzyme, APP, is the major enzyme that degrades des-arg^9-BK. Therefore, acquired (e.g., ACE inhibitor therapy) or constitutive defects (e.g., APP deficiency) are risk factors for the development of anaphylactic and other hypersensitivity reactions that result from activation of the contact system. *Abbreviations*: ACE, angiotensin converting enzyme; APP, aminopeptidase P; AT, antithrombin; BK, bradykinin; CPs, carboxypeptidases; HMWK, high molecular weight kininogen; NO, nitric oxide; OSCS, oversulfated chondroitin sulfate. *Source*: From Warkentin and Greinacher (2009).

(Alban et al., 2011). In March 2008, oversulfated chondroitin sulfate (OSCS; Fig. 7.1B) was identified as the contaminant in the heparin batches responsible for causing these adverse events (Guerrini et al., 2008, 2009). Contaminating OSCS comprised up to 35% of UFH content (Royce, 2008). OSCS prolongs coagulation tests, including the activated thromboplastin time (aPTT) and presumably was added as a cheap semi-synthetic heparin substitute. The pharmacopoeia methods for the quality control of heparin batches were not able to detect the contamination with OSCS (although quality control procedures have subsequently been changed).

Like other sulfated glycans, OSCS exhibits a multitude of effects by interacting with biomolecules. In contrast to heparins, its *in vitro* anticoagulant activity is independent of AT and mainly due to heparin cofactor II-mediated thrombin inhibition (Maruyama et al., 1998; Li et al., 2009). In line with the observed anaphylactoid responses to OSCS-contaminated heparin, OSCS was shown to represent a potent contact activator of factor XII resulting in the activation of the kinin–kallikrein pathway with the formation of both bradykinins and anaphylactic complement fragments C3a and C5a (Kishimoto et al., 2008; Li et al., 2009). Contact activation by OSCS additionally initiates coagulation via the intrinsic pathway as well as by activation of FVII. This procoagulant effect can be recorded by the prothrombin time, which is shortened at low concentrations of OSCS and OSCS-contaminated heparin (Alban and Lühn, 2008; Alban et al., 2011).

Moreover, OSCS forms complexes with PF4, which are potentially more immunogenic than PF4/UFH complexes. From November 2007 to February 2008 (the period anaphylactoid reactions were observed with OSCS-contaminated heparin), a substantial year-over-year increase in HIT cases (compared with the same period in 2007) was observed in one reference laboratory in Germany (increase by 100%)—a country in which OSCS was marketed, but not by a reference laboratory in Canada (increase of HIT by only 13%), where OSCS was not marketed, possibly reflecting greater immunogenicity of OSCS-contaminated heparin (Greinacher and Warkentin, 2008). In addition, OSCS could promote the development of clinical HIT by its overall proinflammatory and procoagulant effects (see above).

IMPLICATIONS FOR THE DEVELOPMENT OF CARBOHYDRATE-BASED HEPARIN ALTERNATIVES
Structural Requirements of Carbohydrate-Based Heparin Alternatives
A carbohydrate-based antithrombotic drug with a reduced risk of inducing HIT antigen(s) should meet the following criteria (Greinacher et al., 1995):

- The molecule should not be branched to reduce its flexibility and to minimize charge clusters.
- Its DS should be lower than 1.0 per monosaccharide, if its chain length exceeds 10 monosaccharides.
- Its MW should be lower than 2.4 kDa (about seven monosaccharides), if its DS is higher than 1.0.
- If the MW is higher than 2.4 kDa and the DS higher than 1.0, then at least the therapeutic concentration must be lower than that exhibiting cross-reactivity with HIT antibodies.

Danaparoid

Danaparoid sodium (Orgaran) is an alternative anticoagulant that is effective for treating patients with HIT (see chap. 16). This heparinoid consists of a depolymerized mixture of GAGs extracted from porcine intestinal mucosa, with an average MW of 4–7 kDa. Its components are approximately 80% low molecular weight heparan sulfate, 8–18% dermatan sulfate, ≤8% chondroitin sulfate, and a small proportion of heparan sulfate (4%) with high affinity for AT (Meuleman, 1992; EDQM, 2012). Apart from the minor AT-binding heparan sulfate component, the constituents of danaparoid have a DS per monosaccharide between 0.5 and 0.7, as well as a low MW. Thus, the two important requirements to form multimolecular complexes with PF4 are not met. This is consistent with the low cross-reactivity rate of danaparoid (about 10%) (Wilde and Markham, 1997) (see chaps. 12 and 16). As danaparoid inhibits platelet activation by HIT antibodies even in the presence of heparin (Chong et al., 1989b), it is possible that the GAG mixture binds to PF4 without producing the antigen. Consequently, less PF4 is available for the small amount of higher-sulfated heparan sulfate molecules responsible for AT binding and, presumably, PF4 binding resulting in cross-reactivity with HIT antibodies (Greinacher et al., 1992). Recently, danaparoid was shown to even displace PF4/H complexes from platelets, to reduce the PF4/H complex size, to inhibit HIT antibody binding to PF4/H complexes, as well as platelet activation by anti-PF4/H antibodies in the presence of heparin (Krauel et al., 2008). This concept has been further developed for partially O-desulfated heparin (see page 198).

Pentasaccharides

Within the scope of developing new carbohydrate-based antithrombotics, fondaparinux, a fully synthetic, chemically defined pentasaccharide (formerly named Org31540/SR90107A, MW = 1728 Da; DS = 1.6; 700 anti-Xa U/mg), has been developed, which corresponds to the AT-binding site of heparin (Petitou et al., 1997) (Fig. 7.8; see also chap. 17). By its highly specific binding to AT, fondaparinux selectively inhibits factor Xa and thus prevents thrombin generation (Bauer et al., 2002).

Fondaparinux does not usually cross-react with HIT antibodies, either in the PF4/H-EIA or in the serotonin release assay (SRA) (Greinacher et al., 1995; Amiral et al., 1997; Ahmad et al., 1999). Immune thrombocytopenia attributable to fondaparinux has not been observed in any of the clinical studies. However, patients treated with fondaparinux in clinical trials generated anti-PF4/H antibodies at a similar frequency as observed in patients treated with LMWH (enoxaparin). These antibodies tested positive in a PF4-dependent EIA and caused platelet activation *in vitro* in the presence of added heparin, although no cross-reactivity with fondaparinux itself could be shown (Warkentin et al., 2005a). It has been hypothesized that PF4 forms only few and potentially relatively unstable multimolecular complexes in the

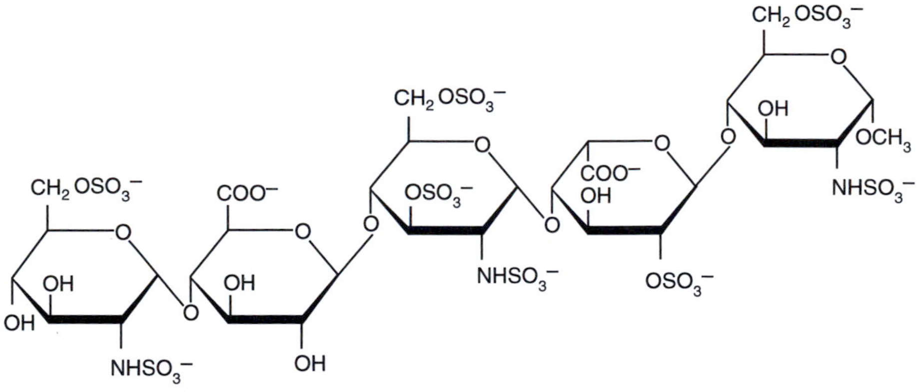

FIGURE 7.8 Chemical structure of the synthetically produced pentasaccharide, fondaparinux (formerly, Org31540/SR90107A; MW = 1728 Da; DS = 1.6; 864 anti-Xa U/mg), with eight sulfate groups corresponding to the natural antithrombin-binding site. *Abbreviations*: DS, degree of sulfation; MW, molecular weight.

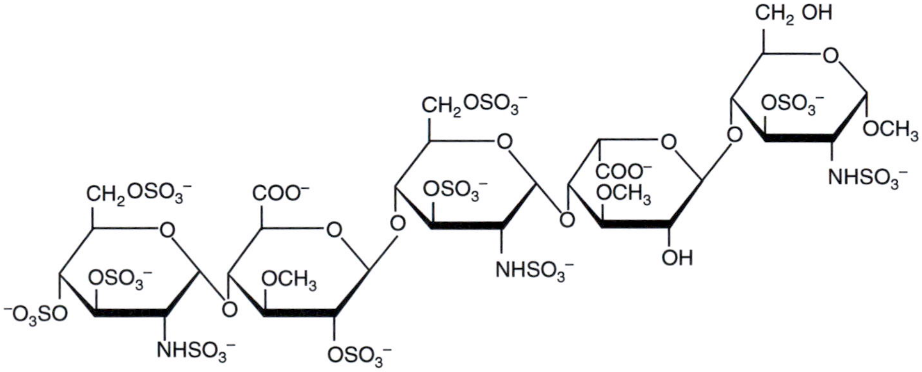

FIGURE 7.9 Chemical structure of the synthetically produced pentasaccharide, Org 32701 (MW = 1991 Da; DS = 2; 1150 anti-Xa U/mg), with a higher degree of sulfation (10 sulfate groups) than the natural antithrombin-binding site. *Abbreviations*: DS, degree of sulfation; MW, molecular weight.

presence of fondaparinux. These few complexes can trigger the immunization but are too sparse to mediate relevant platelet activation (Greinacher et al., 2006).

In support of this concept, we have observed in our laboratory that a more highly sulfated pentasaccharide, Org 32701 (MW = 1991 Da; DS = 2.0) (Herbert et al., 1996) (Fig. 7.9), induces platelet activation in the presence of HIT antibodies. This demonstrates that certain highly sulfated oligosaccharides are indeed able to bind to PF4 and thus to form the HIT neoantigen. But, whether such a highly sulfated pentasaccharide itself could induce clinical HIT cannot yet be answered.

Specifically Designed Oligosaccharides

Pentasaccharides such as fondaparinux or the long-acting idraparinux (Herbert et al., 1998) have minimal, if any, undesirable interactions with blood and vessel components, but their anticoagulant activity is limited to AT-mediated factor Xa inhibition. Additional thrombin inhibitory properties might further improve the anticoagulant efficacy of heparin-related oligosaccharides. Unfortunately, as with heparin, lengthening the sulfated oligosaccharide chain increases nonspecific binding that could have undesirable effects, such as binding to PF4 and associated risk of HIT. Thus, Petitou and coworkers (1999) synthesized "heparin mimetics" that inhibited thrombin, but failed to bind other proteins, particularly PF4. The most promising structure is the hexadecasaccharide SR123781A, which has undergone clinical evaluation (Herbert et al., 2001). It is obtained from glucose through a convergent synthesis and consists of an AT-binding pentasaccharide sequence linked to a thrombin-binding domain via a neutral methylated hexasaccharide "spacer." It specifically catalyzes the AT-mediated inhibition of factor Xa (IC50 = 77 ± 5 ng/mL, 297 ± 13 U/mg) and thrombin (IC50 = 4.0 ± 0.5 ng/mL, 150 ± 30 U/mg), without any effect on heparin cofactor II and without binding to PF4. In the presence of plasma from HIT patients, SR123781A did not activate platelets. Based on its potent antithrombotic activity in animal models, it has been evaluated in phase IIb trials on venous thromboembolism prophylaxis in orthopedic surgery (DRIVE) and therapy of acute coronary syndrome. Despite promising results (Lassen et al., 2008), further development of this parenteral anticoagulant has been stopped.

Low Sulfated Heparin (Partially Desulfated Heparin)

2-O, 3-O desulfated heparin (ODSH) is derived from UFH by selective desulfation at the 2-oxygen (2-O) position on α-L-iduronic acid (2-sulfate) and the 3-O position on D-glucosamine-N-sulfate (3,6-disulfate). Through this chemical modification, ODSH lacks most of the anticoagulant effects of heparin (Rao et al., 2010). It has a low affinity for AT, and therefore low anti-Xa and anti-IIa activities and does not activate factor XII (Rao et al., 2010). ODSH was initially developed to separate the anticoagulant and the anti-inflammatory effects of heparin (Fryer et al., 1997). Using heparin as an anti-inflammatory drug has been shown to be beneficial for inflammatory diseases, such as bronchial asthma, ulcerative colitis, and burns (Young, 2008) due to inhibition of complement activation (Weiler et al., 1992), blockade of L- and P-selectin-initiated cell adhesion (Wang et al., 2002) and reduction of lymphocyte-mediated immune reactions (Lider et al., 1990). The anti-inflammatory effects of heparin are dependent on 6-O-sulfation (Wang et al., 2002) and are almost unaffected by 2-O, 3-O desulfation. Despite partial desulfation, ODSH is still negatively charged sustaining interaction with positively charged proteins such as PF4. Ultra-large complexes (ULCs) of PF4 and ODSH are formed similar to the generation of PF4/UFH ULCs (Joglekar et al., 2012). However, desulfation affects antigenicity of PF4/ODSH complexes as anti-PF4/H antibodies from patients only show minimal cross-reactivity with PF4/ODSH complexes using EIA (Joglekar et al., 2012). Consistently, ODSH does not induce platelet activation in the presence of anti-PF4/H antibodies using either the heparin-induced platelet activation (HIPA) assay (Krauel et al., 2012a) or the SRA (Rao et al., 2010). It is likely that desulfation at the 2-O, 3-O position might prevent close approximation of PF4 tetramers in optimal distances necessary for antigenicity (Greinacher et al., 2006). Nevertheless, ODSH can interfere with relevant reactions in the pathogenesis of HIT. It displaces PF4 and PF4/UFH complexes from cell surfaces, inhibits anti-PF4/H antibody binding to PF4/H complexes and prevents platelet activation by anti-PF4/H antibodies in the presence of platelet-derived PF4 and

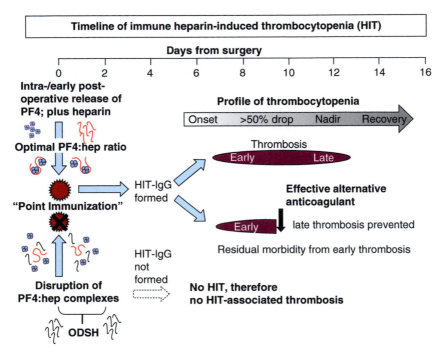

FIGURE 7.10 ODSH as a HIT prevention strategy. The characteristic timeline of HIT begins with intra-/perioperative "point immunization" followed one week later by thrombocytopenia and hyperco-agulability. Whereas "late" HIT-associated thrombosis can be prevented by an effective alternative anticoagulant, only a HIT prevention strategy can avoid morbidity from early HIT-associated throm-bosis. Disruption of immunizing PF4/H complexes by intra-/perioperative coadministration of ODSH with heparin could prevent the anti-PF4/H immune response, and hence HIT and HIT-associated thrombosis. *Abbreviations*: HIT, heparin-induced thrombocytopenia; PF4, platelet factor 4. *Source*: From Warkentin (2012).

heparin (Rao et al., 2010; Joglekar et al., 2012; Krauel et al., 2012a). The inhibitory effect of ODSH is mediated by its ability to disrupt preformed PF4/UFH com-plexes and to prevent PF4/UFH complex formation (Joglekar et al., 2012). As the ODSH concentrations needed for inhibitory effectiveness only show minimal anticoagulant activity (Joglekar et al., 2012; Krauel et al., 2012a), it is an attractive concept to mix UFH or LMWH with ODSH, especially for the application in patients requiring heparin for thrombosis prophylaxis. This might reduce the risk of developing HIT. First experiments using a murine PF4/H immunization model of HIT showed that there is a reduced immunogenicity of PF4/UFH complexes when injected in the presence of ODSH (Joglekar et al., 2012) (see also chap. 10). Figure 7.10 illustrates the concept. Appropriately designed clinical studies are required to further assess this concept in patients.

CONCLUSIONS
From experiments with well-defined GluS, the various structural requirements for a sulfated carbohydrate to form the HIT antigen have become clear. Given this

detailed knowledge, at least three carbohydrate-based anticoagulant options can be proposed that should have a negligible risk for inducing clinical HIT:

- Mixtures of GAGs consisting predominantly of low-sulfated carbohydrates with correspondingly limited capacity to form antigenic complexes with PF4. A prototype of such an anticoagulant is danaparoid, and partially desulfated heparin (ODSH) in combination with UFH or LMWH has great potential in this regard.
- Oligosaccharides with antithrombotic activity similar to the AT-binding pentasaccharide: a prototype is fondaparinux.
- GAGs with highly sulfated, but short, regions that are connected by nonsulfated "spacers": a prototype is the hexadecasaccharide SR123781A (Petitou et al., 1999).

The increasing use of LMWH already seems to have reduced the incidence of HIT. We propose that the problem of HIT can be avoided further by using anticoagulants meeting the foregoing outlined criteria in our treatment arsenal.

ACKNOWLEDGMENTS

Part of this work was supported by Bayerischer Habilitations-Forderpreis 1996/ Hans Zehetmair-Preis (S. A.), Deutsche Forschungsgemeinschaft, DFG Gr 1096/2–1 and Gr 1096/2–2 (A. G.), and Bundesministerium für Bildung und Forschung, Zentrum für Innovationskompetenz ZIK HIKE Förderkennzeichen BMBF FKZ 03Z2CN12 (K. K.).

REFERENCES

Agar C, de Groot PG, Marquart JA, Meijers JC. Evolutionary conservation of the lipopolysaccharide binding site of beta-glycoprotein I. Thromb Haemost 106: 1069–1075, 2011a.

Agar C, de Groot PG, Mörgelin M, Monk SD, van Os G, Levels JH, de Laat B, Urbanus RT, Herwald H, van der Poll T, Meijers JC. β_2-glycoprotein I: a novel component of innate immunity. Blood 117: 6939–6947, 2011b.

Ahmad S, Jeske WP, Walenga JM, Hoppensteadt DA, Wood JJ, Herbert JM, Messmore HL, Fareed J. Synthetic pentasaccharides do not cause platelet activation by antiheparin-platelet factor 4 antibodies. Clin Appl Thromb Haemost 5: 259–266, 1999.

Alban S. Synthese und physiologische Testung neuartiger Heparinoide. Germany: Ph.D. dissertation, University of Regensburg, 1993. [in German]

Alban S. Carbohydrates with anticoagulant and antithrombotic properties. In: Witczak ZJ, Nieforth KA, eds. Carbohydrates in Drug Design. New York: Marcel Dekker, 209–276, 1997.

Alban S, Franz G. Anticoagulant activity of curdlan sulfates in dependence on their molecular weight. Pure Appl Chem 66: 2403–2406, 1994a.

Alban S, Franz G. Gas liquid chromatography-mass spectrometry analysis of anticoagulant active curdlan sulfates. Semin Thromb Hemost 20: 152–158, 1994b.

Alban S, Lühn S. Prothrombin time for detection of contaminated heparins. N Engl J Med 359: 2732–2734, 2008.

Alban S, Jeske W, Welzel D, Franz G, Fareed J. Anticoagulant and antithrombotic actions of a semisynthetic 3–glucan sulfate. Thromb Res 78: 201–210, 1995.

Alban S, Lühn S, Schiemann S, Beyer T, Norwig J, Schilling C, Rädler O, Wolf B, Matz M, Baumann K, Holzgrabe U. Comparison of established and novel purity tests for the quality control of heparin by means of a set of 177 heparin samples. Anal Bioanal Chem 399: 605–620, 2011.

Amiral J. Le facteur 4 plaquettaire, cible des anticorps anti-héparine: application au diagnostic biologique de la thronibopenie induite par héparine (TIH). Ann Med Intern 148: 142–149, 1997. [in French]

Amiral J, Bridey F, Dreyfus M, Vissac AM, Fressinaud E, Wolf M, Meyer D. Platelet factor 4 complexed to heparin is the target for antibodies generated in heparin-induced thrombocytopenia. Thromb Haemost 68: 95–96, 1992.

Amiral J, Bridey F, Wolf M, Boyer-Neumann C, Fressinaud E, Vissac AM, Peynaud-Debayle E, Dreyfus M, Meyer D. Antibodies to macromolecular platelet factor 4-heparin complexes in heparin-induced thrombocytopenia: a study of 44 cases. Thromb Haemost 73: 21–28, 1995.

Amiral J, Peynaud-Debayle E, Wolf M, Bridey F, Vissac AM, Meyer D. Generation of antibodies to heparin-PF4 complexes without thrombocytopenia in patients treated with unfractionated or low molecular weight heparin. Am J Hematol 52: 90–95, 1996a.

Amiral J, Wolf M, Fischer A, Boyer-Neumann C, Vissac A, Meyer D. Pathogenicity of IgA and/or IgM antibodies to heparin-PF4 complexes in patients with heparin-induced thrombocytopenia. Br J Haematol 92: 954–959, 1996b.

Amiral J, Lormeau JC, Marfaing-Koka A, Vissac AM, Wolf M, Boyer-Neumann C, Tardy B, Herbert JM, Meyer D. Absence of cross-reactivity of SR90107A/ORG31540 pentasaccharide with antibodies to heparin-PF4 complexes developed in heparin-induced thrombocytopenia. Blood Coagul Fibrinolysis 8: 114–117, 1997.

Amiral J, Pouplard C, Vissac AM, Walenga JM, Jeske W, Gruel Y. Affinity purification of heparin-dependent antibodies to platelet factor 4 developed in heparin-induced thrombocytopenia: biological characteristics and effects on platelet activation. Br J Haematol 109: 336–341, 2000.

Arepally G, McKenzie SE, Jiang XM, Poncz M, Cines DB. FcγRIIA H/R131 polymorphism, subclass-specific IgG anti-heparin/platelet factor 4 antibodies and clinical course in patients with heparin-induced thrombocytopenia and thrombosis. Blood 89: 370–375, 1997.

Bauer KA, Hawkins DW, Peters PC, Petitou M, Herbert JM, Van Boeckel CA, Meuleman DG. Fondaparinux, a synthetic pentasaccharide: the first in a new class of antithrombotic agents-the selective factor Xa inhibitors. Cardiovasc Drug Rev 20: 37–52, 2002.

Béguin S, Mardiguian J, Lindhout T, Hemker HC. The mode of action of low molecular weight heparin preparation (PK10169) and two of its major components on thrombin generation in plasma. Thromb Haemost 61: 30–34, 1989.

Bendetowicz AV, Kai H, Knebel R, Caplain H, Hemker HC, Lindhout T, Beguin S. The effect of subcutaneous injection of unfractionated and low molecular weight heparin on thrombin generation in platelet rich plasma a study in human volunteers. Thromb Haemost 72: 705–712, 1994.

Beveridge TJ. Structures of gram-negative cell walls and their derived membrane vesicles. J Bacteriol 181: 4725–4733, 1999.

Beyer T, Matz M, Brinz D, Rädler O, Wolf B, Norwig J, Baumann K, Alban S, Holzgrabe U. Composition of OSCS-contaminated heparin occurring in 2008 in batches on the German market. Eur J Pharm Sci 40: 297–304, 2010.

Bianchini P, Liverani L, Spelta F, Mascellani G, Parma B. Variability of heparins and heterogeneity of low molecular weight heparins. Semin Thromb Hemost 33: 496–502, 2007.

Björk I, Olson ST, Shore JD. Molecular mechanisms of the accelerating effect of heparin on the reaction between antithrombin and clotting proteinases. In: Lane DA, Lindahl U, eds. Heparin, Chemical and Biological Properties, Clinical Applications. London: Edward Arnold, 229–255, 1989.

Blossom DB, Kallen AJ, Patel PR, Elward A, Robinson L, Gao G, Langer R, Perkins KM, Jaeger JL, Kurkjian KM, Jones M, Schillie SF, Shehab N, Ketterer D, Venkataraman G, Kishimoto TK, Shriver Z, McMahon AW, Austen KF, Kozlowski S, Srinivasan A, Turabelidze G, Gould CV, Arduino MJ, Sasisekharan R. Outbreak of adverse reactions associated with contaminated heparin. N Engl J Med 359: 2674–2684, 2008.

Bock PE, Luscombe M, Marshall SE, Pepper DS, Holbrook JJ. The multiple complexes formed by the interaction of platelet factor 4 with heparin. Biochem J 191: 769–776, 1980.

Campbell A, Nesheim ME, Doctor VM. Mechanism of potentiation of antithrombin III [AT-III] inhibition by sulfated xylans. Thromb Res 47: 341–352, 1987.

Capitanio AM, Niewiarowski S, Rucinski B, Tuszynski GP, Cierniewski CS, Hershock D, Kornecki E. Interaction of platelet factor 4 with human platelets. Biochim Biophys Acta 839: 161–173, 1985.

Carlsson LE, Santoso S, Baurichter G, Kroll H, Papenberg S, Eichler P, Westerdaal NAC, Kiefel V, van de Winkel JGJ, Greinacher A. Heparin-induced thrombocytopenia: new insights into the impact of the FcγRIIa-R-H131 polymorphism. Blood 92: 1526–1531, 1998.

Casu B. Structure and biological activity of heparin. Adv Carbohydr Chem Biochem 43: 51–134, 1985.

Casu B. Heparin structure. Haemostasis 20(Suppl 1): 62–73, 1990.

Cella G, Scattolo N, Luzzatto G, Stevanato F, Vio C, Girolami ASO. Effects on platelets and on the clotting system of four glycosaminoglycans extracted from hog mucosa and one extracted from aortic intima of the calf. J Med 17: 331–346, 1986.

Choay J. Structure and activity of heparin and its fragments: an overview. Semin Thromb Hemost 15: 359–364, 1989.

Chong BH, Fawaz I, Chestermann CN, Berndt MC. Heparin-induced thrombocytopenia: mechanism of interaction of the heparin-dependent antibody with platelets. Br J Haematol 73: 235–240, 1989a.

Chong BH, Ismail F, Cade J, Gallus AS, Gordon S, Chesterman CN. Heparin induced thrombocytopenia: studies with a new molecular weight heparinoid, org 10172. Blood 73: 1592–1596, 1989b.

Chong BH, Pilgrim RL, Cooley MA, Chesterman CN. Increased expression of platelet IgG Fc receptors in immune heparin-induced thrombocytopenia. Blood 81: 988–993, 1993.

Cines DB, Tomaski A, Tannenbaum S. Immune endothelial-cell injury in heparin-associated thrombocytopenia. N Engl J Med 316: 581–589, 1987.

Dawes J, Pumphrey CW, McLaren KM, Prowse CV, Pepper DS. The in vivo release of human platelet factor 4 by heparin. Thromb Res 27: 65–76, 1982.

de Groot PG, Derksen RH. Pathophysiology of the antiphospholipid syndrome. J Thromb Haemost 3: 1854–1860, 2005.

Denton J, Lane DA, Thunberg L, Slater AM, Lindahl U. Binding of platelet factor 4 to heparin oligosaccharides. Biochem J 209: 455–460, 1983.

EDQM. Monograph No 2090: Danaparoid sodium. European Pharmacopoeia 7.5, 2012.

Fareed J, Walenga JM, Hoppensteadt D, Haun X, Racanelli A. Comparative study on the in vitro and in vivo activities of seven low molecular weight heparins. Haemostasis 18(Suppl 3): 3–15, 1988.

Fondu P. Heparin-associated thrombocytopenia: an update. Acta Clin Belg 50: 343–357, 1995.

Franz G, Alban S. Structure-activity relationship of antithrombotic polysaccharide derivatives. Int J Biol Macromol 17: 311–314, 1995.

Fryer A, Huang YC, Rao G, Jacoby D, Mancilla E, Whorton R, Piantadosi CA, Kennedy T, Hoidal J. Selective O-desulfation produces nonanticoagulant heparin that retains pharmacological activity in the lung. J Pharmacol Exp Ther 282: 208–219, 1997.

Gironell A, Altes A, Arboix A, Fontcuberta J, Munoz Z, Marti-Vilalta JL. Pentosan polysulfate-induced thrombocytopenia: a case diagnosed with an ELISA test used for heparin-induced thrombocytopenia. Ann Hematol 73: 51–62, 1996.

Greinacher A. Antigen generation in heparin-associated thrombocytopenia: the non-immunologic type and the immunologic type are closely linked in their pathogenesis. Semin Thromb Hemost 21: 106–116, 1995.

Greinacher A, Warkentin TE. Contaminated heparin. N Engl J Med 359: 1291–1292, 2008.

Greinacher A, Warkentin TE. Heparin-induced anaphylactic and anaphylactoid reactions: two distinct but overlapping syndromes. Expert Opin Drug Saf 8: 129–144, 2009.

Greinacher A, Michels I, Mueller-Eckhardt C. Heparin-associated thrombocytopenia: the antibody is not heparin specific. Thromb Haemost 67: 545–549, 1992.

Greinacher A, Michels I, Liebenhoff U, Presek P, Mueller-Eckhardt C. Heparin-associated thrombocytopenia: immune complexes are attached to the platelet membrane by the negative charge of highly sulphated oligosaccharides. Br J Haematol 84: 711–716, 1993.

Greinacher A, Amiral J, Dummel V, Vissac AM, Kiefel V, Mueller-Eckhardt C. Laboratory diagnosis of heparin-associated thrombocytopenia, comparison of platelet aggregation test, heparin-induced platelet activation (HIPA) test, and PF4/heparin ELISA. Transfusion 34: 381–385, 1994a.

Greinacher A, Feigl M, Mueller-Eckhardt C. Cross reactivity studies between sera of patients with heparin-associated thrombocytopenia and a new low molecular weight heparin, reviparin. Thromb Haemost 72: 644–645, 1994b.

Greinacher A, Pötzsch B, Amiral J, Dummel V, Eichner A, Mueller-Eckhardt C. Heparin-associated thrombocytopenia: isolation of the antibody and characterization of a multimolecular PF4-Heparin complex as the major antigen. Thromb Haemost 71: 247–251, 1994c.

Greinacher A, Alban S, Dummel V, Franz G, Mueller-Eckhardt C. Characterization of the structural requirements for a carbohydrate based anticoagulant with a reduced risk of inducing the immunological type of heparin-associated thrombocytopenia. Thromb Haemost 74: 886–892, 1995.

Greinacher A, Eichler P, Lubenow N, Luz M. Heparin-induced thrombocytopenia with thromboembolic complications: meta-analysis of two prospective trials to assess the value of parenteral treatment with lepirudin and its therapeutic aPTT range. Blood 96: 846–851, 2000.

Greinacher A, Eichler P, Lietz T, Warkentin TE. Replacement of unfractionated heparin by low molecular weight heparin for postorthopedic surgery antithrombotic prophylaxis lowers the overall risk of symptomatic thrombosis because of a lower frequency of heparin-induced thrombocytopenia. Blood 106: 2921–2922, 2005.

Greinacher A, Gopinadhan M, Günther JU, Omer-Adam MA, Strobel U, Warkentin TE, Papastavrou G, Weitschies W, Helm CA. Close approximation of two platelet factor 4 tetramers by charge neutralization forms the antigens recognized by HIT antibodies. Arterioscler Thromb Vasc Biol 26: 2386–2389, 2006.

Greinacher A, Alban S, Omer-Adam MA, Weitschies W, Warkentin TE. Heparin-induced thrombocytopenia: a stoichiometry-based model to explain the differing immunogenicities of unfractionated heparin, low molecular weight heparin, and fondaparinux in different clinical settings. Thromb Res 122: 211–220, 2008.

Greinacher A, Kohlmann T, Strobel U, Sheppard JA, Warkentin TE. The temporal profile of the anti-PF4/heparin immune response. Blood 113: 4970–4976, 2009.

Greinacher A, Holtfreter B, Krauel K, Gätke D, Weber C, Ittermann T, Hammerschmidt S, Kocher T. Association of natural anti-platelet factor 4/heparin antibodies with periodontal disease. Blood 118: 1395–1401, 2011.

Guerrini M, Beccati D, Shriver Z, Naggi A, Viswanathan K, Bisio A, Capila I, Lansing JC, Guglieri S, Fraser B, Al-Hakim A, Gunay NS, Zhang Z, Robinson L, Buhse L, Nasr M, Woodcock J, Langer R, Venkataraman G, Linhardt RJ, Casu B, Torri G, Sasisekharan R. Oversulfated chondroitin sulfate is a contaminant in heparin associated with adverse clinical events. Nat Biotechnol 26: 669–675, 2008.

Guerrini M, Zhang Z, Shriver Z, Naggi A, Masuko S, Langer R, Casu B, Linhardt RJ, Torri G, Sasisekharan R. Orthogonal analytical approaches to detect potential contaminants in heparin. Proc Nat Acad Sci USA 106, 16956–16961, 2009.

Handin RI, Cohen HJ. Purification and binding properties of human platelet factor four. J Biol Chem 251: 4273–4282, 1976.

Hensel E, Gesch D, Biffar R, Bernhardt O, Kocher T, Splieth C, Born G, John U. Study of Health in Pomerania (SHIP): a health survey in an East German region. Objectives and design of the oral health section. Quintessence Int 34: 370–378, 2003.

Herbert JM, Herault JP, Bernat A, van Amsterdam RG, Vogel GM, Lormeau JC, Petitou M, Meuleman DG. Biochemical and pharmacological properties of SANORG 32701. Comparison with the "synthetic pentasaccharide" (SR 90107/ORG 31540) and standard heparin. Circ Res 79: 590–600, 1996.

Herbert JM, Herault JP, Bernat A, van Amsterdam RG, Lormeau JC, Petitou M, van Boeckel C, Hoffman P, Meuleman DG. Biochemical and pharmacological properties of SANORG 34006, a potent and long-acting synthetic pentasaccharide. Blood 91: 4197–4205, 1998.

Herbert JM, Herault JP, Bernat A, Savi P, Schaeffer P, Driguez PA, Duchaussoy P, Petitou M. SR123781A, a synthetic heparin mimetic. Thromb Haemost 85: 852–860, 2001.

Hirsh J, Raschke R. Heparin and low molecular weight heparin: the Seventh ACCP Conference on Antithrombotic and Thrombolytic Therapy. Chest 126 (3 Suppl): 188S–203S, 2004.

Horne MK III. The effect of secreted heparin-binding proteins on heparin binding to platelets. Thromb Res 70: 91–98, 1993.

Horne MK III, Alkins BR. Platelet binding of IgG from patients with heparin-induced thrombocytopenia. J Lab Clin Med 127: 435–442, 1996.

Horne MK III, Hutchison KJ. Simultaneous binding of heparin and platelet factor-4 to platelets: further insights into the mechanism of heparin-induced thrombocytopenia. Am J Hematol 58: 24–30, 1998.

Horsewood P, Warkentin TE, Hayward CP, Kelton JG. The epitope specificity of heparin-induced thrombocytopenia. Br J Haematol 95: 161–167, 1996.

Joglekar MV, Quintana Diez PM, Marcus S, Qi R, Espinasse B, Wiesner MR, Pempe E, Liu J, Monroe DM, Arepally GM. Disruption of PF4/H multimolecular complex formation with a minimally anticoagulant heparin (ODSH). Thromb Haemost 107: 717–725, 2012.

John U, Greiner B, Hensel E, Ludemann J, Piek M, Sauer S, Adam C, Born G, Alte D, Greiser E, Haertel U, Hense HW, Haerting J, Willich S, Kessler C. Study of Health in Pomerania (SHIP): a health examination survey in an east German region: objectives and design. Soz Praventivmed 46: 186–194, 2001.

Juhl D, Eichler P, Lubenow N, Strobel U, Wessel A, Greinacher A. Incidence and clinical significance of anti-PF4/heparin antibodies of the IgG, IgM, and IgA class in 755 consecutive patient samples referred for diagnostic testing for heparin-induced thrombocytopenia. Eur J Haematol 76: 420–426, 2006.

Kaplan KL, Niewiarowski S. Nomenclature of secreted platelet proteins-report of the working party on secreted platelet proteins of the subcommittee on platelets. Thromb Haemost 53: 282–284, 1985.

Kappers-Klunne MC, Boon DM, Hop WC, Michiels JJ, Stibbe J, van der Zwaan C, Koudstaal PJ, van Vliet HH. Heparin-induced thrombocytopenia and thrombosis: a prospective analysis of the incidence in patients with heart and cerebrovascular diseases. Br J Haematol 96: 442–446, 1997.

Kelton JG, Sheridan D, Santos A, Smith J, Steeves K, Smith C, Brown C, Murphy WG. Heparin-induced thrombocytopenia: laboratory studies. Blood 72: 925–930, 1988.

Kelton JG, Smith JW, Warkentin TE, Hayward CP, Denomme GA, Horsewood P. Immunoglobulin G from patients with heparin-induced thrombocytopenia binds to a complex of heparin and platelet factor 4. Blood 83: 3232–3239, 1994.

Kindness G, Long WF, Williamson FB. Anticoagulant effects of sulphated polysaccharides in normal and antithrombin III-deficient plasmas. Br J Pharmacol 69: 675–677, 1980.

Kishimoto TK, Viswanathan K, Ganguly T, Elankumaran S, Smith S, Pelzer K, Lansing JC, Sriranganathan N, Zhao G, Galcheva-Gargova Z, Al-Hakim A, Bailey GS, Fraser B, Roy S, Rogers-Cotrone T, Buhse L, Whary M, Fox J, Nasr M, Dal Pan GJ, Shriver Z, Langer RS, Venkataraman G, Austen KF, Woodcock J, Sasisekharan R. Contaminated heparin associated with adverse clinical events and activation of the contact system. N Engl J Med 358: 2457–2467, 2008.

Klener P, Kubisz PSO. Platelet heparin-neutralizing activity (platelet factor 4). Acta Univ Carol Med (Praha) 24: 79–86, 1978.

Krauel K, Fürll B, Warkentin TE, Weitschies W, Kohlmann T, Sheppard JI, Greinacher A. Heparin-induced thrombocytopenia--therapeutic concentrations of danaparoid, unlike fondaparinux and direct thrombin inhibitors, inhibit formation of platelet factor 4-heparin complexes. J Thromb Haemost 6: 2160–2167, 2008.

Krauel K, Pötschke C, Weber C, Kessler W, Fürll B, Ittermann T, Maier S, Hammerschmidt S, Broker BM, Greinacher A. Platelet factor 4 binds to bacteria, [corrected] inducing antibodies cross-reacting with the major antigen in heparin-induced thrombocytopenia. Blood 117: 1370–1378, 2011.

Krauel K, Hackbarth C, Fürll B, Greinacher A. Heparin-induced thrombocytopenia: in vitro studies on the interaction of dabigatran, rivaroxaban, and low-sulfated heparin, with platelet factor 4 and anti-PF4/heparin antibodies. Blood 119: 1248–1255, 2012a.

Krauel K, Weber C, Greinacher A, Hammerschmidt S. Endotoxin of gram-negative bacteria contribute to PF4 binding thereby exposing PF4/heparin-like epitopes [abstr]. Hämostaseologie 32: A5, 2012b.

Lane DA, Denton J, Flynn AM, Thunberg L, Lindahl U. Anticoagulant activities of heparin oligosaccharides and their neutralization by platelet factor 4. Biochem J 218: 725–732, 1984.

Lassen MR, Dahl O, Mismetti P, Zielske D, Turpie AG. SR123781A: a new once-daily synthetic oligosaccharide anticoagulant for thromboprophylaxis after total hip replacement surgery: the DRIVE (dose ranging study in elective total hip replacement surgery) study. J Am Coll Cardiol 51: 1498–1504, 2008.

Li ZQ, Liu W, Park KS, Sachais BS, Arepally GM, Cines DB, Poncz M. Defining a second epitope for heparin-induced thrombocytopenia/thrombosis antibodies using KKO, a murine HIT-like monoclonal antibody. Blood 99: 1230–1236, 2002.

Li B, Suwan J, Martin JG, Zhang F, Zhang Z, Hoppensteadt D, Clark M, Fareed J, Linhardt RJ. Oversulfated chondroitin sulfate interaction with heparin-binding proteins: new insights into adverse reactions from contaminated heparins. Biochem Pharmacol 78: 292–300, 2009.

Lider O, Mekori YA, Miller T, Bar-Tana R, Vlodavsky I, Baharav E, Cohen IR, Naparstek Y. Inhibition of T lymphocyte heparanase by heparin prevents T cell migration and T cell-mediated immunity. Eur J Immunol 20: 493–499, 1990.

Linhardt RJ, Toida T. Heparin oligosaccharides: new analogues development and applications. In: Witczak ZJ, Nieforth KA, eds. Carbohydrates in Drug Design. New York: Marcel Dekker, 277–341, 1997.

Linhardt RJ, Rice KM, Kim YS, Lohse DL, Wang HM, Loganathan D. Mapping and quantification of the major oligosaccharide components of heparin. Biochem J 254: 781–787, 1988.

Loscalzo J, Melnick B, Handin RI. The interaction of platelet factor four and glycosaminoglycans. Arch Biochem Biophys 240: 446–455, 1985.

Lubenow N, Hinz P, Thomaschewski S, Lietz T, Vogler M, Ladwig A, Jünger M, Nauck M, Schellong S, Wander K, Engel G, Ekkernkamp A, Greinacher A. The severity of trauma determines the immune response to PF4/heparin and the frequency of heparin-induced thrombocytopenia. Blood 15: 1797–1803, 2010.

Luscher EF, Kaser-Glanzman R. Platelet heparin-neutralizing factor (platelet factor 4). Thromb Diath Haemorrh 33: 66–72, 1975.

Maccarana M, Lindahl U. Mode of interaction between platelet factor 4 and heparin. Glycobiology 3: 271–277, 1993.

Maier S, Traeger T, Entleutner M, Westerholt A, Kleist B, Huser N, Holzmann B, Stier A, Pfeffer K, Heidecke CD. Cecal ligation and puncture versus colon ascendens stent peritonitis: two distinct animal models for polymicrobial sepsis. Shock 21: 505–511, 2004.

Martel N, Lee J, Wells PS. Risk for heparin-induced thrombocytopenia with unfractionated and low molecular weight heparin thromboprophylaxis: a meta-analysis. Blood 106: 2710–2715, 2005.

Maruyama T, Toida T, Imanari T, Yu G, Linhardt RJ. Conformational changes and anticoagulant activity of chondroitin sulfate following its O-sulfonation. Carbohydr Res 306: 35–43, 1998.

Mayo KH, Roongta V, Ilyina E, Milius R, Barker S, Quinlan C, La Rosa G, Daly TJ. NMR solution structure of the 32–kDa platelet factor 4 ELR-motif N-terminal chimera: a symmetric tetramer. Biochemistry 34: 11399–11409, 1995.

Meuleman DG. Orgaran (Org 10172): its pharmacological profile in experimental models. Haemostasis 22: 58–65, 1992.

Mikhailov D, Young HC, Linhardt RJ, Mayo KH. Heparin dodecasaccharide binding to platelet factor-4 and growth-related protein-α: induction of a partially folded state and implications for heparin-induced thrombocytopenia. J Biol Chem 274: 25317–25329, 1999.

Moore S, Pepper DS, Cash JD. Platelet antiheparin activity. The isolation and characterization of platelet factor 4 released from thrombin-aggregated washed human platelets and its dissociation into subunits and the isolation of membrane-bound antiheparin activity. Biochim Biophys Acta 379: 370–384, 1975.

Neuhaus FC, Baddiley J. A continuum of anionic charge: structures and functions of D-alanyl-teichoic acids in gram-positive bacteria. Microbiol Mol Biol Rev 67: 686–723, 2003.

Newman PM, Chong BH. Further characterization of antibody and antigen in heparin-induced thrombocytopenia. Br J Haematol 107: 303–309, 1999.

Newman PM, Chong BH. Heparin-induced thrombocytopenia: new evidence for the dynamic binding of purified anti-PF4-Heparin antibodies to platelets and the resultant platelet activation. Blood 96: 182–187, 2000.

Niewiarowski S. Report of the Working Party on Platelets. Platelet factor 4 (PF4), platelet protein with heparin neutralizing activity. Thromb Haemost 36: 273–276, 1976.

Novotny WF, Maffi T, Mehta RL, Milner PG. Identification of novel heparin releasable proteins, as well as the cytokines midkine and pleiotrophin, in human postheparin plasma. Arterioscler Thromb 13: 1798–1805, 1993.

O'Brien JR, Etherington MD, Pashley MA. The heparin-mobilisable pool of platelet factor 4: a comparison of intravenous and subcutaneous heparin and Kabi heparin fragment 2165. Thromb Haemost 54: 735–738, 1985.

Padilla A, Gray E, Pepper DS, Barrowcliffe TW. Inhibition of thrombin generation by heparin and low molecular weight (LMW) heparins in the absence and presence of platelet factor 4 (PF4). Br J Haematol 82: 406–413, 1992.

Petitou M, Duchaussoy P, Jaurand G, Gourvenec F, Lederman I, Strassel JM, Barzu T, Crepon B, Herault JP, Lormeau JC, Bernat A, Herbert JM. Synthesis and pharmacological properties of a close analogue of an antithrombotic pentasaccharide (SR 90107A/ORG 31540). J Med Chem 40: 1600–1607, 1997.

Petitou M, Herault JP, Bernat A, Driguez PA, Duchaussoy P, Lormeau JC, Herbert JM. Synthesis of thrombin-inhibiting heparin mimetics without side effects. Nature 398: 417–422, 1999.

Prechel MM, McDonald MK, Jeske WP, Messmore HL, Walenga JM. Activation of platelets by heparin-induced thrombocytopenia antibodies in the serotonin release assay is not dependent on the presence of heparin. J Thromb Haemost 3: 2168–2175, 2005.

PROTECT Investigators for the Canadian Critical Care Trials Group and the Australian and New Zealand Intensive Care Society Clinical Trials Group, Cook D, Meade M, Guyatt G, Walter S, Heels-Ansdell D, Warkentin TE, Zytaruk N, Crowther M, Geerts W, Cooper DJ, Vallance S, Qushmaq I, Rocha M, Berwanger O, Vlahakis NE. Dalteparin versus unfractionated heparin in critically ill patients. N Engl J Med 364: 1305–1314, 2011.

Rao NV, Argyle B, Xu X, Reynolds PR, Walenga JM, Prechel M, Prestwich GD, MacArthur RB, Walters BB, Hoidal JR, Kennedy TP. Low anticoagulant heparin targets multiple sites of inflammation, suppresses heparin-induced thrombocytopenia, and inhibits interaction of RAGE with its ligands. Am J Physiol Cell Physiol 299: C97–110, 2010.

Rauova L, Poncz M, McKenzie SE, Reilly MP, Arepally G, Weisel JW, Nagaswami C, Cines DB, Sachais BS. Ultra large complexes of PF4 and heparin are central to the pathogenesis of heparin-induced thrombocytopenia. Blood 105: 131–138, 2005.

Rauova L, Zhai L, Kowalska MA, Arepally GM, Cines DB, Poncz M. Role of platelet surface PF4 antigenic complexes in heparin-induced thrombocytopenia pathogenesis: diagnostic and therapeutic implications. Blood 107: 2346–2353, 2006.

Rosenthal MA, Rischin D, McArthur G, Ribbons K, Chong B, Fareed J, Toner G, Green MD, Basser RL. Treatment with the novel anti-angiogenic agent PI-88 is associated with immune-mediated thrombocytopenia. Ann Oncol 13: 770–776, 2002.

Royce K FDA failures contribute to spread of contaminated drugs. Worldfocus 17.12, 2008, http://worldfocus.org/blog/2008/12/17/fda-failures-contribute-to-spread-of-contaminated-drugs/3287/. [Accessed: 2012, April 10th].

St. Charles R, Walz DA, Edwards BF. The three-dimensional structure of bovine platelet factor 4 at 3.0–a resolution. J Biol Chem 264: 2092–2099, 1989.

Salem HH, van der Weyden MB. Heparin-induced thrombocytopenia. variable platelet-rich plasma reactivity to heparin-dependent platelet aggregating factor. Pathology 15: 297–299, 1983.

Savi P, Chong BH, Greinacher A, Gruel Y, Kelton JG, Warkentin TE, Eichler P, Meuleman D, Petitou M, Herault JP, Cariou R, Herbert JM. Effect of fondaparinux on platelet activation in the presence of heparin-dependent antibodies: a blinded comparative multicenter study with unfractionated heparin. Blood 105: 139–144, 2005.

Sear CH, Poller L. Antiheparin activity of human serum and platelet factor 4. Thromb Diath Haemorrh 30: 93–105, 1973.

Selleng S, Malowsky B, Strobel U, Wessel A, Ittermann T, Wollert HG, Warkentin TE, Greinacher A. Early-onset and persisting thrombocytopenia in post-cardiac surgery patients is rarely due to heparin-induced thrombocytopenia, even when antibody tests are positive. J Thromb Haemost 8: 30–36, 2010.

Sikara MP, Routsias JG, Samiotaki M, Panayotou G, Moutsopoulos HM, Vlachoyiannopoulos PG. β_2 Glycoprotein I (β_2GPI) binds platelet factor 4 (PF4): implications for the pathogenesis of antiphospholipid syndrome. Blood 115: 713–723, 2010.

Stuckey JA, St. Charles R, Edwards BF. A model of the platelet factor 4 complex with heparin. Proteins 14: 277–287, 1992.

Suh JS, Malik MI, Aster RH, Visentin GP. Characterization of the humoral immune response in heparin-induced thrombocytopenia. Am J Hematol 54: 196–201, 1997.

Suh JS, Aster RH, Visentin GP. Antibodies from patients with heparin-induced thrombocytopenia/thrombosis recognize different epitopes on heparin: platelet factor 4. Blood 91: 916–922, 1998.

Suzuki S, Koide M, Sakamoto S, Yamamoto S, Matsuo M, Fujii E, Matsuo T. Early onset of immunological heparin-induced thrombocytopenia in acute myocardial infarction. Blood Coagul Fibrinolysis 8: 13–15, 1997.

Tardy PB, Tardy B, Grelac F, Reynaud J, Mismetti P, Bertrand JC, Guyotat D. Pentosan polysulfate-induced thrombocytopenia and thrombosis. Am J Hematol 88: 803–808, 1994.

Turpie AGG. New therapeutic opportunities for heparins: what does low molecular weight heparin offer? J Thromb Thrombolysis 3: 145–149, 1996.

van Os G, Meijers JC, Agar C, Seron MV, Marquart JA, Åkesson P, Urbanus RT, Derksen RH, Herwald H, Mörgelin M, De Groot PG Induction of anti-β_2-glycoprotein I autoantibodies in mice by protein H of Streptococcus pyogenes. J Thromb Haemost 9: 2447–2456, 2011.

Visentin GP. Heparin-induced thrombocytopenia: molecular pathogenesis. Thromb Haemost 82: 448–456, 1999.

Visentin GP, Ford SE, Scott JP, Aster RH. Antibodies from patients with heparin induced thrombocytopenia/thrombosis are specific for platelet factor 4 complexed with heparin or bound to endothelial cells. J Clin Invest 93: 81–88, 1994.

Visentin GP, Malik M, Cyganiak KA, Aster RH. Patients treated with unfractionated heparin during open heart surgery are at high risk to form antibodies reactive with heparin: platelet factor 4 complexes. J Lab Clin Med 128: 376–383, 1996.

Visentin GP, Moghaddam M, Beery SE, McFarland JG, Aster RH. Heparin is not required for detection of antibodies associated with heparin induced thrombocytopenia/thrombosis. J Lab Clin Med 138: 22–31, 2001.

Viskov C, Just M, Laux V, Mourier P, Lorenz M. Description of the chemical and pharmacological characteristics of a new hemisynthetic ultra-low molecular weight heparin, AVE5026. J Thromb Haemost 7: 1143–1151, 2009.

Wang L, Brown JR, Varki A, Esko JD. Heparin's anti-inflammatory effects require glucosamine 6-O-sulfation and are mediated by blockade of L- and P-selectins. J Clin Invest 110: 127–136, 2002.

Warkentin TE, Bernstein RA. Delayed-onset heparin-induced thrombocytopenia and cerebral thrombosis after a single administration of unfractionated heparin. N Engl J Med 348: 1067–1069, 2003.

Warkentin TE, Kelton JG. Delayed-onset heparin-induced thrombocytopenia and thrombosis. Ann Intern Med 135: 502–506, 2001.

Warkentin TE, Sheppard JI. No significant improvement in diagnostic specificity of an anti-PF4/polyanion immunoassay with use of high heparin confirmatory procedure. J Thromb Haemost 4: 281–282, 2006.

Warkentin TE, Levine MN, Hirsh J, Horsewood P, Roberts RS, Gent M, Kelton JG. Heparin-induced thrombocytopenia in patients treated with low molecular weight heparin or unfractionated heparin. N Engl J Med 332: 1330–1335, 1995.

Warkentin TE, Elavathil LJ, Hayward CPM, Johnston MA, Russett JI, Kelton JG. The pathogenesis of venous limb gangrene associated with heparin-induced thrombocytopenia. Ann Intern Med 127: 804–812, 1997.

Warkentin TE, Cook RJ, Marder VJ, Sheppard JA, Moore JC, Eriksson BI, Greinacher A, Kelton JG. Anti-platelet factor 4/heparin antibodies in orthopedic surgery patients receiving antithrombotic prophylaxis with fondaparinux or enoxaparin. Blood 106: 3791–3796, 2005a.

Warkentin TE, Sheppard JA, Moore JC, Moore KM, Sigouin CS, Kelton JG. Laboratory testing for the antibodies that cause heparin-induced thrombocytopenia: how much class do we need? J Lab Clin Med 146: 341–346, 2005b.

Warkentin TE, Sheppard JI, Sigouin CS, Kohlmann T, Eichler P, Greinacher A. Gender imbalance and risk factor interactions in heparin-induced thrombocytopenia. Blood 108: 2937–2941, 2006.

Warkentin TE, Makris M, Jay RM, Kelton JG. A spontaneous prothrombotic disorder resembling heparin-induced thrombocytopenia. Am J Med 121: 632–636, 2008.

Warkentin TE, Sheppard JA, Moore JC, Cook RJ, Kelton JG. Studies of the immune response in heparin-induced thrombocytopenia. Blood 113: 4963–4969, 2009.

Warkentin TE, Cook RJ, Marder VJ, Greinacher A. Anti-PF4/heparin antibody formation postorthopedic surgery thromboprophylaxis: the role of non-drug risk factors and evidence for a stoichiometry-based model of immunization. J Thromb Haemost 8: 504–512, 2010.

Weiler JM, Edens RE, Linhardt RJ, Kapelanski DP. Heparin and modified heparin inhibit complement activation in vivo. J Immunol 148: 3210–3215, 1992.

Weimann G, Lubenow N, Selleng K, Eichler P, Albrecht D, Greinacher A. Glucosamine sulfate does not cross react with the antibodies of patients with heparin-induced thrombocytopenia. Eur J Haematol 66: 195–199, 2001.

Wilde MI, Markham A. Danaparoid. A review of its pharmacology and clinical use in the management of heparin-induced thrombocytopenia. Drugs 54: 903–924, 1997.

Williams RT, Damaraju LV, Mascelli MA, Barnathan ES, Califf RM, Simoons ML, Deliargyris EN, Sane DC. Anti-platelet factor 4/heparin antibodies: an independent predictor of 30–day myocardial infarction after acute coronary ischemic syndromes. Circulation 107: 2307–2312, 2003.

Young E. The anti-inflammatory effects of heparin and related compounds. Thromb Res 122: 743–752, 2008.

Young E, Prins MH, Levine MN, Hirsh J. Heparin binding to plasma proteins, an important mechanism for heparin resistance. Thromb Haemost 67: 639–643, 1992.

Zantl N, Uebe A, Neumann B, Wagner H, Siewert JR, Holzmann B, Heidecke CD, Pfeffer K. Essential role of gamma interferon in survival of colon ascendens stent peritonitis, a novel murine model of abdominal sepsis. Infect Immun 66: 2300–2309, 1998.

Zhang X, Chen L, Bancroft DP, Lai CK, Maione TE. Crystal structure of recombinant human platelet factor 4. Biochemistry 33: 8361–8366, 1994.

8 Platelet and leukocyte Fcγ receptors in heparin-induced thrombocytopenia

Gregory A. Denomme

INTRODUCTION

Heparin-induced thrombocytopenia (HIT) is a unique immune-mediated disorder. The central paradigm is that HIT is caused by IgG that produces strong platelet activation via interaction with platelet FcγIIa receptors (FcγRIIa). HIT is relatively common, occurring in as many as 5% of certain heparin-treated patient populations. Affected patients have thrombocytopenia, often develop a paradoxical thrombotic episode, with timing consistent with heparin being the causal agent, and without any other obvious cause (Lo et al., 2006). One possible reason for the unique clinical profile is the central role that platelet FcγRIIa plays in mediating platelet activation in HIT. Indirect evidence suggests a crucial role for platelet activation in the pathogenesis of HIT because thrombocytopenia and the presence of HIT antibodies are strongly associated with thrombosis, whereas the formation of antibodies without thrombocytopenia is not (Warkentin et al., 1995). Notwithstanding the role that platelet FcγRIIa plays in platelet activation, leukocyte FcγRs may also contribute to the pathogenesis of HIT (Xiao et al., 2008).

It has been known for several years that HIT results from a predominant IgG immune response to antigenic determinants involving platelet-bound heparin (Green et al., 1978) and platelet factor 4 (PF4) (Amiral et al., 1992). Thus, the pathogenesis of HIT resembles a type II immune reaction, that is, a cytotoxic antibody response (Roitt et al., 1985), and both human T-cell *in vitro* studies and a murine model of HIT support a T-cell dependent immune response (Bacsi et al., 1999; Suvarna et al., 2005). The typical features of a type II immune response, such as phagocytosis, killer-cell activity, or complement-mediated lysis, do not seem to predominate in HIT, but do occur (see next paragraph). Instead, thrombocytopenia results primarily from FcγRIIa-mediated platelet activation, aggregation, and granule release (Chong et al., 1981) as a result of IgG binding to platelet factor 4/heparin (PF4/H) complexes on the platelet surface. Why platelets react this way may be linked to the role platelets play in the innate immune response. Being the first cells that adhere to sites of vessel injury, platelets can be activated by bacteria through interactions with various receptors, namely, integrin, complement, toll-like, and FcγRIIa (Cox et al., 2011). It is thought that the release of antimicrobial molecules—including PF4—as a result of platelet activation after vessel injury, provides some level of host protection from infection (Ford et al., 1997; Krauel et al., 2011). Given the rapid timing of HIT and the innate response of platelet FcγRIIa activation, it is possible that germline immunoglobulins, available to aid in the clearance of bacteria (Casali and Schettino, 1996), or the preexposure to PF4/bacteria complexes (Kottenberg-Assenmacher et al., 2006; Greinacher et al., 2011; Krauel et al., 2011), may induce rapid development of anti-PF4/H antibodies upon exposure to heparin. Certainly, HIT without proximate heparin exposure could be explained by recent bacterial infection (Warkentin et al., 2008; Olah et al., 2012).

HIT antibodies also activate endothelium *in vitro* by interaction with PF4/heparan sulfate complexes (Cines et al., 1987; Greinacher et al., 1994b; Visentin et al., 1994). However, unlike platelets, human endothelium (with the exception of placental villous endothelial cells and a subset of endothelial cells found in the superficial dermal vascular plexus) does not express any FcγRs, either constitutively or in the setting of immune complex diseases (Sedmak et al., 1991; Gröger et al., 1996). Thus, platelet activation and endothelial activation in HIT probably arise from fundamentally distinct processes. Other effects of HIT include the formation of platelet-leukocyte aggregates, the release of tissue factor (TF) from monocytes, and the FcγRIIIa-dependent phagocytosis or natural killer (NK) cell destruction of antibody-sensitized platelets (Khairy et al., 2001; Pouplard et al., 2001; Gruel et al., 2004).

One of the most important unanswered questions in the pathophysiology of this disorder is an explanation for why only a few patients who develop HIT antibodies become thrombocytopenic, or more mechanistically, why only certain anti-PF4/H antibodies activate platelets. This problem has led investigators to study the role of FcγRIIa in explaining, at least partly, the heterogenous clinical sequelae among patients with HIT. This chapter (*i*) reviews the structure and function of the platelet FcγRIIa; (*ii*) describes the mechanism of HIT antibody-induced platelet activation by FcγRIIa; and (*iii*) summarizes the studies that have attempted to identify the role of FcγRs in modifying the clinical manifestations of HIT.

FcγR STRUCTURE, DISTRIBUTION, AND FUNCTION

FcγRIIa is a member of a family of structurally related glycoproteins (GPs), many of which are expressed on hematopoietic cells (Table 8.1). Twelve different transcripts have been reported, derived from eight genes grouped into three different classes: I, II, and III (van de Winkel and Capel, 1993; Rascu et al., 1997; Gessner et al., 1998). Allelic polymorphic variants add yet another level of diversity for FcγRIIa, FcγRIIIa, and FcγRIIIb. The genomic organization of the FcγR genes on chromosome 1q23 was resolved by Su and coworkers (2002). The multigenic region at 1q23 is 1.73 megabase in size, contains two heat shock proteins, and is in the following gene order and orientation:

FCGR2A(5′-3′)-HSPA6-FCGR3A(3′-5′)-FCGR2C(5′-3′)-HSPA7-FCGR3B(3′-5′)-FCGR2B(5′-3′)-…telomer

The affinity for IgG varies among isoforms and variants. FcγRIIa-His[131] has a higher affinity for human IgG2 than FcγRIIa-Arg[131] (Warmerdam et al., 1991). One nonfunctional FcγRIIc variant has a nonsense codon, which results in a null phenotype (Metes et al., 1998). When cross-linked, each isoform participates in biologic activities through distinct signal transduction pathways that affect cell functions, including antigen presentation, immune complex clearance, phagocytosis and the oxidative burst, release of cytokines and intracellular granular mediators, antibody-dependent cellular cytotoxicity, and downregulation of antibody production or phagocytosis.

Only FcγRIIa is expressed on platelets (Rosenfeld et al., 1985; Kelton et al., 1987). The receptor is a single α-chain, 40-kDa GP, with an extracellular region

TABLE 8.1   The Family of Fcγ Receptors: Molecular and Structural Characteristics and Tissue Distribution

	FcγRI (CD64)	FcγRII (CD32)	FcγRIII (CD16)
Genes	IA, IB, IC	IIA, IIB, IIc	IIIA, IIIB
Functional variants[a]	None	IIa: Gln/Lys^{127} IIa: Arg/His^{131} IIc: Gln/stop codon^{13}	IIIa: Leu/Arg/His^{48} IIIa: Phe/Val^{158} IIIb: NA1/NA2 IIIb: Ala/Asp^{60} (SH)
RNA transcripts[b]	IA1 IB1, IB2 IC	IIA1, IIA2 IIB1, IIB2, IIB3 IIC	IIIA IIIB
Glycoprotein expressed[c]	Ia	IIa1, sIIa2 IIb1, sIIb2, IIb3 IIc	IIIa IIIb (GPI linked)
Molecular weight (kDa)	72	40	50–80
Extracellular Ig-like domains	3	2	2
Intracellular tyrosine motif[d]	None	ITAM (IIa, IIc) ITIM (IIb)	None
Noncovalent-associated subunit	γ-chain	None	β-chain, γ-chain, ζ-chain
Affinity constant	10^8 M^{-1}	$<10^7$ M^{-1}	IIIa: 3×10^7 M^{-1} IIIb: $<10^7$ M^{-1}
IgG subclass avidity[e]	3 = 1 > 4 >>>> 2	IIa-Arg^{131} 3 > 1 >>> 2 > 4 IIa-His^{131} 3 > 1 = 2 > 4 IIb1 3 > 1 > 4 >>>> 2	IIIa-Val^{158} 1 > 3 >>> 2,4 IIIa-Val^{158} > Phe^{158} for 1 and 3 IIIb-NA1 > IIIb-NA2 for 1 and 3
Hematopoietic cell distribution	CD34 progenitor cells, monocytes, macrophages, dendritic cells	IIa: platelets, endothelial cells, monocytes, macrophages, eosino-/baso-/neutrophils, Langerhans/dendritic cells IIb: B cells, monocytes IIc: NK cells	IIIa: monocytes, macrophages, NK cells, T cells IIIb: neutrophils

[a]Allelic polymorphisms that show differences in IgG binding; NA1/NA2 variants have multiple amino acid differences (Ory et al., 1989); SH+ individuals (Bux et al., 1997) carry three copies of FcγRIIIb (Koene et al., 1998); the FcγRIIc null phenotype is due to a nonsense mutation (Metes et al., 1998).
[b]Multiple mRNA transcripts from FcγRIb, IIa, and IIb are the result of alternative splicing of primary transcripts.
[c]Soluble forms of FcγRIIa and IIb (sIIa, sIIb) are devoid of the hydrophobic transmembrane exon.
[d]ITAM, immunoreceptor tyrosine-based activation motif; ITIM, immunoreceptor tyrosine-based inhibition motif.
[e]Numbers represent the relative order of IgG subclass binding to variants of FcγRIIa (Warmerdam et al., 1990), FcγRIIIa (Koene et al., 1997; Wu et al., 1997), and FcγRIIIb (Salmon et al., 1990; Bredius et al., 1994b).
Abbreviations: GPI, glycosyl-phosphatidylinositol; NK, natural killer.

consisting of two immunoglobulin-like, disulfide-linked domains responsible for ligand binding, a transmembrane region, and an intracellular domain that incorporates an immunoreceptor tyrosine-based activation motif (ITAM) essential for intracellular signal transduction (Brooks et al., 1989; Qiu et al., 1990). A soluble form of the receptor is produced by alternative splicing of primary RNA transcripts to exclude exon 5 containing the transmembrane region (Rappaport et al., 1993).

The extracellular domain of FcγRIIa shares 96% amino acid identity with FcγRIIb and FcγRIIc (Brooks et al., 1989). The G → A polymorphism at nucleotide position 519 of the cDNA (position 535 in Genbank Reference Sequence NM_021642) is responsible for the Arg/His[131] functional variants (Clark et al., 1989). An additional polymorphism, an A → G at nucleotide 207 of the cDNA, results in a Gln-Trp[27] substitution in the mature polypeptide (Warmerdam et al., 1991). However, the Arg-His[131] position is near or within the binding region for IgG Fc (Hulett et al., 1995), and it is this polymorphism that is associated with the affinity differences for human IgG2 (Warmerdam et al., 1991). More recently, another polymorphism proximal to Arg[131] that affects IgG2 binding has been found in a single healthy individual (Norris et al., 1998): A lysine substitution for glutamine at position 127 demonstrated a significant increase in FcγR-mediated phagocytosis in this homozygous FcγRIIa-Arg[131] individual.

FcγRIIa has a low affinity for IgG ($<10^7 M^{-1}$) and interacts mainly with antigen/antibody complexes (Warmerdam et al., 1991; Parren et al., 1992). The copy number of FcγRIIa expressed on resting platelets varies among healthy individuals but is stable (Rosenfeld et al., 1987). There is roughly a threefold variation among individuals, with the copy number ranging from 600 to 1500 molecules per platelet when assayed using an intact murine monoclonal antibody IV.3 (McCrae et al., 1990) and 1500 to more than 4500 when tested with a Fab preparation (Tomiyama et al., 1992; Brandt et al., 1995). There are no major differences in FcγRIIa copy number between males and females, among platelets from persons of different ages, or for the three genotypic classes of FcγRIIa-Arg/His[131] (Brandt et al., 1995).

IMMUNOGLOBULIN G (IgG) AGONISTS AND PLATELET ACTIVATION
FcγRIIa-Mediated Platelet Activation

Murine monoclonal IgG1 anti-CD9 were among the first studied for their platelet-activating properties. Subsequently, it was determined that monoclonal antibodies to GPIIb/IIIa, β_2-microglobulin, GPIV (CD36), and other selected antigens can activate platelets (for review: Rubinstein et al., 1995). In each instance, platelet activation occurs by a defined mechanism: first, the variable region of the antibody binds to its cognate antigen; then the Fc portion of the antibody interacts with platelet FcγRIIa. Evidence for FcγRIIa dependency includes the inhibition of platelet activation by the murine monoclonal anti-FcγRIIa antibody (IV.3). However, some platelet GPs (e.g., GPIb) do not support activation by monoclonal antibodies; others support activation despite their usual sequestered location within platelets (e.g., GPIa*), and still other GPs (e.g., GPIIb/IIIa) support activation by only certain monoclonal antibodies (Horsewood et al., 1991). These observations suggest that specific factors, such as target protein membrane mobility and localization of the epitope, which permit the formation of multimolecular GP antigen/IgG/FcγRIIa complexes, are crucial for FcγRIIa-mediated platelet activation. The IgG can interact with either FcγRIIa on the same platelet (*intra*platelet activation) or with FcγRIIa located on other platelets in close proximity (*inter*platelet activation) (Anderson et al., 1991; Horsewood et al., 1991).

Complexed human IgG is also a potent stimulator of platelet activation. Karas and coworkers (1982) showed that trimeric human IgG and larger immune complexes had significant affinity for platelet FcγRIIa. King et al. (1990) showed that a minimum of trimeric IgG molecules are necessary for platelet activation. Heat-aggregated IgG also is a potent agonist for platelet activation (Warkentin et al., 1994; Warkentin and Sheppard, 1999), as are streptokinase/antistreptokinase complexes (Lebrazi et al., 1995) and PF4/H immune complexes (Greinacher et al., 1994b).

HIT-IgG causes the generation of thromboxane A_2 and associated platelet granule release (Chong et al., 1981). Indeed, several different "activation assays" have been developed that detect HIT antibodies by their ability to cause resting platelets to aggregate (Greinacher et al., 1991), effect granule release (Sheridan et al., 1986), or generate platelet-derived microparticles (Warkentin et al., 1994) (see chap. 11).

Procoagulant, Platelet-Derived Microparticles

Platelet activation by various agonists leads to procoagulant alterations of the platelet membrane. This includes loss of the usual membrane asymmetry (i.e., with platelet activation, there is increased transbilayer movement of phosphatidylserine from the inner to the outer leaflet of the platelet plasma membrane). The membrane "flip-flop" is a consequence of a calcium-dependent enzyme ("scramblase") that serves to undo the membrane asymmetry actively maintained in resting platelets by other enzymes (aminophospholipid translocase and "floppase") (Bevers et al., 1999). Additionally, platelet activation also leads to profound morphologic changes that include the generation of procoagulant platelet-derived "microparticles" (Sims et al., 1989).

Sera and purified IgG from patients with HIT also generate platelet-derived microparticles via the platelet FcγRIIa (Warkentin et al., 1994). Indeed, HIT serum is superior in generating platelet-derived microparticles and in producing platelet procoagulant activity than thrombin, collagen, and adenosine diphosphate (ADP); only the nonphysiologic agonist calcium ionophore produces greater numbers of microparticles and procoagulant activity than does HIT serum (Warkentin and Sheppard, 1999). Flow cytometry using particle size ("forward scatter") and fluorescein-labeled platelet GP-specific monoclonal antibodies can detect platelet-derived microparticles generated by HIT antibodies (Warkentin et al., 1994; Hughes et al., 2000). This technique has been used as a diagnostic assay for HIT (Lee et al., 1996). Alternatively, Tomer (1997) used fluorescent-labeled annexin V, a protein that binds to phosphatidylserine, to detect activated platelets and microparticles.

There is some uncertainty as to whether the "microparticles" detected by flow cytometry represent true microparticles or rather platelets that have undergone considerable morphologic changes during activation. Use of orthogonal light scatter, combined with fluorescence gating on platelet antigens, detects significant increases in total particle count, suggesting that at least some microparticles are generated (Bode and Hickerson, 2000). Moreover, microparticles being generated by HIT antibodies is suggested by a study that used confocal microscopy and scanning/transmission electron microscopy for their detection (Hughes et al., 2000) (Fig. 8.1).

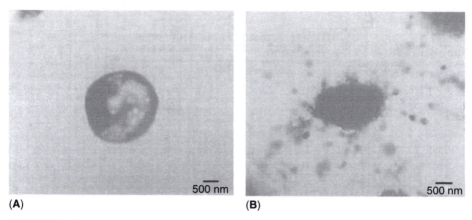

(A)   **(B)**

FIGURE 8.1 Electron microscopy of negatively stained platelets activated *in situ* with HIT serum. Platelets were allowed to settle on bovine albumin-coated Formvar grids and then incubated with **(A)** serum testing negative for HIT antibodies or heparin (not shown) or **(B)** HIT serum in the presence of heparin, 0.1 U/mL. Platelets were then fixed with 2% glutaraldehyde and negatively stained with 2% phosphotungstic acid. Unactivated platelets demonstrated round or discoid shapes (see A), whereas platelets activated by HIT serum demonstrated numerous surrounding microparticles ranging in size from <0.1 to 1.0 μm in diameter. (Original magnification × 13,000.) *Abbreviation:* HIT, heparin-induced thrombocytopenia. *Source:* From Hughes et al., 2000.

ADP Potentiation of Platelet Activation

ADP is an important autocrine stimulator of platelet activation by HIT-IgG (Chong et al., 1981). This observation was confirmed by Anderson and Anderson (1990) who showed that *in vitro* FcγRIIa-mediated platelet activation was augmented by ADP. Moreover, Polgár and coworkers (1998) found that pretreatment of platelets with a potent ADP receptor antagonist completely blocked the activity of HIT sera. This observation indicates that ADP and a functional ADP receptor are crucial to FcγRIIa activation by HIT-IgG. However, it should be pointed out that patients receiving ADP receptor antagonists (e.g., clopidogrel) can still develop HIT and HIT-associated thrombosis (Selleng et al., 2005).

FcγRIIa-Mediated Signal Transduction

FcγRIIa coligation, as a result of IgG binding, leads to activation of phosphatidylinositol 3-kinase (PI 3-kinase) and phospholipase C-γ2 (PLCγ2), with the subsequent release of diacylglycerol (DAG) and inositol triphosphate (IP3), mobilization of internal calcium stores, and platelet aggregation (Anderson and Anderson, 1990). Initially, IgG binding leads to FcγRIIa coligation, resulting in the phosphorylation of FcγRIIa ITAMs by Src family protein tyrosine kinases (Huang et al., 1992; Chacko et al., 1994). Following FcγRIIa phosphorylation, tyrosine kinase (e.g., p72^{syk}) and PI 3-kinase activation occurs through the noncovalent interaction of their SH2 domains with phosphorylated FcγRIIa ITAMs (Greinacher et al., 1994a; Yanaga et al., 1995; Chacko et al., 1996). Subsequently, PLCγ2 is phosphorylated by p72^{syk} (Blake et al., 1994), which is dependent on phosphatidylinositol-trisphosphate (PtdIns[3,4,5]P3) generated by IP 3-kinase (Gratacap et al., 1998). PLCγ2 activation is crucial for the production of DAG and IP3. More recently, the importance of Syk tyrosine kinase in

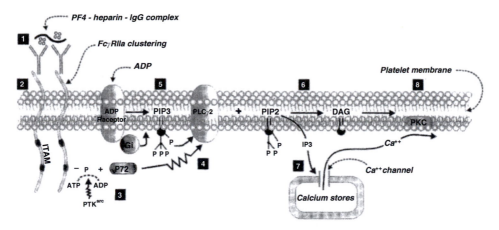

FIGURE 8.2 Fcγ receptor-mediated signal transduction. PF4/heparin/IgG complexes (1) bind to FcγRIIa, causing receptor clustering (2). The ITAMs on FcγRIIa are phosphorylated by PTK[src] (3). The phosphorylated ITAMs interact with SH domains on p72[syk] to phosphorylate PLCγ2 (4). ADP receptors, activated via ADP and Gi proteins, generate PIP3 via PI 3-kinase (not shown) (5), which helps phosphorylate PLCγ2. Activated PLCγ2 acts on PIP2 to generate IP3, and DAG from phosphatidylinositol-bisphosphate (6). IP3 mobilizes Ca++ to the intracellular space via Ca++ channels (7) and together with DAG activates downstream PKC signaling pathways (8). *Abbreviations*: DAG, diacylglycerol; IP3, inositol triphosphate; ITAMs, immunoreceptor tyrosine activation motifs; PF4, platelet factor 4; PKC, protein kinase C; PLCγ2, phospholipase Cγ2; PIP3, phosphatidylinositol-trisphosphate; PTK[src], src protein tyrosine kinases.

HIT has been realized by the inhibition of *in vitro* PF4/H/IgG complex-induced platelet aggregation by the Syk inhibitors (Lhermusier et al., 2011; Reilly et al., 2011). The inhibitor was also evaluated in a murine model of HIT; in theory, Syk inhibitors could prove to be useful therapies for HIT since inhibition of platelet activation was demonstrated in this model (Reilly et al., 2011), and Syk inhibitors can ameliorate platelet activation without otherwise affecting hemostasis (Andre et al., 2011).

FcγRIIa-dependent PI 3-kinase activation does not produce sufficient levels of PtdIns(3,4,5)P3 to phosphorylate PLCγ2, cause platelet granule release, and aggregation (Gratacap et al., 2000). ADP receptor activation by Gi-protein signaling is required to generate PtdIns(3,4,5)P3 via PI 3-kinase, which generates optimal levels of PtdIns(3,4,5)P3 when combined with FcγRIIa activation and leads to efficient PLCγ2 phosphorylation. Phosphorylated PLCγ2 then generates DAG and IP3 from PtdIns(4,5)P2, mobilizing calcium and effecting platelet aggregation (Fig. 8.2). In support of the need for Gi-protein signaling, the stimulation of platelets, using specific agonists (low concentration thrombin or ADP) that target G-protein (PAR1 and PAR4) and G-protein-coupled receptors, result in FcγRIIa phosphorylation by src kinases (Canobbio et al., 2006). Moreover, lipid rafts appear to play an important role in the organization of the FcγRIIa-G-protein signaling pathways leading to PLCγ2 phosphorylation (Bodin et al., 2003; Canobbio et al., 2006). These findings help to explain the previous observations that ADP scavengers (e.g., apyrase) fully inhibit platelet aggregation by HIT-IgG (Polgár et al., 1998). It appears that a small amount of platelet (pre)activation "arms" the cell for subsequent "strong" platelet release and aggregation.

FcγRIIA ACTIVATION IN HIT

Although an association between heparin treatment and paradoxical thrombosis was first suspected over 50 years ago (Weismann and Tobin, 1958), it was Rhodes and colleagues (1973) who first provided evidence that serum from HIT patients contained a substance, most likely IgG, that aggregated normal platelets in the presence of heparin. This observation was confirmed by Fratantoni et al. (1975), who reported a simple indirect aggregation method for detecting HIT antibodies. In 1986, Sheridan and coworkers (1986) reported a washed platelet activation assay, employing radiolabeled serotonin, as an activation endpoint that was sensitive and specific for detecting clinically significant HIT antibodies. This same group later reported that platelet activation by HIT antibodies was platelet FcγRIIa dependent, as it could be completely abrogated by a murine monoclonal anti-FcγRIIa antibody, IV.3 (Kelton et al., 1988). Other workers confirmed the central importance of the platelet FcγRIIa in mediating platelet activation in HIT (Adelman et al., 1989; Chong et al., 1989a,b). Subsequently, Amiral and colleagues (1992) reported that the major target antigen for HIT-IgG was PF4 complexed to heparin, a finding quickly confirmed by other workers (Greinacher et al., 1994b; Kelton et al., 1994; Visentin et al., 1994).

Dynamic Model of Platelet Activation in HIT

The initial event in HIT is the binding of HIT-IgG to PF4/H complexes on the platelet surface. HIT-IgG binds to platelets even if the Fc receptors are blocked (Newman and Chong, 2000). Platelet activation by HIT-IgG is a dynamic process: initially, tiny amounts of PF4/H complexes form on the platelet surface. HIT-IgG binds to these complexes then engaging and cross-linking FcγRIIa by their Fc moiety. FcγRIIa ligation triggers platelet activation and degranulation (including release of the crucial potentiator, ADP). The released PF4 binds heparin and forms more complexes containing antigen on the platelet surface. Thus, positive feedback accelerates platelet activation. HIT-IgG also causes the release of TF and interleukin-8 (IL-8) from monocytes (Arepally and Mayer, 2001). In addition, antibodies to IL-8 (a chemokine structurally related to PF4) have been reported in some HIT patients. It appears that these antibodies can activate platelets (Regnault et al., 2003). FcγRIIa clustering and ITAM phosphorylation also appear to affect GPVI/FcRγ activation (independent of any collagen binding to GPVI), resulting in GPVI ectodomain shedding (Gardiner et al., 2008). Thus, HIT can recruit other signaling pathways.

Platelet FcγRIIa Numbers

Variable expression of FcγRIIa numbers among individuals could affect susceptibility to immune complex diseases (Rosenfeld et al., 1987) or even to HIT. The number of platelet surface-expressed FcγRIIa molecules is increased dramatically in HIT (Chong et al., 1993b). However, increased FcγRIIa expression is also seen after *in vitro* activation of platelets by HIT antibodies. Elevated FcγRIIa numbers may be a consequence of platelet activation in HIT, rather than a proximate cause. This notion is supported by the fact that increased platelet FcγRIIa levels are seen in patients with atherothrombosis and diabetes mellitus (Calverley et al., 2002).

Plasma-Soluble FcγRIIa

Soluble FcγRIIa, which is released from α-granules on platelet activation by thrombin, has been demonstrated in plasma (Gachet et al., 1995). However, the relative amount of membrane versus soluble FcγRIIa is fixed (Keller et al., 1993). Gachet and colleagues (1995) reported that approximately 2 ng of soluble FcγRIIa is produced from 10^9 platelets. This value equals 300 molecules per platelet compared with roughly 5–10 times as many molecules on the platelet surface. Due to the low affinity, a much larger amount of plasma-soluble FcγRIIa would be needed to inhibit significantly PF4/H immune complexes from binding to platelet FcγRIIa. Moreover, plasma levels of soluble FcγRIIa are higher in patients with HIT than in heparin-treated or other nonthrombocytopenic controls, presumably as a marker of *in vivo* platelet activation in HIT (Saffroy et al., 1997).

Plasma IgG Concentrations

Plasma IgG levels appear to influence platelet activation and aggregation by HIT sera. With a platelet-rich plasma (PRP) aggregation test to detect HIT antibodies, Chong et al. (1993a) showed variable platelet sensitivity to aggregation that was stable over time among different platelet donors. Chong and coworkers showed that the addition of purified human IgG to the PRP inhibited platelet aggregation by HIT sera, with complete inhibition at 40 mg/mL. It is possible that the effect of purified IgG is due to the presence of small IgG oligomers, because Karas et al. (1982) demonstrated that monomeric IgG does not bind to the platelet FcγRIIa. Furthermore, Greinacher et al. (1994a) showed that different preparations of intravenous IgG (ivIgG) for therapeutic use varied in their ability to inhibit HIT antibody-induced platelet serotonin release. Although the use of ivIgG to treat HIT does not appear to be common, it has some rationale in certain clinical settings (see chap. 12).

FcγRIIa-Arg/His[131] Polymorphism

The Arg/His amino acid variation at position 131 of FcγRIIa affects the ability of murine monoclonal IgG1 as well as human IgG2 to activate platelets (Horsewood et al., 1991; Parren et al., 1992; Tomiyama et al., 1992; Bachelot et al., 1995). These observations prompted Burgess et al. (1995) to suggest that FcγRIIa variants could be a risk factor for developing HIT. In a small cohort of patients, they found an over-representation of the FcγRIIa-His[131] variant. They hypothesized that IgG2 might be an important IgG subclass among HIT-IgG, as this could explain an apparent association between HIT and the FcγRIIa-His[131] variant. However, subsequent reports argued against this hypothesis: IgG1 rather than IgG2 was the predominant subclass among HIT-IgG (Arepally et al., 1997; Denomme et al., 1997; Suh et al., 1997). Nevertheless, in support of a biologic basis for a possible increased frequency of FcγRIIa-His[131], two groups found that HIT antibodies, including those that were predominantly IgG1, preferentially activated washed platelets of the His[131] variant *in vitro* (Denomme et al., 1997; Bachelot-Loza et al., 1998). However, Brandt et al. (1995) found the opposite activation profile in platelet aggregation studies using citrated PRP (i.e., the FcγRIIa-Arg[131] variant was preferentially activated by HIT plasma). No consensus has emerged from the seven studies that investigated the frequency of FcγRIIa-Arg/His[131] variants for patients with HIT: three studies show an overrepresentation of FcγRIIa-His[131] (Brandt et al., 1995; Burgess et al., 1995; Denomme et al., 1997); two studies found no correlation with either variant

(Arepally et al., 1997; Bachelot-Loza et al., 1998); and two studies (including the largest) showed the reverse correlation (Carlsson et al., 1998; Kroupis et al., 2009).

Animal Model of HIT

Animal models of HIT are discussed in chapter 10. Arepally and coworkers (2000) developed a murine monoclonal antibody, termed KKO, by immunizing mice with PF4/H. This murine IgG$_{2b}\kappa$ monoclonal antibody mimics HIT-IgG, as it requires both PF4 and heparin to activate human platelets through their FcγRIIa. However, besides lacking FcγRIIa, mouse PF4 is not recognized by HIT-IgG or KKO. To overcome these problems, Reilly and colleagues (2001) produced transgenic mice that express both human FcγRIIa and human PF4. In these animals, addition of KKO caused thrombocytopenia and death, including thrombosis of the lung vasculature. This murine model has proven useful to address immunologic questions related to HIT. First, large macromolecular complexes are a necessary component in the development of HIT (Rauova et al., 2005). Second, a preexisting prothrombotic condition may influence the development of HIT. Hypercholesterolemic diet-fed mice had increased platelet and endothelial cell activation and were predisposed to HIT to a greater extent than healthy diet-fed syngeneic control mice (Reilly et al., 2006).

When platelet-activating (anti-CD9) IgG was administered to FcγRIIa transgenic mice, more severe thrombocytopenia resulted, compared with a previously studied (nonactivating) anti-mouse platelet IgG (Taylor et al., 2000). Severe thrombosis, shock, and death developed in FcγRIIa transgenic mice crossed with FcRγ-chain knockout mice (i.e. devoid of functional FcγRIIIa). Moreover, splenectomy facilitated anti-CD9–mediated shock in FcγRIIa transgenic mice. The authors concluded that the clearance of antibody-sensitized platelets by phagocytic cells in the spleen may play a protective role in preventing thrombosis.

Unlike mice, primate platelets do possess FcγRIIa. Thus, a primate model for HIT may be feasible, as suggested by a recent report (Ahmad et al., 2000). The animals (*Macaca mulatto*) used do not express the human Arg-His polymorphism, perhaps explaining why less variability in platelet activation response to HIT-IgG was observed in these *in vitro* studies. The primate model may have value in evaluating therapeutic agents for HIT (Untch et al., 2002).

Monocyte FcγRs in HIT

Monocytes and macrophages possess several different classes of FcγR (Table 8.1), and thus may play a part in influencing the frequency and severity of both thrombocytopenia and thrombosis in HIT. One role, discussed in the previous section, involves their potential to influence the balance between platelet activation and reticuloendothelial-mediated platelet clearance in HIT. Another function recently proposed for monocytes is that of contributing to the procoagulant state in HIT (a role posited previously for endothelial cells). Pouplard and colleagues (2001) found that by adding HIT-IgG and PF4 (or PF4/H) directly to isolated monocytes or to whole blood, the monocytes produced TF, an effect that could be inhibited by high concentrations of heparin. Arepally and Mayer (2001) found that monocytes expressed surface TF when incubated with PF4 in the presence of either HIT-IgG or the HIT-mimicking murine monoclonal antibody, KKO. Because monocytes express sulfated proteoglycans on their surface, PF4 binding to monocytes can occur in the absence of added heparin. These studies raise the possibility that monocytes play an important role in the pathogenesis of the procoagulant state characteristic of HIT, a finding supported by more recent studies by Rauova and colleagues (2010). Animal models (Taylor et al., 2000) also suggest that there may be a balance between platelet activation by HIT-IgG (predisposing one to thrombosis) and clearance of platelets by monocytes-macrophages (protecting somewhat against thrombosis). However, phagocytosis or NK cell destruction of antibody-sensitized platelets likely contribute to the thrombocytopenia since HIT is associated with an overrepresentation of FcγRIIIa-Val[158] (Gruel et al., 2004), an FcγR with higher affinity for IgG1 and IgG3 (Table 8.1).

FcγRIIA POLYMORPHISMS IN DISEASE
Determining the FcγRIIa Polymorphism

The FcγRIIa-Arg/His[131] polymorphism was first identified on the basis of functional differences effected by anti-CD3 monoclonal antibodies of the murine IgG1 subclass (Tax et al., 1983, 1984). Proliferation assays distinguished "high" and "low" responders relative to the effects of these anti-CD3 murine monoclonal antibodies on T-cell-dependent mitogenesis. Subsequently, individuals bearing the FcγRIIa-Arg[131] phenotype were identified as the "high responders" and the functional differences between the two variants were later confirmed using other FcγRIIa-dependent assays, such as erythrocyte antigen-rosetting, phagocytosis, and platelet activation (Clark et al., 1989; Warmerdam et al., 1991; Parren et al., 1992; Salmon et al., 1992). Murine monoclonal IgG1 activates platelets of all three Arg/His[131] phenotypes, but the homozygous FcγRIIa-Arg[131] variant requires less murine monoclonal antibody for platelet activation to occur.

The high-affinity binding of human IgG2 to FcγRIIa results when histidine is substituted at amino acid 131 of the mature protein (Warmerdam et al., 1991). FcγRIIa-His[131] has a greater affinity for human IgG2 but a lower affinity for murine IgG1. Therefore, the terms high and low responder, used historically for the effects of murine monoclonal antibodies on Arg[131] and His[131] FcγRIIa phenotypes, respectively, is confusing, as the opposite reaction profile is observed with human IgG2. The high/low responder terminology has been largely replaced in favor of referring simply to the amino acid polymorphism.

The FcγRIIa-Arg/His[131] variant polymorphism can be determined in three ways: (*i*) by functional assay, such as T-cell-dependent proliferation or murine monoclonal antibody activation; (*ii*) by specific binding using 41H16, a monoclonal antibody that binds exclusively to the FcγRIIa Arg[131] variant; and (*iii*) by molecular genotyping. Several DNA-based methods have been developed to genotype for the FcγRIIa-Arg/His[131] nucleotide substitution (Clark et al., 1991; Osborne et al., 1994; Bachelot et al., 1995; Burgess et al., 1995; Jiang et al., 1996; Denomme et al., 1997; Carlsson et al., 1998; Flesch et al., 1998).

Influence of FcγRIIa Polymorphism in Infectious or Autoimmune Disease

A few early studies have examined whether expression of the FcγRIIa-Arg/His[131] polymorphism influences susceptibility to infectious or autoimmune disease. In theory, the weaker binding of human IgG2 to the FcγRIIa-Arg[131] variant suggests that this gene might be overrepresented among patients with recurrent infections characterized by certain microbes with polysaccharide coats (i.e., involving an IgG2 antibody response) and overrepresented in disease characterized by circulating immune complexes (because phagocytic cells bearing the FcγRIIa-His[131]

TABLE 8.2   Role of FcγRIIa-Arg/His[131] Polymorphism in Disease

Disease	Predominant FcγRIIa variant	Comment
Infections by encapsulated bacteria	Arg[131]	Reduced binding of IgG2 by FcγRIIa-Arg[131]-MPS cells reduces phagocytosis, conferring susceptibility to infections with bacteria bearing polysaccharide capsules (Haemophilus, meningococcus)
Immune complex nephritis (SLE)	Arg[131]	Reduced clearance of IgG-containing immune complexes by FcγRIIa-Arg[131]-MPS cells leads to greater glomerular deposition of immune complexes
HIT with thrombosis	Arg[131]	Reduced clearance of IgG-containing immune complexes by FcγRIIa-Arg[131]-MPS cells leads to greater immune complex-dependent activation of platelets and endothelial cells (Carlsson et al., 1998)
HIT with or without thrombosis	His[131]	Increased activation by HIT-IgG1 and HIT-IgG2 of FcγRIIa-His[131] platelets, without significant role for MPS cells (Denomme et al., 1997)

Abbreviations: Arg, arginine; FcγRIIa, FcγIIa receptor; His, histidine; HIT, heparin-induced thrombocytopenia; MPS, mononuclear phagocytic system (reticuloendothelial system); SLE, systemic lupus erythematosus.

variant would clear these complexes more readily). Certainly, a skewed genotypic distribution favoring the FcγRIIa-Arg[131] variant has been noted in patients with *Haemophilus influenzae* infections (Sanders et al., 1994) and meningococcal septic shock (Bredius et al., 1994a). Furthermore, there is also predominance of FcγRIIa-Arg[131] in patients with elevated levels of immune complexes and glomerulonephritis complicating systemic lupus erythematosus (Duits et al., 1995) (Table 8.2).

FcγRIIa Polymorphism in HIT

It was logical to hypothesize that the platelet FcγRIIa-Arg/His[131] polymorphism would influence the clinical expression of HIT. First, platelets from normal individuals exhibit considerable variability in their activation by HIT sera (Salem and Van der Weyden, 1983; Pfueller and David, 1986; Warkentin et al., 1992). Second, many patients who form HIT antibodies during heparin treatment do not develop thrombocytopenia (Warkentin et al., 1995, 2005; Amiral et al., 1996; Suh et al., 1997). Third, the inciting role of heparin, a sulfated carbohydrate, suggested that there could be an important role for HIT antibodies of IgG2 subclass, which is the subclass with higher affinity for FcγRIIa-His[131] that is predominantly formed in response to carbohydrate antigens (Herrmann et al., 1992). However, HIT epitopes form on the protein PF4 when it undergoes conformation change bound to heparin (see chapters 6, 7, and 9). Consequently, it was speculated that the FcγRIIa variant distribution in HIT would differ significantly from a random control population and especially differ from patients who did not develop thrombocytopenia during heparin treatment (Denomme et al., 1997; Bachelot-Loza et al., 1998).

The seven studies investigating the role of the FcγRIIa-Arg/His[131] variants have not yielded uniform results (Fig. 8.3). Three studies showed a predominance

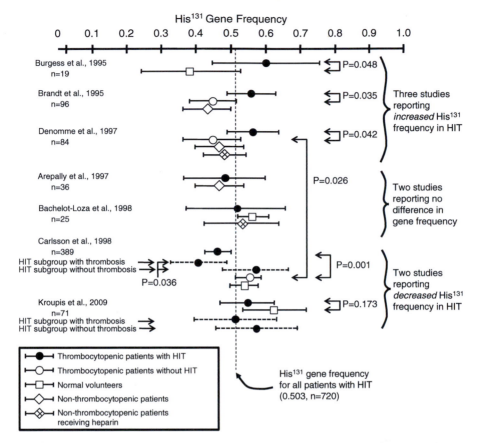

FIGURE 8.3 FcγRIIa-His[131] gene frequencies in seven studies of HIT are shown: The first four studies were from North American centers and the last three from Europe. Although the first three studies showed predominance of His[131] in patients with HIT, the Carlsson et al., study showed predominance of Arg[131] in patients with HIT complicated by thrombosis. A complicating feature is the difference in gene frequencies between control populations. Only two groups (Carlsson et al., 1998 and Kroupis et al., 2009) confirmed alleles using shared reference samples.

of the His[131] variant in patients with HIT that was significant, compared with control patients. Together with evidence that HIT antibodies preferentially activate platelets *in vitro* from individuals bearing the FcγRIIa-His[131] variant (Denomme et al., 1997; Bachelot-Loza et al., 1998), it was suggested that FcγRIIa-His[131] predominance could reflect a greater potential for these platelets to be activated *in vivo* by HIT antibodies (Table 8.2). Two relatively small studies did not show any significant differences in the Arg/His[131] variants between HIT patients and controls.

However, the largest of the seven studies, involving 389 patients (i.e., more than the 331 HIT patients reported in the other six studies combined), showed an increase in the frequency of the Arg[131], rather than the His[131], variant in patients with HIT (Carlsson et al., 1998). Moreover, these workers observed that the increase in FcγRII-Arg[131] variant occurred only in the subset of patients whose HIT was complicated by thrombosis. These investigators proposed that reduced clearance of IgG-containing immune complexes by phagocytic cells bearing FcγRIIa-Arg[131] leads to greater immune complex-dependent activation of platelets, thus predisposing one to thrombosis (Table 8.2). Although Arepally and coworkers (1997) did not observe a significant increase in the FcγRIIa-Arg[131] variant among HIT patients with thrombosis, their subset of HIT patients with thrombosis was much smaller than that reported by Carlsson (23 *vs* 68 patients). On the other hand, when Pouplard and colleagues (1999) examined the FcγRIIa-Arg/His[131] variant frequency among patients who formed antibodies against PF4/H following cardiac surgery, they noted that platelet levels were significantly lower only in the homozygous FcγRIIa-Arg/Arg[131] group, when compared with patients who did not form antibodies.

The explanation for the differences among these various studies is not readily apparent. However, a complicating aspect is noted in Figure 8.3: the frequency of the FcγRIIa-His[131] variant is higher in the European control populations (Bachelot-Loza et al., 1998; Carlsson et al., 1998), compared with the North American and Australian controls (Brandt et al., 1995; Burgess et al., 1995; Denomme et al., 1997; Arepally et al., 1997), an observation consistent with population allele frequencies reported by Rascu et al. (1997). Indeed, pairwise Chi-square analysis for the frequency of the FcγRIIa-His[131] variant among the various controls shows that the control population of Carlsson's study differs from that reported by Denomme and Brandt (Fig. 8.3). The FcγRIIa-Arg/His[131] variants differ among populations: in whites and African Americans, the allele frequencies have roughly a 50:50 balance (Osborne et al., 1994; Lehrnbecher et al., 1999). In contrast, in the Japanese and Chinese populations, the FcγRIIa-His[131] allele frequency is approximately 75% (Rascu et al., 1997; Osborne et al., 1994). It is possible that unrecognized differences in population between HIT patients and controls could be important. For example, whereas samples from HIT patients could be referred from a wider geographic area, control patients might have been obtained from a localized area. None of the seven studies reported on the FcγRIIa-Arg/His[131] variant distribution among heparin-treated patients who formed HIT antibodies but who did not develop thrombocytopenia (i.e., the ideal control group for assessing the influence of the FcγRIIa polymorphism).

In summary, the role of the FcγRIIa-Arg/His[131] variants in contributing to the pathogenesis of HIT remains controversial. Regardless of its ultimate resolution, the elucidation of the biologic basis for differences in frequency of FcγRIIa phenotype between HIT patients, with or without thrombosis, and control subjects will provide new insights into the pathogenesis of immune-mediated disease.

ACKNOWLEDGMENTS

Some of the studies described were supported by a Career Development Fellowship Award of the Canadian Blood Services. The author was a Bayer/Canadian Blood Services/Medical Research Council Scholar.

REFERENCES

Adelman B, Sobel M, Fujimura Y, Ruggeri ZM, Zimmerman TS. Heparin-associated thrombocytopenia: observations on the mechanism of platelet aggregation. J Lab Clin Med 113: 204–210, 1989.

Ahmad S, Jeske WP, Walenga JM, Aldabbagh A, Iqbal O, Fareed J. Human anti-heparin-platelet factor 4 antibodies are capable of activating primate platelets: towards the development of a HIT model in primates. Thromb Res 100: 47–54, 2000.

Amiral J, Bridey F, Dreyfus M, Vissaco AM, Fressinaud E, Wolf M, Meyer D. Platelet factor 4 complexed to heparin is the target for antibodies generated in heparin-induced thrombocytopenia. Thromb Haemost 68: 95–96, 1992.

Amiral J, Peynaud-Debayle E, Wolf M, Bridey F, Vissac AM, Meyer D. Generation of antibodies to heparin-PF4 complexes without thrombocytopenia in patients treated with unfractionated or low molecular weight heparin. Am J Hematol 52: 90–95, 1996.

Anderson GP, Anderson CL. Signal transduction by the platelet Fc receptor. Blood 76: 1165–1172, 1990.

Anderson GP, van de Winkel JGJ, Anderson CL. Anti-GPIIb/IIIa (CD41) monoclonal antibody-induced platelet activation requires Fc receptor-dependent cell-cell interaction. Br J Haematol 79: 75–83, 1991.

Andre P, Morooka T, Sim D, Abe K, Lowell C, Nanda N, Delaney S, Siu G, Yan Y, Hollenbach S, Pandey A, Gao H, Wang Y, Nakajima K, Parikh SA, Shi C, Phillips D, Owen W, Sinha U, Simon DI. Critical role for syk in responses to vascular injury. Blood 118: 5000–5010, 2011.

Arepally GM, Mayer IM. Antibodies from patients with heparin-induced thrombocytopenia stimulate monocytic cells to express tissue factor and secrete interleukin-8. Blood 98: 1252–1254, 2001.

Arepally G, McKenzie SE, Jiang XM, Poncz M, Cines DB. FcγRIIA H/R131 polymorphism, subclass-specific IgG anti-heparin/platelet factor 4 antibodies and clinical course in patients with heparin-induced thrombocytopenia and thrombosis. Blood 89: 370–375, 1997.

Arepally GM, Kamei S, Park KS, Kamei K, Li ZQ, Liu W, Siegel DL, Kisiel W, Cines DB, Poncz M. Characterization of a murine monoclonal antibody that mimics heparin-induced thrombocytopenia antibodies. Blood 95: 1533–1540, 2000.

Bachelot C, Saffroy R, Gandrille S, Aiach M, Rendu F. Role of FcγRIIA gene polymorphism in human platelet activation by monoclonal antibodies. Thromb Haemost 74: 1557–1563, 1995.

Bachelot-Loza C, Saffroy R, Lasne D, Chatellier G, Aiach M, Rendu F. Importance of the FcγRIIa-Arg/His-131 polymorphism in heparin-induced thrombocytopenia diagnosis. Thromb Haemost 79: 523–528, 1998.

Bacsi S, De Palma R, Visentin GP, Gorski J, Aster RH. Complexes of heparin and platelet factor 4 specifically stimulate T cells from patients with heparin-induced thrombocytopenia/thrombosis. Blood 94: 208–215 1999.

Bevers EM, Comfurius P, Dekkers DW, Zwaal RF. Lipid translocation across the plasma membrane of mammalian cells. Biochim Biophys Acta 1439: 317–330, 1999.

Blake RA, Asselin J, Walker T, Watson SP. Fcγ receptor II stimulated formation of inositol phosphates in human platelets is blocked by tyrosine kinase inhibitors and associated with tyrosine phosphorylation of the receptor. FEBS Lett 342: 15–18, 1994.

Bode AP, Hickerson DHM. Characterization and quantitation by flow cytometry of membranous microparticles formed during activation of platelet suspensions with ionophore or thrombin. Platelets 11: 259–271, 2000.

Bodin S, Viala C, Ragab A, Payrastre B. A critical role of lipid rafts in the organization of a key FcγRIIa-mediated signaling pathway in human platelets. Thromb Haemost 89: 318–330, 2003.

Brandt JT, Isenhart CE, Osborne JM, Ahmed A, Anderson CL. On the role of platelet FcγRIIa phenotype in heparin-induced thrombocytopenia. Thromb Haemost 74: 1564–1572, 1995.

Bredius RGM, Derkz BHF, Fijen CAP, de Wit TPM, de Haas M, Weening RS, van de Winkel JGJ, Out TA. FcγIIa (CD32) polymorphism in fulminant meningococcal septic shock in children. J Infect Dis 170: 848–853, 1994a.

Bredius RGM, Fijen CAP, de Haas M, Kuijper EJ, Weening RS, van de Winkel JGJ, Out TA. Role of neutrophil FcγRIII (CD32) and FcγRIII (CD 16) polymorphic forms in phagocytosis of human IgG1- and IgG3–opsonized bacteria and erythrocytes. Immunology 83: 624–630, 1994b.

Brooks DG, Qiu WQ, Luster AD, Ravetch JV. Structure and expression of human IgG FcRII (CD32). functional heterogeneity is encoded by the alternatively spliced products of multiple genes. J Exp Med 170: 1369–1385, 1989.

Burgess JK, Lindeman R, Chesterman CN, Chong BH. Single amino acid mutation of Fcγ
    receptor is associated with the development of heparin-induced thrombocytopenia. Br J
    Haematol 91: 761–766, 1995.
Bux J, Stein EL, Bierling P, Fromont P, Clay ME, Stoncek DF, Santoso S. Characterization of a
    new alloantigen (SH) on the human neutrophil Fcγ receptor IIIb. Blood 89: 1027–1034, 1997.
Calverley DC, Brass E, Hacker MR, Tsao-Wei DD, Espina BM, Pullarkat VA, Hodis HN, Gro-
    shen S. Potential role of platelet FcγRIIA in collagen-mediated platelet activation associ-
    ated with atherothrombosis. Atherosclerosis 164: 261–267, 2002.
Canobbio I, Stefanini L, Guidetti GF, Balduini C, Torti M. A new role for FcγRIIA in the poten-
    tiation of human platelet activation induced by weak stimulation. Cell Signal 18: 861–870,
    2006.
Carlsson LE, Santoso S, Baurichter G, Kroll H, Papenberg S, Eichler P, Westerdaal NAC, Kiefel
    V, van de Winkel JGJ, Greinacher A. Heparin-induced thrombocytopenia: new insights
    into the impact of the FcγRIIa-R-H131 polymorphism. Blood 92: 1526–1531, 1998.
Casali P, Schettino EW. Structure and function of natural antibodies. Curr Top Microbiol
    Immunol 210: 167–179, 1996.
Chacko GW, Duchemin AM, Coggeshall KM, Osborne JM, Brandt JT, Anderson CL. Cluster-
    ing of the platelet Fcγ receptor induces noncovalent association with the tyrosine kinase
    p72syk. J Biol Chem 269: 32435–32440, 1994.
Chacko GW, Brandt JT, Coggeshall KM, Anderson CL. Phosphoinositide 3–kinase and p72syk
    noncovalently associate with the low affinity Fcγ receptor on human platelets through an
    immunoreceptor tyrosine-based activation motif. J Biol Chem 271: 10775–10781, 1996.
Chong BH, Grace CS, Rozenberg MC. Heparin-induced thrombocytopenia: effect of heparin
    platelet antibody on platelets. Br J Haematol 49: 531–540, 1981.
Chong BH, Castaldi PA, Berndt MC. Heparin-induced thrombocytopenia: effect of rabbit IgG,
    and its Fab and Fc fragments on antibody-heparin-platelet interaction. Thromb Res 55:
    291–295, 1989a.
Chong BH, Fawaz I, Chesterman CN, Berndt MC. Heparin-induced thrombocytopenia:
    mechanism of interaction of the heparin-dependent antibody with platelets. Br J Haema-
    tol 73: 235–240, 1989b.
Chong BH, Burgess J, Ismail F. The clinical usefulness of the platelet aggregation test for the
    diagnosis of heparin-induced thrombocytopenia. Thromb Haemost 69: 344–350, 1993a.
Chong BH, Pilgrim RL, Cooley MA, Chesterman CN. Increased expression of platelet IgG Fc
    receptors in immune heparin-induced thrombocytopenia. Blood 81: 988–993, 1993b.
Cines DB, Tomaski A, Tannenbaum S. Immune endothelial-cell injury in heparin associated
    thrombocytopenia. N Engl J Med 316: 581–589, 1987.
Clark MR, Clarkson SB, Ory PA, Stollman N, Goldstein IM. Molecular basis for a polymor-
    phism involving Fc receptor II on human monocytes. J Immunol 143: 1731–1734, 1989.
Clark MR, Stuart SG, Kimberly RP, Ory PA, Goldstein IM. A single amino acid distinguishes
    the high-responder from the low-responder form of Fc receptor II on human monocytes.
    Eur J Immunol 21: 1911–1916, 1991.
Cox D, Kerrigan SW, Watson SP. Platelets and the innate immune system: mechanisms of
    bacterial-induced platelet activation. J Thromb Haemost 9: 1097–1107, 2011.
Denomme GA, Warkentin TE, Horsewood P, Sheppard JI, Warner MN, Kelton JG. Activation
    of platelets by sera containing IgG1 heparin-dependent antibodies: an explanation for the
    predominance of the FcγRIIa "low responder" (his$_{131}$) gene in patients with heparin-
    induced thrombocytopenia. J Lab Clin Med 130: 278–284, 1997.
Duits AJ, Bootsma H, Derksen RHWM, Spronk PE, Kater L, Kallenberg CGM, Capel PJA,
    Westerdaal NAC, Spierenburg GT, Gmelig-Meyling FHJ, van de Winkel JGJ. Skewed dis-
    tribution of IgG Fc receptor IIa (CD32) polymorphism is associated with renal disease in
    systemic lupus erythematosus patients. Arthritis Rheum 39: 1832–1836, 1995.
Flesch BK, Bauer F, Neppert J. Rapid typing of the human Fcγ receptor IIA polymorphism by
    polymerase chain reaction amplification with allele-specific primers. Transfusion 38:
    174–176, 1998.
Ford I, Douglas CW, Cox D, Rees DG, Heath J, Preston FE. The role of immunoglobulin G and
    fibrinogen in platelet aggregation by Streptococcus sanguis. Br J Haematol 97: 737–746,
    1997.

Fratantoni JC, Pollet R, Gralnick HR. Heparin-induced thrombocytopenia: confirmation of diagnosis with in vitro methods. Blood 45: 395–401, 1975.

Gachet C, Astier A, de la Salle H, de la Salle C, Fridman WH, Cazenave JP, Hanau D, Teillaud JL. Release of FcγRIIa2 by activated platelets and inhibition of anti-CD9–mediated platelet aggregation by recombinant FcγRIIa2. Blood 85: 698–704, 1995.

Gardiner EE, Karunakaran D, Arthur JF, Mu FT, Powell MS, Baker RI, Hogarth PM, Kahn ML, Andrews RK, Berndt MC. Dual ITAM-mediated proteolytic pathways for irreversible inactivation of platelet receptors: de-ITAM-izing FcγRIIa. Blood 111: 165–174, 2008.

Gessner JE, Heiken H, Tamm A, Schmidt RE. The IgG Fc receptor family. Ann Hematol 76: 231–248, 1998.

Gratacap MP, Payrastre B, Viala C, Mauco G, Plantavid M, Chap H. Phosphatidylinositol 3, 4, 5–triphosphate-dependent stimulation of phospholipase C-γ2 is an early key event in FcγRIIA-mediated activation of human platelets. J Biol Chem 273: 24314–24321, 1998.

Gratacap MP, Hérault JP, Viala C, Ragab A, Savi P, Herbert JM, Chap H, Plantavid M, Payrastre B. FcγRIIA requires a Gi-dependent pathway for an efficient stimulation of phosphoinositide 3–kinase, calcium mobilization, and platelet aggregation. Blood 96: 3439–3446, 2000.

Green D, Harris K, Reynolds N, Roberts M, Patterson R. Heparin immune thrombocytopenia: evidence for a heparin-platelet complex as the antigenic determinant. J Lab Clin Med 91: 167–175, 1978.

Greinacher A, Michels I, Kiefel V, Mueller-Eckhardt C. A rapid and sensitive test for diagnosing heparin-associated thrombocytopenia. Thromb Haemost 66: 734–736, 1991.

Greinacher A, Liebenhoff U, Kiefel V, Presek P, Mueller-Eckhardt C. Heparin-associated thrombocytopenia: the effects of various intravenous IgG preparations on antibody mediated platelet activation—a possible new indication of high dose i.v. IgG. Thromb Haemost 71: 641–645, 1994a.

Greinacher A, Pötzsch B, Amiral J, Dummel V, Eichner A, Mueller-Eckhardt C. Heparin-associated thrombocytopenia: isolation of the antibody and characterization of a multimolecular PF4-Heparin complex as the major antigen. Thromb Haemost 71: 247–251, 1994b.

Greinacher A, Holtfreter B, Krauel K, Gätke D, Weber C, Ittermann T, Hammerschmidt S, Kocher T. Association of natural anti-platelet factor 4/heparin antibodies with periodontal disease. Blood 118: 1395–1401, 2011.

Gröger M, Sarmay G, Fiebiger E, Wolff K, Petzelbauer P. Dermal microvascular endothelial cells express CD32 receptors in vivo and in vitro. J Immunol 156: 1549–1556, 1996.

Gruel Y, Pouplard C, Lasne D, Magdelaine-Beuzelin C, Charroing C, Watier H. The homozygous FcγRIIIa-158 V genotype is a risk factor for heparin-induced thrombocytopenia in patients with antibodies to heparin-platelet factor 4 complexes. Blood 104: 2791–2793, 2004.

Herrmann DJ, Hamilton RG, Barington T, Frasch CE, Arakere G, Makela O, Mitchell LA, Nagel J, Rijkers GT, Zegers B, Danve B, Ward JI, Brown CS. Quantitation of human IgG subclass antibodies to haemophilus influenzae type b capsular polysaccharide. J Immunol Methods 148: 101–114, 1992.

Horsewood P, Hayward CPM, Warkentin TE, Kelton JG. Investigation of the mechanisms of monoclonal antibody-induced platelet activation. Blood 78: 1019–1026, 1991.

Huang MM, Indik Z, Brass LF, Hoxie JA, Schreiber AD, Brugge JS. Activation of FcγRII induces tyrosine phosphorylation of multiple proteins including FcγRII. J Biol Chem 267: 5467–5473, 1992.

Hughes M, Hayward CPM, Warkentin TE, Horsewood P, Chorneyko KA, Kelton JG. Morphological analysis of microparticle generation in heparin-induced thrombocytopenia. Blood 96: 188–194, 2000.

Hulett MD, Witort E, Brinkworth RI, McKenzie IFC, Hogarth PM. Multiple regions of human FcγRII (CD32) contribute to the binding of IgG. J Biol Chem 270: 21188–21194, 1995.

Jiang XM, Arepally G, Poncz M, McKenzie SE. Rapid detection of the FcγRIIA-H/R131 ligand-binding polymorphism using an allele-specific restriction enzyme digestion (ASRED). J Immunol Methods 199: 55–59, 1996.

Karas SP, Rosse WF, Kurlander RJ. Characterization of the IgG-Fc receptor on human platelets. Blood 60: 1277–1282, 1982.

Keller MA, Cassel DL, Rappaport EF, McKenzie SE, Schwartz E, Surrey S. Fluorescence-based RT PCR analysis: determination of the ratio of soluble to membrane-bound forms of FcγRIIA transcripts in hematopoietic cell lines. PCR Methods Appl 3: 32–38, 1993.

Kelton JG, Smith JW, Santos AV, Murphy WG, Horsewood P. Platelet IgG Fc receptor. Am J Hematol 25: 299–310, 1987.

Kelton JG, Sheridan D, Santos A, Smith J, Steeves K, Smith C, Brown C, Murphy WG. Heparin-induced thrombocytopenia: laboratory studies. Blood 72: 925–930, 1988.

Kelton JG, Smith JW, Warkentin TE, Hayward CPM, Denomme GA, Horsewood P. Immunoglobulin G from patients with heparin-induced thrombocytopenia binds to a complex of heparin and platelet factor 4. Blood 83: 3232–3239, 1994.

Khairy M, Lasne D, Brohard-Bohn B, Aich M, Rendu F, Bachelot-Loza C. A new approach in the study of the molecular and cellular events implicated in heparin-induced thrombocytopenia. formation of leukocyte-platelet aggregates. Thromb Haemost 85: 1090–1096, 2001.

King M, McDermott P, Schreiber AD. Characterization of the Fcγ receptor on human platelets. Cell Immunol 128: 462–479, 1990.

Koene HR, Kleijer M, Algra J, Roos D, von dem Borne AEGK, de Haas M. FcγRIIIa-158V/F polymorphism influences the binding of IgG by natural killer cell FcγRIIIa, independently of the FcγRIIIa-48L/R/H phenotype. Blood 90: 1109–1114, 1997.

Koene HR, Kleijer M, Roos D, de Haas M, von dem Borne AEGK. FcγRIIIB gene duplication: evidence for presence and expression of three distinct FcγRIIIB genes in NA(1+, 2+) SH(+) individuals. Blood 91: 673–679, 1998.

Kottenberg-Assenmacher E, Volbracht L, Jakob H, Greinacher A, Peters J. Disseminated intravascular clotting associated with Fc-receptor IIa-mediated platelet activation in a patient with endocarditis after aortic valve replacement. Br J Anaesth 97: 630–633, 2006.

Krauel K, Pötschke C, Weber C, Kessler W, Fürll B, Ittermann T, Maier S, Hammerschmidt S, Bröker BM, Greinacher A. Platelet factor 4 binds to bacteria, [corrected] inducing antibodies cross-reacting with the major antigen in heparin-induced thrombocytopenia. Blood 117: 1370–1378, 2011. Erratum in: Blood 117: 5783, 2011.

Kroupis C, Theodorou M, Kounavi M, Oliveira SC, Iliopoulou E, Mavri-Vavayanni M, Melissari EN, Degiannis D. Development of a real-time PCR detection method for a FCGR2A polymorphism in the lightcycler and application in the heparin-induced thrombocytopenia syndrome. Clin Biochem 42: 1685–1693, 2009.

Lebrazi J, Helft G, Abdelouahed M, Elalamy I, Mirshahi M, Samama MM, Lecompte T. Human anti-streptokinase antibodies induce platelet aggregation in an Fc receptor (CD32) dependent manner. Thromb Haemost 74: 938–942, 1995.

Lee DP, Warkentin TE, Denomme GA, Hayward CPM, Kelton JG. A diagnostic test for heparin-induced thrombocytopenia: detection of platelet microparticles using flow cytometry. Br J Haematol 95: 724–731, 1996.

Lehrnbecher T, Foster CH, Zhu S, Leitman SF, Goldin LR, Huppi K, Chanock SJ. Variant genotypes of the low-affinity Fcγ receptors in two control populations and a review of low-affinity Fcγ receptor polymorphisms in control and disease populations. Blood 94: 4220–4232, 1999.

Lhermusier T, van Rottem J, Garcia C, Xuereb JM, Ragab A, Martin V, Gratacap MP, Sié P, Payrastre B. The syk-kinase inhibitor R406 impairs platelet activation and monocyte tissue factor expression triggered by heparin-PF4 complex directed antibodies. J Thromb Haemost 9: 2067–2076, 2011.

Lo GK, Juhl D, Warkentin TE, Sigouin CS, Eichler P, Greinacher A. Evaluation of pretest clinical score (4 T's) for the diagnosis of heparin-induced thrombocytopenia in two clinical settings. J Thromb Haemost 4: 759–765, 2006.

McCrae KR, Shattil SJ, Cines DB. Platelet activation induces increased Fcγ receptor expression. J Immunol 144: 3920–3927, 1990.

Metes D, Ernst LK, Chambers WH, Sulica A, Herberman RB, Morel PA. Expression of functional CD32 molecules on human NK cells is determined by an allelic polymorphism of the FcγRIIC gene. Blood 91: 2369–2380, 1998.

Newman PM, Chong BH. Heparin-induced thrombocytopenia: new evidence for the dynamic binding of purified anti-PF4-heparin antibodies to platelets and the resultant platelet activation. Blood 96: 182–187, 2000.

Norris CF, Pricop L, Millard S, Taylor SM, Surrey S, Schwartz E, Salmon JE, McKenzie SE. A naturally occurring mutation in FcγRIIA: a Q to K127 change confers unique IgG binding properties to the R131 allelic form of the receptor. Blood 91: 656–662, 1998.

Olah Z, Kerenyi A, Kappelmayer J, Schlammadinger A, Razso K, Boda Z. Rapid-onset heparin-induced thrombocytopenia without previous heparin exposure. Platelets 23: 495–498, 2012.

Ory PA, Clark MA, Kwoh EE, Clarkson SB, Goldstein IM. Sequences of complementary DNAs that encode the NA1 and NA2 forms of Fc receptor III on human neutrophils. J Clin Invest 84: 1688–1691, 1989.

Osborne JM, Chacko GW, Brandt JT, Anderson CL. Ethnic variation in frequency of an allelic polymorphism of human FcγRIIa determined with allele specific oligonucleotide probes. J Immunol Methods 173: 207–217, 1994.

Parren PWHI, Warmerdam PAM, Boeije LCM, Arts J, Westerdaal NAC, Vlug A, Capel PJA, Aarden LA, van de Winkel JGJ. On the interaction of IgG subclasses with the low affinity FcγRIIa (CD32) on human monocytes, neutrophils, and platelets. Analysis of a functional polymorphism to human IgG2. J Clin Invest 90: 1537–1546, 1992.

Pfueller SL, David R. Different platelet specificities of heparin-dependent platelet aggregating factors in heparin-associated immune thrombocytopenia. Br J Haematol 64: 149–159, 1986.

Polgár J, Eichler P, Greinacher A, Clemetson KJ. Adenosine diphosphate (ADP) and ADP receptor play a major role in platelet activation/aggregation induced by sera from heparin-induced thrombocytopenia patients. Blood 91: 549–554, 1998.

Pouplard C, May MA, Iochmann S, Amiral J, Marchand M, Gruel Y. Antibodies to platelet factor 4-Heparin after cardiopulmonary bypass in patients anticoagulated with unfractionated heparin or a low molecular weight heparin: clinical implications for heparin-induced thrombocytopenia. Circulation 99: 2530–2536, 1999.

Pouplard C, Iochmann S, Renard B, Hérault O, Gruel Y. Induction of monocyte tissue factor expression by antibodies to heparin-platelet factor 4 complexes developed in heparin-induced thrombocytopenia. Blood 97: 3300–3302, 2001.

Qiu WQ, de Bruin D, Brownstein BH, Pearse R, Ravetch JV. Organization of the human and mouse low-affinity FcγR genes: duplication and recombination. Science 248: 732–735, 1990.

Rappaport EF, Cassel DL, Walterhouse DO, McKenzie SE, Surrey S, Keller MA, Schreiber AD, Schwartz E. A soluble form of the human Fc receptor FcγRIIa: cloning, transcript analysis and detection. Exp Hematol 21: 689–696, 1993.

Rascu A, Repp R, Westerdaal NAC, Kalden JR, van de Winkel JGJ. Clinical relevance of Fcγ receptor polymorphisms. Ann NY Acad Sci 815: 282–295, 1997.

Rauova L, Poncz M, McKenzie SE, Reilly MP, Arepally G, Weisel JW, Nagaswami C, Cines DB, Sachais BS. Ultralarge complexes of PF4 and heparin are central to the pathogenesis of heparin-induced thrombocytopenia. Blood 105: 131–138, 2005.

Rauova L, Hirsch JD, Greene TK, Zhai L, Hayes VM, Kowalska MA, Cines DB, Poncz M. Monocyte-bound PF4 in the pathogenesis of heparin-induced thrombocytopenia. Blood 116:5021–5031, 2010.

Regnault V, de Maistre E, Carteaux JP, Gruel Y, Nguyen P, Tardy B, Lecompte T. Platelet activation induced by antibodies to interleukin-8. Blood 101: 1419–1421, 2003.

Reilly MP, Taylor SM, Hartman NK, Arepally GM, Cines DB, Poncz M, McKenzie SE. Heparin-induced thrombocytopenia/thrombosis in a transgenic mouse model requires human platelet factor 4 and platelet activation through FcγRIIA. Blood 98: 2442–2447, 2001.

Reilly MP, Taylor SM, Franklin C, Sachais BS, Cines DB, Williams KJ, McKenzie SE. Prothrombotic factors enhance heparin-induced thrombocytopenia and thrombosis in vivo in a mouse model. J Thromb Haemost 4: 2687–2694, 2006.

Reilly MP, Sinha U, André P, Taylor SM, Pak Y, Deguzman FR, Nanda N, Pandey A, Stolla M, Bergmeier W, McKenzie SE. PRT-060318, a novel syk inhibitor, prevents heparin-induced thrombocytopenia and thrombosis in a transgenic mouse model. Blood 117: 2241–2246, 2011.

Rhodes GR, Dixon RH, Silver D. Heparin induced thrombocytopenia with thrombotic and hemorrhagic manifestations. Surg Gynecol Obstet 136: 409–416, 1973.

Roitt I, Brostoff J, Male D, eds. Immunology. London: Gower Medical Publishing, 1985.

Rosenfeld SI, Looney RJ, Leddy JP, Phipps DC, Abraham GN, Anderson CL. Human platelet Fc receptor for immunoglobulin G identification as a 40,000–molecular-weight membrane protein shared by monocytes. J Clin Invest 76: 2317–2322, 1985.

Rosenfeld SI, Ryan DH, Looney RJ, Anderson CL, Abraham GN, Leddy JP. Human Fcγ receptors: stable inter-donor variation in quantitative expression on platelets correlates with functional responses. J Immunol 144: 3920–3927, 1987.

Rubinstein E, Boucheix C, Worthington RE, Carroll RC. Anti-platelet antibody interactions with Fcγ receptor. Semin Thromb Hemost 21: 10–22, 1995.

Saffroy R, Bachelot-Loza C, Fridman WH, Aiach M, Teillaud JL, Rendu F. Plasma levels of soluble Fcγ receptors II (sCD32) and III (sCD16) in patients with heparin-induced thrombocytopenia. Thromb Haemost 78: 970–971, 1997.

Salem HH, Van der Weyden MB. Heparin-induced thrombocytopenia. Variable platelet-rich plasma reactivity to heparin-dependent aggregating factor. Pathology 15: 297–299, 1983.

Salmon JE, Edberg JC, Kimberly RP. Fcγ receptor III on human neutrophils. J Clin Invest 85: 1287–1295, 1990.

Salmon JE, Edberg JC, Brogle NL, Kimberly RP. Allelic polymorphism of human Fcγ receptor IIA and Fcγ receptor IIIB. Independent mechanisms for differences in human phagocyte function. J Clin Invest 89: 1274–1281, 1992.

Sanders LAM, van de Winkel JGJ, Rijkers GT, Voorhorst-Ogink MM, de Haas M, Capel PJA, Zegers BJM. Fcγ receptor IIa (CD32) heterogeneity in patients with recurrent bacterial respiratory tract infections. J Infect Dis 170: 854–861, 1994.

Sedmak DD, Davis DH, Singh U, van de Winkel JG, Anderson CL. Expression of IgG Fc receptor antigens in placenta and on endothelial cells in humans. an immunohistochemical study. Am J Pathol 138: 175–181, 1991.

Selleng K, Selleng S, Raschke R, Schmidt CO, Rosenblood GS, Greinacher A, Warkentin TE. Immune heparin-induced thrombocytopenia can occur in patients receiving clopidogrel and aspirin. Am J Hematol 78: 188–192, 2005.

Sheridan D, Carter C, Kelton JG. A diagnostic test for heparin-induced thrombocytopenia. Blood 67: 27–30, 1986.

Sims PJ, Wiedmer T, Esmon CT, Weiss HJ, Shattil SJ. Assembly of the platelet prothrombinase complex is linked to vesiculation of the platelet plasma membrane. Studies in Scott syndrome: an isolated defect in platelet procoagulant activity. J Biol Chem 264: 17049–17057, 1989.

Su K, Wu J, Edberg JC, McKenzie SE, Kimberly RP. Genomic organization of classical human low-affinity Fcγ receptor genes. Genes Immun 3(Suppl 1): S51–S56, 2002.

Suh JS, Malik MI, Aster RH, Visentin GP. Characterization of the humoral response in heparin-induced thrombocytopenia. Am J Hematol 54: 196–201, 1997.

Suvarna S, Rauova L, McCracken EK, Goss CM, Sachais BS, McKenzie SE, Reilly MP, Gunn MD, Cines DB, Poncz M, Arepally G. PF4/heparin complexes are T cell-dependent antigens. Blood 106: 929–931, 2005.

Taylor SM, Reilly MP, Schreiber AD, Chien P, Tuckosh JR, McKenzie SE. Thrombosis and shock induced by activating antiplatelet antibodies in human FcγRIIA transgenic mice: the interplay among antibody, spleen, and Fc receptor. Blood 96: 4254–4260, 2000.

Tax WJM, Williams HW, Reckers PPM, Capel PJA, Keone RAP. Polymorphism in mitogenic effect of IgG1 monoclonal antibodies against T3 antigen on human T cells. Nature 304: 445, 1983.

Tax WJM, Hermes FFM, Willems RW, Capel JA, Koene RAP. Fc receptors for mouse IgG1 on human monocytes: polymorphism and role in antibody-induced T cell proliferation. J Immunol 133: 1185–1189, 1984.

Tomer A. A sensitive and specific functional flow cytometric assay for the diagnosis of heparin-induced thrombocytopenia. Br J Haematol 98: 648–656, 1997.

Tomiyama Y, Kunicki TJ, Zipf TF, Ford SB, Aster RH. Response of human platelets to activating monoclonal antibodies: importance of FcγRII (CD32) phenotype and level of expression. Blood 80: 2261–2268, 1992.

Untch B, Ahmad S, Messmore HL, Schultz CL, Ma Q, Hoppensteadt DA, Walenga JM, Fareed J. Development of a non-human primate subclinical model of heparin-induced thrombocytopenia: platelet response to human anti-heparin-platelet factor 4 antibodies. Thromb Res 106: 149–156, 2002.

van de Winkel JGJ, Capel PJA. Human IgG Fc receptor heterogeneity: molecular aspects and clinical implications. Immunol Today 14: 215–221, 1993.

Visentin GP, Ford SE, Scott JP, Aster RH. Antibodies from patients with heparin-induced thrombocytopenia/thrombosis are specific for platelet factor 4 complexed with heparin or bound to endothelial cells. J Clin Invest 93: 81–88, 1994.

Warkentin TE, Sheppard JI. Generation of platelet-derived microparticles and procoagulant activity by heparin-induced thrombocytopenia IgG/serum and other IgG platelet agonists: a comparison with standard platelet agonists. Platelets 10: 319–326, 1999.

Warkentin TE, Hayward CPM, Smith CA, Kelly PM, Kelton JG. Determinants of donor platelet variability when testing for heparin-induced thrombocytopenia. J Lab Clin Med 120: 371–379, 1992.

Warkentin TE, Hayward CPM, Boshkov LK, Santos AV, Sheppard JI, Bode AP, Kelton JG. Sera from patients with heparin-induced thrombocytopenia generate platelet-derived microparticles with procoagulant activity: an explanation for the thrombotic complications of heparin-induced thrombocytopenia. Blood 84: 3691–3699, 1994.

Warkentin TE, Levine MN, Hirsh J, Horsewood P, Roberts RS, Tech M, Gent M, Kelton JG. Heparin-induced thrombocytopenia in patients treated with low molecular weight heparin or unfractionated heparin. N Engl J Med 332: 1330–1335, 1995.

Warkentin TE, Sheppard JI, Moore JC, Moore KM, Sigouin CS, Kelton JG. Laboratory testing for the antibodies that cause heparin-induced thrombocytopenia: how much class do we need? J Lab Clin Med 146: 341–346, 2005.

Warkentin TE, Makris M, Jay RM, Kelton JG. A spontaneous prothrombotic disorder resembling heparin-induced thrombocytopenia. Am J Med 121: 632–636, 2008.

Warmerdam PAM, van de Winkel JGJ, Gosselin EJ, Capel PJA. Molecular basis for a polymorphism of human Fcγ receptor II (CD32w). J Exp Med 172: 19–25, 1990.

Warmerdam PAM, van de Winkel JGJ, Vlug A, Westerdaal NAC, Capel PJA. A single amino acid in the second domain of the human Fcγ receptor II is critical for human IgG2 binding. J Immunol 147: 1338–1343, 1991.

Weismann RE, Tobin RW. Arterial embolism occurring during systemic heparin therapy. Arch Surg 76: 219–227, 1958.

Wu J, Edberg JC, Redecha PB, Bansal V, Guyre PM, Coleman K, Salmon JE, Kimberly RP. A novel polymorphism of FcγRIIIa (CD 16) alters receptor function and predisposes to autoimmune disease. J Clin Invest 100: 1059–1070, 1997.

Xiao Z, Visentin GP, Dayananda KM, Neelamegham S. Immune complexes formed following the binding of anti-platelet factor 4 (CXCL4) antibodies to CXCL4 stimulate human neutrophil activation and cell adhesion. Blood 112: 1091–100, 2008.

Yanaga F, Poole A, Asselin J, Blake R, Schieven GL, Clark EA, Law CL, Watson SP. Syk interacts with tyrosine-phosphorylated proteins in human platelets activated by collagen and cross-linking of the Fcγ-IIA receptor. Biochem J 313: 471–478, 1995.

9 Cellular and molecular immunopathogenesis of heparin-induced thrombocytopenia

Lubica Rauova, Gowthami M. Arepally, Douglas B. Cines, and Mortimer Poncz

INTRODUCTION

Unfractionated heparin (UFH) remains an important anticoagulant in a number of clinical settings. Because of its rapid onset and complete reversibility with protamine sulfate, it is the primary anticoagulant used for cardiopulmonary bypass (CPB) and other forms of vascular surgery and in patients at a high risk for bleeding (Weitz and Weitz, 2010). However, the paradox of thrombosis caused by the infusion of UFH was recognized more than 50 years ago (Weismann and Tobin, 1958) and a distinct syndrome called heparin-induced thrombocytopenia (HIT) was identified by the early 1970s (Natelson et al., 1969; Rhodes et al., 1973). Later, it was shown that antibodies formed by these patients caused platelet activation in the presence of heparin (Fratantoni et al., 1975; Cines et al., 1980), and subsequently it was appreciated that these antibodies were directed against a protein released from activated platelets—platelet factor 4 (PF4)—complexed to heparin (Amiral et al., 1992). Our current understanding of this syndrome is that HIT is caused by antibodies against PF4/heparin (PF4/H) immune complexes that crosslink or otherwise engage FcγIIA receptors (FcγRIIA) on platelets and related Fc receptors on monocytes and possibly other vascular cells. This promotes platelet activation and generation of thrombin, leading to an explosive feed-forward, prothrombotic loop.

Despite these advances in our understanding of its pathogenesis, HIT remains an all-too-frequent complication of heparin therapy, which may be accompanied by devastating limb- and life-threatening complications. It is unclear how antibody formation is initiated and why only a small subset of patients developing HIT antibodies progress to the clinical manifestations of thrombocytopenia and thrombosis.

PLATELET FACTOR 4

Human PF4 (hPF4) is a member of a large family of small (~8–10 kDa in their monomeric form) proteins that typically contain four cysteine residues in conserved locations, called chemokines (or chemokine ligands). Thus far, 48 chemokines and 19 chemokine receptors have been identified and classified into four families (CC, CXC, CX3C, and XC) based on the sequence pattern of the first two cysteine residues in the ligands. PF4 (CXCL4) belongs to the CXC subfamily of chemokines, characterized by one amino acid separating the first two of four conserved cysteines (Baggiolini, 1998). PF4 is expressed predominantly in megakaryocytes and stored in platelet α-granules, where it constitutes ~2% of the total platelet α-granular content on a molar basis, making it one of the most abundant proteins retained within these granules (Holt and Niewiarowski, 1985; Rucinski et al., 1990). Synthesis of low levels of PF4 has also been reported in activated human monocytes (El-Gedaily et al., 2004; Schaffner et al., 2005), microglia (de Jong et al., 2008), and human T cells (Lasagni et al., 2007), but its biologic role in these cells remains uncertain. Other CXC chemokines released from platelet α-granules include CXCL1 (Gro-α), CXCL5 (epithelial neutrophil-activating protein 78, ENA78), CXCL8 (interleukin-8, IL-8), and CXCL7, which includes platelet basic protein (PBP) and N-terminally truncated PBP-derived proteins: connective tissue-activating peptide-III (CTAP-III), β-thromboglobulin (β-TG) and neutrophil-activating protein-2 (NAP-2) (for review see Lambert et al., 2007b). CXC chemokines with an N-terminal Glu-Leu-Arg sequence (ELR+) bind to a distinct subset of the G-protein coupled receptors (GPCRs) that trigger intracellular signaling. PF4 lacks the ELR motif critical for binding to GPCRs and its activity appears to be reliant on binding to surface glycosaminoglycans (GAGs) (Hoogewerf et al., 1997; Petersen et al., 1999). An alternatively spliced CXCR3 receptor, designated CXCR3-B, has been described in humans. Both the variants of CXCR3, CXCR3-A and CXCR3-B, bind CXCL9, CXCL10, and CXCL11 chemokines, but only CXCR3-B binds and is activated by PF4 as well (Lasagni et al., 2003). CXCR3-B has been identified only on human T-lymphocytes and microvascular endothelial cells (ECs) *in vitro*. However, the expression of CXCR3-B *in vivo* is less firmly established and PF4 exerts broad biologic effects on virtually every nucleated cell in the vasculature (for review see Kasper and Petersen, 2011). PF4 also plays auxiliary roles in regulating thrombosis (Eslin et al., 2004; Kowalska et al., 2010), megakaryocytopoiesis (Lambert et al., 2007a, 2009), immune modulation (Fleischer et al., 2002; Liu et al., 2005; Romagnani et al., 2005; Kasper and Petersen, 2011), angiogenesis (Aidoudi and Bikfalvi, 2010), and atherosclerosis (Sachais et al., 2007; Koenen et al., 2009).

Because of its relative abundance, hPF4 was the first chemokine to be sequenced (Deuel et al., 1977) and cloned (Poncz et al., 1987). Native hPF4 is a globular tetramer composed of identical 7.8 kDa subunits that are asymmetrically associated (Mayo and Chen, 1989; Zhang et al., 1994) and stabilized by electrostatic interactions. Crystallographic- and NMR-based analyses support a model in which heparin wraps around the tetramer by binding to an equatorial ring of cationic charges running perpendicular to the lysine containing α-helices (Stuckey et al., 1992; Zhang et al., 1994). This distribution is of significance in the pathogenesis of HIT and possibly in at least some of its other biologic functions (Kowalska et al., 2011).

HIT ANTIGENIC COMPLEX

Heparin is usually required to trigger the anti-PF4/H immune response. However, the antigenic epitope is not found on heparin itself, but rather requires heparin (or a chemically related molecule) plus a cofactor found in platelet lysates (Green et al., 1978), later identified as PF4 (Amiral et al., 1992). Three binding sites for HIT antibodies have been identified in the PF4 molecule (Suh et al., 1998; Ziporen et al., 1998; Li et al., 2002) (Fig. 9.1). It was first proposed that the epitopes recognized by HIT antibodies might be composed of either

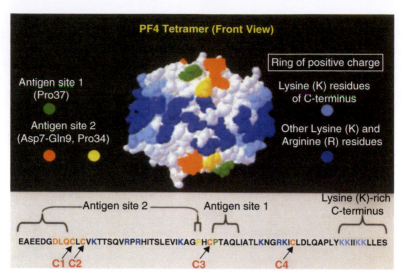

FIGURE 9.1 Structural localization of HIT antigenic sites. The crystal structure and amino acid sequence of the human platelet factor 4 tetramer are shown. (*Top*) Three-dimensional representation of the PF4 tetramer, indicating two epitopes. The "ring of positive charge" is formed by lysine residues in the C-terminus (*light blue*) and by other lysine and arginine residues (*dark blue*). (*Bottom*) The linear sequence of the 70-amino acid polypeptide of a single PF4 molecule is shown. *Source*: From Li et al. (2002).

combinatorial epitopes, consisting partly of heparin and partly of PF4, or conformational epitopes on the PF4 molecule induced by heparin. However, many structurally distinct, linear molecules having in common appropriately spaced, strong anionic charges closely fixed to the molecular backbone and of a sufficient length can modify PF4 to become antigenic (see also chap. 7). Such unrelated molecules as polyvinyl sulfate, polyvinyl sulfonate, polyvinyl phosphate, polyvinyl phosphonate, and polyanethole sulfonate all react with PF4 to produce complexes recognized by HIT antibodies (Visentin et al., 2001). This argues against a combinatorial epitope comprised in part by heparin. Moreover, studies using atomic force microscopy revealed that heparin approximates PF4 tetramers (Greinacher et al., 2006), which may enhance the avidity of HIT antibodies. Lastly, recent studies indicate that small molecule inhibitors of PF4 oligomerization by heparin block the binding of HIT antibodies and their capacity to cause platelet activation (Sachais et al., 2012).

So how does PF4, a "self"-protein, come to be recognized as "nonself" when combined with heparin? As mentioned, PF4 is stored in the α-granules of platelets in complex with the chondroitin sulfate (CS)-containing proteoglycan, serglycin (Perin et al., 1988; Kolset et al., 1996). Serglycin, most probably the predominant proteoglycan found within platelet α-granules (Woulfe et al., 2008), is crucial for trafficking and storage of specific secretory proteins. Serglycin knockout mice do not express CS-containing proteoglycans in their platelets, which contain profoundly reduced α-granule proteins, such as PF4, β-TG, and platelet-derived growth factor (Woulfe et al., 2008).

When platelets are activated, PF4/CS complexes are released from the granules and rebind to the platelet cell surface (George and Onofre, 1982) through CS (Horne, 1993). It is theorized that the low affinity of PF4 to CS permits facile transfer of PF4 to cell surfaces expressing GAGs with higher affinity, especially heparan sulfate (HS) on monocytes and ECs. Heparin, by virtue of its higher affinity for PF4, may foster this process by displacing PF4 from the platelet membrane CS (Loscalzo et al., 1985) and by promoting the formation of large, stable, soluble PF4 complexes through electrostatic interactions. In solution, heparin and PF4 form complexes that vary in size depending on their molar ratio (Bock et al., 1980; Rauova et al., 2005). Binding of HIT antibodies to PF4/H or PF4/GAGs, activation of platelets by HIT antibodies, and *in vivo* immunogenicity in animal models (see chap. 10) all follow a similar bell-shaped curve, which peaks at a very narrow (close to equimolar) ratio of PF4 tetramers to heparin monomers in UFH (estimated mean molecular weight, ~15 kDa) (Hirsh et al., 2001). At this ratio, PF4 and UFH form ultralarge (>670 kDa) complexes (ULCs) that are remarkably stable (Rauova et al., 2005); their surface charge approaches zero (due to charge neutralization) and they acquire the capacity to induce a robust anti-PF4/H immune response in mice (Suvarna et al., 2005, 2007) (Fig. 9.2). ULCs are also capable of binding multiple antibody molecules per complex, which may help sustain interactions with FcγRIIA, leading to platelet activation (Rauova et al., 2005).

Similar principles apply to PF4 bound to other sulfated GAGs at different molar ratios. GAGs consist of repeating disaccharide units with sequences that vary by saccharide composition, linkage, acetylation, and N- and O-sulfation. Additionally, their chain lengths range from 1 to 25,000 disaccharide units (Handel et al., 2005). The antigenicity of the PF4/GAG complex depends not only on the molar ratio of the reactants but also on the length, chemical composition, and structure of the GAG itself (Greinacher et al., 1995). The most abundant GAG is HS, a polysaccharide that is expressed on almost every cell in the body and that comprises 50–90% of the total GAGs associated with endothelial proteoglycans (Irhcke et al., 1993). The structures of HS are highly variable, due largely to great diversity in sequence, patterns of sulfation, and size, ranging from 5 to 70 kDa (Turnbull et al., 2001). Other major classes of GAGs found on cell surfaces include CS and dermatan sulfate (DS), both of which are less anionic than HS (Sugahara et al., 2003). Many chemokines bind to heparin and other GAGs (Lortat-Jacob et al., 2002), but PF4 binds with 10- to 100-fold higher affinity (Witt and Lander, 1994). Binding of PF4 to the CS domain of thrombomodulin (TM) potentiates the activation of protein C (PC) (Kowalska et al., 2011). This probably involves the formation of ULC-like structures, as HIT antibodies recognize this PF4/CS complex. This observation supports two general theses: (*i*) that PF4 released from activated platelets modulates physiologic processes in the process of forming HIT-like antigenic complexes, and (*ii*) that binding of HIT antibodies to these complexes may contribute to the pathogenic mechanisms underlying the prothrombotic state (Kowalska et al., 2011).

PF4 forms antigenic complexes with endogenous GAGs on the surface of platelets (Rauova et al., 2006) and monocytes (Rauova et al., 2010) and likely other hematopoietic and vascular cells (Cines et al., 1987; Visentin et al., 1994; Petersen et al., 1999; Xiao et al., 2008). The fact that HIT-IgG and the HIT-like monoclonal antibody, KKO (Arepally et al., 2000), bind to cultured ECs and CHO cells in the presence of exogenous PF4, but not to CHO cells lacking HS- or CS-containing proteoglycans (Ahmad et al., 1999; Arepally and Mayer, 2001) and that the binding of

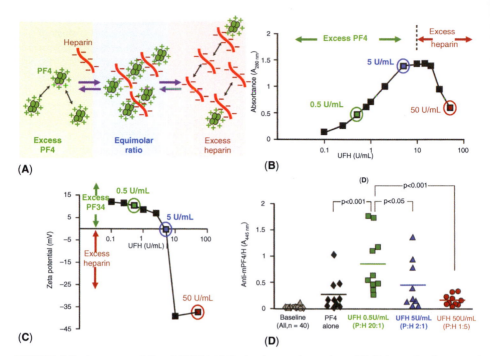

FIGURE 9.2 Immunogenicity of PF4/H ULCs is charge dependent. (**A**) Schematic diagram of studies. Mouse (m) PF4 was mixed with increasing concentrations of heparin to yield a molar excess of PF4 on the left (green), to an equimolar ratio shown in the middle (blue), or to a molar excess of heparin on the right (red). In (**B**) and (**C**), increasing amounts of UFH (0–50 U/mL) were added to a fixed dose of mPF4 (200 µg/mL) and light absorbance (B) or surface charge (ζ-potential) (**C**) were measured. Green, blue, and red encircled data refer to the molar ratio of mPF4 to UFH as in (**A**). In (**D**), 100 µL of mPF4/H complexes containing mPF4 (200 µg/mL) with the indicated amounts of UFH were infused into BL6 mice and serum anti-mPF4/H antibodies were measured on day 15. *Source*: Adapted from Suvarna et al. (2007).

KKO to platelets is inhibited by pretreatment with chondroitinase ABC (Rauova et al., 2006), demonstrate the critical role that surface GAGs play in the formation of cell-associated PF4 complexes. Formation of cell surface antigenic complexes follows a bell-shaped curve as PF4/H complexes in solution, with peak binding of KKO and activation by HIT antibodies over a narrow range of added PF4. This implies that a subset of PF4 might be reorganized into large antigenic complexes on cell surfaces by GAGs at specific molar ratios of reactants, as in solution, while at higher or lower PF4 concentration, the formation of antigenic complexes is less efficient (Cines et al., 2007). The pattern and reactivity of these complexes is highly dependent on the specific composition of the membrane GAGs. There is a significantly greater increase in binding of KKO to PF4 on monocytes (which express high-affinity HS and DS) than to platelets (which express low-affinity CS almost exclusively) (Rauova et al., 2009, 2010). Binding of KKO to activated macrophages increases further when surface GAGs undergo hypersulfation (Petricevich and Michelacci, 1990).

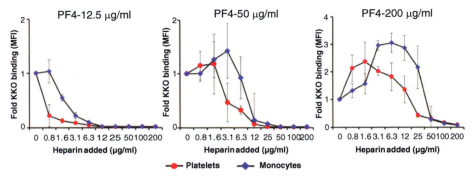

FIGURE 9.3 Monocytes retain more surface HIT antigenic complexes after heparinization. The graphs show the fold-increase in MFI of antibody binding in the presence of the concentrations of PF4 and heparin noted on the X-axis compared with MFI in its absence; the results are normalized to account for the difference in surface area of monocytes and platelets. The Y-axis indicates fold change in antibody binding to human platelets (red circles) and monocytes (blue diamonds) at PF4 concentrations of 12.5, 50, and 200 µg/mL from baseline (absence of added heparin) relative to binding with heparin added at the concentrations shown. *Abbreviations*: MFI, mean fluorescence intensity; PF4, platelet factor 4. *Source*: Adapted from Rauova et al. (2010).

The effect of heparin on the recognition of PF4/GAG complexes on cell surfaces by HIT antibodies is also concentration-dependent. Heparin dissociates PF4 from the cell and reduces antibody binding when added to cells at or below PF4 concentrations optimal for antigenic complex formation (Rauova et al., 2009, 2010). At high concentrations of added PF4, antigenicity actually increases initially as UFH is added, consistent with reorganization of residual nondissociated PF4 into antigenic complexes. Alternatively, the initial increase in antibody binding may be attributable to UFH removing excess PF4 from the cell surface until the optimal PF4/GAG ratio is reached, at which point large antigenic complexes predominate. Antibody binding falls as the UFH concentration is increased further, due to dissociation of the complexes and PF4 from the cell surface. Heparin displaces PF4 from platelet CS at two to four times lower concentrations than is required to remove PF4 from monocytes, which express higher affinity HS and DS in addition to CS (Rauova et al., 2009, 2010) (Fig. 9.3). Together, these data place the focus on cell surface-bound PF4/GAG complexes in the effector response and suggest circulating soluble HIT complexes may participate in PF4 transfer among cells and/or help initiate the production of pathogenic antibodies.

IMMUNE RESPONSE IN HIT

Anti-PF4/H antibodies are a hallmark of the immune response in HIT, but little is known about the cellular basis of PF4/H antibody production. Heparin and PF4 have independent effects on the immune system. Heparin can exert an "adjuvant"-like effect on the immune response to several cationic proteins, such as protamine sulfate, which is used to reverse heparin in patients undergoing CPB (Chudasama et al., 2010). This may occur through structural modifications of the proteins and formation of multimolecular complexes with immunostimulatory properties. The immune response to protamine sulfate/heparin complexes shares a number of similarities to anti-PF4/H seroconversion, including the temporal course of antibody production, stoichiometric requirements and dose-dependence on heparin, and an antibody response that is specific for the immunizing protein (Chudasama et al., 2010). These studies raise the possibility that GAG–protein complexes may stimulate a conserved pathway that is a component of the innate immune response system.

PF4 has important immunomodulatory functions *in vitro*, too. PF4 strongly inhibits T-cell proliferation, interferon-γ (IFN-γ), and IL-2 release from isolated T cells (Fleischer et al., 2002), and the proliferative response of human CD4+CD25- T cells, while inducing the expansion of CD4+CD25+ T regulatory (Tr) cells (Liu et al., 2005). CD4+CD25+ Tr cells comprise 5–10% of the endogenous CD4+ T-cell subset and are able to suppress CD4+ and CD8+ T-cell responses *in vitro* and *in vivo* upon TCR engagement. However, CD4+CD25+ Tr cells lose their potent suppressor function *in vitro* in the presence of PF4 (Liu et al., 2005). PF4 also modulates the production of TH1 and TH2 cytokines (Romagnani et al., 2005) and modulates innate immunity by affecting the stimulation, survival, and differentiation of monocyte/macrophages (Kasper and Petersen, 2011). However, the *in vivo* implications of these regulatory roles of PF4 are unclear, and PF4 bound to GAGs may form surface ULCs with potent immunostimulatory properties.

Some of the serologic characteristics of the antibody response to PF4/H have received extensive study. Antibodies associated with clinical disease are predominantly of the IgG isotype (Warkentin et al., 2005) and may be detected in heparin-naïve patients as early as four days after drug exposure without notable antecedent IgM antibodies (Greinacher et al., 2009; Warkentin et al., 2009). Titers of anti-PF4/H antibodies typically wane over time, often becoming undetectable by three to four months (Warkentin and Kelton, 2001), but antibodies may persist for years on occasion. Consistent with the often transient nature of antibody response, fewer circulating PF4/H memory B cells were found in seropositive HIT patients (6.7%) than in patients immunized with tetanus-toxin (50%). This finding that PF4/H did not induce a robust and durable increase in memory B cells in the peripheral blood (Selleng et al., 2010) may help to explain how patients fail to seroconvert or develop HIT when reexposed to heparin months to years later (Pötzsch et al., 2000; Warkentin and Kelton, 2001; Lubenow and Greinacher, 2002). However, differences in the extent of PF4 release, heparin exposure, and cytokine milieu may contribute as well. The pattern of isotype development, the finding of anti-PF4/H antibodies in the general population (Hursting et al., 2010; Krauel et al., 2011) and evidence of PF4-binding to bacterial cell surfaces (Greinacher et al., 2011; Krauel et al., 2011) have led to a proposal that the immune response to PF4/H is "primed" by prior exposure to PF4 as a result of infections and/or platelet activation at sites where sufficient antigen presenting cells (APCs) are present. However, the apparent lack of immune recall (Warkentin and Kelton, 2001), requirement for a narrow stoichiometric ratio of PF4 and heparin to develop an *in vivo* immune response and the serologic features of antibody responses in naïve mice suggests that alternative explanations are plausible.

Studies in humans and in mice provide some evidence of T-cell involvement in anti-PF4/H antibody production. Culture of peripheral blood mononuclear cells (PBMCs) from patients with HIT incubated with irradiated autologous PBMCs as a source of APCs, IL-2, and antigen (PF4 plus heparin, PF4 alone, heparin alone or media) led to selective expansion of T cells with similar CDR3 motifs only in response to PF4/H complexes (Bacsi et al., 2001). Evidence of skewed rearrangements involving the TCR β chains, βV 5.1, βV11 (Bacsi et al., 1999), and βV17 (Bacsi et al., 2001) was found; however, control patients, PF4/H dosing, and cytokine analysis were not studied (Bacsi et al., 1999). T cells are indispensible for production of platelet-activating anti-PF4/H antibodies in mice (Suvarna et al., 2005) and T cell help requires CD4 cells, but not TLR signaling through MyD88 (Survarna et al., 2008) (see chap. 10).

CELL ACTIVATION IN HIT

The predominant clinical feature of HIT is that, unlike most other drug-induced or autoantibody-mediated thrombocytopenias, anti–PF4/H antibodies predispose to thrombosis. HIT antibodies initiate cellular activation by engaging cellular IgG-Fc receptors. Activation of human platelets via FcγRIIA is a well-recognized feature of HIT (Kelton et al., 1988; Chong et al., 1989). This is most clearly exemplified by the development of a HIT-like thrombotic/thrombocytopenic phenotype in mice double transgenic for hPF4 and FcγRIIA (which are not present on normal mouse platelets) (Reilly et al., 2001) (see also chap. 10). Signal transduction leading to cell activation has been attributed to cross-linking of this low-affinity receptor by multivalent immune complexes (chap. 8). As mentioned in section "HIT antigenic complex", PF4 forms antigenic complexes with endogenous GAGs on the surface of platelets similar to ULCs that form between heparin and PF4 in solution (Rauova et al., 2006). Binding of multiple HIT antibodies to each of these ULCs assembled on cell surfaces may facilitate configuration of an array of multiple IgG antibodies with greater opportunity to stably crosslink FcγRIIA, thus leading to platelet activation. The pathogenic relevance of surface PF4 expression is supported by *in vivo* studies in transgenic mice expressing varying amounts of PF4, in which the severity of KKO-induced thrombocytopenia is proportionate to total platelet (and surface) hPF4 (Fig. 9.4) in the absence of exogenous heparin, establishing that cellular GAGs are sufficient to induce the antigen target for HIT antibodies (Rauova et al., 2006). Variation in PF4 content (Lambert et al., 2007a) and the extent of platelet activation (e.g., post-CPB surgery) may contribute to risk by permitting retention of antigenic cell-associated PF4/GAG complexes at therapeutic concentrations of heparin. This is consistent with results in a murine model, in which high doses of heparin that fully protected mice expressing intermediate levels of PF4 (twofold human platelets) from KKO-induced thrombocytopenia, but did not protect high-PF4 expressing (sixfold human platelets) mice. In contrast, disruption of PF4/GAG complex by protamine sulfate prevented thrombocytopenia almost completely in both lines (Rauova et al., 2010).

Binding of HIT antibodies to platelets results in activation accompanied by the release of procoagulant microparticles, likely increased binding of activated platelets to endothelium, and rapid clearance of antibody-bound platelets from the circulation (Warkentin, 1996; Hughes et al., 2000). The mechanism(s) that cause thrombocytopenia may change over the clinical course of HIT. Initially, hepatosplenic clearance may predominate, offering a protective mechanism to clear the triggering antigen and antibody from the circulation. With disease progression, activation of monocytes, ECs, and possibly other cell types contributes to thrombin generation (Greinacher et al., 2000), and platelet consumption within thrombi may predominate.

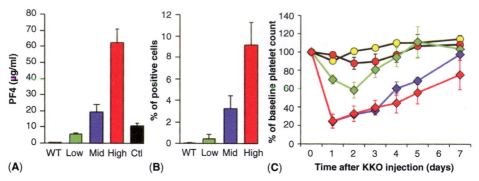

FIGURE 9.4 Severity of thrombocytopenia in a murine model of HIT is proportionate to total platelet and surface human PF4 (hPF4). (**A**) Total platelet-associated hPF4 expressed per milliliter of blood in wild-type (WT) animals and the three hPF4 transgenic mice lines studied. Controls (Ctl) were platelets from four human donors. (**B**) Flow cytometric measurement of platelet-bound FITC-KKO in the same animals as in panel A measured 10 min after intravenous injection of FITC-KKO. (**C**) Platelet counts in mice after intraperitoneal injection of KKO. All animals received 200 µg KKO. (Red circles) mice expressing high levels of hPF4; (yellow circles) FcγRIIA transgenic mice not expressing hPF4; (green diamonds) mice expressing FcγRIIA and low levels of hPF4; (blue diamonds) mice expressing FcγRIIA and moderately elevated levels of hPF4; (red diamonds) mice expressing FcγRIIA and high levels of hPF4. *Source*: Adapted from Rauova et al., 2006.

Monocytes play an important role in thrombosis and fibrin deposition in part through the synthesis and surface expression of tissue factor (TF), the physiologic initiator of normal coagulation and a major initiator of clotting in thrombotic diseases. TF functions as an essential cofactor for factor (F) VIIa to efficiently cleave its substrates, FIX and FX, to their active forms (FIXa and FXa, respectively). The formation of the TF–FVIIa complex is crucial for initiation of coagulation, leading to thrombin generation and fibrin formation. Monocytes express GAGs with a high affinity for PF4, sensitizing them to antibody binding, which stimulates expression of TF (Arepally and Mayer, 2001; Pouplard et al., 2001; Rauova et al., 2010) and release of TF-expressing microparticles (Kasthuri et al., 2012). In addition to low affinity FcγRIIA, which is the only FcR expressed on human platelets, monocytes constitutively express high-affinity FcγRI. Blocking FcγRI, but not FcγRIIA, on monocytes prevented TF expression by HIT antibodies *in vitro* (Kasthuri et al., 2012). ECs, monocytes, and other cells in contact with blood do not constitutively express functional TF. Therefore, the induction of TF expression by HIT antibodies may initiate intravascular coagulation, with the resultant generation of thrombin, leading to an explosive feed-forward system of platelet, EC, and leukocyte activation, and formation of fibrin.

As mentioned, monocytes bind PF4 and form HIT antigenic complexes at lower concentrations of PF4 than platelets. Because of their higher natural affinity, PF4 complexed with monocyte-HS and DS is more resistant to dissociation by heparin (Fig. 9.3); this implies that monocytes remain targets for pathogenic antibodies when the levels of available PF4 drop below those needed to form antigenic complexes on platelets. In addition, activation of monocytes by proinflammatory agents, such as bacterial lipopolysaccharide and IL-1α triggers hypersulfation of monocyte GAGs, along with inducing expression of HS-proteoglycans with side-chains that differ in length and structure that may further increase PF4 binding (Parish, 2006), underlining the link between inflammation and manifestation of HIT. Monocytes or monocyte-derived particles are incorporated into thrombi, especially on the arterial side of the circulation, where they might contribute significantly to thrombus development (see chap. 10, Fig. 10.2). Depletion of monocytes from circulation in a murine model of HIT attenuates thrombosis, but exacerbates thrombocytopenia (Rauova et al., 2010). In the absence of monocytes, more PF4, and consequently more HIT antibodies, may target the platelet surface, enhance their hepatosplenic clearance and reduce platelet availability to promote intravascular thrombosis. On the other hand, dual activation of platelets by (i) monocyte TF/thrombin generation and (ii) HIT antibody-induced platelet activation via FcγRIIA leads to formation of highly procoagulant "coated platelets" (Andre et al., 2011) and promotes thrombosis and platelet consumption within thrombi. Coated platelets (formerly called COAT – COllagen And Thrombin activated platelets) form after dual stimulation via a G-protein pathway—especially by thrombin—and by an ITAM pathway, including activation by FcγRIIA (Batar and Dale, 2001; Dale et al., 2002; Munnix et al., 2009). The main characteristics of coated platelets are exposure of phosphatidylserine (PS) and retention of high levels of several procoagulant proteins on their surface, including FV, fibrinogen, fibronectin, thrombospondin, and von Willebrand factor, thus supporting robust prothrombinase activity.

IMMUNE VASCULAR INJURY IN HIT

The most important complication of HIT is thrombosis. Clinically overt arterial or venous thrombi have been observed in 50% or more of patients with HIT in some series (see chaps. 2 and 4), a frequency that far exceeds any other drug-induced immune platelet disorder. The propensity for thrombosis is only in part attributable to platelet and monocyte activation described in section "Cell activation in HIT". In addition, significant amounts of PF4 are normally associated with EC proteoglycans (Rao et al., 1983) where it becomes a target for HIT antibodies (Cines et al., 1987; Visentin et al., 1994). Alterations in the local vascular milieu and endothelial dysfunction enhance adhesion of activated platelets and monocytes, with accrual of PF4 and other chemokines, thus promoting proinflammatory and prothrombotic processes that are likely to be part of the propensity for thrombosis. Localization of clotting observed in HIT relates to antigen expression and response to injury at the level of the vessel wall itself.

The Endothelium in Hemostasis

Under physiologic conditions, the endothelial surface is covered with a relatively thick sheath of glycosylated molecules, referred to as the glycocalyx (Chappell et al., 2009), made up predominantly of HS, which has high affinity for PF4. A major role of the endothelium is to regulate blood fluidity and trafficking of circulating hematopoietic cells (for review see Cines et al., 1998; Celie et al., 2009). ECs express a variety of factors that inhibit coagulation, including soluble substances, such as nitric oxide and prostacyclin (acting to inhibit platelet activation), and tissue-type plasminogen activator (tPA, acting to promote fibrinolysis), among many others. EC surface-bound molecules with anticoagulant activity include TM, complement regulatory proteins, receptors for activated protein C (aPC), urokinase, and plasminogen.

Unperturbed ECs also do not express soluble and cell-associated molecules that promote platelet and leukocyte adhesion, such as endothelial leukocyte adhesion molecule (ELAM), P-selectin, and platelet-activating factor. Each is induced, however, when the cells are stimulated by agonists such as cytokines and thrombin (Drake et al., 1993; Kaplanski et al., 1998), or when injured by immune factors, atherosclerosis, or shear stress (Yu et al., 2005). Additionally, injured ECs express less HS and TM, internalize and degrade aPC, elaborate TF, and secrete abundant plasminogen activator inhibitor-1 (PAI-1), each of which promote thrombus formation (Cines et al., 1998). Histochemical studies of the endothelium in murine models of inflammation have confirmed many of these observations predicated in cell culture (Fries et al., 1993), affirming the notion that the endothelium undergoes multifaceted changes from an antithrombotic to a procoagulant phenotype in response to injury.

Also relevant to the pathogenesis of HIT is the remarkable heterogeneity of ECs, within and among different vascular beds, owing to genetic differences and acquired changes in phenotype (for reviews see Cines et al., 1998; Aird, 2003). For example, in vivo, only a small fraction of ECs constitutively express tPA (Levin and del Zoppo, 1994), whereas distinct subsets of ECs express TF and E-selectin when exposed to endotoxin (Drake et al., 1993). ECs from different organs express tissue-specific promoters that regulate the expression of von Willebrand factor in vivo (Aird et al., 1997). ECs also show regional variation in the synthesis of prostacyclin and expression of leukocyte adhesion molecules and Fcγ receptors, among many other phenotypic differences.

There is also evidence to indicate that PC activation on macrovascular ECs is mediated predominantly through the endothelial protein C receptor (EPCR), whereas TM may predominate in the microvasculature (Laszik et al., 1997; Van de Wouwer et al., 2004). Activation of PC by thrombin is accelerated 20-fold after binding to EPCR, but it is TM that changes thrombin from a procoagulant to an anticoagulant enzyme. Binding of thrombin to TM on the cell membrane surface catalyzes activation of PC more than 1000-fold (Esmon, 2001). The anticoagulant function of TM is tightly linked to its anti-inflammatory properties via the PC–TM–EPCR system, which effectively switches the substrate specificity and functional properties of thrombin from a procoagulant/proinflammatory to an anticoagulant/anti-inflammatory molecule (for review see Conway, 2012).

The behavior of ECs can also be modified during the evolution of vascular disease. For example, atherosclerotic vessels produce less nitric oxide in response to a variety of stimuli than do healthy vessels (Shaul, 2003). Atherosclerotic vessels may also undergo alterations in expression of GAGs (Talusan et al., 2005) and an increase in expression of various cell adhesion molecules (for review see Fuster et al., 1998). Binding of advanced glycation end products to specific EC receptors during normal aging and diabetes mellitus increases vascular permeability, exposing the subendothelial matrix to lipoproteins and other injurious substances (Basta et al., 2004). It is also likely that genetic variation in EC behavior contributes to the host response to antibody- and platelet-mediated EC injury, although the methods to identify or monitor such risk factors in the clinical setting remain to be fully developed. Thus, any inquiry into the reason why only a subset of patients who develop anti-PF4/H antibodies develop thrombosis, or why thrombi occur at restricted vascular sites, must take into consideration the specific attributes of the affected endothelial vascular bed as well as its extent of preactivation.

The expression and anticoagulant function of HS-type proteoglycans (HSPGs) by ECs appears to be a major component in the pathogenesis of vascular thrombosis in patients with HIT. HSPGs expressed by ECs bind antithrombin III (AT) *in vitro* and *in vivo*, and accelerate the inactivation of thrombin and FXa approximately 20-fold, an effect that is biologically equivalent to 0.1–0.5 U/mL of heparin (Marcum and Rosenberg, 1984). Microheterogeneity in the composition of HSPG in arteries, veins, and capillaries has been noted (Lowe-Krentz and Joyce, 1991), but the significance of these differences is unknown. Expression of HSPG by ECs also undergoes developmental changes (David et al., 1992), and its composition varies after the cells are exposed to thrombin (Benezra et al., 1993), homocysteine (Nishinaga et al., 1993), heparin (Nader et al., 1989), wounding and migration (Kinsella and Wight, 1986), and after induction by activated platelets (Yahalom et al., 1984), among other stimuli. ECs also bind heparin (for review see Patton et al., 1995), which alters their proliferation, matrix composition, and many other vascular functions. It has also been reported that AT is displaced from ECs by heparin, and its binding is inhibited by PF4 (Stern et al., 1985). Whether HIT antibodies promote the capacity of PF4 to neutralize AT activity has not been reported.

PF4 and the Endothelium

Cultured ECs bind approximately 50 pmol PF4/10^5 cells (Rybak et al., 1989). Since the glycocalyx is considerably thicker and contains more GAGs *in vivo* (Chappell et al., 2009), the capacity of healthy endothelium to bind PF4 is remarkable. Several classes of binding sites have been identified, including a high-capacity, low-affinity site on HSPG, as well as higher-affinity binding sites consistent with specific chemokine receptors (CXCR3-B—see section "Platelet Factor 4") and coagulant proteins (see below). Binding of PF4 to the endothelium is attenuated by pretreatment with heparinase (Marcum and Rosenberg, 1984), and plasma concentrations are increased 10- to 20-fold after heparin is infused intravenously (Dawes et al., 1982). Binding of PF4 to EC GAGs is independent of the pentasaccharide involved in the binding of AT (Loscalzo et al., 1985). PF4 has 10- to 100-fold greater affinity for EC HSPG than does AT (Jordan et al., 1982) and thus markedly attenuates the antiprotease cofactor activity of AT on intact vessels (Busch et al., 1980; Stern et al., 1985). The affinity of PF4 for ECs is lower compared with that toward purified heparin (K_d = 2–3 μmol/L *vs* 2 nmol/L, respectively) (Rybak et al., 1989).

The involvement of PF4 in hemostasis is mediated in part by charge-dependent interactions with EC GAGs (Eslin et al., 2004; see chap. 10). Similar to the other vascular cells, the amount of PF4 on the vasculature may affect antigen assembly and thereby contribute to the clinical variability seen in patients with anti-PF4/H antibodies. Thrombosis may be fostered in patients who release relatively large amounts of PF4 from their platelets, either due to constitutive overexpression or due to platelet-activating effects of atherosclerosis and vascular injury. Heparin may stabilize or propagate thrombosis by neutralizing the charge effects of "excess" cell-surface PF4. Assembly of cell-surface antigenic complexes capable of binding HIT antibodies in the absence of circulating drug may contribute to the development of HIT when only low-sensitizing doses of heparin are employed and to the persistent hypercoagulable state after heparin has been withdrawn.

The anticoagulant properties of PF4 on the vasculature are mediated in part through PC mentioned above. TM is posttranslationally modified by the addition of a CS A-like GAG, which invests it with the capacity to bind cationic peptides at physiologic pH. Binding studies using surface plasmon resonance (Dudek et al., 1997) confirmed a strong interaction between PF4 and TM containing CS as well as PF4 and the Gla domain of PC. The binding of PF4 (but not β-TG or thrombospondin) increases PC cofactor activity 25-fold in a cell-free system, whereas the binding of eosinophilic cationic protein, major basic protein, and histidine-rich glycoprotein to these GAG residues inhibits the function of TM (Slungaard and Key, 1994; Dudek et al., 1997). Both the Gla domain of PC and CS side chain of TM are necessary for PF4 to increase aPC generation. Addition of PF4 to cultured ECs accelerates aPC generation approximately 5- to 10-fold depending on vascular origin (Slungaard et al., 2003). Injection of PF4 into primates infused with thrombin increases aPC generation 2- to 3-fold and prolongs the baseline activated partial thromboplastin time (Slungaard et al., 2003). In addition, PF4 released from platelets in mice enhanced aPC generation in a model of thrombin infusion and increased survival of mice following lipopolysaccharide (LPS)-induced endotoxemia (Kowalska et al., 2007). The PF4-mediated acceleration of aPC activity via CS bound to TM exhibits the same bell-shaped profile seen with the formation of HIT antigenic complexes of PF4 with heparin in solution or with GAGs on cell surfaces described in section "HIT antigenic complex". The ability of HIT antibodies to block PF4 enhancement of aPC generation may contribute to the prothrombotic state (Kowalska et al., 2011).

A pathogenic role of PF4 in atherogenesis has been recently elucidated. Human atherosclerotic lesions are invested with PF4 (Pitsilos et al., 2003). PF4 is found not only along the overlying endothelium, but also in foam cells and acellular portions of the plaque. *In vitro*, PF4 binds to the low-density lipoprotein (LDL) receptor and to proteoglycans, forming ternary complexes with limited migration into clathrin-coated pits, thereby retarding endocytosis and catabolism of LDL (Sachais et al., 2002). PF4 binds directly to oxidized LDL, promoting foam cell formation (Nassar et al., 2003) and upregulating expression of E-selectin, an adhesion molecule implicated in atherogenesis (Yu et al., 2005). In mice, activated platelets deposit PF4 on endothelium and monocytes, potentiating the effects of P-selectin on platelet–leukocyte aggregate formation and development of atherosclerosis (Huo et al., 2003). In a murine model of HIT, a hypercholesterolemic diet increased platelet reactivity and EC activation, as indicated by elevated levels of soluble vascular cell adhesion molecule (Reilly et al., 2006). Antibodies to PF4/H complexes have been identified as an independent predictor of myocardial infarction at 30 days in patients presenting with acute coronary ischemic syndromes (Williams et al., 2003).

HIT antibodies may modify the interactions of PF4 with diseased endothelium by (i) binding to PF4/proteoglycan complexes in atherosclerotic lesions, (ii) inducing formation of platelet–leukocyte aggregates (Khairy et al., 2001), or (iii) binding to circulating monocytes (Arepally and Mayer, 2001; Pouplard et al., 2001), thereby increasing local inflammation and stimulating procoagulant processes. Binding of HIT antibodies to ECs and their activation was described over 25 years ago (Cines et al., 1987). Binding was reduced when the cells were pretreated with enzymes that degrade heparin or HS, whereas addition of chondroitinase was without effect. HIT sera induced ECs to express TF, and the expression of procoagulant activity was enhanced further in the presence of platelets. These observations were confirmed and extended by Visentin and colleagues (1994), who demonstrated that the binding of HIT antibodies to human umbilical venous ECs was dependent on PF4, but not on exogenous heparin, in contrast to the requirement for both to be added for antibody binding to platelets. This is consistent with the concept that PF4 released from activated platelets can form a competent antigenic complex on the pericellular matrix of the endothelium (Hayes et al., 2011).

IMPLICATIONS

Our current understanding of the pathogenesis of HIT is shown in Figure 9.5. The amount of PF4 that is deposited on the vascular endothelium and/or bound to the surface of platelets, monocytes, and other vascular cells varies depending on the expression levels and extent of intravascular platelet activation. Infused heparin displaces a proportion of cell-bound PF4, leading to the formation of soluble PF4/H complexes. Depending on the ratio of PF4 and heparin, residual cell-bound PF4/GAG or PF4/H complexes may become immunogenic and trigger antibody

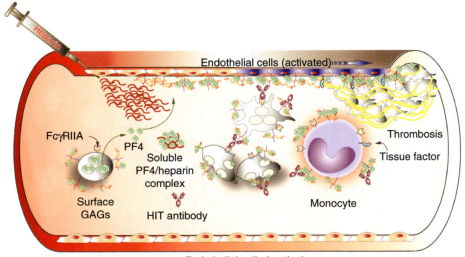

FIGURE 9.5 Surface PF4/GAGs on cells underlie pathogenesis in HIT. PF4 is deposited on the vascular endothelium and bound to the surface of platelets, monocytes, and other vascular cells. Infused heparin displaces a proportion of cell-bound PF4, leading to the formation of soluble PF4/H complexes. Depending on the ratio of PF4 and heparin, residual cell-bound PF4/GAG or PF4/H complexes may become immunogenic and trigger antibody production. PF4 rapidly dissociates from cell-associated GAGs and in most of the patients heparin removes all PF4 from the cell surface. Therefore, there is no target for these antibodies on cell surfaces, and HIT does not occur. In patients with residual PF4 bound to the surface of platelets, it becomes a target for circulating antibodies causing thrombocytopenia, platelet activation through FcγRIIA with additional release of PF4, setting up a positive feed-forward loop of platelet, monocyte, and EC sensitization, and antibody binding and activation. PF4 binds with even greater avidity to monocyte and endothelial GAGs. Binding of HIT antibodies to monocytes leads to TF expression, which may contribute to the development of intravascular thrombosis. Activated platelets also adhere to the activated endothelium, especially at sites of focal injury (atherosclerosis, inflammation, trauma). PF4 released from activated platelets binds to the surface of ECs, which then bind HIT antibodies, leading to EC activation, TF expression, and thrombin generation. Thrombin activates additional platelets, leading to the next round of PF4 release, more extensive endothelial cell activation and platelet recruitment into thrombi, all eventuating in extensive thrombosis.

production. PF4 rapidly dissociates from cell-associated GAGs and in most of the patients heparin removes all PF4 from the cell surface. Therefore, there is no target for these antibodies on cell surfaces, and HIT does not occur. In patients with ongoing platelet activation, possibly affected by greater stores in their α-granules, PF4/CS is continuously translocated to the surface of platelets, where it is a target for circulating antibodies causing thrombocytopenia. Platelet activation through FcγIIA promotes additional release of PF4, setting up a positive feed-forward loop of platelet, monocytes, and EC sensitization, antibody binding, and activation. Activated platelets also form heterotypic aggregates with leukocytes and endothelium. PF4 binds with even greater avidity to monocyte and endothelial GAGs, which is further increased by oversulfation as a result of inflammation, leading to persistent antigen expression beyond the period when platelets are the prime target. Binding of HIT antibodies to monocytes and endothelium leads to TF expression and release of IL-8 (and likely diverse other proinflammatory and procoagulant effects), which may contribute to the development of intravascular thrombosis. Activated platelets also adhere to the activated endothelium, especially at sites of focal injury (atherosclerosis, inflammation, trauma). PF4 released from activated platelets binds to the surface of ECs, which then bind HIT antibodies, leading to EC activation. Activated ECs express TF, culminating in the generation of thrombin. Thrombin activates additional platelets, leading to the next round of PF4 release, more extensive EC activation and platelet recruitment into thrombi, all eventuating in extensive thrombosis.

The distinguishing features of this model, with its focus on cell-associated antigen formation, help to explain the seemingly paradoxical occurrence of thrombocytopenia and thrombosis, and why the procoagulant state may persist after heparin has been discontinued and thrombocytopenia has resolved. This model also suggests that steps proximal to the generation of thrombin, including prevention of PF4 oligomerization, thereby preventing antigen formation on cell surfaces, and inhibition of Fc receptor-mediated platelet and monocyte activation, may be more rational targets for intervention than systemic administration of thrombin inhibitors.

REFERENCES

Ahmad S, Walenga JM, Jeske WP, Cella G, Fareed J. Functional heterogeneity of antiheparin-platelet factor 4 antibodies: implications in the pathogenesis of the HIT syndrome. Clin Appl Thromb Hemost 5(Suppl 1): S32–S37, 1999.

Aidoudi S, Bikfalvi A. Interaction of PF4 (CXCL4) with the vasculature: a role in atherosclerosis and angiogenesis. Thromb Haemost 104: 941–948, 2010.

Aird WC. Endothelial cell heterogeneity. Crit Care Med 31: S221–S230, 2003.

Aird WC, Edelberg JM, Weiler-Guettler H, Simmons WW, Smith TW, Rosenberg RD. Vascular bed-specific expression of an endothelial cell gene is programmed by the tissue microenvironment. J Cell Biol 138: 1117–1124, 1997.

Amiral J, Bridey F, Dreyfus M, Vissoc AM, Fressinaud E, Wolf M, Meyer D. Platelet factor 4 complexed to heparin is the target for antibodies generated in heparin-induced thrombocytopenia. Thromb Haemost 68: 95–96, 1992.

Andre P, Stolla M, Woulfe D, Chavez M, Bergmeier W, Rauova L, Cines DB, Poncz M, McKenzie S. Formation of procoagulant platelets in heparin-induced thrombocytopenia (HIT) follows a unique signaling pathway [abstr]. Blood 118(Suppl): 197, 2011.

Arepally GM, Mayer IM. Antibodies from patients with heparin-induced thrombocytopenia stimulate monocytic cells to express tissue factor and secrete interleukin-8. Blood 98: 1252–1254, 2001.

Arepally GM, Kamei S, Park KS, Kamei K, Li ZQ, Liu W, Siegel DL, Kisiel W, Cines DB, Poncz M. Characterization of a murine monoclonal antibody that mimics heparin-induced thrombocytopenia antibodies. Blood 95: 1533–1540, 2000.

Bacsi S, De Palma R, Visentin GP, Gorski J, Aster RH. Complexes of heparin and platelet factor 4 specifically stimulate T cells from patients with heparin-induced thrombocytopenia/thrombosis. Blood 94: 208–215, 1999.

Bacsi S, Geoffrey R, Visentin G, De Palma R, Aster R, Gorski J. Identification of T cells responding to a self-protein modified by an external agent. Hum Immunol 62: 113–124, 2001.

Baggiolini M. Chemokines and leukocyte traffic. Nature 392: 565–568, 1998.

Basta G, Schmidt AM, De Caterina R. Advanced glycation end products and vascular inflammation: implications for accelerated atherosclerosis in diabetes. Cardiovasc Res 63: 582–592, 2004.

Batar P, Dale GL. Simultaneous engagement of thrombin and FcγRIIA receptors results in platelets expressing high levels of procoagulant proteins. J Lab Clin Med 138: 393–402, 2001.

Benezra M, Vlodavsky I, Ishai-Michaeli R, Neufeld G, Bar-Shavit R. Thrombin-induced release of active basic fibroblast growth factor-heparan sulfate complexes from subendothelial extracellular matrix. Blood 81: 3324–3331, 1993.

Bock PE, Luscombe M, Marshall SE, Pepper DS, Holbrook JJ. The multiple complexes formed by the interaction of platelet factor 4 with heparin. Biochem J 191: 769–776, 1980.

Busch C, Dawes J, Pepper DS, Wasteson A. Binding of platelet factor 4 to cultured human umbilical vein endothelial cells. Thromb Res 19: 129–137, 1980.

Celie JW, Beelen RH, van den Born J. Heparan sulfate proteoglycans in extravasation: assisting leukocyte guidance. Front Biosci 14: 4932–4949, 2009.

Chappell D, Jacob M, Paul O, Rehm M, Welsch U, Stoeckelhuber M, Conzen P, Becker BF. The glycocalyx of the human umbilical vein endothelial cell: an impressive structure ex vivo but not in culture. Circ Res 104: 1313–1317, 2009.

Chong BH, Castaldi PA, Berndt MC. Heparin-induced thrombocytopenia: effects of rabbit IgG, and its Fab and FC fragments on antibody-heparin-platelet interaction. Thromb Res 55: 291–295, 1989.

Chudasama SL, Espinasse B, Hwang F, Qi R, Joglekar M, Afonina G, Wiesner MR, Welsby IJ, Ortel TL, Arepally GM. Heparin modifies the immunogenicity of positively charged proteins. Blood 116: 6046–6053, 2010.

Cines DB, Kaywin P, Bina M, Tomaski A, Schreiber AD. Heparin-associated thrombocytopenia. N Engl J Med 303: 788–795, 1980.

Cines DB, Tomaski A, Tannenbaum S. Immune endothelial-cell injury in heparin-associated thrombocytopenia. N Engl J Med 316: 581–589, 1987.

Cines DB, Pollak ES, Buck CA, Loscalzo J, Zimmerman GA, McEver RP, Pober JS, Wick TM, Konkle BA, Schwartz BS, Barnathan ES, McCrae KR, Hug BA, Schmidt AM, Stern DM. Endothelial cells in physiology and in the pathophysiology of vascular disorders. Blood 91: 3527–3561, 1998.

Cines DB, Rauova L, Arepally G, Reilly MP, McKenzie SE, Sachais BS, Poncz M. Heparin-induced thrombocytopenia: an autoimmune disorder regulated through dynamic autoantigen assembly/disassembly. J Clin Apher 22: 31–36, 2007.

Conway EM. Thrombomodulin and its role in inflammation. Semin Immunopathol 34: 107–125, 2012.

Dale GL, Friese P, Batar P, Hamilton SF, Reed GL, Jackson KW, Clemetson KJ, Alberio L. Stimulated platelets use serotonin to enhance their retention of procoagulant proteins on the cell surface. Nature 415: 175–179, 2002.

David G, Bai XM, Van der Schueren B, Cassiman JJ, Van den Berghe H. Developmental changes in heparan sulfate expression: in situ detection with mAbs. J Cell Biol 119: 961–975, 1992.

Dawes J, Pumphrey CW, McLaren KM, Prowse CV, Pepper DS. The in vivo release of human platelet factor 4 by heparin. Thromb Res 27: 65–76, 1982.

de Jong EK, de Haas AH, Brouwer N, van Weering HR, Hensens M, Bechmann I, Pratley P, Wesseling E, Boddeke HW, Biber K. Expression of CXCL4 in microglia in vitro and in vivo and its possible signaling through CXCR3. J Neurochem 105: 1726–1736, 2008.

Deuel TF, Keim PS, Farmer M, Heinrikson RL. Amino acid sequence of human platelet factor 4. Proc Natl Acad Sci U S A 74: 2256–2258, 1977.

Drake TA, Cheng J, Chang A, Taylor FB Jr. Expression of tissue factor, thrombomodulin, and e-selectin in baboons with lethal Escherichia coli sepsis. Am J Pathol 142: 1458–1470, 1993.

Dudek AZ, Pennell CA, Decker TD, Young TA, Key NS, Slungaard A. Platelet factor 4 binds to glycanated forms of thrombomodulin and to protein C, a potential mechanism for enhancing generation of activated protein C. J Biol Chem 272: 31785–31792, 1997.

El-Gedaily A, Schoedon G, Schneemann M, Schaffner A. Constitutive and regulated expression of platelet basic protein in human monocytes. J Leukoc Biol 75: 495–503, 2004.

Eslin DE, Zhang C, Samuels KJ, Rauova L, Zhai L, Niewiarowski S, Cines DB, Poncz M, Kowalska MA. Transgenic mice studies demonstrate a role for platelet factor 4 in thrombosis: dissociation between anticoagulant and antithrombotic effect of heparin. Blood 104: 3173–3180, 2004.

Esmon CT. Protein C anticoagulant pathway and its role in controlling microvascular thrombosis and inflammation. Crit Care Med 29: S48–S51; 51–42, 2001.

Fleischer J, Grage-Griebenow E, Kasper B, Heine H, Ernst M, Brandt E, Flad HD, Petersen F. Platelet factor 4 inhibits proliferation and cytokine release of activated human T cells. J Immunol 169: 770–777, 2002.

Fratantoni JC, Pollet R, Gralnick HR. Heparin-induced thrombocytopenia: confirmation of diagnosis with in vitro methods. Blood 45: 395–401, 1975.

Fries JW, Williams AJ, Atkins RC, Newman W, Lipscomb MF, Collins T. Expression of VCAM-1 and e-selectin in an in vivo model of endothelial activation. Am J Pathol 143: 725–737, 1993.

Fuster V, Poon M, Willerson JT. Learning from the transgenic mouse: endothelium, adhesive molecules, and neointimal formation. Circulation 97: 16–18, 1998.

George JN, Onofre AR. Human platelet surface binding of endogenous secreted factor VIII-von Willebrand factor and platelet factor 4. Blood 59: 194–197, 1982.

Green D, Harris K, Reynolds N, Roberts M, Patterson R. Heparin immune thrombocytopenia: evidence for a heparin-platelet complex as the antigenic determinant. J Lab Clin Med 91: 167–175, 1978.

Greinacher A, Alban S, Dummel V, Franz G, Mueller-Eckhardt C. Characterization of the structural requirements for a carbohydrate based anticoagulant with a reduced risk of inducing the immunological type of heparin-associated thrombocytopenia. Thromb Haemost 74: 886–892, 1995.

Greinacher A, Eichler P, Lubenow N, Kwasny H, Luz M. Heparin-induced thrombocytopenia with thromboembolic complications: meta-analysis of 2 prospective trials to assess the value of parenteral treatment with lepirudin and its therapeutic aPTT range. Blood 96: 846–851, 2000.

Greinacher A, Gopinadhan M, Günther JU, Omer-Adam MA, Strobel U, Warkentin TE, Papastavrou G, Weitschies W, Helm CA. Close approximation of two platelet factor 4 tetramers by charge neutralization forms the antigens recognized by HIT antibodies. Arterioscler Thromb Vasc Biol 26: 2386–2393, 2006.

Greinacher A, Kohlmann T, Strobel U, Sheppard JI, Warkentin TE. The temporal profile of the anti-PF4/heparin immune response. Blood 113: 4970–4976, 2009.

Greinacher A, Holtfreter B, Krauel K, Gatke D, Weber C, Ittermann T, Hammerschmidt S, Kocher T. Association of natural anti-platelet factor 4/heparin antibodies with periodontal disease. Blood 118: 1395–1401, 2011.

Handel TM, Johnson Z, Crown SE, Lau EK, Proudfoot AE. Regulation of protein function by glycosaminoglycans-as exemplified by chemokines. Annu Rev Biochem 74: 385–410, 2005.

Hayes VM, Cines DB, Poncz M, Rauova L. Rolling recruitment of endothelial cell (EC) activation in the prothrombotic nature of heparin-induced thrombocytopenia (HIT) [abstr]. Blood 118(Suppl): 536, 2011.

Hirsh J, Anand SS, Halperin JL, Fuster V. Mechanism of action and pharmacology of unfractionated heparin. Arterioscler Thromb Vasc Biol 21: 1094–1096, 2001.

Holt JC, Niewiarowski S. Biochemistry of alpha granule proteins. Semin Hematol 22: 151–163, 1985.

Hoogewerf AJ, Kuschert GS, Proudfoot AE, Borlat F, Clark-Lewis I, Power CA, Wells TN. Glycosaminoglycans mediate cell surface oligomerization of chemokines. Biochemistry 36: 13570–13578, 1997.

Horne MK 3rd. The effect of secreted heparin-binding proteins on heparin binding to platelets. Thromb Res 70: 91–98, 1993.

Hughes M, Hayward CP, Warkentin TE, Horsewood P, Chorneyko KA, Kelton JG. Morphological analysis of microparticle generation in heparin-induced thrombocytopenia. Blood 96: 188–194, 2000.

Huo Y, Schober A, Forlow SB, Smith DF, Hyman MC, Jung S, Littman DR, Weber C, Ley K. Circulating activated platelets exacerbate atherosclerosis in mice deficient in apolipoprotein E. Nat Med 9: 61–67, 2003.

Hursting MJ, Pai PJ, McCracken JE, Hwang F, Suvarna S, Lokhnygina Y, Bandarenko N, Arepally GM. Platelet factor 4/heparin antibodies in blood bank donors. Am J Clin Pathol 134: 774–780, 2010.

Ihrcke NS, Wrenshall LE, Lindman BJ, Platt JL. Role of heparan sulfate in immune system-blood vessel interactions. Immunol Today 14: 500–505, 1993.

Jordan RE, Favreau LV, Braswell EH, Rosenberg RD. Heparin with two binding sites for antithrombin or platelet factor 4. J Biol Chem 257: 400–406, 1982.

Kaplanski G, Marin V, Fabrigoule M, Boulay V, Benoliel AM, Bongrand P, Kaplanski S, Farnarier C. Thrombin-activated human endothelial cells support monocyte adhesion in vitro following expression of intercellular adhesion molecule-1 (ICAM-1; CD54) and vascular cell adhesion molecule-1 (VCAM-1; CD106). Blood 92: 1259–1267, 1998.

Kasper B, Petersen F. Molecular pathways of platelet factor 4/CXCL4 signaling. Eur J of Cell Biol 90: 521–526, 2011.

Kasthuri RS, Glover SL, Jonas W, McEachron T, Pawlinski R, Arepally GM, Key NS, Mackman N. PF4/heparin-antibody complex induces monocyte tissue factor expression and release of tissue factor positive microparticles by activation of FcγRI. Blood 119: 5285–5293, 2012.

Kelton JG, Sheridan D, Santos A, Smith J, Steeves K, Smith C, Brown C, Murphy WG. Heparin-induced thrombocytopenia: laboratory studies. Blood 72: 925–930, 1988.

Khairy M, Lasne D, Brohard-Bohn B, Aiach M, Rendu F, Bachelot-Loza C. A new approach in the study of the molecular and cellular events implicated in heparin-induced thrombocytopenia, formation of leukocyte-platelet aggregates. Thromb Haemost 85: 1090–1096, 2001.

Kinsella MG, Wight TN. Modulation of sulfated proteoglycan synthesis by bovine aortic endothelial cells during migration. J Cell Biol 102: 679–687, 1986.

Koenen RR, von Hundelshausen P, Nesmelova IV, Zernecke A, Liehn EA, Sarabi A, Kramp BK, Piccinini AM, Paludan SR, Kowalska MA, Kungl AJ, Hackeng TM, Mayo KH, Weber C. Disrupting functional interactions between platelet chemokines inhibits atherosclerosis in hyperlipidemic mice. Nat Med 15: 97–103, 2009.

Kolset SO, Mann DM, Uhlin-Hansen L, Winberg JO, Ruoslahti E. Serglycin-binding proteins in activated macrophages and platelets. J Leukoc Biol 59: 545–554, 1996.

Kowalska MA, Mahmud SA, Lambert MP, Poncz M, Slungaard A. Endogenous platelet factor 4 stimulates activated protein C generation in vivo and improves survival after thrombin or lipopolysaccharide challenge. Blood 110: 1903–1905, 2007.

Kowalska MA, Rauova L, Poncz M. Role of the platelet chemokine platelet factor 4 (PF4) in hemostasis and thrombosis. Thromb Res 125: 292–296, 2010.

Kowalska MA, Krishnaswamy S, Rauova L, Zhai L, Hayes V, Amirikian K, Esko JD, Bougie DW, Aster RH, Cines DB, Poncz M. Antibodies associated with heparin-induced thrombocytopenia (HIT) inhibit activated protein C generation: new insights into the prothrombotic nature of HIT. Blood 118: 2882–2888, 2011.

Krauel K, Potschke C, Weber C, Kessler W, Fürll B, Ittermann T, Maier S, Hammerschmidt S, Broker BM, Greinacher A. Platelet factor 4 binds to bacteria, [corrected] inducing antibodies cross-reacting with the major antigen in heparin-induced thrombocytopenia. Blood 117: 1370–1378, 2011.

Lambert MP, Rauova L, Bailey M, Sola-Visner MC, Kowalska MA, Poncz M. Platelet factor 4 is a negative autocrine in vivo regulator of megakaryopoiesis: clinical and therapeutic implications. Blood 110: 1153–1160, 2007a.

Lambert MP, Sachais BS, Kowalska MA. Chemokines and thrombogenicity. Thromb Haemost 97: 722–729, 2007b.

Lambert MP, Wang Y, Bdeir KH, Nguyen Y, Kowalska MA, Poncz M. Platelet factor 4 regulates megakaryopoiesis through low-density lipoprotein receptor-related protein 1 (LRP1) on megakaryocytes. Blood 114: 2290–2298, 2009.

Lasagni L, Francalanci M, Annunziato F, Lazzeri E, Giannini S, Cosmi L, Sagrinati C, Mazzinghi B, Orlando C, Maggi E, Marra F, Romagnani S, Serio M, Romagnani P. An alternatively spliced variant of CXCR3 mediates the inhibition of endothelial cell growth induced by IP-10, Mig, and I-TAC, and acts as functional receptor for platelet factor 4. J Exp Med 197: 1537–1549, 2003.

Lasagni L, Grepin R, Mazzinghi B, Lazzeri E, Meini C, Sagrinati C, Liotta F, Frosali F, Ronconi E, Alain-Courtois N, Ballerini L, Netti GS, Maggi E, Annunziato F, Serio M, Romagnani S, Bikfalvi A, Romagnani P. PF-4/CXCL4 and CXCL4L1 exhibit distinct subcellular localization and a differentially regulated mechanism of secretion. Blood 109: 4127–4134, 2007.

Laszik Z, Mitro A, Taylor FB Jr, Ferrell G, Esmon CT. Human protein C receptor is present primarily on endothelium of large blood vessels: implications for the control of the protein C pathway. Circulation 96: 3633–3640, 1997.

Levin EG, del Zoppo GJ. Localization of tissue plasminogen activator in the endothelium of a limited number of vessels. Am J Pathol 144: 855–861, 1994.

Li ZQ, Liu W, Park KS, Sachais BS, Arepally GM, Cines DB, Poncz M. Defining a second epitope for heparin-induced thrombocytopenia/thrombosis antibodies using KKO, a murine HIT-like monoclonal antibody. Blood 99: 1230–1236, 2002.

Liu CY, Battaglia M, Lee SH, Sun QH, Aster RH, Visentin GP. Platelet factor 4 differentially modulates CD4+CD25+ (regulatory) versus CD4+CD25- (nonregulatory) T cells. J Immunol 174: 2680–2686, 2005.

Lortat-Jacob H, Grosdidier A, Imberty A. Structural diversity of heparan sulfate binding domains in chemokines. Proc Natl Acad Sci U S A 99: 1229–1234, 2002.

Loscalzo J, Melnick B, Handin RI. The interaction of platelet factor four and glycosaminoglycans. Arch Biochem Biophys 240: 446–455, 1985.

Lowe-Krentz LJ, Joyce JG. Venous and aortic porcine endothelial cells cultured under standardized conditions synthesize heparan sulfate chains which differ in charge. Anal Biochem 193: 155–163, 1991.

Lubenow N, Greinacher A. Hirudin in heparin-induced thrombocytopenia. Semin Thromb Hemost 28: 431–438, 2002.

Marcum JA, Rosenberg RD. Anticoagulantly active heparin-like molecules from vascular tissue. Biochemistry 23: 1730–1737, 1984.

Mayo KH, Chen MJ. Human platelet factor 4 monomer-dimer-tetramer equilibria investigated by 1H NMR spectroscopy. Biochemistry 28: 9469–9478, 1989.

Munnix IC, Cosemans JM, Auger JM, Heemskerk JW. Platelet response heterogeneity in thrombus formation. Thromb Haemost 102: 1149–1156, 2009.

Nader HB, Buonassisi V, Colburn P, Dietrich CP. Heparin stimulates the synthesis and modifies the sulfation pattern of heparan sulfate proteoglycan from endothelial cells. J Cell Physiol 140: 305–310, 1989.

Nassar T, Sachais BS, Akkawi S, Kowalska MA, Bdeir K, Leitersdorf E, Hiss E, Ziporen L, Aviram M, Cines D, Poncz M, Higazi AA. Platelet factor 4 enhances the binding of oxidized low-density lipoprotein to vascular wall cells. J Biol Chem 278: 6187–6193, 2003.

Natelson EA, Lynch EC, Alfrey CP Jr, Gross JB. Heparin-induced thrombocytopenia, An unexpected response to treatment of consumption coagulopathy. Ann Intern Med 71: 1121–1125, 1969.

Nishinaga M, Ozawa T, Shimada K. Homocysteine, a thrombogenic agent, suppresses anticoagulant heparan sulfate expression in cultured porcine aortic endothelial cells. J Clin Invest 92: 1381–1386, 1993.

Parish CR. The role of heparan sulphate in inflammation. Nat Rev Immunol 6: 633–643, 2006.

Patton WA II, Granzow CA, Getts LA, Thomas SC, Zotter LM, Gunzel KA, Lowe-Krentz LJ. Identification of a heparin-binding protein using monoclonal antibodies that block heparin binding to porcine aortic endothelial cells. Biochem J 311 (Pt 2): 461–469, 1995.

Perin JP, Bonnet F, Maillet P, Jolles P. Characterization and N-terminal sequence of human platelet proteoglycan. Biochem J 255: 1007–1013, 1988.

Petersen F, Brandt E, Lindahl U, Spillmann D. Characterization of a neutrophil cell surface glycosaminoglycan that mediates binding of platelet factor 4. J Biol Chem 274: 12376–12382, 1999.

Petricevich VL, Michelacci YM. Proteoglycans synthesized in vitro by nude and normal mouse peritoneal macrophages. Biochim Biophys Acta 1053: 135–143, 1990.

Pitsilos S, Hunt J, Mohler ER, Prabhakar AM, Poncz M, Dawicki J, Khalapyan TZ, Wolfe ML, Fairman R, Mitchell M, Carpenter J, Golden MA, Cines DB, Sachais BS. Platelet factor 4 localization in carotid atherosclerotic plaques: correlation with clinical parameters. Thromb Haemost 90: 1112–1120, 2003.

Poncz M, Surrey S, LaRocco P, Weiss MJ, Rappaport EF, Conway TM, Schwartz E. Cloning and characterization of platelet factor 4 cDNA derived from a human erythroleukemic cell line. Blood 69: 219–223, 1987.

Pötzsch B, Klövekorn W-P, Madlener K. Use of heparin during cardiopulmonary bypass in patients with a history of heparin-induced thrombocytopenia. N Engl J Med 343: 515–515, 2000.

Pouplard C, Iochmann S, Renard B, Herault O, Colombat P, Amiral J, Gruel Y. Induction of monocyte tissue factor expression by antibodies to heparin-platelet factor 4 complexes developed in heparin-induced thrombocytopenia. Blood 97: 3300–3302, 2001.

Rao AK, Niewiarowski S, James P, Holt JC, Harris M, Elfenbein B, Bastl C. Effect of heparin on the in vivo release and clearance of human platelet factor 4. Blood 61: 1208–1214, 1983.

Rauova L, Poncz M, McKenzie SE, Reilly MP, Arepally G, Weisel JW, Nagaswami C, Cines DB, Sachais BS. Ultralarge complexes of PF4 and heparin are central to the pathogenesis of heparin-induced thrombocytopenia. Blood 105: 131–138, 2005.

Rauova L, Zhai L, Kowalska MA, Arepally GM, Cines DB, Poncz M. Role of platelet surface PF4 antigenic complexes in heparin-induced thrombocytopenia pathogenesis: diagnostic and therapeutic implications. Blood 107: 2346–2353, 2006.

Rauova L, Arepally G, McKenzie SE, Konkle BA, Cines DB, Poncz M. Platelet and monocyte antigenic complexes in the pathogenesis of heparin-induced thrombocytopenia (HIT). J Thromb Haemost 7(Suppl 1): 249–252, 2009.

Rauova L, Hirsch JD, Greene TK, Zhai L, Hayes VM, Kowalska MA, Cines DB, Poncz M. Monocyte-bound PF4 in the pathogenesis of heparin-induced thrombocytopenia. Blood 116: 5021–5031, 2010.

Reilly MP, Taylor SM, Hartman NK, Arepally GM, Sachais BS, Cines DB, Poncz M, McKenzie SE. Heparin-induced thrombocytopenia/thrombosis in a transgenic mouse model requires human platelet factor 4 and platelet activation through FcγRIIA. Blood 98: 2442–2447, 2001.

Reilly MP, Taylor SM, Franklin C, Sachais BS, Cines DB, Williams KJ, McKenzie SE. Prothrombotic factors enhance heparin-induced thrombocytopenia and thrombosis in vivo in a mouse model. J Thromb Haemost 4: 2687–2694, 2006.

Rhodes GR, Dixon RH, Silver D. Heparin induced thrombocytopenia with thrombotic and hemorrhagic manifestations. Surg Gynecol Obstet 136: 409–416, 1973.

Romagnani P, Maggi L, Mazzinghi B, Cosmi L, Lasagni L, Liotta F, Lazzeri E, Angeli R, Rotondi M, Filì L, Parronchi P, Serio M, Maggi E, Romagnani S, Annunziato F. CXCR3-mediated opposite effects of CXCL10 and CXCL4 on TH1 or TH2 cytokine production. J Allergy Clin Immunol 116: 1372–1379, 2005.

Rucinski B, Niewiarowski S, Strzyzewski M, Holt JC, Mayo KH. Human platelet factor 4 and its C-terminal peptides: heparin binding and clearance from the circulation. Thromb Haemost 63: 493–498, 1990.

Rybak ME, Gimbrone MA Jr, Davies PF, Handin RI. Interaction of platelet factor four with cultured vascular endothelial cells. Blood 73: 1534–1539, 1989.

Sachais BS, Kuo A, Nassar T, Morgan J, Kariko K, Williams KJ, Feldman M, Aviram M, Shah N, Jarett L, Poncz M, Cines DB, Higazi AA. Platelet factor 4 binds to low-density lipoprotein receptors and disrupts the endocytic machinery, resulting in retention of low-density lipoprotein on the cell surface. Blood 99: 3613–3622, 2002.

Sachais BS, Turrentine T, Dawicki McKenna JM, Rux AH, Rader D, Kowalska MA. Elimination of platelet factor 4 (PF4) from platelets reduces atherosclerosis in C57Bl/6 and apoE–/– mice. Thromb Haemost 98: 1108–1113, 2007.

Sachais BS, Rux AH, Cines DB, Yarovoi SV, Garner LI, Watson SP, Hinds J, Rux JJ. Rational design and characterization of platelet factor 4 antagonists for the study of heparin-induced thrombocytopenia. Blood 119: 5955–5962, 2012.

Schaffner A, Rhyn P, Schoedon G, Schaer DJ. Regulated expression of platelet factor 4 in human monocytes--role of PARs as a quantitatively important monocyte activation pathway. J Leukoc Biol 78: 202–209, 2005.

Selleng K, Schutt A, Selleng S, Warkentin TE, Greinacher A. Studies of the anti-platelet factor 4/heparin immune response: adapting the enzyme-linked immunosorbent spot assay for detection of memory B cells against complex antigens. Transfusion 50: 32–39, 2010.

Shaul PW. Endothelial nitric oxide synthase, caveolae and the development of atherosclerosis. J Physiol 547: 21–33, 2003.

Slungaard A, Key NS. Platelet factor 4 stimulates thrombomodulin protein C-activating cofactor activity, a structure-function analysis. J Biol Chem 269: 25549–25556, 1994.

Slungaard A, Fernandez JA, Griffin JH, Key NS, Long JR, Piegors DJ, Lentz SR. Platelet factor 4 enhances generation of activated protein C in vitro and in vivo. Blood 102: 146–151, 2003.

Stern D, Nawroth P, Marcum J, Handley D, Kisiel W, Rosenberg R, Stern K. Interaction of antithrombin III with bovine aortic segments, role of heparin in binding and enhanced anticoagulant activity. J Clin Invest 75: 272–279, 1985.

Stuckey JA, St Charles R, Edwards BF. A model of the platelet factor 4 complex with heparin. Proteins 14: 277–287, 1992.

Sugahara K, Mikami T, Uyama T, Mizuguchi S, Nomura K, Kitagawa H. Recent advances in the structural biology of chondroitin sulfate and dermatan sulfate. Curr Opin Struct Biol 13: 612–620, 2003.

Suh JS, Aster RH, Visentin GP. Antibodies from patients with heparin-induced thrombocytopenia/thrombosis recognize different epitopes on heparin: platelet factor 4. Blood 91: 916–922, 1998.

Suvarna S, Rauova L, McCracken EK, Goss CM, Sachais BS, McKenzie SE, Reilly MP, Gunn MD, Cines DB, Poncz M, Arepally G. PF4/heparin complexes are T cell-dependent antigens. Blood 106: 929–931, 2005.

Suvarna S, Espinasse B, Qi R, Lubica R, Poncz M, Cines DB, Wiesner MR, Arepally GM. Determinants of PF4/heparin immunogenicity. Blood 110: 4253–4260, 2007.

Suvarna S, Qi R, Hollingsworth JW, Arepally GM. Platelet factor 4-heparin complexes trigger immune responses independently of the MyD88 pathway. Br J Haematol 142: 671–673, 2008.

Talusan P, Bedri S, Yang S, Kattapuram T, Silva N, Roughley PJ, Stone JR. Analysis of intimal proteoglycans in atherosclerosis-prone and atherosclerosis-resistant human arteries by mass spectrometry. Mol Cell Proteomics 4: 1350–1357, 2005.

Turnbull J, Powell A, Guimond S. Heparan sulfate: decoding a dynamic multifunctional cell regulator. Trends Cell Biol 11: 75–82, 2001.

Van de Wouwer M, Collen D, Conway EM. Thrombomodulin-protein C-EPCR system: integrated to regulate coagulation and inflammation. Arterioscler Thromb Vasc Biol 24: 1374–1383, 2004.

Visentin GP, Ford SE, Scott JP, Aster RH. Antibodies from patients with heparin-induced thrombocytopenia/thrombosis are specific for platelet factor 4 complexed with heparin or bound to endothelial cells. J Clin Invest 93: 81–88, 1994.

Visentin GP, Moghaddam M, Beery SE, McFarland JG, Aster RH. Heparin is not required for detection of antibodies associated with heparin-induced thrombocytopenia/thrombosis. J Lab Clin Med 138: 22–31, 2001.

Warkentin TE. Heparin-induced thrombocytopenia: IgG-mediated platelet activation, platelet microparticle generation, and altered procoagulant/anticoagulant balance in the pathogenesis of thrombosis and venous limb gangrene complicating heparin-induced thrombocytopenia. Transfus Med Rev 10: 249–258, 1996.

Warkentin TE, Kelton JG. Temporal aspects of heparin-induced thrombocytopenia. N Engl J Med 344: 1286–1292, 2001.

Warkentin TE, Sheppard JI, Moore JC, Moore KM, Sigouin CS, Kelton JG. Laboratory testing for the antibodies that cause heparin-induced thrombocytopenia: how much class do we need? J Lab Clin Med 146: 341–346, 2005.

Warkentin TE, Sheppard JI, Moore JC, Cook RJ, Kelton JG. Studies of the immune response in heparin-induced thrombocytopenia. Blood 113: 4963–4969, 2009.

Weismann RE, Tobin RW. Arterial embolism occurring during systemic heparin therapy. AMA Arch Surg 76: 219–225, 1958.

Weitz DS, Weitz JI. Update on heparin: what do we need to know? J Thromb Thrombolysis 29: 199–207, 2010.

Williams RT, Damaraju LV, Mascelli MA, Barnathan ES, Califf RM, Simoons ML, Deliargyris EN, Sane DC. Anti-platelet factor 4/heparin antibodies: an independent predictor of 30-day myocardial infarction after acute coronary ischemic syndromes. Circulation 107: 2307–2312, 2003.

Witt DP, Lander AD. Differential binding of chemokines to glycosaminoglycan subpopulations. Curr Biol 4: 394–400, 1994.

Woulfe DS, Lilliendahl JK, August S, Rauova L, Kowalska MA, Abrink M, Pejler G, White JG, Schick BP. Serglycin proteoglycan deletion induces defects in platelet aggregation and thrombus formation in mice. Blood 111: 3458–3467, 2008.

Xiao Z, Visentin GP, Dayananda KM, Neelamegham S. Immune complexes formed following the binding of anti-platelet factor 4 (CXCL4) antibodies to CXCL4 stimulate human neutrophil activation and cell adhesion. Blood 112: 1091–1100, 2008.

Yahalom J, Eldor A, Fuks Z, Vlodavsky I. Degradation of sulfated proteoglycans in the subendothelial extracellular matrix by human platelet heparitinase. J Clin Invest 74: 1842–1849, 1984.

Yu G, Rux AH, Ma P, Bdeir K, Sachais BS. Endothelial expression of e-selectin is induced by the platelet-specific chemokine platelet factor 4 through LRP in an NF-kappaB-dependent manner. Blood 105: 3545–3551, 2005.

Zhang X, Chen L, Bancroft DP, Lai CK, Maione TE. Crystal structure of recombinant human platelet factor 4. Biochemistry 33: 8361–8366, 1994.

Ziporen L, Li ZQ, Park KS, Sabnekar P, Liu WY, Arepally G, Shoenfeld Y, Kieber-Emmons T, Cines DB, Poncz M. Defining an antigenic epitope on platelet factor 4 associated with heparin-induced thrombocytopenia. Blood 92: 3250–3259, 1998.

10 Murine models of heparin-induced thrombocytopenia

Gowthami M. Arepally, Bruce S. Sachais, Douglas B. Cines,
Mortimer Poncz, Lubica Rauova, and Steven E. McKenzie

INTRODUCTION

Heparin-induced thrombocytopenia (HIT) is the most common drug-induced allergy in the western world. Yet, the clinical disorder has little in common with other drug-induced allergic reactions, such as penicillin or sulfa-containing medications. Although hypersensitivity responses to these drugs are rare, idiosyncratic, and long-lived, antibody responses triggered by heparin are common in certain clinical settings (Visentin et al., 1996; Bauer et al., 1997; Pouplard et al., 1999) yet are short-lived (Pötzsch et al., 2000; Warkentin and Kelton, 2001). Presently, it is not known why an immune response occurs so commonly after heparin exposure, why only a subset of antibody-positive patients develop thrombocytopenia and why others develop fulminant thrombotic complications.

Animal models of HIT have been developed in recent years to help address these fundamental biological questions. These studies have been facilitated by the development of reagents (recombinant proteins and monoclonal antibodies) and murine knockout and transgenic mice involving mutations that affect platelet factor 4 (PF4) and Fcγ receptor (FcγR) biology. The first section of this chapter summarizes biological insights gained from individual murine strains with disruption and/or variant expression of components involved in HIT, namely, heparin, PF4, and FcγRs. In the second section, we describe the three defined animal models of HIT, their technical features, strengths, and limitations, and their application to understanding the pathogenesis of HIT.

MURINE STRAINS FOR THE STUDY OF HEPARIN, PF4, AND Fcγ RECEPTOR BIOLOGY

Murine Strains of Heparin Biology

Heparin and related glycosaminoglycans (GAGs), such as heparan sulfate (HS) and chondroitin sulfate (CS) bind PF4 with high affinity and form antigenic complexes that initiate and propagate HIT. The biochemical synthesis of heparin and related GAGs is complex (see chap. 7) and involves a series of enzymatic pathways that regulate synthesis of proteoglycan core protein (Syndecan-1, −2, −3, −4) or contribute to the synthesis or modification of the polysaccharide chain (>7 classes of enzymes are involved in the modification of heparin/HS polysaccharide chains). With the description of the first two murine knockouts of mast cell heparin in 1999 (Forsberg et al., 1999; Humphries et al., 1999), a number of murine strains have been developed to examine the contribution of various HS enzymes to *in vivo* heparin/HS biology.

Due to space limitations, only general descriptions of these animal models will be provided below. For a more comprehensive review of available murine mutant models of HS biosynthesis, the reader is referred to a recent summary by Sarrazin and colleagues (2011).

Strains and Phenotype

Mice lacking mast cell heparin were the first mutant models examining defects in heparin biosynthesis (Forsberg et al., 1999; Humphries et al., 1999). These mice were developed through targeted disruption of N-deacetylase/N-sulfotransferase-2 (*NDST-2*), a sulfotransferase that is required early in the biosynthesis of heparin. NDST-2-null mice are viable and show normal growth and fertility and do not manifest structural abnormalities of heparin/HS or have defective hemostasis, suggesting that other enzymes involved in GAG synthesis can compensate for NDST-2 function. Phenotypic abnormalities in NSDT-2 null mice were restricted to the mast cell lineage, with abnormalities in granule formation and mast cell protease function.

Since these original descriptions, most of the genes involved in HS proteoglycan (HSPG) or polysaccharide biosynthesis have been deleted or mutated in mice. Of the HSPG core proteins, targeted disruptions of genes encoding betaglycan (*Tgfbr3*), perlecan (*Hspg2*), and agrin (*Agrn*) are lethal *in utero* (Sarrazin et al., 2011). Selective deletion of syndecan (–1, –3, or –4), glypican (–1, –3, –4, or 6), or collagen XVIII (*Coll18a1*) produces viable animals, which express a wide-array of phenotypic abnormalities ranging from defective angiogenesis and wound healing, to immune abnormalities and impaired organogenesis (cardiac, neural, renal, and musculoskeletal) (Forsberg and Kjellen, 2001; Sarrazin et al., 2011). Of the enzymes involved in the biosynthesis of heparin/HS polysaccharide chains, genetic deletion of glucuronyltransferase I (*Glcat1*), HS copolymerase (*Ext1/Ext2*), N-deacetylase/N-sulfotransferase-1 (*NDST-1*), uronyl C5 epimerase (*Glce*), uronyl 2-O-sulfotransferase (*H2st*) and glucosaminyl 6-O-sulfotransferase 1 (*H6st1*) lead to embryonic or perinatal lethality. Conditional or tissue-specific knockout strains have also been developed using flox/Cre-recombinase methodology (Orban et al., 1992). Disruption of endothelial specific HS was achieved using mice expressing an endothelial-specific Cre recombinase (*Tie2Cre+*) crossed with mice expressing floxed *Ndst1*$^{f/f}$ gene (Wang et al., 2005). These Ndst1$^{f/f}$/Tie2Cre$^+$ mice exhibit reduced expression of sulfated residues on endothelium [42% in wildtype (WT) *vs* 18% Ndst1$^{f/f}$/Tie2Cre$^+$ mice] and show impairments in chemokine-induced neutrophil infiltration. Relevant to HIT biology, recent studies employed the Ndst1$^{f/f}$/Tie2Cre$^+$ mice show that activated protein C (aPC) generation in the presence of human PF4 (hPF4) did not differ significantly from control murine PF4$^{-/-}$ (mPF4$^{-/-}$) mice, suggesting that endothelial HS is not critical for aPC generation *in vivo* (Kowalska et al., 2011).

Murine Strains of PF4 Biology

PF4 (CXCL4) is a 7.8-kDa chemokine primarily synthesized by megakaryocytes and stored in the platelet α-granules (see chap. 6). PF4 is an essential component of the antigenic complex recognized by HIT antibodies (Amiral et al., 1992; Greinacher et al., 1994). PF4 has been shown to interact with at least two members of the LDL receptor superfamily of receptors (Sachais et al., 2002; Yu et al., 2005), the LDL receptor (LDL-R) and the LDL receptor-related protein (LRP), as well as the chemokine receptor CXCR3B (Lasagni et al., 2003; Struyf et al., 2011). PF4 binding to LDL-R results in retention of LDL on the surface of cells (Sachais et al., 2002), whereas interaction with LRP leads to activation of the transcription factor NF-κB (Yu et al., 2005). While CXCR3B, an alternatively spliced form of the CXCR3 receptor, was also recently identified as a low-affinity functional receptor for PF4 (Lasagni et al., 2003; Struyf et al., 2011), PF4's biological and functional activity is primarily dictated by its high avidity for cell-surface GAGs.

Murine strains lacking mPF4 or overexpressing hPF4 (hPF4^{low}, hPF4^{mid}, and hPF4^{high}) have been developed jointly by the Poncz and McKenzie Laboratories and used extensively to study the pathogenesis of HIT (Reilly et al., 2001; Zhang et al., 2001). These mice are presently available only through the Poncz Laboratory.

The mPF4$^{-/-}$ and hPF4-overexpressing animals are viable and have normal growth and fertility. Neither mPF4$^{-/-}$ mice nor hPF4 overexpressing animals display a spontaneous bleeding or thrombotic tendency or changes *in vitro* hemostatic parameters (tail bleeding time, whole blood clotting time, activated partial thromboplastin time [aPTT], and response to high-dose platelet agonists). An inverse relationship between PF4 expression and circulating platelet counts/megakaryocyte colony numbers is notable in both strains. Mice lacking mPF4 exhibit higher platelet counts (15% as compared with WT) and generate increased numbers of megakaryocyte colonies (40% greater than WT) (Lambert et al., 2007), whereas hPF4 overexpressing transgenic animals show a dose-dependent decrease in platelet counts and megakaryocyte numbers. hPF4^{high} animals have 22 copies of hPF4 transgene/haploid genome and express six times the platelet content of PF4 as human control subjects (Rauova et al., 2006), but have 50% lower platelet counts and megakaryocyte colonies (Lambert et al., 2007). Similarly, hPF4^{mid} (carrying six copies/haploid genome) and hPF4^{low} animals (carrying one transgene/haploid genome) express proportionately reduced PF4 content compared with healthy subjects (twice and half the amount of PF4 relative to healthy subjects, respectively) and manifest milder degree of thrombocytopenia. This inverse relationship between PF4 expression and platelet counts is not due to shortened lifespan, but rather from an inhibitory effect of intramedullary PF4 on megakaryopoiesis (Lambert et al., 2007).

Both knockout and transgenic strains show abnormal responses to vascular injury in response to FeCl$_3$ injury (Eslin et al., 2004). Knockout mice are slower to initiate an occlusive thrombus (10.6 ± 2.9 *vs* 8.7 ± 1.9 minutes for WT mice) and form unstable thrombi (<20% stable occlusive thrombi for mPF4$^{-/-}$ *vs* 85% for WT mice). Infusion of hPF4 (2.5 mg/kg) or another small positively charged protein, protamine sulfate (PS, 1.5–3.0 mg/kg), into mPF4$^{-/-}$ mice restores stable thrombus formation. The hPF4 overexpressing animals also have prolonged times to occlusion and form unstable thrombi (25% stable thrombi *vs* 85% in WT animals) (Eslin et al., 2004). Unlike mPF4$^{-/-}$ mice, which show the expected sensitivity to the anticoagulant effects of heparin, the hPF4 overexpressing animals display unusual dose-dependent responses to heparin. Therapeutic doses of heparin, leading to expected increases in aPTT, enhance thrombus stability in hPF4^{high} animals rather than prolonging the time to occlusion. In these mice, "supratherapeutic" heparin doses are required to impede thrombus formation. One possible explanation is that the formation of stable occlusive thrombi is mediated in large part through charge–charge interactions by the released PF4 neutralizing the anticoagulant (e.g., antithrombin cofactor activity) effects of negatively charged endothelium. When platelets are activated at sites of vascular injury, released PF4 also neutralizes the negatively charged surfaces of platelets and endothelial cells, which may allow closer approximation of platelets to each other and to the endothelial lining, thereby enhancing thrombus formation. In the absence of PF4, cell surfaces retain sufficient negative charge and repulsive forces between endothelial cells and platelets to prevent stable thrombus formation. Conversely, in the presence of excess PF4, endothelial cells may become highly cationic and once again, repulsive forces prevent close approximation of PF4-coated platelets with endothelial cells. In this latter scenario, a therapeutic dose of heparin promotes charge neutralization and affects thrombus stability. As described below ("Murine HITT Model" [p. 260]), the hPF4$^{+/+}$ overexpressing strains have been pivotal in the development of the murine model of HIT (Reilly et al., 2001) and for characterizing the effects of PF4 concentration on disease manifestations.

Murine Strains of FcγR Biology
Some of the important effector functions of IgG antibodies are mediated through binding and cross-linking cell-surface FcγR. FcγRs are highly conserved proteins in mammals and, in humans, are expressed on all hematopoietic cells, with the exception of red cells (Nimmerjahn and Ravetch, 2007) (see chap. 8). Three general classes of FcγRs are expressed on human cells: FcγRI, FcγRII [FcγRIIa (CD32A), FcγRIIB (CD32B), FcγRIIC], FcγRIII [FcγRIIIA (CD16) and FcγRIIIB]. Rodent FcγRs, while similar, are subdivided into four classes: FcγRI, FcγRIIB (CD32B), FcγRIII and FcγRIV (Nimmerjahn and Ravetch, 2007). Murine strains with targeted disruption of the common FcγR γ-chain (Takai et al., 1994), individual receptors (FcγRI) (Barnes et al., 2002; Ioan-Facsinay et al., 2002), FcγRIIB (Takai et al., 1996), FcγRIII (Hazenbos et al., 1996), and FcγRIV (Nimmerjahn et al., 2010) and combined receptors, for example, FcγRI/FcγRIII (Tarzi et al., 2003) and FcγRIV/FcγRIIB (Li and Ravetch, 2011) have been described. Descriptions of each of the phenotypic alterations in these murine strains are beyond the scope of this review. The reader is referred to recent reviews by Nimmerjahn and Ravetch (2007, 2011), summarizing the biological insights gained from *in vivo* disruption or modifications of these genes.

Activation of platelet FcγRIIa is required for the development of HIT (Sheridan et al., 1986; Kelton et al., 1994; Reilly et al., 2001) (see chap. 8). Human platelets express FcγRIIa, but not other FcγRs (FcγRI, III, or FcγRII isoforms, B or C) (Cassel et al., 1993; McKenzie et al., 1999). Because mice do not express platelet FcγRIIa (CD32A) (McKenzie et al., 1999), transgenic mice expressing hFcγRIIA on platelets and macrophages were developed by McKenzie and colleagues (1999) to examine mechanisms of immune-mediated thrombocytopenia and HIT. The human FcγRIIa (hFcγRIIA) mice, expressing the R^{131} isoform, were developed on a C57BL/6J × SJL F1 background and express hFcγRIIA on macrophages and platelets (McKenzie et al., 1999). Platelets from hFcγRIIA mice aggregate in response to cross-linking by immune complexes (McKenzie et al., 1999), whereas platelets from WT mice do not. Injections of antiplatelet antibodies induce severe thrombocytopenia in hFcγRIIA mice, but not in WT or FcR γ-chain deficient mice (γ-KO) (McKenzie et al., 1999). Thrombocytopenia induced by antiplatelet antibodies in hFcγRIIA mice is comparable with mice expressing hFcγRIIA mice on a FcR γ-chain background (hFcγRIIA/γ-KO), suggesting that the contributions of FcγRI, FcγRIII, and FcγRIV to immune-mediated thrombocytopenia *in vivo* can be overcome (McKenzie et al., 1999). When hFcγRIIA/γ-KO mice are injected with a platelet activating antibody (anti-CD9), these mice unlike hFcγRIIA, γ-KO, or WT mice, experience severe thrombocytopenia, shock, and increased mortality in response to anti-CD9. Double-mutant hFcγRIIA/γ-KO or WT mice succumbing to shock from anti-CD9 and evidence of thrombosis and cellular/fibrin aggregates in the pulmonary vasculature (Taylor et al., 2000). The hFcγRIIA transgenic mice are available through Jackson Laboratories (Bar Harbor, Maine). The hFcγRIIA transgenic mice were mated with the various hPF4+/+ overexpressing lines to generate the murine HIT models described below (see section "Murine HITT Model").

DEFINED ANIMAL MODELS OF HIT

Animal models provide insights into *in vivo* disease pathogenesis that could not otherwise be obtained through study of humans. This is clearly the case in HIT, where purposeful manipulation of the PF4/heparin (PF4/H) immune response is not possible in the clinical setting, due to the life-threatening nature of antibodies. Whereas clinical studies provide correlative information and inform hypotheses, animal models allow direct investigation of cause and effect. For HIT, an animal model was the first to provide definitive evidence that PF4/H antibodies are pathogenic and cause both thrombocytopenia and thrombosis *in vivo* (Reilly et al., 2001). Furthermore, HIT models also have permitted systematic investigation of the risk factors contributing to disease pathogenesis, including contributions of PF4 dose, heparin concentrations, hypercholesterolemia, and monocyte activation as disease modifiers in HIT. Finally, HIT models are an excellent platform for investigation of novel therapeutics (Reilly et al., 2012). The following section provides a summary of the three models of HIT that have been described to date, technical considerations, and the major studies that devolved from these murine models. Figure 10.1 provides an overview of the three models

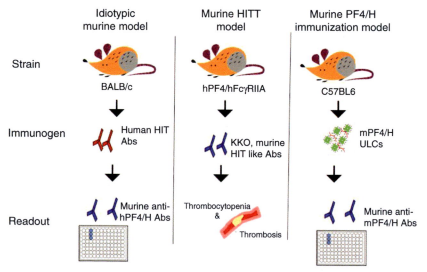

FIGURE 10.1 Salient features of murine models for study of HIT pathogenesis. Diagram shows strains used, primary immunogen, and experimental readout. See Table 10.1 for additional technical details for utilizing murine models. *Abbreviations*: Ab(s), antibody(ies); hFcγRIIA, human Fcγ receptor; HIT, heparin-induced thrombocytopenia; hPF4, human platelet factor 4; hPF4/H, human PF4/heparin; mPF4/H ULCs, murine PF4/heparin ultra-large complexes.

TABLE 10.1 Murine Models of Heparin-induced Thrombocytopenia

Animal model (Original description)	Description	Strain (s)	Immunogen/ stimulant	Optimized immunization strategy	Technical notes	Relevant findings with the model
Idiotypic murine model (Blank et al., 1997)	Based on disruption of idiotypic networks	BALB/c (14 wk age)	Human polyclonal IgG from human HIT patients and/or control subjects	Optimized strategy based on following report (Blank et al., 1997): *Immunization strategy:* • 1st Immunization: 20 µg IgG in CFA intradermal injections (hind foot pads) • Booster 14 days later with 20 µg IgG in PBS *To elicit clinical disease after PF4/H antibodies develop:* • UFH (5 U/mouse) sc daily for 4 days or • LMWH (Clexane) 0.02 mg/mouse sc	• Mouse anti-hPF4/H (Ab3) detected 2 mo after booster immunization • mice develop thrombocytopenia upon UFH, but not with LMWH • No thrombosis described	• Ab3 specific for hPF4/H • Mice develop thrombocytopenia with UFH but not LMWH (Blank et al., 1997).
Murine HITT model (Reilly et al., 2001)	Infusion of a HIT-like antibody to induce thrombocytopenia and thrombosis	Double transgenic mice (hPF4+/ hFcγRIIA+) on a mPF4 null C57BL/6J x SJL F1 background	KKO, a murine HIT-like monoclonal antibody + heparin	Optimized strategy based on following reports (Rauova et al., 2006; Reilly et al., 2012): • KKO 20–40 mg/kg (~200–400 µg/mouse) diluted in 200 µL sterile PBS, IP once on day 0. • Heparin 1200–1600 mg/ kg (~20–30 U/mouse) injected sc X 4 days, starting day 0.	• Clinical phenotype for thrombocytopenia and thrombosis requires KKO, hPF4, hFcγRIIA and heparin. • Thrombocytopenia with KKO can occur in the absence of heparin in hPF4^high/hFcγRIIA mice. • Heparin exacerbates thrombocytopenia and thrombosis	• Degree of thrombocytopenia is dependent on platelet hPF4 expression (Rauova et al., 2006) • Monocyte depletion results in exacerbation of thrombocytopenia; prothrombotic effects of HIT antibodies require monocytes (Rauova et al., 2010)

(continued)

TABLE 10.1 *(continued)* Murine Models of Heparin-induced Thrombocytopenia

Animal model (Original description)	Description	Strain (s)	Immunogen/ stimulant	Optimed immunization strategy	Technical notes	Relevant findings with the model
						• Inhibition of FcγRIIa signalling via syk abrogates thrombocytopenia and thrombosis (Reilly et al., 2012)
Murine PF4/H immunization model (Suvarna et al., 2005)	Immunization with mPF4/H complexes to elicit anti-mPF4/H Abs	BALB/c and C57BL/6J	mPF4/H complexes	Optimized strategy based on following report (Suvarna et al., 2009): • mPF4 100 µg/mL mixed with 5 U/mL heparin in sterile HBSS and injected into mice daily by RO × 5 days	• Development of murine anti-PF4/H Abs seen at 8–15 days from start of immunization • Abs are specific for mPF4/H and activate hFcγRIIA platelets • Mice do not develop thrombocytopenia or thrombosis	• T-cells are required for anti-PF4/H Ab production *in vivo* • PF4/H immune response not MyD88 dependent • Immune response is heparin-dependent

Abbreviations: Ab, antibody; CFA, complete Freund's adjuvant; HBSS, Hank's balanced salt solution; IP, intraperitoneal; LMWH, low molecular weight heparin; PF4/H, PF4/ heparin; PBS, phosphate-buffered saline; RO, retroorbital; sc, subcutaneous; UFH, unfractionated heparin.

and Table 10.1 provides a detailed summary with technical notes and applications of the various models.

Two distinct approaches have been described for modeling HIT *in vivo*. The first approach, which was used in the idiotypic immunization model and the murine HITT model, relies on passive administration of HIT or HIT-like antibodies to study the pathogenesis of thrombocytopenia and thrombosis. The second approach utilizes intravenous injections of mPF4/H complexes to study mechanisms of HIT antibody induction. At present, no model recapitulates the full disease spectrum from antibody induction to clinical manifestations of thrombocytopenia and thrombosis.

Idiotype Immunization Model
Description of the Model
The first murine model of HIT was developed by Shoenfeld and colleagues (Blank et al., 1997) and relied on manipulation of the immune idiotypic network (Jerne, 1974) using human HIT antibodies. The idiotypic network is a regulatory network of antibodies that arise in response to antigenic determinants on a given immunoglobulin variable region (idiotype). An idiotype occurring on one antibody (Ab1) elicits an antibody (anti-idiotype or Ab2) that recognizes determinants expressed on Ab1. This may generate anti–anti-idiotype antibodies (Ab3 and so on) that mirror the idiotypes on Ab1. Shoenfeld and colleagues have shown that the idiotypic network can be experimentally manipulated in animals by injecting human autoantibodies (Ab1) from patients with systemic lupus erythematosus (SLE) (Mendlovic et al., 1990) or Wegener's granulomatosis (Shoenfeld et al., 1995) to generate murine autoantibodies (Ab3) with the specificities of the immunizing human autoantibody (Ab1). This strategy was applied to HIT by injecting BALB/c mice with human HIT IgG repetitively over several weeks (Table 10.1). Murine anti-hPF4/H antibodies developed 1–2 months after initial/booster immunization with HIT-IgG, but not control IgG, bound to hPF4/H specifically, and were competitively inhibited by the immunizing HIT-IgG (Blank et al., 1997). When seropositive mice were given unfractionated heparin (UFH, 5 U/mouse/day × 4 days) or low molecular weight heparin (LMWH, 20 µg/mouse/day × 4 days), UFH, but not LMWH, elicited thrombocytopenia (40% decline relative to WT animals) in sensitized mice (Blank et al., 1997).

Strengths and Limitations of the Idiotype Model
The idiotype model was the first to demonstrate, albeit indirectly, the pathogenicity of HIT antibodies *in vivo*. However, a number of theoretical and technical limitations have limited its further development. The role of idiotypic regulation in the generation of antigen-specific immunity remains controversial (Cohn, 1986) and to what extent anti-idiotypic antibodies in this model mirror the specificities of primary pathogenic antibodies remains unknown. Second, as WT mice lack platelet FcγRIIa, the mechanism for thrombocytopenia in this model cannot be fully explained. Finally, several technical limitations of this murine model limit its utility and applicability in HIT, including use of polyclonal IgG from HIT patients, rather than antigen-specific IgG; use of Freund's adjuvant to boost antibody production; and the time required for *in vivo* antibody production (more than two months).

Applications of This Model for Understanding HIT Pathogenesis
After the original description, there have been no reported studies using this model for studies of HIT pathogenesis. The idiotype model has been supplanted by the murine HIT-thrombosis (HITT) model described below.

Murine HITT Model

Description of Model

The murine HITT model was developed to study the pathogenic effects of HIT antibodies *in vivo*. First described in 2001 by the McKenzie Laboratory (Reilly et al., 2001), the model has undergone additional modifications in collaboration with the Poncz Laboratory. The murine HITT model was developed by crossing two humanized transgenic lines (the hPF4 overexpressing strain crossed with the hFcγRIIA strain) on a C57BL6/J × SJL F1 background to create a double transgenic line expressing both hPF4/hFcγRII. These double transgenic mice are viable and show no abnormal developmental features. In later studies, both groups have developed the mice on an mPF4 null background to remove the confounding effects of mPF4 co-expression. Double transgenic mice are given injections of a murine HIT-like monoclonal antibody (KKO, 200 µg/mL) (Arepally et al., 2000) or isotype control intraperitoneally on first day of immunization (D0). Platelet counts are measured at baseline and days 1, 2, 3, 4, and 7 following antibody injection. Mild-to-moderate thrombocytopenia (30–40% reduction from baseline platelet counts) can be induced in the absence of heparin in strains overexpressing intermediate to high levels of hPF4 (hPF4^{high}/hFcγRIIA). Exposure to subcutaneous heparin (20 U/day) daily for five days exacerbates and extends the duration of thrombocytopenia (>80% compared with WT) 1–3 days after initiation of heparin therapy) (Reilly et al., 2001). Exposure to higher doses of heparin generates thrombi in the pulmonary vasculature (Reilly et al., 2001). By contrast, injections of KKO into single transgenic mice (hPF4$^{+/+}$ alone or hFcγRIIA alone) or WT mice does not elicit thrombocytopenia or thrombosis.

Strengths and Limitations of the Murine HITT Model

The murine HITT model was the first animal model to unequivocally demonstrate the pathogenicity of anti-PF4/H antibodies (Arepally et al., 2000) *in vivo*. Specifically, this model showed the critical importance of antigen (hPF4 and heparin), the platelet FcγRIIa, and HIT antibodies in recapitulating disease biology. One limitation of this model is its reliance on preformed HIT antibodies, especially the monoclonal HIT-like antibody, KKO, in studying manifestations of thrombocytopenia and thrombosis (Rauova et al., 2006, 2010; Reilly et al., 2006). Injection of polyclonal human HIT antibodies purified from well-characterized patients also causes thrombocytopenia and thrombosis in these mice, but the availability and volumes of patient derived material is often limiting (unpublished observations). Due to the need for passive infusion of HIT antibodies, this model has not been used to study the ontogeny of the immune response to explain how antibodies evolve in the host pathologically.

Applications of This Model for Understanding HIT Pathogenesis

The murine HITT model has been utilized extensively in recent years to study the contribution of host risk factors in the sentinel clinical manifestations of thrombocytopenia and thrombosis:

a) Role of PF4 level: HIT antibodies recognize antigenic complexes that form on various cell surfaces through binding of PF4 to GAGs, such as CS and HS (Tannenbaum et al., 1986; Horne, 1993; Visentin et al., 1994; Arepally et al., 2000; Rauova et al., 2006). Using the murine HITT model, Rauova and colleagues (2006) demonstrated the importance of cell surface–bound PF4 and PF4 levels on HIT antibody- mediated effects *in vivo*. To examine the role of surface-bound PF4 and PF4 levels, double transgenic mice expressing hFcγRIIA and varying amounts of hPF4 (hPF4^{low}, hPF4^{mid}, and hPF4^{high}) were developed. When these transgenic lines, expressing different levels of hPF4, were exposed to the same dose of the murine HIT-like antibody, KKO, without heparin, clear dose-dependent effects were seen. PF4^{high}/hFcγRIIA mice developed severe thrombocytopenia (80% decline from baseline platelet counts) within three hours of antibody administration, whereas hPF4^{mid}/hFcγRIIA developed the same nadir (80% decline from BL platelet counts), but manifested a shorter duration of thrombocytopenia (4 days *vs* 5–7 days for hPF4^{high}/hFcγRIIA). hPF4^{low}/hFcγRIIA, on the other hand, developed more moderate thrombocytopenia (40% decline from baseline platelet counts), in the absence of heparin, and had a shorter duration of thrombocytopenia (three to four days). Heparin administration (20 U/day × 4 days) along with KKO prolonged the duration of thrombocytopenia in hPF4^{mid}/hFcγRIIA (from 4 to >7 days). Pre-treatment of these same animals with high dose heparin (100 U/kg) or protamine sulfate (PS, 2 mg/kg) prior to KKO abrogated the thrombocytopenia, suggesting that charge-dependent interactions of PF4 with cell-surface GAGs (Lambert et al., 2007) contributes significantly to the pathogenicity of HIT antibodies *in vivo*.

b) Role of hypercholesterolemia: Host factors, such as arterial/venous injury (Boshkov et al., 1993; Hong et al., 2003) and cardiovascular disease (Boshkov et al., 1993; Williams et al., 2003) predispose individuals to complications of HIT. To examine the contribution of vascular disease in HIT, Reilly and colleagues (2006) studied the effects of a proatherogenic diet in the murine HITT model. Murine HIT mice (hPF4^{mid}/hFcγRIIA) were given a standard diet (SD) or a hypercholesterolemic diet (HD) for four weeks to induce hypercholesterolemia. Mice given a HD developed the expected threefold increase in plasma cholesterol, which was accompanied by increased platelet reactivity and endothelial cell activation. Specifically, hypercholesterolemic hPF4^{mid}/hFcγRIIA mice injected with KKO and heparin developed more profound thrombocytopenia, higher thrombin–antithrombin (TAT) levels and histological evidence of thrombosis, whereas murine HIT mice on a standard chow developed moderate thrombocytopenia (43% ± 5% *vs* 17.4% ± 3.3% of baseline platelet counts) and no evidence of thrombosis was seen. These studies suggest that hypercholesterolemia and the resultant vascular hyperreactivity exacerbate the prothrombotic effects of HIT antibodies *in vivo*.

c) Role of monocytes: Activated monocytes express cellular tissue factor (TF), a physiological source of thrombin generation (Gregory and Edgington, 1985). Although HIT antibodies from patients can bind to monocytes and trigger TF activity *in vitro* (Arepally and Mayer, 2001; Pouplard et al., 2001), the extent to which monocytes contribute to the *in vivo* pathogenesis of HIT was not known, until studies were performed in the murine HIT model (Rauova et al., 2010). The relative binding of KKO and PF4 to monocytes was more than eightfold higher than to platelets, even after adjusting for differences in surface area. These *in vitro* differences in HIT antibody binding were accompanied by profound biological consequences. When murine HITT mice are injected with liposomal clodronate (an intracellular toxin, which causes transient depletion of monocytes for three days; Sunderkötter et al., 2004), mice develop profound and protracted thrombocytopenia in response to KKO (nadir of >80% reduction from baseline platelet counts from 3 to 48 hours after KKO injection) compared with animals injected with KKO and control liposomes (nadir of ~30% reduction from baseline platelet counts) (Rauova et al., 2010). Similar findings were seen using gadolinium chloride to selectively inactivate macrophage function. The finding of more severe thrombocytopenia in the murine HITT model when monocytes were depleted was unexpected, as monocytes were predicted to enhance platelet clearance. These findings may be explained by the *in vitro* observations of enhanced binding of HIT antibodies to monocytes relative to platelets, suggesting that monocytes provide an important *in vivo* cellular reservoir for binding of HIT antibodies. Elimination of this important cellular reservoir leads to increased antibody binding to platelets and more profound thrombocytopenia.

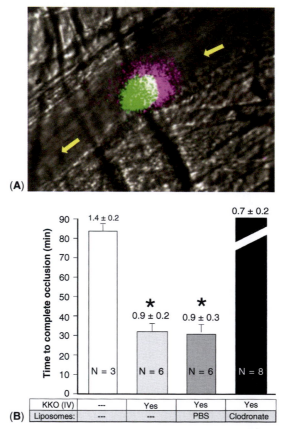

FIGURE 10.2 Role of monocytes in heparin-induced thrombocytopenia. **(A)** Intravital microscopy of arteriole injury for showing the accumulation of CD115-labeled monocytes and/or microparticles at the upstream end of a growing thrombus. Platelets appear green, monocytes pink, and the overlap white. The yellow arrow denotes the direction of blood flow. **(B)** Times to complete occlusion in a photochemical carotid artery model in FcγRIIa/hPF4 mice after clodronate- or PBS-laden liposomes infusion in the presence or absence of KKO. The platelet counts at the time of study are indicated above each bar and is per 10^9/mL. *N* values are noted in the figures. *$P < 0.001$ for time to occlusion relative to mice not receiving either KKO or liposomes. Abbreviations: IV, intravenous; PBS, phosphate-buffered saline *Source*: From Rauova et al. (2010).

Monocyte depletion also had surprising effects on prothrombotic tendency as evident in the murine HITT model. As shown in Figure 10.2A, monocytes are recruited to growing thrombi in the presence of KKO. Therefore, monocyte depletion was expected to enhance KKO binding to platelets and enhance thrombus formation. However, a contrary outcome was seen. These findings were demonstrated through studies of photochemical injury using rose bengal in mice with or depleted of monocytes. When double transgenic HIT mice at baseline are subjected to photochemical injury, thrombus formation—as measured by time to occlusion of a Doppler probe—occurs in 86 ± 10 minutes (Fig. 10.2B). KKO infusion in these same mice significantly shortens the occlusion time (35 ± 8 minutes, $P < 0.0005$ for baseline *vs* KKO infusion; Figure 10.2B), despite a 60% reduction in platelet count. However, if monocytes are depleted from the double transgenic mice with clodronate, KKO infusion results in severe thrombocytopenia and marked prolongation of occlusion time (>90 minutes). The prolongation of occlusion time in the setting of monocyte depletion was not due to thrombocytopenia, as other HIT mice developed a similar degree of thrombocytopenia after KKO infusion and manifested a shortened occlusion time, suggesting that monocytes

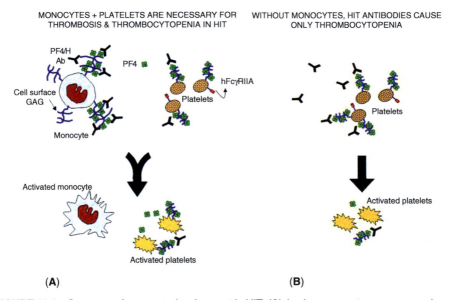

(A)　　　　　　　　　　　　　　　　　(B)

FIGURE 10.3 Summary of monocyte involvement in HIT: (**A**) *In vivo*, monocytes serve as an important cellular reservoir for HIT antibody binding. Monocytes express abundant cell-surface GAGs, which can form antigenic complexes that preferentially bind HIT antibodies. HIT antibodies also bind to PF4 bound to platelet cell-surface GAGs. HIT antibody binding triggers monocyte activation with subsequent upregulation of TF activity and contributes to thrombin generation seen in HIT. Platelet activation by HIT antibodies leads to platelet activation and consumption and contributes to thrombocytopenia alone. (**B**) Monocyte depletion leads to removal of an important cellular reservoir for HIT antibody binding. Circulating HIT antibodies now only bind to platelets, leading to platelet activation/consumption. There is no thrombin generation in the absence of monocytes. Abbreviations: Ab, antibody; GAG, glycosaminoglycans; hFcγRIIA, human FcγIIa receptor; HIT, heparin-induced thrombocytopenia; PF4, platelet factor 4; PBS, phosphate-buffered saline; PF4/H, platelet factor 4/heparin; TF, tissue factor.

account for the differences in prothrombotic tendency in the presence of KKO. Taken together, these findings indicate a major role for monocytes in the pathogenesis of HIT (Fig. 10.3). Monocytes not only provide a cellular reservoir for binding of HIT antibodies, but also serve as a critical cellular intermediary for thrombin generation (Rauova et al., 2010).

d) Effects of Syk inhibition: As described above, the murine HITT model definitively established the importance of the human receptor FcγRIIa in the pathogenesis of HIT. Binding of HIT antibodies to platelet FcγRIIa initiates intracellular signaling through a variety of nonreceptor protein tyrosine kinases, including spleen tyrosine kinase (Syk) (Poole et al., 1997). The role of Syk inhibition was examined recently in the murine HIT model using PRT-060318 (PRT318, Portola Pharmaceuticals, S. San Francisco, California, U.S.A.), a novel and highly specific Syk inhibitor (Reilly et al., 2012). PRT318 potently inhibited platelet activation *in vitro* by diverse agonists that act through FcγRIIa, including convulxin (via GPVI/FcRγ), anti-CD9 (a murine platelet activating antibody) and KKO. PRT318, however, did not inhibit platelet activation by adenosine diphosphate (ADP) or thrombin, which signal through G-protein coupled receptors. The effects of Syk inhibition were examined *in vivo* using the murine HIT model in the presence of KKO and heparin. Vehicle-treated mice, developed the expected thrombocytopenia after injection of KKO and heparin, but PRT318-treated mice showed no significant change in platelet counts (47.8% ± 10.1% of baseline platelet counts for vehicle treated vs 89.7% ± 3.69% of baseline for PRT318 mice; $P < 0.004$). Near-infrared imaging of lung tissue showed dramatic differences in thrombus development (Fig. 10.4). As shown in Figure 10.4, vehicle treated mice showed widely dispersed thrombi of different sizes in the lung vasculature as compared with

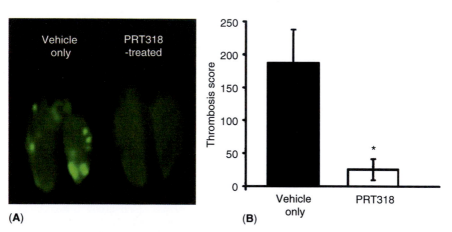

(A)   (B)

FIGURE 10.4 HIT immune complex-mediated thrombosis *in vivo*. HITT model mice treated with the HIT-like antibody KKO with Syk inhibitor, PRT318 or vehicle. Platelets from donor mice were isolated, labeled with Alexa750-labeled antibodies to GPIX and injected into HITT model mice 1 hr before challenge with heparin (1400 U/kg, subcutaneously). Lungs were extracted and scanned on a Li-COR Odyssey at 780 nm. **(B)** The Thrombosis Score reflects the product of the mean thrombus area (square pixels) and the mean number of thrombi (defined by a signal intensity that is 1.5-fold above the background). The Thrombosis Score is significantly different in vehicle only-treated mice (score 186.9) *versus* PRT318-treated mice (score 25.7). *P <0.03. Abbreviations: HIT, heparin-induced thrombocytopenia; HITT, HIT-thrombosis. *Source*: From Reilly et al. (2012).

mice treated with PRT318. These studies demonstrate that inhibition of FcγRIIa-Syk signaling with PRT318 or related compounds might serve as a therapeutic target for human HIT.

Murine PF4/heparin Immunization Model
Description of the Model
The mPF4/H immunization model was developed to understand the cellular basis of the anti-PF4/H immune response *in vivo*. This model was based on the rationale that anti-PF4/H antibodies in humans develop upon exposure to endogenous hPF4 complexed to heparin (Amiral et al., 1992), that sensitization is dramatically enhanced in settings associated with high circulating levels of PF4 and heparin, such as cardiopulmonary bypass (CPB) (Bauer et al., 1997) and that mPF4 shares significant homology with hPF4 (>75%) (Arepally et al., 2000). As described in Table 10.1, the optimized murine model utilizes WT BL6 mice (lacking platelet FcγRIIa) receiving daily injections of mPF4/H (100 µg/mL PF4 and 5 U/mL heparin) for five days (D1–5) without use of adjuvant. Antibodies to mPF4/H develop 8–15 days (D8–15) from the start of immunization, are transient and share a number of relevant biological properties with human anti-PF4/H antibodies (anti-hPF4/H), including antigen specificity, heparin-dependent binding, and capacity to activate platelets expressing FcγRIIa *in vitro* (Suvarna et al., 2005, 2009).

Strengths and Limitations of the Murine PF4/H Immunization Model
The strengths of the murine immunization model are in its ability to recapitulate essential features of the affector limb of the HIT immune response. In so doing, this model allows investigators to examine the cellular and antigenic basis that initiates and sustains immune response and facilitates fundamental studies of the immune response that are not possible in humans. However, a major limitation of this model is that seropositive mice do not develop thrombocytopenia. These findings are presumed to be due to lack of the hFcγIIA receptor, as the immunization model was developed in WT mice (Suvarna et al., 2009). However, additional risk factors, possibly the presence of circulating antigenic complexes, inflammation and/or vascular disease, are critical to develop thrombocytopenia and thrombosis.

Applications of This Model for Understanding HIT Immune Pathogenesis
As shown in Table 10.1, this novel animal model has been instrumental in studying various antigenic properties and cellular requirements to generate anti-PF4/H antibodies.

a) Cellular requirements for HIT antibody formation: Although HIT is a drug-induced immunological disorder, it has certain atypical features in that the immune response against PF4/H occurs commonly, often shows dose-dependence, and is immunologically transient. These atypical features have led to the speculation about the cellular origins of HIT, and specifically whether T-cells are essential for the immune response. The first application of the model was to address the role of T-cells in the HIT immune response. Nude mice, congenitally lacking T-cells, and WT animals were injected with mPF4/H complexes or DNP-Ficoll, a T-cell independent antigen that triggers anti-DNP antibodies in the absence of T-cells. WT mice injected with mPF4/H complexes developed anti-mPF4/H antibodies, but nude mice did not. By contrast, both athymic and euthymic mice injected with DNP-Ficoll developed antigen-specific responses

(Suvarna et al., 2005), providing strong preliminary support for a T-cell requirement in HIT. The murine immunization model has also facilitated studies of the mechanisms of cellular activation by PF4/H complexes. Specifically, the role of Toll-like receptors (TLRs), a family of pattern recognition receptors (PRRs), was examined through studies of MyD88 deficient mice. Engaging TLRs on antigen-presenting cells (APCs) activates various intracellular signaling cascades through a common adaptor protein, myeloid differentiation primary response gene 88 (MyD88) (Takeda et al., 2003). To determine if TLRs contribute to anti-PF4/H antibody production *in vivo*, MyD88$^{-/-}$, MyD88$^{+/-}$, and WT mice were immunized with mPF4/H complexes and antibody production was followed over time. There were no differences in frequency or intensity of seroconversion among the various cohorts, suggesting that PF4/H complexes do not trigger immune activation through MyD88-dependent TLRs. Finally, recent studies demonstrate that PF4/H complexes, but not PF4 alone, trigger dendritic cells to express increased levels of the cytokines IL-12 (Chudasama et al., 2010) and interferon-γ (unpublished studies from the Arepally Laboratory).

b) Heparin dependence of the immune response: As described in chapters 6, 7, and 9, recent studies have shown that cationic PF4 and anionic heparin assemble to form ultra-large complexes (ULCs) through electrostatic interactions—optimal complex formation occurs at PF4/H molar ratios associated with charge neutralization (Rauova et al., 2005; Greinacher et al., 2006; Suvarna et al., 2007). However, if either compound is in molar excess, complex size is diminished in proportion to the amount of excess net repulsive forces present in solution (Rauova et al., 2005; Greinacher et al., 2006; Suvarna et al., 2007). To determine if HIT antibody formation was similarly dependent on heparin and ULCs, Suvarna and colleagues (2007) used the murine immunization model to study the immunizing effects of mPF4/H complexes formed at various PF4/H molar ratios. Mice were injected with a fixed concentration of mPF4 (100 μg/mL) and varying amounts of heparin (0.25, 0.5, 5, or 50 U/mL) to yield PF4:H molar ratios of 20:1, 10:1, 1:1, and 1:10. Robust seroconversions were seen with PF4 in molar excess (20:1 and 10:1>1:1), but not when heparin was in molar excess (1:10; see Figure 10.5) (Suvarna et al., 2007). These studies were the first to demonstrate that the immunogenicity of PF4/H complexes *in vivo* was heparin-dependent and that the variability seen in human seroconversions may be explained, in part, by differences in the composition of PF4/H complexes.

c) Immunostimulatory effects of heparin-containing complexes: The murine immunization model has also been successfully applied to studying the immunizing effects of other heparin-binding proteins, such as PS and lysozyme (LYS). PS (MW 4100 and pI = 12) (Balhorn, 2007) and LYS (MW 14 kDa, pI = 10.5) (Blake et al., 1965) are two basic proteins that bind heparin with high affinity and form heparin-dependent complexes (Rossmann et al., 1982; van de Weert et al., 2004). Mice immunized with PS/heparin (PS/H) and LYS-heparin (LYS/H) complexes using the immunization strategy for mPF4/H complexes (Chudasama et al., 2010) developed antigen-specific antibodies (to PS/H or LYS/H, respectively), whereas animals did not mount a response to soluble antigen PS or LYS alone. The murine antibodies to PS/H or LYS/H were specific for each antigen and were not cross-reactive with other heparin-dependent complexes [e.g., anti-PS/H did not bind to PF4/H, Lys/H, or bovine serum albumin (BSA), and others]. The similarity in the *in vivo* responses to PF4/H, PS/H, and LYS/H

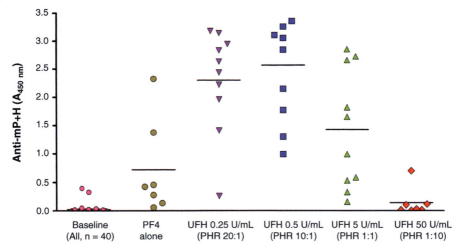

FIGURE 10.5 Immune response to PF4/H complexes is heparin-dependent. BL6 mice were injected with mPF4 and UFH at various concentrations and antibodies to mPF4/H (mP + H) were assayed. Cohorts (n = 7/cohort for PF4 alone, and UFH 50 U/mL; n = 10/cohort for other conditions) were injected with mPF4 (100 μg/mL) alone or in combination with heparin at various PF4:H molar ratios (PHRs, from left to right after PF4 alone, 20:1, 10:1, 1:1, and 1:10). *Abbreviations*: UFH, unfractionated heparin. *Source*: From Suvarna et al. (2007).

complexes suggest that heparin's immunostimulatory effect is in large part mediated by the biophysical attributes of heparin-containing ULCs. The murine studies with PS/H suggested the possibility that humans exposed to PS/H complexes could become similarly sensitized to this antigen. Because humans undergoing CPB receive large doses of PS and heparin, patients undergoing CPB were examined for the development of antibodies to PS/H. Plasma from normal subjects (n = 45) and CPB patients (n = 15) prior to surgery and five days after surgery showed minimal reactivity in the PS/H enzyme immunoassay. However, anti-PS/H antibody levels were significantly elevated in ~27% by 30 days after CPB (Chudasama et al., 2010). Similar to the outcome of the murine studies, seropositive patients recognized PS/H preferentially over PS alone (p = ns) and showed minimal cross-reactivity with other heparin-containing antigens ($P < 0.001$ for PS/H *vs* BSA, LYS, LYS/H, or hPF4/H). The discovery of this new class of anti-PS/H antibodies in humans highlights the translational potential of murine models in studying human disease.

SUMMARY

Studies of murine HIT models have provided insights into the pathogenesis of HIT that could otherwise not be modeled in humans. Reagents, such as KKO, a murine monoclonal HIT-like antibody and availability of murine knockout and transgenic (hPF4 and hFcγRIIA) mice have facilitated the development of a murine HITT model to study the mechanisms underlying thrombocytopenia and thrombosis. Studies with this HITT model have shown the importance of hPF4 dose, hypercholesterolemia, and monocyte activation in the pathogenesis of thrombocytopenia and thrombosis. The parallel development of an active immunization model has facilitated studies of host responses to antigen and investigations of the cellular basis of the HIT immune response. As yet, existing murine models do not model the full biology of HIT disease (from immune induction to thrombocytopenia/ thrombosis). However, given the availability of reagents, techniques and various murine strains, it is expected that this limitation will be overcome in the near future and will likely provide additional insights into the pathogenesis of HIT.

REFERENCES

Amiral J, Bridey F, Dreyfus M, Vissoc AM, Fressinaud E, Wolf M, Meyer D. Platelet factor 4 complexed to heparin is the target for antibodies generated in heparin-induced thrombocytopenia. Thromb Haemost 68: 95–96, 1992.

Arepally GM, Mayer IM. Antibodies from patients with heparin-induced thrombocytopenia stimulate monocytic cells to express tissue factor and secrete interleukin-8. Blood 98: 1252–1254, 2001.

Arepally GM, Kamei S, Park KS, Kamei K, Li ZQ, Liu W, Siegel DL, Kisiel W, Cines DB, Poncz M. Characterization of a murine monoclonal antibody that mimics heparin-induced thrombocytopenia antibodies. Blood 95: 1533–1540, 2000.

Balhorn R. The protamine family of sperm nuclear proteins. Genome Biol 8: 227, 2007.

Barnes N, Gavin AL, Tan PS, Mottram P, Koentgen F, Hogarth PM. FcγRI-deficient mice show multiple alterations to inflammatory and immune responses. Immunity 16: 379–389, 2002.

Bauer TL, Arepally G, Konkle BA, Mestichelli B, Shapiro SS, Cines DB, Poncz M, McNulty S, Amiral J, Hauck WW, Edie RN, Mannion JD. Prevalence of heparin-associated antibodies without thrombosis in patients undergoing cardiopulmonary bypass surgery. Circulation 95: 1242–1246, 1997.

Blake CC, Koenig DF, Mair GA, North AC, Phillips DC, Sarma VR. Structure of hen egg-white lysozyme. a three-dimensional Fourier synthesis at 2 Angstrom resolution. Nature 206: 757–761, 1965.

Blank M, Cines DB, Arepally G, Eldor A, Afek A, Shoenfeld Y. Pathogenicity of human anti-platelet factor 4 (PF4)/heparin in vivo: generation of mouse anti-PF4/heparin and induction of thrombocytopenia by heparin. Clin Exp Immunol 108: 333–339, 1997.

Boshkov LK, Warkentin TE, Hayward CPM, Andrew M, Kelton JG. Heparin-induced thrombocytopenia and thrombosis: clinical and laboratory studies. Br J Haematol 84: 322–328, 1993.

Cassel DL, Keller MA, Surrey S, Schwartz E, Schreiber AD, Rappaport EF, McKenzie SE. Differential expression of FcγRIIA, FcγRIIB and FcγRIIC in hematopoietic cells: analysis of transcripts. Mol Immunol 30: 451–460, 1993.

Chudasama SL, Espinasse B, Hwang F, Qi R, Joglekar M, Afonina G, Wiesner MR, Welsby IJ, Ortel TJ, Arepally GM. Heparin modifies the immunogenicity of positively-charged proteins. Blood 116: 6046–6053, 2010.

Cohn M. The concept of functional idiotype network for immune regulation mocks all and comforts none. Ann Inst Pasteur Immunol 137C: 64–76, 1986.

Eslin DE, Zhang C, Samuels KJ, Rauova L, Zhai L, Niewiarowski S, Cines DB, Poncz M, Kowalska MA. Transgenic mice studies demonstrate a role for platelet factor 4 in thrombosis: dissociation between anticoagulant and antithrombotic effect of heparin. Blood 104: 3173–3180, 2004.

Forsberg E, Kjellen L. Heparan sulfate: lessons from knockout mice. J Clin Invest 108: 175–180, 2001.

Forsberg E, Pejler G, Ringvall M, Lunderius C, Tomasini-Johansson B, Kusche-Gullberg M, Eriksson I, Ledin J, Hellman L, Kjellén L. Abnormal mast cells in mice deficient in a heparin-synthesizing enzyme. Nature 400: 773–776, 1999.

Gregory SA, Edgington TS. Tissue factor induction in human monocytes. Two distinct mechanisms displayed by different alloantigen-responsive T cell clones. J Clin Invest 76: 2440–2445, 1985.

Greinacher A, Pötzsch B, Amiral J, Dummel V, Eichner A, Mueller-Eckhardt C. Heparin-associated thrombocytopenia: isolation of the antibody and characterization of a multi-molecular PF4-heparin complex as the major antigen. Thromb Haemost 71: 247–251, 1994.

Greinacher A, Gopinadhan M, Günther JU, Omer-Adam MA, Strobel U, Warkentin TE, Papastavrou G, Weitschies W, Helm CA. Close approximation of two platelet factor 4 tetramers by charge neutralization forms the antigens recognized by HIT antibodies. Arterioscler Thromb Vasc Biol 26: 2386–2393, 2006.

Hazenbos WLW, Gessner JE, Hofhuis FMA, Kuipers H, Meyer D, Heijnen IA, Schmidt RE, Sandor M, Capel PJ, Daëron M, van de Winkel JG, Verbeek JS. Impaired IgG-dependent anaphylaxis and Arthus reaction in FcγRIII (CD16) deficient mice. Immunity 5: 181–188, 1996.

Hong AP, Cook DJ, Sigouin CS, Warkentin TE. Central venous catheters and upper-extremity deep-vein thrombosis complicating immune heparin-induced thrombocytopenia. Blood 101: 3049–3051, 2003.

Horne MKD. The effect of secreted heparin-binding proteins on heparin binding to platelets. Thromb Res 70: 91–98, 1993.

Humphries DE, Wong GW, Friend DS, Gurish MF, Qiu WT, Huang C, Sharpe AH, Stevens RL. Heparin is essential for the storage of specific granule proteases in mast cells. Nature, 400: 769–772, 1999.

Ioan-Facsinay A, De Kimpe SJ, Hellwig SMM, Van Lent PL, Hofhuis FM, Van Ojik HH, Sedlik C, da Silveira SA, Gerber J, De Jong YF, Roozendaal R, Aarden LA, Van den Berg WB, Saito T, Mosser D, Amigorena S, Izui S, Van Ommen GJ, Van Vugt M, Van der Winkel JG, Verbeek JS. FcγRI (CD64) contributes substantially to severity of arthritis, hypersensitivity responses, and protection from bacterial infection. Immunity 16: 391–402, 2002.

Jerne NK. Towards a network theory of the immune system. Ann Immunol (Paris) 125C: 373–389, 1974.

Kelton JG, Smith JW, Warkentin TE, Hayward CPM, Denomme GA, Horsewood P. Immuno-globulin G from patients with heparin-induced thrombocytopenia binds to a complex of heparin and platelet factor 4. Blood 83: 3232–3239, 1994.

Kowalska MA, Krishnaswamy S, Rauova L, Zhai L, Hayes V, Amirikian K, Esko JD, Bougie DW, Aster RH, Cines DB, Poncz M. Antibodies associated with heparin-induced thrombocyto-penia (HIT) inhibit activated protein C generation: new insights into the prothrombotic nature of HIT. Blood 118: 2882–2888, 2011.

Lambert MP, Rauova L, Bailey M, Sola-Visner MC, Kowalska MA, Poncz M. Platelet factor 4 is a negative autocrine in vivo regulator of megakaryopoiesis: clinical and therapeutic implications. Blood 110: 1153–1160, 2007.

Lasagni L, Francalanci M, Annunziato F, Lazzeri E, Giannini S, Cosmi L, Sagrinati C, Mazzin-ghi B, Orlando C, Maggi E, Marra F, Romagnani S, Serio M, Romagnani P. An alternatively spliced variant of CXCR3 mediates the inhibition of endothelial cell growth induced by IP-10, Mig, and I-TAC, and acts as functional receptor for platelet factor 4. J Exp Med 197: 1537–1549, 2003.

Li F, Ravetch JV. Inhibitory Fcγ receptor engagement drives adjuvant and anti-tumor activities of agonistic CD40 antibodies. Science 333: 1030–1034, 2011.

Mckenzie SE, Taylor SM, Malladi P, Yuhan H, Cassel DL, Chien P, Schwartz E, Schreiber AD, Surrey S, Reilly MP. The role of the human Fc receptor FcγRIIA in the immune clearance of platelets: a transgenic mouse model. J Immunol 162: 4311–4318, 1999.

Mendlovic S, Brocke S, Fricke H, Shoenfeld Y, Bakimer R, Mozes E. The genetic regulation of the induction of experimental SLE. Immunology 69: 228–236, 1990.

Nimmerjahn F, Ravetch JV. Fc-receptors as regulators of immunity. Adv Immunol 96: 179–204, 2007.

Nimmerjahn F, Ravetch JV. FcγRs in health and disease. Curr Top Microbiol Immunol 350: 105–125, 2011.

Nimmerjahn F, Lux A, Albert H, Woigk M, Lehmann C, Dudziak D, Smith P, Ravetch JV. FcγRIV deletion reveals its central role for IgG2a and IgG2b activity in vivo. Proc Natl Acad Sci U S A 107: 19396–19401, 2010.

Orban PC, Chui D, Marth JD. Tissue- and site-specific DNA recombination in transgenic mice. Proc Natl Acad Sci U S A 89: 6861–6865, 1992.

Poole A, Gibbins JM, Turner M, Van Vugt MJ, Van de Winkel JG, Saito T, Tybulewicz VL, Watson SP. The Fc receptor γ-chain and the tyrosine kinase Syk are essential for activation of mouse platelets by collagen. EMBO J 16: 2333–2341, 1997.

Pötzsch B, Klovekorn WP, Madlener K. Use of heparin during cardiopulmonary bypass in patients with a history of heparin-induced thrombocytopenia. New Engl J Med 343: 515, 2000.

Pouplard C, May MA, Iochmann S, Amiral J, Vissac AM, Marchand M, Gruel Y. Antibodies to platelet factor 4-heparin after cardiopulmonary bypass in patients anticoagulated with unfractionated heparin or a low molecular weight heparin: clinical implications for heparin-induced thrombocytopenia. Circulation 99: 2530–2536, 1999.

Pouplard C, Iochmann S, Renard B, Herault O, Colombat P, Amiral J, Gruel Y. Induction of monocyte tissue factor expression by antibodies to heparin-platelet factor 4 complexes developed in heparin-induced thrombocytopenia. Blood 97: 3300–3302, 2001.

Rauova L, Poncz M, Mckenzie SE, Reilly MP, Arepally G, Weisel JW, Nagaswami C, Cines DB, Sachais BS. 2005. Ultralarge complexes of PF4 and heparin are central to the pathogenesis of heparin-induced thrombocytopenia. Blood 105: 131–138, 2005.

Rauova L, Zhai L, Kowalska MA, Arepally GM, Cines DB, Poncz M. Role of platelet surface PF4 antigenic complexes in heparin-induced thrombocytopenia pathogenesis: diagnostic and therapeutic implications. Blood 107: 2346–2353, 2006.

Rauova L, Hirsch JD, Greene TK, Zhai L, Hayes VM, Kowalska MA, Cines DB, Poncz M. Monocyte-bound PF4 in the pathogenesis of heparin-induced thrombocytopenia. Blood 116: 5021–5031, 2010.

Reilly MP, Taylor SM, Hartman NK, Arepally GM, Sachais BS, Cines DB, Poncz M, McKenzie SE. Heparin-induced thrombocytopenia/thrombosis in a transgenic mouse model requires human platelet factor 4 and platelet activation through FcγRIIA. Blood 98: 2442–2447, 2001.

Reilly MP, Taylor SM, Franklin C, Sachais BS, Cines DB, Williams KJ, McKenzie SE.. Pro-thrombotic factors enhance heparin-induced thrombocytopenia and thrombosis in vivo in a mouse model. J Thromb Haemost 4: 2687–2694, 2006.

Reilly MP, Sinha U, André P, Taylor SM, Pak Y, DeGuzman FR, Nanda N, Pandey A, Stolla M, Bergmeier W, McKenzie SE. PRT-060318, a novel syk inhibitor, prevents heparin-induced thrombocytopenia and thrombosis in a transgenic mouse model. Blood 117: 2241–2246, 2012.

Rossmann P, Matousovic K, Horacek V. Protamine-heparin aggregates. their fine structure, histochemistry, and renal deposition. Virchows Archiv B Cell Pathol Incl Mol Pathol 40: 81–98, 1982.

Sachais BS, Kuo A, Nassar T, Morgan J, Kariko K, Williams KJ, Feldman M, Aviram M, Shah N, Jarett L, Poncz M, Cines DB, Higazi AA. Platelet factor 4 binds to low-density lipoprotein receptors and disrupts the endocytic itinerary, resulting in retention of low-density lipoprotein on the cell surface. Blood 99: 3613–3622, 2002.

Sarrazin S, Lamanna WC, Esko JD. Heparan sulfate proteoglycans. Cold Spring Harb Perspect Biol Cold Spring Harb Perspect Biol 3: a004952, 2011.

Sheridan D, Carter C, Kelton JG. A diagnostic test for heparin-induced thrombocytopenia. Blood 67: 27–30, 1986.

Shoenfeld Y, Tomer Y, Blank M. A new experimental model for Wegener's granulomatosis. Isr J Med Sci 31: 13–16, 1995.

Struyf S, Salogni L, Burdick MD, Vandercappellen J, Gouwy M, Noppen S, Proost P, Opdena-kker G, Parmentier M, Gerard C, Sozzani S, Strieter RM, Van Damme J. Angiostatic and chemotactic activities of the CXC chemokine CXCL4L1 (platelet factor-4 variant) are mediated by CXCR3. Blood 117: 480–488, 2011.

Sunderkötter C, Nikolic T, Dillon MJ, Van Rooijen N, Stehling M, Drevets DA, Leenen PJ. Subpopulations of mouse blood monocytes differ in maturation stage and inflammatory response. J Immunol 172: 4410–4417, 2004.

Suvarna S, Rauova L, McCracken EK, Goss CM, Sachais BS, McKenzie SE, Reilly MP, Gunn MD, Cines DB, Poncz M, Arepally G. PF4/heparin complexes are T cell-dependent antigens. Blood 106: 929–931, 2005.

Suvarna S, Espinasse B, Qi R, Lubica R, Poncz M, Cines DB, Wiesner MR, Arepally GM. Determinants of PF4/heparin immunogeneicity Blood 110: 4253–4260, 2007.

Suvarna S, Qi R, Arepally G. Optimization of a murine immunization model for study of PF4/heparin antibodies. J Thromb Haemost 7: 857–864, 2009.

Takai T, Li M, Sylvestre D, Clynes R, Ravetch JV. FcR γ-chain deletion results in pleiotrophic effector cell defects. Cell 76: 519–529, 1994.

Takai T, Ono M, Hikida M, Ohmori H, Ravetch JV. Augmented humoral and anaphylactic responses in FcγRII-deficient mice. Nature 379: 346–349, 1996.

Takeda K, Kaisho T, Akira S. Toll-like receptors. Ann Rev Immunol 21: 335–376, 2003.

Tannenbaum SH, Finko R, Cines DB. Antibody and immune complexes induce tissue factor production by human endothelial cells. J Immunol 137: 1532–1537, 1986.

Tarzi RM, Davies KA, Claassens JW, Verbeek JS, Walport MJ, Cook HT. Both Fcγ receptor I and Fcγ receptor III mediate disease in accelerated nephrotoxic nephritis. Am J Pathol 162: 1677–1683, 2003.

Taylor SM, Reilly MP, Schreiber AD, Chien P, Tuckosh JR, McKenzie SE. Thrombosis and shock induced by activating antiplatelet antibodies in human FcγRIIA transgenic mice: the interplay among antibody, spleen, and Fc receptor. Blood 96: 4254–4260, 2000.

Van de Weert M, Andersen MB, Frokjaer S. Complex coacervation of lysozyme and heparin: complex characterization and protein stability. Pharm Res 21: 2354–2359, 2004.

Visentin GP, Ford SE, Scott JP, Aster RH. Antibodies from patients with heparin-induced thrombocytopenia/thrombosis are specific for platelet factor 4 complexed with heparin or bound to endothelial cells. J Clin Invest 93: 81–88, 1994.

Visentin GP, Malik M, Cyganiak KA, Aster RH. Patients treated with unfractionated heparin during open heart surgery are at high risk to form antibodies reactive with heparin: platelet factor 4 complexes J Lab Clin Med 128: 376–383, 1996.

Wang L, Fuster M, Sriramarao P, Esko JD. Endothelial heparan sulfate deficiency impairs l-selectin- and chemokine-mediated neutrophil trafficking during inflammatory responses. Nat Immunol 6: 902–910, 2005.

Warkentin TE, Kelton JG. Temporal aspects of heparin-induced thrombocytopenia. New Engl J Med 344: 1286–1292, 2001.

Williams RT, Damaraju LV, Mascelli MA, Barnathan ES, Califf RM, Simoons ML, Deliargyris EN, Sane DC. Anti-platelet factor 4/heparin antibodies: an independent predictor of 30-day myocardial infarction after acute coronary ischemic syndromes. Circulation 107: 2307–2312, 2003.

Yu G, Rux AH, Ma P, Bdeir K, Sachais BS. Endothelial expression of E-selectin is induced by the platelet-specific chemokine platelet factor 4 through LRP in an NF-κB-dependent manner. Blood 105: 3545–3551, 2005.

Zhang C, Thornton MA, Kowalska MA, Sachais BS, Feldman M, Poncz M, McKenzie SE, Reilly MP. Localization of distal regulatory domains in the megakaryocyte-specific platelet basic protein/platelet factor 4 gene locus. Blood, 98: 610–617, 2001.

Laboratory testing for heparin-induced thrombocytopenia

Theodore E. Warkentin and Andreas Greinacher

INTRODUCTION

Heparin-induced thrombocytopenia (HIT) is caused by heparin-dependent antibodies that usually recognize multimolecular complexes of platelet factor 4/heparin (PF4/H). HIT can be viewed as a clinicopathologic syndrome (Warkentin et al., 1998, 2011b). Thus, a diagnosis of HIT should be based on two criteria: (*i*) clinically evident abnormalities, most commonly thrombocytopenia with or without thrombosis (see chap. 2), and (*ii*) detection of HIT antibodies.

Two major classes of assays—platelet activation (functional) and PF4-dependent (antigen) immunoassays—have been developed to detect HIT antibodies (Warkentin and Sheppard, 2006a) (Table 11.1).

PLATELET ACTIVATION ASSAYS FOR HIT ANTIBODIES
Washed Platelet Assays

The classic washed platelet assay for HIT is the serotonin release assay (SRA) (Sheridan et al., 1986; Warkentin et al., 1992). This assay was a modification of a platelet-washing technique in use at McMaster University that resuspended washed platelets in buffer containing physiological concentrations of calcium. The purpose was to avoid platelet activation artifacts associated with low calcium concentrations (Mustard et al., 1972; Kinlough-Rathbone et al., 1983) (see chap. 1). The use of washed platelets is also central to certain other functional assays, such as the heparin-induced platelet activation (HIPA) assay (Greinacher et al., 1991). Figure 11.1 summarizes washed platelet assays for HIT.

Preparation of Platelets for Washed Platelet Assays

1. Collect 8.4 volumes of blood from a normal donor into 1.6 volumes of acid–citrate–dextrose (ACD).

Comment. Aspirin-free normal blood donors whose platelets are known to respond well to HIT sera should be selected, as there is considerable heterogeneity to platelet activation by HIT sera among platelets obtained from different normal individuals (Warkentin et al., 1992). In Hamilton, platelets from two donors are combined. In Greifswald, platelets from four different donors selected randomly are prepared and tested individually. ABO blood group discrepancies do not affect the results of these assays (Greinacher et al., 1991).

TABLE 11.1   Classification of Laboratory Tests for Heparin-induced Thrombocytopenia

---

Platelet activation (functional) assays
  Washed platelet assays
    Serotonin release assay (SRA): quantitation of ^{14}C-radiolabeled serotonin released from dense
      granules of activated platelets (Sheridan et al., 1986); chemical and chromatographic
      detection of serotonin also described (Koch et al., 2002; Fouassier et al., 2006)
    Heparin-induced platelet activation (HIPA) test: visual assessment of platelet aggregation
      (Greinacher et al., 1991; Eichler et al., 1999)
    Adenosine triphosphate (ATP) release detected by luminography (Stewart et al., 1995)
    Platelet microparticle assay: quantitation of platelet-derived microparticles by flow cytometry
      (Lee et al., 1996)
  Platelets in citrated platelet-rich plasma (c-PRP)
Platelet aggregation test (PAT): assessment of platelet aggregation using conventional
    aggregometry (Fratantoni et al., 1975; Chong et al., 1993a)
    Annexin V-binding assay: quantitation by flow cytometry of annexin V binding to anionic
      phospholipids expressed by activated platelets (Tomer, 1997; Tomer et al., 1999)
    Serotonin release detected by flow cytometry (Gobbi et al., 2003)
  Whole blood impedance platelet aggregometry (Multiplate® analyzer, Verum Diagnostica,
    subsidiary of Dynabyte Medical [Roche]) (Elalamy et al., 2009; Morel-Kopp et al., 2010, 2012)
Antigen assays (PF4-dependent)
  Enzyme immunoassays (EIAs)
    Target antigen: PF4/H complexes (Amiral et al., 1992; Horsewood et al., 1996; Juhl et al., 2006)
      (several in-house assays; also Asserachrom® HPIA; HPIA-IgG, Diagnostica Stago)
    Target antigen: PF4/polyvinylsulfonate complexes (Visentin et al., 2001; Warkentin
      et al., 2010) (LIFECODES® PF4 Enhanced®; LIFECODES® PF4 IgG; Gen-Probe GTI
      Diagnostics)
    Target antigen: PF4 (and/or other protein)/heparin complexes (Warkentin et al., 2010;
      Pouplard et al., 2010; Morel-Kopp et al., 2011) (Zymutest HIA, HYPHEN BioMed; Sysmex)
    Fluid-phase enzyme immunoassay (Newman et al., 1998; Warkentin et al., 2005a)
  Rapid assays (based on PF4- or PF4/heparin-coated particle agglutination)
    Lateral flow immunoassay (LFI) using gold nanoparticles (Milenia® QuickLine HIT, Milenia
      Biotec) (Sachs et al., 2011)
    Particle gel immunoassay (PaGIA) (Meyer et al., 1999) [ID-PaGIA Heparin/PF4, DiaMed
      (Bio-Rad Laboratories)]
    Particle immunofiltration assay (PIFA® Heparin/PF4 Rapid Assay, Akers BioSciences)
      (Warkentin et al., 2007)
  Rapid assays (automated instrument-based)
    Target antigen: PF4/polyvinylsulfonate complexes
      ACL TOP® family analyzer: latex particle-based assay (HemosIL HIT-Ab$_{(PF4-H)}$)
      ACL AcuStar® analyzer: chemiluminescence-based assays (HemosIL AcuStar HIT-IgG$_{(PF4-H)}$
        and HemosIL AcuStar HIT-Ab$_{(PF4-H)}$)

---

2. Perform differential centrifugation to obtain ACD-anticoagulated platelet–rich plasma (PRP).

Comment. Low-speed centrifugation prepares ACD-anticoagulated PRP. Additional ACD (111 µL/mL PRP) is added (Greifswald) to ensure that the pH of the PRP is sufficiently low (<6.5) to prevent platelet aggregation that otherwise would occur during platelet pelleting: the platelet release reaction is triggered by close platelet contact in low calcium concentrations at physiological pH

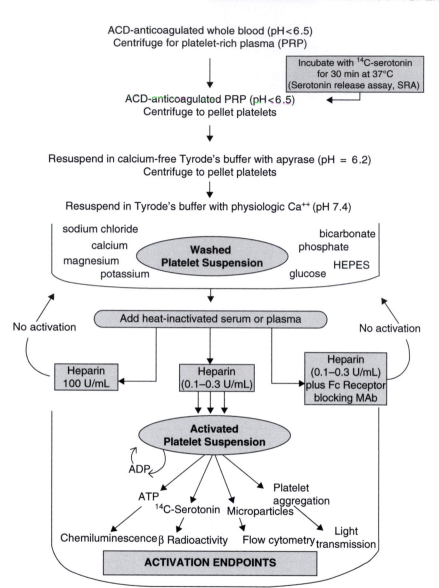

FIGURE 11.1   Schematic overview of washed platelet assays: HIT serum causes platelet activation at therapeutic (0.1–0.3 U/mL) heparin concentrations, but not in the presence of Fc receptor-blocking monoclonal antibody or high (100 U/mL) heparin concentrations. Platelet activation by HIT serum is potentiated by ADP release from platelet dense granules. Various platelet activation endpoints can be used. False-positive results can be avoided if typical reaction profiles of non-HIT platelet activation triggers are recognized: e.g., (*i*) residual thrombin (activation at low but not high heparin concentrations, including activation in the presence of Fc receptor-blocking monoclonal antibody); (*ii*) immune complexes (activation at low and high heparin concentrations, both of which are inhibited by Fc receptor-blocking monoclonal antibody); and (*iii*) TTP serum (variable activation in the presence of heparin that is not inhibited by Fc receptor-blocking monoclonal antibody). *Abbreviations*: ACD, acid–citrate–dextrose; ADP, adenosine diphosphate; ATP, adenosine triphosphate; PRP, platelet-rich plasma; TTP, thrombotic thrombocytopenic purpura.

(Kinlough-Rathbone et al., 1983). If the serotonin release method is used, the PRP is incubated at 37°C for 30 minutes with [^{14}C]serotonin (0.1 μCi/mL of PRP added from a stock solution of 50 μCi/mL of [^{14}C]serotonin) (Lee et al., 1996).

3. Wash the platelets by pelleting them from PRP, then gently resuspend the platelets in calcium- and magnesium-free Tyrode's buffer, pH 6.3, containing glucose (5.6 mmol/L) and apyrase (2.5 U/mL).

Comment. Tyrode's buffer consists of physiological concentrations of sodium chloride (NaCl, 137 mmol/L), potassium chloride (2.7 mmol/L), calcium chloride (CaCl$_2$, 2 mmol/L), magnesium chloride (MgCl$_2$, 1.0 mmol/L), and sodium dihydrogen phosphate (NaH$_2$PO$_4$, 3.3 mmol/L); however, calcium-free and magnesium-free Tyrode's is used in this wash step to avoid activating the coagulation factors and platelets. The low pH prevents platelets from aggregating during pelleting. Apyrase is an enzyme that degrades adenine nucleotides (i.e., accumulation of the ADP from the platelets is prevented). Azide-free bovine serum albumin (3.5 mg/mL) and hirudin (1 U/mL) are included in the wash buffer in Greifswald, but not Hamilton, although HEPES (5 mmol/L) is added to this buffer in Hamilton. Following resuspension, the platelets are incubated for 15 minutes at 37°C (Greifswald).

4. Pellet the washed platelets as before, and then gently resuspend the platelets into calcium- and magnesium-containing Tyrode's buffer, pH 7.4, without apyrase or hirudin.

Comment. Following resuspension, the platelets should "rest" for 45 minutes at 37°C (Greifswald). The final resuspension buffer (Tyrode's buffer at physiological pH) contains calcium (2 mmol/L) and magnesium (1 mmol/L Hamilton; 2 mmol/L Greifswald). The platelet count is adjusted to a minimum of 300×10^9/L; thus, after the addition of washed platelets (75 μL) to the microtiter wells containing test serum (20 μL) and heparin/buffer (5 μL in Hamilton, 10 μL in Greifswald), the final platelet concentration will be at least 215×10^9/L. Apyrase must not be included in this buffer, as the ADP released during assessment of HIT-induced platelet activation is an important potentiator of platelet Fc receptor-mediated platelet activation (Polgár et al., 1998).

Test Conditions of Heparin-Dependent Platelet Activation: Perform Platelet Activation Studies Under Various Test Conditions

Comment. In Hamilton, sera are studied using six different reaction conditions: (*i*) buffer; (*ii*) unfractionated heparin (UFH), 0.1 U/mL; (*iii*) UFH, 0.3 U/mL; (*iv*) UFH, 100 U/mL; (*v*) low molecular weight heparin (LMWH), enoxaparin, 0.1 U/mL; and (*vi*) UFH, 0.3 U/mL plus a monoclonal antibody (IV.3) that inhibits platelet Fc receptor-mediated platelet activation. In Greifswald, routine testing is performed using (*i*) buffer; (*ii*) LMWH (reviparin), 0.2 U/mL; (*iii*) UFH, 100 U/mL; and (*iv*) sometimes LMWH 0.2 U/mL plus IV.3 is performed to resolve unclear results. In Greifswald, the LMWH preparation reviparin (Clivarine) is used because of its narrow molecular weight (MW) range (80% of its chains have molecular mass of 2.4–7.2 kDa, i.e., 4–12 disaccharide units) (Jeske et al., 1997); this results in more consistent formation of PF4/H complexes, enhancing sensitivity of the assay (Greinacher et al., 1994b). Platelets are incubated with various test and positive and negative control sera under these various reaction conditions for up to 30 minutes (Greifswald) or 60 minutes (Hamilton). Addition of hirudin avoids thrombin-dependent platelet activation. The order of pipetting is important in optimizing assay results (Eichler et al., 1999)

TABLE 11.2   Pipette Scheme for the HIPA Test

	Add first	Add second	Add third	Add fourth	Add last		
	Hirudin (50 U/mL)	Heat-inactivated patient or control serum	UFH 1050 U/mL = 100 U/mL (final)	Washed platelet suspension (300×10⁹/L)	Suspension buffer	LMWH (2.1 anti-Xa U/mL) = 0.2 U/mL (final)	Danaparoid^a (2.1 anti-Xa U/mL) = 0.2 U/mL (final)
Control with buffer	10 µL	20 µL	–	75 µL	10 µL	–	–
Low heparin concentration	10 µL	20 µL	–	75 µL	–	10 µL	–
High heparin concentration	10 µL	20 µL	10 µL	75 µL	–	–	–
Cross-reactivity with danaparoid	10 µL	20 µL		75 µL	–	–	10 µL

^aTesting for danaparoid cross reactivity is no longer routinely performed.
Abbreviations: LMWH, low molecular weight heparin; HIPA, heparin-induced platelet activation; UFH, unfractionated heparin.

(Table 11.2). After adding serum to the microtiter plate wells, high heparin concentrations are added to the appropriate wells: this will disrupt PF4/H complexes that may be present in the serum. After adding washed platelets, buffer and LMWH (low concentrations) are added. If inhibition by monoclonal antibody IV. 3 is tested, this reagent is added before addition of the washed platelet suspension. In Hamilton, the pipetting order for the SRA is (*i*) addition of buffer/heparin, (*ii*) serum, and (*iii*) platelets.

Interpretation of the Obtained Test and Control Data
Comment. Several techniques can be used to assess the activation of washed platelets (Fig. 11.1). The actual method of detection of platelet activation is probably less important than the technique of platelet preparation itself, including the selection of suitable platelet donors.

A positive test result is one in which heparin-dependent platelet activation occurs at therapeutic concentrations of heparin (0.1–0.3 U/mL) but is inhibited at very high (100 U/mL) heparin concentrations and in the presence of platelet Fc receptor-blocking monoclonal antibody. By assessing activation in the presence of different LMWH compounds or danaparoid, studies of *in vitro* cross-reactivity can be performed. It is important to ensure that control HIT sera, including one or more weak positive controls, react as expected. Given the experience from a workshop on testing for HIT antibodies (Eichler et al., 1999), we recommend exchange of weak positive control sera among laboratories for quality control.

Platelet Activation Endpoints
[¹⁴C]Serotonin release was the first activation endpoint described using washed platelets (Sheridan et al., 1986). In this method, the washed platelets are incubated with test and control serum or plasma and heparin/buffer in flat-bottomed

polystyrene microtiter wells (in duplicate or triplicate), performed on a plate shaker (shaken, not stirred). After 1 hour, the reaction is halted with 100 μL of 0.5% EDTA in phosphate-buffered saline (PBS). The microtiter plates are centrifuged at 1000 g for 5 minutes, and 50 μL of supernatant fluid is transferred to tubes containing scintillation fluid for detection of [^{14}C]serotonin released during platelet activation.

Carbon-14 is a radioisotope with a long half-life (5730 years) that emits β-particles (electrons). Laboratories require special licenses to handle radioisotopes, thus limiting widespread use of this platelet-activation marker. However, it is also possible to quantitate serotonin by nonradioactive analysis (Koch et al., 2002; Gobbi et al., 2003; Fouassier et al., 2006). Results are expressed as percentage of serotonin released. This is calculated based on comparison with maximal possible release (determined following detergent-induced platelet lysis), and adjusted for background release (determined by quantitating serotonin release from a sample incubated with buffer alone). Acceptable experiments should have less than 5% background release, with both buffer and negative control serum being negative for (platelet-activating) HIT antibodies.

Aggregation of Washed Platelets
A convenient and useful activation endpoint—platelet aggregation—was reported in the HIPA assay (Greinacher et al., 1991, 1994a; Eichler et al., 1999). Test serum and heparin buffer are placed in U-bottomed polystyrene microtiter wells containing two stainless steel spheres, and the platelets are stirred at approximately 500 rpm, using a magnetic stirrer. At 5-minute intervals, the wells are examined against an indirect light source: a change in appearance of the reaction mixture from turbidity (nonaggregated platelets) to transparency (aggregated platelets) is considered a positive result. Although the activation endpoint is evaluated subjectively, interobserver agreement is good. A further advantage of this technique is its repeated evaluation of platelet activation over time. Thus, strong HIT sera that cause the typical activation profile of HIT (i.e., activation at low, but not high, heparin concentrations) within 15–30 minutes are readily identified. A strong HIT serum could eventually cause platelet activation even at the high heparin concentration; this reaction is typically delayed and therefore recognized by repeated evaluation, but can cause an "indeterminate" reaction pattern (activation at both low and high heparin concentrations) if activation is assessed at a later time point only. Occasionally there is interference with visual interpretation (e.g., a lipemic serum).

Luminography
Stewart et al. (1995) reported luminography to detect platelet activation, using a commercially available lumiaggregometer. Adenosine triphosphate (ATP) is released from platelet-dense granules during platelet activation. In the presence of luciferin–luciferase reagent, a light flash is generated in the presence of ATP, which is detected and quantitated. Another group reported similar results using a standard scintillation counter (Teitel et al., 1996). It is uncertain how the sensitivity and specificity of these assays compare with other markers of platelet activation.

Platelet-Derived Microparticle Generation

Generation of platelet-derived microparticles occurs when washed platelets are activated by HIT sera (Warkentin et al., 1994). With the use of a fluorescein-labeled anti-GPIα murine monoclonal antibody, a method for quantitating microparticles using flow cytometry was reported by Lee et al. (1996). Although both platelets and microparticles bind fluorescein-labeled anti-GPIα monoclonal antibodies, they can be distinguished by their size and scatter parameters using flow cytometry, with microparticles quantitated in relation to platelet numbers (Lee et al., 1996).

Heat Inactivation of Patient Serum or Plasma

To avoid thrombin-induced platelet activation in buffer containing physiological calcium, steps are taken to inactivate residual thrombin. Thus, plasma and serum must first be heat inactivated before use in these assays. Heating at 56°C for 30–45 minutes inactivates thrombin and complement. Fibrin and other precipitates are removed by high-speed centrifugation (8000 g for 5 minutes). More intense heating of serum (63°C for 20 minutes) forms platelet-activating immune complexes (Warkentin et al., 1994); thus, if a patient sample shows heparin-independent platelet activation ("indeterminate" result), another sample aliquot should be heat inactivated, and the HIT assay repeated. Often, this will result in the disappearance of the initial artifact that presumably was caused by too intense heat inactivation (Moore et al., 2008). Serum is preferred for use in functional HIT assays in our laboratories, as serum contains more PF4, thereby facilitating initial formation of the antigen.

Biological Basis for High Sensitivity of Washed Platelets
to Activation by HIT Antibodies

Table 11.3 lists differences between using washed platelets and platelets suspended in citrate-anticoagulated plasma to study HIT antibody-mediated platelet activation. Some of these differences may be important in explaining the greater sensitivity and specificity of washed platelets in detecting HIT antibodies.

1. Baseline platelet activation, including platelet-granule release, occurs during preparation of washed platelets. This enhances the platelet-binding capacity of heparin (Horne and Chao, 1989) and may also increase the availability of PF4 to form the target antigen.

2. Apyrase is used to prevent the accumulation of ADP during platelet washing. This prevents platelets from becoming refractory to subsequent ADP-mediated platelet activation (Ardlie et al., 1970). Empirically, apyrase grade III (Sigma, St. Louis, MO, USA) is acceptable for use: grades I and II are too impure, and grades IV and higher are expensive.

3. Physiological calcium concentrations are preferred when washed platelets are used. Under these conditions, ADP produces only primary platelet aggregation. However, as observed by Packham et al. (1971), traces of immunoglobulin complexes in amounts too low to cause aggregation themselves will cause secondary aggregation to occur following the addition of ADP. The importance of ADP in mediating HIT antibody-induced platelet activation has been reported by Polgár and colleagues (1998). Thus, the reaction conditions that exist when washed platelets are used appear to maximize HIT antibody-induced platelet activation because the platelets retain sensitivity to ADP-mediated platelet activation.

TABLE 11.3 Comparison Between Citrated Platelet-Rich Plasma and Washed Platelet Assays

Technical aspects	Washed platelet assay	Platelet-rich plasma assay	Comments
Platelet preparation	High *g* centrifugation during washing: increased baseline platelet activation	Low *g* centrifugation: less baseline platelet activation	Availability of PF4 may be higher using washed platelets (greater formation of PF4/heparin antigen complexes)
Apyrase	Apyrase added to wash solution, but not to the final resuspension (reaction) buffer	No apyrase used (no wash steps)	Apyrase degrades ADP, and prevents its accumulation; thus, platelet refractoriness to ADP-mediated potentiation of HIT serum-induced platelet activation is avoided by apyrase
Reaction milieu	Physiological calcium concentration (2 mmol/L)	Low (micromolar) calcium owing to citrate	IgG-mediated platelet activation optimal with physiological calcium concentrations
IgG levels	Reduced IgG levels during final reaction	Normal plasma IgG levels	Reduced inhibition of Fc receptor-mediated platelet activation by IgG in washed platelet assays
Plasma protein	Reduced plasma protein levels	Normal plasma protein levels	Reduced nonidiosyncratic platelet activation by heparin using washed platelets (?)
Reaction assessment	Microtiter plates	Conventional aggregometer	Many assays performed simultaneously using microtiter plates
Temperature	Room temperature	37°C	Unknown significance

Note: See text for further details on differences between washed platelet and citrated plasma assays (pp. 278–280).

4. Low concentrations of IgG are present in the final washed platelet reaction mixture: there is a fivefold reduction in IgG compared with citrated platelet-rich plasma (c-PRP) assays, because only IgG from the test serum is present in the final reaction mixture. Chong and colleagues (1993a) showed that high plasma IgG levels in one platelet donor's blood seemed to explain the discrepancy between studies using donor c-PRP (poor reactivity) and donor washed platelets (good reactivity). These and other investigators (Greinacher et al., 1994c) also observed that addition of IgG inhibits HIT serum-induced activation of washed platelets in a dose-dependent fashion.

5. Low concentrations of fibrinogen and other plasma proteins could reduce the potential for nonidiosyncratic heparin-induced platelet aggregation (Salzman

et al., 1980; Chong et al., 1993a). In contrast, low concentrations of heparin rarely cause significant activation of washed platelets. It is possible that acute-phase reactant proteins such as fibrinogen could lead to false-positive activation assays for HIT using c-PRP.

6. Room temperature conditions are used for washed platelet assays; in contrast, c-PRP studies are performed at 37°C. Although this is a major difference between the assays, it is unknown whether there are advantages or disadvantages of performing washed platelet assays at room temperature. In Greifswald, all buffers are warmed to 37°C, and all incubation steps are performed at this temperature; only the final incubation on the microtiter plates is performed at room temperature.

7. Multiple serum–platelet reactions in microtiter plates can be performed, and even several hundred reactions studied in parallel. Quality control is thereby enhanced by the large number of control and test reaction conditions that can be analyzed, and the long incubation period employed (up to 60 minutes). The incubation period in HIT assays should be at least 20–30 minutes (Stewart et al., 1995).

Quality Control in Washed Platelet Assays for HIT
The variable reactivity of donor platelets to HIT sera is an important issue in activation assays for HIT. It has long been recognized that inconsistent results can be obtained using these assays (Salem and van der Weyden, 1983; Pfueller and David, 1986; Warkentin et al., 1992).

Hierarchical vs Idiosyncratic Platelet Activation by HIT Sera
The results of a systematic investigation, summarized in Table 11.4, showed that both HIT sera and platelet donors exhibit variable reactivity in a hierarchical, rather than an idiosyncratic, manner. The strongest reactions were produced by strong HIT sera against strongly reactive platelet donors. All of the negative reactions occurred when the weakest sera were mixed with the weakest platelets. Importantly, no unexpected negative reactions occurred elsewhere in the 10 × 10 serum–platelet grid (Table 11.4). Furthermore, the relative ranking of platelet donors appeared to be stable over time, an observation also reported by Chong and colleagues (1993a) in their study of platelet donor variability using c-PRP.

The finding of a hierarchical pattern of reactivity has important implications for quality control in diagnostic testing for HIT using activation assays. First, it indicates that platelets from certain donors who tend to respond well to HIT sera should be chosen. Second, relatively weak HIT sera should be included as positive controls (~20–50% serotonin release, or 25 minutes lag time in the HIPA).

Heparin-Independent Platelet Activation: Indeterminate Results
About 5% of patient sera yield an indeterminate result in an activation assay. This is defined as platelet activation that occurs at both therapeutic (0.1–0.3 U/mL) and supratherapeutic (10–100 U/mL) heparin concentrations. Often an interpretable result is obtained when the assay is repeated using another heat-inactivated aliquot (Moore et al., 2008). This suggests that the first result may have been an artifact caused by heat-aggregated IgG generated *ex vivo*. However, some serum and plasma samples repeatedly demonstrate heparin-independent platelet activation.

TABLE 11.4   Reactivities of 10 HIT Sera with Platelets from 10 Normal Donors

HIT sera	Normal platelet donors: Strongest (P_1) to Weakest (P_{10})									
(S_1–S_{10})	P_1 84.3	P_2 71.2	P_3 68.4	P_4 53.6	P_5 52.5	P_6 41.3	P_7 39.7	P_8 38.9	P_9 36.9	P_{10} 29.9
S_1 85.4	++++	++++	++++	++++	++++	++++	+++	++++	++	+++
S_2 84.4	++++	++++	++++	++++	++++	+++	+++	++++	+++	+++
S_3 69.1	++++	++++	++++	+++	+++	++	+++	++	++	++
S_4 61.0	++++	++++	+++	+++	+++	++	++	++	++	+
S_5 56.4	++++	+++	+++	++	+++	++	++	+	+	+
S_6 50.7	+++	+++	+++	+++	++	++	++	++	+	+
S_7 44.1	++++	+++	+++	+	++	+	+	+	++	−
S_8 30.1	++++	++	+++	+	+	+	−	−	−	−
S_9 24.2	+++	++	+	++	+	−	−	−	−	−
S_{10} 11.3	++	+	+	−	−	−	−	−	−	−

Serum samples and platelet donors are ranked from strongest to weakest (S_1 – S_{10} and P_1 – P_{10}, respectively), according to the mean percentage of [^{14}C]serotonin release when considering all 100 serum–platelet donor pairs (10 pairs corresponding to each HIT serum and each normal platelet donor). For each serum–platelet donor pair, the individual amount of serotonin release is summarized as follows: 80–100% release, + + + +; 60–79.9% release, + + +; 40–59.9% release, + +; 20–39.9% release, +; <20% release, −. Overall, there is a graded pattern of reactivity among the individual reaction pairs that is hierarchical (i.e., there are no unexpected weak or strong reactions among the pairs). All negative reactions (<20% release) were found in the lower right portion of the table. Conversely, the strongest reactions (>80% release) were found in the upper left portion of the table.
Source: From Warkentin et al., 1992.

Biologic explanations include circulating immune complexes (e.g., systemic lupus erythematosus), high-titer HLA class I alloantibodies, and, possibly, other platelet-activating factors (e.g., thrombotic thrombocytopenic purpura). An antigen assay is required for further investigation when an indeterminate result is consistently obtained; in these circumstances, HIT should only be considered probable if a strong enzyme immunoassay (EIA) result is obtained [e.g., >1.5 units of optical density (OD)] (discussed subsequently).

Inhibition by High Heparin Concentrations

Sheridan and colleagues (1986) first emphasized that there was a relatively specific activation profile triggered by HIT sera and plasmas: activation at therapeutic heparin concentrations (maximal at 0.1–0.3 U/mL) that progressively diminished with increasing heparin concentrations, typically falling to background activation at very high (100 U/mL) heparin concentrations. Classically, a positive test was deemed as greater than 20% serotonin release at 0.1 U/mL heparin and less than 20% serotonin release at 100 U/mL heparin. These criteria should not be applied indiscriminately, however. For example, a very strong HIT serum could produce more than a 90% release at 0.1 U/mL heparin and 25% release at 100 U/mL heparin. Alternatively, a serum or plasma sample that was not adequately heat-inactivated could produce a similar reaction profile (i.e., residual thrombin is inhibited by the high, but not low, heparin concentration). The strength of reactivity caused by patient serum can be helpful: clinically significant HIT antibodies almost always cause more than 50% serotonin release using optimally reactive platelets (Warkentin et al., 2000). In the HIPA test, differences in the lag time to platelet aggregation provide useful information.

Inhibition by Fc Receptor Blockade

Platelet activation by HIT antibodies is inhibited in the presence of a murine IgG2b monoclonal antibody (IV.3) that recognizes the platelet FcγIIa receptor (Kelton et al., 1988; Chong et al., 1989) and can be used to enhance test specificity.

Interpretation of Platelet Activation by HIT Serum in the Absence of Added Heparin

With activation assays, it is not uncommon for HIT serum or plasma to cause substantial platelet activation even in the *absence* of added heparin (Warkentin and Kelton, 2001a; Prechel et al., 2005; Socher et al., 2008; Linkins and Warkentin, 2011). However, even greater platelet activation occurs in the presence of added heparin. When strong serum-dependent platelet activation occurs with buffer and at a 0.1–0.3 U/mL heparin concentration, it is important to ensure that the other reactions (at 100 U/mL heparin, and 0.1–0.3 U/mL heparin together with Fc receptor blockade) are as expected. This is because residual thrombin could produce strong platelet activation in both the absence and presence of low heparin concentration, thereby causing the potential for a false-positive result.

There are at least two potential explanations for strong platelet activation in the absence of added heparin. First, there may be residual heparin in the sample (White et al., 1992; Pötzsch et al., 1996). However, this phenomenon usually persists despite attempts to remove heparin using binding resins. Furthermore, heparin-independent platelet activation can be a feature of serum obtained from patients with "delayed-onset HIT," in which the presence of residual heparin is unlikely because onset of thrombocytopenia and thrombosis begins several days after the patient's last exposure to heparin (Warkentin and Kelton, 2001a) (see chap. 2). These observations better support the second explanation, which is that some (perhaps many) HIT antibodies recognize platelet-bound PF4 in the absence of an exogenous source of heparin, perhaps by PF4 bound to platelet glycosaminoglycans, such as chondroitin sulfate (Rauova et al., 2006). Alternatively, as HIT antibodies are heterogenous, there may be pathogenic antibody subpopulations that bind relatively well to PF4 even in the absence of heparin or heparin-like molecules (Newman and Chong, 1999; Amiral et al., 2000). This phenomenon has implications for the interpretation of tests of cross-reactivity of LMWH and danaparoid, as discussed later.

Advantages and Disadvantages of Washed Platelet Assays

High sensitivity and specificity is the major advantage of the washed platelet activation assays. In our hands, utilizing "weak positive" control HIT sera for quality control, the sensitivity of the SRA for clinical HIT is very high (>97%) (Warkentin et al., 2000, 2005b), and only reduced by the small number (<3%) of patient samples that yield "indeterminate" results (Moore et al., 2008). The diagnostic specificity is also high in most clinical settings, especially if the test gives a very strong result (>80% serotonin release) and all the controls react as expected. Indeed, the SRA can be considered as a "dichotomotizing" assay: sera usually yield either negative or very strong results (>80% serotonin release), with relatively few samples showing intermediate levels of platelet activation (Fig. 11.2).

The major disadvantage of washed platelet assays for detecting HIT antibodies is that they are technically demanding and labor intensive. A workshop that compared a washed platelet assay (the HIPA test) and an antigen assay showed

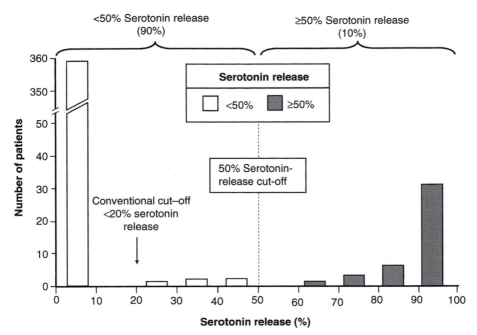

FIGURE 11.2 Dichotomization of results of SRA testing for HIT antibodies (*n* = 405 patients tested). The data are shown as deciles of mean percent serotonin release (at 0.1 and 0.3 U/mL) unfractionated heparin). The conventional cutoff defining a positive SRA test result is 20%; however, the Author (T. E. W.) generally uses 50% as the cutoff (assuming all controls react as expected, including weak positive control serum), as this better discriminates between HIT and non-HIT thrombocytopenia. Only ~10% of patients investigated for HIT achieved a positive test result at this cutoff. Overall, >97% of patients in this data set tested either clearly negative (<20% serotonin release) or strongly positive (>80% serotonin release). *Abbreviations*: HIT, heparin-induced thrombocytopenia; SRA, serotonin release assay. *Source*: Warkentin et al. (2008).

greater variability in activation assay results among the participating laboratories (Eichler et al., 1999). Washed platelet activation assays are best suited for reference laboratories assessing many HIT sera, as this facilitates acquisition of sufficient technical experience to perform the assay successfully on a consistent basis. Assay-specific disadvantages include the requirement for radioactivity (SRA), the use of a subjective, visual endpoint (HIPA), and expensive equipment (flow cytometry-based assays).

Activation Assays Using Citrate-Anticoagulated Platelet-Rich Plasma

The first reports describing the use of normal donor c-PRP to detect platelet activation caused by HIT serum or plasma appeared in the 1970s (Rhodes et al., 1973; Fratantoni et al., 1975; Babcock et al., 1976). A ratio of serum (or plasma) to c-PRP between 0.66 and 1.0 was used (e.g., 200 μL serum added to 200–300 μL c-PRP). No standardized method has evolved, however, although a survey of 54 laboratories in France (Nguyen et al., 1994) found some practices to be more common. For example, most laboratories test patient citrated platelet-poor plasma (c-PPP) rather than heat-inactivated serum. Variable heparin concentrations are used, most commonly between 0.5 and 1.0 U/mL. The ratio of patient c-PPP to donor c-PRP is usually 1:1, and ABO discrepancies are usually ignored. About 75% of the laboratories use at least two platelet donors for diagnostic testing.

Testing for HIT Antibodies Using c-PRP

The following description of the assay taken from Chong and colleagues (1989, 1993a) has the highest reported sensitivity and specificity among c-PRP methods. Blood is obtained from normal blood donors whose platelets respond well to serum or plasma from HIT patients, and c-PRP is prepared. Testing involves addition of 150 μL of patient heat-inactivated c-PPP or serum to 340 μL of c-PRP (final platelet concentration, 250–350 × 10⁹/L) at 37°C. The platelets are monitored for a few minutes to exclude nonspecific platelet aggregation. After addition of 10 μL heparin/saline, aggregation is monitored over the next 15 minutes or until aggregation has occurred. A positive result is an increase in light transmission of more than 25% above baseline in the presence of therapeutic-dose heparin (0.5 U/mL) and patient serum or c-PPP and inhibition of aggregation in the presence of patient serum or plasma and supratherapeutic-dose heparin (100 U/mL). Use of such a two-point assay reduced the false-positive rate, as serum or plasma from some patients without HIT caused platelet aggregation at all heparin concentrations tested. To ensure that the platelets are functional, platelets are also tested with collagen (2 μg/mL). Details on methodology of c-PRP assays are also given elsewhere (Kapsch and Silver, 1981; Almeida et al., 1998).

Some workers report that platelets from a patient with HIT are very reactive to heparin-dependent activation by their own serum or plasma (Kappa et al., 1987; Chong et al., 1993b). Use of autologous c-PRP can sometimes be limited by the patient's thrombocytopenia, however. Potential explanations for the high sensitivity of autologous platelets include persisting high Fc receptor expression on platelets of patients with acute HIT (Chong et al., 1993b) and baseline platelet activation (Chong et al., 1994), with the potential for higher PF4 availability.

Disadvantages of c-PRP Aggregation Assays

Problems with these assays include (i) potential for false-positive interpretation if heparin produces nonspecific aggregation of donor platelets, an effect that could be enhanced nonspecifically by proaggregatory factors in the patient serum or plasma, and (ii) risk of false-negative interpretation if HIT serum-induced platelet aggregation begins even before addition of heparin.

Nonspecific activation of platelets by heparin occurs with some normal donor c-PRP (Chong et al., 1993a), rendering these donors unsuitable for diagnostic testing. Plasma from very sick patients is more likely to cause nonspecific aggregation of platelets in c-PRP in the presence of heparin, leading to potential for false-positive platelet aggregation test results (Goodfellow et al., 1998; Trehel-Tursis et al., 2012; Warkentin, 2012).

An important practical disadvantage is that only a limited number of platelet aggregation tracings can be performed using conventional aggregometers. Thus, relatively few reactions with a limited number of patient and control samples can be evaluated.

Other Assays Using Citrated-Anticoagulated Whole Blood or PRP

Tomer (1997) reported a c-PRP activation assay for HIT antibodies in which the activation endpoint is quantitation of binding of fluorescein-labeled recombinant annexin V to platelets, as detected using flow cytometry. Annexin V, a placental protein, interacts with the prothrombinase-binding anionic phospholipids expressed on the surface of activated platelets and correlates with platelet procoagulant activity. It is uncertain whether the reaction conditions employed (e.g., 30-minute incubation at 26°C) or the high sensitivity of annexin V binding (300-fold increase over baseline) overcomes the inherent limitations of sensitivity observed with other assays using c-PRP. Gobbi and colleagues (2003) developed a flow cytometry assay modeled after that of Tomer (1997), except that loss of serotonin from platelet granules was used as the platelet activation endpoint. Vitale et al. (2001) found P-selectin to be a better marker of platelet activation than annexin V, and Mullier et al. (2010) used platelet microparticle formation as a readout.

Comparison of Washed Platelet and c-PRP Activation Assays

It became evident during the mid-1980s that the sensitivity of c-PRP aggregation assays for HIT was relatively poor (Kelton et al., 1984; Pfueller and David, 1986). Favaloro and colleagues (1992) first compared the c-PRP aggregation assay with the washed platelet SRA. They observed that only 6 of 13 HIT sera or plasmas that tested positive in the SRA also tested positive in the c-PRP aggregation assay. In contrast, no sample was identified that tested positive only in the aggregation assay. Chong and colleagues (1993a) also found a higher sensitivity for the SRA method. However, considerable variability in sensitivity for HIT antibodies among the various platelet donors was seen, ranging from 39–81% (c-PRP assay) to 65–94% (washed platelet SRA).

Strong evidence in favor of a higher sensitivity for washed platelet assays was provided by direct comparison using platelets prepared and tested in parallel that were obtained simultaneously from the same platelet donors (Greinacher et al., 1994a). Only 23 of 70 HIT sera that tested positive by the HIPA assay also tested positive using c-PRP aggregation. In contrast, all but one of 24 sera testing positive in the c-PRP aggregation assay also tested positive in the HIPA test.

More recently, Walenga and colleagues (1999) also found a lower sensitivity of the c-PRP aggregation test compared with the SRA. In contrast, Pouplard et al., (1999) reported a similar high sensitivity of the c-PRP as the SRA (91% *vs* 88%), but with a lower specificity (77% *vs* 100%).

The biologic basis for the superior operating characteristics (sensitivity–specificity profile) of the washed platelet activation assays *vis-à-vis* c-PRP-based assays for HIT diagnosis remains uncertain.

Whole Blood Impedance Aggregometry

A multiple electrode platelet aggregometer, known as Multiplate® (Dynabyte Medical, Munich, Germany), can be used to test patient serum or c-PPP against citrate-anticoagulated whole blood obtained from a normal platelet donor, thus avoiding platelet handling and preparation as required for other platelet activation assays. Per the manufacturer, the term Multiplate® derives from "multiple platelet function analyzer"; multiple also refers to the multiple electrodes in the disposable test cell (four electrodes form two independent sensor units, which detect platelet aggregation), multiple channels of the instrument (five) as well as multiple test procedures available for comprehensively assessing platelet function.

Three studies (Elalamy et al., 2009; Morel-Kopp et al., 2010, 2012) reported use of whole blood impedance aggregometry (WBIA) for detecting HIT antibodies; one study (Elalamy et al., 2009) noted sensitivity to be lower than that of a washed platelet SRA, but similar to that of standard platelet aggregometry. In contrast, Morel-Kopp et al. (2012) found broadly similar sensitivity between the SRA and WBIA.

ANTIGEN ASSAYS FOR HIT ANTIBODIES

"Antigen assays" are essentially synonymous with "PF4-dependent" immunoassays, as >99% of sera that contain heparin-dependent platelet-activating antibodies also recognize PF4/H complexes in an EIA (Greinacher et al., 2007; Warkentin et al., 2008). Although a theoretical disadvantage of PF4-dependent immunoassays is that they will fail to detect HIT antibodies that target non–PF4-dependent antigens [e.g., interleukin-8, neutrophil-activating peptide-2 (see chap. 6)], in practice, these appear to be rarely responsible for HIT, and well-documented supporting clinical studies implicating these putative "minor" HIT antigens are sparse. Use of either patient serum or plasma (EDTA- or citrate-anticoagulated) yields similar results (Krakow et al., 2007), although high levels of heparin in lithium heparin-anticoagulated chemistry tubes cause false-negative anti-PF4/H EIA results by inhibiting antibody binding (Warkentin and Sheppard, 2007).

Solid-Phase PF4-H Enzyme Immunoassay

The solid-phase EIA has been described in detail (Amiral et al., 1992; Greinacher et al., 1994a; Visentin et al., 1994; Amiral et al., 1995; Horsewood et al., 1996; Juhl et al., 2006). The first commercial EIA was from Diagnostic Stago (Asnières-sur-Seine, France). Methods differ in the way that PF4/H complexes are coated on the microtiter wells. A general scheme is shown in Figure 11.3. In this assay, stoichiometric concentrations

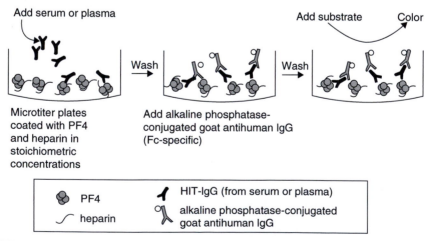

FIGURE 11.3 Schematic figure of solid-phase PF4/heparin-EIA. *Abbreviations*: EIA, enzyme immunoassay; HIT, heparin-induced thrombocytopenia; PF4, platelet factor 4.

of PF4 and heparin (e.g., 50 μL each of 20 μg/mL PF4 and 1 U/mL UFH) dissolved in PBS are added together to the wells of a microtiter plate and incubated at 4°C overnight. After washing with PBS Tween 20 (PBS-Tw), the wells are "blocked" with a protein-containing solution, such as PBS-Tw containing either 10% normal goat serum (NGS) or 20% fetal calf serum, followed by washing with PBS-Tw. To perform the assay, 50–100 μL of test or control plasma or serum diluted 1:50 in PBS containing 2% NGS is added to duplicate wells for 1 hour at room temperature. After thorough washing with PBS-Tw, bound immunoglobulin is detected by adding alkaline phosphatase-conjugated goat antihuman immunoglobulin (e.g., affinity-purified goat antihuman IgG Fc diluted 1:1000 in PBS-Tw-2% NGS) followed by incubation for 1 hour at room temperature. After thorough washing, *p*-nitrophenyl phosphate in 1 M diethanolamine buffer is added. After incubation in the dark, the reaction is stopped with 1 N NaOH, and absorbance is read at 405 nm using an automated microplate reader. The upper limit of the normal range is usually set at the mean +3 SD obtained using normal sera. Some laboratories set an indeterminate range for samples that are only minimally above the upper normal range (e.g., up to 1.0 units).

Solid-Phase PF4–Polyvinylsulfonate Antigen Assay
Several negatively charged substances can cause the cryptic autoepitope(s) within PF4 to become recognizable to HIT antibodies (see chaps. 5 and 6). Indeed, a commercial assay for HIT using PF4 complexed with polyvinylsulfonate has been developed (Visentin et al., 2001). Sensitivity and reproducibility were high using polyvinylsulfonate that had been fractionated to a relatively uniform MW (5000 ± 500 Da). Some technical advantages of this assay include the observation that the ratio of PF4/PVS is not critical (cf. PF4/H), with acceptable concentrations of PVS ranging from 0.1 to 100 mmol/L for a corresponding concentration of 10 μg/mL PF4. The antigen complex is also stable for long periods.

The manufacturer of the PF4/polyvinylsulfonate EIA (Gen-Probe GTI Diagnostics, Waukesha, Wisconsin, U.S.A.) recommends that a confirmatory step be performed, in which inhibition by 50% or more in the presence of high heparin (100 IU/mL) is considered supportive of a positive test result. However, as discussed later, this maneuver does not distinguish between clinically relevant and irrelevant anti-PF4/H antibodies, so test specificity is only modestly increased.

Solid-Phase PF4 (and/or other protein)/heparin complexes
HYPHEN Biomed (Neuville-sur-Oise, France) has commercialized several assays, collectively known as Zymutest HIA, which utilize PF4 (and potentially other heparin-binding proteins) obtained from platelet lysate to form antigen complexes to which HIT antibodies bind. In this assay, heparin is covalently linked to the microtiter plate in a way that still allows for binding to proteins, and a lysate of platelets and leukocytes is added, providing heparin-binding proteins, which form the antigenic complexes. Marketed are monospecific assays (detecting individually IgG, IgA, or IgM), as well as an assay that detects all three immunoglobulin classes (Zymutest HIA-IgG/A/M).

Pouplard and colleagues (2010) reported high sensitivity of the Zymutest HIA-IgG/A/M for SRA-positive HIT, with much higher diagnostic specificity observed for the IgG-specific assay. Two groups (Warkentin et al., 2010; Bakchoul et al., 2011) compared the Zymutest-IgG against another commercially available

IgG-specific EIA (from Gen-Probe GTI Diagnostics); both assays had very good operating characteristics, with somewhat better specificity observed with the latter assay. Both groups also found many EIA-positive samples that yielded negative results in the washed platelet activation assay.

COMPARISON OF SOLID-PHASE ENZYME IMMUNOASSAYS

Table 11.5 compares three commercial EIAs, as well as the two "in-house" EIAs used in the Authors' laboratories. Discrepant results between corresponding poly-specific or IgG-specific assays are observed in approximately 10–20% of patient samples tested, usually with weakly reacting samples. However, on rare occasions, more strongly reacting HIT antibodies within a particular patient's serum test negative in one of the assays, suggesting that there are subtle differences in conformation of HIT antigens between the assays that could result in very occasional false-negative results (<1% of sera testing EIA-negative despite clear positive testing in a washed platelet activation assay).

All three commercial EIAs now offer IgG-specific versions. The primary advantage is that detection of the IgG class alone greatly improves diagnostic specificity without substantial loss of sensitivity (Lindhoff-Last et al., 2001; Untch et al., 2002; Warkentin et al., 2005b, 2010; Bakchoul et al., 2009; Pouplard et al., 2010; Morel-Kopp et al., 2011). This improves test specificity because PF4/H-reactive IgA and IgM class antibodies (which are detected in the polyspecific EIAs) are unlikely to cause HIT.

High Heparin Inhibition Maneuver

PF4 and heparin form immunogenic, multimolecular complexes only when both are present at stoichiometrically optimal concentrations (PF4:heparin molar ratio, approximately 1:1 to 2:1). Very high concentrations of heparin (10–100 U/mL) disrupt these complexes. This property is exploited in laboratory diagnostic

TABLE 11.5 Comparison of Three Commercial and Two In-House EIAs for Detecting HIT Antibodies

Manufacturer	PF4 (source)	Polyanion	Assay	Ab classes
Diagnostica Stago	Recombinant	Heparin	1. Asserachrom HPIA; 2. Asserachrom HPIA-IgG	1. IgG/A/M 2. IgG
Gen-Probe GTI Diagnostics	Platelets (outdated)	Polyvinylsulfonate (PVS)	1. PF4 Enhanced 2. PF4 IgG	1. IgG/A/M 2. IgG
HYPHEN BioMed	Platelet lysate	Heparin bound to protamine	Zymutest HIA	IgG/A/M; IgG IgA IgM
McMaster Platelet Immunology Laboratory	Platelets (outdated)	Heparin	"In-house"	IgG IgA IgM
Greifswald Platelet Laboratory	Platelets (fresh or outdated)	Heparin	"In-house"	IgG IgA IgM

testing: addition of high heparin inhibits platelet activation (Sheridan et al., 1986) and PF4-dependent immunoassays (Greinacher et al., 1994d).

Some investigators—and one manufacturer (Gen-Probe GTI Diagnostics)—recommend performing a high heparin maneuver to increase diagnostic specificity (Whitlatch et al., 2008, 2010). In this "confirmatory procedure," a positive EIA result is performed in parallel with very high heparin concentrations, usually 100 U/mL heparin. Such high heparin levels disrupt the antigenic PF4/H complexes, with reactivity usually inhibited by >50%. However, this maneuver only increases diagnostic specificity to a minor degree, since both pathogenic and nonpathogenic anti-PF4/H antibodies are usually inhibited by high heparin. Also, in practice, relatively few EIA-"positive" samples are not inhibited by high heparin. Of concern, occasionally a true-positive HIT serum/plasma will fail to be inhibited by the high heparin procedure (perhaps because of very high antibody titers), thus risking sample misclassification (Warkentin and Sheppard, 2006b; Bakchoul et al., 2011; Selleng et al., 2011). For this reason, we suggest using the high heparin procedure only when the OD is weakly positive (<1.0 OD units): in this situation, failure of high heparin to inhibit binding indicates that heparin-dependent platelet-activating antibodies are unlikely to be present, without the risk of sample misclassification that can result when the high heparin step is used for samples yielding higher reactivity in the EIA (Althaus et al., 2011). However, PF4-dependent EIAs appear to differ with respect to effects of the high heparin inhibition step, and further work is needed to clarify this issue. Another consideration: including the high heparin step will either double test costs (by requiring that each assay be performed both in the absence and in the presence of high heparin), or will delay the reporting of a positive test result (in case an algorithm is used in which a tentative positive test result is subsequently "confirmed" by this maneuver) (Warkentin and Sheppard, 2006b).

Fluid-Phase EIA

The fluid-phase EIA for HIT antibodies (Newman et al., 1998) is an adaptation of a staphylococcal protein A antibody-capture EIA method (Nagi et al., 1993). By permitting antibody–antigen interactions to occur in a fluid phase, problems of protein (antigen) denaturation inherent in solid-phase assays are avoided.

PF4 (5% biotinylated) is mixed with an optimal concentration of heparin, and this antigen mixture is incubated with diluted patient serum or plasma (Fig. 11.4). Subsequently, the antigen–antibody mixture is incubated with protein G-Sepharose in a microcentrifuge tube. Biotinylated antigen–antibody complexes become bound to the protein G-Sepharose by antibody Fc, and the complexes are separated from unbound antigen by centrifugation and washing. The amount of biotin-PF4/H/antibody complexes immobilized to the beads is measured using peroxidase substrate after initial incubation with streptavidin-conjugated peroxidase.

The fluid-phase EIA appears to have a lower rate of false-positive reactions. This may be because in the solid-phase-EIA, nonspecific binding of IgG to the microtiter wells can occur. Furthermore, the cryptic antigen site of PF4 can be exposed when the molecule comes into close contact with the plastic surface, even in the absence of heparin (Newman and Chong, 1999). The fluid-phase assay avoids these problems by first precipitating all reactive IgG antibodies, then detecting the antigen specifically bound to the IgG. Thus, higher concentrations of patient serum or plasma can be tested without increasing nonspecific reactivity. The advantages of this assay in performing *in vitro* cross-reactivity are discussed

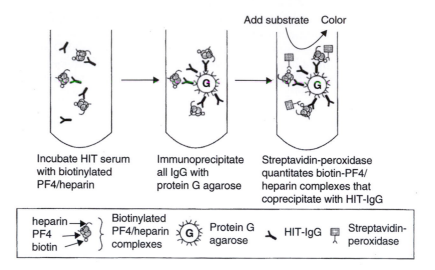

FIGURE 11.4 Schematic figure of fluid-phase PF4/heparin-EIA. *Abbreviations*: EIA, enzyme immunoassay; HIT, heparin-induced thrombocytopenia; PF4, platelet factor 4.

later. Because antibody is bound using protein G-Sepharose, IgM and IgA anti-PF4/H antibodies are not detected in this assay.

Wang and coworkers (1999a,b) used protein A to capture IgG antibodies from HIT patient serum. The immobilized antibodies were then incubated with normal serum (presumed to contain PF4) and fluorescence-labeled heparin. The amount of fluorescence dye bound to the protein A Sepharose was used to detect HIT antibodies. The major drawbacks of this approach include the initial capturing of IgG other than HIT-IgG, as well as the unpredictable PF4/heparin ratios.

A newly developed assay, the gold nanoparticle-based lateral flow immunoassay, is also a fluid-phase assay, and is discussed subsequently under the classification of a "rapid assay."

Rapid Assay: Lateral Flow Immunoassay Using Gold Nanoparticles

A rapid nanoparticle-based fluid-phase EIA is marketed in Europe by Milenia Biotec (Giessen, Germany) (Kolde et al., 2011; Sachs et al., 2011). In this "lateral-flow immunoassay" (LFI), capillary action causes the test sample to flow laterally along a solid phase (test strip) (Fig. 11.5). Flow commences after 5 μL of patient serum and two drops of reagent (ligand-labeled PF4/polyanion complexes) are added to the sample pad. During their migration through the test strip, the ligand-labeled PF4/polyanion complexes come into contact with (red-colored) gold nanoparticles, which are coated with antiligand. At the same time, anti-PF4/polyanion antibodies (if present) bind to the PF4/polyanion complexes. These complexes continue to migrate to the test line, where immobilized goat anti-human IgG captures the IgG/PF4/polyanion complexes to which the gold nanoparticles are also bound (through the ligand–antiligand interaction). A positive reaction is a bold-colored line. A control antibody (antiligand antibody) is included on each test strip and should result in a bold line at the end of the test strip, irrespective of test sample positivity or

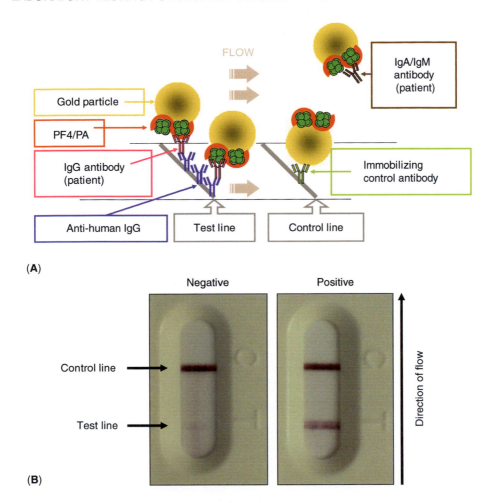

FIGURE 11.5 Gold nanoparticle-based lateral-flow immunoassay. This assay can be classified both as a "fluid-phase" immunoassay, as well as a "rapid assay." (**A**) Schematic drawing. The test kit includes two test cassettes with the inserted strips. In the "test line," strips are coated with a goat anti-human IgG antibody (blue) embedded onto the membrane, which will capture human anti-PF4/H antibodies of IgG class (red) that have bound to PF4/polyanion (PF4/PA) complexes on gold nanoparticles. The control line contains antibodies (green) that bind to and thereby immobilize the free (unused) conjugate/gold nanoparticles. Anti-PF4/H antibodies of IgA and/or IgM classes (black) are not detected. (**B**) Appearance of a representative negative and positive assay result. See text for further details. *Source*: Courtesy of T. Bakchoul and U. Sachs.

negativity; this ensures that proper reagent application and sample migration has occurred. The turnaround time for the LFI (after preparation of patient serum) is only 15 minutes; further, the single-assay design facilitates on-demand testing (Cuker, 2011). Results can be read visually, or quantitatively with a reader.

In an evaluation of this assay by the Platelet Immunology Laboratory in Giessen, Germany, the investigators found the HIT-LFI to have high sensitivity for

Particle Gel Immunoassay
(DiaMed ID-PaGIA Heparin/PF4 antibody test)

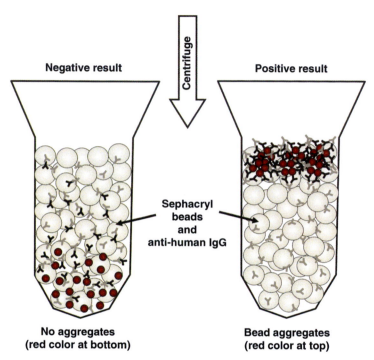

FIGURE 11.6   Schematic drawing showing the PaGIA using gel centrifugation technology. A secondary anti-antibody is used to facilitate particle gel agglutination. Unlike the EIA, which reaches an equilibrium state of antibody–antigen reaction, the PaGIA is a dynamic immunoassay. *Abbreviations*: HIT, heparin-induced thrombocytopenia; PaGIA, particle gel immunoassay; PF4, platelet factor 4. *Source*: From Warkentin and Sheppard (2006a).

detecting platelet-activating HIT antibodies, but with the additional advantage of fewer false-positive results compared with the PaGIA and two other commercial IgG-specific EIAs (Sachs et al., 2011).

Rapid Assay: Particle Gel Immunoassay (ID-H/PF4 Test)

Figure 11.6 illustrates a rapid assay for anti-PF4/H antibodies, the particle gel immunoassay [(PaGIA], ID-H/PF4–PaGIA) (DiaMed, Cressier sur Morat, Switzerland). This assay utilizes PF4/H complexes bound to red, high-density polystyrene particles; after addition of patient serum or plasma, the anti-PF4/H antibodies bind to the antigen-coated beads (Meyer et al., 1999; Eichler et al., 2002). However, IgG class antibodies do not agglutinate the polystyrene beads well, and therefore a secondary antihuman immunoglobulin antibody is added into the sephacryl gel. The principle of this (and other gel centrifugation assays) is that upon centrifugation, the agglutinated beads (indicating the presence of anti-PF4/H antibodies) do not migrate through the sephacryl gel (strong positive result), whereas nonagglutinated beads (indicating absence of antibodies) pass through the gel (negative result), thus forming a red band at the bottom. A weak positive result is indicated by dispersal of the particles throughout the gel. The assay is technically easy, can be performed rapidly, and is readily automated. Results are read visually. The method is available to blood banks that utilize a gel centrifugation technology system. The PaGIA has been in use in Europe, Asia, and Canada for several years, but is not available in the United States.

Eichler and colleagues (2002) compared this assay with two functional assays (HIPA test; SRA) and two commercially available solid-phase PF4-dependent EIAs. In preselected samples, the H/PF4–PaGIA had a sensitivity intermediate between that of the functional and commercial antigen assays. The specificity appeared to resemble that of the functional assays.

In contrast, Risch and coworkers (2003) found many more sera to test positive using the H/PF4–PaGIA, compared with a commercial EIA (Asserochrom®), among 42 patients sampled 10–18 days following cardiac surgery (69% *vs* 26%). Since none of the patients had clinical evidence of HIT, this suggested that the diagnostic specificity of the H/PF4–PaGIA was far less than the solid-phase EIA. These authors did not test sera from patients with HIT, and therefore were unable to assess test sensitivity.

The manufacturer's instructions indicate that the assay is to be read as "positive" (any agglutination within the gel), "negative" (no agglutination) using neat (undiluted) serum, or "borderline." However, when a positive or borderline test result was obtained, Alberio et al., (2003) repeated the assay with undiluted and serially diluted plasma (up to one in 1024) until the result was negative. The reported titer was the last positive result followed by either borderline or negative results. Patients judged clinically to have had "probable" or "highly probable/definite" HIT had antibody titers of four or more in 39 of 54 (72%) cases, compared with only two of 85 (2%) judged "unlikely" to have had HIT. Furthermore, all 19 of the patient samples that tested positive in a c-PRP aggregation assay tested positive in the PaGIA (generally, in a titer of eight or higher). Among all patients studied, the percentage with associated thrombotic complications increased from 8% (negative or low titer) to 55% (positive titer 4–16) to 74% (positive titer 32–256). This study suggests that reporting quantitatively the results of the H/PF4–PaGIA—with a titer of four or more being clinically significant—may increase diagnostic usefulness.

The PaGIA will occasionally "miss" a true-positive HIT result, and thus its sensitivity (~95%) is not as high as that of the EIA (~99%). In some cases, faulty lots may have accounted for suboptimal sensitivity (Schneiter et al., 2009). We later summarize a comprehensive comparative study (Bakchoul et al., 2009) of the PaGIA that integrated clinical information (4Ts score), IgG- and polyspecific PF4-dependent assays (from Gen-Probe GTI Diagnostics), and a functional test (HIPA) in the section, "Comparison of Activation and Antigen Assays."

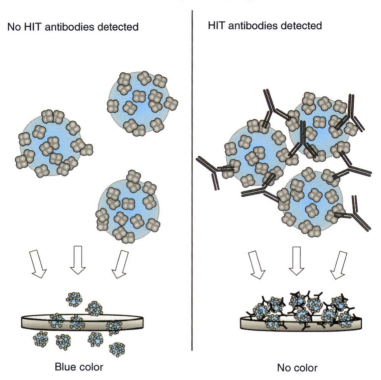

PIFA® (Particle ImmunoFiltration Assay)
PF4-coated polystyrene microspheres

No HIT antibodies detected   HIT antibodies detected

Blue color   No color

FIGURE 11.7   Schematic drawing showing the PIFA. *Abbreviations*: HIT, heparin-induced throm-bocytopenia; PIFA, particle immunofiltration assay; PF4, platelet factor 4. *Source*: From Warkentin and Sheppard (2006a).

Rapid Assay: Particle Immunofiltration Assay

More recently, another rapid immunoassay for anti-PF4/H antibodies, the "PIFA®
Heparin/PF4 Rapid Assay" (Akers BioSciences, Thorofare, New Jersey, U.S.A.) has
been approved by the U.S. Food and Drug Administration (Fig. 11.7). This assay
utilizes a system known as "particle immunofiltration assay" (PIFA®), wherein
patient serum (fresh not frozen/thawed) is added to a reaction well containing
dyed particles coated with PF4 (*not* PF4/heparin). The lack of requirement for heparin presumably reflects formation of the HIT antigens through close approximation of PF4 tetramers achieved under the conditions of PF4 binding to the particles
(Greinacher et al., 2006). Subsequently, nonagglutinated—but not agglutinated—
particles—will migrate through the membrane filter. Thus, a negative test is shown
by a blue color in the result well, whereas no color indicates a positive test. FDA
approval was based on the assay being judged by the FDA as substantially equivalent to the solid-phase EIA available from GTI. However, in a preliminary report
(Francis et al., 2006), and in the laboratories of both authors (Warkentin et al., 2007),

this assay showed unacceptable sensitivity and specificity for detecting anti-PF4/H antibodies, and its use is not recommended.

Rapid Assays: Instrumentation-Based Assays

Two automated assays that utilize proprietary instruments, one based on agglutination of latex particles and the other on chemiluminescence, have recently been developed by Instrumentation Laboratory (Bedford, Massachusetts, U.S.A.).

Latex Particle-Enhanced Immunoturbidimetric Assay

The HemosIL HIT-Ab$_{(PF4-H)}$, which is performed using an ACL TOP® Family system, is a latex particle enhanced immunoturbidimetric assay that detects anti-PF4/H antibodies of all immunoglobulin classes (Davidson et al., 2011). In this assay, a suspension of polystyrene latex particles coated with mouse monoclonal anti-PF4/H reacts with a solution containing PF4/polyvinylsulfonate (PVS) (the reaction buffer also contains a blocking agent against human antimouse antibodies to minimize this interference on the assay results). To this is added patient sample (citrated plasma); if patient anti-PF4/H antibodies are not present, the HIT-mimicking monoclonal antibody coated onto the latex particles will bind with the PF4/PVS reagent, and agglutination will occur. However, if the patient plasma contains anti-PF4/H antibodies, then agglutination will be inhibited by binding competition. In this competitive agglutination system, the degree of agglutination is inversely proportional to the level of antibodies in the patient sample, as assessed by decrease in light transmittance. (The assay is calibrated using a buffer containing monoclonal anti-PF4/H.) Thus, a positive sample will result in a *lower* absorbance (turbidimetric) than negative samples. The software automatically reports the results in units per milliliter as the inverse proportion to absorbance. If a strong positive result measures outside the test range (0–5.7U/mL), the instrument automatically reruns the test after making an on-board dilution and correcting the final result for the dilution factor; thus, the effective measuring range is up to 16.0U/mL. A positive test is a result ≥1.0U/mL. The technology allows for on-demand single-patient testing, so that a result can be provided within 15 minutes of sample preparation.

In a study of 414 patient samples that compared the HemosIL HIT-Ab$_{(PF4-H)}$ with the Stago EIA (IgG/A/M), overall agreement was seen in 88% of samples (co-negativity, 95%, co-positivity 60%) (Davidson et al., 2011). However, patient information was not available, and no platelet activation assay was used, so implications of discrepant results could not be ascertained.

The HemosIL HIT-Ab$_{(PF4-H)}$ assay is not currently available in the United States or China but is available elsewhere.

Chemiluminenscence Assays

The chemiluminescence assays (HemosIL AcuStar HIT-IgG$_{(PF4-H)}$, HemosIL AcuStar HIT-Ab$_{(PF4-H)}$), which are performed using the ACL AcuStar® hemostasis testing system, are also based on binding of anti-PF4/H antibodies to PF4/PVS (Legnani et al., 2010). Here, magnetic particles coated with PF4/PVS capture anti-PF4/H antibodies present within a patient sample. After incubation, magnetic separation, and a wash step, a tracer consisting of an isoluminol-labeled anti-human IgG antibody (or a mixture of three isoluminol-labeled monoclonal antibodies [anti-IgG, -IgA, and -IgM]) is added, which binds to the captured anti-PF4/H antibodies on the particles. After a second incubation, magnetic separation, and a wash step, reagents that trigger the luminescence reaction are added, and the emitted light is measured as relative light units (RLUs) by the instrument's optical system. The RLUs are directly proportional to the concentration of anti-PF4/H antibodies in the sample. A positive test is a result ≥1.00 U/mL for both the total antibody and IgG-specific assay. This assay can be performed with serum or plasma and can distinguish between different immunoglobulin classes. It shows a wide range of reactivity, and thus stronger results may indicate a higher likelihood of HIT (Legnani et al., 2010). The fully automated random access analyzer also allows for single-patient testing, providing test results in approximately 30 minutes.

COMPARISON OF ACTIVATION AND ANTIGEN ASSAYS

Both PF4/H-EIAs and washed platelet activation assays have approximately equal (high) sensitivity for clinical HIT (Greinacher et al., 1994a; Warkentin et al., 2000, 2005b). For serum or plasma samples that are known to be positive by one sensitive washed platelet activation assay (e.g., SRA or HIPA), the corresponding probability of the PF4/H-EIA for confirming the positive result is at least 75–90% (Greinacher et al., 1994a; Arepally et al., 1995), with more recent studies suggesting ~99% sensitivity of the EIA (Warkentin et al., 2005b, 2008; Juhl et al., 2006; Greinacher et al., 2007). Conversely, a similar percentage of referred samples with high clinical probability of HIT that test positive in the EIA will also test positive using a washed platelet activation assay (Greinacher et al., 1994a; Lo et al., 2006; Schenk et al., 2006, 2007). The sensitivity of both EIA and SRA was very high for detecting antibodies that caused HIT in prospectively collected serial blood samples in postoperative orthopedic patients exhibiting a high frequency of HIT (Warkentin et al., 2000, 2005b, 2009).

Although both antigen and activation assays have a similar high sensitivity for clinical HIT, there is considerable evidence that antigen assays have far greater sensitivity for detecting anti-PF4/H antibodies not associated with thrombocytopenia or other clinical events (Amiral et al., 1995; Arepally et al., 1995; Bauer et al., 1997; Warkentin et al., 2000, 2005b, 2009; Juhl et al., 2006; Schenk et al., 2006, 2007; Warkentin, 2011) (Table 11.6; Fig. 11.8). Stated another way, the functional assays are more diagnostically specific for clinically evident HIT than are the antigen assays. The biologic explanation for greater specificity of a sensitive activation assay for clinical HIT, compared with an antigen assay, could relate to the functional heterogeneity of HIT antibodies against antigenic determinants on PF4, only some of which activate platelets strongly (Amiral et al., 2000). Data reported by Visentin and colleagues (1994) also support a higher sensitivity of antigen assays for detecting platelet-activating anti-PF4/H antibodies. These workers studied 12 HIT plasmas that tested positive in both SRA and PF4/H-EIA. However, at a 1:100 sample dilution, only two of the 12 samples still tested positive in the activation assay. In contrast, even at a 1:200 dilution, all 12 plasmas still tested positive in the EIA. Bachelot and colleagues (1998) observed that HIT plasmas that tested only weakly positive in the PF4/H-EIA tended to give negative washed platelet SRA results when using platelets with the least reactive FcγIIa receptor phenotype, Arg[131].

The difference in sensitivity for HIT antibodies between the PF4/H-EIA and aggregation studies using c-PRP is considerable. Only about 33–64% of samples

TABLE 11.6 Frequency of Thrombocytopenia (>50% Platelet Count Fall) Among Anti-PF4/H EIA-Positive (EIA+) Patients (Polyspecific or IgG-Specific Assay) Who Received Heparin (UFH or LMWH): a Comparison of SRA+ vs SRA-Negative (SRA−) Status

	Frequency of thrombocytopenia	
SRA status	**Positive in polyspecific EIA (IgG/A/M)**	**Positive in IgG-specific EIA**
A. Postorthopedic surgery patients[a]		
SRA+	12/24	12/24
SRA−	0/58	0/16
P	<0.0001	0.0009
B. Venous thromboembolism patients[a,b]		
SRA+	4/4	4/4
SRA−	0/15	0/6
P	0.0003	0.0048
C. Postcardiac surgery patients		
SRA+	4/11	NA
SRA−	0/152	NA
P	<0.0001	NA

Data to construct this Table were obtained from published literature (Warkentin et al., 1995, 2005b, 2011a; Lee and Warkentin, 2007; Pouplard et al., 2005).
[a]For the data shown, the cutoff for a positive SRA was 20% serotonin release. For study A (postorthopedic surgery), if instead a 50% serotonin release cutoff is used, the comparisons (polyspecific EIA) yield similar results: 11/20 vs 1/62 (P < 0.0001), and unchanged data for study B (venous thromboembolism patients).
[b]For the venous thromboembolism study, all positive EIA results shown were ≥1.0 units of optical density.
Source: From Warkentin (2011).
Abbreviations: EIA, enzyme immunoassay; LMWH, low molecular weight heparin; NA, not available; SRA+, positive in the serotonin release assay; SRA−, negative in the serotonin release assay; UFH, unfractionated heparin.

that test positive in the PF4/H-EIA also test positive using c-PRP aggregation (Greinacher et al., 1994a; Nguyen et al., 1995; Rugeri et al., 1999). Although one laboratory reported a greater sensitivity using c-PRP aggregation than the EIA (Look et al., 1997), these workers did not employ a two-point method, and so may have observed false-positive results using the aggregation assay.

Bakchoul and colleagues (2009) published a comprehensive comparison of the PaGIA in comparison with IgG- and polyspecific EIAs, as well as the (washed platelet) HIPA. Moreover, these authors presented clinical information using the 4Ts scoring system (see chap. 3). Figure 11.9 depicts the interrelationship of these assays. Of note, occasional HIT cases are missed by the PaGIA (sensitivity, ~95%), although its diagnostic specificity is better than that of the EIAs. The data also support the "iceberg" model of HIT, wherein platelet-activating antibodies comprise a subset of anti-PF4/H antibodies, and with both types of assays (functional and immunoassays) having very high sensitivity for HIT, but with the HIPA having greater diagnostic specificity than the EIA-IgG, and the latter having greater specificity than the polyspecific EIA.

To date, relatively few comparative data are available between washed platelet activation assays and the newer immunoassays, such as the lateral flow immunoassay and the instrumentation-based assays.

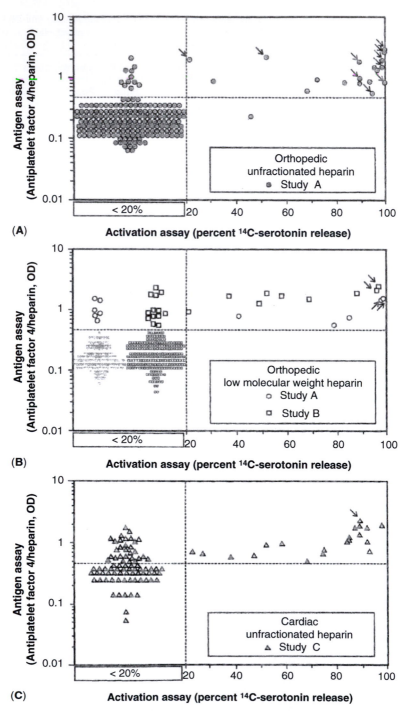

FIGURE 11.8 Comparison of activation and antigen assays for HIT-IgG: analysis of prospective studies. (*Continued*)

FIGURE 11.8 (*Continued*) Quantitative results of an activation assay, the SRA, are shown on the *x*-axis [although samples that gave <20% serotonin release are shown without reference to the actual quantitative result obtained (see box designated <20%)]; quantitative results of the antigen assay (which detected only IgG anti-PF4/H antibodies) are shown on the *y*-axis. (**A**) Orthopedic surgery patients who received UFH; (**B**) orthopedic surgery patients who received LMWH; and (**C**) cardiac surgery patients who also received postoperative UFH. The arrows indicate the data points corresponding to the 15 patients who developed clinical HIT (>50% platelet count fall from the postoperative peak). The data show similarly high sensitivity of the activation and antigen assays for clinical HIT; however, the activation assay had higher specificity for clinical HIT. Most sera (13/15, 87%) from patients with clinical HIT strongly activated platelets (>80% serotonin release). *Abbreviations*: HIT, heparin-induced thrombocytopenia; LMWH, low molecular weight heparin; PF4, platelet factor 4; SRA, serotonin release assay; UFH, unfractionated heparin. *Source*: From Warkentin et al. (2000).

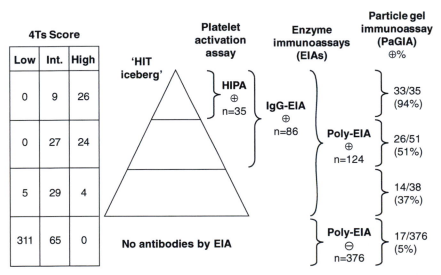

FIGURE 11.9 Key data from the article by Bakchoul and colleagues (2009) when viewed per the "iceberg model" of HIT. The central "iceberg" depicts three different antibody reaction profiles, as defined by the platelet activation test (HIPA assay) and two EIAs [IgG-EIA (IgG-specific EIA); poly-EIA (polyspecific EIA, i.e., detects IgG, IgA, and/or IgM class anti-PF4/H antibodies; both assays from Gen-Probe GTI Diagnostics)]. The table on the far left shows the pretest probability scores (4Ts) for the three different antibody reaction profiles, as well as for patients who tested negative in both EIAs (bottom row of 4Ts table). On the far right, the corresponding results in the particle gel immunoassay (PaGIA) are shown. The data demonstrate that the sensitivity of the PaGIA for definite HIT (35 patients depicted as the "tip of the iceberg") is only 94% (33/35). At the other extreme, ~5% of the patients who have no antibodies by EIA will test positive in the PaGIA (17/376). *Abbreviations*: EIA, enzyme immunoassay; HIPA, heparin-induced platelet activation; HIT, heparin-induced thrombocytopenia; Int., intermediate; PaGIA, particle gel immunoassay. *Source*: From Warkentin and Linkins (2009).

INTERPRETATION OF HIT TEST RESULTS

It is important to incorporate clinical information into the interpretation of any laboratory result for HIT. This is because thrombocytopenia, whether or not caused by HIT, is common in hospitalized patients receiving heparin, and because nonpathogenic HIT antibodies are often detected by sensitive assays in patients who have received heparin five or more days ago. Indeed, Bayesian approaches that integrate pretest probability of HIT with the results of testing for HIT antibodies have been described (Warkentin, 2005; Warkentin and Cook, 2011; Nellen et al., 2012).

How Should Clinical HIT Be Defined?

HIT is a clinicopathologic syndrome, and thus is defined as a patient with a clinical profile consistent with HIT, and in whom heparin-dependent, platelet-activating antibodies can be detected. From an operational point-of-view, this corresponds to at least an "intermediate" pretest probability score (e.g., >4 points in the 4Ts scoring system) and having a positive washed platelet activation assay for "strong" heparin-dependent platelet-activating antibodies (generally >50% serotonin release; or <25 min lag time in the HIPA in at least two out of four platelet donors) (Warkentin et al., 2011b). If a positive EIA is used to support the presence of antibodies, the clinician should be aware that non–platelet-activating antibodies could give a "false-positive" test result, and so if the clinical picture suggests alternative diagnoses, requesting the more specific washed platelet assay may be helpful. Another relevant issue, discussed in the section "Diagnostic Interpretation of Laboratory Results," is that a higher "strength" of a positive washed platelet activation assay or solid-phase EIA increases the likelihood of the patient having HIT (Warkentin et al., 2000, 2005b, 2008, 2009; Warkentin, 2005).

Laboratory testing for HIT antibodies is often performed in clinical situations suggesting a low probability for HIT, presumably because physicians wish to "rule out" this diagnosis (Lo et al., 2006). Nellen and coworkers (2012), summarizing seven studies of the 4Ts scoring system, found that only 0.5% of patients with a low probability 4Ts score had HIT. Furthermore, we have found that only about 7–10% of patients who undergo testing for HIT antibodies have a serologic profile consistent with the diagnosis (Juhl et al., 2006; Warkentin and Sheppard, 2006a; Greinacher et al., 2007; Warkentin et al., 2008). These observations suggest that patients judged to be at low probability for HIT ought not to undergo testing, particularly using low-specificity assays.

Rapid vs Typical Onset of Thrombocytopenia

We discuss the diagnostic approach to HIT based on the timing of onset of thrombocytopenia, either rapid (<5 days) or typical (≥5 days) (see chap. 2).

In general, there are two broad pretest probabilities for patients with rapid thrombocytopenia: low and high. Patients with low pretest probability for HIT are those who have not recently been exposed to heparin (thus, they would not be expected to have circulating HIT antibodies, or to have generated them so quickly), or who have another good explanation for thrombocytopenia (most often, early postoperative thrombocytopenia). (An important caveat is that sometimes a recent heparin exposure is not known to the patient or has not been documented in the medical records.) With a low pretest probability for HIT, any of the sensitive assays for HIT (e.g., washed platelet activation assay, EIA, PaGIA) can reliably rule out HIT (Pouplard et al., 2007). However, an unexpected negative result in a patient with a high pretest probability, or an unexpected positive result in a patient with a low pretest probability, should lead to repeating the test or performance of the complementary activation or antigen assay. Additionally, further clinical information should be sought. (For example, has another explanation for the thrombocytopenia become apparent? Could the patient have had an unrecognized recent heparin exposure?) But the central tenet of HIT remains that if two sensitive and complementary tests for HIT antibodies (washed platelet activation assay, PF4-dependent antigen test) both give negative test results, the diagnosis of HIT is excluded—even in a patient with a high pretest probability (Warkentin et al., 2011b).

In contrast, for patients with the typical temporal onset of thrombocytopenia (i.e., a platelet count fall that begins 5–10 days after beginning heparin treatment), we believe that, in general, there are two different pretest probabilities for HIT: moderate and high. Because HIT is a relatively common explanation for thrombocytopenia that begins during this characteristic time period, it should be considered a plausible diagnosis even if another possible explanation for thrombocytopenia is identified (hence, a moderate pretest probability). In a patient without another apparent explanation for thrombocytopenia, or one in whom an unexplained new thrombotic event has occurred, the pretest probability for HIT would be considered to be high. However, a critically ill patient who has early-onset and persisting thrombocytopenia—without a "superimposed" additional platelet count decline or thrombotic event occurring within the day 5–10 (or 14) "window" characteristic of HIT—is unlikely to have "true" HIT, even if heparin-dependent platelet-activating antibodies become detectable (Selleng et al., 2010).

Diagnostic Interpretation of Laboratory Results

In patients with a high pretest probability of HIT who have a negative screening test, and in whom no other plausible diagnosis becomes apparent, the test should be repeated and the complementary activation or antigen assay should be performed (either from the same or a different blood sample). The diagnosis of HIT is very unlikely if both activation and antigen assays are negative, and is also unlikely if the EIA is positive but a well-performed washed platelet activation assay is negative (Warkentin et al., 2011b). It is uncertain whether a patient who tests EIA-negative but (washed platelet) activation assay-positive is more likely to have HIT related to a "minor" (i.e., non–PF4-dependent) antigen or whether this simply represents a false-positive functional assay due to a non-HIT platelet-activating factor.

In patients with a moderate pretest probability who test positive for HIT, the final diagnosis may well rest on the overall clinical picture, rather than on the test result alone. This conclusion results from two clinical realities: (*i*) sensitive HIT assays frequently detect clinically insignificant anti-PF4/H antibodies in patients who have received heparin for more than five days, and (*ii*) thrombocytopenia, whether caused by HIT or not, is common in clinical practice. There is strong evidence that positive washed platelet activation assays for HIT have greater diagnostic specificity for clinical HIT (Warkentin et al., 2000, 2005b; Lo et al., 2007; Warkentin, 2011; see Table 11.6), especially when strong, rapid platelet activation is produced by patient serum. Regardless, these considerations underscore the importance of conceptualizing HIT as a clinicopathologic syndrome, in which both clinical information and results of HIT antibody testing are used for diagnosis.

The diagnostic usefulness of certain laboratory tests for HIT is shown in Figure 11.10 (Warkentin, 2003). Both the SRA and an in-house EIA that detects only HIT-IgG were very sensitive and specific for clinical HIT in postorthopedic surgery patients. The diagnostic usefulness of these assays was somewhat less in a postcardiac surgery population. For example, among postcardiac surgery patients, the

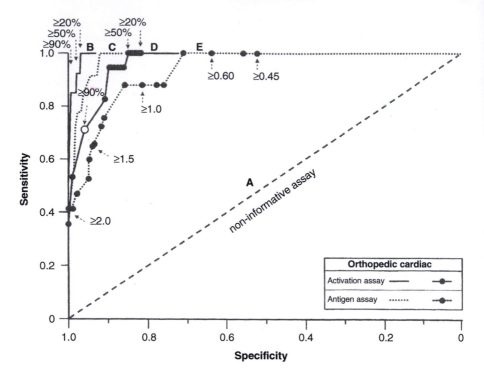

FIGURE 11.10 Sensitivity–specificity tradeoffs for diagnosis of HIT (receiver–operating characteristic curve analysis). The arrows indicate various cutoffs between positive and negative test results; e.g., the open circle indicates 90% serotonin release (postcardiac surgery patient) using a washed platelet activation assay (serotonin release assay). The likelihood ratio for HIT for a given positive test result can be estimated from the graph, using the formula: likelihood ratio = sensitivity/(1 − specificity). Thus, for 90% serotonin release (postcardiac surgery), the estimated likelihood ratio is 0.7/(1 − 0.965) = 20. *Source*: From Warkentin (2003).

likelihood ratio of a strong-positive SRA result (90% serotonin release; see open circle in Fig. 11.10) is about 20. The likelihood ratio, which is defined as the extent to which a given test result alters the physician's estimate of the pretest probability of HIT, is defined as sensitivity/(1 − specificity). In this example, the corresponding likelihood ratio is 0.70/(1 − 0.965) = 20. Thus, if the physician had estimated a pretest probability of 50% (odds of 0.5:0.5), then this test result would increase the posttest probability of having HIT to more than 95% (0.5:0.5 × 20:1 = 20:1, or 95.2%). In contrast, the high sensitivity of this assay to detect clinically important HIT antibodies (>95%) means that a negative test result lowers the posttest probability to less than 5%.

The diagnostic impact of such a strong-positive SRA result (90% serotonin release) is even greater in postorthopedic surgery patients, for whom the corresponding likelihood ratio is about 85, that is, 0.85/(1 − 0.99). As before, a negative test result essentially rules out HIT.

Although a PF4-dependent EIA that detects only HIT-IgG antibodies has lower diagnostic specificity than the SRA, it remains a very useful assay. The likelihood ratios for a strong positive test result (e.g., OD > 1.5) range from about 10 to 40 for postcardiac and postorthopedic surgery patients, respectively. Also, its high sensitivity (~99%) means that a negative test generally rules out HIT (Greinacher et al., 2007; Warkentin et al., 2008, 2011b). The combination of a positive EIA and a negative functional assay, however, does not support a diagnosis of HIT (Lo et al., 2007; Warkentin and Cook, 2011).

Thus, HIT antibody testing is among the most useful of platelet immunology assays. For comparison, Figure 11.10 also shows the profile of a "noninformative assay" (see line A). This is the profile for various tests of "platelet-associated IgG" for the diagnosis of autoimmune thrombocytopenia. Certain glycoprotein-specific platelet antibody tests have operating characteristics intermediate between those for HIT and a noninformative assay. For example, the monoclonal antibody immobilization of platelet antigens (MAIPA) assay has only moderate sensitivity but high specificity for diagnosis of autoimmune thrombocytopenia.

Figure 11.10 shows the operating characteristics for two assays: the SRA and a PF4/H-EIA that detects only IgG antibodies. Warkentin and coworkers (2005b) used archived plasma samples to compare the operating characteristics of a commercial EIA (PF4/PVS-EIA, Gen-Probe GTI Diagnostics) that detects antibodies of all three major immunoglobulin classes (IgG, IgA, IgM) (Fig. 11.11). This study showed that the additional detection of IgA and IgM class antibodies *worsened* the EIA's operating characteristics, by detecting clinically insignificant IgA and IgM antibodies without any offsetting improvement in test sensitivity. These data are consistent with the view that HIT is usually (perhaps invariably) caused by IgG antibodies, that is, the only antibody class able to activate platelets via their IgG (Fcγ) receptors.

Optical Density Levels and Prediction of a Positive Functional Assay

A practical implication of Figures 11.10 and 11.11 is that the *magnitude* of a positive HIT antibody test provides diagnostically useful information, with a strong positive result associated with a greater likelihood of a patient having clinical HIT compared with a weak positive result (Warkentin, 2003; Warkentin et al., 2008). This is illustrated more clearly in Figure 11.12, which shows the probability of a positive washed platelet activation assay (SRA) in relation to the magnitude of a positive IgG-specific EIA, expressed in OD units. The relationship is striking: for every 1.0 U increase in OD in the IgG-specific EIA, the probability of a positive SRA increases by 40 (odds ratio), or, expressed another way, from ~5% to ~25% to ~95% for corresponding OD values of 0.5, 1.5, and 2.5, respectively (Warkentin et al., 2008). Similar relationships are also seen for the polyspecific EIA (Warkentin et al., 2008), as well as with other PF4-dependent EIAs (Greinacher et al., 2010). However, OD measurements are not standardized, and these relationships may not necessarily apply in any given laboratory.

Given that higher OD values predict for greater risk of platelet-activating antibodies being present and hence a higher risk of HIT, one might predict that higher ODs would also predict for higher frequency of thrombosis. Indeed, several groups have reported a strong association between increasing OD values and greater frequency of thrombotic outcomes (Zwicker et al., 2004; Altuntas et al., 2008; Baroletti et al., 2012). Other authors without immediate access to functional assays have used OD values in a treatment algorithm to help determine their therapeutic approach (Ruf et al., 2011).

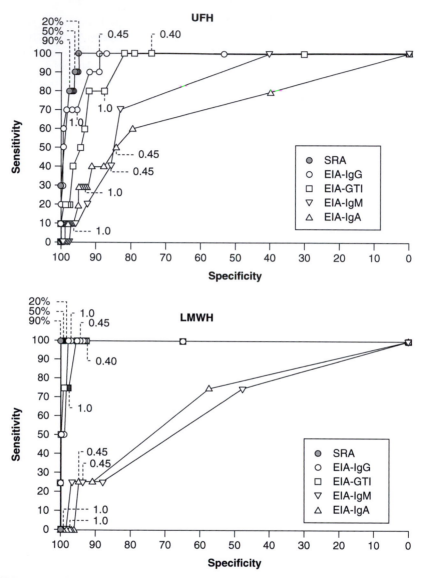

FIGURE 11.11 Comparisons of ROC curves among five different assays for anti-PF4/H antibodies. (*Top*) UFH-treated patients (*n* = 192). (*Bottom*) LMWH-treated patients (*n* = 256). The sensitivity–specificity tradeoffs at different diagnostic cutoffs for clinical HIT are shown. For the SRA, the points represent stepwise 10% changes in percent serotonin release. For the EIA-IgG and EIA-GTI, the points represent stepwise 0.20 units of OD, except for the point labeled 0.45, which represents the usual diagnostic cutoff for the three EIAs shown (EIA-IgG, EIA-IgA, and EIA-IgM). For both UFH- and LMWH-treated patients, the ROC curves show that the operating characteristics rank as follows for the diagnosis of clinical HIT: SRA > EIA-IgG > EIA-GTI (poly-specific EIA) > EIA-IgA ~ EIA-IgM. *Abbreviations*: EIA, enzyme immunoassay; LMWH, low molecular weight heparin; ROC, receiver–operating characteristic; UFH, unfractionated heparin. *Source*: From Warkentin et al. (2005b).

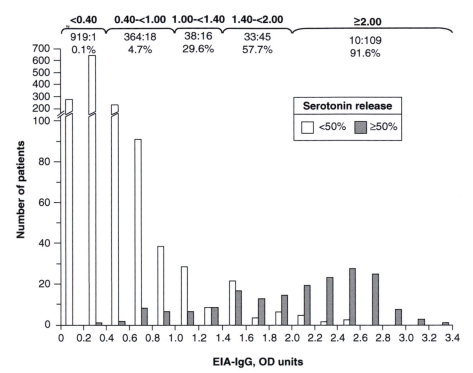

FIGURE 11.12   Predictivity of the EIA-IgG for a positive SRA. For each of five groups of quantitative EIA-IgG data (<0.40, 0.40 to <1.00, 1.00 to <1.40, 1.40 to <2.00, and ≥2.00 OD units), the percent of samples yielding a positive SRA result (≥50% serotonin release) is shown. The probability of a positive SRA result varied considerably, in relation to the magnitude of the EIA result, expressed in OD units. For the particular EIA-IgG depicted (the "in-house" assay of the McMaster Platelet Immunology Laboratory), the probability of a positive SRA result did not reach 50% or greater until the OD value was approximately 1.20–1.50 units or greater. *Abbreviations*: OD, optical density. *Source*: From Warkentin et al. (2008).

Routine Repeat Testing for HIT Antibodies with Initial Negative Results

Some investigators advocate routine repeat testing for HIT antibodies by EIA when an initial test result is negative (Refaai et al., 2003; Chan et al., 2008). However, we do not recommend this practice. The high sensitivity (~99%) of the EIA for HIT—including when samples are tested from the earliest phase of the HIT-related platelet count decline (Warkentin et al., 2009)—means that the clinical events (e.g., thrombocytopenia) that led to initial testing almost certainly are *not* due to HIT. Thus, in the absence of progressive or recurrent thrombocytopenia, or subsequent development of thrombosis, a subsequent positive EIA obtained on a routine basis is much more likely to represent a seroconversion event involving nonpathogenic anti-PF4/H (Selleng et al., 2010). When HIT is strongly suspected—despite a negative EIA—there may be greater utility in performing an EIA from a different manufacturer (as rare false-negative EIAs can occur even when anti-PF4/H antibodies are present) or in performing the complementary platelet activation assay (as it in theory can detect pathologic antibodies against non–PF4-dependent antigens) than in repeating the test using a later blood sample.

Transience of HIT Antibodies
It is important to perform tests for HIT antibodies using blood samples obtained during or soon after resolution of HIT-related thrombocytopenia. The reason is that HIT antibodies are remarkably transient, and decline to weak or nondetectable levels within weeks or a few months (Warkentin and Kelton, 2001b). On some occasions, antibodies levels decline markedly even within days, an observation that helps explain the intriguing phenomenon of resolution of thrombocytopenia in some patients with HIT even if heparin is continued (Greinacher et al., 2009). Repeated testing using a functional assay at one- to two-week intervals is recommended when the patient with recent HIT is awaiting surgery for which heparin use is desired (e.g., cardiac or vascular surgery) (see chaps. 12 and 19).

IN VITRO CROSS-REACTIVITY
Cross-Reactivity Using Activation Assays
Cross-reactivity studies have been performed most frequently using activation assays. However, there are no standard methods for, or even a standard definition of, in vitro cross-reactivity. In one study of LMWH and danaparoid cross-reactivity, an increase in platelet activation in the presence of the drug over baseline was used to determine cross-reactivity (Warkentin, 1996). This definition was used to avoid falsely attributing cross-reactivity to drug-independent platelet activation that is produced by some patients' sera. The reason for this definition was the common phenomenon that platelet activation can be caused by a patient's serum even in the absence of added heparin (although inhibited by high concentrations of heparin). In the HIPA test, comparison of the lag time to aggregation can be used to judge cross-reactivity: if a sample shows platelet aggregation with danaparoid or LMWH earlier than in the presence of buffer, then cross-reactivity is present. In general, in vitro cross-reactivity with danaparoid is usually clinically insignificant (Warkentin, 1996; Newman et al., 1998), and routine testing for cross-reactivity is not recommended (see chaps. 12 and 16).

Comparison of c-PRP vs Washed Platelet Assays
Sensitive washed platelet assays generally show almost 100% cross-reactivity of HIT antibodies for LMWH (Greinacher et al., 1992; Warkentin et al., 1995). Indeed, LMWH is somewhat better than UFH for detecting weakly activating HIT antibodies using washed platelet assays (Greinacher et al., 1994b). However, very different results have been reported by investigators using c-PRP assays (Makhoul et al., 1986; Chong et al., 1989; Kikta et al., 1993; Vun et al., 1996). Here, LMWH consistently shows less cross-reactivity compared with UFH. It is possible that differences in nonidiosyncratic heparin-induced platelet activation underlie these observations (see chap. 5): UFH is more likely to result in weak platelet activation, including some PF4 release, which leads to amplification of the platelet activation response in the presence of PF4/H-reactive HIT antibodies. In contrast, in washed platelet assays, IgG-mediated platelet activation, but not nonidiosyncratic HIPA, occurs.

Cross-Reactivity Using Antigen Assays

Although it is theoretically possible to perform a solid-phase EIA to assess cross-reactivity (Amiral et al., 1995), this is complicated because the antigen has to be coated as a complex to the solid phase. This problem has been overcome in a fluid-phase EIA described by Newman and colleagues (1998). Because this assay detects binding to a defined quantity of labeled PF4-containing antigen, the assay is able to determine *in vitro* cross-reactivity more accurately than the solid-phase EIA. These investigators observed an *in vitro* cross-reactivity rate of 88% for LMWH; about half the HIT samples reacted weakly against danaparoid in their study. The fluid-phase EIA has also been used to show that the antithrombin-binding pentasaccharide, fondaparinux, usually does not cross-react with HIT-IgG antibodies (Warkentin et al., 2005a).

ACKNOWLEDGMENTS

Studies described in this chapter were supported by the Heart and Stroke Foundation of Ontario (operating grants A2449, T2967, B3763, T4502, T5207, T6157, and T6950), and by the Deutsche Forschungsgemeinschaft Gir 1096/2–1 and Gir 1096/2–2. Dr. Warkentin was a Research Scholar of the Heart and Stroke Foundation of Canada. We thank Prof. Tamam Bakchoul for careful review of the manuscript.

REFERENCES

Alberio L, Kimmerle S, Baumann A, Taleghani BM, Biasiutti FD, Lämmle B. Rapid determination of anti-heparin/platelet factor 4 antibody titers in the diagnosis of heparin-induced thrombocytopenia. Am J Med 114: 528–536, 2003.

Almeida JI, Coats R, Liem TK, Silver D. Reduced morbidity and mortality rates of the heparin-induced thrombocytopenia syndrome. J Vasc Surg 27: 309–316, 1998.

Althaus K, Strobel U, Warkentin TE, Greinacher A. Combined use of the high heparin step and optical density to optimize diagnostic sensitivity and specificity of an anti-PF4/heparin enzyme-immunoassay. Thromb Res 128: 256–260, 2011.

Altuntas F, Matevosyan K, Burner J, Shen YM, Sarode R. Higher optical density of an antigen assay predicts thrombosis in patients with heparin-induced thrombocytopenia. Eur J Haematol 80: 429–435, 2008.

Amiral J, Bridey F, Dreyfus M, Vissac AM, Fressinaud E, Wolf M, Meyer D. Platelet factor 4 complexed to heparin is the target for antibodies generated in heparin-induced thrombocytopenia. Thromb Haemost 68: 95–96, 1992.

Amiral J, Bridey F, Wolf M, Boyer-Neumann C, Fressinaud E, Vissac AM, Peynaud-Debayle E, Dreyfus M, Meyer D. Antibodies to macromolecular platelet factor 4-Heparin complexes in heparin-induced thrombocytopenia: a study of 44 cases. Thromb Haemost 73: 21–28, 1995.

Amiral J, Pouplard C, Vissac AM, Walenga JM, Jeske W, Gruel Y. Affinity purification of heparin-dependent antibodies to platelet factor 4 developed in heparin-induced thrombocytopenia: biological characteristics and effects on platelet activation. Br J Haematol 109: 336–341, 2000.

Ardlie NG, Packham MA, Mustard JF. Adenosine diphosphate-induced platelet aggregation in suspensions of washed rabbit platelets. Br J Haematol 19: 7–17, 1970.

Arepally G, Reynolds C, Tomaski A, Amiral J, Jawad A, Poncz M, Cines DB. Comparison of the PF4/heparin ELISA assay with the 14C-serotonin assay in the diagnosis of heparin-induced thrombocytopenia. Am J Clin Pathol 104: 648–654, 1995.

Babcock RB, Dumper CW, Scharfman WB. Heparin-induced immune thrombocytopenia. N Engl J Med 295: 237–241, 1976.

Bachelot-Loza C, Saffroy R, Lasne D, Chatellier G, Aiach M, Rendu F. Importance of the FcγRIIa-Arg/His-131 polymorphism in heparin-induced thrombocytopenia diagnosis. Thromb Haemost 79: 523–528, 1998.

Bakchoul T, Giptner A, Najaoui A, Bein G, Santoso S, Sachs UJ. Prospective evaluation of PF4/heparin immunoassays for the diagnosis of heparin-induced thrombocytopenia. J Thromb Haemost 7: 1260–1265, 2009.

Bakchoul T, Giptner A, Bein G, Santoso S, Sachs UJ. Performance characteristics of two commercially available IgG-specific immunoassays in the assessment of heparin-induced thrombocytopenia (HIT). Thromb Res 127: 345–348, 2011.

Bauer TL, Arepally G, Konkle BA, Mestichelli B, Shapiro SS, Cines DB, Poncz M, McNulty S, Amiral J, Hauck WW, Edie RN, Mannion JD. Prevalence of heparinassociated antibodies without thrombosis in patients undergoing cardiopulmonary bypass surgery. Circulation 95: 1242–1246, 1997.

Baroletti S, Hurwitz S, Conti NA, Fanikos J, Piazza G, Goldhaber SZ. Thrombosis in suspected heparin-induced thrombocytopenia occurs more often with high antibody levels. Am J Med 125: 44–49, 2012.

Chan M, Malynn E, Shaz B, Uhl L. Utility of consecutive repeat HIT ELISA testing for heparin-induced thrombocytopenia. Am J Hematol 83: 212–217, 2008.

Chong BH, Ismail F, Cade J, Gallus AS, Gordon S, Chesterman CN. Heparin-induced thrombocytopenia: studies with a new molecular weight heparinoid, Org 10172. Blood 73: 1592–1596, 1989.

Chong BH, Burgess J, Ismail F. The clinical usefulness of the platelet aggregation test for the diagnosis of heparin-induced thrombocytopenia. Thromb Haemost 69: 344–350, 1993a.

Chong BH, Pilgrim RL, Cooley MA, Chesterman CN. Increased expression of platelet IgG Fc receptors in immune heparin-induced thrombocytopenia. Blood 81: 988–993, 1993b.

Chong BH, Murray B, Berndt MC, Dunlop LC, Brighton T, Chesterman CN. Plasma P-selectin is increased in thrombotic consumptive platelet disorders. Blood 83: 1535–1541, 1994.

Cuker A. Heparin-induced thrombocytopenia (HIT) in 2011: an epidemic of overdiagnosis. Thromb Haemost 106: 993–994, 2011.

Davidson SJ, Ortel TL, Smith LJ. Performance of a new, rapid, automated immunoassay for the detection of anti-platelet factor 4/heparin complex antibodies. Blood Coagul Fibrinolysis 22: 340–344, 2011.

Eichler P, Budde U, Haas S, Kroll H, Loreth RM, Meyer O, Pachmann U, Potzsch B, Schabel A, Albrecht D, Greinacher A. First workshop for detection of heparin-induced antibodies: validation of the heparin-induced platelet activation test (HIPA) in comparison with a PF4/heparin ELISA. Thromb Haemost 81: 625–629, 1999.

Eichler P, Raschke R, Lubenow N, Meyer O, Schwind P, Greinacher A. The new ID-heparin/PF4 antibody test for rapid detection of heparin-induced antibodies in comparison with functional and antigenic assays. Br J Haematol 116: 887–891, 2002.

Elalamy I, Galea V, Hatmi M, Gerotziafas GT. Heparin-induced multiple electrode aggregometry: a potential tool for improvement of heparin-induced thrombocytopenia diagnosis. J Thromb Haemost 7: 1932–1934, 2009.

Favaloro EJ, Bernal-Hoyos E, Exner T, Koutts J. Heparin-induced thrombocytopenia laboratory investigation and confirmation of diagnosis. Pathology 24: 177–183, 1992.

Fouassier M, Bourgerette E, Libert F, Pouplard C, Marques-Verdier A. Determination of serotonin release from platelets by HPLC and ELISA in the diagnosis of heparin-induced thrombocytopenia: comparison with reference method by [14C]-serotonin release assay. J Thromb Haemost 4: 1136–1139, 2006.

Francis JL, Drexler A, Duncan MK, Desai H, Amaya M, Robson T, Meyer TV, Reyes E, Rathmann K, Amirkhosravi A. Prospective evaluation of laboratory tests for the diagnosis of heparin-induced thrombocytopenia [abstr]. Blood 108: 312a, 2006.

Fratantoni JC, Pollet R, Gralnick HR. Heparin-induced thrombocytopenia: confirmation of diagnosis with in vitro methods. Blood 45: 395–401, 1975.

Gobbi G, Mirandola P, Tazzari PL, Ricci F, Caimi L, Cacchioli A, Papa S, Conte R, Vitale M. Flow cytometry detection of serotonin content and release in resting and activated platelets. Br J Haematol 121: 892–896, 2003.

Goodfellow KJ, Brown P, Malia RG, Hampton KK. A comparison of laboratory tests for the diagnosis of heparin-induced thrombocytopenia [abstr]. Br J Haematol 101(Suppl 1): 89, 1998.

Greinacher A, Michels I, Kiefel V, Mueller-Eckhardt C. A rapid and sensitive test for diagnosing heparin-associated thrombocytopenia. Thromb Haemost 66: 734–736, 1991.

Greinacher A, Michels I, Mueller-Eckhardt C. Heparin-associated thrombocytopenia: the antibody is not heparin specific. Thromb Haemost 67: 545–549, 1992.

Greinacher A, Amiral J, Dummel V, Vissac A, Kiefel B, Mueller-Eckhardt C. Laboratory diagnosis of heparin-associated thrombocytopenia and comparison of platelet aggregation test, heparin-induced platelet activation test, and platelet factor 4/heparin enzyme-linked immunosorbent assay. Transfusion 34: 381–385, 1994a.

Greinacher A, Feigl M, Mueller-Eckhardt C. Crossreactivity studies between sera of patients with heparin associated thrombocytopenia and a new low molecular weight heparin, reviparin. Thromb Haemost 72: 644–645, 1994b.

Greinacher A, Liebenhoff U, Kiefel V, Presek P, Mueller-Eckhardt C. Heparin-associated thrombocytopenia: the effects of various intravenous IgG preparations on antibody mediated platelet activation—a possible new indication for high dose i.v. IgG. Thromb Haemost 71: 641–645, 1994c.

Greinacher A, Pötzsch B, Amiral J, Dummel V, Eichner A, Mueller-Eckhardt C. Heparin-associated thrombocytopenia: isolation of the antibody and characterization of a multimolecular PF4-heparin complex as the major antigen. Thromb Haemost 71: 247–251, 1994d.

Greinacher A, Gopinadhan M, Gunther JU, Omer-Adam MA, Strobel U, Warkentin TE, Papastavrou G, Weitschies W, Helm CA. Close approximation of two platelet factor 4 tetramers by charge neutralization forms the antigens recognized by HIT antibodies. Arterioscler Thromb Vasc Biol 26: 2386–2393, 2006.

Greinacher A, Strobel U, Wessel A, Lubenow N, Selleng K, Eichler P, Warkentin TE. Heparin-induced thrombocytopenia: a prospective study on the incidence, platelet-activating capacity and clinical significance of anti-PF4/heparin antibodies of the IgG, IgM, and IgA classes. J Thromb Haemost 5: 1666–1673, 2007.

Greinacher A, Kohlmann T, Strobel U, Sheppard JI, Warkentin TE. The temporal profile of the anti-PF4/heparin immune response. Blood 113: 4970–4976, 2009.

Greinacher A, Ittermann T, Bagemühl J, Althaus K, Fürll B, Selleng S, Lubenow N, Schellong S, Sheppard JI, Warkentin TE. Heparin-induced thrombocytopenia: towards standardization of platelet factor 4/heparin antigen tests. J Thromb Haemost 8: 2025–2031, 2010.

Horne MK III, Chao ES. Heparin binding to resting and activated platelets. Blood 74: 238–243, 1989.

Horsewood P, Warkentin TE, Hayward CPM, Kelton JG. The epitope specificity of heparin-induced thrombocytopenia. Br J Haematol 95: 161–167, 1996.

Jeske W, Fareed J, Eschenfelder V, Iqbal O, Hoppensteadt D, Ahsan A. Biochemical and pharmacologic characteristics of reviparin, a low molecular mass heparin. Semin Thromb Hemost 23: 119–128, 1997.

Juhl D, Eichler P, Lubenow N, Strobel U, Wessel A, Greinacher A. Incidence and clinical significance of anti-PF4/heparin antibodies of the IgG, IgM, and IgA class in 755 consecutive patient samples referred for diagnostic testing for heparin-induced thrombocytopenia. Eur J Haematol 76: 420–426, 2006.

Kappa JR, Fisher CA, Berkowitz HD, Cottrell ED, Addonizio VP Jr. Heparin-induced platelet activation in sixteen surgical patients: diagnosis and management. J Vasc Surg 5: 101–109, 1987.

Kapsch D, Silver D. Heparin-induced thrombocytopenia with thrombosis and hemorrhage. Arch Surg 116: 1423–1427, 1981.

Kelton JG, Sheridan D, Brain H, Powers PJ, Turpie AG, Carter CJ. Clinical usefulness of testing for a heparin-dependent platelet-aggregating factor in patients with suspected heparin-associated thrombocytopenia. J Lab Clin Med 103: 606–612, 1984.

Kelton JG, Sheridan D, Santos A, Smith J, Steeves K, Smith C, Brown C, Murphy WG. Heparin-induced thrombocytopenia: laboratory studies. Blood 72: 925–930, 1988.

Kikta MJ, Keller MP, Humphrey PW, Silver D. Can low molecular weight heparins and heparinoids be safely given to patients with heparin-induced thrombocytopenia syndrome? Surgery 114: 705–710, 1993.

Kinlough-Rathbone RL, Packham MA, Mustard JF. Platelet aggregation. In: Harker LA, Zimmerman TS, eds. Methods in Hematology: Measurements of Platelet Function. Edinburgh: Churchill Livingstone, 64–91, 1983.

Koch S, Harenberg J, Ödel M, Schmidt-Gayk H, Walch S, Budde U. Development of a high-pressure liquid chromatography method for diagnosis of heparin-induced thrombocytopenia. Am J Clin Pathol 117: 900–904, 2002.

Kolde HJ, Dostatni R, Mauracher S. Rapid and simple IgG specific test for the exclusion of heparin induced thrombocytopenia. Clin Chem Lab Med 49: 2065–2068, 2011.

Krakow EF, Goudar R, Petzold E, Suvarna S, Last M, Welsby IJ, Ortel TL, Arepally GM. Influence of sample collection and storage on the detection of platelet factor 4-heparin antibodies. Am J Clin Pathol 128: 150–155, 2007.

Lee DH, Warkentin TE. Frequency of heparin-induced thrombocytopenia. In: Warkentin TE, Greinacher A, eds. Heparin-Induced Thrombocytopenia, 4th edn. New York: Informa Healthcare USA, 2007, 67–116.

Lee DH, Warkentin TE, Denomme GA, Hayward CPM, Kelton JG. A diagnostic test for heparin-induced thrombocytopenia: detection of platelet microparticles using flow cytometry. Br J Haematol 95: 724–731, 1996.

Legnani C, Cini M, Pili C, Boggian O, Frascaro M, Palareti G. Evaluation of a new automated panel of assays for the detection of anti-PF4/heparin antibodies in patients suspected of having heparin-induced thrombocytopenia. Thromb Haemost 104: 402–409, 2010.

Lindhoff-Last E, Gerdsen F, Ackermann H, Bauersachs R. Determination of heparin-platelet factor 4–IgG antibodies improves diagnosis of heparin-induced thrombocytopenia. Br J Haematol 113: 886–890, 2001.

Linkins LA, Warkentin TE. Heparin-induced thrombocytopenia: real world issues. Semin Thromb Hemost 37: 653–663, 2011.

Lo GK, Juhl D, Warkentin TE, Sigouin CS, Eichler P, Greinacher A. Evaluation of pretest clinical score (4 T's) for the diagnosis of heparin-induced thrombocytopenia in two clinical settings. J Thromb Haemost 4: 759–765, 2006.

Lo GK, Sigouin CS, Warkentin TE. What is the potential for overdiagnosis of HIT? Am J Hematol 82: 1037–1043, 2007.

Look KA, Sahud M, Flaherty S, Zehnder JL. Heparin-induced platelet aggregation vs. platelet factor 4 enzyme-linked immunosorbent assay in the diagnosis of heparin-induced thrombocytopenia-thrombosis. Am J Clin Pathol 108: 78–82, 1997.

Makhoul RG, Greenberg CS, McCann RL. Heparin-induced thrombocytopenia and thrombosis: a serious clinical problem and potential solution. J Vasc Surg 4: 522–528, 1986.

Meyer O, Salama A, Pittet N, Schwind P. Rapid detection of heparin-induced platelet antibodies with particle gel immunoassay (ID-HPF4). Lancet 354: 1525–1526, 1999.

Moore JC, Arnold DM, Warkentin TE, Warkentin AE, Kelton JG. An algorithm for resolving 'indeterminate' test results in the platelet serotonin release assay for investigation of heparin-induced thrombocytopenia. J Thromb Haemost 6: 1595–1597, 2008.

Morel-Kopp MC, Aboud M, Tan CW, Kulathilake C, Ward C. Whole blood impedance aggregometry detects heparin-induced thrombocytopenia antibodies. Thromb Res 125: e234–e239, 2010.

Morel-Kopp MC, Aboud M, Tan CW, Kulathilake C, Ward C. Heparin-induced thrombocytopenia: evaluation of IgG and IgGAM ELISA assays. Int J Lab Hematol 33: 245–250, 2011.

Morel-Kopp MC, Tan CW, Brighton TA, McRae S, Baker R, Tran H, Mollee P, Kershaw G, Joseph J, Ward C; ASTH Clinical Trials Group. Validation of whole blood impedance aggregometry as a new diagnostic tool for HIT. results of a large Australian study. Thromb Haemost 107: 575–583, 2012.

Mullier F, Bailly N, Cornet Y, Dubuc E, Robert S, Osselaer JC, Chatelain C, Dogné JM, Chatelain B. Contribution of platelet microparticles generation assay to the diagnosis of type II heparin-induced thrombocytopenia. Thromb Haemost 103: 1277–1281, 2010.

Mustard JF, Perry DW, Ardlie NG, Packham MA. Preparation of suspensions of washed platelets from humans. Br J Haematol 22: 193–204, 1972.

Nagi PK, Ackermann F, Wendt H, Savoca R, Bosshard HR. Protein A antibody-capture ELISA (PACE): an ELISA format to avoid denaturation of surface-adsorbed antigens. J Immunol Methods 158: 267–276, 1993.

Nellen V, Sulzer I, Barizzi G, Lämmle B, Alberio L. Rapid exclusion or confirmation of heparin-induced thrombocytopenia: a single-center experience with 1,291 patients. Haematologica 97: 89–97, 2012.

Newman PM, Chong BH. Further characterization of antibody and antigen in heparin-induced thrombocytopenia. Br J Haematol 107: 303–309, 1999.

Newman PM, Swanson RL, Chong BH. Heparin-induced thrombocytopenia: IgG binding to PF4-Heparin complexes in the fluid phase and cross-reactivity with low molecular weight heparin and heparinoid. Thromb Haemost 80: 292–297, 1998.

Nguyen P, Lecompte T. And Groupe d'Etude sur l'Hemostase et la Thromboses (GEHT) de la Societe Franchise d'Hematologie. Heparin-induced thrombocytopenia: a survey of tests employed and attitudes in haematology laboratories. Nouv Rev Fr Hematol 36: 353–357, 1994.

Nguyen P, Droulle C, Potron G. Comparison between platelet factor 4/heparin complexes ELISA and platelet aggregation test in heparin-induced thrombocytopenia. Thromb Haemost 74: 793–810, 1995.

Packham MA, Guccione MA, Perry DW. ADP does not release platelet granule contents in a plasma-free system [abstr]. Fed Proc 30: 201, 1971.

Pfueller SL, David R. Different platelet specificities of heparin-dependent platelet aggregating factors in heparin-induced thrombocytopenia. Br J Haematol 64: 149159, 1986.

Polgár J, Eichler P, Greinacher A, Clemetson KJ. Adenosine diphosphate (ADP) and ADP receptor play a major role in platelet activation/aggregation induced by sera from heparin-induced thrombocytopenia patients. Blood 91: 549–554, 1998.

Pötzsch B, Keller M, Madlener K, Muller-Berghaus G. The use of heparinase improves the specificity of crossreactivity testing in heparin-induced thrombocytopenia. Thromb Haemost 76: 1118–1122, 1996.

Pouplard C, Amiral J, Borg JY, Laporte-Simitsidis S, Delahousse B, Gruel Y. Decision analysis for use of platelet aggregation test, carbon 14–serotonin release assay, and heparin-platelet factor 4 enzyme-linked immunosorbent assay for diagnosis of heparin-induced thrombocytopenia. Am J Clin Pathol 111: 700–706, 1999.

Pouplard C, May MA, Regina S, Marchand M, Fusciardi J, Gruel Y. Changes in platelet count after cardiac surgery can effectively predict the development of pathogenic heparin-dependent antibodies. Br J Haematol 128: 837–841, 2005.

Pouplard C, Gueret P, Fouassier M, Ternisien C, Trossaert M, Régina S, Gruel Y. Prospective evaluation of the '4Ts' score and particle gel immunoassay specific for the diagnosis of heparin-induced thrombocytopenia. J Thromb Haemost 5: 1373–1379, 2007.

Pouplard C, Leroux D, Regina S, Rollin J, Gruel Y. Effectiveness of a new immunoassay for the diagnosis of heparin-induced thrombocytopenia and improved specificity when detecting IgG antibodies. Thromb Haemost 103: 145–150, 2010.

Prechel MM, McDonald MK, Jeske WP, Messmore HL, Walenga JM. Activation of platelets by heparin-induced thrombocytopenia antibodies in the serotonin release assay is not dependent on the presence of heparin. J Thromb Haemost 3: 2168–2175, 2005.

Rauova L, Zhai L, Kowalska MA. Aepally GM, Cines DB, Poncz M. Role of platelet surface PF4 antigenic complexes in heparin-induced thrombocytopenia pathogenesis: diagnostic and therapeutic implications. Blood 107: 2346–2353, 2006.

Refaai MA, Laposata M, Van Cott EM. Clinical significance of a borderline titer in a negative ELISA test for heparin-induced thrombocytopenia. Am J Clin Pathol 119: 6l–65, 2003.

Rhodes GR, Dixon RH, Silver D. Heparin induced thrombocytopenia with thrombotic and hemorrhagic manifestations. Surg Gynecol Obstet 136: 409–416, 1973.

Risch L, Bertschmann W, Heijnen IAFM, Huber AR. A differentiated approach to assess the diagnostic usefulness of a rapid particle gel immunoassay for the detection of antibodies against heparin-platelet factor 4 in cardiac surgery patients. Blood Coagul Fibrinolysis 14: 99–106, 2003.

Ruf KM, Bensadoun ES, Davis GA, Flynn JD, Lewis DA. A clinical-laboratory algorithm incorporating optical density value to predict heparin-induced thrombocytopenia. Thromb Haemost 105: 553–559, 2011.

Rugeri L, Bauters A, Trillot N, Susen S, Decoen C, Watel A, Jude B. Clinical usefulness of combined use of platelet aggregation test and anti PF4-H antibodies ELISA test for the diagnosis of heparin-induced thrombocytopenia. Hematology 4: 367–372, 1999.

Sachs UJ, von Hesberg J, Santoso S, Bein G, Bakchoul T. Evaluation of a new nanoparticle-based lateral-flow immunoassay for the exclusion of heparin-induced thrombocytopenia (HIT). Thromb Haemost 106: 1197–1202, 2011.

Salem HH, van der Weyden MB. Heparin-induced thrombocytopenia. Variable platelet-rich plasma reactivity to heparin dependent platelet aggregating factor. Pathology 15: 297–299, 1983.

Salzman EW, Rosenberg RD, Smith MH, Lindon JN, Favreau L. Effect of heparin and heparin fractions on platelet aggregation. J Clin Invest 65: 64–73, 1980.

Schenk S, El-Banayosy A, Prohaska W, Arusoglu L, Morshuis M, Koester-Eiserfunke W, Kizner L, Murray E, Eichler P, Koerfer R, Greinacher A. Heparin-induced thrombocytopenia in patients receiving circulatory support. J Thorac Cardiovasc Surg 131: 1373–1381, 2006.

Schenk S, El-Banayosy A, Morshuis M, Arusoglu L Eichler P, Lubenow N, Tenderich G, Koerfer R, Greinacher A, Prohaska W. IgG classification of anti-PF4/heparin antibodies to identify patients with heparin-induced thrombocytopenia during mechanical circulatory support. J Thromb Haemost 5: 235–241, 2007.

Schneiter S, Colucci G, Sulzer I, Barizzi G, Lämmle B, Alberio L. Variability of anti-PF4/heparin antibody results obtained by the rapid testing system ID-H/PF4-PaGIA. J Thromb Haemost 7: 1649–1655, 2009.

Selleng S, Malowsky B, Strobel U, Wessel A, Ittermann T, Wollert HG, Warkentin TE, Greinacher A. Early-onset and persisting thrombocytopenia in post-cardiac surgery patients is rarely due to heparin-induced thrombocytopenia even when antibody tests are positive. J Thromb Haemost 8: 30–36, 2010.

Selleng S, Schreier N, Wollert HG, Greinacher A. The diagnostic value of the anti-PF4/heparin immunoassay high-dose heparin confirmatory test in cardiac surgery patients. Anesth Analg 112: 774–776, 2011.

Sheridan D, Carter C, Kelton JG. A diagnostic test for heparin-induced thrombocytopenia. Blood 67: 27–30, 1986.

Socher I, Kroll H, Jorks S, Santoso S, Sachs UJ. Heparin-independent activation of platelets by heparin-induced thrombocytopenia antibodies: a common occurrence. J Thromb Haemost 6: 197–2000, 2008.

Stewart MW, Etches WS, Boshkov LK, Gordon PA. Heparin-induced thrombocytopenia: an improved method of detection based on lumiaggregometry. Br J Haematol 91: 173–177, 1995.

Teitel JM, Gross P, Blake P, Garvey MB. A bioluminescent adenosine nucleotide release assay for the diagnosis of heparin-induced thrombocytopenia. Thromb Haemost 76: 479, 1996.

Tomer A. A sensitive and specific functional flow cytometric assay for the diagnosis of heparin-induced thrombocytopenia. Br J Haematol 98: 648–656, 1997.

Tomer A, Masalunga C, Abshire TC. Determination of heparin-induced thrombocytopenia: a rapid flow cytometric assay for direct demonstration of antibody-mediated platelet activation. Am J Hematol 61: 53–61, 1999.

Trehel-Tursis V, Louvain-Quintard V, Zarrouki Y, Imbert A, Doubine S, Stéphan F. Clinical and biological features of patients suspected or confirmed to have heparin-induced thrombocytopenia in a cardiothoracic surgical ICU. Chest 8 Mar 2012. [Epub ahead of print]

Untch B, Ahmad S, Jeske WP, Messmore HL, Hoppensteadt DA, Walenga JM, Lietz H, Fareed J. Prevalence, isotype, and functionality of antiheparin-platelet factor 4 antibodies in patients treated with heparin and clinically suspected for heparin-induced thrombocytopenia. Thromb Res 105: 117–123, 2002.

Visentin GP, Ford SE, Scott JP, Aster RH. Antibodies from patients with heparin-induced thrombocytopenia/thrombosis are specific for platelet factor 4 complexed with heparin or bound to endothelial cells. J Clin Invest 93: 81–88, 1994.

Visentin GP, Moghaddam M, Beery SE, McFarland JG, Aster RH. Heparin is not required for detection of antibodies associated with heparin-induced thrombocytopenia/thrombosis. J Lab Clin Med 138: 22–31, 2001.

Vitale M, Tazzari P, Ricci F, Mazza MA, Zauli G, Martini G, Caimi L, Manzoli FA, Conte R. Comparison between different laboratory tests for the detection and prevention of heparin-induced thrombocytopenia. Cytometry 46: 290–295, 2001.

Vun CH, Evans S, Chong BH. Cross-reactivity study of low molecular weight heparin and heparinoid in heparin-induced thrombocytopenia. Thromb Res 81: 525–532, 1996.

Walenga JM, Jeske WP, Fasanella AR, Wood JJ, Ahmad S, Bakhos M. Laboratory diagnosis of heparin-induced thrombocytopenia. Clin Appl Thrombosis/Hemostasis 5 (Suppl 1): S21–S27, 1999.

Wang L, Huhle G, Malsch R, Hoffmann U, Song X, Harenberg J. Determination of heparin-induced IgG antibody by fluorescence-linked immunofiltration assay (FLIFA). J Immunol Meth 222: 93–99, 1999a.

Wang L, Huhle G, Malsch R, Hoffmann U, Song X, Harenberg J. Determination of heparin-induced IgG antibody in heparin-induced thrombocytopenia type II. Eur J Clin Invest 29: 232–237, 1999b.

Warkentin TE. Danaparoid (Orgaran) for the treatment of heparin-induced thrombocytopenia (HIT) and thrombosis: effects on in vivo thrombin and cross-linked fibrin generation, and evaluation of the clinical significance of in vitro cross-reactivity (XR) of danaparoid for HIT-IgG [abstr]. Blood 88(Suppl 1): 626a, 1996.

Warkentin TE. Platelet count monitoring and laboratory testing for heparin-induced thrombocytopenia. Arch Pathol Lab Med 127: 783, 2003.

Warkentin TE. New approaches to the diagnosis of heparin-induced thrombocytopenia. Chest 127 (2 Suppl): 35S–45S, 2005.

Warkentin TE. How I diagnose and manage heparin-induced thrombocytopenia. Hematology Am Soc Hematol Educ Program 2011: 143–149, 2011.

Warkentin TE. HIT in the ICU: a transatlantic perspective. Chest 2012; in press.

Warkentin TE, Cook RJ. Impact of laboratory testing for heparin-induced antibodies: using Bayes' rule to prevent overdiagnosis of heparin-induced thrombocytopenia. [Bedeutung von Laboruntersuchungen von Heparin-induzierten Antikörpern: Einsatz des Bayes Wahrscheinlichkeitstheorems zur Prävention der Überdiagnose einer Heparin-induzierten Thrombozytopenie]. J Lab Med 35: 45–54, 2011.

Warkentin TE, Kelton JG. Delayed-onset heparin-induced thrombocytopenia and thrombosis. Ann Intern Med 135: 502–506, 2001a.

Warkentin TE, Kelton JG. Temporal aspects of heparin-induced thrombocytopenia. N Engl J Med 344: 1286–1292, 2001b.

Warkentin TE, Linkins LA. Immunoassays are not created equal. J Thromb Haemost 7: 1256–1259, 2009.

Warkentin TE, Sheppard JI. Testing for heparin-induced thrombocytopenia antibodies. Transfus Med Rev 20: 259–272, 2006a.

Warkentin TE, Sheppard JI. No significant improvement in diagnostic specificity of an anti-PF4/polyanion immunoassay with use of high heparin confirmatory procedure. J Thromb Haemost 4: 281–282, 2006b.

Warkentin TE, Sheppard JI. Clinical sample investigation (CSI) hematology: pinpointing the precise onset of heparin-induced thrombocytopenia (HIT). J Thromb Haemost 5: 636–637, 2007.

Warkentin TE, Hayward CPM, Smith CA, Kelly PM, Kelton JG. Determinants of platelet variability when testing for heparin-induced thrombocytopenia. J Lab Clin Med 120: 371–379, 1992.

Warkentin TE, Hayward CPM, Boshkov LK, Santos AV, Sheppard JI, Bode AP, Kelton JG. Sera from patients with heparin-induced thrombocytopenia generate platelet-derived microparticles with procoagulant activity: an explanation for the thrombotic complications of heparin-induced thrombocytopenia. Blood 84: 3691–3699, 1994.

Warkentin TE, Levine MN, Hirsh J, Horsewood P, Roberts RS, Gent M, Kelton JG. Heparin-induced thrombocytopenia in patients treated with low molecular weight heparin or unfractionated heparin. N Engl J Med 332: 1330–1335, 1995.

Warkentin TE, Chong BH, Greinacher A. Heparin-induced thrombocytopenia: towards consensus. Thromb Haemost 79: 1–7, 1998.

Warkentin TE, Sheppard JI, Horsewood P, Simpson PJ, Moore JC, Kelton JG. Impact of the patient population on the risk for heparin-induced thrombocytopenia. Blood 96: 1703–1708, 2000.

Warkentin TE, Cook RJ Marder VJ, Sheppard JI Moore JC Eriksson BI Greinacher A, Kelton JG. Anti-platelet factor 4/heparin antibodies in orthopedic surgery patients receiving antithrombotic prophylaxis with fondaparinux or enoxaparin. Blood 106: 3791–3796, 2005a.

Warkentin TE, Sheppard JA, Moore JC, Moore KM, Sigouin CS, Kelton JG. Laboratory testing for the antibodies that cause heparin-induced thrombocytopenia: how much class do we need? J Lab Clin Med 146: 341–346, 2005b.

Warkentin TE, Sheppard JI, Raschke R, Greinacher A. Performance characteristics of a rapid assay for anti-PF4/heparin antibodies, the Particle ImmunoFiltration Assay. J Thromb Haemost 5: 2308–2310, 2007.

Warkentin TE, Sheppard JI, Moore JC, Sigouin CS, Kelton JG. Quantitative interpretation of optical density measurements using PF4-dependent enzyme-immunoassays. J Thromb Haemost 6: 1304–1312, 2008.

Warkentin TE, Sheppard JI, Moore JC, Cook RJ, Kelton JG. Studies of the immune response in heparin-induced thrombocytopenia. Blood 113: 4963–4969, 2009.

Warkentin TE, Sheppard JI, Moore JC, Kelton JG. The use of well-characterized sera for the assessment of new diagnostic enzyme-immunoassays for the diagnosis of heparin-induced thrombocytopenia. J Thromb Haemost 8: 216–218, 2010.

Warkentin TE, Davidson BL, Büller HR, Gallus A, Gent M, Lensing AWA, Piovella F, Prins MH, Segers AEM, Kelton JG. Prevalence and risk of preexisting heparin-induced thrombocytopenia antibodies in patients with acute VTE. Chest 140: 366–373, 2011a.

Warkentin TE, Greinacher A, Gruel Y, Aster RH, Chong BH. on behalf of the Scientific and Standardization Committee of the International Society on Thrombosis and Haemostasis. Laboratory testing for heparin-induced thrombocytopenia: a conceptual framework and implications for diagnosis. J Thromb Haemost 9: 2498–2500, 2011b.

White MM, Siders L, Jennings LK, White FL. The effect of residual heparin on the interpretation of heparin-induced platelet aggregation in the diagnosis of heparin-associated thrombocytopenia. Thromb Haemost 68: 88, 1992.

Whitlatch NL, Perry SL, Ortel TL. Anti-heparin/platelet factor 4 antibody optical density values and the confirmatory procedure in the diagnosis of heparin-induced thrombocytopenia. Thromb Haemost 100: 678–684, 2008.

Whitlatch NL, Kong DF, Metjian AD, Arepally GM, Ortel TL. Validation of the high-dose heparin confirmatory step for the diagnosis of heparin-induced thrombocytopenia. Blood 116: 1761–1766, 2010.

Zwicker JI, Uhl L, Huang WY, Shaz BH, Baucer KA. Thrombosis and ELISA optical density values in hospitalized patients with heparin-induced thrombocytopenia. Thromb Haemost 2: 2133–2137, 2004.

12 Treatment of heparin-induced thrombocytopenia: An overview

Andreas Greinacher and Theodore E. Warkentin

INTRODUCTION

Heparin-induced thrombocytopenia (HIT) presents a unique situation: heparin causes the very complications that its use was intended to prevent, for example, pulmonary embolism, stroke, and limb gangrene. Furthermore, several treatment paradoxes pose serious management pitfalls (Table 12.1). This chapter summarizes our treatment approaches, with emphasis on practical management issues. We wish to highlight two important issues. First, HIT is a syndrome of increased thrombin generation ("hypercoagulability state"). Accordingly, we emphasize the use of rapidly acting anticoagulant drugs that control thrombin generation in HIT. Second, there is increasing evidence that in most patients in whom testing for HIT antibodies is requested, a non-HIT diagnosis ultimately is made (Lo et al., 2006; Greinacher et al., 2007). Thus, the risk of failing to prevent a HIT-associated thrombosis (through timely use of a nonheparin anticoagulant) must be balanced against the risk of inducing adverse effects from using another anticoagulant, for example, bleeding complications (for which no antidote exists).

Regarding studies of HIT, there are only two small randomized controlled trials (RCTs) (Chong et al., 2001; Boyce et al., 2011). As there are no definitive studies that have directly compared two different treatment options for HIT, any recommendation for use of one of these drugs does not imply any proven or consistent advantage over any of the others. However, there are important pharmacologic differences, which might well favor use of one in the particular circumstances of an individual patient situation (see chaps. 13–17). In our evaluations of nonrandomized studies (e.g., against historical controls) or uncontrolled case-series, we have also taken into account whether the diagnosis of HIT was supported by testing for HIT antibodies.

Disclaimer

There are several challenging treatment issues. Patients with HIT are not clinically homogeneous; they represent a complex mix of varying initial indications for heparin, location, and severity of HIT-associated thrombosis, and, not infrequently, dysfunction of one or more vital organs. This presents difficulties both for performing clinical studies as well as in the application of treatment recommendations for individual patients. Furthermore, there are important differences among countries in the approval or availability status of certain recommended treatment approaches. *Thus, the treatment recommendations we make cannot be indiscriminately applied to all patients with suspected or confirmed HIT.*

TABLE 12.1 Treatment Paradoxes of HIT Management

Treatment for HIT	Paradoxical effect of treatment	Comments
Discontinue heparin	Potential for increase in thrombin generation; high frequency of thrombosis despite stopping heparin	Use an alternative, rapid-acting anticoagulant in therapeutic doses[a] when heparin is stopped because of strongly suspected HIT
Coumarin (e.g., warfarin, phenprocoumon)	High frequency of thrombosis; potential for coumarin necrosis (venous limb gangrene and skin necrosis syndromes)	Control thrombin generation with an alternative anticoagulant[a]; postpone coumarin pending substantial platelet count recovery
LMWH	High frequency of exacerbating thrombocytopenia when given to patients with acute HIT	Although LMWH is less likely than UFH to cause HIT, LMWH is likely to maintain or worsen acute HIT caused by UFH
Low-dose danaparoid[b]	High frequency of thrombosis if low-dose danaparoid is given to patients with "isolated HIT"	High (therapeutic)-dose danaparoid recommended for patients strongly suspected (or confirmed) to have isolated HIT or HIT-thrombosis
Platelet transfusions	May increase risk for platelet-mediated thrombosis	Spontaneous bleeding is uncommon in HIT; thus, prophylactic platelet transfusions are relatively contraindicated (however, platelet transfusions are appropriate in bleeding patients or for an invasive procedure with a high bleeding risk or with diagnostic uncertainty)
IVC filters	May increase risk for IVC thrombosis, pulmonary embolism, limb ischemia/necrosis	IVC filters should be avoided in acute HIT; if used, concomitant anticoagulation in therapeutic doses should be given
Use low-dose alternative anticoagulation or heparin in patients with low probability for HIT	Risk of bleeding outweighs risk of thrombosis in patients with thrombocytopenia due to other reasons than HIT	The risk–benefit ratio of therapeutic-dose nonheparin anticoagulation is not favorable for non-HIT thrombocytopenia, given the high risk of bleeding and lower risk of thrombosis (overall, only 5–10% of patients evaluated serologically for HIT are shown to have heparin-dependent, platelet-activating antibodies)

(Continued)

TABLE 12.1 (*Continued*) Treatment Paradoxes of HIT Management

Treatment for HIT	Paradoxical effect of treatment	Comments
Use heparin for cardiovascular surgery despite previous history of HIT	In patients with a history of HIT who subsequently test negative for HIT antibodies, heparin is safer for intravascular anticoagulation than alternative anticoagulants	HIT antibodies usually disappear quickly (within a few weeks or months), and are not regenerated within five days following reexposure to heparin, thus allowing heparin use during surgery

[a]Rapidly acting alternative anticoagulants include danaparoid, fondaparinux, recombinant hirudin (lepirudin, desirudin), argatroban, bivalirudin, and likely also the new oral anticoagulants, such as dabigatran and rivaroxaban.
[b]Low-dose danaparoid (750 U two or three times a day) is approved for prevention of thrombosis in acute HIT in some jurisdictions.
Abbreviations: HIT, heparin-induced thrombocytopenia; IVC, inferior vena cava; LMWH, low molecular weight heparin; UFH, unfractionated heparin.

A further practical problem is that the major treatment options for HIT include relatively new and, for some physicians, unfamiliar or even unapproved anticoagulant agents. This presents extra challenges to physicians and also to laboratories asked to monitor anticoagulant treatment effects, as the treatment "learning curve" may occur in emergency situations. Also, immediate results of reliable laboratory tests for HIT are usually unavailable. Difficult management decisions may be needed amid diagnostic uncertainty: A diagnosis of HIT that seems obvious in retrospect may not have been so clear during its early evolution.

As an iatrogenic illness that occurs unpredictably and unexpectedly, often in a setting of antithrombotic prophylaxis, medicolegal aspects must also be considered (McIntyre and Warkentin, 2004; Ulsenheimer, 2004). Thus, once HIT is entertained as part of a differential diagnosis, we suggest that physicians document carefully the various diagnostic and treatment considerations as events unfold.

As a *common, rare disease* [we acknowledge Prof. R. Hull (Calgary, Canada) for this description of HIT] that physicians only occasionally manage and that only rarely enters into clinical studies, we need to acknowledge that no final answer for treatment is likely to emerge. Therefore, even in this fifth edition, this chapter should be viewed as a basis for further discussion and study of the treatment of HIT patients.

NONIMMUNE HEPARIN-ASSOCIATED THROMBOCYTOPENIA

In some patients, especially those with comorbid conditions associated with platelet activation (burns and anorexia nervosa), heparin treatment can result in a transient decrease in platelet count (Reininger et al., 1996; Burgess and Chong, 1997) (see chap. 5). Unfractionated heparin (UFH) activates platelets directly (Salzman et al., 1980; Gao et al., 2011), an effect observed less frequently with low molecular weight heparin (LMWH) (Brace and Fareed, 1990). Known as nonimmune heparin-associated thrombocytopenia (nonimmune HAT), this direct proaggregatory effect of heparin occurs predominantly in patients receiving high-dose, intravenous (IV) UFH therapy. Typically, platelet counts decrease within the first one to two days of treatment and then recover over the next three to four days. There are no data indicating that these patients are at increased risk for adverse outcomes, including thrombosis. Indeed, it is possible that inappropriate discontinuation of heparin for nonimmune HAT could *increase* the risk for thrombosis, owing to the underlying clinical condition for which heparin is being given.

Management of patients in whom HIT is a potential reason for the decrease in platelet count, but judged nevertheless to be at low probability of having HIT, is discussed in section "Management of the Patient with a Low or Intermediate Probability of HIT (Pending Results of HIT Antibody Testing)".

THERAPY OF (IMMUNE) HIT
Pathogenesis of HIT: Treatment Implications

HIT is caused by antibodies that usually recognize multimolecular complexes of platelet factor 4 (PF4) and heparin (PF4/H). HIT can be viewed as a syndrome of *in vivo* thrombin generation that results from the activation of platelets, endothelium, monocytes, and coagulation pathways (Warkentin and Kelton, 1994; Greinacher, 1995; Warkentin et al., 1998; Warkentin, 2003) (Fig. 12.1) (see chaps. 5–10). Given this model of pathogenesis, therapy for acute HIT should focus on the following issues: (*i*) rapid reduction of increased thrombin generation; (*ii*) treatment of HIT-associated thrombosis; and (*iii*) interruption of heparin-dependent platelet activation (i.e., discontinuation of heparin). In most patients with HIT, effective pharmacologic therapy for thrombosis will involve an agent that rapidly controls thrombin generation, although in some situations, additional adjunctive treatments may be necessary (e.g., surgical thromboembolectomy, high-dose IV IgG).

With increased testing for HIT antibodies, it is now clear that many patients develop anti-PF4/H antibodies without developing clinical HIT (see chaps. 4 and 11). In these patients, it seems acceptable to continue heparin treatment but to monitor the platelet counts carefully ("watch-and-wait" strategy). An open issue is whether in patients who test positive in an antigen assay only, but negative in a sensitive functional assay using washed platelets, heparin can be continued. It is the practice of the authors to continue heparin in these patients, especially if the antigen assay shows a low reactivity [e.g., optical density (OD) <1.0 unit].

Several studies of heparin administration in the contexts of acute coronary syndrome, cardiac surgery, and hemodialysis have suggested that presence of anti-PF4/H antibodies confers adverse prognosis (e.g., increased cardiovascular events or increased length-of-hospital-stay) even in the absence of clinically evident HIT (Mattioli et al., 2000, 2009; Williams et al., 2003; Mascelli et al., 2004a,b; Bennett-Guerrero et al., 2005; Pena de la Vega et al., 2005; Kress et al., 2007; Selleng et al., 2010). However, whether this reflects true pathogenicity of these antibodies in the presence of heparin ("forme fruste" HIT) or whether the presence of antibodies represents simply a surrogate marker for other adverse prognostic markers (e.g., inflammation) is an important unresolved question (Warkentin and Sheppard, 2006). Only one study (Selleng et al., 2010) evaluated the role of different anti-PF4/H antibody classes, and found that IgM (but not IgG) antibodies detected preoperatively correlated with nonthrombotic adverse events postcardiac surgery. In all, these observations would suggest that classic HIT-related mechanisms are not likely responsible for adverse prognosis of anti-PF4/H antibodies (Yusuf et al., 2012).

Discontinuation of Heparin for Clinically Suspected HIT

Numerous case reports describe the occurrence of new, progressive, or recurrent thromboembolic events during continued or repeated use of heparin in patients

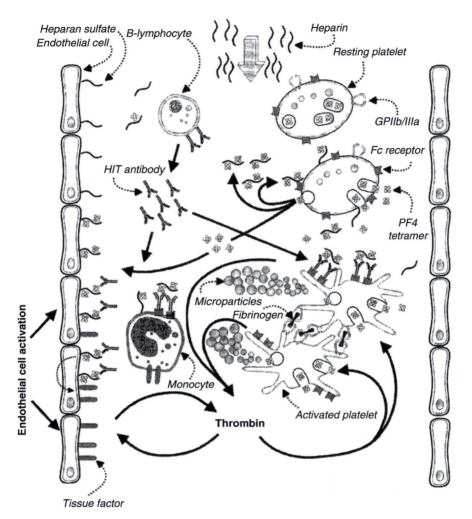

FIGURE 12.1   Pathogenesis of HIT; a central role for thrombin generation: HIT-IgG antibodies bind to several identical epitopes on the same antigen complex, thus forming immune complexes that become localized to the platelet surface. The IgG immune complexes can cross-link the platelet Fcγlla receptors, resulting in Fcγlla receptor-dependent platelet activation (Kelton et al., 1988). The GPIIb/IIIa complex is not required for platelet activation (Greinacher et al., 1994a). The activated platelets trigger a cascade of events that ultimately lead to activation of the coagulation pathways, resulting in thrombin generation. Activated platelets release their α-granule proteins (Chong et al., 1994), including PF4, leading to the formation of more multimolecular PF4/heparin complexes, setting up a vicious cycle of platelet activation, triggering even more platelet activation (Greinacher, 1995). The activated platelets bind fibrinogen, recruit other platelets, and begin to form a primary clot. During shape change, procoagulant, platelet-derived microparticles are released, providing a phospholipid surface for amplifying thrombin generation (Warkentin et al., 1994). The released PF4 also binds to endothelial cell heparan sulfate, forming local antigen complexes to which HIT antibodies bind (Cines et al., 1987; Greinacher et al., 1994b; Visentin et al., 1994). Tissue factor expression on activated endothelial cells and monocytes (Arepally and Mayer, 2001; Pouplard et al., 2001) further enhances thrombin generation. *Abbreviations*: GP, glycoprotein; HIT, heparin-induced thrombocytopenia; PF4, platelet factor 4.

with acute HIT. Moreover, the thrombocytopenia usually (but not always) persists if heparin is not stopped. Thus, all heparin treatment should be discontinued in patients strongly suspected of having HIT and usually substituted by another anticoagulant, while awaiting results of HIT antibody testing. There are two reasons for substituting heparin with another anticoagulant. The first is that the potential benefit of stopping heparin (e.g., less antibody-induced heparin-dependent platelet activation) might be outweighed in some patients by a "rebound" in thrombin generation following loss of heparin's anticoagulant action. The second is that a substantial proportion of acute HIT sera (~50%) can cause platelet activation even in the absence of pharmacologic heparin, that is, HIT has features of an autoimmune disorder.

> *Recommendation.* All heparin administration should be discontinued in patients clinically suspected of having (immune) HIT.

The routine use of heparin (e.g., line flushing) is pervasive in hospitals. Thus, based on our experience, it can be helpful to institute methods to reduce the risk for inadvertent heparin use in hospitalized patients with HIT.

> *Recommendation.* A clearly visible note should be placed above the patient's bed stating "NO HEPARIN: HIT."

Not infrequently, patients in whom heparin administration has been stopped because of clinically suspected HIT subsequently are found to have negative laboratory tests for HIT antibodies. In our experience, it is reasonable and safe to restart heparin therapy in these patients, provided the intervening clinical events are consistent with an alternative explanation for thrombocytopenia (see chap. 3) and provided the laboratory has adequately excluded the presence of HIT antibodies (see chap. 11).

> *Recommendation.* Heparin can be restarted in patients proved not to have HIT antibodies by a sensitive platelet activation assay or a PF4-dependent antigen assay.

It remains somewhat unclear how to manage patients with discrepant results in the antigen test and in the functional assay, although our view is that a patient who tests negative in a suitable functional assay can safely be treated by heparin despite testing positive by an IgG-specific antigen test.

Anticoagulation of the HIT Patient with Thrombosis
The Need for Anticoagulation of HIT-Associated Thrombosis
HIT is a strong, independent risk factor for venous and arterial thrombosis (Warkentin et al., 1995, 2003). HIT can be complicated by thrombosis in several ways: (*i*) a preceding thrombosis, leading to the heparin treatment that caused HIT (this is usually *not* considered to be HIT-associated thrombosis); (*ii*) new, progressive, or recurrent thrombosis resulting from HIT itself; or (*iii*) both reasons. The relationship between thrombocytopenia and thrombosis in HIT is variable: thrombosis can both precede (or coincide with) the onset of thrombocytopenia or thrombosis can occur several days (or even a few weeks) later (Warkentin and Kelton, 1996; Greinacher et al., 2005).

For a HIT patient with thrombosis in whom heparin administration has been discontinued, there is a high risk for subsequent thrombosis. It is increasingly clear that many—perhaps most—HIT patients' sera contain antibodies with heparin-independent platelet-activating properties (Warkentin and Kelton, 2001a; Prechel et al., 2005; Socher et al., 2008; Linkins and Warkentin, 2011); thus, ongoing

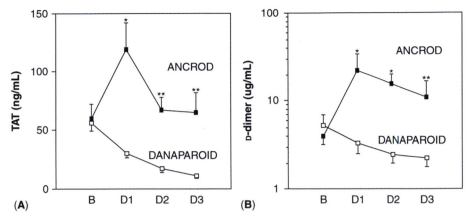

FIGURE 12.2 Thrombin generation and fibrin formation in acute HIT. (**A**) Thrombin generation, as assessed by TAT complexes, is markedly increased in acute HIT (mean, 55ng/mL; normal, <4.1ng/mL). Whereas danaparoid reduces thrombin generation in these patients, the defibrinogenating snake venom, ancrod, does not. (**B**) Levels of cross-linked fibrin degradation products (D-dimer) are increased in patients with acute HIT (mean, 4–5µg/mL; normal, <0.5µg/mL). Whereas danaparoid reduces D-dimer levels, ancrod increases their levels. Baseline (**B**) samples were obtained at diagnosis of HIT and before treatment with danaparoid or ancrod; subsequent values are shown for day 1 (D1, 1–24hr postinitiation of treatment), day 2 (D2, 25–48hr), and day 3 (D3, 49–72hr). *$P < 0.001$, **$P < 0.002$. *Abbreviations*: HIT, heparin-induced thrombocytopenia; TAT, thrombin-antithrombin. *Source*: From Warkentin (1998).

antibody-induced platelet activation will continue for some time, even if heparin is stopped. That this phenomenon may be biologically relevant is suggested by three prospective treatment cohort studies (Greinacher et al., 1999a,b; Lubenow et al., 2005), in which the initial incidence of thrombotic events ranged from 5% to 10% per patient day (see chap. 14). This high event rate (5.1% per day in the meta-analysis) occurred after stopping heparin therapy and after laboratory confirmation of HIT but before the institution of alternative anticoagulation with lepirudin (mean period of treatment delay: 1.3 days) (Greinacher et al., 2000; Lubenow et al., 2005). This experience suggests that alternative anticoagulant therapy should not be delayed for results of HIT antibody testing in patients strongly suspected of having HIT.

Anticoagulants Evaluated for Treatment of HIT: Indirect Factor Xa Inhibitors and Direct Thrombin Inhibitors

Current treatment of HIT focuses on agents that rapidly control thrombin generation (Fig. 12.2) (see chaps. 13–17). There are two broad categories of anticoagulants that have been used to treat HIT: (*i*) indirect antifactor Xa inhibitors; and (*ii*) direct thrombin inhibitors (DTIs). Table 12.2 lists several key differences between these two categories of rapidly acting, nonheparin anticoagulants.

Danaparoid and fondaparinux are *indirect* (antithrombin-dependent) inhibitors of factor Xa (danaparoid also has some anti-thrombin activity in addition), whereas lepirudin, desirudin, argatroban, and bivalirudin inhibit thrombin directly and without the need for a cofactor, that is, they are classified as *direct* thrombin inhibitors.

TABLE 12.2   A Comparison of Two Classes of Anticoagulant Used to Treat HIT

	Indirect (AT-dependent) factor Xa inhibitors: Danaparoid, Fondaparinux	Direct thrombin inhibitors: r-Hirudin [Lepirudin, Desirudin], Argatroban, Bivalirudin
Half-life	√ Long (danaparoid, 25 hr[a]; fondaparinux, 17 hr): reduces risk of rebound hypercoagulability	Short (<2 hr): potential for rebound hypercoagulability
Dosing	√ Both prophylactic- and therapeutic-dose regimens[b]	Prophylactic-dose regimens are not established (exception: subcutaneous desirudin)
Monitoring	√ Direct (antifactor Xa levels): accurate drug levels obtained	Indirect (PTT): risk for DTI underdosing due to PTT elevation caused by non-DTI factors (PTT confounding)
Effect on INR	√ No significant effect: thus, simplifies overlap with warfarin	Increases INR: argatroban > bivalirudin > r-hirudin; complicates warfarin overlap
Protein C pathway	√ No significant effect	Thrombin inhibition could impair activation of protein C pathway
Reversibility of action	√ Irreversible inhibition: AT forms covalent bond with factor Xa	Irreversible inhibition only with r-hirudin
Efficacy and safety established for non-HIT indications	√ Treatment and prophylaxis of VTE (danaparoid, fondaparinux) and ACS (fondaparinux[c])	Not established for most non-HIT settings
Platelet activation	√ Danaparoid (but not fondaparinux) inhibits platelet activation by HIT antibodies	No effect
Inhibition of clot-bound thrombin	No effect	√ Inhibition of both free and clot-bound thrombin
Drug clearance	Predominantly renal	Variable (predominantly hepatobiliary: argatroban); predominantly renal: r-hirudin)
Approved for HIT treatment	Danaparoid[d]	Lepirudin, argatroban, (bivalirudin[e])

Check mark (√) indicates favorable feature in comparison of drug classes (in Authors' opinions).
[a]For danaparoid, half-lives of its anti-thrombin and its thrombin generation inhibition activities (2–4 hr and 3–7 hr, respectively) are shorter than for its anti-Xa activity (~25 hr).
[b]Although therapeutic dosing is recommended for HIT, availability of prophylactic-dose regimens increases flexibility when managing potential non-HIT situations.
[c]Fondaparinux is approved for treatment of ACS in Canada but not in the United States.
[d]Danaparoid is neither approved nor available in the United States for treatment of HIT.
[e]Bivalirudin is approved for percutaneous coronary intervention in the setting of HIT.
Abbreviations: ACS, acute coronary syndrome; AT, antithrombin; DTI, direct thrombin inhibitor; HIT, heparin-induced thrombocytopenia; INR, international normalized ratio; PTT, partial thromboplastin time; VTE, venous thromboembolism.

Recommendation. Therapeutic-dose anticoagulation with a rapidly acting alternative, nonheparin anticoagulant should be given to a patient with thrombosis complicating acute HIT. Treatment should not be delayed pending laboratory confirmation in a patient strongly suspected to have HIT. The specific choice of anticoagulant depends on many factors, including drug availability, physician experience with any particular agent, and pharmacologic considerations (especially regarding renal and hepatic function).

Availability and approval status of anticoagulants varies in different countries. Fondaparinux and argatroban are likely the most widely available alternative anticoagulants. Although danaparoid had been the alternative anticoagulant agent available in most countries worldwide, manufacturing problems substantially restricted its supply in recent years. Bivalirudin, desirudin, and the new oral anticoagulants are also potential options for managing some patients with HIT, but current information is still too preliminary to allow for broad recommendations (see chaps. 14, 15, and 17).

A general problem of new anticoagulants in HIT is that it is very difficult, or even impossible, to perform large enough prospective RCTs in acute HIT. Thus, it is unlikely that these drugs will ever receive a formal approval for this indication. For example, there is considerable experience supporting the use of fondaparinux as an effective treatment of HIT. However, it is unlikely that definitive studies of this anticoagulant for HIT that would lead to regulatory approval will ever be done. The same considerations will likely apply to all other new anticoagulants.

An advantage of danaparoid and fondaparinux is that they can be given on an outpatient basis by subcutaneous (sc) injection. Thus, following normalization of the platelet counts, the transition to vitamin K antagonists (if desired) can be performed without the need for a prolonged in-hospital treatment period.

Pharmacologic and Pharmacokinetic Considerations in Anticoagulant Selection

The lack of prospective comparative studies between any of the alternative anticoagulants precludes definitive conclusions about relative efficacy and safety. However, there are several pharmacologic and pharmacokinetic differences that physicians should consider when determining which drug might be preferred in an individual patient (Tables 12.3, 12.4, 12.5, 12.6). For example, in a patient with vital organ or limb ischemia or infarction, who might need urgent surgical intervention, an agent with a short half-life may be desirable. But, in a patient with venous thromboembolism in whom an uncomplicated overlap with (longer-term) warfarin anticoagulation is anticipated or who requires outpatient treatment by sc injections, danaparoid or fondaparinux use is advantageous. Argatroban (which undergoes hepatobiliary clearance) is suited for patients with renal insufficiency, as dose reduction is generally not required (in this regard, argatroban differs from all other alternative anticoagulants currently available). Conversely, desirudin or bivalirudin may be more suitable than argatroban for patients with hepatobiliary dysfunction, including reduced liver perfusion due to cardiac insufficiency.

As the key therapeutic goal of anticoagulation during acute HIT is to achieve effective inhibition of thrombin or its generation, the ability to determine accurately the drug anticoagulant levels is an important issue. In the case of danaparoid, drug levels can be measured *directly* (via antifactor Xa levels), whereas in most medical centers, the anticoagulant levels of the DTIs are measured *indirectly,*

TABLE 12.3 Main Characteristics of Danaparoid Sodium

Mechanism of action, pharmacokinetics	Monitoring	Undesirable effects	Comments
Catalyzes the inactivation of factor Xa by AT, and of thrombin (IIa) by AT and HCII Bioavailability after sc injection ~100%; peak anti-Xa levels, 4–5 hr after injection (Danhof et al., 1992) Mean plasma distribution time following IV bolus, ~2.3 hr Plasma $t_{1/2}$ of anti-Xa activity, 17–28 hr (mean, 25 hr); $t_{1/2}$ of anti-IIa activity, 2–4 hr (Danhof et al., 1992)	Anti-Xa levels during treatment by an amidolytic assay using danaparoid reference curve Monitoring recommended in patients with: (*i*) significant renal impairment; (*ii*) body weight < 45 kg or >110 kg; (*iii*) life- or limb-threatening thrombosis; (*iv*) unexpected bleeding; (*v*) critically ill or unstable patient	XR with HIT antibodies: *in vitro* XR usually not associated with adverse effects; patients should be monitored for *in vivo* XR (unexplained platelet count fall, progressive new TECs); *in vivo* XR is estimated to occur in ~3% of patients (Magnani and Gallus, 2006) Bleeding complications in compassionate-release study (Ortel and Chong, 1998): fatal (0.9%), major nonfatal bleeding (6.5%); no major bleeds in RCT (Chong et al., 2001) Skin hypersensitivity: rare	Anticoagulant effect depends on adequate AT levels Does not significantly prolong the PTT, ACT, PT/INR (does not interfere with monitoring of overlapping oral anticoagulants) Reduce dosage if serum creatinine >265 µmol/L *No antidote*: in case of overdosage, stop the drug and treat bleeding with blood products as indicated

Abbreviations: ACT, activated clotting time; PTT, partial thromboplastin time; AT, antithrombin III; HCII, heparin cofactor II; HIT, heparin-induced thrombocytopenia; IV, intravenous; PT/INR, prothrombin time/international normalized ratio; RCT, randomized controlled trial; sc, subcutaneous; TEC, thromboembolic complication; $t_{1/2}$, drug half-life; XR, cross-reactivity.

using the (activated) partial thromboplastin time (PTT). This can cause underdosing in patients with prothrombin deficiency or other coagulopathies ("PTT confounding"), as a "therapeutic" PTT may not necessarily indicate adequate dosing of the DTI (see chap. 2). Other factors to consider include drug availability to, and prior experience of, the physician and availability and turnaround time of laboratory monitoring.

DTI Dosing
The approved dosing regimens of the DTIs—as presented within the product monographs—were often too high, especially with lepirudin (Lubenow et al., 2005; Tardy et al., 2006; see also chap. 14). Accordingly, it is recommended that for most situations using hirudins, the IV infusion rate be reduced, even in patients with normal renal function (the dose is reduced substantially more in the presence of renal dysfunction) (Warkentin et al., 2008; Linkins et al., 2012). Moreover, PTT

TABLE 12.4 Main Characteristics of Fondaparinux

Mechanism of action, pharmacokinetics	Monitoring	Undesirable effects	Comments
Catalyzes the inactivation of factor Xa by AT Bioavailability after sc injection ~100%; peak anti-Xa levels, 2–3 hr after injection Plasma $t_{1/2}$ of anti-Xa activity, ~17–21 hr, greatly prolonged in renal impairment	Anti-factor Xa levels during treatment by an amidolytic assay[a] Monitoring recommended in patients with: (*i*) significant renal impairment; (*ii*) body weight < 45 kg or >110 kg; (*iii*) life- or limb-threatening thrombosis; (*iv*) unexpected bleeding; (*v*) critically ill or unstable patient	Induce anti-PF4/H antibodies (similar frequency as with LMWH); rarely may induce autoimmune HIT (<1:10,000); XR with HIT antibodies *in vitro* and/or *in vivo* (rare)	Anticoagulant effect depends on adequate AT levels; does not significantly prolong the PTT, ACT, PT/INR (does not interfere with monitoring of overlapping oral anticoagulants) Reduce dosage in renal impairment *No antidote*: in case of overdosage, stop the drug and treat bleeding with blood products as indicated

[a]Monitoring is not performed routinely.
Abbreviations: ACT, activated clotting time; PTT, partial thromboplastin time; AT, antithrombin III; HCII, heparin cofactor II; HIT, heparin-induced thrombocytopenia; IV, intravenous; PT/INR, prothrombin time/international normalized ratio; sc, subcutaneous; TEC, thromboembolic complication; $t_{1/2}$, drug half-life; XR, cross-reactivity.

monitoring should be performed at 4-hour intervals until stable anticoagulation within the therapeutic range is observed (whereupon once-daily monitoring is appropriate). For argatroban, postmarketing studies indicate that it is increasingly common to reduce the initial infusion rate from the approved dose (2 µg/kg/min) to 0.5–1.2 µg/kg/min (Tables 12.6 and 12.7), especially in critically ill patients or in patients with cardiac dysfunction, even when hepatic dysfunction is not clinically apparent (Alatri et al., 2012) (see chap. 13).

PTT Confounding

The PTT, a global coagulation assay, is most often used for monitoring of DTI therapy. However, when baseline PTT values are elevated because of HIT-associated coagulopathies—including disseminated intravascular coagulation (DIC) as a complication of HIT—then PTT values may not accurately reflect DTI plasma levels. This can result in the phenomenon known as "PTT confounding," whereby supratherapeutic PTTs result in inappropriate DTI dose interruptions or reductions—not because the elevated PTT values reflect supratherapeutic DTI levels (in which case reduced dosing would be appropriate), but rather because of the combined effects of the underlying coagulopathy and the PTT-prolonging effects of the DTI (Greinacher and Warkentin, 2008; Warkentin, 2011a,b).

PTT confounding was first recognized in the setting of initiating DTI therapy in patients with HIT who were already receiving warfarin (vitamin K antagonists such as warfarin will prolong the PTT); shortly after starting DTI therapy, supratherapeutic PTT levels were reached, and DTI therapy was interrupted with rapid progression of microvascular thrombosis and multiple limb necrosis (Warkentin, 2006). Subsequently, this phenomenon has also been recognized in the absence of

TABLE 12.5   Main Characteristics of the r-Hirudins, Lepirudin, and Desirudin

Mechanism of action, pharmacokinetics	Monitoring	Undesirable effects	Comments
Direct, noncovalent, irreversible inhibitor of free and clot-bound thrombin Bioavailability after sc injection, ~100%; peak effect, 2–3 hr Mean plasma distribution time after IV bolus, ~2 hr Mean plasma $t_{1/2}$, 1.3 hr; $t_{1/2}$ greatly prolonged in renal failure (~200 hr in nephrectomized patients)	PTT during treatment; a more precise monitoring is possible by the ECT (see chaps. 14 and 19) Daily PTT monitoring is recommended in all patients (see comments re: antihirudin antibodies) Monitoring by ECT recommended: (i) During CPB (ii) Unexpected bleeding Monitoring by quantitative hirudin EIA or ECA recommended: when prothrombin levels are decreased (Lindhoff-Last et al., 2000; see chap. 14)	Development of antihirudin antibodies in ~40% of patients. In about 3% of patients, these antibodies enhance the anticoagulant effect of hirudin, and require a substantial dose reduction Anaphylactic reactions: ~0.015% (first exposure) ~0.15% (reexposure) associated with IV bolus injection (Greinacher et al., 2003) Reduce dosage if serum creatinine >90 µmol/L (see chap. 14) Allergic reactions: rare Skin hypersensitivity: rare Bleeding complications in HIT patients in prospective studies: major bleeding in two prospective studies, 13.4, 17% (see chap. 14)	~40% of patients develop antihirudin antibodies on day 5 or later of treatment; in only ~5% of these patients is a dose reduction or increase needed; risk of anaphylactic reactions post-IV bolus No major effect on PT/INR (Greinacher et al., 2000) *No antidote*: In case of overdosage, stop the drug and treat bleeding with blood products as indicated (hemofiltration with a high-flux membrane is a possible treatment for life-threatening bleeding)

Abbreviations: PTT, partial thromboplastin time; CPB, cardiopulmonary bypass; ECA, ecarin chromogenic assay; ECT, ecarin clotting time; EIA, enzyme immunoassay; HIT, heparin-induced thrombocytopenia; IV, intravenous; PT/INR, prothrombin time/international normalized ratio; sc, subcutaneous; $t_{1/2}$, drug half-life.

vitamin K antagonism, including in the setting of severe HIT-associated DIC (Greinacher and Warkentin, 2008; Warkentin, 2010a, 2011a,b; Linkins and Warkentin, 2011; see chap. 2). PTT confounding is not specific for HIT, and has also observed in non-HIT settings, such as critically ill patients with coagulopathies (Warkentin, 2011a; see chap. 3).

Figure 12.3 shows a case where the patient had an elevated PTT secondary to HIT-associated DIC prior to initiation of a DTI. This patient case illustrates several features of PTT confounding, including (i) baseline (pre-DTI) coagulopathy (e.g., elevated PTT or INR, low-normal fibrinogen); (ii) abrupt increase in PTT values to supratherapeutic levels soon after commencing DTI therapy; (iii) usually, several supratherapeutic PTT values in succession, resulting in a prolonged period of dose

TABLE 12.6   Main Characteristics of the Direct Thrombin Inhibitor, Argatroban

Mechanism of action, pharmacokinetics	Monitoring	Undesirable effects	Comments
Direct, noncovalent, reversible inhibitor of free and clot-bound thrombin	PTT during treatment; few data exist as to whether more precise monitoring at higher doses would be achieved using other methods, such as ECT	No major side effects besides bleeding complications	Only IV use of argatroban has been tested in HIT
~50% of the drug is plasma protein bound		Argatroban makes all functional clotting assays unreliable	Reduce dosage by 75% in case of liver impairment
Steady state is reached 1–3 hr after starting IV infusion	Target INR is >4.0 when warfarin is overlapped with argatroban (however, following discontinuation of argatroban, the usual target INR of 2.0–3.0 applies during further warfarin treatment)		No dose reduction in renal failure
Mean plasma $t_{1/2}$ is 40–50 min; $t_{1/2}$ is prolonged 4- to 5-fold in moderate liver impairment			*No antidote*: in case of overdosage or severe bleeding, stop the drug and treat bleeding with blood products as indicated
	Note: in case of prothrombin deficiency, PTT gives falsely high values		Argatroban prolongs the INR and requires a strategy adopted to the INR reagent used for overlapping treatment with warfarin (see chap. 13)

Abbreviations: PTT, partial thromboplastin time; ECT, ecarin-clotting time; HIT, heparin-induced thrombocytopenia; INR, international normalized ratio; IV, intravenous; $t_{1/2}$, drug half-life.

interruptions and/or reductions; and (*iv*) progression or new development of macro- and/or microvascular thrombosis.

Patients with HIT-associated DIC are at high risk for treatment failure due to PTT confounding, not only because of their underlying coagulopathy, but also because these patients usually have features of "delayed-onset" (or "autoimmune") HIT, whereby their thrombocytopenia and associated hypercoagulability state intensifies for several days despite stopping heparin (Warkentin, 2010a). Figure 12.4 illustrates the general picture of patients who have severe HIT-associated hyperco-agulability in the setting of HIT that begins after stopping heparin, or that worsens despite stopping heparin. Very few laboratories routinely test for heparin-independent platelet-activating features of HIT antibodies, and thus this syndrome is underrecognized. As a general rule, blood from such patients will yield high OD values in the PF4-dependent EIAs.

> *Recommendation.* In patients with underlying coagulopathy (e.g., DIC or warfarin-related), DTI monitoring ideally should be performed by an assay that is independent of prothrombin concentrations (more widely available in Europe), especially when early post-treatment PTT values seem higher than expected for the DTI dose given.

Danaparoid Cross-Reactivity
Danaparoid is a mixture of nonheparin anticoagulant glycosaminoglycans, pre-dominantly (low-sulfated) heparan sulfate, dermatan sulfate, and chondroitin

TABLE 12.7 Dosing of Argatroban Recommended by a European Consensus Group

Patient group		Initial dose [μg/kg/min]	Bolus [μg/kg]	Monitoring parameter and frequency	Target range to be achieved by titration
Patients with HIT or suspicion of HIT					
Intensive care unit (i.e., critically ill patients, post-cardiac surgery)	With acute life-threatening TE	2.0	–	PTT 2 hr after every dose adjustment or at least once daily	PTT 1.5–3.0 times baseline not exceeding 100 sec
	With acute non–life-threatening TE	1.0	–		
	Without TE	0.5[a]	–		
Non–intensive care unit	Without hepatic impairment	2.0	–		
	With hepatic impairment	0.5	–		
Pediatric	Without hepatic impairment	0.75	–		
	With hepatic impairment	0.2	–		
Renal replacement therapy					
Continuous RRT		0.5[a]	100[b]	PTT	PTT see above
Intermittent RRT (outpatients)		2.0	250	ACT	ACT 170–230 sec[d]
Percutaneous coronary intervention		25.0	350	ACT[c]	ACT 300–450 sec

[a]Further dose adjustment can be made based on extent of critical illness (see Alatri et al., 2012).
[b]No bolus is required if the patient is already receiving argatroban.
[c]ACT should be checked 5–10 min after completing the bolus dose.
[d]The infusion should be stopped one hour before the end of hemodialysis.
Abbreviations: ACT, activated clotting time; PTT, (activated) partial thromboplastin time; HIT, heparin-induced thrombocytopenia; RRT, renal replacement therapy; TE, thromboembolism.
Source: From Alatri et al. (2012).

sulfate (see chap. 16). About 10–40% of HIT patient sera "cross-react" *in vitro* with danaparoid, depending on the assay used (lower cross-reactivity rates by platelet aggregometry, higher rates with fluid-phase PF4/H immunoassays) (Vun et al., 1996; Warkentin et al., 2005a; Magnani and Gallus, 2006). The majority of patients with detectable *in vitro* cross-reactivity have favorable clinical courses that do not differ significantly (either in clinical outcomes or in time to platelet count recovery) from patients without cross-reactivity (Warkentin, 1996). Furthermore, in many patients, therapeutic concentrations of danaparoid *disrupt* PF4/heparin/IgG immune complexes, thereby inhibiting HIT antibody-induced platelet activation (Chong et al., 1989; Krauel et al., 2008); this is a unique pharmacologic attribute not shared by any other anticoagulant. For all of these reasons, we do not advise testing for *in vitro* cross-reactivity in patients in whom danaparoid treatment is planned.

> *Recommendation. In vitro* cross-reactivity testing for danaparoid using HIT patient serum or plasma is not recommended prior to danaparoid administration.

Figure 12.5 illustrates the clinical course of a critically ill patient with severe thrombocytopenia (platelet count nadir, 2×10^9/L) and DIC complicating postcardiac surgery HIT who was successfully managed by danaparoid. The case illustrates the

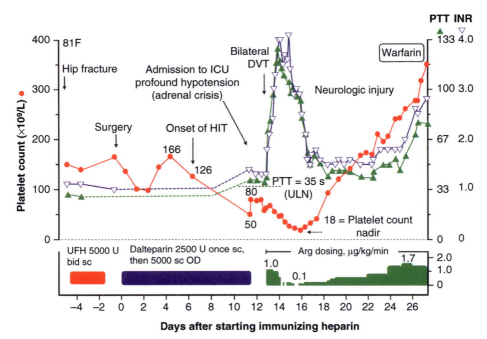

FIGURE 12.3 Shows PTT confounding secondary to HIT-associated consumptive coagulopathy. The patient developed HIT six days after starting dalteparin thromboprophylaxis post–hip fracture surgery. On day 11, the patient was admitted to the ICU for severe hypotension secondary to adrenal failure (flat ACTH stimulation test; bilateral adrenal infarction by imaging). HIT-associated bilateral lower-limb DVT was treated with argatroban begun at 1 µg/kg/min. Despite stopping all heparin, the platelet count fell over four days from 80 to 18 ×10⁹/L (nadir). Five PTT measurements preargatroban were all elevated (range, 38–41 sec; normal, 22–35 sec). Postinitiating argatroban, persisting supratherapeutic PTT values resulted in multiple argatroban dose reductions and interruptions; when HIT was most intense (as judged by platelet count nadir), argatroban dosing was <0.1 µg/kg/min. The laboratory and clinical profile is consistent with intense HIT-associated consumptive coagulopathy, with confounding of PTT monitoring of argatroban therapy and associated underdosing despite supratherapeutic PTT values. *Abbreviations*: ACTH, adrenocorticotropic hormone; Arg, argatroban; bid, twice daily; DVT, deep vein thrombosis; F, female; HIT, heparin-induced thrombocytopenia; ICU, intensive care unit; INR, international normalized ratio; OD, once daily; PTT, partial thromboplastin time; sc, subcutaneous; U, units; ULN, upper limit of normal. *Source*: From Linkins and Warkentin (2011).

usefulness of being able to obtain antifactor Xa levels (thus avoiding PTT confounding in the setting of HIT-associated DIC) and the advantage of a long pharmacologic half-life (thus, avoiding rebound hypercoagulability when the danaparoid infusion) was temporarily held.

Fondaparinux for Treating HIT

Fondaparinux (Arixtra) is a synthetic pentasaccharide that catalyzes the inactivation of factor Xa by antithrombin. In several case series (Kuo and Kovacs, 2005; Lobo et al., 2008; Grouzi et al., 2010; Pappalardo et al., 2010; Goldarb and Blostein, 2011; Warkentin et al., 2011) describing a total of 71 patients, no new thrombotic events occurred after initiating treatment with fondaparinux (95% CI, 0–5.1%). This

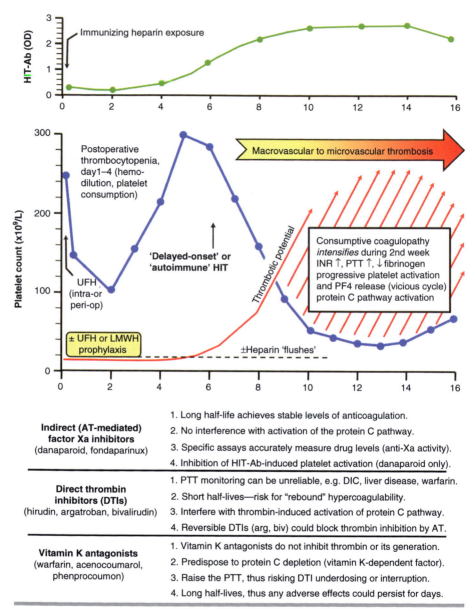

FIGURE 12.4   Conceptual framework of HIT: focus on heparin-independent platelet activation and delayed-onset ("autoimmune") HIT. (*Upper panel*) The timeline of HIT antibody (HIT-Ab) formation, as judged by OD units in an anti-PF4/polyanion EIA; (*middle panel*) illustration of a platelet count decline in the absence of heparin (or with small amounts of heparin, e.g., "flushes") indicating "delayed-onset" HIT, with intensification of HIT-associated hypercoagulability from day 7 to 14, especially after stopping heparin. (*Lower panel*) Comparing different classes of anticoagulant for expected effects on HIT-associated hypercoagulability. (*Continued*)

FIGURE 12.4 (*Continued*) *Abbreviations*: PTT, (activated) partial thromboplastin time; arg, argatroban; AT, antithrombin; biv, bivalirudin; DIC, disseminated intravascular coagulation; DTI, direct thrombin inhibitor; HIT, heparin-induced thrombocytopenia; HIT-Ab, HIT antibodies; LMWH, low molecular weight heparin; INR, international normalized ratio; OD, optical density; periop, perioperative; PF4, platelet factor 4; UFH, unfractionated heparin. Source: From Warkentin (2010a).

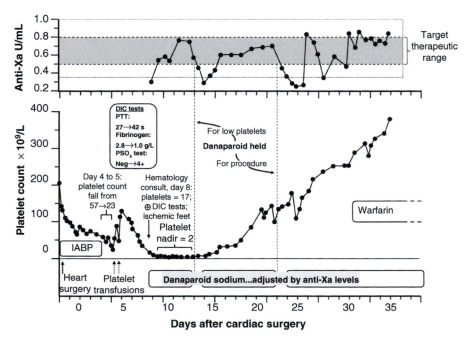

FIGURE 12.5 Danaparoid for severe HIT. Despite overt DIC, bilateral limb ischemia, and the lowest platelet count (2 × 10⁹/L) due to HIT encountered by one of the Authors (T. E. W.), this patient fully recovered from HIT and without loss of limb or any other permanent sequelae. The evidence for overt DIC included elevated PTT, reduced fibrinogen, and strongly positive (4+) protamine sulfate (PSO$_4$) paracoagulation assay at day 8, which represents changes from normal values at day 5. *Abbreviations*: DIC, disseminated intravascular coagulation; IABP, intra-aortic balloon pump; PSO$_4$, protamine sulfate; PTT, (activated) partial thromboplastin time. *Source*: From Warkentin (2010a).

favorable experience indicates that fondaparinux likely provides effective anticoagulation in most patients with HIT. The pharmacokinetics of fondaparinux, however, depend on renal function. Major bleeding occurred in approximately 5% of the patients (4/71), and appeared to be more common in patients who were critically ill and/or with renal dysfunction.

Monitoring of the drug levels may help to avoid under- or overdosing. In this regard, monitoring of danaparoid and fondaparinux by antifactor Xa assays is more reliable than monitoring of DTIs with the PTT or the ECT (see above). The antifactor Xa assays do not depend on individual patient factors.

Fondaparinux can be monitored 4 hours after the first and second injection with a target peak antifactor Xa level of ~1.5 U/mL; and before the next injection with a target trough level of ~0.7 anti-Xa U/mL to avoid underdosage. If the peak level is not reached, a second dose of the drug should be given (depending on the aFXa-level, 1.5 or 2.5 mg); if the trough level is too high, the dose given at the next day should be reduced.

Fondaparinux has been shown to induce anti-PF4/H antibodies approximately as frequently as LMWH (Warkentin et al., 2005a); consistent with its immunogenic capacity, presumably antigenic multimolecular complexes of PF4 and fondaparinux have been visualized directly at a molecular level (Greinacher et al., 2006); and, most important, a few cases of fondaparinux-associated HIT have been reported (Warkentin et al., 2007; Warkentin, 2010b; see chap. 17).

However, fondaparinux appears to form relatively few multimolecular complexes with PF4 (Greinacher et al., 2006). These few complexes appear to be sufficient to induce an immune response, but not enough to activate many platelets (Savi et al., 2005). To date, none of the patients reported in the case series have developed apparent worsening of their HIT when treated with fondaparinux.

The anti-PF4/H immune response varies considerably among different patients. Some patients form antibodies that can activate platelets in the presence of buffer alone (i.e., in the complete absence of heparin) during the acute phase of HIT (Warkentin and Kelton, 2001a; Prechel et al., 2005; Socher et al., 2008). These antibodies, which behave like platelet-activating autoantibodies, have been detected in a few cases of fondaparinux-associated HIT. These rare patients require high-dose anticoagulation until platelet recovery occurs.

A major advantage of fondaparinux is that it can be given sc on an outpatient basis, which allows for postdischarge overlap with vitamin K antagonists after normalization of the platelet count (potentially avoiding a one-week prolongation of hospitalization required for DTI-warfarin overlap).

Other Drugs that Reduce Thrombin Generation in HIT

Other drugs with antithrombotic activity described anecdotally as treatment for HIT include bivalirudin (see chap. 15) and dermatan sulfate (Agnelli et al., 1994; Taliani et al., 1999; Imberti et al., 2003). Dabigatran, rivaroxaban, and apixaban may well emerge as alternative anticoagulants appropriate for treatment of HIT, as they are effective anticoagulants that do not interact with PF4 (Krauel et al., 2012). Dabigatran use was described in one postoperative patient who had anti-PF4/H antibodies, but who did not have HIT (Fieland and Taylor, 2012).

Anticoagulation of the HIT Patient Without Thrombosis

Approximately 50% of patients with HIT do not have a new HIT-associated thrombosis at the time HIT is first clinically suspected on the basis of thrombocytopenia alone (Warkentin and Kelton, 1996; Greinacher et al., 1999a,b, 2005). In a retrospective cohort study of 62 such patients with "isolated HIT," the subsequent 30-day cumulative thrombotic event rate was high (52.8%) (see Fig. 4.5 in chap. 4). The rate of thrombosis was similar in the two largest patient subgroups: patients treated with discontinuation of heparin therapy alone (20/36, 56%) and patients treated with substitution of warfarin for heparin (10/21, 48%). The majority of events involved the venous circulation (4:1 ratio), with six of the 62 patients developing pulmonary embolism (two fatal); another patient who died suddenly may also have had a fatal pulmonary embolism.

In a subsequent large retrospective cohort study of serologically confirmed HIT performed by Wallis and coworkers (1999), a 38% thrombotic event rate was observed in patients with isolated HIT managed by cessation of heparin. Furthermore, early cessation of heparin was not associated with a reduction in the rate of thrombosis. In another study, Zwicker and colleagues (2004) observed that five (36%) of 14 patients with clinically suspected HIT who tested strongly positive (>1.00 units of OD) for anti-PF4/H antibodies by anti-PF4/H enzyme immunoassay (EIA) developed symptomatic thrombosis. The high symptomatic thrombotic event rates observed in these three retrospective cohort studies are consistent with prospective treatment cohort studies that also observed a high rate of thrombosis (5–10%/day over the first one to two days) soon after the diagnosis of HIT (Greinacher et al., 1999a,b, 2000).

These high thrombotic event rates among patients with isolated HIT suggest that many patients may have had subclinical deep vein thrombosis (DVT) at the time that HIT was first suspected. Indeed, Tardy and colleagues (1999) found that eight of 16 patients identified as having isolated HIT had subclinical DVT identified by systematic duplex ultrasound investigations.

> *Recommendation.* Patients strongly suspected (or confirmed) to have acute HIT should undergo imaging studies for lower limb DVT, especially those at highest risk for venous thromboembolism, such as postoperative patients.

There is evidence that therapeutic-dose anticoagulant therapy of isolated HIT is effective. In a retrospective analysis of patients with isolated HIT comparing treatment with danaparoid and lepirudin, it was observed that patients who received *prophylactic-dose* danaparoid (750 U sc b.i.d. or t.i.d.) had a trend to a higher rate of thrombosis than patients treated with lepirudin (0.1 mg/kg body weight/hr, PTT-adjusted) (Farner et al., 2001). In contrast, patients with HIT-associated thrombosis had similar outcomes when treated with therapeutic doses of either drug. This indicates that *therapeutic*, rather than prophylactic, doses of danaparoid may be more effective for patients with isolated HIT (Farner et al., 2001; Warkentin, 2001). Further evidence supporting the use of therapeutic-dose anticoagulation for isolated HIT includes the results of (PTT-adjusted) therapy with the DTIs, lepirudin, and argatroban (Lewis et al., 2001, 2003, 2006; Lubenow et al., 2004).

We usually prescribe an alternative anticoagulant in *therapeutic* doses in this situation of strongly suspected (or confirmed) HIT. However, prophylactic-dose anticoagulation is a reasonable option in patients with a low or intermediate likelihood of having HIT or in HIT patients judged to be at high risk for bleeding complications. Another option could be regular screening for venous thrombosis without anticoagulation in a patient at very high bleeding risk. Thrombocytopenia itself should not be considered a contraindication to anticoagulation in patients with HIT, as petechiae and other spontaneous hemorrhagic manifestations are not usually seen in these patients (see chap. 2). However, if the platelet count is less than 20×10^9/L and bleeding signs, but not thrombosis, are observed, then alternative diagnoses, such as posttransfusion purpura or other drug-dependent immune thrombocytopenic disorders, should be considered (see chap. 3).

> *Recommendation.* Therapeutic-dose anticoagulation with a rapidly acting alternative, nonheparin anticoagulant should be considered in patients strongly suspected (or confirmed) to have HIT even in the absence of symptomatic thrombosis. Anticoagulation should be continued at least until recovery of the platelet counts to a stable plateau.

It is uncertain whether anticoagulation of isolated HIT beyond the time to platelet count recovery (to a stable plateau) is required, if there are no ongoing risk factors for thrombosis, such as atrial fibrillation or prolonged immobility. In the prospective lepirudin studies (Lubenow et al., 2004), the risk of subsequent thrombosis (35 day follow-up) among patients with isolated HIT treated until full platelet count recovery was low. We therefore do not usually give prolonged anticoagulation in our own clinical practice. (See also sections "Longer-Term Anticoagulant Management of the HIT Patient with Thrombosis" and "Vitamin K Antagonists" regarding *contraindication* to the use of vitamin K antagonists during the acute thrombocytopenic phase of HIT). It is reasonable to repeat a duplex ultrasound of the lower extremities prior to discharging a patient to home when ongoing anticoagulation will not be given.

Longer-Term Anticoagulant Management of the HIT Patient with Thrombosis

Acute HIT by itself is not an indication for longer-term anticoagulation (i.e., three to six months). However, HIT-associated thrombosis, or the underlying disease itself, often is. For longer-term control of thrombosis, oral anticoagulants of the coumarin class (e.g., warfarin or phenprocoumon) are still the most widely used treatments. However, as discussed subsequently, special precautions are needed for managing transition to vitamin K antagonist therapy. Besides transitioning to vitamin K antagonists, other options include the following: continuing fondaparinux or danaparoid by sc injection or transitioning to one of the newer oral anticoagulants, for example, dabigatran or rivaroxaban.

Transition to Vitamin K Antagonist (Coumarin) Therapy

Generally, it takes at least five days of vitamin K antagonist therapy before therapeutic functional hypoprothrombinemia is achieved (Harrison et al., 1997). It is important that thrombin generation be controlled in patients with acute HIT before and during initiation of coumarin treatment, particularly in patients with severe HIT-associated DVT, because otherwise coumarin-induced necrosis (venous limb gangrene and skin necrosis syndromes) can be induced (Warkentin et al., 1997; Srinivasan et al., 2004) (see chap. 2). This proscription against coumarin use applies particularly during the acute thrombocytopenic phase of HIT, as coumarins fail to inhibit the marked hypercoagulability state of HIT, while at the same time they can cause severe depletion of the vitamin K-dependent natural anticoagulant, protein C. These are the circumstances predisposing to the disturbed procoagulant–anticoagulant balance characteristic of the coumarin necrosis syndromes in HIT. Thus, it is important to *postpone* starting administration of coumarin anticoagulants until therapeutic anticoagulation is achieved with danaparoid, fondaparinux, r-hirudin, bivalirudin, or argatroban *and* until there has been substantial platelet count recovery (usually to at least $150 \times 10^9/L$, indicating that the platelet-activating effects of the HIT antibodies have largely resolved).

> *Recommendation.* To minimize the risk of coumarin necrosis in a patient with acute HIT, vitamin K antagonist (coumarin) therapy should be delayed until the patient is adequately anticoagulated with a rapidly acting parenteral anticoagulant, and not until there has been substantial platelet count recovery (at least $>150 \times 10^9/L$). The vitamin K antagonist should be started in low maintenance doses (e.g., ≤ 5 mg warfarin), with at least five days of overlap with the parenteral anticoagulant (including at least two days in the target-therapeutic range), and the parenteral anticoagulant should not be stopped until the platelet count has reached a stable plateau.

Besides minimizing the risk of coumarin-induced microthrombosis/necrosis, there are two other important reasons for postponing coumarin anticoagulation in a patient with acute HIT. First, since coumarins increase the PTT, and since the PTT is usually used to monitor the anticoagulant effect of the DTIs, the patient is at risk of receiving insufficient dosing of the DTI if coumarin has already been given (PTT confounding). This phenomenon has been implicated in some patients who have developed venous limb gangrene during overlapping DTI—coumarin therapy (Warkentin, 2006). Second, the DTIs have varying effects on the global clotting assays, in particular, the prothrombin time/international normalized ratio (PT/INR), as follows: argatroban > bivalirudin > lepirudin (Gosselin et al., 2004; Warkentin et al., 2005b; see Fig. 15.3 in chap. 15). Because the INR is used to guide coumarin therapy, there is a special issue during the management of DTI—coumarin overlap, namely the effect of the DTI on the INR, especially with argatroban. Once the anticoagulant effect of the DTI has dissipated (usually within a few hours of stopping the DTI), the circumstances favoring microvascular thrombosis—and, hence, coumarin-induced necrosis—might well be present, that is, ongoing thrombin generation from acute HIT, warfarin-induced protein C depletion, and active DVT (Warkentin et al., 1997; Smythe et al., 2002; Srinivasan et al., 2004). Thus, postponing coumarin therapy in a patient with acute HIT until the platelet count has normalized will reduce the risk that premature discontinuation of the DTI could occur at a time when HIT antibodies are still causing substantial activation of platelets and the clotting system.

A corollary to the above considerations is that it is important to reverse with vitamin K the effects of coumarin, if HIT is recognized *after* coumarin therapy has already been begun (e.g., 10 mg vitamin K by slow IV infusion over 30–60 minutes) (Warkentin, 2006; Warkentin et al., 2008; Linkins et al., 2012). This is particularly important if a DTI will be used to manage anticoagulation (in contrast to the DTIs, danaparoid and fondaparinux prolong neither the PTT nor INR to any significant extent).

> *Recommendation.* Oral or IV vitamin K should be given to reverse coumarin anticoagulation in a patient recognized as having acute HIT after coumarin has been commenced.

In case of coumarin overdose and severe bleeding during the first three months after an episode of HIT, prothrombin complex concentrates should only be used with extreme caution to "reverse" coumarin anticoagulation. This is because these concentrates contain heparin and have been associated with recurrent thrombocytopenia and thrombosis in patients with circulating HIT antibodies (Greinacher et al., 1992).

> *Recommendation.* Prothrombin complex concentrates should not be used to reverse coumarin anticoagulation in a patient with acute or recent HIT unless bleeding is otherwise unmanageable.

Transition from the alternative nonheparin anticoagulants (danaparoid, fondaparinux, argatroban, r-hirudin, bivalirudin) to the new oral anticoagulants (rivaroxaban, dabigatran, apixaban) is a theoretically attractive option for long-term anticoagulation after recovery from acute HIT, but experience to date has not been reported.

Management of the Patient with a Low or Intermediate Probability of HIT (Pending Results of HIT Antibody Testing)

In patients with HIT without thrombosis, the risk of major bleeding with therapeutic-dose DTI therapy per patient-day has been reported to be as high as 1.0% for lepirudin (i.e., 14.3% major bleeding over a mean treatment period of 13.9 days) (Lubenow et al., 2004) and for argatroban it was 0.6% and 1.0% (3.1% and 5.3% major bleeding over a mean treatment period of 5.3 and 5.1 days, respectively) (Lewis et al., 2001, 2003). In the large case series of HIT patients treated with danaparoid (Magnani and Gallus, 2006), the risk for major bleeding was 0.4% per day for prophylactic-dose therapy (3.2% major bleeding over a median treatment duration of six days) (Dr H. Magnani, personal communication).

These relatively high risks for bleeding (especially with DTIs) should be contrasted with the much lower expected rate of thrombosis (~0.3–0.5% per patient day) among all patients investigated for HIT by ordering laboratory testing for HIT antibodies. This calculation is based on the estimated initial thrombotic event-rate per day (~5%) multiplied by the relatively low overall risk of obtaining a positive test result using a functional test for platelet-activating heparin-dependent antibodies (~6–10%) (Warkentin and Sheppard, 2006; Greinacher et al., 2007). Thus, the high risk of bleeding with therapeutic-dose anticoagulation suggests that such therapy is justified only if the clinical likelihood is judged to be at least intermediate, if not high, based on the clinical picture, prior to obtaining the results of laboratory testing for HIT antibodies. Unless otherwise dictated by the patient's clinical condition, the use of an alternative anticoagulant in *prophylactic doses* might be safer in this situation. This could be achieved in several ways: for example, danaparoid 750 U t.i.d. sc, a dosing regimen that is approved for prophylaxis of new thrombosis in several jurisdictions. Another option is prophylactic-dose fondaparinux (2.5 mg once-daily sc).

Desirudin has been assessed in patients with suspected HIT in an open-label trial. Sixteen patients were randomized to receive either argatroban in therapeutic dose or desirudin in prophylactic dose (15 mg sc every 12 hours) in patients without thrombosis, and desirudin at higher doses (30 mg sc every 12 hours) in patients with thrombosis (Boyce et al., 2011). The authors found that the efficacy of the two drugs appeared comparable. As desirudin is also renally excreted, there is still a risk of accumulation if the renal function is impaired. These results require further investigation in a larger cohort to determine if fixed sc dosing of desirudin with minimal monitoring is safe.

> *Recommendation.* In a patient with a low probability for HIT (e.g., 4Ts score ≤ 3) pending the results of laboratory testing for HIT antibodies, we suggest either continuing the use of heparin or using alternative, nonheparin anticoagulation in prophylactic, rather than in therapeutic, doses (assuming there is no other reason for therapeutic-dose anticoagulation).

> *Recommendation.* In a patient with an intermediate probability for HIT (e.g., 4Ts score of 4 or 5), who has an alternative explanation for thrombocytopenia and who does not require therapeutic-dose anticoagulation for other reasons, we suggest alternative anticoagulation in prophylactic, rather than in therapeutic, doses.

Regardless of the pretest probability of HIT, if a sensitive laboratory test excludes the presence of HIT antibodies, then use of heparin is appropriate.

Reexposure of the HIT Patient to Heparin
Heparin Reexposure of the Patient with Acute or Recent HIT
Deliberate or accidental readministration of heparin to a patient with acute or recent HIT can cause an abrupt platelet count fall, sometimes complicated by thrombosis or acute systemic (anaphylactoid) reactions (see chap. 2). Accordingly, deliberate

heparin rechallenge for diagnostic purposes is not recommended, especially because sensitive assays for HIT antibodies are available. This is a strong recommendation because the diagnostic usefulness of laboratory assays for HIT has been established in controlled studies (see chap. 11).

> *Recommendation.* Deliberate reexposure to heparin of a patient with acute or recent HIT for diagnostic purposes is not recommended. Rather, the diagnosis should first be excluded or confirmed in most situations by testing acute patient serum or plasma for HIT antibodies using a sensitive activation or antigen assay.

Heparin Reexposure of the Patient with a History of Remote HIT

HIT antibodies decrease rapidly after the acute phase of HIT and are usually not detectable three months after an episode of HIT (Warkentin and Kelton, 2001b). There are few data describing the clinical and serologic outcomes of patients reexposed with heparin with previously documented HIT in the remote past (arbitrarily, more than three months ago, or sooner, if HIT antibodies have disappeared). One patient who developed fatal HIT on day 15 of UFH treatment had a history of HIT complicated by thrombosis six years earlier (Gruel et al., 1990). However, several patients with previous remote HIT have been observed in whom repeat heparin use caused neither HIT nor HIT antibody formation (Pötzsch et al., 2000; Warkentin and Kelton, 2001b). More recently, hemodialysis patients with HIT—following disappearance of their HIT antibodies—were deliberately reexposed to either LMWH or UFH on a regular ongoing basis for hemodialysis; none of the eight rechallenged patients described developed recurrence of HIT (Hartman et al., 2006; Wanaka et al., 2010).

Because there are acceptable alternative anticoagulant options for most prophylactic and therapeutic indications, both UFH and LMWH usually should be avoided in patients with a previous history of HIT. As discussed in the following section, however, there are special circumstances, such as cardiac or vascular surgery or hemodialysis, during which it is reasonable to use heparin for a patient with a previous history of HIT.

> *Recommendation.* Heparin should not be used for antithrombotic prophylaxis or therapy in a patient with a previous history of HIT, except under special circumstances (e.g., cardiac or vascular surgery, or hemodialysis).

HIT IN SPECIAL CLINICAL SITUATIONS
Cardiac or Vascular Surgery
Management of the Patient with Acute or Recent HIT

For patients with acute HIT who require heart surgery, or with recent HIT and persistence of circulating HIT antibodies, it is possible to use alternative anticoagulants during cardiopulmonary bypass (CPB) (see chap. 19). The major option for alternative anticoagulation for such patients is bivalirudin, as this has the greatest experience and an established protocol. Unfortunately, there is no specific antidote, and it therefore is not ideal for managing CPB. Other options, for example, co-administration of UFH with an antiplatelet agent, such as tirofiban (GPIIb/IIIa antagonist) or epoprostenol (prostacyclin analogue), or danaparoid, or argatroban, are either not well established or have certain important drawbacks. This special topic of managing cardiac surgery patients with acute or previous HIT is discussed in chap. 19.

There is less experience using alternative anticoagulants for intraoperative anticoagulation of vascular surgery. Danaparoid and lepirudin have also been used to provide intraoperative anticoagulation, as well as to "flush" blood vessels during vascular surgery in patients with acute HIT [for review, see Warkentin (2004)]. There is some experience using argatroban for vascular surgery, and bivalirudin is another option (see chap. 19).

> *Recommendation.* Alternative anticoagulation should be used for heart or vascular surgery in a patient with acute or recent HIT with detectable heparin-dependent, platelet-activating antibodies. Bivalirudin is an appropriate alternative for intraoperative anticoagulation.

Management of the Patient Following Disappearance of HIT Antibodies

The drawbacks of alternative anticoagulants for CPB provide a rationale for the use of heparin in two groups of patients with a previous history of HIT: (*i*) a patient with a history of HIT, but who no longer has circulating HIT antibodies detected by a sensitive (washed platelet) activation assay; and (*ii*) a patient with acute or recent HIT who requires elective heart surgery. In the latter situation, it is reasonable to delay cardiac surgery until HIT antibodies become undetectable, which usually occurs in a few weeks or months (Warkentin and Kelton, 2001b; Warkentin and Greinacher, 2003).

It is feasible to give UFH for cardiac or vascular surgery in a patient with a previous history of HIT, provided that HIT antibodies are not detectable at the time of surgery (Olinger et al., 1984; Smith et al., 1985; Makhoul et al., 1987; Pötzsch et al., 2000; Warkentin and Kelton, 2001b; Warkentin and Greinacher, 2003). Although sufficient experience has been gained to strongly recommend using heparin in a patient testing negative for anti-PF4/H antibodies, less data exist on the use of heparin in patients who have a negative functional assay but still test positive for anti-PF4/H IgG. In our view, this is a feasible approach, provided that a sensitive platelet activation is used. This approach is especially important in patients on ventricular assist devices who are awaiting cardiac transplant (Selleng et al., 2008).

We recommend that heparin be avoided completely both before surgery (to prevent potential for restimulation of HIT antibodies) and after surgery (thus making HIT unlikely even if HIT antibodies are reformed). Current evidence suggests that there is a minimum time (five days) to formation of clinically significant HIT antibodies even in patients who have a previous history of HIT (Cadroy et al., 1994; Warkentin and Kelton, 2001b; Lubenow et al., 2002). The patient should receive routine doses of UFH for the surgical procedure itself. Preoperative anticoagulation (e.g., for heart catheterization) and postoperative antithrombotic prophylaxis can be achieved with a nonheparin agent, such as danaparoid (750 U b.i.d. or t.i.d.) or desirudin (15 mg b.i.d. sc) (Eriksson et al., 1997) (see chaps. 14 and 16).

> *Recommendation.* In a patient with a previous history of HIT, heart or vascular surgery can be performed using heparin, provided that (platelet-activating) HIT antibodies are absent (by sensitive functional assay) and heparin use is restricted to the surgical procedure itself.

HIT During Pregnancy

There are a few reports describing HIT during pregnancy (Henny et al., 1986; Meytes et al., 1986; Calhoun and Hesser, 1987; Copplestone and Oscier, 1987; van Besien et al., 1991; Greinacher et al., 1993a). Danaparoid has been used in at least

91 pregnancies using dosing schedules similar to those in nonpregnant patients (Lindhoff-Last et al., 2005; Magnani, 2010). Danaparoid does not cross the placenta, based on cord blood assessment (Magnani and Gallus, 2006) (see chap. 16). Fondaparinux also does not undergo significant placental transfer (judged by a dually perfused *in vitro* human cotyledon model) (Lagrange et al., 2002), whereas about 10% of the maternal concentration of fondaparinux was found in the cord blood of a newborn (Harenberg, 2007). Few reports describe the use of lepirudin during pregnancy (Huhle et al., 2000; Furlan et al., 2006). Hirudin can cross the placenta in low doses (Markwardt et al., 1988) and has caused embryopathy in rabbits given high doses of hirudin (Lubenow and Greinacher, 2000). Furthermore, a zebrafish model reveals that thrombin plays a role in embryogenesis (Jagadeeswaran et al., 1997). Thus, danaparoid and fondaparinux are preferred for treatment of HIT during (early) pregnancy (Warkentin et al., 2008; Linkins et al., 2012).

> *Recommendation.* If available, danaparoid (and possibly fondaparinux) is preferred for parenteral anticoagulation of pregnant patients with HIT, or in those who have a previous history of HIT.

Treatment of HIT in Children

There are only a few reports describing the management of HIT in children [for review, see Klenner et al. (2004); Takemoto and Streiff (2011)] (see chap. 21); therefore, no clear treatment recommendations can be made. Experience from small case series suggests that lepirudin, argatroban, and danaparoid can be used successfully in children. A recent prospective study of fondaparinux use in children included patients with HIT (Young et al., 2011). The dosing schedules for adults (appropriately weight-adjusted for the child) can be used as a guideline, but careful monitoring is recommended.

ADJUNCTIVE THERAPIES
Medical Thrombolysis

Thrombocytopenia is not a contraindication to thrombolytic therapy in patients with HIT. Streptokinase (Fiessinger et al., 1984; Cohen et al., 1985; Bounameaux et al., 1986; Cummings et al., 1986; Mehta et al., 1991), urokinase (Krueger et al., 1985; Leroy et al., 1985; Clifton and Smith, 1986; Nitta et al., 2011), and tissue plasminogen activator (t-PA) (Dieck et al., 1990; Schiffman et al., 1997; Turba et al., 2007) have been used both systemically and by local infusion (Quinones-Baldrich et al., 1989). In patients at high bleeding risk, an ultra-low-dose t-PA (2 mg/hr over 12 hours) was successfully applied without bleeding complications (Olbrich et al., 1998). As thrombin generation is not inhibited by thrombolysis, concomitant non-heparin anticoagulation should be given, in reduced dose, until the fibrinolytic effects have waned.

> *Recommendation.* Regional or systemic pharmacologic thrombolysis should be considered as a treatment adjunct in selected patients with limb-threatening thrombosis or pulmonary embolism with severe cardiovascular compromise.

Surgical Thromboembolectomy and Fasciotomies

Vascular surgery is often needed to salvage an ischemic limb threatened by HIT-associated acute arterial thromboembolism involving large arteries (Sobel et al., 1988; Warkentin et al., 2012). When performing vascular surgery during acute HIT, it is appropriate to maintain anticoagulation at least in the lower therapeutic range, if possible, before, during, and after surgery, until platelet count recovery. In patients with latent HIT (i.e., no longer thrombocytopenic, but with clinically significant levels of HIT antibodies still present), the intensity of anticoagulation depends on the perceived risk of vessel (or graft) occlusion. In patients at high risk of occlusion (e.g., surgery involving below-knee vessels), the patient should be therapeutically anticoagulated before vessel clamping (in addition to receiving intraoperative flushes with anticoagulant), with therapeutic anticoagulation maintained for several days after surgery. In surgery involving larger vessels, the use of intraoperative flushes alone, followed by postoperative prophylactic-dose anticoagulation, might be sufficient.

Either danaparoid, lepirudin, bivalirudin, or argatroban can provide intraoperative anticoagulation. One author (A. G.) uses one of the following solutions to flush the vessel postembolectomy: (i) r-hirudin, 0.1 mg/mL saline (one 20 mg ampule in 200 mL saline), using up to 250 mL in a normal-weight patient, and assessing the PTT before giving more lepirudin to avoid overdosage (the r-hirudin flushes thus can achieve therapeutic intraoperative anticoagulation; see chap. 14); (ii) danaparoid, 3.0 anti-Xa U/mL (i.e., one 750 U ampule in 250 mL saline), using up to 50 mL in a normal-weight patient (this small flush dose is used because systemic anticoagulation is achieved by giving a 2250 U bolus of danaparoid preoperatively (see chap. 16). Chapter 19 discusses the use of bivalirudin for this indication.

In one small study, eight of 10 patients with acute HIT successfully received UFH for intraoperative anticoagulation—without the need for limb amputation—indicating that catastrophic intraoperative thrombosis does not always result even when UFH is used for intraoperative anticoagulation for acute thromboembolectomy (Warkentin et al., 2012). In these patients, UFH was used because of the urgent need for surgery and because the diagnosis of HIT was either not apparent or not considered at the time of clinical presentation. In contrast, three of four patients who received alternative (nonheparin) anticoagulation because HIT was diagnosed preoperatively required limb amputation. This small study highlights that the optimal approach for intraoperative anticoagulation remains unknown.

> *Recommendation.* Surgical thromboembolectomy is an appropriate adjunctive treatment for selected patients with limb-threatening large-vessel arterial thromboembolism. Thrombocytopenia is not a contraindication to surgery. An alternative anticoagulant to heparin should preferably be used for intraoperative anticoagulation, although choice of anticoagulant and dosing remain unknown.

In contrast to large artery thrombosis, a surgical role for severe venous or microvascular limb ischemia is less certain (Warkentin, 2007). Fasciotomy is sometimes performed in patients with severe venous limb ischemia and suspected compartment syndrome, but this procedure may delay or interrupt much-needed anticoagulation. Furthermore, it is uncertain to what extent compartment syndromes contribute to limb ischemia/necrosis in patients with HIT-associated DVT and associated microvascular thrombosis, including those related to severe DIC and/or coumarin-induced protein C depletion. In our view, therapy should focus on intensive medical therapy, including aggressive anticoagulation and (when appropriate) reversal of coumarin anticoagulation with IV vitamin K.

Intravenous Gammaglobulin

In vitro, both intact IgG and its Fc fragments inhibit HIT antibody-induced platelet activation, an effect that depends somewhat on the method of immunoglobulin preparation (Greinacher et al., 1994a) (see chap. 8). Case reports describe rapid increase in the platelet counts after high-dose IV IgG (Vender et al., 1986; Frame et al., 1989; Nurden et al., 1991; Grau et al., 1992; Prull et al., 1992; Warkentin and Kelton, 1994; Winder et al., 1998). A consensus conference (Anderson et al., 2007) has recommended that IV IgG be considered contraindicated for treatment for HIT. However, in our view, the evidence that IV IgG treatment interrupts platelet activation by HIT antibodies, and the favorable (albeit limited) experience provides a rationale for its use as an adjunct to anticoagulant therapy in certain life- or limb-threatening situations, or in the setting of persisting HIT. The dose should be 1 g/kg body weight, possibly repeated one or two days later.

> *Recommendation.* IV IgG is a possible adjunctive treatment in selected patients requiring rapid blockade of the Fc receptor-dependent platelet-activating effects of HIT antibodies (e.g., management of patients with cerebral venous thrombosis, severe limb ischemia, or severe and/or persisting thrombocytopenia).

Plasmapheresis

Plasmapheresis has been associated with successful treatment outcomes in uncontrolled studies of patients with severe HIT (Vender et al., 1986; Bouvier et al., 1988; Nand and Robinson, 1988; Manzano et al., 1990; Thorp et al., 1990; Brady et al., 1991; Poullin et al., 1998; Kramer et al., 2009). Whether this is due to removal of HIT antibodies or pathogenic immune complexes, or even correction of acquired natural anticoagulant deficiencies by normal plasma replacement, is unresolved. For example, a patient with warfarin-induced acquired protein C deficiency and severe venous limb ischemia may have benefited from correction of the protein C deficiency with apheresis using plasma replacement (Warkentin et al., 1997). More recently, intraoperative plasmapheresis has been described as a strategy to decrease antibody levels in patients awaiting cardiac surgery so that UFH could be given for intraoperative anticoagulation (Welsby et al., 2010; Jaben et al., 2011).

> *Recommendation.* Plasmapheresis, using plasma as replacement fluid, may be a useful adjunctive therapy in selected patients with acute HIT and life- or limb-threatening thrombosis who are suspected or proved to have acquired deficiency of one or more natural anticoagulant proteins, as well as for pre- or intraoperative removal of HIT antibodies when UFH is planned for intraoperative anticoagulation.

Antiplatelet Agents

Dextran

High molecular weight dextran in high concentrations inhibits platelet function and fibrinogen polymerization; it also inhibits HIT antibody-mediated platelet aggregation (Sobel et al., 1986). However, an RCT (Chong et al., 2001) (see chap. 16) showed that in patients with severe HIT-associated thrombosis, dextran 70 was less effective therapy than danaparoid. It is unknown whether dextran would provide additional clinical benefit if combined with another anticoagulant. We do not advocate dextran for the management of HIT.

Recommendation. Dextran should not be used as primary therapy for acute HIT complicated by thrombosis.

Acetylsalicylic Acid, Dipyridamole, and Clopidogrel

Both acetylsalicylic acid (aspirin, ASA) and dipyridamole have been used in HIT patients with variable success (Janson et al., 1983; Makhoul et al., 1986; Kappa et al., 1987, 1989; Laster et al., 1989; Gruel et al., 1991; Hall et al., 1992; Almeida et al., 1998). Sometimes the platelet count appeared to rise promptly with the application of antiplatelet therapy (Warkentin, 1997). However, HIT antibodies are potent platelet activators, and their effect cannot always be blocked *in vitro* by ASA or dipyridamole—indeed, HIT has occurred in patients who receive dual antiplatelet therapy with ASA and clopidogrel) (Selleng et al., 2005). These antiplatelet agents may be used as *adjunctive* therapy (to anticoagulant therapy), particularly in patients with arteriopathy. A potential drawback is increased bleeding (especially when combined with other antithrombotic agents).

> *Recommendation.* Antiplatelet agents, such as aspirin or clopidogrel, may be used as adjuncts to anticoagulant therapy of HIT, particularly in selected (arteriopathic) patients at high risk for arterial thromboembolism. The possible benefit in preventing arterial thrombosis should be weighed against the potential for increased bleeding.

Platelet Glycoprotein IIb/IIIa Inhibitors

Several platelet glycoprotein (GP) IIb/IIIa inhibitors potently block fibrinogen binding to platelets. They also can reduce thrombin generation by inhibiting the exposure of procoagulant phospholipid surfaces on platelets (Herault et al., 1998; Keularts et al., 1998; Pedicord et al., 1998). *In vitro*, GPIIb/IIIa antagonists inhibit platelet aggregation (Herault et al., 1997), endothelial cell activation (Herbert et al., 1998), and platelet microparticle generation (Mak et al., 1998) by HIT antibodies. However, Fc receptor-dependent platelet activation by HIT antibodies is independent of the GPIIb/IIIa complex (Greinacher et al., 1994a); therefore, GPIIb/IIIa inhibitors do not inhibit platelet granule release (Tsao et al., 1997; Polgár et al., 1998). As these agents do not have a direct anticoagulant effect, they probably need to be combined with an anticoagulant (danaparoid, r-hirudin, or argatroban) to treat HIT. Because there are no data available on the interaction of these nonheparin anticoagulants with the GPIIb/IIIa inhibitors, and because a synergistic effect on bleeding is likely, combined use for the management of HIT should be considered experimental. Theoretically, synthetic GPIIb/IIIa inhibitors with a short half-life could be safer than agents with a long half-life (e.g., abciximab).

> *Recommendation.* GPIIb/IIIa inhibitors should be considered as experimental treatment in HIT and used with caution if combined with anticoagulant drugs.

CAVEATS FOR THE TREATMENT OF HIT
Low Molecular Weight Heparin

LMWH is less likely than UFH to cause HIT antibody formation as well as clinical HIT (Warkentin et al., 1995, 2003). Furthermore, LMWH binds less avidly to platelets than does UFH (Greinacher et al., 1993b). With functional assays employing platelet-rich plasma, several investigators reported a reduced cross-reactivity of HIT antibodies with LMWH compared with UFH (Ramakrishna et al., 1995; Slocum et al., 1996; Vun et al., 1996); however, with sensitive washed platelet functional assays, the cross-reactivity rate of LMWH is nearly 100% (Greinacher et al., 1992; Warkentin et al., 1995, 2005a).

Owing to the unavailability of other anticoagulant options during the 1980s, LMWH preparations were often used in Europe for further parenteral anticoagulation of HIT patients. No prospective cohort studies are available, but case reports (Roussi et al., 1984; Leroy et al., 1985; Vitoux et al., 1986; Gouault-Heilmann et al., 1987; Bauriedel et al., 1988; Kirchmaier and Bender, 1988) and a review (Reuter, 1987) suggest that LMWH may benefit some patients. Other case series, however, clearly show that LMWH is associated with disastrous complications in HIT patients (Horellou et al., 1984; Leroy et al., 1985; Gouault-Heilmann et al., 1987; Greinacher et al., 1992; Kleinschmidt et al., 1993). Unfortunately, no laboratory assay reliably predicts these differing treatment responses.

Treatment of HIT with LMWH is frequently unsuccessful. Of eight consecutive HIT patients who received LMWH, thrombocytopenia persisted in all, and new thromboembolic events occurred in two patients (Greinacher et al., 1992). After LMWH became available in North America, a similar experience was observed in seven HIT patients treated with LMWH (Warkentin, 1997). Another study has also shown a relatively high risk of adverse outcomes of treating HIT with LMWH (Ranze et al., 2000).

Recommendation. LMWH should not be used to treat patients with acute HIT.

Vitamin K Antagonists

Although vitamin K antagonists, such as warfarin, phenprocoumon, and other coumarin agents, are an important option for the longer-term management of patients with HIT-associated thrombosis, they are ineffective, and potentially dangerous, when given to patients with acute HIT as single therapy, or even in combination with DTIs (Warkentin et al., 1997; Smythe et al., 2002; Srinivasan et al., 2004) (see chap. 2). In patients with active DVT, oral anticoagulants may cause thrombosis to progress to involve even the microvasculature, leading to coumarin-induced venous limb gangrene. This syndrome appears to result from a transient disturbance in procoagulant–anticoagulant balance: increased thrombin generation associated with HIT remains high during early warfarin treatment, while simultaneously there is severe, acquired deficiency in the natural anticoagulant protein C. Although high doses of oral anticoagulants may be more likely to cause this syndrome, even relatively low doses that produce a rise in the INR (especially to >4.0) can cause limb gangrene in some patients, particularly in patients with severe HIT-associated hypercoagulability and overt (decompensated) DIC. Thus, warfarin and phenprocoumon should always be given in combination with an agent that reduces thrombin generation in patients with acute HIT, and must only be started once the acute HIT has largely subsided, as judged by substantial recovery of the platelet count (in general, $>150 \times 10^9/L$). Furthermore, anticoagulant—coumarin overlap should occur over at least five days, and the alternative anticoagulant should not be stopped until the platelet count has reached a stable plateau (see also section, "Longer-term anticoagulant management of the HIT patient with thrombosis)."

Recommendation. Vitamin K antagonist (coumarin) therapy is *contraindicated* during the acute (thrombocytopenic) phase of HIT. In patients who have already received coumarin when HIT is diagnosed, reversal with vitamin K is recommended. (See pp. 334–335 for specific details of managing coumarin therapy in HIT.)

Ancrod

Ancrod, a defibrinogenating thrombin-like enzyme (Malayan pit viper venom), cleaves fibrinopeptide A but not fibrinopeptide B from fibrinogen (Bell, 1997), without binding to platelets or proteolyzing platelet surface proteins (Kelton et al., 1999). Ancrod was previously used to treat HIT, especially in Canada (Teasdale et al., 1989; Cole et al., 1990; Demers et al., 1991). However, ancrod does not inhibit—and may even increase—thrombin generation in HIT (Fig. 12.2) (Warkentin, 1998). Furthermore, its use might predispose to coumarin-induced venous limb gangrene (Warkentin et al., 1997; Gupta et al., 1998). Also, ancrod was less effective than danaparoid in a historically controlled study (Lubenow et al., 2006). The manufacturer discontinued ancrod in 2002.

Platelet Transfusions

Usually there is no need to treat thrombocytopenia with platelet transfusions, as patients with HIT rarely evince petechiae or bleed spontaneously. Indeed, in theory, platelet transfusions should be avoided because the transfused platelets can be activated by the same immune mechanisms as the patient's own platelets. Anecdotal experience describes thrombotic events soon after platelet transfusions given to patients with acute HIT (Babcock et al., 1976; Cimo et al., 1979). Several consensus conferences (Contreras, 1998; Hirsh et al., 2001; British Committee for Standards in Haematology, 2003; Warkentin and Greinacher, 2004; Warkentin et al., 2008; Linkins et al., 2012) have stated that thrombotic thrombocytopenic purpura (TTP) and HIT are two disorders in which prophylactic platelet transfusions are not recommended because of the theoretical risk of precipitating thrombosis.

However, very low platelet counts, bleeding for other reasons, such as surgery, or periprocedural considerations—particularly in the setting of diagnostic uncertainly—may require the transfusion of platelet concentrates. Two retrospective chart reviews identified four patients in whom HIT was proved by functional assay (Hopkins and Goldfinger, 2008) and 37 patients in whom HIT was suspected due to a positive screening assay (Refaai, et al., 2010); platelet transfusions were given for prophylactic reasons ($n = 25$) and for bleeding ($n = 16$). However, none of these patients developed new thromboembolism, and bleeding was controlled in 10 of 16 patients. According to a consensus conference (Linkins et al., 2012): "In summary, there is no direct evidence supporting an increased risk of thrombosis in patients with HIT who are given platelet transfusions. However, the evidence is also too limited to support the safety of platelet transfusions." It is likely that platelet transfusions are not very (if at all) prothrombotic, and so they may constitute a reasonable therapeutic option in certain clinical settings, particularly very severe thrombocytopenia ($<20 \times 10^9/L$), bleeding, before a major invasive procedure (Linkins et al., 2012), or when the diagnosis of HIT seems unlikely.

> *Recommendation.* Prophylactic platelet transfusions are relatively contraindicated in patients with acute HIT, but may be appropriate with very severe thrombocytopenia, bleeding, major invasive procedure, or in the context of diagnostic uncertainty.

Vena Cava Filters

Vena cava (Greenfield) filters are sometimes used to manage patients judged to be at high risk for life-threatening pulmonary embolism. However, their use can be complicated by massive vena cava thrombosis, including the renal veins, and serious progression of venous thromboembolism (including risk of venous limb gangrene), especially if pharmacologic anticoagulation is not given (Sobel et al., 1988; Jouanny et al., 1993; Ishibashi et al., 2005; Jung et al., 2011; Nitta et al., 2011). In our opinion, these devices are risky in the setting of acute HIT, and we do not advocate their use.

> *Recommendation.* Inferior vena cava filters should be considered relatively contraindicated in patients with acute HIT.

REFERENCES

Agnelli G, Iorio A, De Angelis V, Nenci GG. Dermatan sulphate in heparin-induced thrombocytopenia. Lancet 344: 1295–1296, 1994.

Alatri A, Armstrong AE, Greinacher A, Koster A, Kozek-Langenecker SA, Lancé MD, Link A, Nielsen JD, Sandset PM, Spanjersberg AJ, Spannagl M. Results of a consensus meeting on the use of argatroban in patients with heparin-induced thrombocytopenia requiring antithrombotic therapy—a European perspective. Thromb Res 129: 426–433, 2012.

Almeida JI, Coats R, Liem TK, Silver D. Reduced morbidity and mortality rates of the heparin-induced thrombocytopenia syndrome. J Vasc Surg 27: 309–316, 1998.

Anderson D, Ali K, Blanchette V, Brouwers M, Couban S, Radmoor P, Huebsch L, Hume H, McLeod A, Meyer R, Moltzan C, Nahirniak S, Nantel S, Pineo G, Rock G. Guidelines on the use of intravenous immune globulin for hematologic conditions. Transfus Med Rev 21(2 Suppl 1): S9–S56, 2007.

Arepally GM, Mayer IM. Antibodies from patients with heparin-induced thrombocytopenia stimulate monocytic cells to express tissue factor and secrete interleukin-8. Blood 98: 1252–1254, 2001.

Babcock RB, Dumper CW, Scharfman WB. Heparin-induced thrombocytopenia. N Engl J Med 295: 237–241, 1976.

Bauriedel G, Gerbig H, Riess H, Samtleben W, Steinbeck G. Heparin-induzierte thrombozytopenie. weiterbehandlung mit niedermolekularem Heparin. Munch Med Wochenschr 8: 133–134, 1988. [in German]

Bell WR Jr. Defibrinogenating enzymes. Drugs 54(Suppl 3): 18–31, 1997.

Bennett-Guerrero E, Slaughter TF, White WD, Welsby IJ, Greenberg CS, El-Moalem H, Ortel TL. Preoperative anti-PF4/heparin antibody level predicts adverse outcome after cardiac surgery. J Thorac Cardiovasc Surg 130: 1567–1572, 2005.

Bounameaux H, de Moerloose P, Schneider PA, Leuenberger A, Krahenbuhl B, Bouvier CA. Thrombose arterielle femorale associee a une thrombopenie induit parl'heparin. Schweiz Med Wochenschr 116: 1576–1579, 1986. [in French]

Bouvier JL, Lefevre P, Villain P, Elias A, Durand JM, Juhan I, Serradimigni A. Treatment of serious heparin-induced thrombocytopenia by plasma exchange: report on 4 cases. Thromb Res 51: 335–336, 1988.

Boyce SW, Bandyk DF, Bartholomew JR, Frame JN, Rice L. A randomized, open-label pilot study comparing desirudin and argatroban in patients with suspected heparin-induced thrombocytopenia with or without thrombosis: PREVENT-HIT study. Am J Ther 18: 14–22, 2011.

Brace LD, Fareed J. Heparin-induced platelet aggregation. II. Dose/response relationships for two low molecular weight heparin fractions (CY 216 and CY 222). Thromb Res 59: 1–14, 1990.

Brady J, Riccio JA, Yumen OH, Makary AZ, Greenwood SM. Plasmapheresis: a therapeutic option in the management of heparin-associated thrombocytopenia with thrombosis. Am J Clin Pathol 96: 394–397, 1991.

British Committee for Standards in Haematology. Blood Transfusion Task Force. Guidelines for the use of platelet transfusions. Br J Haematol 122: 10–23, 2003.

Burgess JK, Chong BH. The platelet proaggregating and potentiating effects of unfractionated heparin, low molecular weight heparin and heparinoid in intensive care patients and healthy controls. Eur J Haematol 58: 279–285, 1997.

Cadroy Y, Amiral J, Raynaud H, Brunei P, Mazaleyrat A, Sauer M, Sie P. Evolution of antibodies anti-PF4/heparin in a patient with a history of heparin-induced thrombocytopenia reexposed to heparin. Thromb Haemost 72: 783–784, 1994.

Calhoun BC, Hesser JW. Heparin-associated antibody with pregnancy: discussion of two cases. Am J Obstet Gynecol 156: 964–966, 1987.

Chong BH, Ismail F, Cade J, Gallus AS, Gordon S, Chesterman CN. Heparin-induced thrombocytopenia: studies with a new low molecular weight heparinoid, Org 10172. Blood 73: 1592–1596, 1989.

Chong BH, Murray B, Berndt MC, Dunlop LC, Brighton T, Chesterman CN. Plasma P-selectin is increased in thrombotic consumptive platelet disorders. Blood 83: 1535–1541, 1994.

Chong BH, Gallus AS, Cade JF, Magnani H, Manoharan A, Oldmeadow M, Arthur C, Rickard K, Gallo J, Lloyd J, Seshadri P, Chesterman CN. Prospective randomised open-label comparison of danaparoid with dextran 70 in the treatment of heparin-induced thrombocytopenia with thrombosis. A clinical outcome study. Thromb Haemost 86: 1170–1175, 2001.

Cimo PL, Moake JL, Weinger RS, Ben-Menachem Y, Khalil KG. Heparin-induced thrombocytopenia: association with a platelet aggregating factor and arterial thromboses. Am J Hematol 6: 125–133, 1979.

Cines DB, Tomaski A, Tannenbaum S. Immune endothelial-cell injury in heparin-associated thrombocytopenia. N Engl J Med 316: 581–589, 1987.

Clifton GD, Smith MD. Thrombolytic therapy in heparin-associated thrombocytopenia with thrombosis. Clin Pharm 5: 597–601, 1986.

Cohen JI, Cooper MR, Greenberg CS. Streptokinase therapy of pulmonary emboli with heparin-associated thrombocytopenia. Arch Intern Med 145: 1725–1726, 1985.

Cole CW, Fournier LM, Bormanis J. Heparin-associated thrombocytopenia and thrombosis: optimal therapy with ancrod. Can J Surg 33: 207–210, 1990.

Contreras M. The appropriate use of platelets: an update from the edinburgh consensus conference. Br J Haematol 101(Suppl 1): 10–12, 1998.

Copplestone A, Oscier DG. Heparin-induced thrombocytopenia in pregnancy. Br J Haematol 65: 248, 1987.

Cummings JM, Mason TJ, Chomka EV, Pouget JM. Fibrinolytic therapy of acute myocardial infarction in the heparin thrombosis syndrome. Am Heart J 112: 407–409, 1986.

Danhof M, de Boer A, Magnani HN, Stiekema JCJ. Pharmacokinetic considerations on orgaran (Org 10172) therapy. Hemostasis 22: 73–84, 1992.

Demers C, Ginsberg JS, Brill-Edwards P, Panju A, Warkentin TE, Anderson DR, Turner C, Kelton JG. Rapid anticoagulation using ancrod for heparin-induced thrombocytopenia. Blood 78: 2194–2197, 1991.

Dieck JA, Rizo-Patron C, Unisa A, Mathur V, Massumi GA. A new manifestation and treatment alternative for heparin-induced thrombosis. Chest 98: 1524–1526, 1990.

Eriksson BI, Wille-Jorgensen P, Kalebo P, Mouret P, Rosencher N, Bosch P, Baur M, Ekman S, Bach D, Lindbratt S, Close P. A comparison of recombinant hirudin with a low molecular weight heparin to prevent thromboembolic complications after total hip replacement. N Engl J Med 337: 1329–1335, 1997.

Farner B, Eichler P, Kroll H, Greinacher A. A comparison of danaparoid and lepirudin in heparin-induced thrombocytopenia. Thromb Haemost 85: 950–957, 2001.

Fieland D, Taylor M. Dabigatran use in a postoperative coronary artery bypass patient with nonvalvular atrial fibrillation and heparin-PF4 antibodies. Ann Pharmacother 46: e3, 2012.

Fiessinger JN, Aiach M, Rocanto M, Debure C, Gaux JC. Critical ischemia during heparin-induced thrombocytopenia. treatment by intra-arterial streptokinase. Thromb Res 33: 235–238, 1984.

Frame JN, Mulvey KP, Phares JC, Anderson MJ. Correction of severe heparin-associated thrombocytopenia with intravenous immunoglobulin. Ann Intern Med 111: 946–947, 1989.

Furlan A, Vianello F, Clementi M, Prandoni P. Heparin-induced thrombocytopenia occurring in the first trimester of pregnancy: successful treatment with lepirudin. a case report. Haematologica 91(8 Suppl): ECR40, 2006.

Gao C, Boylan B, Fang J, Wilcox DA, Newman DK, Newman PJ. Heparin promotes platelet responsiveness by potentiating $\alpha IIb\beta 3$-mediated outside-in signaling. Blood 117: 4946–4952, 2011.

Goldfarb MJ, Blostein MD. Fondaparinux in acute heparin-induced thrombocytopenia: a case series. J Thromb Haemost 9: 2501–2503, 2011.

Gosselin RC, Dager WE, King JH, Janatpour KA, Mahackian KA, Larkin EC, Owings JT. Effect of direct thrombin inhibitors, bivalirudin, lepirudin, and argatroban, on prothrombin time and INR values. Am J Clin Pathol 121: 593–599, 2004.

Gouault-Heilmann M, Huet Y, Adnot S, Contant G, Bonnet F, Intrator L, Payen D, Levent M. Low molecular weight heparin fractions as an alternative therapy in heparin-induced thrombocytopenia. Haemostasis 17: 134–140, 1987.

Grau E, Linares M, Olaso MA, Ruvira J, Sanchis J. Heparin-induced thrombocytopenia—response to intravenous immunoglobulin in vivo and in vitro. Am J Hematol 39: 312–313, 1992.

Greinacher A. Antigen generation in heparin-associated thrombocytopenia: the non-immunologic type and the immunologic type are closely linked in their pathogenesis. Semin Thromb Hemost 21: 106–116, 1995.

Greinacher A, Warkentin TE. The direct thrombin inhibitor hirudin. Thromb Haemost 99: 819–829, 2008.

Greinacher A, Michels I, Mueller-Eckhardt C. Heparin-associated thrombocytopenia: the antibody is not heparin-specific. Thromb Haemost 67: 545–549, 1992.

Greinacher A, Eckhardt T, Mussmann J, Mueller-Eckhardt C. Pregnancy complicated by heparin-associated thrombocytopenia: management by a prospectively in vitro selected heparinoid (Org 10172). Thromb Res 71: 123–126, 1993a.

Greinacher A, Michels I, Liebenhoff U, Presek P, Mueller-Eckhardt C. Heparin-associated thrombocytopenia: immune complexes are attached to the platelet membrane by the negative charge of highly sulfated oligosaccharides. Br J Haematol 84: 711–716, 1993b.

Greinacher A, Liebenhoff U, Kiefel V, Presek P, Mueller-Eckhardt C. Heparin-associated thrombocytopenia: the effects of various intravenous IgG preparations on antibody mediated platelet activation—a possible new indication for high dose i.v. IgG. Thromb Haemost 71: 641–645, 1994a.

Greinacher A, Pötzsch B, Amiral J, Dummel V, Eichner A, Mueller-Eckhard C. Heparin-associated thrombocytopenia: isolation of the antibody and characterization of a multimolecular PF4-Heparin complex as the major antigen. Thromb Haemost 71: 247–251, 1994b.

Greinacher A, Völpel H, Janssens U, Hach-Wunderle V, Kemkes-Matthes B, Eichler P, Mueller-Velten HG, Pötzsch B. Recombinant hirudin (lepirudin) provides safe and effective anticoagulation in patients with the immunologic type of heparin-induced thrombocytopenia: a prospective study. Circulation 99: 73–80, 1999a.

Greinacher A, Janssens U, Berg G, Böck M, Kwasny H, Kemkes-Matthes B, Eichler P, Völpel H, Pötzsch B, Luz M. Lepirudin (recombinant hirudin) for parenteral anticoagulation in patients with heparin-induced thrombocytopenia. Circulation 100: 587–593, 1999b.

Greinacher A, Eichler P, Lubenow N, Kwasny H, Luz H. Heparin-induced thrombocytopenia with thromboembolic complications: meta-analysis of two prospective trials to assess the value of parenteral treatment with lepirudin and its therapeutic aPTT range. Blood 96: 846–851, 2000.

Greinacher A, Lubenow N, Eichler P. Anaphylactic and anaphylactoid reactions associated with lepirudin in patients with heparin-induced thrombocytopenia. Circulation 108: 2062–2065, 2003.

Greinacher A, Farner B, Kroll H, Kohlmann T, Warkentin TE, Eichler P. Clinical features of heparin-induced thrombocytopenia including risk factors for thrombosis. A retrospective analysis of 408 patients. J Thromb Haemost 94: 132–135, 2005.

Greinacher A, Gopinadhan M, Günther JU, Omer-Adam MA, Strobel U, Warkentin TE, Papastavrou G, Weitschies W, Helm CA. Close approximation of two platelet factor 4 tetramers by charge neutralization forms the antigens recognized by HIT antibodies. Arterioscler Thromb Vasc Biol 26: 2386–2393, 2006.

Greinacher A, Juhl D, Strobel V, Wessel A, Lubenow N, Selleng K, Eichler P, Warkentin TE. Heparin-induced thrombocytopenia: a prospective study on the incidence, platelet-activating capacity and clinical significance of anti-PF4/heparin antibodies of the IgG, IgM, and IgA classes. J Thromb Haemost 5: 1666–1673, 2007.

Grouzi E, Kyriakou E, Panagou I, Spiliotopoulou I. Fondaparinux for the treatment of acute heparin-induced thrombocytopenia: a single-center experience. Clin Appl Thromb Hemost 16: 663–667, 2010.

Gruel Y, Lang M, Darnige L, Pacouret G, Dreyfus X, Leroy J, Charbonnier B. Fatal effect of re-exposure to heparin after previous heparin-associated thrombocytopenia and thrombosis. Lancet 336: 1077–1078, 1990.

Gruel Y, Lermusiaux P, Lang M, Darnige L, Rupin A, Delahousse B, Guilmot JL, Leroy J. Usefulness of antiplatelet drugs in the management of heparin-associated thrombocytopenia and thrombosis. Ann Vasc Surg 5: 552–555, 1991.

Gupta AK, Kovacs MJ, Sauder DN. Heparin-induced thrombocytopenia. Ann Pharmacother 32: 55–59, 1998.

Hall AV, Clark WF, Parbtani A. Heparin-induced thrombocytopenia in renal failure. Clin Nephrol 38: 86–89, 1992.

Harenberg J. Treatment of a woman with lupus and thromboembolism and cutaneous intolerance to heparins using fondaparinux during pregnancy. Thromb Res 119: 385–388, 2007.

Harrison L, Johnston M, Massicotte MP, Crowther M, Moffat K, Hirsh J. Comparison of 5–mg and 10–mg loading doses in initiation of warfarin therapy. Ann Intern Med 126: 133–136, 1997.

Hartman V, Malbrain M, Daelemans R, Meersman P, Zachée P. Pseudo-pulmonary embolism as a sign of acute heparin-induced thrombocytopenia in hemodialysis patients: safety of resuming heparin after disappearance of HIT antibodies. Nephron Clin Pract 104: c143–c148, 2006.

Henny CHP, ten Cate H, ten Cate JW, Prummel MF, Peters M, Büller HR. Thrombosis prophylaxis in an AT III deficient pregnant women: application of a low molecular weight heparinoid. Thromb Haemost 55: 301, 1986.

Herault JP, Lale A, Savi P, Pflieger AM, Herbert JM. In vitro inhibition of heparin-induced platelet aggregation in plasma from patients with HIT by SR 121566, a newly developed Gp IIb/IIIa antagonist. Blood Coagul Fibrinolysis 8: 206–207, 1997.

Herault JP, Peyrou V, Savi P, Bernat A, Herbert JM. Effect of SR121566A, a potent GP IIb-IIIa antagonist on platelet-mediated thrombin generation in vitro and in vivo. Thromb Haemost 79: 383–388, 1998.

Herbert JM, Savi P, Jeske WP, Walenga JM. Effect of SR 121566A, a potent GP IIb-IIIa antagonist, on the HIT serum/heparin-induced platelet mediated activation of human endothelial cells. Thromb Haemost 80: 326–331, 1998.

Hirsh J, Warkentin TE, Shaughnessy SG, Anand SS, Halperin JL, Raschke R, Granger C, Ohman EM, Dalen JE. Heparin and low molecular weight heparin. mechanisms of action, pharmacokinetics, dosing, monitoring, efficacy, and safety. Chest 119(Suppl): 64S–94S, 2001.

Hopkins CK, Goldfinger D. Platelet transfusions in heparin-induced thrombocytopenia: a report of four cases and review of the literature. Transfusion 48: 2128–2132, 2008.

Horellou MH, Conard J, Lecrubier C, Samama M, Roque-D'Orbcastel O, de Fenoyl O, Di Maria G, Bernadou A. Persistent heparin-induced thrombocytopenia despite therapy with low molecular weight heparin. Thromb Haemost 51: 134, 1984.

Huhle G, Geberth M, Hoffmann U, Heene DL, Harenberg J. Management of heparin-associated thrombocytopenia in pregnancy with subcutaneous r-hirudin. Gynecol Obstet Invest 49: 67–69, 2000.

Imberti D, Verso M, Silvestrini E, Taliani MR, Agnelli G. Successful treatment with dermatan sulphate in six patients with heparin-induced thrombocytopenia and acute venous thromboembolism. J Thromb Haemost 1: 2696–2697, 2003.

Ishibashi H, Takashi O, Hosaka M, Sugimoto I, Takahashi M, Nihei T, Kawanishi J, Ishiguchi T. Heparin-induced thrombocytopenia complicated with massive thrombosis of the inferior vena cava after filter placement. Int Angiol 24: 387–390, 2005.

Jaben EA, Torloni AS, Pruthi RK, Winters JL. Use of plasma exchange in patients with heparin-induced thrombocytopenia: a report of two cases and a review of the literature. J Clin Apher 26: 219–224, 2011.

Jagadeeswaran P, Liu YC, Eddy CA. Effects of hirudin (thrombin specific inhibitor) in zebrafish embryos: a developmental role for thrombin. Blood Cells Mol Dis 23: 410–414, 1997.

Janson PA, Moake JL, Garpinito C. Aspirin prevents heparin-induced platelet aggregation in vivo. Br J Haematol 53: 166–168, 1983.

Jouanny P, Jeandel C, Laurain MC, Penin F, Cuny G. Thrombopenie a l'heparine et filtre cave. difficultes du traitement. J Mal Vasc 18: 320–322, 1993. [in French]

Jung M, McCarthy JJ, Baker KR, Rice L. Safety of IVC filters with heparin-induced thrombocytopenia: a retrospective study [abstr]. Blood 118: abstract 2225, 2011.

Kappa JR, Horn MK III, Fisher CA, Cottrell ED, Ellison A, Addonizio VP Jr. Efficacy ofiloprost (ZK36374) versus aspirin in preventing heparin-induced platelet activation during cardiac operations. J Thorac Cardiovasc Surg 97: 405–413, 1987.

Kappa JR, Fisher CA, Addonizio VP. Heparin-induced platelet activation: the role of thromboxane A2 synthesis and the extent of granule release in two patients. J Vasc Surg 9: 574–579, 1989.

Kelton JG, Sheridan D, Santos A, Smith J, Steeves K, Smith C, Brown C, Murphy WG. Heparin-induced thrombocytopenia: laboratory studies. Blood 72: 925–930, 1988.

Kelton JG, Smith JW, Moffatt D, Santos A, Horsewood P. The interaction of ancrod with human platelets. Platelets 10: 24–29, 1999.

Keularts IMLW, Béguin S, de Zwaan C, Hemker HC. Treatment with a GPIIb/III antagonist inhibits thrombin generation in platelet rich plasma from patients. Thromb Haemost 80: 370–371, 1998.

Kirchmaier CM, Bender N. Heparin-induzierte Thrombozytopenie mit arterieller undvenoser Thrombose. Inn Med 15: 174–178, 1988.

Kleinschmidt S, Ziegenfuss T, Seyfert UT, Greinacher A. Septisch toxisches Herz Kreislauf Versagen als Folge einer Heparin-induzierten Thrombozytopenie mit "White Clot Syndrome". Anaesthesiol Intensivmed Notfallmed Schmerzther 28: 58–60, 1993. [in German]

Klenner AF, Lubenow N, Raschke R, Greinacher A. Heparin-induced thrombocytopenia in children: 12 new cases and review of the literature. Thromb Haemost 91: 719–724, 2004.

Kramer R, Oberg-Higgins P, Russo L, Braxton JH. Heparin-induced thrombocytopenia with thrombosis syndrome managed with plasmapheresis. Interact Cardiovasc Thorac Surg 8: 439–441, 2009.

Krauel K, Fürll B, Warkentin TE, Weitschies W, Kohlmann T, Sheppard JI, Greinacher A. Heparin-induced thrombocytopenia—therapeutic concentrations of danaparoid, unlike fondaparinux and direct thrombin inhibitors, inhibit formation of platelet factor 4-heparin complexes. J Thromb Haemost 6: 2160–2167, 2008.

Krauel K, Hackbarth C, Fürll B, Greinacher A. Heparin-induced thrombocytopenia: in vitro studies on the interaction of dabigatran, rivaroxaban, and low-sulfated heparin, with platelet factor 4 and anti-PF4/heparin antibodies. Blood 119: 1248–1255, 2012.

Kress DC, Aronson S, McDonald ML, Malik MI, Divgi AB, Tector AJ, Downey FX III, Anderson AJ, Stone M, Clancy C. Positive heparin-platelet factor 4 antibody complex and cardiac surgical outcomes. Ann Thorac Surg 83: 1737–1743, 2007.

Krueger SK, Andreas E, Weinand E. Thrombolysis in heparin-induced thrombocytopenia with thrombosis. Ann Intern Med 103: 159, 1985.

Kuo KHM, Kovacs MJ. Successful treatment of heparin induced thrombocytopenia (HIT) with fondaparinux. Thromb Haemost 93: 999–1000, 2005.

Lagrange F, Vergnes C, Bran JL, Paolucci F, Nadal T, Leng JJ, Saux MC, Banwarth B. Absence of placental transfer of pentasaccharide (fondaparinux, Arixtra) in the dually perfused human cotyledon in vitro. Thromb Haemost 87: 831–835, 2002.

Laster JL, Elfrink R, Silver D. Reexposure to heparin of patients with heparin-associated antibodies. J Vasc Surg 9: 677–681, 1989.

Leroy J, Leclerc MH, Delahousse B, Guerois C, Foloppe P, Gruel Y, Toulemonde F. Treatment of heparin-associated thrombocytopenia and thrombosis with low molecular weight heparin (CY 216). Semin Thromb Hemost 11: 326–329, 1985.

Lewis BE, Wallis DE, Berkowitz SD, Matthai WH, Fareed J, Walenga JM, Bartholomew J, Sham R, Lerner RG, Zeigler ZR, Rustagi PK, Jang IK, Rifkin SD, Moran J, Hursting MJ, Kelton JG, For the ARG-911 Study Investigators. Argatroban anticoagulant therapy in patients with heparin-induced thrombocytopenia. Circulation 103: 1838–1843, 2001.

Lewis BE, Wallis DE, Leya F, Hursting MJ, Kelton JG. Argatroban anticoagulation in patients with heparin-induced thrombocytopenia. Arch Intern Med 163: 1849–1856, 2003.

Lewis BE, Wallis DE, Hursting MJ, Levine RL, Leya F. Effects of argatroban therapy, demographic variables, and platelet count on thrombotic risks in heparin-induced thrombocytopenia. Chest 129: 1407–1416, 2006.

Lindhoff-Last E, Piechottka GP, Rabe F, Bauersachs R. Hirudin determination in plasma can be strongly influenced by the prothrombin level. Thromb Res 100: 55–60, 2000.

Lindhoff-Last E, Magnani HN, Kreutzenbeck HJ. Treatment of 51 pregnancies with danaparoid because of heparin intolerance. Thromb Haemost 93: 63–69, 2005.

Linkins LA, Warkentin TE. Heparin-induced thrombocytopenia: real world issues. Semin Thromb Hemost 37: 653–663, 2011.

Linkins LA, Dans AL, Moores LK, Bona R, Davidson BL, Schulman S, Crowther M. Treatment and prevention of heparin-induced thrombocytopenia: antithrombotic therapy and prevention of thrombosis, ninth edition: American College of Chest Physicians evidence-based clinical practice guidelines. Chest 141(2 Suppl): e495S–530S, 2012.

Lo GK, Juhl D, Warkentin TE, Sigouin CS, Eichler P, Greinacher A. Evaluation of pretest clinical score (4 T's) for the diagnosis of heparin-induced thrombocytopenia in two clinical settings. J Thromb Haemost 4: 759–765, 2006.

Lobo B, Finch C, Howard A, Minhas S. Fondaparinux for the treatment of patients with acute heparin-induced thrombocytopenia. Thromb Haemost 99: 208–14, 2008.

Lubenow N, Greinacher A. Heparin-induced thrombocytopenia. Recommendations for optimal use of recombinant hirudin. BioDrugs 14: 109–125, 2000.

Lubenow N, Kempf R, Eichner A, Eichler P, Carlsson LE, Greinacher A. Heparin-induced thrombocytopenia: temporal pattern of thrombocytopenia in relation to initial use or reexposure to heparin. Chest 122: 37–42, 2002.

Lubenow N, Eichler P, Lietz T, Farner B, Greinacher A. Lepirudin for prophylaxis of thrombosis in patients with acute isolated heparin-induced thrombocytopenia: an analysis of 3 prospective studies. Blood 104: 3072–3077, 2004.

Lubenow N, Eichler P, Lietz T, Greinacher A, and the HIT Investigators Group. Lepirudin in patients with heparin-induced thrombocytopenia—results of the third prospective study (HAT-3) and a combined analysis of HAT-1, HAT-2, and HAT-3. J Thromb Haemost 3: 2428–2436, 2005.

Lubenow N, Warkentin TE, Greinacher A, Wessel A, Sloane DA, Krahn EL, Magnani HN. Results of a systematic evaluation of treatment outcomes for heparin-induced thrombocytopenia in patients receiving danaparoid, ancrod, and/or coumarin explain the rapid shift in clinical practice during the 1990s. Thromb Res 117: 507–515, 2006.

Magnani HN. An analysis of clinical outcomes of 91 pregnancies in 83 women treated with danaparoid (Orgaran®). Thromb Res 125: 297–302, 2010.

Magnani HN, Gallus A. Heparin-induced thrombocytopenia (HIT). A report of 1,478 clinical outcomes of patients treated with danaparoid (Orgaran) from 1982 to mid- 2004. Thromb Haemost 95: 967–981, 2006.

Mak KH, Kottke-Marchant K, Brooks LM, Topol EJ. In vitro efficacy of platelet glycoprotein IIb/IIIa antagonist in blocking platelet function in plasma of patients with heparin-induced thrombocytopenia. Thromb Haemost 80: 989–993, 1998.

Makhoul RG, Greenberg CS, McCann RL. Heparin-associated thrombocytopenia and thrombosis: a serious clinical problem and potential solution. J Vasc Surg 4: 522–528, 1986.

Makhoul RG, McCann RL, Austin EH, Greenberg CS, Lowe JE. Management of patients with heparin-associated thrombocytopenia and thrombosis requiring cardiac surgery. Ann Thorac Surg 43: 617–621, 1987.

Manzano L, Yebra M, Vargas JA, Barbolla L, Alvarez-Mon M. Plasmapheresis in heparin-induced thrombocytopenia and thrombosis. Stroke 21: 1236, 1990.

Markwardt F, Fink G, Kaiser B, Klocking HP, Nowak G, Richter M, Sturzebecher J. Pharmacological survey of recombinant hirudin. Pharmazie 43: 202–207, 1988.

Mascelli MA, Deliargyris EN, Damaraju LV, Barnathan ES, Califf RM, Simoons ML, Sane DC. Antibodies to platelet factor 4/heparin are associated with elevated endothelial cell activation markers in patients with acute coronary ischemic syndromes. J Thromb Thrombolysis 18: 171–175, 2004a.

Mascelli MA, Deliargyris EN, Damaraju LV, Barnathan ES, Sane DC. Role of anti-PF4/heparin antibodies in recurrent thrombotic events after coronary syndromes. Semin Thromb Hemost 30: 347–350, 2004b.

Mattioli AV, Bonetti L, Sternieri S, Mattioli G. Heparin-induced thrombocytopenia in patients treated with unfractionated heparin: prevalence of thrombosis in a 1 year follow-up. Ital Heart J 1: 39–42, 2000.

Mattioli AV, Bonetti L, Zennaro M, Ambrosio G, Mattioli G. Heparin/PF4 antibodies formation after heparin treatment: temporal aspects and long-term follow-up. Am Heart J 157: 589–595, 2009.

McIntyre KM, Warkentin TE. Legal aspects of heparin-induced thrombocytopenia: U.S. perspectives. In: Warkentin TE, Greinacher, eds. Heparin-Induced Thrombocytopenia, 3rd edn. New York: Marcel Dekker, 573–585, 2004.

Mehta DP, Yoder EL, Appel J, Bergsman KL. Heparin-induced thrombocytopenia and thrombosis: reversal with streptokinase. A case report and review of literature. Am J Hematol 36: 275–279, 1991.

Meytes D, Ayalon H, Virag I, Weisbort Y, Zakut H. Heparin-induced thrombocytopenia and recurrent thrombosis in pregnancy. A case report. J Reprod Med 31: 993–996, 1986.

Nand S, Robinson JA. Plasmapheresis in the management of heparin-associated thrombocytopenia with thrombosis. Am J Hematol 28: 204–206, 1988.

Nitta N, Shitara S, Nozaki K. Heparin-induced thrombocytopenia in a glioblastoma multiforme patient with inferior vena cava filter placement for deep venous thrombosis. Neurol Med Chir (Tokyo) 51: 445–448, 2011.

Nurden AT, Laroche-Traineau J, Jallu V, Broult J, Durrieu C, Besse P, Brossel C, Hourdille P. Heparin-induced thrombocytopenia: observation of the nature of the antibody activities and on the use of gammaglobulin concentrates in a patient with thrombotic complications [abstr]. Thromb Haemost 65: 796, 1991.

Olbrich K, Wiersbitzky M, Wacke W, Eichler P, Zinke H, Schwock M, Mox B, Kraatz G, Motz W, Greinacher A. Atypical heparin-induced thrombocytopenia complicated by intracardiac thrombus, effectively treated with ultra-low-dose rt-PA lysis and recombinant hirudin (lepirudin). Blood Coagul Fibrinolysis 9: 273–277, 1998.

Olinger GN, Hussey CV, Olive JA, Malik MI. Cardiopulmonary bypass for patients with previously documented heparin-induced platelet aggregation. J Thorac Cardiovasc Surg 87: 673–677, 1984.

Ortel TL, Chong BH. New treatment options for heparin-induced thrombocytopenia. Semin Hematol 35: 26–34, 1998.

Pappalardo F, Scandroglio A, Maj G, Zangrillo A, D'Angelo A. Treatment of heparin-induced thrombocytopenia after cardiac surgery: preliminary experience with fondaparinux. J Thorac Cardiovasc Surg 139: 790–792, 2010.

Pedicord DL, Thomas BE, Mousa SA, Dicker IB. Glycoprotein IIb/IIIa receptor antagonists inhibit the development of platelet procoagulant activity. Thromb Res 90: 247–258, 1998.

Pena de la Vega L, Miller RS, Benda MM, Grill DE, Johnson MG, McCarthy JT, McBane RD II. Association of heparin-dependent antibodies and adverse outcomes in hemodialysis patients: a population-based study. J Lab Clin Med 80: 995–1000, 2005.

Polgár J, Eichler P, Greinacher A, Clemetson KJ. Adenosine diphosphate (ADP) and ADP receptor play a major role in platelet activation/aggregation induced by sera from heparin-induced thrombocytopenia patients. Blood 91: 549–554, 1998.

Pötzsch B, Klovekorn WP, Madlener K. Use of heparin during cardiopulmonary bypass in patients with a history of heparin-induced thrombocytopenia. N Engl J Med 343: 515, 2000.

Poullin P, Pietri P, Lefevre P. Heparin-induced thrombocytopenia with thrombosis: successful treatment with plasma exchange. Br J Haematol 102: 630–631, 1998.

Pouplard C, Iochmann S, Renard B, Herault O, Colombat P, Amiral J, Gruel Y. Induction of monocyte tissue factor expression by antibodies to heparin-platelet factor 4 complexes developed in heparin-induced thrombocytopenia. Blood 97: 3300–3302, 2001.

Prechel MM, McDonald MK, Jeske WP, Messmore HL, Walenga JM. Activation of platelets by heparin-induced thrombocytopenia antibodies in the serotonin release assay is not dependent on the presence of heparin. J Thromb Haemost 3: 2168–2175, 2005.

Prull A, Nechwatal R, Riedel H, Maurer W. Therapie des heparin-induzierten thrombose-thrombozytopenie syndroms mit immunglobulinen. Dtsch Med Wochenschr 117: 1838–1842, 1992. [in German]

Quinones-Baldrich WJ, Baker JD, Busuttil RW, Machleder HI, Moore WS. Intraoperative infusion of lytic drug for thrombotic complications of revascularisation. J Vasc Surg 10: 408–417, 1989.

Ramakrishna R, Manoharan A, Kwan YL, Kyle PW. Heparin-induced thrombocytopenia: cross-reactivity between standard heparin, low molecular weight heparin, dalteparin (Fragmin) and heparinoid, danaparoid (Orgaran). Br J Haematol 91: 736–738, 1995.

Ranze O, Eichner A, Lubenow N, Kempf R, Greinacher A. The use of low molecular weight heparins in heparin-induced thrombocytopenia (HIT): a cohort study [abstr]. Ann Hematol 79(Suppl 1): P198, 2000.

Refaai MA, Chuang C, Menegus M, Blumberg N, Francis CW. Outcomes after platelet transfusion in patients with heparin-induced thrombocytopenia. J Thromb Haemost 8: 1419–1421, 2010.

Reininger CB, Greinacher A, Graf J, Lasser R, Steckmeier B, Schweiberer L. Platelets of patients with peripheral arterial disease are hypersensitive to heparin. Thromb Res 81: 641–649, 1996.

Reuter HD. Niedermolekulares heparin in der therapie der heparininduzierten thrombozytopenie. Med Klin 82: 115–118, 1987. [in German]

Roussi JH, Houboyan LL, Goguel AF. Use of low molecular weight heparin in heparin-induced thrombocytopenia with thrombotic complications. Lancet 1: 1183, 1984.

Salzman EW, Rosenberg RD, Smith MH, Lindon JN, Favreau L. Effect of heparin and heparin fractions on platelet aggregation. J Clin Invest 65: 64–73, 1980.

Savi P, Chong BH, Greinacher A, Gruel Y, Kelton JG, Warkentin TE, Eichler P, Meuleman D, Petitou M, Herault JP, Cariou R, Herbert JM. Effect of fondaparinux on platelet activation in the presence of heparin-dependent antibodies: a blinded comparative multicenter study with unfractionated heparin. Blood 105: 139–144, 2005.

Schiffman H, Unterhalt M, Harms K, Figulla HR, Völpel H, Greinacher A. Erfolgreiche behandlung einer heparin-induzierten thrombozytopenie typ II im kindesalter mit rekombinantem hirudin. Monat Kinderheilkd 145: 606–612, 1997. [in German]

Selleng K, Selleng S, Raschke R, Schmidt CO, Rosenblood GS, Greinacher A, Warkentin TE. Immune heparin-induced thrombocytopenia can occur in patients receiving clopidogrel and aspirin. Am J Hematol 78: 188–192, 2005.

Selleng S, Haneya A, Hirt S, Selleng K, Schmid C, Greinacher A. Management of anticoagulation in patients with subacute heparin-induced thrombocytopenia scheduled for heart transplantation. Blood 112: 4024–4027, 2008.

Selleng S, Malowsky B, Itterman T, Bagemühl J, Wessel A, Wollert HG, Warkentin TE, Greinacher A. Incidence and clinical relevance of anti-platelet factor 4/heparin antibodies before cardiac surgery. Am Heart J 160: 362–369, 2010.

Slocum MM, Adams JG Jr, Teel R, Spadone DP, Silver D. Use of enoxaparin in patients with heparin-induced thrombocytopenia syndrome. J Vasc Surg 23: 839–849, 1996.

Smith JP, Walls JT, Muscato MS, McCord ES, Worth ER, Curtis JJ, Silver D. Extracorporeal circulation in a patient with heparin-induced thrombocytopenia. Anaesthesiology 62: 363–365, 1985.

Smythe MA, Warkentin TE, Stephens JL, Zakalik D, Mattson JC. Venous limb gangrene during overlapping therapy with warfarin and a direct thrombin inhibitor for immune heparin-induced thrombocytopenia. Am J Hematol 71: 50–52, 2002.

Sobel M, Adelman B, Greenfield LJ. Dextran 40 reduces heparin-mediated platelet aggregation. J Surg Res 40: 382–387, 1986.

Sobel M, Adelman B, Szentpeterey S, Hofmann M, Posner MP, Jenvey W. Surgical management of heparin-associated thrombocytopenia. Strategies in the treatment of venous and arterial thromboembolism. J Vasc Surg 8: 395–401, 1988.

Socher I, Kroll H, Jorks S, Santoso S, Sachs UJ. Heparin-independent activation of platelets by heparin-induced thrombocytopenia antibodies: a common occurrence. J Thromb Haemost 6: 197–200, 2008.

Srinivasan AF, Rice L, Bartholomew JR, Rangaswamy C, La Perna L, Thompson JE, Murphy S, Baker KR. Warfarin-induced skin necrosis and venous limb gangrene in the setting of heparin-induced thrombocytopenia. Arch Intern Med 164: 66–70, 2004.

Takemoto CM, Streiff MB. Heparin-induced thrombocytopenia screening and management in pediatric patients. Hematology Am Soc Hematol Educ Program 2011: 162–169, 2011.

Taliani MR, Agnelli G, Nenci GG, Gianese F. Dermatan sulphate in patients with heparin-induced thrombocytopenia. Br J Haematol 104: 87–89, 1999.

Tardy B, Tardy-Poncet B, Fournel P, Venet C, Jospe R, Dacosta A. Lower limb veins should be systematically explored in patients with isolated heparin-induced thrombocytopenia. Thromb Haemost 82: 1199–1200, 1999.

Tardy B, Lecompte T, Boelhen F, Tardy-Poncet B, Elalamy I, Morange P, Gruel Y, Wolf M, Francois D, Racadot E, Camarasa P, Blouch MT, Nguyen F, Doubine S, Dutrillaux F, Alhenc-Gelas M, Martin-Toutain I Bauters A, Ffrench P, de Maistre E, Grunebaum L, Mouton C, Huisse MG, Gouault-Heilmann M, Lucke V, And the GEHT-HIT Study Group. Predictive factors for thrombosis and major bleeding in an observational study in 181 patients with heparin-induced thrombocytopenia treated with lepirudin. Blood 108: 1492–1496, 2006.

Teasdale SJ, Zulys VJ, Mycyk T, Baird RJ, Glynn MF. Ancrod anticoagulation for cardiopulmonary bypass in heparin-induced thrombocytopenia and thrombosis. Ann Thorac Surg 48: 712–713, 1989.

Thorp D, Canty A, Whiting J, Dart G, Lloyd JV, Duncan E, Gallus A. Plasma exchange and heparin-induced thrombocytopenia. Prog Clin Biol Res 337: 521–522, 1990.

Tsao PW, Forsythe MS, Mousa SA. Dissociation between the anti-aggregatory and anti-secretory effects of platelet integrin αIIbβ3 (GPIIb/IIIa) antagonists, c7E3 and DMP728. Thromb Res 89: 137–146, 1997.

Turba UC, Bozlar U, Simsek S. Catheter-directed thrombolysis of acute lower extremity arterial thrombosis in a patient with heparin-induced thrombocytopenia. Catheter Cardiovasc Interv 70: 1046–1050, 2007.

Ulsenheimer K. Legal aspects of heparin-induced thrombocytopenia: European perspectives. In: Warkentin TE, Greinacher, eds. Heparin-Induced Thrombocytopenia, 3rd edn. New York: Marcel Dekker, 587–593, 2004.

Van Besien K, Hoffman R, Golichowski A. Pregnancy associated with lupus anticoagulant and heparin-induced thrombocytopenia: management with a low molecular weight heparinoid. Thromb Res 62: 23–29, 1991.

Vender JS, Matthew EB, Silverman IM, Konowitz H, Dau PC. Heparin-associated thrombocytopenia: alternative managements. Anesth Analg 65: 520–522, 1986.

Visentin GP, Ford SE, Scott PJ, Aster RH. Antibodies from patients with heparin-induced thrombocytopenia/thrombosis are specific for platelet factor 4 complexed with heparin or bound to endothelial cells. J Clin Invest 93: 81–88, 1994.

Vitoux JF, Mathieu JF, Roncato M, Fiessinger JN, Aiach M. Heparin-associated thrombocytopenia treatment with low molecular weight heparin. Thromb Haemost 55: 37–39, 1986.

Vun CM, Evans S, Chong BH. Cross-reactivity study of low molecular weight heparins and heparinoid in heparin-induced thrombocytopenia. Thromb Res 81: 525–532, 1996.

Wallis DE, Workman KL, Lewis BE, Steen L, Pifarre R, Moran JF. Failure of early heparin cessation as treatment for heparin-induced thrombocytopenia. Am J Med 106: 629–635, 1999.

Wanaka K, Matsuo T, Matsuo M, Kaneko C, Miyashita K, Asada R, Matsushima H, Nakajima Y. Re-exposure to heparin in uremic patients requiring hemodialysis with heparin-induced thrombocytopenia. J Thromb Haemost 8: 616–618, 2010.

Warkentin TE. Danaparoid (Orgaran) for the treatment of heparin-induced thrombocytopenia (HIT) and thrombosis: effects on in vivo thrombin and cross-linked fibrin generation, and evaluation of the clinical significance of in vitro cross-reactivity (XR) of danaparoid for HIT-IgG [abstr]. Blood 88(Suppl 1): 626a, 1996.

Warkentin TE. Heparin-induced thrombocytopenia. Pathogenesis, frequency, avoidance and management. Drug Saf 17: 325–341, 1997.

Warkentin TE. Limitations of conventional treatment options for heparin-induced thrombocytopenia. Semin Hematol 35(Suppl 5): 17–25, 1998.

Warkentin TE. Heparin-induced thrombocytopenia: yet another treatment paradox? Thromb Haemost 85: 947–949, 2001.

Warkentin TE. Heparin-induced thrombocytopenia: pathogenesis and management. Br J Haematol 121: 535–555, 2003.

Warkentin TE. Heparin-induced thrombocytopenia and vascular surgery. Acta Chir Belg 104: 257–265, 2004.

Warkentin TE. Should vitamin K be administered when HIT is diagnosed after administration of coumarin? J Thromb Haemost 4: 894–896, 2006.

Warkentin TE. The diagnosis and management of heparin-induced thrombocytopenia. In: Bergan JJ, ed. The Vein Book. Amsterdam: Elsevier, Inc., 395–403, 2007.

Warkentin TE. Agents for the treatment of heparin-induced thrombocytopenia. Hematol/Oncol Clin N Am 24: 755–775, 2010a.

Warkentin TE. Fondaparinux: does it cause HIT? can it treat HIT? Expert Rev Hematol 3: 567–581, 2010b.

Warkentin TE. Heparin-induced thrombocytopenia in critically ill patients. Crit Care Clin 27; 805–823, 2011a.

Warkentin TE. HIT paradigms and paradoxes. J Thromb Haemost 9(Suppl 1): 105–117, 2011b.

Warkentin TE, Greinacher A. Heparin-induced thrombocytopenia and cardiac surgery. Ann Thorac Surg 76: 2121–2131, 2003.

Warkentin TE, Greinacher A. Heparin-induced thrombocytopenia: recognition, treatment, and prevention: the seventh ACCP conference on antithrombotic and thrombolytic therapy. Chest 126(3 Suppl): 311S–337S, 2004.

Warkentin TE, Kelton JG. Interaction of heparin with platelets, including heparin-induced thrombocytopenia. In: Bounameaux H, ed. Low Molecular Weight Hepar-ins in Prophylaxis and Therapy of Thromboembolic Diseases. New York: Marcel Dekker, 75–127, 1994.

Warkentin TE, Kelton JG. A 14–year study of heparin-induced thrombocytopenia. Am J Med 101: 502–507, 1996.

Warkentin TE, Kelton JG. Delayed-onset heparin-induced thrombocytopenia and thrombosis. Ann Intern Med 135: 502–506, 2001a.

Warkentin TE, Kelton JG. Temporal aspects of heparin-induced thrombocytopenia. N Engl J Med 344: 1286–1292, 2001b.

Warkentin TE, Sheppard JI. Testing for heparin-induced thrombocytopenia antibodies. Transf Med Rev 20: 259–272, 2006.

Warkentin TE, Hayward CPM, Boshkov LK, Santos AV, Sheppard JI, Bode AP, Kelton JG. Sera from patients with heparin-induced thrombocytopenia generate platelet-derived microparticles with procoagulant activity: an explanation for the thrombotic complications of heparin-induced thrombocytopenia. Blood 84: 3691–3699, 1994.

Warkentin TE, Levine MN, Hirsh J, Horsewood P, Roberts RS, Gent M, Kelton JG. Heparin-induced thrombocytopenia in patients treated with low molecular weight heparin or unfractionated heparin. N Engl J Med 332: 1330–1335, 1995.

Warkentin TE, Elavathil LJ, Hayward CPM, Johnston MA, Russett JI, Kelton JG. The pathogenesis of venous limb gangrene associated with heparin-induced thrombocytopenia. Ann Intern Med 127: 804–812, 1997.

Warkentin TE, Chong BH, Greinacher A. Heparin-induced thrombocytopenia: towards consensus. Thromb Haemost 79: 1–7, 1998.

Warkentin TE, Roberts RS, Hirsh J, Kelton JG. An improved definition of immune heparin-induced thrombocytopenia in postoperative orthopedic patients. Arch Intern Med 263: 2518–2524, 2003.

Warkentin TE, Cook RJ, Marder VJ, Sheppard JI, Moore JC, Eriksson BI, Greinacher A, Kelton JG. Anti-platelet factor 4/heparin antibodies in orthopedic surgery patients receiving antithrombotic prophylaxis with fondaparinux or enoxaparin. Blood 106: 3791–3996, 2005a.

Warkentin TE, Greinacher A, Craven S, Dewar L, Sheppard JI, Ofosu FA. Differences in the clinically effective molar concentrations of four direct thrombin inhibitors explain their variable prothrombin time prolongation. Thromb Haemost 94: 958–964, 2005b.

Warkentin TE, Maurer BT, Aster RH. Heparin-induced thrombocytopenia associated with fondaparinux. N Engl J Med 356: 2653–2654, 2007.

Warkentin TE, Greinacher A, Koster A, Lincoff AM. Treatment and prevention of heparin-induced thrombocytopenia. American College of Chest Physicians evidence-based clinical practice guidelines (8th edition). Chest 133(6 Suppl): 340S–380S, 2008.

Warkentin TE, Pai M, Sheppard JI, Schulman S, Spyropoulos AC, Eikelboom JW. Fondaparinux treatment of acute heparin-induced thrombocytopenia confirmed by the serotonin-release assay: a 30-month, 16-patient case series. J Thromb Haemost 9: 2389–2396, 2011.

Warkentin TE, Pai M, Cook RJ. Intraoperative anticoagulation and limb amputations in patients with immune heparin-induced thrombocytopenia who require vascular surgery. J Thromb Haemost 10: 148–150, 2012.

Welsby IJ, Um J, Milano CA, Ortel TL, Arepally G. Plasmapheresis and heparin reexposure as a management strategy for cardiac surgical patients with heparin-induced thrombocytopenia. Anesth Analg 110: 30–35, 2010.

Williams RT, Damaraju LV, Mascelli MA, Barnathan ES, Califf RM, Simoons ML, Deliargyris EN, Sane DC. Anti-platelet factor 4/heparin antibodies. An independent predictor of 30–day myocardial infarction after acute coronary ischemic syndromes. Circulation 107: 2307–2312, 2003.

Winder A, Schoenfeld Y, Hochman R, Keren G, Levy Y, Eldor A. High-dose intravenous gammaglobulins for heparin-induced thrombocytopenia: a prompt response. J Clin Immunol 18: 330–334, 1998.

Young G, Yee DL, O'Brien SH, Khanna R, Barbour A, Nugent DJ. FondaKIDS: a prospective pharmacokinetic and safety study of fondaparinux in children between 1 and 18 years of age. Pediatr Blood Cancer 57: 1049–1054, 2011.

Yusuf AM, Warkentin TE, Arsenault KA, Whitlock R, Eikelboom JW. Prognostic importance of preoperative anti-PF4/heparin antibodies in patients undergoing cardiac surgery. a systematic review. Thromb Haemost 107: 8–14, 2012.

Zwicker JI, Uhl L, Huang WY, Shaz BH, Bauer KA. Thrombosis and ELISA optical density values in hospitalized patients with heparin-induced thrombocytopenia. J Thromb Haemost 2: 2133–2137, 2004.

13 Argatroban therapy in heparin-induced thrombocytopenia

Lawrence Rice, Martin Beiderlinden, and Marcie J. Hursting

INTRODUCTION

When heparin-induced thrombocytopenia (HIT) is reasonably suspected, all heparin exposures should be eliminated and an alternative nonheparin anticoagulant expeditiously initiated (Warkentin et al., 2008; Linkins et al., 2012). Alternative anticoagulation is mandated, regardless of whether there is a complicating thrombosis or other ongoing need for anticoagulation, because of the high risk for new clots (Warkentin and Kelton, 1996; Rice, 2004). In the United States, two alternative anticoagulants (argatroban and lepirudin) have been Food and Drug Administration (FDA)-approved for HIT; one of these (lepirudin) has been withdrawn from production by the manufacturer as of 2012. Argatroban, a parenteral direct thrombin inhibitor (DTI), has been the drug of first choice for HIT at many institutions, and is now the only FDA-approved medication for the treatment of HIT in the United States. Formally approved indications for argatroban are for prophylaxis or treatment of thrombosis in patients with HIT (United States and Japan), for patients with or at risk for HIT undergoing percutaneous coronary intervention (PCI) (United States and Japan), for patients with HIT undergoing hemodialysis (Japan), and for adult patients with HIT who require parenteral antithrombotic therapy (Austria, Canada, Denmark, Finland, France, Germany, Iceland, Italy, Netherlands, Norway, Spain, and Sweden). This chapter reviews the pharmacology of argatroban, its efficacy and safety in HIT, and practical aspects of dosing, monitoring, and use in special populations.

PHARMACOLOGY AND DESCRIPTIVE FEATURES

Chemical and Product Descriptions

Argatroban (molecular weight, 526.66) is a synthetic DTI derived from L-arginine (Fig. 13.1) and consists of a mixture of 21-(R) and 21-(S) stereoisomers in an approximate 65:35 ratio with no interconversion between stereoisomers (Okamoto and Hijikata, 1981; Kikumoto et al., 1984; Rawson et al., 1993). The drug has been marketed under the name Argatroban (with a capital A; GlaxoSmithKline) in the United States and under the trademarks Novastan, Argatra, Arganova, and Slonnen (Mitsubishi Tanabe Pharma Group) elsewhere. Under these names/trademarks, argatroban is typically supplied as a concentrated (100 mg/mL) solution in a 2.5-mL, single-use vial that should be diluted in saline, 5% dextrose, or lactated Ringer's solution to 1 mg/mL, final concentration, before use. Some countries (e.g., Germany, Austria, and Finland) have a multidose option, wherein an as-needed volume of the concentrate may be removed from the vial for dilution to 1 mg/mL, final concentration, before use. In

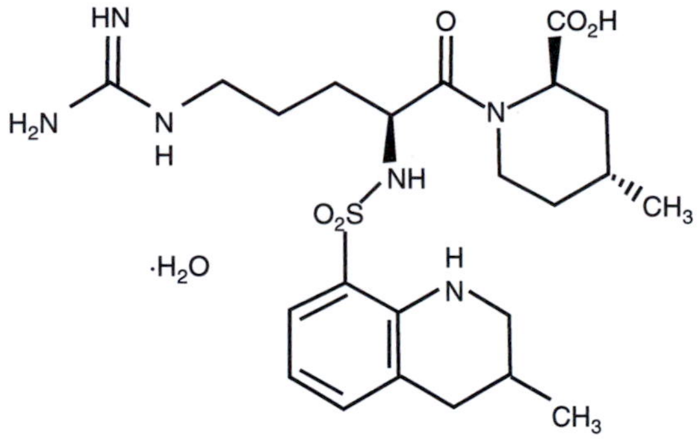

FIGURE 13.1 Chemical structure of argatroban. Its chemical name is 1-[5-[(aminoiminomethyl) amino]-1-oxo-2-[[(1,2,3,4-tetrahydro-3-methyl-8-quinolinyl)sulfonyl]amino]-pentyl]-4-methyl-2-piperidinecarboxylic acid, monohydrate, and its molecular weight is 526.66.

2011 and early 2012, generic versions of argatroban in ready-to-use, single-use vials (125 mg/125 mL in saline, Sandoz; and 50 mg/50 mL in aqueous solution, Medicines Company) and as a concentrate (100 mg/mL, Hikma) were approved in the United States.

Clinical Pharmacology
Mechanism of Action
Argatroban is a potent, selective inhibitor of thrombin, developed by rational drug design through mimicry of thrombin substrates (Okamoto and Hijikata, 1981; Kikumoto et al., 1984). Argatroban displays an inhibitory constant of 0.04 μmol/L for thrombin with little or no effect on related serine proteases (Kikumoto et al., 1984). The anticoagulant effects are exerted without the need of a cofactor by inhibiting thrombin-catalyzed or -induced reactions, such as fibrin formation, activation of factors V, VIII, and XIII, and platelet aggregation. Argatroban binds tightly and reversibly to thrombin (Fig. 13.2) by inserting the dual hydrophobic moieties on its arginine backbone into deep clefts near the thrombin active site (Banner and Hadvary, 1991). Thus, physiologic substrates of thrombin are sterically hindered from access to the catalytic pocket. Argatroban effectively inhibits both free and clot-bound thrombin (Berry et al., 1994; Hantgan et al., 1998) and delays clot formation without reducing clot strength (Nielson et al., 2006; Young et al., 2007).

Distribution, Metabolism, and Excretion
Argatroban distributes mainly in the extracellular fluid, with a steady state volume of distribution of 174 mL/kg (Swan and Hursting, 2000). It is 54% serum protein-bound (Tatsuno et al., 1986). Metabolism is primarily hepatic, with hydroxylation and aromatization of the 3-methyltetrahydroquinoline ring (Izawa et al., 1986). Cytochrome P450 3A4/5 catalyzes the formation of each of four known metabolites *in vitro*, yet this is not a major elimination path *in vivo*. In plasma, unchanged argatroban is the major component, and the primary metabolite (M1, three- to fivefold less active than argatroban) is present at 0–20% of the parent drug (Ahsan et al., 1997). Other metabolites are found only in very low quantities in urine, but not in

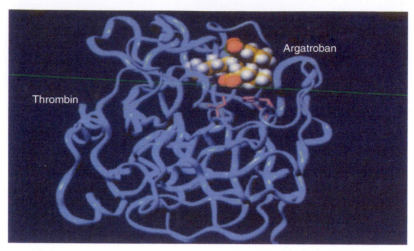

FIGURE 13.2   Model of the interaction between argatroban and thrombin.

plasma or feces. Systemic clearance of argatroban is approximately 5.1 mL/min/kg for infusion doses up to 40 μg/kg/min in healthy volunteers (Swan et al., 2000). The elimination half-life is 39–51 minutes (Swan and Hursting, 2000), with excretion primarily via the feces, presumably by biliary secretion. Urinary recovery of unchanged drug averages 16–23% within 24 hours in healthy volunteers (Izawa et al., 1986; Argatroban Prescribing Information, U.S.A., 2009).

Pharmacokinetic–Pharmacodynamic Relationship
The pharmacokinetic and pharmacodynamic profiles of intravenous (iv) argatroban are consistent with an anticoagulant that is predictable, has a fast onset of action, and is rapidly eliminated (Swan and Hursting, 2000; Swan et al., 2000). Anticoagulant effects are routinely monitored using the activated partial thromboplastin time (aPTT). The aPTT measured using most commercial reagents is prolonged to approximately 2.25 times the normal control at plasma argatroban 0.53–0.67 μg/mL (Francis and Hursting, 2005). Higher levels of anticoagulation, such as required during PCI, are monitored using the activated clotting time (ACT). Argatroban also increases in a dose-dependent fashion the prothrombin time (PT)/ international normalized ratio (INR), thrombin time, ecarin clotting time, and ecarin chromogenic assay (Clark et al., 1991; Walenga et al., 1999; Swan et al., 2000; Harder et al., 2004; Siegmund et al., 2008). Ecarin-based assays are suggested as preferred alternatives for monitoring argatroban and may warrant further evaluation to establish target ranges (Gosselin et al., 2004; Harder et al., 2004; Siegmund et al., 2008; Kuczka et al., 2011). High-performance liquid chromatography (Rawson et al., 1993; Walenga et al., 1999) and liquid chromatography/tandem mass spectrometry (Tran et al., 1999; Molinaro, 2010) are described but not practical (or needed) for routine monitoring.

Immediately upon initiation of argatroban infusion, anticoagulant effects are measureable. Steady-state levels of both drug and anticoagulant effect typically are attained within 1–3 hours (faster when a loading bolus is administered) and maintained with low intra- and intersubject variability until the infusion is

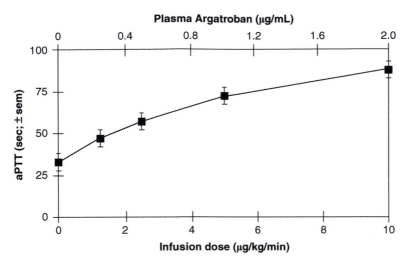

FIGURE 13.3 Relationship at steady state between argatroban dose, plasma argatroban concentration, and anticoagulant effect (aPTT). Mean (SEM) steady-state plasma argatroban concentrations and aPTT values are for healthy subjects (n = 9) administered iv argatroban at doses between 1.25 and 10 µg/kg/min. *Abbreviations*: aPTT, activated partial thromboplastin time; SEM, standard error of mean. *Source*: Data from Swan et al. (2000).

discontinued or the dosage adjusted. Plasma drug levels increase proportionally with doses up to 40 µg/kg/min and correlate well with the steady-state anticoagulant effects. Figure 13.3 shows the relationship at steady state between argatroban dose up to 10 µg/kg/min, plasma argatroban concentration, and aPTT. When infusion is stopped, plasma argatroban concentrations decline rapidly (half-life of 39–51 minutes), and anticoagulant effects return to pretreatment values (Swan et al., 2000).

Special Populations
Pharmacokinetic studies in adults reveal no clinically significant effects on the pharmacokinetics or pharmacodynamics of argatroban with age, sex, or renal function (Swan and Hursting, 2000; Murray et al., 2004; Tang et al., 2005). No dose adjustment is required for patients with renal impairment. Among 644 patients (446 with HIT) with varying degrees of renal dysfunction reported in the literature before 2008, argatroban consistently was well tolerated, provided adequate anticoagulation, and enabled renal replacement therapy (RRT) modalities with no or few thrombotic or bleeding complications (Hursting and Murray, 2008).

Adult patients with at least moderate hepatic impairment (Child–Pugh score >6), compared with healthy volunteers, have an approximate fourfold decrease in drug clearance (to 1.5 mL/min/kg) and an approximate threefold increase in elimination half-life (to 152 minutes) (Swan and Hursting, 2000). Clearance is approximately twofold less in seriously ill pediatric patients than healthy adults and is further reduced when serum bilirubin levels are elevated (Madabushi et al., 2011). Downward dose adjustment is thus required in patients with hepatic impairment and in seriously ill pediatric patients.

This appears to also pertain to seriously ill adult patients. The aPTT response to argatroban is often enhanced, with decreased doses needed (even in the absence of apparent significant liver disease or injury) in critically ill patients with multiple organ system failure, postcardiac surgery, or with conditions that may indirectly affect hepatic function/perfusion, such as severe anasarca or heart failure (de Denus and Spinler, 2003; Reichert et al., 2003; Williamson et al., 2004; Koster et al., 2006, 2007; Levine et al., 2006; Beiderlinden et al., 2007a,b; Begelman et al., 2008; Brand et al., 2008; Hoffman et al., 2008; Link et al., 2009a,b; Smythe et al., 2009; Keegan et al., 2009; Saugel et al., 2010; Yoon et al., 2010). Decreased clearance is suspected, although the reasons for this effect are unclear, are likely multifactorial and await pharmacokinetic study (Murray, 2009). Downward dose adjustment is advised.

In patients without hepatic dysfunction undergoing PCI, argatroban pharmacokinetics are similar to those reported in healthy volunteers; clearance is unaffected by age, sex, or race; and the relationship between plasma argatroban and ACT is predictable with low interindividual variability (Cox et al., 2004; Akimoto et al., 2011).

Drug–Drug Interactions

Concomitant use of argatroban with antiplatelet, thrombolytic, or other anticoagulant drugs may increase the risk of bleeding (Cruz-Gonzalez et al., 2008a; Hursting and Verme-Gibboney, 2008).

No pharmacokinetic interactions have been demonstrated between argatroban and warfarin (Brown and Hursting, 2002). However, the established ("traditional") relationship between PT/INR and bleeding risk is altered during argatroban combination therapy with warfarin [or another vitamin K antagonist (VKA)]. Argatroban/VKA cotherapy prolongs the INR beyond that produced by the VKA alone, without exerting additional effects on vitamin K-dependent factor X levels, and INRs >5 commonly occur during cotherapy (and sometimes during argatroban monotherapy) without bleeding (Sheth et al., 2001; Harder et al., 2004; Bartholomew and Hursting, 2005; Hursting et al., 2005). The section "Argatroban Dosing and Monitoring" presents guidelines for the argatroban-to-VKA transition.

No pharmacokinetic or pharmacodynamic interactions have been demonstrated between argatroban and aspirin (Clark et al., 1991), erythromycin (Tran et al., 1999), acetaminophen, digoxin, or lidocaine (Inglis et al., 2002). Their coadministration should require no dosage adjustments. In support of simultaneous administration via Y-site injection, argatroban, and eptifibatide or tirofiban are chemically and physically compatible, and argatroban and many commonly used medications are physically and visually compatible (Hartman et al., 2002; Honikso et al., 2004; Patel and Hursting, 2005). By exception, argatroban and amiodarone should not be infused through the same iv line because precipitation may occur (Honikso et al., 2004).

Drug–Antibody Interactions

Argatroban does not cross-react with HIT antibodies or potentiate HIT (Walenga et al., 1996). Argatroban does not cross-react with antihirudin antibodies and may be used in patients who have them (Harenberg et al., 2005). Prolonged or repeated exposure to argatroban does not result in the generation of antibodies that alter its anticoagulant activity (Walenga et al., 2002).

Reversing Argatroban Effects

Argatroban has a gentle dose–response relationship that offers a wide margin of safety during dose titration (Fig. 13.3). However, as with any anticoagulant, bleeding is a major safety concern. In postmarketing experience with argatroban in HIT, clinically significant bleeding rates are 0–10% in the noninterventional setting and 0–6% in the interventional setting (Rice and Hursting, 2008). The bleeding risk is increased when the aPTT exceeds 100 seconds in the noninterventional setting or the ACT exceeds 450 seconds during PCI (Cruz-Gonzalez et al., 2008b; Hursting and Verme-Gibboney, 2008). Excessive anticoagulation, with or without bleeding, may be controlled by discontinuing argatroban or decreasing its infusion dose. Anticoagulant parameters generally return to baseline within 2 hours after discontinuation of argatroban (Swan and Hursting, 2000; Swan et al., 2000). This reversal takes longer (at least 6 hours and may be more than 24 hours) in patients with hepatic impairment. Argatroban has no antidote. If life-threatening bleeding occurs and excessive plasma argatroban levels are suspected, argatroban should be discontinued immediately, and the patient should be provided symptomatic and supportive therapy. Argatroban clearance by high-flux dialysis membranes is clinically insignificant (Murray et al., 2004; Tang et al., 2005). Recombinant factor VIIa or fresh frozen plasma has been used, with varied results, to treat argatroban-treated patients with supratherapeutic aPTTs, severe bleeding, or overdose (Alsoufi et al., 2004; Malherbe et al., 2004; Yee and Kuter, 2006; Brand et al., 2008). The use of smart infusion technology pumps that intercept keypad entry errors reduces the likelihood of accidental argatroban overdose (Fanikos et al., 2007).

Clinical Uses of Argatroban

Besides HIT, argatroban therapy has been evaluated in acute myocardial infarction (Theroux, 1997; Jang et al., 1999; Vermeer et al., 2000), unstable angina (Gold et al., 1993), peripheral arterial obstructive disease (Matsuo et al., 1995), stroke (Kobayashi and Tazaki, 1997; LaMonte et al., 2004b; Barreto et al., 2012), PCI (Herrman et al., 1996; Jang et al., 2004; Rössig et al., 2011), and RRT (Murray et al., 2004; Sun et al., 2011). Argatroban produces predictable anticoagulant effects and is well tolerated. Along with its indications in HIT, argatroban is approved for use in acute cerebral thrombosis (Japan and South Korea), chronic arterial occlusion (Japan, South Korea, and China), and hemodialysis of antithrombin-deficient patients (Japan).

ARGATROBAN THERAPY OF HIT
Overview of Studies

The efficacy and safety of argatroban therapy in patients with clinically diagnosed HIT were evaluated in the following prospective, multicenter, open-label studies:

- ARG-911, a historical controlled study
- ARG-915, a follow-on study that also used the historical control group from ARG-911 as comparator
- ARG-915X, a Phase III extension of study ARG-915 that allowed physicians continued access to argatroban while it was under regulatory review.

Study ARG-911 has been reported in full (Lewis et al., 2001). Topline data from study ARG-915 (without its extension) and safety summaries from ARG-911 plus

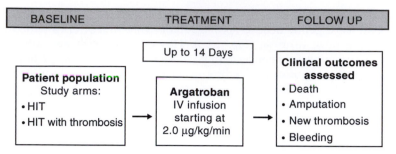

FIGURE 13.4 Schematic of the study design for ARG-911, ARG-915, and ARG-915X. Patients with a clinical diagnosis of HIT with or without thrombosis were eligible. The starting dose of argatroban, 2.0 µg/kg/min, was titrated to achieve an aPTT 1.5–3.0 times the baseline aPTT (not to exceed 100 sec). Outcomes over a 37-day period were compared with those of a historical control group. *Abbreviations*: aPTT, activated partial thromboplastin time; HIT, heparin-induced thrombocytopenia; iv, intravenous.

ARG-915 appear in the product labeling information (Argatroban Prescribing Information, U.S.A., 2009). Outcomes of patients with acute HIT from study ARG-915 plus its extension, together referred to as "Argatroban-915," have also been reported in full (Lewis et al., 2003). Across these studies, 754 patients received argatroban therapy on 809 separate occasions (Lewis et al., 2000).

When these studies were conducted between 1995 and 1998, no approved alternative agent was available for use as an active comparator, and a randomized, placebo-controlled design was deemed unethical; thus, historical controls were used for comparison. The studies were similar in design with regard to objectives, inclusion and exclusion criteria, the argatroban dosing regimen, and assessments. In each study, patients were assigned at enrollment to one of two prospectively defined study arms: HIT (with isolated thrombocytopenia) or HIT with thrombosis (also referred to as "HIT with thrombosis syndrome" or "HITTS"). Figure 13.4 presents the study design.

Study Objectives
The objective of study ARG-911 was to evaluate the use of argatroban as an anticoagulant for the prophylaxis of thrombosis in HIT patients and the treatment of HIT patients with thrombosis. Similarly, the objective of studies ARG-915 and ARG-915X was to evaluate the safety and efficacy of argatroban in HIT patients, with or without thrombosis, requiring anticoagulation.

Study Population
Adult patients were eligible if they had a clinical diagnosis of HIT with or without thrombosis. HIT was defined as a platelet count $<100 \times 10^9/L$, or a 50% decrease in the platelet count after initiation of heparin therapy, with no apparent explanation other than HIT. Patients with a documented history of a positive HIT antibody test who needed anticoagulation were also eligible for the HIT study arm in the absence of thrombocytopenia. Patients were excluded if they had an unexplained aPTT greater than two times control at baseline, documented coagulation disorder, or bleeding diathesis unrelated to HIT, a lumbar puncture within the prior seven days,

or a history of previous aneurysm, hemorrhagic stroke, or recent (within 6 months) thrombotic stroke unrelated to HIT. Re-entry of patients into studies ARG-915 and ARG-915X was allowed, although outcomes from initial entries only were included in the primary analyses to avoid potential bias.

The historical control group of ARG-911 consisted of patients at the participating centers (maximum of three controls per center, identified from laboratory logs of patients who were tested for HIT) who met the same inclusion–exclusion criteria for the study and who were seen prior to the initiation of the study. Controls were treated according to the local standard of practice at the time of HIT diagnosis, with typical treatments being heparin discontinuation and/or oral anticoagulation (Lewis et al., 2001).

Treatment

The treatment group received an initial dose of argatroban 2 µg/kg/min via continuous iv infusion. The aPTT was measured at least 2 hours later, and the dosage was adjusted (up to 10 µg/kg/min, maximum) until the aPTT was 1.5–3 times the baseline aPTT value (not to exceed 100 sec). The aPTT was measured daily and 2 hours after each dosage adjustment. Patients remained on argatroban for up to 14 days, until the underlying condition resolved or appropriate anticoagulation was provided with other agents.

Assessments

The primary efficacy assessment was a composite endpoint of all-cause death, all-cause amputation, or new thrombosis within a 37-day study period. Additional analyses included the evaluation of event rates for the components of the composite endpoint and death due to thrombosis. Secondary efficacy endpoints included the achievement of adequate anticoagulation (i.e., an aPTT >1.5 times baseline) and resolution of thrombocytopenia (i.e., platelet count $>100 \times 10^9$/L or >1.5 times baseline by study day 3). Major bleeding was defined as overt and associated with a hemoglobin decrease >2 g/dL that led to a transfusion of >2 units or that was intracranial, retroperitoneal, or into a major prosthetic joint. Other overt bleeding was considered minor.

Argatroban-911

In study ARG-911, 304 patients having clinically diagnosed HIT $(n = 160)$ or HITTS $(n = 144)$ received argatroban at a mean dose of 2.0 µg/kg/min for an average of six days. This study also enrolled 193 historical controls (HIT, $n = 147$; HITTS, $n = 46$). Although not required for enrollment, laboratory confirmation of HIT antibodies occurred in 57% of the argatroban-treated patients and 77% of controls; the remaining individuals were either never tested or had a negative result (Lewis et al., 2001).

Efficacy

As seen in Table 13.1, the composite endpoint was reduced significantly in argatroban-treated patients *versus* controls with HIT (25.6% *vs* 38.8%, $P = 0.014$). In HITTS, the composite endpoint occurred in 43.8% of argatroban-treated patients compared with 56.5% of controls ($P = 0.13$). Significant between-group differences by time-to-event analysis of the composite endpoint favored argatroban treatment in HIT ($P = 0.010$, hazard ratio = 0.60; 95% CI, 0.40–0.89) (Fig. 13.5A) and HITTS ($P = 0.014$, hazard ratio = 0.57; 95% CI, 0.36–0.90) (Fig. 13.5B).

TABLE 13.1 Comparisons of Argatroban-Treated Patients with Historical Controls in ARG-911

Parameter	HIT, n (%)			HIT with thrombosis, n (%)		
	Control (n = 147)	Argatroban (n = 160)	P	Control (n = 46)	Argatroban (n = 144)	P
Composite endpoint[a]	57 (38.8)	41 (25.6)	0.014	26 (56.5)	63 (43.8)	0.13
	Odds ratio = 0.54 (95% CI, 0.33–0.88)			Odds ratio = 0.60 (95% CI, 0.31–1.17)		
Components by severity[b]						
Death (all causes)	32 (21.8)	27 (16.9)	0.31	13 (28.3)	26 (18.1)	0.15
Amputation (all causes)	3 (2.0)	3 (1.9)	1.00	4 (8.7)	16 (11.1)	0.79
New thrombosis	22 (15.0)	11 (6.9)	0.027	9 (19.6)	21 (14.6)	0.49
Death due to thrombosis	7 (4.8)	0 (0.0)	0.005	7 (15.2)	1 (0.7)	<0.001
Any new thrombosis[c]	33 (22.4)	13 (8.1)	<0.001	16 (34.8)	28 (19.4)	0.044

[a]All-cause death, all-cause amputation, or new thrombosis within 37-day study period.
[b]Severity ranking: all-cause death > all-cause amputation > new thrombosis; patients with multiple outcomes counted once.
[c]Patient counted only once if multiple events occurred.
Abbreviations: ARG, argatroban; HIT, heparin-induced thrombocytopenia.
Source: From Lewis et al. (2001).

Argatroban therapy, compared with control, significantly reduced death due to thrombosis in each study arm (HIT, $P = 0.005$; HITTS, $P < 0.001$). There were no between-group differences in all-cause mortality. The incidence of amputation (as the most severe outcome) was similar between groups. Argatroban therapy also significantly reduced new thrombosis in each study arm (HIT, $P < 0.001$; HITTS, $P = 0.044$).

Argatroban-treated patients achieved therapeutic aPTTs generally at first measure (i.e., within 4–5 hours of starting therapy) and maintained these levels throughout infusion. Compared with controls, argatroban-treated patients had a significantly more rapid rise in platelet counts, with resolution of thrombocytopenia by day 3 in 53% of argatroban-treated patients with HIT and 58% of patients with HITTS.

Safety
Major bleeding occurred in 6.9% (21/304) of argatroban-treated patients, compared with 6.7% (13/193) of historical controls. In each group, there were two fatal bleeding events. One patient experienced a fatal intracranial hemorrhage four days after discontinuation of argatroban and following urokinase and warfarin therapy; one historical control patient also experienced a fatal intracranial hemorrhage. Minor bleeding rates were similar between the groups (41%). The most common adverse events among argatroban-treated patients with HIT or HITTS, respectively, were diarrhea (11%) and pain (9%).

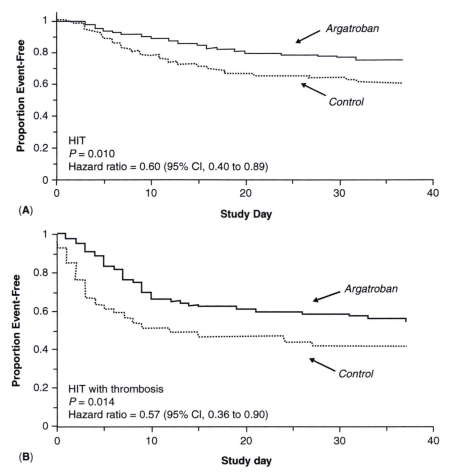

FIGURE 13.5 Time to first event for the composite endpoint through day 37 in study ARG-911. Significant differences in favor of argatroban therapy were detected in (**A**) the HIT study arm (argatroban group, $n = 160$; historical controls, $n = 147$) and (**B**) the HIT with thrombosis study arm (argatroban group, $n = 144$; historical controls, $n = 46$). *Abbreviations*: ARG, argatroban; HIT, heparin-induced thrombocytopenia. *Source*: Data from Lewis et al. (2001).

Argatroban-915

A total of 418 patients with acute HIT ($n = 189$) or HITTS ($n = 229$) were prospectively treated with argatroban in study ARG-915 or its extension (together referred to as "Argatroban-915") (Lewis et al., 2003). The mean argatroban dose was 1.8 µg/kg/min, and the mean duration of therapy was six days. Comparisons were made with 185 historical controls with acute HIT with or without thrombosis (obtained from ARG-911).

Efficacy

Efficacy results (Table 13.2) confirmed those from ARG-911. There were improvements in the composite endpoint for argatroban-treated patients *versus* controls

TABLE 13.2 Comparisons of Argatroban-Treated Patients and Historical Controls with Acute HIT in Argatroban-915

	HIT, n (%)			HIT with thrombosis, n (%)		
Outcome	Control (n = 139)	Argatroban (n = 189)	Pa	Control (n = 46)	Argatroban (n = 229)	Pa
Composite endpoint[b]	54 (38.8)	53 (28.0)	0.04	26 (56.5)	95 (41.5)	0.07
Death (all causes)[c]	29 (20.9)	36 (19.0)	0.78	13 (28.3)	53 (23.1)	0.45
Death due to thrombosis	6 (4.3)	1 (0.5)	0.04	7 (15.2)	6 (2.6)	0.002
Amputation (all causes)[c]	4 (2.9)	8 (4.2)	0.57	5 (10.9)	34 (14.8)	0.64
New thrombosis[c]	32 (23.0)	11 (5.8)	<0.001	16 (34.8)	30 (13.1)	<0.001
Major bleeding[d]	12 (8.6)	10 (5.3)	0.27	1 (2.2)	14 (6.1)	0.48
Minor bleeding[d]	57 (41.0)	59 (31.2)	0.08	19 (41.3)	87 (38.0)	0.74

[a]Significance level of $P < 0.05$ for the primary endpoint (composite) and bleeding and $P < 0.0125$ for secondary endpoints (components of composite, and death due to thrombosis).
[b]All-cause death, all-cause amputation, or new thrombosis within 37-day study period.
[c]Outcome categories are not mutually exclusive; within a given category, a patient is counted only once if >1 event.
[d]Patients with >1 event are counted only once.
Abbreviation: HIT, heparin-induced thrombocytopenia.

among those with HIT (28.0% *vs* 38.8%, $P = 0.04$) or HITTS (41.5% *vs* 56.5%, $P = 0.07$). Argatroban treatment was significantly favored, compared with control, by time-to-event analysis of the composite endpoint in HIT ($P = 0.02$, hazard ratio = 0.64, 95% CI, 0.43–0.93) or HITTS ($P = 0.008$, hazard ratio = 0.56, 95% CI, 0.36–0.87).

Consistent with ARG-911, the positive benefits on the composite endpoint were driven largely by significant reductions in new thrombosis ($P < 0.001$ in each study arm) (Table 13.2). There were no significant between-group differences in all-cause mortality or amputation. Argatroban therapy significantly reduced the incidence of death due to thrombosis in patients having HITTS ($P = 0.002$).

Similar, predictable aPTT responses occurred in patients with HIT or HITTS. The target aPTT was typically achieved by first assessment, and mean aPTT values remained generally constant throughout the infusion. Platelet counts recovered more rapidly in argatroban-treated patients than controls ($P < 0.001$ for each study arm).

Safety

Major bleeding rates were not different between argatroban-treated patients and controls in either study arm (Table 13.2). Twenty-four (5.7%) argatroban-treated patients experienced major bleeding, including a single fatal event in a patient hospitalized for rectal bleeding who received urokinase. No patient experienced an intracranial hemorrhage. Minor bleeding rates were not different between the groups and were similar to those in ARG-911.

Combined Analysis of the Prospective Studies

A secondary, combined analysis of the ARG-911, ARG-915, and ARG-915X studies evaluated the effect of argatroban *versus* historical control on thrombosis-related

TABLE 13.3 Cox Proportional Hazard Analysis of Argatroban-Treated Patients Versus Historical Control: Combined Data from ARG-911 and ARG-915/X

Outcome	HIT		HIT with thrombosis	
	Hazard ratio (95% CI)	P	Hazard ratio (95% CI)	P
Thrombotic composite[a]	0.33 (0.20–0.54)	<0.001	0.39 (0.25–0.62)	<0.001
Death due to thrombosis	0.072 (0.009–0.60)	0.015	0.13 (0.045–0.40)	<0.001
Amputation secondary to HIT-associated thrombosis	0.54 (0.15–2.03)	0.36	1.22 (0.44–3.39)	0.71
New thrombosis	0.29 (0.17–0.50)	<0.001	0.32 (0.18–0.55)	<0.001

[a]Death due to thrombosis, amputation secondary to HIT-associated thrombosis, or new thrombosis within a 37-day study period.
Abbreviations: ARG, argatroban; HIT, heparin-induced thrombocytopenia.

(rather than all-cause) outcomes in clinically diagnosed HIT (Lewis et al., 2006). The analysis population included 882 patients (697 argatroban-treated and 185 historical controls), presenting with either HIT or HITTS. The primary endpoint was a 37-day composite of death due to thrombosis, amputation secondary to HIT-associated thrombosis, or new thrombosis.

Argatroban therapy, compared with control, significantly reduced the risk for the thrombotic composite in HIT (hazard ratio, 0.33; 95% CI, 0.20–0.54; $P < 0.001$) and HITTS (hazard ratio, 0.39; 95% CI, 0.25–0.62; $P < 0.001$) (Table 13.3). The anti-thrombotic benefits remained significant after adjusting for patient age, sex, race, weight, and baseline platelet count. In each HIT presentation, the positive antithrombotic effect was driven by significant risk reductions in new thrombosis and death due to thrombosis (Table 13.3). The risk of amputation secondary to HIT-associated thrombosis was not different between groups.

Patients with a History of HIT Requiring Acute Anticoagulation

The prospective studies of argatroban in HIT included 36 patients with a history of serologically confirmed HIT who had fully recovered from their initial episode of HIT, had a normal platelet count, and had no exposure to heparin or other parenteral anticoagulants (except argatroban) during their hospitalization (Matthai et al., 2005). Each patient required acute anticoagulation, most often for venous thromboembolism or acute coronary syndrome (12 had previously received argatroban). All evaluable patients were successfully anticoagulated with no new thromboembolic events or major bleeding. No adverse events were related to reexposure.

Argatroban Reexposure

Across the prospective studies of HIT, 55 patients underwent therapy with argatroban on more than one occasion. The argatroban dosing and duration were similar between these patients (repeat group) and patients upon their first exposure (initial group, $n = 754$). Event rates were less in the repeat group than in the initial group for the composite endpoint (20% vs 34%), new thrombosis (3.6% vs 11.1%), and major bleeding (3.6% vs 6.6%). In contrast to what has been seen with lepirudin (Greinacher et al., 2003), patients reexposed to argatroban had no allergic reactions or apparent differences, relative to the initial group, in adverse experiences (Lewis et al., 2000).

Discussion of Prospective Studies of Argatroban Therapy in HIT

Consistently in these studies, argatroban therapy, compared with historical control, produced significant benefits in clinical outcomes in patients having HIT with or without thrombosis. Argatroban was effective in reducing the all-cause composite of death, amputation, or new thrombosis as well as the thrombosis-related composite of death due to thrombosis, amputation secondary to HIT-associated thrombosis, or new thrombosis; lowering mortality from thrombosis and preventing new thrombotic events—without increasing bleeding. Also, as shown in a retrospective analysis of study patient records, argatroban reduced the risk of new stroke and stroke-associated mortality, without increasing intracranial hemorrhage (LaMonte et al., 2004a). Although argatroban therapy had no benefit on amputation rate in the prospective studies, retrospective analysis of study patient records revealed that prior to receiving argatroban, 46% of the amputees received warfarin and 98% had severe ischemia or gangrene (Haas and Lewis, 2011). In other subgroup analyses, argatroban provided effective anticoagulation and was well tolerated in patients in the prospective studies with acute illness (Gray et al., 2007), coronary artery disease (Jang et al., 2008), venous thromboembolism (Begelman et al., 2005), renal impairment (Guzzi et al., 2006), renal failure (Reddy et al., 2005; Murray and Hursting, 2006), and hepatic impairment (Levine et al., 2006). Across the prospective studies, the overall major bleeding rate was 6% in argatroban-treated patients, similar to that (7%, $P = 0.74$) in controls (Lewis et al., 2006), and no patient had an intracranial hemorrhage while on argatroban therapy.

Study patients had clinically diagnosed HIT, and laboratory confirmation of HIT was not required for their treatment. This study design simulated the "real world" of managing HIT, wherein guidelines recommend initiating alternative anticoagulation upon strong clinical suspicion, without delay for laboratory confirmation of HIT (Warkentin et al., 2008). In study ARG-911, HIT antibodies were demonstrated in most, but not all, patients. Argatroban therefore is an effective antithrombotic agent in clinically suspected as well as laboratory-confirmed HIT. Argatroban also provided effective anticoagulation in patients with a history of HIT who required acute anticoagulation for a variety of indications and was well tolerated upon reexposure.

Besides these studies, prospective data comparing argatroban with other therapies in HIT are limited. A small, randomized, open-label study evaluated argatroban ($n = 8$) and subcutaneous desirudin (a DTI not approved in HIT; $n = 8$) in patients with confirmed or suspected HIT. During therapy, no one died or required amputation; one argatroban-treated patient had worsening thrombosis and two had major bleeding, whereas no desirudin-treated patient had thrombosis or major bleeding (Boyce et al., 2011). A prospective, randomized, double-blinded trial of argatroban and lepirudin in critically ill patients with confirmed or suspected HIT was terminated March 2012 when lepirudin supply ended (ClinTrials.gov, 2012).

The prospective, historical controlled studies supported the approval of argatroban as an anticoagulant for the prophylaxis or treatment of thrombosis in patients with HIT. The US FDA (and later, EU regulatory agencies) adopted the per-protocol dosing regimen for recommendation. More than a decade worth of post-marketing experience with argatroban has led to some dosing guidance refinements aimed to further optimize patient safety, as discussed in section "Argatroban Dosing and Monitoring". Argatroban has been the preferred anticoagulant for treating many patients, including those with renal insufficiency (Linkins et al., 2012). Its delivery by iv infusion, short half-life, predominant hepatic elimination (and limited effect of renal clearance), ease of monitoring, and positive safety and efficacy profiles make argatroban particularly advantageous for the sickest patients, that is, those treated in intensive care units, which account for two-thirds of clinically suspected HIT patients in some series (Kodityal et al., 2006; Skrupky et al., 2010; Alatri et al., 2012; Kiser et al., 2011).

ARGATROBAN DOSING AND MONITORING
Duration of Therapy
Argatroban should be initiated upon reasonable clinical suspicion of HIT (means for assessing pretest probability of HIT are published) without delay for laboratory testing (Warkentin et al., 2008; Cuker et al., 2010). Later, once laboratory results are known and the post-test probability of HIT is determined, nonheparin therapy may be reconsidered (Keeling et al., 2006; NCCN, 2011). In patients with confirmed HIT, nonheparin anticoagulation should be maintained for at least 4 weeks, or at least 3 months after an episode of HIT-associated thrombosis (NCCN, 2011; Linkins et al., 2012). According to HIT treatment guidelines (Linkins et al., 2012), argatroban should be continued at least until the platelet count substantially recovers (usually at least to $150 \times 10^9/L$) and is stable. After that (and only after that), if VKA therapy is desired, argatroban should be overlapped with the VKA (initiated at the intended maintenance dose) for a minimum of five days and until the desired VKA effect level is achieved (see section "Conversion to VKA Therapy"). These guidelines are important to ensure continuous anticoagulation and avoid warfarin-induced venous limb gangrene or skin necrosis syndromes (see chaps. 2 and 12). In argatroban-treated patients in study Argatroban-915, mean platelet counts were $>150 \times 10^9/L$ after four days of therapy (Lewis et al., 2003). In postmarketing experience, typical durations of argatroban therapy are between five and 16 days (Hursting and Soffer, 2009).

Dosing and Dosage Adjustments
For prophylaxis or treatment of thrombosis in HIT (Table 13.4), the recommended initial dose (by the FDA and EU regulatory agencies) of argatroban in adults is $2\,\mu g/kg/min$ (Argatroban Prescribing Information, U.S.A., 2009; Argatroban Summary of Product Characteristics, 2011). Because hepatic impairment decreases argatroban clearance, a reduced initial dose, that is, $0.5\,\mu g/kg/min$, is recommended for adult patients with at least moderate hepatic impairment, defined as a Child–Pugh score >6 (Swan and Hursting, 2000), and is also appropriate for patients with hepatic impairment defined as serum bilirubin $>1.5\,mg/dL$ (Levine et al., 2006). In the EU, argatroban is contraindicated in patients with severe liver impairment. A reduced initial dose is also advised for patients who are critically ill with multiple organ system failure, are postcardiac surgery, or have heart failure, severe anasarca, or other conditions that may indirectly affect hepatic function and possibly diminish argatroban clearance (Beiderlinden et al., 2007a,b; Begelman et al., 2008; Hoffman et al., 2008; Warkentin et al., 2008; Keegan et al., 2009; Link et al., 2009a,b; Smythe et al., 2009; Saugel et al., 2010; Yoon et al., 2010). The recommended initial

TABLE 13.4 Argatroban Therapy in HIT (Recommendations by the FDA and/or EU Regulatory Agencies)

Clinical use	IV Argatroban (Based on patient's body weight)	Monitoring and adjusting therapy
Prophylaxis or treatment of thrombosis[a]	*Recommended by FDA and EU regulatory agencies* Adults: 2 µg/kg/min Renal impairment: 2 µg/kg/min Moderate hepatic impairment: 0.5 µg/kg/min[b] Seriously ill pediatric patients[c]: Normal hepatic function: 0.75 µg/kg/min Hepatic impairment: 0.2 µg/kg/min *Additional recommendations by EU regulatory agencies for other adult special populations:* Critically ill with (multiple) organ system failure: 0.5 µg/kg/min Postoperative cardiac surgery: 0.5 µg/kg/min Hemodialysis (if not already receiving argatroban): 250 µg/kg bolus then 2 µg/kg/min	Check aPTT at least 2 hr after initiating therapy or any dose change[d] Adjust dose (not to exceed 10 µg/kg/min) to achieve steady state aPTT 1.5–3 times the baseline value (not to exceed 100 sec)
PCI[e,f]	*Recommended by FDA and EU regulatory agencies* Bolus of 350 µg/kg (given over 3–5 min) and infusion dose of 25 µg/kg/min	Check ACT 5–10 min after initial bolus, any additional bolus or any change in infusion dose Adjust infusion dose (15–40 µg/kg/min) to achieve an ACT of 300–450 sec As needed, give additional bolus of 150 µg/kg

[a]For patients with HIT (with or without thrombosis), and patients with a documented history of HIT who are no longer thrombocytopenic but require anticoagulation. Outside the United States, the precise indication wording may vary by country, e.g., argatroban is approved in some countries as an anticoagulant in adult patients with HIT who require parenteral antithrombotic therapy.

[b]Clinical experience informs that a reduced dose is also needed for patients who are critically ill with multiple organ system failure, or underwent cardiac surgery, or have heart failure, severe anasarca, or other conditions that might indirectly affect hepatic function/perfusion (see text and additional recommendations by EU regulatory agencies for special populations). In some countries, argatroban is contraindicated in patients with severe hepatic impairment.

[c]The safety and effectiveness of argatroban have not been fully established in pediatric patients.

[d]In patients with hepatic impairment, check aPTT at least 4–5 hr after initiating therapy or any dose change (Levine et al., 2006).

[e]Includes patients with or at risk for HIT. PCI includes angioplasty, stent implantation, and atherectomy. Oral aspirin 325 mg should be given 2–24 hr before PCI. Argatroban should be avoided in PCI patients with clinically significant hepatic disease.

[f]These recommendations do not consider the combination use of argatroban with GPIIb/IIIa antagonists or other contemporary PCI practices, wherein lower doses of argatroban (e.g., 250–300 µg/kg bolus followed by infusion of 15–20 µg/kg/min) have provided effective anticoagulation with acceptable bleeding risk (Jang et al., 2004; Cruz-Gonzalez et al., 2008a; Rössig et al., 2011).

Abbreviations: ACT, activated clotting time; aPTT, activated partial thromboplastin time; GP, glycoprotein; HIT, heparin-induced thrombocytopenia; IV, intravenous; PCI, percutaneous coronary intervention.

dose by EU regulatory agencies for critically ill patients with (multiple) organ system failure and for postoperative cardiac surgery patients is 0.5 μg/kg/min. No initial dose adjustment is needed for patients with renal impairment. For hemodialysis in patients not already receiving argatroban, EU regulatory agencies recommend a 250 μg/kg initial bolus, then a 2 μg/kg/min infusion dose. Based on pharmacometric analysis of a small prospective study, the recommended initial dose (by the FDA and EU regulatory agencies) for seriously ill pediatric patients is 0.75 μg/kg/min if hepatic function is normal, and 0.2 μg/kg/min if hepatic function is impaired (Madabushi et al., 2011; Young et al., 2011).

The initial dose should be adjusted, as needed, to achieve a target aPTT 1.5–3 times the baseline value. The aPTT should be checked 2 hours after initiating therapy or any dose adjustment (and at least daily). Because achievement of steady-state anticoagulation will be delayed in many patients with hepatic impairment, it would be prudent to check their aPTT after at least 4–5 hours (Levine et al., 2006). Approximately one in six patients in study ARG-911 maintained the initial dose for the duration of therapy, indicating that adjustment may be unnecessary (Verme-Gibboney and Hursting, 2003). When adjustment is necessary, the patient's current dose, aPTT, and clinical status (e.g., hepatic function) should be considered. A reasonable increment is 0.5 μg/kg/min; smaller increments (e.g., 0.25 μg/kg/min or less) are appropriate when the dose is already reduced (Verme-Gibboney and Hursting, 2003; Madabushi et al., 2011).

In single-center postmarketing experience (Arpino and Hallisey, 2004; Kiser et al., 2005; Smythe et al., 2005; Kodityal et al., 2006; Skrupky et al., 2010; Yoon et al., 2010; Shepherd et al., 2011) and in a multicenter HIT registry (Bartholomew et al., 2007; Rice et al., 2007), doses of 0.5–1.2 μg/kg/min typically yielded target aPTTs. The reasons for the relatively lower dose requirement in these patients, as compared with the ARG-911 and ARG-915 patients, remain unclear and may reflect more "real world" (nontrial) or contemporary practices, such as possible preference for the lower range of goal aPTTs. Patient body mass index (BMI) and sex do not affect the dose required to achieve target aPTTs (Jang et al., 2007; Rice et al., 2007). The aPTT-adjusted, maintenance dose has been shown to decrease by 0.1–0.6 μg/kg/min for each 30 mL/min decrease in creatinine clearance (Arpino and Hallisey, 2004; Guzzi et al., 2006); to be lesser in patients with hepatic and renal dysfunction than hepatic dysfunction alone (Reddy et al., 2005; Levine et al., 2006); and to decrease with increasing severity scores of critical illness (Keegan et al., 2009; Link et al., 2009a,b), or the number of failed organ systems (Begelman et al., 2008).

Standardized argatroban dosing protocols, including ones for patients with hepatic impairment or critical illness, are published and appear useful in shortening the time to achieve target aPTTs, shortening the time to dose stabilization, and improving the percentage of aPTTs in target range (Cypher, 2006; Fugate and Chiappe, 2008; Ansara et al., 2009; Bradley and Branan, 2011; Kiser et al., 2011). To minimize the time of titration, the target appropriate infusion rate (in μg/kg/min) for a critically ill patient may also be calculated using a severity score of illness, such as the sequential organ failure assessment (SOFA) [infusion rate $= 2.18 - 0.09 \times$ (SOFA score)], acute physiology and chronic health evaluation (APACHE)-II [infusion rate $= 2.15 - 0.06 \times$ (APACHE-II score)], or the simplified acute physiology score (SAPS)-II [infusion rate $= 2.06 - 0.03 \times$ (SAPS-II score)] (Alatri et al., 2012).

Conversion to VKA Therapy

Conversion from argatroban to VKA therapy should be initiated only after the platelet count has substantially recovered and reached a stable plateau (see section "Duration of Therapy"). Concomitant use of argatroban and a VKA (e.g., warfarin, phenprocoumon, or acenocoumarol) prolongs the PT/INR beyond that produced by the VKA alone, and INRs >5 commonly occur during argatroban/VKA cotherapy without major bleeding (Sheth et al., 2001; Harder et al., 2004; Bartholomew and Hursting, 2005; Hursting et al., 2005). Figure 13.6 presents a guideline for the conversion from argatroban to warfarin therapy (Sheth et al., 2001). Typically for argatroban 1–2 μg/kg/min, a cotherapy INR >4 predicts a warfarin monotherapy INR between approximately 2.0 and 3.0, that is, in the therapeutic range for warfarin monotherapy. In general, after at least five days of coadministration of warfarin and argatroban at doses up to 2 μg/kg/min, argatroban can be discontinued when the cotherapy INR is >4 (and ideally has been for two days). When the INR is assessed using the Owren type PT assay (Scandinavian countries), a target cotherapy INR of 3 is suggested (Alatri et al., 2012). Also, because argatroban monotherapy prolongs the INR (sometimes to >4), a practical suggestion is to note what the INR is on argatroban monotherapy (before warfarin initiation) and to target a cotherapy INR that is higher. Upon cessation of argatroban, the INR should be checked 4–6 hours later, when the effect of argatroban is negligible, to ensure an actual therapeutic value reflective of warfarin monotherapy. Guidelines are similar for the conversion from argatroban to phenprocoumon or acenocoumarol therapy (Harder et al., 2004).

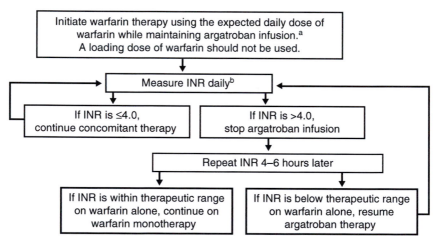

FIGURE 13.6 Guidelines for conversion from argatroban to warfarin anticoagulation. Warfarin should be initiated only once there has been substantial resolution of the thrombocytopenia, and beginning only with anticipated maintenance doses (≤5 mg/day). Argatroban and warfarin should be overlapped for at least five days before discontinuing argatroban. Ideally, the INR should be within the target therapeutic range (i.e., >4.0 during cotherapy for argatroban doses up to 2 μg/kg/min) for at least the last two days of overlap.
[a]For argatroban infusion at ≤2 μg/kg/min, the INR on monotherapy may be estimated from the INR on cotherapy.
[b]If the dose of argatroban is >2 μg/kg/min, temporarily reduce to a dose of 2 μg/kg/min 4–6 hours prior to measuring the INR.
Abbreviation: INR, international normalized ratio.

Factor assays that are insensitive to argatroban interference, such as the two-stage chromogenic factor X assay, may also be used for monitoring VKA effects during the transition (Hoppensteadt et al., 1997; Sheth et al., 2001) and may be particularly useful if the INR is >4 on argatroban monotherapy. A chromogenic factor X level of 45% or less is a reliable predictor that the INR will be therapeutic when argatroban therapy is discontinued (Arpino et al., 2005). Assays that are insensitive to VKA effects, such as the ecarin clotting time or plasma diluted thrombin time, may be used as alternatives to the aPTT, if needed, for monitoring argatroban during the transition (Harder et al., 2004; Love et al., 2007). Although not systematically studied, a proposed approach for facilitating conversion to VKA therapy involves avoiding the argatroban–VKA overlap by first switching from argatroban to fondaparinux therapy after the platelet count has recovered, and then introducing the VKA (Warkentin et al., 2008).

SPECIAL CLINICAL CIRCUMSTANCES
Percutaneous Coronary Intervention
Clinical Studies
Argatroban anticoagulation was evaluated in three multicenter, open-label prospective studies in patients with or at risk for HIT undergoing PCI, including percutaneous transluminal coronary angioplasty, stent implantation, or rotational atherectomy. The studies (ARG-216, ARG-310, and ARG-311) were similar in design with respect to eligibility criteria, argatroban dosing regimen, and main outcome assessments, and their pooled analysis has been reported (Lewis et al., 2002). Overall, 91 patients with or at risk for HIT underwent 112 PCIs on argatroban anticoagulation. Patients received 325 mg oral aspirin 2–24 hours before PCI. In the catheterization laboratory, patients received iv argatroban at 25 μg/kg/min (initial bolus dose of 350 μg/kg) titrated to achieve an ACT of 300–450 seconds during PCI (mean infusion dose, 23 μg/kg/min). Additional bolus doses of 150 μg/kg to achieve or maintain the target ACT were allowed, although usually not needed. Target ACT values were achieved typically within 10 minutes of initiating argatroban and were maintained throughout the infusion. When argatroban was discontinued after the procedure, ACTs rapidly returned to baseline. The sheath was removed when the ACT was <160 seconds.

Primary efficacy endpoints were subjective assessment of the satisfactory outcome of the procedure and adequate anticoagulation, which occurred in 94.5% and 97.8%, respectively, of patients undergoing their initial PCI with argatroban (n = 91) (Table 13.5). Death (no patients), myocardial infarction (four patients), and revascularization at 24 hours after PCI (four patients) occurred in seven (7.7%) patients. Other efficacy endpoints were also consistent with argatroban enabling a satisfactory outcome (Table 13.5). One patient (1%) experienced major periprocedural bleeding (nonfatal retroperitoneal hemorrhage). No unsatisfactory outcomes occurred during repeat PCIs with argatroban (n = 21; mean separation of 150 days from the initial PCI). Overall, the clinical outcomes compared favorably with those reported historically for heparin anticoagulation during PCI.

More recently, a retrospective study evaluated the efficacy and safety of argatroban in 102 patients with confirmed or suspected HIT undergoing PCI for acute coronary syndrome (Cruz-Gonzalez et al., 2008a). Argatroban was administered at a mean infusion dose of 17 μg/kg/min (mean initial bolus of

TABLE 13.5 Efficacy Assessments in Patients with or at Risk of HIT Undergoing PCI Using Argatroban Anticoagulation

	Number of patients with outcome/total *n* (%)	
Outcome	**Initial group**	**Repeat group**
Satisfactory outcome of procedure[a]	86/91 (94.5%)	21/21 (100%)
Adequate anticoagulation[a]	89/91 (97.8%)	21/21 (100%)
Lack of major acute complications[b]	89/91 (97.8%)	21/21 (100%)
Angiographic success[c]	86/88 (97.7%)	20/20 (100%)
Clinical success[d]	86/88 (97.7%)	20/20 (100%)

[a]Primary, subjective outcomes.
[b]No death, emergent coronary artery bypass graft surgery, or Q-wave myocardial infarction during argatroban infusion or 24 hr of its cessation (or discharge, whichever came first).
[c]Final stenosis of <50% in at least one lesion attempted, for patients with angiographic data available.
[d]Angiographic success plus the lack of major acute complications.
Abbreviations: HIT, heparin-induced thrombocytopenia; PCI, percutaneous coronary intervention.

239 µg/kg), and 52 patients simultaneously received a glycoprotein (GP) IIb/ IIIa inhibitor. No difference was detected between patients who did, *versus* who did not, receive GPIIb/IIIa inhibition in the composite endpoint of death, myocardial infarction or urgent revascularization within 30 days (17% *versus* 16%) or major bleeding (6% *vs* 0%).

Although argatroban is not approved for use in non-HIT patients during PCI, prospective, multicenter studies have been conducted. In one study (Jang et al., 2004), 152 patients received argatroban (initial bolus of 250 or 300 µg/kg followed by an infusion of 15 µg/kg/min) in combination with a GPIIb/IIIa inhibitor during PCI. An additional argatroban bolus of 150 µg/kg was administered if ACTs 5–15 minutes after initiating argatroban were <275 seconds. Median ACTs achieved were approximately 300 seconds. The primary efficacy composite endpoint of death, myocardial infarction, and urgent revascularization at 30 days occurred in four (2.6%) patients. Two (1.3%) patients had major bleeding. In another study (Rössig et al., 2011), 140 patients were randomized to receive argatroban (initial bolus of 250, 300, or 350 µg/kg followed, respectively, by 15, 20, or 25 µg/kg/min infusion) or heparin (70–100 IU/kg bolus) in combination with dual antiplatelet therapy during PCI. The minimum target ACT of 250 seconds was reached after the initial bolus in 86–97% of patients in the argatroban groups (46% in the heparin group). The composite endpoint of death, myocardial infarction, and urgent revascularization at 30 days was not different between groups (0–3.2% for argatroban and 3.0% for heparin). No argatroban-treated patient had major bleeding.

Argatroban Dosing and Monitoring During PCI

The FDA and EU regulatory agencies recommend that for patients with or at risk for HIT undergoing PCI, argatroban should be started at an infusion dose of 25 µg/kg/ min and a bolus of 350 µg/kg given over 3–5 minutes (Table 13.4). The ACT should be checked 5–10 minutes after the bolus dose is completed. If the ACT is >300 seconds, the PCI may proceed. If the ACT is <300 seconds, an additional bolus dose of

150 µg/kg should be given and the infusion dose increased to 30 µg/kg/min. If the ACT is >450 seconds after the initial bolus, then the infusion dose should be reduced to 15 µg/kg/min. After any additional bolus or dosage adjustment, the ACT should be checked again after 5–10 minutes to confirm the patient attained a therapeutic ACT. During a prolonged procedure, additional ACTs should be obtained every 20–30 minutes. For patients requiring anticoagulation after the procedure, argatroban infusion may be continued at a reduced dose such as that recommended for the prophylaxis or treatment of thrombosis in HIT.

These recommendations do not consider the possible combination use of argatroban with GPIIb/IIIa antagonists or more contemporary PCI practices, wherein target ACTs <300 seconds (e.g., 250 sec) may be preferred. Lower doses of argatroban, for example, bolus dose of 250–300 µg/kg followed by an infusion dose of 15–20 µg/kg/min, have provided adequate anticoagulation for contemporary PCI, with an acceptable bleeding risk in patients with or at risk for HIT (Cruz-Gonzalez et al., 2008a) or without HIT (Jang et al., 2004; Rössig et al., 2011). High doses of argatroban should be avoided in patients with clinically significant hepatic disease, including laboratory evidence, such as aspartate aminotransferase or alanine aminotransferase at least three times the upper limit of normal. Argatroban use during PCI has not been studied in such patients. Initial dosage adjustment for obesity (BMI up to $51 \, kg/m^2$) or renal dysfunction appears unnecessary in PCI (Hursting and Jang, 2008b; Hursting and Jang, 2010).

Because argatroban equally prolongs the Hemochron ACT and HemoTec ACT (Iqbal et al., 2002), investigators in the earlier PCI trials effectively used whichever ACT method was available at the site to monitor anticoagulation (Lewis et al., 2002; Jang et al., 2004). In a more recent study in patients undergoing cardiac catheterization, argatroban prolonged the Hemochron ACT less than the Medtronic Plus ACT (e.g., paired ACTs of 248 and 275 sec), with excellent correlation between paired values (Chia et al., 2009). Users should thus be aware of the potential for differences in ACT response to argatroban in association with evolving ACT technologies.

Peripheral Intervention
A single-center, retrospective study evaluated the efficacy and safety of argatroban during percutaneous peripheral intervention in 48 patients with confirmed or suspected HIT (Baron et al., 2008). Lower extremity revascularization was performed using argatroban anticoagulation (mean bolus dose of 173 µg/kg, followed by a mean infusion dose of 11 µg/kg/min). There were no thrombotic complications during the procedure. The composite of death, urgent revascularization, and amputation within 30 days occurred in 12 (25%) patients. The major bleeding rate was 6%.

Renal Replacement Therapy
Argatroban administration by bolus alone, infusion alone, or bolus plus infusion was evaluated in a prospective three-way cross-over study of 13 patients with end-stage renal disease who underwent a total of 38 hemodialysis sessions of 3- or 4-hour duration (Murray et al., 2004). Dialysis dose was effectively delivered using each regimen. The most satisfactory intradialysis anticoagulation was achieved using a steady-state infusion of argatroban (2 µg/kg/min begun approximately 4 hours before dialysis), or a 250 µg/kg bolus dose at the start of dialysis followed by a continuous 2 µg/kg/min infusion; mean ACTs increased from 131 seconds at

baseline to 200 and 197 seconds, respectively, after 60 minutes of dialysis. No dialysis membrane required changing. One session was shortened by 15 minutes owing to circuit clotting. There were no thrombotic or bleeding events. Argatroban dialytic clearance was clinically insignificant. Although the study was conducted in patients without HIT, similar regimens may be adequate for inpatients with HIT already at steady-state argatroban levels or outpatients with a history of HIT who require RRT.

The pharmacokinetics, pharmacodynamics, and safety of argatroban during a single RRT session were prospectively evaluated in five patients with or at risk for HIT (Tang et al., 2005). Patients underwent hemodialysis or continuous venovenous hemofiltration while receiving continuous iv argatroban 0.5–2 µg/kg/min. ACTs, aPTTs, and plasma argatroban levels remained stable during RRT. Effective RRT was evidenced by the urea reduction ratio. No patient experienced bleeding or thrombosis. Argatroban clearance by the high-flux membranes was clinically insignificant.

Argatroban use during RRT was also prospectively evaluated in critically ill patients with HIT or without HIT. In a randomized study (Sun et al., 2011), critically ill non-HIT patients with acute renal failure undergoing intermittent venovenous hemofiltration received either saline/heparin flush in the dialyzer circuit ($n = 44$) or argatroban anticoagulation (75 µg/kg bolus, followed by 0.4–0.6 µg/kg/min infusion; $n = 57$). All argatroban-treated patients completed treatment (185 sessions); clotting in the circuit occurred in 16% of the other patients. No major bleeding occurred. In a study of 10 patients with HIT and acute renal failure after cardiovascular surgery (Koster et al., 2007), patients typically received continuous venovenous hemofiltration, then intermittent hemodialysis when hemodynamics were stable. Argatroban 1 µg/kg/min was infused for 1 hour before RRT and adjusted to achieve target aPTTs of 50–80 seconds during RRT or 40–60 seconds during periods without RRT (mean doses, 0.06–0.29 µg/kg/min). Filter patency was good for approximately 30 hours, no filter system had to be exchanged due to premature filter thrombosis, and no bleeding was attributed to problems with anticoagulation. In a study of 30 intensive care patients with HIT and acute renal failure undergoing continuous RRT (Link et al., 2009a,b), the maintenance argatroban dose inversely correlated with severity scores of critical illness, including SOFA and SAPS-II scores. Mean filter patency at 24 hours was 98%. No patient had severe bleeding. The use of severity scores for predicting dose requirements in this setting warrants further study (Link et al., 2009a,b; Murray, 2009).

A retrospective study of the prospective ARG-911 and ARG-915 studies evaluated the safety, outcomes, and argatroban dosing patterns in 47 HIT patients requiring RRT (Reddy et al., 2005). Patients with renal and hepatic impairment required median lower doses (0.7 µg/kg/min) than patients without hepatic impairment (1.7 µg/kg/min). Two (4%) patients experienced thrombosis while on argatroban. Major bleeding occurred in three (6%) of 50 treatment courses in a 37-day follow-up period. Argatroban provided effective anticoagulation and was well tolerated, upon initial and repeat administration.

Critical Illness

Argatroban therapy was prospectively evaluated in 24 critically ill patients (defined as SAPSII score ≥30 points) with multiple organ dysfunction (defined as SOFA score ≥7) and suspected or confirmed HIT (Beiderlinden et al., 2007a). Argatroban was administered as an initial infusion dose of 2 µg/kg/min (first five patients only) or 0.2 µg/kg/min, adjusted to achieve aPTTs 1.5–3 times normal or 50–60 seconds. The higher initial dose led to aPTT overshoot within 4 hours and in three patients, bleeding, whereas the reduced initial dose provided sufficient anticoagulation without bleeding. The mean maintenance dose was 0.22 µg/kg/min in both groups. No thromboembolic complications occurred during therapy. Prospective evaluations of argatroban use in critically ill patients undergoing RRT have also been conducted and are discussed in section "Renal Replacement Therapy".

Several retrospective, single-center studies have also evaluated argatroban in critically ill patients with suspected or confirmed HIT. In 65 intensive care patients (Begelman et al., 2008), therapeutic doses (adjusted to achieve aPTTs 1.5–3 times baseline) were lower in patients with heart failure (0.58 vs 0.97 µg/kg/min) and decreased as the number of failed organ systems increased from 1 to 2 to 3 or more (1.1 vs 0.87 vs 0.58 µg/kg/min). In a comparison of 38 intensive care patients and 43 non–intensive care patients (Smythe et al., 2009), mean aPTT-adjusted argatroban doses were 0.8 and 1.3 µg/kg/min, respectively. In a comparison of 34 critically ill patients and 19 non–critically ill patients (Keegan et al., 2009), the mean aPTT-adjusted doses were 0.6 and 1.4 µg/kg/min, respectively, and an inverse relationship existed between the SOFA score and argatroban doses <0.75 µg/kg/min. In 12 intensive care patients with multiple organ dysfunction syndrome (Saugel et al., 2010), the mean final argatroban dose was 0.32 µg/kg/min, and doses were lower in patients with, *versus* without, hepatic insufficiency. In each study, argatroban provided effective anticoagulation and was well tolerated. Although retrospective analysis of the ARG-911 and ARG-915 studies found no substantial dose reduction in acutely ill patients (mean dose 1.9 µg/kg/min; $n = 390$) (Gray et al., 2007), these more contemporary experiences consistently indicate that reduced doses are needed.

Critically ill patients in intensive care units represent the majority of patients treated for suspected or confirmed HIT in many medical centers (Kodityal et al., 2006; Skrupky et al., 2010; Alatri et al., 2012; Kiser et al., 2011). As previously mentioned, dosing nomograms for these patients are available (Ansara et al., 2009; Alatri et al., 2012; Kiser et al., 2011), and experts encourage reducing the time of titration by calculating the patient's target dose (see section "Dosing and Dosage Adjustments" for formulas) using the SOFA, APACHE-II, or SAPS-II score (Alatri et al., 2012).

Cardiovascular Surgery

The safety and efficacy of argatroban anticoagulation during cardiovascular surgery are not established in patients with or at risk for HIT. Guidelines have been proposed based on retrospective analysis of 21 published cases and suggest an initial dose of 5 µg/kg/min (and a 100 µg/kg bolus for on-pump surgery), adjusted to target ACTs of 300–500 seconds for off-pump surgery and 400–600 seconds for on-pump surgery, with the ACT checked every 15 minutes (Martin et al., 2007). Prolonged coagulopathy and prolonged argatroban elimination following cardiopulmonary bypass (Gasparovic et al., 2004; Genzen et al., 2010), thrombosis during off-pump cardiac surgery (Cannon et al., 2004), and a high bleeding risk in pediatric patients (Hursting et al., 2006) are reported safety concerns.

Postcardiac Surgery

In a prospective, multicenter, open-label study (Koster et al., 2006), 14 patients with a history of HIT or suspected HIT following cardiovascular surgery with cardiopulmonary bypass (CPB) received argatroban 0.8–1.0 µg/kg/min initially, adjusted to achieve aPTTs of 50–70 seconds (mean final dose, 0.3–0.4 µg/kg/min) for a mean of 3.0 days. One patient had increased postoperative bleeding (with an aPTT >80 sec) for which argatroban was temporarily discontinued until bleeding stopped. The other patients had unremarkable clinical courses. A reduced initial dose was used because two earlier patients had aPTT overshoot when administered 2 µg/kg/min initially. Prospective study (see description in section "Renal Replacement Therapy") also showed that target aPTTs were achieved at reduced argatroban doses (mean doses, 0.06–0.29 µg/kg/min) in 10 postcardiac surgery patients requiring RRT (Koster et al., 2007).

Other experiences support the need for reduced doses in this setting. In a single-center, retrospective study of 39 postoperative cardiac surgery patients with presumed or previous HIT (Hoffman et al., 2008), median argatroban doses were 0.5 µg/kg/min initially and 0.6 µg/kg/min during a median 5.3-day duration of therapy (target aPTT, 45–90 sec). One patient developed thrombosis, one underwent finger amputation, seven died (five after argatroban cessation), and four had significant bleeding. In another retrospective study (Yoon et al., 2010), 31 postoperative cardiac surgery patients with suspected HIT received a median argatroban dose of 0.7 µg/kg/min for a median duration of 5.9 days. No new thromboembolic complications occurred. Blood transfusion was required in 20 patients and associated with longer operation times and increased use of an intra-aortic balloon pump. In a case series of four patients with HIT after cardiac surgery (Reichert et al., 2003), argatroban therapy was initiated at a dose of 2 µg/kg/min ($n = 3$) or 1 µg/kg/min ($n = 1$), and the resultant aPTT was supratherapeutic in each patient (and >100 sec in three patients). Reduced dosages may be associated with decreased cardiac output, hepatic perfusion, and drug clearance, and upward adjustments may be needed as organ systems recover after surgery; however, this remains to be established (Dager, 2008).

Extracorporeal Life Support
In nine consecutive patients with suspected HIT undergoing extracorporeal membrane oxygenation (ECMO) for severe acute respiratory distress syndrome (Beiderlinden et al., 2007b), argatroban was administered at a mean maintenance dose of 0.15 µg/kg/min (target aPTT, 50–60 sec) for a mean four days. Eight patients simultaneously received continuous RRT. An initial dose of 2 µg/kg/min was used in the first patient only and resulted in excessive anticoagulation and bleeding. All other patients received an initial dose of 0.2 µg/kg/min, achieved target aPTTs within 8 hours, and had no bleeding. No clotting in the oxygenator or extracorporeal system occurred.

Argatroban as a primary ($n = 20$) or secondary ($n = 8$) postoperative anticoagulant was retrospectively evaluated in patients (some with suspected HIT) implanted with ventricular assist devices (VADs) (Samuels et al., 2008). Argatroban was started at 1.0 µg/kg/min (or 0.5 µg/kg/min if hepatic dysfunction was present) and adjusted without difficulty to achieve target aPTTs (60–90 sec). No patient had argatroban discontinued due to coagulopathy. Antithrombotic effectiveness of argatroban was similar to that of heparin ($n = 5$), with less postoperative bleeding.

A case series described five patients with suspected HIT administered argatroban while on ECMO or VAD support (Cornell et al., 2007). Starting doses of 0.2–2 µg/kg/min were adjusted to achieve ACTs of 210–230 seconds, and maximum doses were 0.2–3.5 µg/kg/min. No visible thrombi were detected in the circuits while patients received argatroban (6–184 hours). No one had an adverse reaction directly attributed to argatroban.

Race/Ethnicity
In prospective, multicenter studies of argatroban therapy in HIT, argatroban provided effective antithrombotic therapy irrespective of patient race/ethnicity, yet thrombotic risk was twice as great in nonwhites as whites (Lewis et al., 2006). Among nonwhites, the median argatroban dose was less in Asians (1.0 μg/kg/min) than African Americans or Hispanics (1.9 μg/kg/min, each group), and thrombotic complication rates were less in Asians than African Americans or Hispanics (8%, 27%, and 29%, respectively); however group sizes were small ($n = 13$–52), some baseline differences existed, and further study is needed (Hursting and Jang, 2008a).

Obesity
Obese ($n = 32$; BMI >30 kg/m^2 and up to 51 kg/m^2) and nonobese ($n = 51$) patients in a multicenter HIT registry had similar argatroban dosing requirements, aPTT responses, and thrombotic and bleeding event rates (Rice et al., 2007). Among 225 patients (85 obese) from previous studies of argatroban in PCI, periprocedural ischemic and bleeding complication rates were similar between obese and nonobese patients, and no association was detected between BMI (up to 51 kg/m^2) and the first ACT after argatroban bolus administration, the mean infusion dose, the need for additional bolus doses, or the time to ACTs ≤ 160 seconds after stopping infusion (Hursting and Jang, 2008b).

Women, Including Pregnant or Nursing Women
Argatroban provided effective antithrombotic therapy irrespective of patient sex in the prospective, multicenter studies of argatroban therapy in HIT; however, the thrombotic risk was almost twice as great in women as men (Lewis et al., 2006). For patients in a multicenter HIT registry, the initial and maintenance argatroban doses, duration of therapy, and aPTT responses were comparable between women ($n = 42$) and men ($n = 50$); 24% of women (16% of men) experienced the composite endpoint of death, amputation, or new thrombosis within 37 days; and the major bleeding rate was 2% for each sex (Jang et al., 2007).

Argatroban anticoagulation in pregnant or nursing women has not been studied. A few case reports describe successful argatroban therapy in pregnant women with HIT (Francis, 2004; Young et al., 2008; Ekbatani et al., 2010). Teratology studies in rats reveal no evidence of impaired fertility or fetal harm due to argatroban (Argatroban Prescribing Information, U.S.A., 2009). Because animal reproductive studies are not always predictive of human response, it is recommended that the drug be used during pregnancy only if clearly needed.

Argatroban is detected in rat milk (Iida et al., 1986). It is unknown whether argatroban is excreted in human milk, although many drugs are. Hence, it is recommended that a decision be made either to discontinue nursing or discontinue the drug.

Geriatric Patients
The pharmacokinetic parameters of argatroban are similar between young adults and elderly volunteers (Swan and Hursting, 2000), and no dosage adjustment is required for the elderly. The effectiveness of argatroban in HIT was not influenced

by patient age (range, 17–91 years) in the ARG-911 and ARG-915 studies (Lewis et al., 2001, 2006). Age was also not a significant factor determining therapeutic argatroban doses or thrombotic risk for elderly patients 65–93 years of age in a multicenter HIT registry (Bartholomew et al., 2007).

Pediatric Patients

The safety and effectiveness of argatroban in pediatric patients have not been fully established. However, argatroban was well tolerated and provided adequate anticoagulation in a multicenter, open-label study of 18 seriously ill pediatric patients (age, 1.6 weeks to 16 years) requiring nonheparin anticoagulation typically for suspected or confirmed HIT (Young et al., 2011). Thirteen patients received argatroban as a continuous infusion, most often initiated at $1\,\mu g/kg/min$, adjusted to achieve aPTTs 1.5–3 times the baseline value. Within 30 days, five patients experienced thrombosis (two during therapy). Two patients had major bleeding. Based on pharmacometric analyses, an initial argatroban dose of $0.75\,\mu g/kg/min$ (if hepatic function is normal) or $0.2\,\mu g/kg/min$ (if hepatic function is impaired) is recommended for seriously ill pediatric patients (Madabushi et al., 2011; Young et al., 2011).

A literature review described 34 pediatric patients aged one week to 16 years, most with or at risk for HIT, administered argatroban for prophylaxis or treatment of thrombosis or during a variety of procedures, including cardiac catheterization, RRT, ECMO or VAD support, and CPB (Hursting et al., 2006). Argatroban generally provided therapeutic levels of anticoagulation; by exception, the bleeding risk during CPB was unacceptably high.

CONCLUSION

Argatroban, an effective DTI with a predictable dose–response effect, offers several theoretical advantages as an anticoagulant for patients with HIT: it inhibits free and bound thrombin, it does not cross-react with HIT antibodies, its anticoagulant effects are rapidly active and also rapidly reversible, and it is well tolerated upon prolonged or repeated administration. Argatroban is also unique among nonheparin anticoagulants in that it is predominantly hepatically metabolized with minimal renal clearance, and hence is well suited for use in patients with renal insufficiency or failure that is common in critically ill patients. Indeed, the majority of patients with suspected HIT in many institutions are in intensive care or otherwise very ill, generally with a high risk of bleeding, and commonly require procedural interventions (sometimes urgently), so there is a need for a short-acting anticoagulant that is easily monitored and controlled. With its short half-life, delivery by iv infusion, easy monitoring, predominantly nonrenal clearance, and established efficacy and safety record, argatroban offers unique advantages in such very sick patients. Other nonheparin anticoagulants, such as fondaparinux and desirudin, can be problematic in this situation due to a long half-life, renal clearance, and/or difficulty in monitoring. Prospective multicenter studies, additional supportive clinical investigations, and over a decade worth of postmarketing experiences consistently demonstrate that argatroban provides rapid, adequate anticoagulation with an acceptable safety profile in patients with or risk for HIT in both noninterventional and interventional settings. Experiences continue to inform dosing refinements aimed to optimize its safety in patients in special populations (e.g., reduced initial dosing in seriously ill pediatric patients, critically ill patients, and postcardiac surgery patients) and/or requiring procedures (e.g., RRT, contemporary PCI, peripheral intervention, or extracorporeal life support). Argatroban therefore offers a versatile therapeutic option for the management of patients with or at risk for HIT in diverse clinical settings, with special advantages to those in the intensive care unit.

REFERENCES

Ahsan A, Ahmad S, Iqbal O, Schwarz R, Knappenberger G, Joffrion J, Becker JC, Messmore H. Comparative studies on the biochemical and pharmacological properties of a major metabolite of argatroban (MI): potential clinical implications. Thromb Haemost 78(Suppl 2): 370, 1997.

Akimoto K, Klinkhardt U, Zeiher A, Niethammer M, Harder S. Anticoagulation with argatroban for elective percutaneous coronary intervention: population pharmacokinetics and pharmacokinetic-pharmacodynamic relationship of coagulation parameters. J Clin Pharmacol 51: 805–818, 2011.

Alatri A, Armstrong A, Greinacher A, Koster A, Kozek-Langenecker SA, Lancé MD, Link A, Nielsen JD, Sandset PM, Spanjersberg AJ, Spannagl M. Results of a consensus meeting on the use of argatroban in patients with heparin-induced thrombocytopenia requiring antithrombotic therapy—an European perspective. Thromb Res 129: 426–433, 2012.

Alsoufi B, Boshkov LK, Kirby A, Ibsen L, Dower N, Shen I, Underlierder R. Heparin-induced thrombocytopenia (HIT) in pediatric cardiac surgery: an emerging cause of morbidity and mortality. Semin Thorac Cardiovasc Surg Pediatr Card Surg Annu 7: 155–171, 2004.

Ansara AJ, Arif S, Warhurst RD. Weight-based argatroban dosing nomogram for treatment of heparin-induced thrombocytopenia. Ann Pharmacother 43: 9–18, 2009.

Argatroban Prescribing Information. Research Triangle Park, U.S.A.: GlaxoSmithKline, 2009.

Argatroban Summary of Product Characteristics. London, UK: Mitsubishi Pharma Europe Ltd, 2011.

Arpino PA, Hallisey RK. Effect of renal function on the pharmacodynamics of argatroban. Ann Pharmacother 38: 25–29, 2004.

Arpino PA, Demirjian Z, Van Cott EM. Use of the chromogenic factor X assay to predict the international normalized ratio in patients transitioning from argatroban to warfarin. Pharmacotherapy 25: 157–164, 2005.

Banner DW, Hadvary P. Crystallographic analysis at 3.0—a resolution of the binding to human thrombia of four active site-directed inhibitors. J Biol Chem 266: 20085–20093, 1991.

Baron SJ, Yeh RW, Cruz-Gonzalez I, Healy JL, Pomerantsev E, Garasic J, Drachman D, Rosenfield K, Jang IK. Efficacy and safety of argatroban in patients with heparin-induced thrombocytopenia undergoing endovascular intervention for peripheral arterial disease. Catheter Cardiovasc Interv 72: 116–120, 2008.

Barreto AD, Alexandrov AV, Lyden P, Lee J, Martin-Schild S, Shen L, Wu TC, Sisson A, Pandurengan R, Chen Z, Rahbar MH, Balucani C, Barlinn K, Sugg RM, Garami Z, Tsivgoulis G, Gonzales NR, Savitz SI, Mikulik R, Demchuk AM, Grotta JC. The argatroban and tissue-type plasminogen activator stroke study: final results of a pilot safety study. Stroke 43: 770–775, 2012.

Bartholomew JR, Hursting MJ. Transitioning from argatroban to warfarin in heparin-induced thrombocytopenia: an analysis of outcomes in patients with elevated international normalized ratio (INR). J Thromb Thrombolysis 19: 179–184, 2005.

Bartholomew JR, Pietrangeli CE, Hursting MJ. Argatroban anticoagulation for heparin-induced thrombocytopenia in elderly patients. Drugs Aging 24: 489–499, 2007.

Begelman SM, Hursting MJ, Aghababian RV, McCollum D. Heparin-induced thrombocytopenia from venous thromboembolism treatment. J Intern Med 258: 563–572, 2005.

Begelman SM, Baghdasarian SB, Singh IM, Militello MA, Hursting MJ, Bartholomew JR. Argatroban anticoagulation in intensive care patients: effects of heart failure and multiple organ system failure. J Intensive Care Med 23: 313–320, 2008.

Beiderlinden M, Treschan TA, Görlinger K, Peters J. Argatroban anticoagulation in critically ill patients. Ann Pharmacother 41: 749–754, 2007a.

Beiderlinden M, Treschan TA, Görlinger K, Peters J. Argatroban in extracorporeal membrane oxygenation. Artif Organs 31: 461–465, 2007b.

Berry CN, Girardot C, Lecoffre C, Lunven C. Effects of the synthetic thrombin inhibitor argatroban on fibrin- or clot-incorporated thrombin: comparison with heparin and recombinant hirudin. Thromb Haemost 72: 381–386, 1994.

Boyce SW, Bandyk DF, Bartholomew JR, Frame JN, Rice L. A randomized, open-label pilot study comparing desirudin and argatroban in patients with suspected heparin-induced thrombocytopenia with or without thrombosis. Am J Ther 18: 14–22, 2011.

Bradley AM, Branan T. Implementation of an individualized argatroban protocol in an academic medical center. Am J Health-Syst Pharm 68: 1292–1293, 2011.

Brand PA, Egberts JH, Scholz J, Weiler N, Bein B. Argatroban therapy in patients with hepatic and renal impairment. Eur J Anaesthesiol 25: 344–346, 2008.

Brown PM, Hursting MJ. Lack of pharmacokinetic interactions between argatroban and warfarin. Am J Health Syst Pharm 59: 2078–2083, 2002.

Cannon MA, Butterworth J, Riley RD, Hyland JM. Failure of argatroban anticoagulation during off-pump coronary artery bypass surgery. Ann Thorac Surg 77: 711–713, 2004.

Chia S, Van Cott EM, Raffel OC, Jang IK. Comparison of activated clotting times obtained using Hemochron and Medtronic analyzers in patients receiving antithrombin therapy during cardiac catheterization. Thromb Haemost 101: 535–540, 2009.

Clark RJ, Mayo G, Fitzgerald GA, Fitzgerald DJ. Combined administration of aspirin and a specific thrombin inhibitor in man. Circulation 83: 1510–1518, 1991.

ClinTrials.gov. Argatroban versus lepirudin in critically ill patients (ALiCia), ClinTrials Identifier NCT00798525. Accessed 5 July 2012.

Cornell T, Wyrick P, Fleming G, Pasko D, Han Y, Custer J, Haft J, Annich G. A case series describing the use of argatroban in patients on extracorporeal circulation. ASAIO J 53: 460–463, 2007.

Cox DS, Kleinman NS, Boyle DA, Aluri J, Parchman LG, Holdbrook F, Fossler MJ. Pharmacokinetics and pharmacodynamics of argatroban in combination with a platelet glycoprotein IIb/IIIa receptor antagonist in patients undergoing percutaneous coronary intervention. J Clin Pharmacol 44: 981–990, 2004.

Cruz-Gonzalez I, Sanchez-Ledesma M, Baron SJ, Healy JL, Watanabe H, Osakabe M, Yeh RW, Jang IK. Efficacy and safety of argatroban with or without glycoprotein IIb/IIIa inhbitor in patients with heparin-induced thrombocytopenia undergoing percutaneous coronary intervention for acute coronary syndrome. J Thromb Thrombolysis 25: 214–218, 2008a.

Cruz-Gonzalez I, Sanchez-Ledesma M, Osakabe M, Watanabe H, Baron SJ, Healy JL, Yeh RW, Jang IK. What is the optimal anticoagulation level with argatroban during percutaneous coronary intervention? Blood Coag Fibinolysis 19: 401–404, 2008b.

Cuker A, Arepally G, Crowther MA, Rice L, Datko F, Hook K, Propert KJ, Kuter DJ, Ortel TL, Konkle BA, Cines DB. The HIT expert probability (HEP) score: a novel pre-test probability model for heparin-induced thrombocytopenia based on broad expert opinion. J Thromb Haemost 8: 2642–2650, 2010.

Cypher S. Treatment of heparin-induced thrombocytopenia: a practical argatroban dosing protocol for nurses. J Infus Nurs 29: 318–325, 2006.

Dager WE. Considerations for drug dosing post coronary artery bypass graft surgery. Ann Pharmacother 42: 421–424, 2008.

De Denus S, Spinler SA. Decreased argatroban clearance unaffected by hemodialysis in anasarca. Ann Pharmacother 37: 1237–1240, 2003.

Ekbatani A, Asaro LR, Malinow AW. Anticoagulation with argatroban in a parturient with heparin-induced thrombocytopenia. Int J Obstet Anesth 19: 82–87, 2010.

Fanikos J, Fiumara K, Baroletti S, Luppi C, Saniuk C, Mehta A, Silverman J, Goldhaber SZ. Impact of smart infusion technology on administration of anticoagulants (unfractionated heparin, argatroban, lepirudin, and bivalirudin). Am J Cardiol 99: 1002–1005, 2007.

Francis JL. Pregnant woman presents with red toe: case study 2. Thrombin Times Newsletter. CME sponsor, University of Kentucky. Publisher, CTI Clinical Trial and Consulting Services. December 15, 7–9, 2004.

Francis JL, Hursting MJ. Effect of argatroban on the activated partial thromboplastin time: a comparison of 21 commercial reagents. Blood Coagul Fibrinolysis 16: 251–257, 2005.

Fugate S, Chiappe J. Standardizing the management of heparin-induced thrombocytopenia. Am J Health-Syst Pharm 65: 334–339, 2008.

Gasparovic H, Nathan NS, Fitzgerald D, Aranki SF. Severe argatroban-induced coagulopathy in a patient with history of heparin-induced thrombocytopenia. Ann Thorac Surg 78: e89–e91, 2004.

Genzen JR, Fareed J, Hoppensteadt D, Kurup V, Barash P, Coady M, Wu YY. Prolonged elevation of plasma argatroban in a cardiac transplant patient with suspected history of heparin-induced thrombocytopenia with thrombosis. Transfusion 50: 801–807, 2010.

Gold HK, Torres FW, Garabedian HD, Werner W, Jang IK, Khan A, Hagstrom JN, Yasuda T, Leinbach RC, Newell JB, Bovill EG, Stump DC, Collen D. Evidence for a rebound coagulation phenomenon after cessation of a 4-hour infusion of a specific thrombin inhibitor in patients with unstable angina pectoris. J Am Coll Cardiol 21: 1039–1047, 1993.

Gosselin RC, King JH, Janatpour KA, Dager WE, Larkin EC, Owings JT. Comparing direct thrombin inhibitors using aPTT, ecarin clotting times, and thrombin inhibitor management testing. Ann Pharmacother 38: 1383–1388, 2004.

Gray A, Wallis DE, Hursting MJ, Katz E, Lewis BE. Argatroban therapy for heparin-induced thrombocytopenia in acutely ill patients. Clin Appl Thromb Hemost 13: 353–361, 2007.

Greinacher A, Lubenow N, Eichler P. Anaphylactic and anaphylactoid reactions associated with lepirudin in patients with heparin-induced thrombocytopenia. Circulation 108: 2062–2065, 2003.

Guzzi LM, McCollum DA, Hursting MJ. Effect of renal function on argatroban therapy in heparin-induced thrombocytopenia. J Thromb Thrombolysis 22: 169–176, 2006.

Haas S, Lewis B. Identifying patient- and treatment-related factors related to amputation risk in cases of heparin-induced thrombocytopenia treated with argatroban. Int Angiol 30: 541–546, 2011.

Hantgan RR, Jerome WG, Hursting MJ. No effect of clot age or thrombolysis on argatroban's inhibition of thrombin. Blood 92: 2064–2074, 1998.

Harder S, Graff J, Klinkhardt U, von Hentig N, Walenga JM, Watanabe H, Osakabe M, Breddin HK. Transition from argatroban to oral anticoagulation with phenprocoumon or acenocoumarol: effects on prothrombin time, activated partial thromboplastin time, and ecarin clotting time. Thromb Haemost 91: 1137–1145, 2004.

Harenberg J, Jorg I, Fenyvesi T, Piazolo L. Treatment of patients with a history of heparin-induced thrombocytopenia and anti-lepirudin antibodies with argatroban. J Thromb Thrombolysis 19: 65–69, 2005.

Hartman CA, Baroletti SA, Churchill WW, Patel P. Visual compatibility of argatroban with selected drugs. Am J Health Syst Pharm 59: 1784–1785, 2002.

Herrman J-P, Suryapranata H, den Heijer P Gabriel L, Kutryk MJB, Serruys PW. Argatroban during percutaneous transluminal coronary angioplasty: results of a dose-verification study. J Thromb Thrombolysis 3: 367–375, 1996.

Hoffman WD, Czyz Y, McCollum DA, Hursting MJ. Reduced argatroban doses after coronary artery bypass graft surgery. Ann Pharmacother 42: 309–316, 2008.

Honikso ME, Fink JM, Militello MA, Mauro VF, Alexander KS. Compatibility of argatroban with selected cardiovascular agents. Am J Health Syst Pharm 61: 2415–2418, 2004.

Hoppensteadt DA, Kahn S, Fareed J. Factor X values as a means to assess the extent of oral anticoagulation in patients receiving antithrombin drugs. Clin Chem 43: 1786–1788, 1997.

Hursting MJ, Jang IK. Dosing patterns and outcomes in African American, Asian, and Hispanic patients with heparin-induced thrombocytopenia treated with argatroban. J Thromb Thrombolysis 28: 10–15, 2008a.

Hursting MJ, Jang IK. Effect of body mass index on argatroban therapy during percutaneous coronary intervention. J Thromb Thrombolysis 25: 273–279, 2008b.

Hursting MJ, Jang IK. Impact of renal function on argatroban therapy during percutaneous coronary intervention. J Thromb Thrombolysis 29: 1–7, 2010.

Hursting MJ, Murray PT. Argatroban anticoagulation in renal dysfunction: a literature analysis. Nephron Clin Pract 109: c80–c94, 2008.

Hursting MJ, Soffer J. Reducing harm associated with anticoagulation: practical considerations of argatroban therapy in heparin-induced thrombocytopenia. Drug Saf 32: 203–218, 2009.

Hursting MJ, Verme-Gibboney CN. Risk factors for major bleeding in patients with heparin-induced thrombocytopenia: a retrospective study. J Cardiovasc Pharmacol 52: 561–566, 2008.

Hursting MJ, Lewis BE, Macfarlane DE. Transitioning from argatroban to warfarin therapy in patients with heparin-induced thrombocytopenia. Clin Appl Thromb Hemost 11: 279–287, 2005.

Hursting MJ, Dubb J, Verme-Gibboney CN. Argatroban anticoagulation in pediatric patients: a literature analysis. J Pediatr Hematol Oncol 28: 4–10, 2006.

Iida S, Komatsu T, Sato T, Hayashi K, Inokuchi T. Pharmacokinetic studies of argatroban. (MD-805) in rats: excretion into milk and foeto-placental transfer. Jpn Pharmacol Ther 14: 229–235, 1986.

Inglis AML, Sheth SB, Hursting MJ, Tenero DM, Graham AM, DiCicco R. Investigation of the interaction between argatroban and acetaminophen, lidocaine or digoxin. Am J Health Syst Pharm 59: 1258–1266, 2002.

Iqbal O, Ahmad S, Lewis BE, Walenga JM, Rangel Y, Fareed J. Monitoring of argatroban in ARG310 study: potential recommendations for its use in interventional cardiology. Clin Appl Thromb Hemost 8: 217–224, 2002.

Izawa O, Katsuki M, Komatsu T, Iida S. Pharmacokinetic studies of argatroban (MD-805) in human: concentrations of argatroban and its metabolites in plasma, urine, and feces during and after drip intravenous infusion. Jpn Pharmacol Ther 14: 251–263, 1986.

Jang IK, Brown DFM, Giugliao RP, Anderson HV, Losordo D, Nicolau JC, Dutra OP, Bazzino O, Viamonte VM, Norbady R, Liprandi S, Massey TJ, Dinsmore R. Schwarz RP, and the MINT Investigators. A multicenter, randomized study of argatroban versus heparin as adjunct to tissue plasminogen activator (TPA) in acute myocardial infarction: myocardial infarction with Novastan and TPA (MINT) trial. J Am Coll Cardiol 33: 1879–1885, 1999.

Jang IK, Lewis BE, Matthai WH, Kleiman NS. Argatroban anticoagulation in conjunction with glycoprotein IIb/IIIa inhibition in patients undergoing percutaneous coronary intervention: an open-label, nonrandomized pilot study. J Thromb Thrombolysis 18: 31–37, 2004.

Jang IK, Baron SJ, Hursting MJ, Anglade E. Argatroban therapy in women with heparin-induced thrombocytopenia. J Women's Health (Larchmt) 16: 895–901, 2007.

Jang IK, Hursting MJ, McCollum D. Argatroban therapy in patients with coronary artery disease and heparin-induced thrombocytopenia. Cardiology 109: 172–176, 2008.

Keegan SP, Gallagher EM, Ernst NE, Young EJ, Mueller EW. Effects of critical illness and organ failure on therapeutic argatroban dosage requirements in patients with suspected or confirmed heparin-induced thrombocytopenia. Ann Pharmacother 43: 19–27, 2009.

Keeling D, Davidson S, Watson H. The management of heparin-induced thrombocytopenia. Br J Haematol 133: 259–269, 2006.

Kikumoto R, Tamao Y, Tezeka T, Tonomura S, Hara H, Ninomiya K, Kijikata A, Okamoto S. Selective inhibition of thrombin by (2R, 4R)-4-methyl-l-[N2-[(3–methyl-1,2,3,4–tetrahydro-8–quinolinyl)sulfonyl]-L-arginyl)]-2–piperidinecarboxylic acid. Biochemistry 23: 85–90, 1984.

Kiser TH, Jung R, MacLaren R, Fish DN. Evaluation of diagnostic tests and argatroban or lepirudin therapy in patients with suspected heparin-induced thrombocytopenia. Pharmacotherapy 25: 1736–1745, 2005.

Kiser TH, Mann AM, Trujillo TC, Hassell KL. Evaluation of empiric versus nomogram-based direct thrombin inhibitor management in patients with heparin-induced thrombocytopenia. Am J Hematol 86: 267–272, 2011.

Kobayashi W, Tazaki Y. Effect of the thrombin inhibitor argatroban in acute cerebral thrombosis. Semin Thromb Hemost 23: 531–534, 1997.

Kodityal S, Nguyen PH, Kodityal A, Sherer J, Hursting MJ, Rice L. Argatroban for suspected heparin-induced thrombocytopenia: contemporary experience at a large teaching hospital. J Intensive Care Med 21: 86–92, 2006.

Koster A, Buz S, Hetzer R, Kuppe H, Breddin K, Harder S. Anticoagulation with argatroban in patients with heparin-induced thrombocytopenia antibodies after cardiovascular surgery with cardiopulmonary bypass: first results from the ARGE03 trial. J Thorac Cardiovasc Surg 132: 699–700, 2006.

Koster A, Hentschel T, Groman T, Kuppe H, Hetzer R, Harder S, Fischer KG. Argatroban anticoagulation for renal replacement therapy in patients with heparin-induced thrombocytopenia after cardiovascular surgery. J Thorac Cardiovasc Surg 133: 1376–1377, 2007.

Kuczka K, Weber C, Betz C, Picard-Willems B, Poplutz A, Beiderlinden M, Farker K, Merkel U, Harder S. Observations on argatroban dosage and coagulation parameters in ICU patients. Br J Clin Pharmacol 72(Suppl 1): 18–19, 2011.

LaMonte MP, Brown PM, Hursting MJ. Stroke in patients with heparin-induced thrombocytopenia and the effect of argatroban therapy. Crit Care Med 32: 976–980, 2004a.

LaMonte MP, Nash ML, Wang DZ, Woolfenden AR, Schultz J, Hursting MJ, Brown PM. Argatroban anticoagulation in patients with acute ischemic stroke (ARGIS-1): a randomized, placebo-controlled safety study. Stroke 35: 1677–1682, 2004b.

Levine RL, Hursting MJ, McCollum D. Argatroban therapy in heparin-induced thrombocytopenia with hepatic dysfunction. Chest 129: 1167–1175, 2006.

Lewis BE, Wallis DE, Zehnder JL, Barton JC; For the ARG-911/915/915X Investigators. Argatroban reexposure in patients with heparin-induced thrombocytopenia. Blood 96: 52a, 2000.

Lewis BE, Wallis DE, Berkowitz SD, Matthai WH, Fareed J, Walenga JM, Bartholomew J, Sham R, Lerner RG, Zeigler ZR, Rustagi PK, Jang IK, Rifkin SD, Moran J, Hursting MJ, Kelton JG; For the ARG-911 Study Investigators. Argatroban anticoagulant therapy in patients with heparin-induced thrombocytopenia. Circulation 103: 1838–1843, 2001.

Lewis B, Matthai WH, Cohen M, Moses JW, Hursting MJ, Leya F; For the ARG-216/310/311 Investigators. Argatroban anticoagulation during percutaneous coronary intervention in patients with heparin-induced thrombocytopenia. Catheter Cardiovasc Interv 57: 177–184, 2002.

Lewis BE, Wallis DE, Leya F, Hursting MJ, Kelton JG; For the ARG-915 Investigators. Argatroban anticoagulation in patients with heparin-induced thrombocytopenia. Arch Intern Med 163: 1849–1856, 2003.

Lewis BE, Wallis DE, Hursting MJ, Levine RL, Leya F. Effects of argatroban therapy, demographic variables, and platelet count on thrombotic risks in heparin-induced thrombocytopenia. Chest 129: 1407–1416, 2006.

Link A, Girndt M, Selejan S, Mathes A, Böhm M, Rensing H. Argatroban for anticoagulation in continuous renal replacement therapy. Crit Care Med 37: 105–110, 2009a.

Link A, Selejan S, Mathes A, Böhm M, Rensing H. Argatroban for anticoagulation in continuous renal replacement therapy: the authors reply. Crit Care Med 37: 2139–2140, 2009b.

Linkins LA, Dans AL, Moores LK, Bona R, Davidson BL, Schulman S, Crowther M. Treatment and prevention of heparin-induced thrombocytopenia: American college of chest physicians evidence-based clinical practice guidelines (9th ed). 141: e495S–e530S, 2012.

Love JE, Ferrell C, Chandler W. Monitoring direct thrombin inhibitors with a plasma diluted thrombin time. Thromb Haemost 98: 234–242, 2007.

Madabushi R, Cox DS, Hossain M, Boyle DA, Patel BR, Young G, Choi YM, Gobburu JV. Pharmacokinetic and pharmacodynamic basis for effective argatroban dosing in pediatrics. J Clin Pharmacol 51: 19–28, 2011.

Malherbe S, Tsui B, Stobart K, Koller J. Argatroban as anticoagulant in cardiopulmonary bypass in an infant and attempted reversal with recombinant activated factor VII. Anesthesiology 100: 443–445, 2004.

Martin ME, Kloecker GH, Laber DA. Argatroban for anticoagulation during cardiac surgery. Eur J Haematol 78: 161–166, 2007.

Matsuo T, Kario K, Matsuda S, Yamaguchi N, Kakishita E. Effect of thrombin inhibition on patients with peripheral arterial obstructive disease: a multi-center clinical trial of argatroban. J Thromb Thrombolysis 2: 131–136, 1995.

Matthai WH, Hursting MJ, Lewis BE, Kelton JG. Argatroban anticoagulation in patients with a history of heparin-induced thrombocytopenia. Thromb Res 116: 121–126, 2005.

Molinaro RJ. Quantitation of argatroban in plasma using liquid chromatography electrospray tandem mass spectrometry (UPLC-ESI-MS/MS). Methods Mol Biol 603: 57–63, 2010.

Murray PT. Drug dosing in the intensive care unit: the critically ill are a special population too. Crit Care Med 37: 342–343, 2009.

Murray PT, Hursting MJ. Heparin-induced thrombocytopenia in patients administered heparin solely for hemodialysis. Ren Fail 28: 537–539, 2006.

Murray PT, Reddy BV, Grossman EJ, Hammes MS, Trevino S, Ferrell J, Tang I, Hursting MJ, Shamp TR, Swan SK. A prospective study of three argatroban treatment regimens during hemodialysis in end-stage renal disease. Kidney Int 66: 2446–2453, 2004.

NCCN (National Comprehensive Cancer Network) Clinical Practice Guidelines in Oncology. Venous thromboembolic disease version.2.2011. [Available from: http://www.nccn.org/professionals/physician_gls/pdf/vte.pdf, April 7, 2011].

Nielson VG, Steenwyk BL, Gurley WQ, Pereira SJ, Lell WA, Kirklin JK. Argatroban, bivalirudin, and lepirudin do not decrease clot propagation and strength as effectively as heparin-activated antithrombin in vitro. J Heart Lung Transplant 25: 653–663, 2006.

Okamoto S, Hijikata A. Potent inhibition of thrombin by the newly synthesized arginine derivative no. 805. the importance of stereostructure of its hydrophobic carboxamide portion. Biochem Biophys Res Commun 101: 440–446, 1981.

Patel K, Hursting MJ. Compatibility of argatroban with abciximab, eptifibatide, or tirofiban during simulated Y-site administration. Am J Health Syst Pharm 62: 1381–1384, 2005.

Rawson TE, VanGorp KA, Yang J, Kogan TP. Separation of 2l-(R)- and 2l-(S)-argatroban: solubility and activity of the individual diastereoisomers. J Pharm Sci 82: 672–673, 1993.

Reddy BV, Grossman EJ, Trevino SA, Hursting MJ, Murray PT. Argatroban anticoagulation in patients with heparin-induced thrombocytopenia requiring renal replacement therapy. Ann Pharmacother 39: 1601–1605, 2005.

Reichert MG, MacGregor DA, Kincaid EH, Dolinski SY. Excessive argatroban anticoagulation for heparin-induced thrombocytopenia. Ann Pharmacother 37: 652–654, 2003.

Rice L. Heparin-induced thrombocytopenia. Myths and misconceptions (that will cause trouble for you and your patient). Arch Intern Med 164: 1961–1964, 2004.

Rice L, Hursting MJ. Argatroban therapy in heparin-induced thrombocytopenia. Exp Rev Clin Pharmacol 1: 357–367, 2008.

Rice L, Hursting MJ, Baillie GM, McCollum DA. Argatroban anticoagulation in obese versus nonobese patients: implications for treating heparin-induced thrombocytopenia. J Clin Pharmacol 47: 1028–1034, 2007.

Rössig L, Genth-Zotz S, Rau M, Heyndrickx GR, Schneider T, Gulba DC, Desaga M, Buerke M, Harder S, Zeiher AM; ARG-E04 Study Group. Argatroban for elective percutaneous coronary intervention: the ARG-E04 multi-center study. Int J Cardol 148: 214–219, 2011.

Samuels LE, Kohout J, Casanova-Ghosh E, Hagan K, Garwood P, Ferdinand F, Goldman SM. Argatroban as a primary or secondary postoperative anticoagulant in patients implanted with ventricular assist devices. Ann Thorac Surg 85: 1651–1655, 2008.

Saugel B, Phillip V, Moessmer G, Schmid RM, Huber W. Argatroban therapy for heparin-induced thrombocytopenia in ICU patients with multiple organ dysfunction syndrome: a retrospective study. Crit Care 14: R90, 2010.

Shepherd MF, Jacobsen JM, Rosborough TK. Argatroban therapy using enzymatic anti-factor IIa monitoring. Ann Pharmacother 45: 422–423, 2011.

Sheth SB, DiCicco RA, Hursting MJ, Montague T, Jorkasky DK. Interpreting the International Normalized Ratio (INR) in individuals receiving argatroban and warfarin. Thromb Haemost 85: 435–440, 2001.

Siegmund R, Boer K, Poeschel K, Wolf G, Deufel T, Kiehntopf M. Comparison of the ecarin chromogenic assay and different aPTT assays for the measurement of argatroban concentrations in plasma from healthy individuals and from coagulation factor deficient patients. Thromb Res 123: 159–165, 2008.

Skrupky LP, Smith JR, Deal EN, Arnold H, Hollands JM, Martinez EJ, Micek ST. Comparison of bivalirudin and argatroban for the management of heparin-induced thrombocytopenia. Pharmacotherapy 30: 1229–1238, 2010.

Smythe M, Stephens JL, Koerber JM, Mattson JC. A comparison of lepirudin and argatroban outcomes. Clin Appl Thromb Hemost 11: 371–374, 2005.

Smythe MA, Koerber JM, Forsyth LL, Priziola JL, Balasubramaniam M, Mattson JC. Argatroban dosage requirements and outcomes in intensive care versus non-intensive care patients. Pharmacotherapy 29: 1073–1081, 2009.

Sun X, Chen Y, Xiao Q, Wang Y, Zhou J, Ma Z, Xiang J, Chen X. Effects of argatroban as an anticoagulant for intermittent venovenous hemofiltration in patients at high risk of bleeding. Nephrol Dial Transplant 26: 2954–2959, 2011.

Swan SK, Hursting MJ. The pharmacokinetics and pharmacodynamics of argatroban: effects of age, gender, and hepatic or renal dysfunction. Pharmacotherapy 20: 318–329, 2000.

Swan SK, St. Peter JV, Lambrecht LJ, Hursting MJ. Comparison of anticoagulant effects and safety of argatroban and heparin in healthy subjects. Pharmacotherapy 20: 756–770, 2000.

Tang IY, Cox DS, Patel K, Reddy BV, Nahlik L, Trevino S, Murray PT. Argatroban and renal replacement therapy in patients with heparin-induced thrombocytopenia. Ann Pharmacother 39: 231–236, 2005.

Tatsuno J, Komatsu T, Iida S. Pharmacokinetic studies of argatroban (MD-805): protein binding and blood cell binding. Jpn Pharmacol Ther 14(Suppl 5): 243–249, 1986.

Theroux P. The Argatroban Myocardial Infarction (AMI) study. Scientific Session News of the American College of Cardiology 15: 6, 1997.

Tran JQ, DiCicco RA, Sheth SB, Tucci M, Pend L, Jorkasky DK, Hursting MJ, Benincosa LJ. Assessment of the potential pharmacokinetic and pharmacodynamic interactions between erythromycin and argatroban. J Clin Pharmacol 39: 513–519, 1999.

Verme-Gibboney CN, Hursting MJ. Argatroban dosing in patients with heparin-induced thrombocytopenia. Ann Pharmacother 37: 970–975, 2003.

Vermeer F, Vahanian A, Fels PW, Besse P, Muller E, Van de Werf F, Fitzgerald D, Darius H, Puel J, Garrigou D, Simoons ML; For the ARGAMI Study Group. Argatroban and alteplase in patients with acute myocardial infarction: the ARGAMI study. J Thromb Thrombolysis 10: 233–240, 2000.

Walenga JM, Koza MJ, Lewis BE, Pifarre R. Relative heparin-induced thrombocytopenic potential of low molecular weight heparins and new antithrombotic agents. Clin Appl Thromb Hemost 2(Suppl 1): S21–S27, 1996.

Walenga JM, Fasanella AR, Iqbal O, Hoppensteadt DA, Ahman S, Wallis DE, Bakhos M. Coagulation laboratory testing patients treated with argatroban. Semin Thromb Hemost 25(Suppl 1): 61–66, 1999.

Walenga JM, Ahmad S, Hoppensteadt DA, Iqbal O, Hursting MJ, Lewis BE. Argatroban therapy does not generate antibodies that alter its anticoagulant activity in patients with heparin-induced thrombocytopenia. Thromb Res 105: 401–405, 2002.

Warkentin TE, Kelton JG. A 14-year study of heparin-induced thrombocytopenia. Am J Med 101: 502–507, 1996.

Warkentin TE, Greinacher A, Koster A, Linkoff AM. Treatment and prevention of heparin-induced thrombocytopenia: American College of Chest Physicians Evidence-Based Clinical Practice Guidelines, 8th edition. Chest 133: 340S–380S, 2008.

Williamson DR, Boulanger I, Tardif M, Albert M, Gregoire G. Argatroban dosing in intensive care patients with acute renal failure and liver dysfunction. Pharmacotherapy 24: 409–414, 2004.

Yee AJ, Kuter DJ. Successful recovery after an overdose of argatroban. Ann Pharmacother 40: 336–339, 2006.

Yoon JH, Yeh RW, Nam KH, Hoffman WD, Agnihotri AK, Jang IK. Safety and efficacy of argatroban therapy during the early postcardiac surgery period. J Thromb Thrombolysis 30: 276–280, 2010.

Young G, Yonekawa KE, Nakagawa PA, Blain RV, Lovejoy AE, Nugent DJ. Differential effects of direct thrombin inhibitors and antithrombin-dependent anticoagulants on the dynamics of clot formation. Blood Coagul Fibrinolysis 18: 97–103, 2007.

Young G, Boshkov LK, Sullivan JE, Raffini LJ, Cox DS, Boyle DA, Kallender H, Tarka EA, Soffer J, Hursting MJ. Argatroban therapy in pediatric patients requiring nonheparin anticoagulation: an open-label, safety, efficacy, and pharmacokinetic study. Pediatr Blood Cancer 56: 1103–1109, 2011.

Young SK, Al-Mondhiry HA, Vaida SJ, Ambrose A, Botti AJ. Successful use of argatroban during the third trimester of pregnancy: case report and review of the literature. Pharmacotherapy 28: 1531–1536, 2008.

14 Recombinant hirudin for the treatment of heparin-induced thrombocytopenia

Andreas Greinacher

INTRODUCTION

Lepirudin (Refludan, produced by Cellgene, U.K.) became the first direct thrombin inhibitor (DTI) available for treating heparin-induced thrombocytopenia (HIT) in 1997. While in early 2012 the Bayer Group stopped marketing lepirudin, smaller companies took over the marketing rights in some countries (e.g., Pharmore in Germany). At the time this chapter was finalized it remained unclear in which jurisdictions lepirudin will be available. There are two other recombinant hirudins (r-hirudins) available, desirudin (Revasc/Iprivask, Canyon Pharmaceuticals, Basel, Switzerland; available in Europe and North America) and RB variant-hirudin (Thrombexx, Rhein-Minapharm, Cairo, Egypt; available in many countries in Asia and Africa). The pharmacokinetics and biologic activities of the different r-hirudins are very similar. Thus the data obtained in preclinical and clinical studies with lepirudin in HIT may help guide the use of other r-hirudins, especially in countries where lepirudin is not/no longer available.

HIRUDIN AND ITS DERIVATIVES
Chemistry

Hirudin, the most potent natural thrombin inhibitor identified to date, is a 65-amino acid polypeptide (molecular mass, approximately 7 kDa) produced by the parapharyngeal glands of the medicinal leech, *Hirudo medicinalis*. The NH_2-terminal part of the molecule (residues 1–39) is stabilized by three disulfide bridges integral to its function. The COOH-terminal moiety (residues 40–65) is highly acidic. In the 3D structure of hirudin (Clore et al., 1987; Sukumaran et al., 1987), three areas are distinguished: a central core (residues 3–30, 37–46, 56–57), a "finger" (residues 31–36), and a loop (residues 47–55). Hirudin is very stable at extremes of pH (1.5–13.0) and at high temperatures (up to 90°C). It is soluble in water but insoluble in alcohol or acetone. The isoelectric point of hirudin is approximately 4.

Hirudins for therapeutic use are now produced by recombinant biotechnology, using the yeast *Saccharomyces cerevisiae*, yielding the r-hirudins, lepirudin and desirudin. Lepirudin, a desulfatohirudin, differs from natural hirudin by lacking the sulfate group at Tyr-63 and also has an NH_2-terminal leucine residue in place of the isoleucine. Desirudin differs from lepirudin in the N-termini: desirudin possesses a valine-valine and lepirudin a leucine-threonine structure. Otherwise, the two hirudin derivatives are very similar, with molecular weights of 6.96 and 6.98 kDa, respectively. RB-variant hirudin is produced in *Hansenula polymorpha* but otherwise is very similar to the two other r-hirudins.

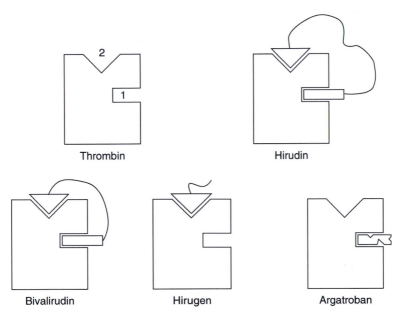

FIGURE 14.1 Schematic representation of the thrombin molecule and its inhibition by hirudin, bivalirudin (formerly, Hirulog), hirugen, and argatroban: (*i*) active-site pocket; (*ii*) fibrinogen-binding site. The active-site pocket catalyzes most of the functions of the thrombin molecule, whereas the fibrinogen-binding exosite mediates the binding of thrombin to fibrinogen. Hirudin is a 7000 Da (7 kDa) protein composed of 65 amino acids, which binds to the active-site pocket and the fibrinogen-binding exosite of thrombin, i.e., it is a *bivalent* direct thrombin inhibitor. Bivalirudin is a small synthetic peptide (20 amino acids) designed also to block both of these sites on thrombin. Hirugen, a synthetic peptide, mimics the binding site of fibrinogen to thrombin, thereby inhibiting binding of thrombin to fibrinogen and, therefore, fibrinogen cleavage by thrombin. The arginine derivative argatroban binds competitively to only the active binding site pocket of thrombin. Hirugen and argatroban are *univalent* direct thrombin inhibitors. *Source*: Adapted from Hermann et al. (1997).

Although these structural differences result in a 10-fold reduction in the dissociation constant of r-hirudin, as compared with natural hirudin, r-hirudins remain highly selective inhibitors of thrombin, with an inhibition constant for thrombin in the picomolar range (Stone and Hofsteenge, 1986).

Pharmacology

r-Hirudins act independently of the cofactors antithrombin and heparin cofactor II (Markwardt, 1992) and form tight, noncovalent 1:1 complexes with thrombin. Interacting with both binding sites, r-hirudins are *bivalent* inhibitors of thrombin (Fig. 14.1), inhibiting all the biologic activities of thrombin.

Three amino acids (residues 46–48) near the NH$_2$-terminus of hirudin bind to the active site cleft of thrombin, while the core of the hirudin molecule closes off the active site pocket of thrombin. The COOH-terminal tail of hirudin interacts with the fibrinogen anion-binding site, helping to block thrombin-catalyzed fibrinogen cleavage. Hirudin inhibits the feedback loop whereby thrombin enhances its own generation via activation of factors Va and VIIIa (Kaiser and Markwardt, 1986;

Pieters et al., 1989). In addition to inhibiting free thrombin, hirudin inhibits clot-bound thrombin (Hogg and Jackson, 1989; Weitz et al., 1990) and thrombin bound to fibrin split products (Weitz et al., 1998). By contrast, heparin–antithrombin complexes are unable to access and inactivate clot-bound thrombin. This important difference between hirudin and heparin might explain why hirudin is more effective than heparin in promoting dissolution of mural thrombi in experimental models (Meyer et al., 1998). Hirudin shows virtually no interaction with plasma proteins (Glusa and Markwardt, 1990), and its activity is standardized in thrombin inhibitory units (TIU): 1 TIU is the amount of hirudin inhibiting 1 U of thrombin at 37°C. The specific activity of lepirudin is 16,000 TIU/mg, the specific activities of desirudin and RB-variant hirudin are about 20,000 TIU/mg.

Pharmacokinetics

r-Hirudins are administered parenterally. Studies of plasma pharmacokinetics in healthy subjects reveal a two-compartment model. The initial plasma half-life $(t_{1/2})$ of r-hirudin is 8–12 minutes, after which it is distributed in the extracellular space. Only 20% of r-hirudin is found in the plasma, while the remaining 80% is in the extravascular compartment (Glusa, 1998). r-hirudins are not transported into the cerebrospinal fluid or breast milk (Lindhoff-Last et al., 2000a; Refludan Package Insert, 2002).

The terminal plasma elimination half-life $(t_{1/2}\beta)$ ranges from 0.8 to 1.7 hours (mean, ~1.3 hr or 80 min) after intravenous (iv) injection of bolus doses of 0.01–0.5 mg/kg and 1.1–2.0 hours after continuous iv infusions over 6 hours. Maximum activated partial thromboplastin time (aPTT) ratios occur about 10 minutes after iv bolus, 3–6 hours following start of continuous iv infusion, and 2–3 hours after subcutaneous (sc) administration (in patients with normal renal function). During iv infusion, therapeutic levels are usually reached within 30–60 minutes. This correlates well with the peak plasma r-hirudin concentrations achieved with these different modes of application. The approved dose for lepirudin in patients with HIT and acute thrombosis (with normal renal function) is an iv bolus of 0.40 mg/kg, followed by an iv infusion of 0.15 mg/kg/hr (Table 14.1). However, there is consistent experience that this dose is too high in most HIT patients (Lubenow et al., 2004, 2005; Hacquard et al., 2005; Tardy et al., 2006). Especially in elderly patients the bolus should be omitted and an initial infusion rate of 0.05–0.10 mg/kg/hr commenced so as to avoid overdosage in case of unrecognized renal insufficiency. The infusion rate should then be adjusted according to aPTT every 4 hours until a steady state is reached (Lubenow et al., 2004) (Fig. 14.2). The main indication for application of the bolus is acute life- or limb-threatening thrombosis.

Renal clearance (160–200 mL/min for an adult with normal body surface area (BSA) of 1.73 m²) and degradation account for approximately 90% of the systemic clearance of r-hirudins. The $t_{1/2}\beta$ of r-hirudin lengthens with deterioration of renal function (Markwardt, 1989; Nowak et al., 1991, 1992, 1997; Vanholder et al., 1994, 1997); in nephrectomized patients, it can be up to 120 hours (Wittkowsky and Kondo, 2000; Dager and White, 2001; Fischer, 2002; Shepherd, 2002).

A clinically important observation is that renal blood flow decreases during anesthesia, so that the elimination half-life is prolonged to 3–5 hours. If r-hirudins are used intraoperatively, the dose should be reduced by 30–50%, and close monitoring is mandatory.

TABLE 14.1 Dosing Schedules for Lepirudin Treatment of Patients with HIT

	Bolus[a,b]	IV Infusion[a,b]	Target aPTT ratio[c]
Dose recommended in all HIT patients without renal impairment	None[d]	0.05–0.10 mg/kg b.w./hr[d]	1.5–2.5 (0.6–1.0 µg/mL)
HIT with isolated thrombocytopenia (dose regimen B in HAT trials)	None[e]	0.10 mg/kg b.w./hr[e]	1.5–2.5 (0.6–1.0 µg/mL)
HIT and thrombosis (dose regimen A1 in HAT trials)	(0.40 mg/kg[e] b.w. iv)	0.15 mg/kg b.w./hr[e]	1.5–2.5 (0.6–1.0 µg/mL)
Thrombosis prophylaxis in patients with a history of HIT	15 mg sc b.i.d.[f]	–	–
HIT with thrombosis and concomitant thrombolysis (dose regimen A2 in HAT trials)	(0.20 mg/kg b.w. iv[e])	0.10 mg/kg b.w./hr[e]	1.5–2.5
Renal dialysis every alternate day	0.10 mg/kg b.w. iv predialysis	–	2.0–2.5
CVVH	–	0.005 mg/kg b.w./hr (initial rate)	1.5–2.5
PCI (Mehta et al., 2002); UA or acute MI without ST elevation (OASIS-2, 1999)	0.40 mg/kg b.w. iv	0.15 mg/kg b.w./hr	1.5–2.5
Vascular surgery (Hach-Wunderle, 2001)	0.40 mg/kg b.w. iv	0.10 mg/kg b.w./hr	1.5–2.5
Vascular surgery (intraoperative vessel flushes)	Use up to 250 mL (0.1 mg/mL solution)	–	–
Postoperative anticoagulation	–	0.10 mg/kg b.w/hr	1.5–2.5
Cardiac surgery using CPB (dose regimen C in HAT trials) (see also chap. 19)	0.25 mg/kg b.w. iv[e] (0.20 mg/kg b.w. in the priming fluid)	0.50 mg/min[a,g]	Monitored by ECT: >2.5 µg/mL before start of CPB; 3.5–4.5 µg/mL during CPB[h]

Note: Repeat aPTT determinations should be made 4–6 hr after any dose adjustment.
[a]A maximum b.w. of 100 kg should be used for dose calculations.
[b]Adjust for renal insufficiency.
[c]The ratio is based on comparison with the normal laboratory mean aPTT. If Actin FS or neothromtin reagents are used, the aPTT target range is usually 1.5–3.0.
[d]This is the author's recommended starting dose in all HIT patients, unless life- or limb-threatening thrombosis is present.
[e]Used in the HAT-1, -2, and -3 trials.
[f]Tested in a prospective, randomized trial after orthopedic surgery with desirudin (Eriksson et al., 1996, 1997b).
[g]Stop 15 min before and after CPB; put 5 mg into CPB after disconnection to avoid clotting of pump.
[h]The target lepirudin level pre-CPB (>2.5 µg/mL) is lower than the level sought during CPB (3.4–4.5 µg/mL) because of the addition of lepirudin to the pump priming fluid (0.2 mg/kg b.w.).
Abbreviations: aPTT, (activated) partial thromboplastin time; b.w., body weight; CPB, cardiopulmonary bypass; CVVH, continuous venovenous hemofiltration; ECT, ecarin clotting time; HIT, heparin-induced thrombocytopenia; iv, intravenous; MI, myocardial infarction; PCI, percutaneous coronary intervention; UA, unstable angina.

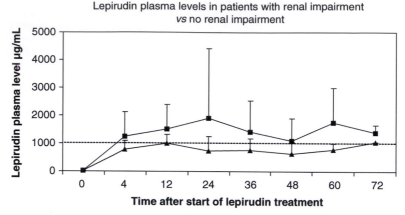

FIGURE 14.2 Time course of lepirudin plasma levels when lepirudin is given in therapeutic dose in patients with normal creatinine levels (lower line) and patients with increased creatinine levels (upper line). The dotted line indicates the upper therapeutic level. Both groups showed similar plasma concentrations after 4 hours, which further increased in patients with renal impairment. Therefore aPTT should be also assessed in all patients every 4 hours after start of treatment, until a steady state is reached, to identify those with drug accumulation. *Abbreviation*: aPTT, activated partial thromboplastin time. *Source*: From Lubenow et al. (2004).

 With sc administration, bioavailability of r-hirudins is nearly 100%. Dose-ranging studies of lepirudin have shown that its concentration in the blood reaches 0.3–0.5 µg/mL after an sc dose of lepirudin of 0.5 µg/kg and about 0.7 µg/mL after an sc dose of 0.75 µg/kg, making twice-daily injections effective (Schiele et al., 1994; Huhle et al., 2000b; Nowak, 2001). When administered subcutaneously, r-hirudins are usually injected into an abdominal skin fold and reach their peak concentration after 2–3 hours.

 The absorption of desirudin is complete when administered sc at doses of 0.3 or 0.5 mg/kg. Following sc administration of single doses of 0.1–0.75 mg/kg, plasma concentrations of desirudin increased to a maximum level (C_{max}) between 1 and 3 hours. Both C_{max} and area-under-the-curve (AUC) values are dose proportional (Fig. 14.3). Desirudin has been administered sc in two major prospective trials for thrombosis prophylaxis after major orthopedic joint-replacement surgery (Eriksson et al., 1996, 1997b) and in a small trial in patients suspected to have HIT (Boyce et al., 2011) and in patients who had HIT or a history of HIT who required thrombosis prophylaxis (Levy et al., 2011) and in intensive care patients in the DESIRABLE trial (Bergese et al., 2012). The pharmacology of desirudin is summarized by Graetz and coworkers (2011).

 Lepirudin has been administered sc for long-term prophylaxis in HIT after the acute disease has been controlled (Huhle et al., 2000b). In one patient the drug was safely administered sc twice daily for eight months for antithrombotic therapy in the setting of malignant disease. Lepirudin has been administered sc as an adjunct to streptokinase in patients with acute myocardial infarction (MI) (Neuhaus et al., 1999) and in the outpatient management of acute MI (Begelman and Deitcher, 2002).

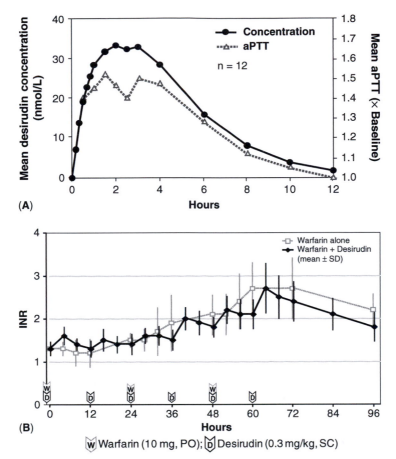

FIGURE 14.3 (**A**) Mean desirudin plasma concentration and corresponding aPTT ratios (aPTT:baseline aPTT) after sc injection of 15 mg desirudin in healthy individuals. *Source*: Canyon Pharmaceuticals and US NDA 21–71. (**B**) Effect of desirudin on INR during the transition to warfarin. Application of the drugs are indicated by symbols W = warfarin 10 mg; D = desirudin 0.3 mg/kg, sc. *Abbreviations*: aPTT, activated partial thromboplastin time; INR, international normalized ratio; sc, subcutaneous. *Source*: From Levy et al. (2009).

Tests for Monitoring Anticoagulation

Numerous tests have been evaluated for monitoring anticoagulation by DTIs, ranging from the ubiquitous aPTT to the newer ecarin clotting time (ECT), enzyme immunoassay (EIA) techniques for directly measuring the hirudin concentration (Hafner et al., 2002), and the ecarin chromogenic assay (ECA) (Lange et al., 2003, 2005).

The aPTT is a global coagulation assay and is the current method of choice for monitoring r-hirudin therapy in most situations. In patients who require higher levels of plasma hirudin and aPTT values above ~70 seconds (depending on the reagent), the hirudin concentration–aPTT curve flattens, and even major changes in plasma levels cause only a minor change in the aPTT. Because the sensitivities of different aPTT reagents vary (Gosselin et al., 2004), it is strongly recommended that

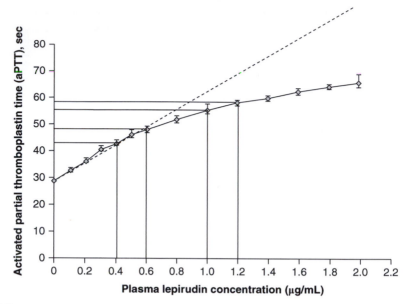

FIGURE 14.4   Lepirudin standard curve. This curve was generated using seven normal plasmas spiked with various concentrations of lepirudin (µg/mL) using reagent Actin FS and the BCS analyzer (Dade-Behring, Germany). Note that incremental changes in aPTT are much smaller as the dose–response curve flattens at greater plasma lepirudin concentrations. *Abbreviation*: aPTT, activated partial thromboplastin time.

each laboratory involved in monitoring of DTIs should generate its own standard dose–response curve for their aPTT reagent using "spiked" normal pooled plasma samples, for example, with 0.25, 0.50, 0.75, 1.0, 1.25, 1.5, and 2.0 µg/mL lepirudin (Fig. 14.4). This will define the expected range over which the aPTT reliably reflects changes in the DTI plasma concentration. At concentrations above this range, the ECT is more reliable for DTI monitoring. This is especially true for very high doses, such as those used during cardiopulmonary bypass (CPB) surgery.

Unlike global coagulation tests, the ECT monitors prolongation of clotting time caused by thrombin inhibition alone (Callas et al., 1995; Nowak and Bucha, 1996; Pötzsch et al., 1997a,b; Koster et al., 2000a; Fabrizio, 2001; de Denus and Spinier, 2002; Liu et al., 2002). Ecarin, which is obtained from snake venom, catalyzes the cleavage of prothrombin to meizothrombin (Kornalik and Blomback, 1975; Novoa and Seegers, 1980; Nishida et al., 1995). Meizothrombin is biologically similar to thrombin, except that it cleaves fibrinogen much more slowly than thrombin. The interaction of meizothrombin with hirudin, however, is similar to that of thrombin. Thus, when all the hirudin present in a blood sample has been neutralized by meizothrombin, thrombin will no longer be inhibited, and clotting will occur.

The ECT shows a linear correlation to lepirudin plasma levels over a wide range. At present, this assay is recommended for monitoring anticoagulation when higher concentrations of lepirudin are used. It is mandatory for monitoring of lepirudin during CPB.

The automated ECA assay provides a linear dose–response curve for all DTIs independently of the patient's prothrombin and fibrinogen levels (Lange et al., 2003, 2005).

In 2005, a workshop compared several methods for monitoring DTIs: aPTT using local reagents and methods (Actin FS, Thrombosil I, Pathromtin SL, Synthasil aPTT, Automated aPTT, STA-PTT, STA—CK Prest 5); aPTT using a common reagent (C-aPTT; Actin FS; Aventis Pharma, Marburg, Germany); anti-IIa chromogenic assay with the S2238 chromogenic substrate from Instrumentation Laboratory/Haemochrom Diagnostica (Essen, Germany); ECT—wet chemistry (Wet ECT) reagents (University Jena, Germany); ECT—dry chemistry reagent (Cardiovascular Diagnostics Inc., Raleigh, North Carolina, U.S.A.) with two ecarin concentrations (low ecarin reagent card: dry ECT; higher concentration ecarin card: TIM); EIA kit (Immuno Bind, Hirudin Elisa kit, American Diagnostica Inc., Greenwich, Connecticut, U.S.A.). The interlaboratory variations for measurement of lepirudin were (from lowest to highest): TIM < C-aPTT < Dry ECT < L-aPTT < wet ECT < anti-IIa < EIA (Gray and Harenberg, 2005).

Limitations of Functional Monitoring Tests
Results obtained with the aPTT or ECT may be inaccurate in patients whose plasma has a reduced concentration of prothrombin [e.g., severe liver disease, disseminated intravascular coagulation (DIC), treatment with vitamin K antagonists] or in patients with fibrinogen depletion (e.g., post-thrombolysis, hemodilution during CPB) (Lindhoff-Last et al., 2000b; de Denus and Spinier, 2002). This is especially problematic during CPB. In the ECT, this can be overcome by addition of normal plasma 1:1 to the assay (Koster et al., 2000a). Also in patients with "lupus anticoagulant" the functional assays are often inaccurate (Salmela et al., 2010).

EIAs measure the plasma concentration of r-hirudin independent of prothrombin concentration and the presence of a lupus anticoagulant. Plasma concentrations for r-hirudin are 0.2–0.4 µg/mL for thrombosis prophylaxis, and 0.6–1.0 µg/mL for therapeutic dose anticoagulation.

The ECA also overcomes the problems associated with monitoring of DTIs by aPTT and ECT, with faster turnaround time than the EIA.

Dose Adjustments
In r-hirudin-treated patients, laboratory values to monitor the anticoagulant effect should be obtained prior to treatment, 4 hours after the start of iv infusion, and then every 4 hours until a steady state is reached (Lubenow et al., 2004, 2005) (Fig. 14.2). Also, 4 hours after every change in dose, monitoring should be repeated. For most patients, the primary laboratory parameter used is the aPTT, with testing performed at least once daily during treatment with lepirudin. If the target range is exceeded, the infusion should be stopped for 2 hours and restarted at a 50% lower dose once the therapeutic range has been reached (Greinacher et al., 1999a,b). When the dose is subtherapeutic, the infusion rate should be increased by 20%.

Renal Impairment–Lepirudin
Lepirudin has been studied in patients with varying degrees of renal impairment. It can be used safely and effectively if started at a very low dose of 0.005–0.01 mg/kg/hr, if there is evidence for renal compromise. If renal function is normal, the starting dose should be 0.05–0.10 mg/kg/hr. In both situations the initial lepirudin

TABLE 14.2   Initial Lepirudin Dosing in Renal Dysfunction

Serum creatinine, mg/dL (μmol/L)	Initial iv infusion rate (Subsequently adjusted to aPTT) (mg/kg/hr)
1–1.58 (90–140)	0.05
1.58–4.52 (140–400)	0.01
>4.52 (>400)	0.005

Abbreviations: aPTT, (activated) partial thromboplastin time; iv, intravenous.

bolus should be omitted (Table 14.2). In case of transient renal failure close monitoring of aPTT is mandatory. Even when renal function appears normal, the potential for unrecognized compensated renal dysfunction exists, so the initial lepirudin bolus should be avoided (unless severe thrombosis is present) and a lower infusion rate of 0.05–0.10 mg/kg/hr iv started, with subsequent adjustments by aPTT.

Renal Impairment–Desirudin

In a pharmacokinetic study, renally impaired subjects with mild [creatinine clearance (CrCl) between 61 and 90 mL/min/1.73 m2 BSA], moderate (CrCl between 31 and 60 mL/min/1.73 m² BSA), and severe (CrCl < 31 mL/min/1.73 m² BSA) renal insuffi ciency, were administered a single iv dose of 0.5, 0.25, or 0.125 mg/kg desirudin, respectively. This resulted in mean dose-normalized effect on the area under the curve (AUC). The AUC increased approximately three- and ninefold for the moderate and severe renally impaired subjects, respectively, compared with healthy individuals. In subjects with mild renal impairment, there was no increase in AUC effect compared with healthy individuals. In subjects with severe renal insuffi ciency, terminal elimination half-lives of desirudin were prolonged up to 12 hours compared with 2–4 hours in normal volunteers or subjects with mild to moderate renal insuffi ciency (desirudin package insert, 2012).

Desirudin was used in a prophylactic dose of 15 mg sc b.i.d. (Eriksson et al., 1997b) without adjustment for renal function (although patients with CrCl <30 mL/min were excluded). Shorr et al. (2012) restratified these patients according to their renal function (Table 14.3). For the "major bleeding" endpoint (which included all perioperative bleeding), 700 patients had normal renal function (351 were treated with the LMWH, enoxaparin, 40 mg sc/day; 349 with desirudin); 758 patients had moderate renal impairment (CrCl, 45–60 mL/min; 365 enoxaparin; 393 desirudin) and 569 patients had more pronounced renal impairment (CrCl, 30–45 mL/min; 294 enoxaparin; 275 desirudin). Table 14.3 shows no significant increase in major bleeding with desirudin compared with enoxaparin.

Because desirudin was administered within 30 minutes before surgery *versus* 12 hours prior to surgery for enoxaparin, a further analysis was conducted to evaluate bleeding during the postoperative period only (beginning 12 hr postop). The "bleeding index" (BI) was calculated for the 1106 patients (555 enoxaparin, 551 desirudin) for whom data were available. As shown in Table 14.3, the postoperative BI was lower for desirudin than for enoxaparin, a result which appears to be driven primarily by differences among patients with greater renal impairment (Shorr et al., 2012).

This is in contrast to current labeling of desirudin in the United States, which recommends reducing the dose of desirudin to 5 mg sc b.i.d. in patients

TABLE 14.3 Major Bleeding and Postoperative Bleeding Index by Renal Function

	CrCl ≥ 60 mL/min		CrCl 45-<60 mL/min		CrCl 30-<45 mL/min		Overall	
	LMWH	Desirudin	LMWH	Desirudin	LMWH	Desirudin	LMWH	Desirudin
Major bleed[a]	0/351 (0%)	2/349 (0.57%)	1/365 (0.27%)	1/393 (0.25%)	1/294 (0.34%)	5/275 (1.82%)	2/1026 (0.19%)	8/1032 (0.78%)
P	0.248		>0.999		0.112		0.109	
Postop BI ≥ 2[b]	24/188 (12.8%)	23/189 (12.2%)	33/197 (16.8%)	25/205 (12.2%)	24/156 (15.4%)	13/147 (8.8%)	84/555 (15.1%)	61/551 (11.1%)
P	0.805		0.205		0.054		0.042	

[a] Frequencies and percentages based on the safety population patients for whom either presence or absence of major bleeding was recorded. (Baseline CrCl was not available for 16 LMWH-treated patients and for 15 desirudin-treated patients, and these are therefore only included in the "overall" column.)
[b] Frequencies and percentages based on operated patients with a valid value for the postoperative bleeding index (BI). The BI was based on the fall in hemoglobin (g/dL) adjusted for red blood transfusions occurring from 12 hr postop (post-operatively) through day 6 inclusive (where day 0 is the day of operation).
Abbreviations: CrCl, creatinine clearance; LMWH, low molecular weight heparin (enoxaparin).
Source: Shorr et al. (2012).

with a CrCl <60 mL/min. Nafziger and Bertino (2010) extracted desirudin plasma concentrations and aPTT data from six studies. Participants with normal renal function or moderate renal impairment (CrCl, 31–60 mL/min) were included in their analysis of pharmacokinetics under different simulation models. After administration of desirudin 15 mg sc every 12 hours to steady state, peak desirudin concentrations were 35 and 47 nmol/L in the normal and moderately impaired renal function groups, respectively. Monte Carlo simulations found median 2-hour C_{max} concentrations of 51.7 nmol/L in normal renal function and 52.4 nmol/L in moderate renal impairment. These authors conclude that dosing of desirudin at 15 mg sc b.i.d. without aPTT monitoring in patients with moderate renal impairment is appropriate and that the dose of 5 mg sc b.i.d. might be too low.

r-Hirudin and Vitamin K Antagonists

Long-term treatment of HIT patients often involves a transition from DTI to oral anticoagulation. Initiation of the transition to vitamin K antagonist (coumarin) therapy should begin only after the platelet count has substantially recovered (preferably, >150 × 10⁹/L), with a minimum of five days of overlapping therapy with an alternative anticoagulant, and with the last two days stably within the target therapeutic range (Warkentin and Greinacher, 2004). In patients with deep vein thrombosis (DVT) associated with acute HIT, the use of vitamin K antagonist can be associated with venous limb gangrene, which typically occurs when this anticoagulant is used alone for treatment of HIT, or when overlapping therapy with DTIs is not managed appropriately, for example, early initiation of coumarin and premature discontinuation of the DTI.

Patients in whom venous limb gangrene occurs typically have an elevated international normalized ratio (INR)—which represents a "surrogate marker" for greatly reduced protein C levels—and thrombocytopenia (surrogate marker for persistent thrombin generation in HIT). Prevention of limb gangrene can be accomplished through careful management of the DTI—warfarin transition, particularly the postponement of coumarin therapy pending substantial platelet count recovery. Patients with suspected coumarin-associated venous limb gangrene should immediately receive vitamin K (e.g., 10 mg iv over 30–60 minutes or 20 mg per os).

In patients who receive vitamin K antagonists before or concomitant with the commencement of lepirudin, this can cause elevated aPTT values (due to coumarin-induced prothrombin level reduction) with the potential for inappropriate lepirudin dose reductions (Warkentin, 2006). Therefore, vitamin K should be given to HIT patients who have received vitamin K antagonists when lepirudin is started (Warkentin and Greinacher, 2004; Greinacher and Warkentin, 2006) (see chap. 12).

Lepirudin

In prospective trials, lepirudin caused minimal prolongation of the prothrombin time (PT) (or INR) once the therapeutic range had been reached. However, Stephens et al. (2005) reported that lepirudin elevates the INR in the absence of warfarin if a thromboplastin with a relatively high international sensitivity index (ISI) of ≥ 2 is used. A systematic laboratory study on the effects of different DTIs on the INR (Warkentin et al., 2005) revealed that the differing effects of the DTIs on PT prolongation are primarily driven by their respective molar plasma concentrations required for clinical effect. DTIs with a relatively low affinity for thrombin (e.g., argatroban) require high plasma concentrations to double the aPTT compared with those with a higher affinity for thrombin (e.g., lepirudin). These higher plasma concentrations, in turn, quench more of the thrombin generated in the PT, thereby prolonging the PT to a greater extent.

In general, the transition from lepirudin to warfarin therapy is usually less complicated than the transition from argatroban (Greinacher et al., 2000) (see chap. 13). Notably, following start of vitamin K antagonist therapy in the prospective lepirudin studies, not a single case of venous limb gangrene occurred.

Desirudin

When given in prophylactic dose of 15 mg sc b.i.d. transition from desirudin to vitamin K antagonists does not differ from the procedure known from prophylactic-dose low molecular weight heparin (LMWH), that is, desirudin is continued until the INR has reached 2.0 with a minimum of a five days overlap (Levy et al., 2009). The effect of desirudin in this low dose on the INR is minimal (Fig. 14.3).

Reversal/Removal of r-Hirudin

Bleeding is an important and potentially severe consequence of hirudin treatment (Antman, 1994; Neuhaus et al., 1994; Frank et al., 1999; Lubenow et al., 2005). As with all DTIs, no specific antidote is available. In a patient with minor bleeding and normal renal function, stopping the drug may be sufficient, since the drug concentration drops quickly. However, when bleeding is life-threatening or the patient has renal failure, cessation alone may not be adequate.

Hemodialysis or hemofiltration can reduce plasma levels of r-hirudin (Riess et al., 1995). However, only some filters are effective, for example, polysulfone F80 (Fresenius, Germany) (Bucha et al., 1999; Frank et al., 1999). Variable efficacy of filters in removing lepirudin could explain conflicting results (Vanholder et al., 1997). Clinical data are limited, and hemofiltration is not always a practical option in emergency situations.

Hirudin overdosage may also be treated pharmacologically by administration of desmopressin (Ibbotson et al., 1991; Butler et al., 1993; Bove et al., 1996), or von Willebrand factor (vWF), or vWF-containing factor VIII concentrates (Dickneite et al., 1996, 1998). Irami and coworkers (1995) described a patient in whom r-hirudin-induced bleeding was treated by the administration of prothrombin complex concentrates, a method previously used in animal models (Diehl et al., 1995). However, since these concentrates can contain heparin, they could be dangerous for a patient with acute HIT. Recombinant factor VIIa is another "panhemostatic" treatment option (Oh et al., 2006). Meizothrombin could also be a potential antidote, but it is not available for use in humans (Nowak and Bucha, 1995).

Clinical Use of r-Hirudin
Lepirudin
Besides its use in patients with HIT, lepirudin has been investigated extensively in controlled clinical trials for acute coronary syndrome (ACS) (n > 14,000), including MI (Antman, 1994; Neuhaus et al., 1994) and unstable angina pectoris (Rupprecht et al., 1995; Organization to Assess Strategies for Ischemic Syndromes [OASIS-2], 1999); and in pilot studies for prophylaxis and treatment of DVT (Parent et al., 1993; Schiele et al., 1997). In patients undergoing hemodialysis (see chap. 18) or cardiac surgery (see chap. 19), there is observational evidence indicating safe and effective use of lepirudin. Results of three prospective clinical trials with lepirudin and an extensive postmarketing drug monitoring study in HIT patients treated in the "real-world" setting are described in the next section.

Desirudin
Desirudin given by sc and iv routes has been extensively assessed in patients requiring thromboprophylaxis after surgery (Eriksson et al., 1996; Eriksson 1997b) with cardiac disease including percutaneous intervention (Serruys et al., 1995) and in the GUSTO IIb trial for acute coronary syndrome (The global use of strategies to open occluded coronary arteries (GUSTO) IIb investigators, 1996; Metz et al., 1998).

CLINICAL STUDIES WITH R-HIRUDIN IN HIT
Desirudin
Desirudin has been assessed in patients with HIT in a prospective, randomized, open-label, exploratory study, the PREVENT-HIT trial, comparing sc desirudin *versus* argatroban in patients with suspected or laboratory-confirmed HIT, with or without thrombosis. Sixteen patients were randomized to treatment with fixed-dose desirudin, 15 mg sc b.i.d. in patients without thrombosis ($n = 7$) and 30 mg sc b.i.d. in patients with thombosis ($n = 1$) or aPTT-adjusted argatroban by iv infusion ($n = 8$) (Frame et al., 2010). The primary efficacy measure was the composite of new or worsening thrombosis (objectively documented), amputation, or death. Other endpoints included major and minor bleeding while on drug therapy, time to platelet count recovery, and pharmacoeconomics. No amputations or deaths occurred. One patient randomized to argatroban had worsening of an existing thrombosis. Major bleeding occurred in two patients on argatroban and in none during desirudin treatment. There was one minor bleed in each treatment group (Boyce et al., 2011). Thus, desirudin might be an option to treat patients suspected to have HIT, especially for bridging the time until results of the HIT antibody test are available in patients with a moderate pretest likelihood for HIT (see chap. 3). The authors also

included pharmacoeconomic analyses and found the average medication cost per course of treatment substantially lower for desirudin compared with argatroban. The numbers of patients enrolled into this study are too small to draw any firm conclusions but desirudin warrants further study as a potentially cost-effective treatment in patients with suspected HIT.

Three Prospective Clinical Trials with Lepirudin: Heparin-Associated Thrombocytopenia-1, -2, and -3

Three prospective studies with lepirudin for HIT were designated heparin-associated thrombocytopenia (HAT)-1, -2, and -3 (Greinacher et al., 1999a,b, 2000; Lubenow and Greinacher, 2002; Lubenow et al., 2005). There was no approved nonheparin alternative anticoagulant during the 3 years in which the HAT studies were conducted (March 1994 to April 1996), and thus for ethical reasons, a placebo control was not appropriate. The HAT studies therefore included comparisons of clinical outcomes with a historical control group treated before lepirudin became available.

A meta-analysis of HAT-1 and -2 was performed to evaluate patients given lepirudin for treatment of HIT with thrombosis (Greinacher et al., 2000). A second meta-analysis of the HAT-1, -2, and -3 studies was performed to evaluate the effects of lepirudin in patients with HIT and isolated thrombocytopenia ("isolated HIT") (Lubenow et al., 2004). In addition, an observational study termed the drug-monitoring program (DMP) was carried out to determine the effects of lepirudin in a large cohort of patients treated in routine clinical settings (Lubenow et al., 2002).

Objectives

The three HAT trials examined whether lepirudin administered iv to patients with serologically confirmed HIT would safely reduce the risk of new arterial or venous thrombosis, limb amputations, and death (composite endpoint). The laboratory objective was to determine whether the drug would allow an increase in the platelet count in thrombocytopenic patients or maintain the baseline platelet values (in non-thrombocytopenic patients), while providing effective anticoagulation. The latter was defined as a prolongation of the aPTT by 1.5- to 2.5-fold over baseline values with no more than two dose increases. (*Note*: If Actin FS or neothromtin reagents were used, the aPTT target range was a 1.5- to 3.0-fold prolongation.)

Patients

Patients were eligible for study if their platelet count fell by more than 50% or to fewer than $100 \times 10^9/L$ or if they exhibited new thrombosis while receiving heparin. A strict criterion for study entry was laboratory confirmation of the clinical diagnosis of HIT by the heparin-induced platelet activation (HIPA) test (Greinacher et al., 1991; Eichler et al., 1999) (see chap. 11).

Clinical outcomes included a composite endpoint (new thrombosis, limb amputation, death) as well as each individual endpoint. Clinical events that occurred between diagnosis and start of treatment with lepirudin were included, as were all clinical events that occurred up to day 14 after stopping lepirudin treatment. Clinical outcomes for lepirudin were compared by Kaplan–Meier time-to-event analysis with a historical control group treated conventionally, beginning at laboratory confirmation of HIT for lepirudin-treated patients and one day after laboratory confirmation for controls.

TABLE 14.4   Patient Characteristics in the HAT Studies

Patient characteristics	All HAT studies $n = 403$	Historical control $(n = 120)^a$	P Value
Age, yr; median (range)	62 (11–90)	67 (19–90)	<0.0001
Male/Female, *n/n*	181/222	41/79	0.037
Field of underlying disease, *n* (%)			<0.0001
Internal medicine	168 (41.7)	41 (34.2)	
Orthopedic surgery	64 (15.9)	38 (31.7)	
Traumatology	30 (7.4)	23 (19.2)	
Cardiovascular surgery	43 (10.7)	9 (7.5)	
Other	98 (24.3)	9 (7.5)	
Median baseline platelet count	79×10^9/L	60×10^9/L	0.030
Patients with TEC during heparin treatment *n* (%)	233/403 (57.8)	80/119 (67.2)	0.066
Type of TEC[b], *n* (%)			0.0821
Venous-distal	127 (54.5)	53 (66.3)	
Venous-proximal	113 (48.5)	23 (28.8)	
Pulmonary embolism	110 (47.2)	35 (43.8)	
Arterial-peripheral	56 (24.0)	17 (21.3)	
Venous other[c]	34 (14.6)	–	

[a]Used for comparison in all HAT-studies.
[b]A patient could have suffered multiple TECs of different types.
[c]Pelvic veins, 11; vena cava, eight; iliac vein, six; subclavian vein, three; portal vein, two; brachiocephalic vein, one; thrombosis leg (unspecified), three.
Abbreviations: HAT, heparin-associated thrombocytopenia; TEC, thromboembolic complication.

Laboratory response was defined as (*i*) the maintenance of an on-treatment aPTT ratio higher than 1.5 in at least 80% of measurements and requiring no more than two dose increases; and (*ii*) an increase in the platelet count to more than 30% from the nadir and to more than 100×10^9/L by day 10 of lepirudin treatment (thrombocytopenic patients), or maintenance of normal platelet counts on days 3 and 10 (nonthrombocytopenic patients). Patient characteristics are given in Table 14.4.

Historical Control Group
The historical control patients (*n* = 120; Table 14.4) also had a diagnosis of HIT confirmed by a positive HIPA test in our laboratory (Greinacher et al., 1999b). They were treated according to hospital protocol with danaparoid (*n* = 36), oral anticoagulants [e.g., phenprocoumon (*n* = 27)], no anticoagulation (*n* = 23), or miscellaneous treatments [e.g., aspirin (*n* = 5), LMWH (*n* = 8), or thrombolytics (*n* = 4)]. Incomplete data for 17 patients in the control group precluded treatment assignment.

HAT-1 Study
The HAT-1 study involved 82 patients with confirmed HIT: 51 patients were assigned to dose regimen A1, five to regimen A2, 18 to regimen B, and eight to regimen C (Tables 14.1, 14.5a, and 14.5b) (Greinacher et al., 1999a). The median duration of treatment was 10 days (range, 3–47 days) for regimen A1, 9 days (7–29 days) for A2, 15 days (2–58 days) for B, and 9 days (3–25 days) for C.

TABLE 14.5a Outcomes from Diagnosis of HIT

Treatment	HAT-1, n = 82					HAT-2, n = 116					HAT-3, n = 205					All HAT-studies, n = 403					Hist. control, n = 120	P^a	Risk reduction%
	A1	A2	B	C	Total	A1	A2	B	C	Total	A1	A2	B	C	Total	A1	A2	B	C	Total			
n =	51	5	18	8	82	65	4	43	4[b,c]	116	98	12	84	10	205	214	21	145	22	403	120	—	—
Death	3	—	3	—	6 (7.3)	8	1	2	—	11 (9.5)	14	2	11	3	30 (14.6)	25	3	16	3	47 (11.2)	21 (17.5)	0.095	36.0
Limb amputation	2	—	2	—	4 (4.9)	4	1	5	—	10 (8.6)	7	—	5	—	12 (5.9)	13	1	12	—	26 (6.5)	8 (6.7)	0.933	3.0
New TEC	3	—	5	—	8 (9.8)	8	1	3	—	12 (10.3)	15	4	9	—	28 (13.7)	26	5	17	—	48 (11.9)	37 (30.8)	<0.0001	61.4
Composite[c]	7	—	8	—	15 (18.3)	17	2	7	—	26 (22.4)	29	6	23	3	61 (29.8)	53	8	38	3	102 (25.3)	53 (44.2)	0.0001	42.8
Major bleeding	7	—	2	2	11 (13.4)	6	1	11	2	20 (17.2)	20	1	12	7	40 (19.5)	33	2	25	11	71 (17.6)	7 (5.8)	0.0015	−67.0

Note: Details of treatment regimens A1, A2, B, and C are given in Table 14.1.

[a] Comparing all patients in the HAT 1–3 studies with the historical control group by categorical analysis.

[b] The four patients receiving regimen C were not reported in the HAT-2 publication.

[c] Composite of death, limb amputation, and new TEC (maximum, one event per patient).

Abbreviations: HAT, heparin-associated thrombocytopenia; TEC, thromboembolic complication.

TABLE 14.5b Outcomes from Start of Treatment

Treatment	HAT-1, n = 82					HAT-2, n = 116					HAT-3, n = 205					All HAT-studies, n = 403					Hist. control, n = 120	$P^a =$	Risk reduction %
n =	A1 51	A2 5	B 18	C 8	Total 82	A1 65	A2 24	B 43	C 4[b]	Total 116	A1 98	A2 12	B 84	C 10	Total 205	A1 214	A2 21	B 145	C 22	Total 403	120		
Death	3	–	3	–	6 (7.3)	8	1	2	–	11 (9.5)	14	2	11	3	30 (14.6)	25	3	16	3	47 (11.2)	21 (17.5)	0.095	36.0
Limb amputation	2	–	1	–	3 (3.7)	4	1	4	–	9 (7.8)	6	–	4	–	10 (4.9)	12	1	9	–	22 (5.5)	8 (6.7)	0.618	17.9
New TEC	3	–	5	–	8 (9.8)	7	1	3	–	11 (9.5)	5	–	6	–	11 (5.4)	15	1	14	–	30 (7.4)	30 (25.0)	<0.0001	70.4
Composite[c]	7	–	8	–	15 (18.3)	16	2	6	–	24 (20.7)	18	2	20	3	43 (21.0)	41	4	34	3	82 (20.3)	52 (43.3)	<0.0001	53.1
Major bleeding	7	–	2	2	11 (13.4)	6	1	11	2	20 (17.2)	20	1	12	7	40 (19.5)	33	2	25	11	71 (17.6)	7 (5.8)	0.0015	–67.0

Note: Details of treatment regimens A1, A2, B, and C are given in Table 14.1.

[a]Comparing all patients in the HAT 1–3 studies with the historical control group by categorical analysis.

[b]The four patients receiving regimen C were not reported in the HAT-2 publication.

[c]Composite of death, limb amputation, and new TEC (maximum, one event per patient).

Abbreviations: HAT, heparin-associated thrombocytopenia; TEC, thromboembolic complication.

HAT-2 Study

The HAT-2 study involved 112 patients with confirmed HIT: 65 patients were assigned to dose regimen A1, four to regimen A2, and 43 to regimen B (Tables 14.5a and 14.5b) (Greinacher et al., 1999b). The overall median duration of treatment was 11 days (range, 0–104 days); for regimen A1, it was 13 days (0–104 days); for A2, 10 days (1–58 days); and for B, eight days (1–67 days).

HAT-3 Study

The third prospective trial, HAT-3, was the largest and involved 205 patients: 98 patients were assigned to dose regimen A1, 12 to regimen A2, and 84 to regimen B (Lubenow et al., 2005). Ten patients received lepirudin for CPB (regimen C), and one received lepirudin by the sc route. Seventeen patients received more than one treatment cycle. For the efficacy parameters only the first treatment cycle was calculated. For safety analysis, especially allergic reactions, all treatment cycles were included.

All 110 patients in treatment groups A1 and A2 had developed at least one thromboembolic complication (TEC) before the start of lepirudin treatment. The ratio of venous:arterial thrombosis in this patient group was 12:1. The median duration of treatment across all treatment arms was 10.0 days: A1, nine days (1–197); A2, 12 days (5–21); B, 10 days (1–47); and C (followed by regimen B post-CPB surgery), seven days (1–37). Mean lepirudin doses were 0.11, 0.08, and 0.07 mg/kg/hr in groups A1, A2, and B, respectively. During the study, phenprocoumon was given to 121 (59%) patients.

Synopsis of HAT-1, -2, and -3

The patient characteristics for all patients enrolled in the HAT studies are given in Table 14.4. Categorical data for the 403 patients from diagnosis of HIT and from start of lepirudin treatment are shown in Tables 14.5a and 14.5b. In all three studies, patients had a highly elevated risk of new TECs in the time period between diagnosis of HIT and start of lepirudin. The risk for a new TEC was decreased by 92.9%—from 5.1% per patient day during the 1.3-day period between diagnosis of HIT and start of lepirudin treatment to 0.4% during active treatment (Fig. 14.5). These data support treatment recommendations that alternative anticoagulation should be started as soon as there is strong clinical suspicion of HIT (Warkentin and Greinacher, 2004).

Bleeding was the most important adverse effect of lepirudin treatment. The overall rate of major bleeding among the 403 patients in the three trials was 17.6% [95% confidence interval (CI): 14.0–21.7%]. However, this included the 22 patients requiring CPB (treatment group C), in whom 11 major bleeds occurred during cardiac surgery. The major bleeding rate was 15.7% if the CPB patients were excluded. In contrast to the efficacy endpoints, all major bleeding episodes occurred during treatment with lepirudin. Five (1.2%) lepirudin-treated patients died from bleeding complications.

There were no major differences in bleeding rates between younger (<65 years of age) and older (≥65 years) patients ($P = 0.520$), or between female and male patients ($P = 0.150$). However, renal impairment was associated with an increased rate of bleeding, when comparing patients with serum creatinine values above and below 90 μmol/L ($P < 0.001$).

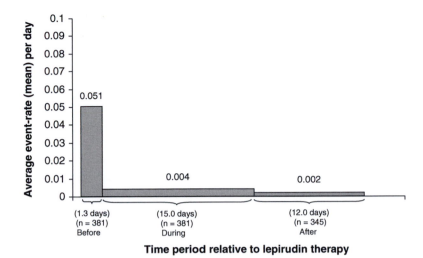

FIGURE 14.5 Average rate of new thromboembolic complications per day in the HAT-1,-2, -3 studies ($n = 381$ patients). The bar width indicates the mean duration of the observation period (days) and is shown for three time periods: before, during, and after lepirudin therapy. The high average event rate [0.051 (5.1%) event per day during a mean period of 1.3 days] from diagnosis of HIT until start of lepirudin therapy indicates that cessation of heparin alone is insufficient to prevent HIT-associated thrombosis, thus warranting treatment with an alternative anticoagulant if HIT is strongly suspected. *Abbreviations*: HAT, heparin-associated thrombocytopenia; HIT, heparin-induced thrombocytopenia. *Source*: From Lubenow et al. (2005).

Antihirudin antibodies were present in 30% of patients at the end of the first treatment cycle and in 70% of reexposed patients. In the three studies, 17 patients (4.2%) experienced allergic reactions. In nine of these, a potential relationship to lepirudin was considered plausible; antihirudin antibodies were detected in five of these nine patients. One of these patients required discontinuation of study drug. No anaphylactic reactions were observed.

Comparison with Historical Control Group
A comparison of the composite and individual efficacy endpoints, as well as the major bleeding endpoint, for the lepirudin and control patients groups (categorical data), was performed from time of HIT diagnosis to end-of-observation period (Table 14.5a), as well as from time of start of treatment (Table 14.5b). (The latter time frame was also used for the analysis of the argatroban treatment studies; see chap. 13). No patients were excluded from the categorical analysis.

The composite and single endpoints were also compared with the historical controls from start of treatment using time-to-event analyses (Fig. 14.6). The composite endpoint occurred less often in the lepirudin-treated patients as compared with controls ($P = 0.04$), primarily due to a reduction in new thrombotic events ($P < 0.001$), whereas the risk for limb amputation ($P = 0.79$) and death ($P = 0.43$) did not differ significantly (however, the studies were not powered to detect differences in these endpoints). However, the risk for major bleeding was increased in the lepirudin-treated patients ($P = 0.015$), even when the 22 patients who underwent

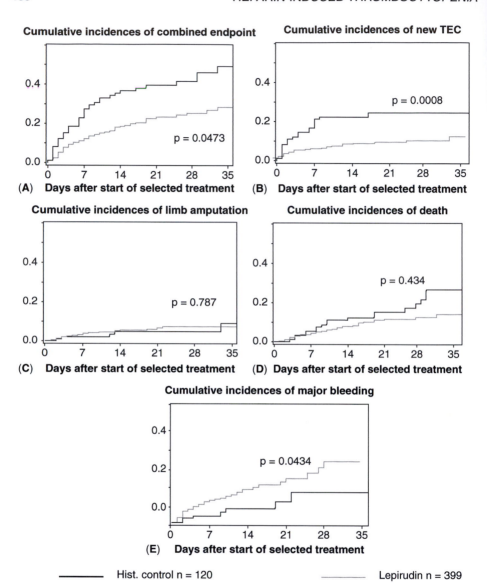

FIGURE 14.6 Time-to-event analyses of efficacy and safety endpoints in the HAT-1, -2, and -3 studies (combined) in comparison with the historical control group. (**A**) Composite endpoint (new thromboembolic complication, limb amputation, or death); (**B**) new thromboembolic complication; (**C**) limb amputation; (**D**) death; and (**E**) major bleeding. *Abbreviation*: HAT, heparin-associated thrombocytopenia. *Source*: From Lubenow et al. (2005).

CPB were excluded. Furthermore, 42 patients (11 from HAT-1, 17 from HAT-2, and 14 from HAT-3) were excluded from the time-to-event comparison because the date of HIT confirmation was >21 days before start of treatment ($n = 29$), or because of missing HIT confirmation date or missing date of stopping of lepirudin therapy ($n = 13$).

TABLE 14.6 Incidences of Composite and Individual Clinical Endpoints in the HAT Studies and the Drug-Monitoring Program

Study and endpoint[a]	Observation period	Lepirudin (%)[b]	Historical control (%)[b]	P Value (Categorical analysis)	P Value (Time to event analysis)	Risk reduction (%)
HIT with thrombosis	Start of treatment to d 35	N = 235	N = 75			
HAT-1, -2, -3						
Composite	–	19.1	40.0	0.002	0.518	52.3
New thrombosis	–	6.8	25.3	0.001	<0.001	73.1
Limb amputation	–	5.5	8.0	0.438	0.458	31.3
Death	–	11.9	12.0	0.984	0.166	0.8
HIT with thrombosis, DMP (Lubenow et al., 2002)	Start to end of Lepirudin treatment	N = 496				
Composite	–	21.9	–	–	–	
New thrombosis	–	5.2	–	–	–	–
Limb amputation	–	5.8	–	–	–	–
Death	–	10.9	–	–	–	–
Isolated HIT, HAT-1, -2, -3 (Lubenow et al., 2004)	Start of treatment to d 35	N = 91	N = 47			
Composite	–	19.8	29.8	0.187	0.028	33.6
New thrombosis	–	4.4	14.9	0.045	0.020	70.5
Limb amputation	–	3.3	0	0.551	0.242	–
Death	–	14.3	21.3	0.296	0.094	32.9
Isolated HIT, DMP (Lubenow et al., 2002)	Start to end of Lepirudin treatment	N = 612				
Composite	–	15.7	–	–	–	–
New thrombosis	–	2.1	–	–	–	–
Limb amputation	–	1.3	–	–	–	–
Death	–	12.3	–	–	–	–

[a]Each patient could contribute only once to the composite endpoint (any one of the individual endpoints of new thrombosis, limb amputation, or death).
[b]Number of patients eligible for comparison.
Abbreviations: d, day; DMP, drug-monitoring program; HAT, heparin-associated thrombocytopenia; HIT, heparin-induced thrombocytopenia

Meta-Analysis of HAT-1, -2, and -3: Patients with HIT and Thrombosis

Table 14.6 summarizes the results of a meta-analysis of the three HAT studies performed to determine the efficacy and safety of lepirudin in 235 patients with HIT complicated by thrombosis. As in the HAT-1, -2, and -3 studies, the risk for new thrombotic complications (per day) was highest between diagnosis of HIT and start of treatment: 26.2% of all such events occurred during this pretreatment period.

Efficacy Outcomes

When outcomes were assessed from the start of lepirudin treatment, the combined endpoint for new thrombosis, limb amputation, and death was significantly lower in the lepirudin-treated patients (n = 235) than in the controls (n = 75) (19.1% *vs* 40.0%; P = 0.002). This difference was primarily due to a reduction in the number of new thrombosis (6.8% *vs* 25.3%; P = 0.001). Incidences of limb amputation (5.5% *vs* 8.0%; P = 0.44) and death (11.9% *vs* 12.0%; P = 0.98) did not differ between the lepirudin group and the historical controls (Table 14.6).

Safety Outcomes

The cumulative incidence of major bleeding was higher in the lepirudin group than in the control group (14.9% *vs* 6.7%; P = 0.064). The mean treatment duration was 14.2 days corresponding to a risk for major bleeding of 1.05% per patient day.

In a previous meta-analysis of HAT-1 and -2 patients (Greinacher et al., 2000), one of the more important points to emerge was the relationship of aPTT ratios with lepirudin safety and efficacy. For low aPTT ratios (<1.5), the incidence of the combined endpoint was not significantly reduced compared with the control (RR = 0.86; 95% CI, 0.38–1.94; P = 0.72). In addition, the risk of bleeding was not significantly greater in the lepirudin group than in the control group (RR = 1.57; 95% CI, 0.52–4.72; P = 0.42). At medium aPTT ratios (1.5–2.5), efficacy was significantly greater for the lepirudin-treated patients than for the controls (RR = 0.42; 95% CI, 0.22–0.80; P = 0.009), but there was also an increased risk of bleeding (RR = 3.21; 95% CI, 1.72–6.02; P = 0.0003). At higher aPTT ratios (>2.5), the efficacy of lepirudin was not enhanced compared with medium aPTT ratios (RR = 0.70; 95% CI, 0.21–2.32; P = 0.56). However, there was a marked increase in bleedings with high aPTT ratios (RR = 6.03; 95% CI, 2.34–15.54; P = 0.0002).

Meta-Analysis of HAT-1, -2, and -3: Patients with Isolated HIT

Each of the HAT trials examined the effects of lepirudin in patients with HIT and isolated thrombocytopenia and in HIT patients with thrombosis. The meta-analysis of HAT-1 and -2 showed that lepirudin was effective in patients with HIT plus thrombosis (Greinacher et al., 2000). In a meta-analysis of HAT-1, -2, and -3, the safety and efficacy of lepirudin in patients with HIT in the absence of known thrombosis was demonstrated (Lubenow et al., 2004). This meta-analysis included 91 patients treated according to dosing regimen B; of these, 20 had a history of HIT (*not* acute HIT). Patients with recent thrombosis at baseline were excluded from this analysis. Mean duration of treatment was 11.0 days (range, 1–68 days). The mean steady state dose was 0.062 ± 0.037 mg/kg/hr.

Efficacy Outcomes

Of the 91 patients in this study during treatment with lepirudin, four (4.4%) experienced new thromboses, three (3.3%) underwent limb amputation, and 13 (14.3%) deaths occurred. Most of the deaths were related to underlying disease, not to HIT or treatment with lepirudin. Since patients were counted only once if multiple events occurred, the incidence of the composite endpoint was 18/91 (19.8%) (Table 14.6). The median platelet count rebounded to 150×10^9/L within four days of beginning lepirudin treatment.

Safety Outcomes

Episodes of major bleeding occurred in 13/91 (14.3%) of patients in this meta-analysis (risk for major bleeding per treatment day 1.3%). aPTT ratios above 2.5 were associated with an increased risk of bleeding, and bleeding rates were significantly lower in patients with aPTT <60 seconds ($P < 0.001$). Nearly all patients with bleeding complications had impaired renal function. Antihirudin antibodies were detected in 26 of the 66 (39.4%) evaluable patients. There were no differences in adverse events or outcomes between patients with and without antihirudin antibodies. No anaphylaxis was observed.

Postmarketing Drug Monitoring Program

Results from 1329 patients treated with lepirudin in a DMP are reported (Lubenow et al., 2002): 496 patients had HIT and thrombosis and 612 patients had isolated HIT. This postmarketing study evaluated the same clinical endpoints as were used in HAT-1, -2, and -3. In this DMP, lepirudin could be started immediately upon clinical diagnosis of HIT, thus avoiding the inherent delay awaiting laboratory confirmation. A total of 382 (77.0%) of the 496 patients with HIT and thrombosis were positive in the HIPA test, whereas 406 (66.3%) of the 612 patients with isolated HIT were positive in the HIPA test.

Efficacy Outcomes

In the routine clinical settings of the DMP, lepirudin-treated patients with isolated HIT and HIT with thrombosis had the lowest incidence of all clinical endpoints reported with any agent. The incidence of the combined clinical endpoint in the 496 patients with HIT and thrombosis was 21.9%: 26 patients (5.2%) experienced new thrombosis, 29 (5.8%) underwent limb amputation, and 54 patients (10.9%) died. The most common cause of death was multiorgan failure [23/54 patients (42.6%)], emphasizing the serious underlying medical condition of these patients. The incidence of new thrombosis in this study (5.2%) was lower than that observed in the HAT-1 and -2 meta-analysis (10.1%). This may be because of physicians' increased clinical experience with lepirudin, as illustrated by the decision to begin lepirudin treatment immediately upon clinical diagnosis of HIT, thereby improving efficacy and safety outcomes.

The combined endpoint of new thrombosis, limb amputation, and death occurred in 96 (15.7%) of the 612 patients with isolated HIT; 13 patients (2.1%) experienced new thrombosis, eight (1.3%) underwent limb amputation, and 75 patients (12.3%) died. As seen in the group of patients with HIT plus thrombosis, the largest cause of death in this group was multiorgan failure (39/75 patients, 52.0%).

The overall mortality rate due to new thrombosis in the group of 1108 patients treated with regimen A1 or B (thus, excluding patients receiving "miscellaneous" treatments) (Table 14.6) was low (15 patients, or 1.4%). Efficacy variables in the DMP were even more favorable than those seen in the meta-analyses of the HAT studies. This DMP thus confirms the efficacy of lepirudin in routine clinical practice for both the prophylaxis and the treatment of thromboembolism in patients with HIT.

There were no differences in the mean infusion rates in patients with HIT and thrombosis (0.12 mg/kg/hr) and those with isolated HIT (0.11 mg/kg/hr) in the DMP. As lepirudin dose is adjusted based on aPTT, the major difference between the two regimens is the initial bolus in HIT patients with acute thrombosis. However, as discussed earlier, in the view of the author the bolus should be avoided in most situations to prevent overdosing.

Safety Outcomes

In the DMP, the incidence of bleeding was greatly decreased when compared with the HAT clinical trials. In the group of 496 patients with HIT plus thrombosis, there were 27 (5.4%) major bleeding episodes, and among the 612 patients with isolated HIT, 36 (5.9%) had major bleeding. Allergic reactions were reported in four (0.8%) patients in the HIT plus thrombosis group and in one (0.2%) patient with isolated HIT. No anaphylaxis was reported.

The decreased incidence of bleeding events in the DMP can most likely be attributed to physicians' greater experience with administering lepirudin and monitoring its effects.

Experience with Lepirudin in a Large Case Series in France

Tardy and colleagues (2006) reported a retrospective observational analysis involving 181 patients (median age, 67 years) with HIT, in whom the diagnosis was confirmed in 89.5% by a laboratory assay. The mean treatment dose was only $0.06 \pm 0.04 \, \text{mg/kg/hr}$, which was much less than the approved dose ($0.15 \, \text{mg/kg/hr}$), as well as the mean doses given in the HAT studies ($0.11 \, \text{mg/kg/hr}$ for HIT with thrombosis and $0.07 \, \text{mg/kg/hr}$ for isolated thrombocytopenia). In the HAT 1–3 studies the rate of new thrombosis was 7.4%, whereas it was somewhat greater (13.8%) in the French cohort. The rate of major bleeding, however, was similar in both the studies: 20.4% in the French cohort and 17.6% in HAT 1–3 (although a somewhat broader definition of major bleeding was used in the French study). As in the HAT studies, Tardy et al. also found that moderate to severe impairment of renal function strongly enhanced bleeding risk ($P < 0.001$). They also found that prolonged treatment with lepirudin and a mean dose exceeding $0.07 \, \text{mg/kg/hr}$ were independent risk factors for bleeding. In the context of the HAT 1–3 studies, this is further evidence that the approved dose for lepirudin is too high and that especially in elderly patients, initial lepirudin dosing should be reduced to 0.05–$0.10 \, \text{mg/kg/hr}$ iv. In patients with known impairment of renal function, dosing should be reduced even further (Table 14.2).

Comparison with Other Treatments for HIT

Mortality rates in patients with HIT remained at approximately 20–30% for more than a decade (King and Kelton, 1984; AbuRahma et al., 1991; Warkentin and Kelton, 1996; Nand et al., 1997). Notably, these rates are two to three times higher than those observed in the HAT studies. In addition to lepirudin, other drugs with anti-thrombin activity (e.g., argatroban) or antifactor Xa activity (e.g., danaparoid, fondaparinux) may be appropriate for management of HIT (see chaps. 14–16).

Comparisons of the various clinical trials of agents used to treat HIT need to be interpreted with caution, because there have been no direct comparative trials and the studies employed different designs. Trials of lepirudin and argatroban, however, utilized similar clinical endpoints and historical controls for comparison. The most obvious differences between the lepirudin and the argatroban trials are (*i*) the need for laboratory confirmation of HIT in the lepirudin trials; (*ii*) treatment duration, which was consistently longer than 10 days in the lepirudin-treated patients but less than seven days in the argatroban-treated patients (potential to increase apparent efficacy and also bleeding with lepirudin); (*iii*) the observation period, which started at the time of diagnosis in lepirudin-treated patients compared with the time of treatment initiation in the argatroban trials (potential to underestimate the efficacy of lepirudin); and (*iv*) a considerable proportion of patients in the historical control group of the HAT trials had been treated with danaparoid (potential to underestimate the efficacy of lepirudin). To allow a more direct comparison, we reanalyzed the data of the HAT trials as per the argatroban trials, that is, analyzing those events occurring from start of active treatment only (Tables 14.5b and 14.6).

The rates for the combined endpoint were consistently lower in the lepirudin trials than in the two argatroban studies. For patients with isolated HIT, the composite event rate was 19.8% in the HAT-1, -2, and -3 meta-analysis (Lubenow et al., 2004), compared with 25.6% and 28.0% in the two argatroban trials. For patients with HIT and thrombosis, the combined endpoint occurred in 19.1% (meta-analysis) with lepirudin (Lubenow et al., 2005), and in 43.8% and 41.5% of patients treated in the two argatroban trials.

Because of the often critical condition of the patient population under study, the rate of deaths observed for both DTIs is not likely to be solely attributable to treatment failure and may vary considerably with different patient populations. As the argatroban trials included many patients who most likely did not have HIT, the death rate associated with HIT might have been overestimated, as non-HIT patients with a decrease of platelet count are often very sick (e.g., septicemia, DIC). Death rates were 14.3% (meta-analysis) and 12.3% (DMP) for patients with isolated HIT treated with lepirudin, but 18.1% and 23.1% in those treated in the two argatroban trials. In patients with HIT complicated by thrombosis, death rates with lepirudin were 11.9% (meta-analysis) and 10.9% (DMP), compared with 18.0% and 23.1% in the argatroban trials.

Among patients with isolated HIT, limb amputation occurred in 3.3% (meta-analysis) and 1.3% (DMP) when treated with lepirudin, and in 1.9% and 4.2% of those treated with argatroban. The amputation rates were higher in HIT with thrombosis; 5.5% (meta-analysis) and 5.8% (DMP) in those treated with lepirudin, *versus* 11.1% and 14.8% in those treated with argatroban.

There was also a difference in the incidences of new thrombosis, which is arguably the most important parameter for assessing efficacy of an alternative anticoagulant in HIT. In those with isolated HIT, it was 4.4% (meta-analysis) and 2.1% (DMP) with lepirudin, and 6.9% and 5.8% in those treated with argatroban. In HIT with thrombosis it was 6.8% (meta-analysis) and 5.2% (DMP) for lepirudin, and 14.6% and 13.1% for argatroban-treated patients.

The risk of major bleeding between lepirudin and argatroban appears similar if treatment duration is taken into account. In the lepirudin trials, 17.6% of patients experienced major bleeding (Table 14.5b) over a mean treatment period of 15 days, that is, a risk for major bleeding of 1.17% per treatment day. In the argatroban trials, major bleeding occurred in 6.9% (Arg-911) and 5.7% (Arg-915) with a mean treatment period of six days in both trials, that is, a risk for major bleeding of 1.05% per treatment day.

Similar rates of efficacy and safety for the two drugs were also observed in a retrospective chart analysis enrolling 61 lepirudin-treated and 29 argatroban-treated

HIT patients in a single center (Smythe et al., 2005). Effective anticoagulation was achieved in 77.8% of argatroban patients and 69.5% of lepirudin patients ($P = 0.61$). Major bleeding occurred in 10.3% and 11.5% of argatroban and lepirudin patients, respectively ($P = 1.0$).

Because there are no prospective data comparing lepirudin and danaparoid for treatment of HIT, we retrospectively compared 126 danaparoid-treated patients with 175 lepirudin-treated patients who fulfilled the same inclusion and exclusion criteria (Farner et al., 2001). In the patients with HIT without TECs at baseline, a time-to-event analysis showed that the cumulative risk of the combined endpoint was higher in danaparoid-treated patients than in the lepirudin-treated patients [$P = 0.02$ by log rank test; hazard ratio (HR) = 2.9 (95% CI, 1.1–7.6); $P = 0.027$]. This was due primarily to an increased incidence of new TECs [20% (95% CI, 8.4–36.9) for danaparoid vs 6.3% (95% CI, 1.3–17.2) for lepirudin; $P = 0.087$]. Of note, patients with isolated HIT usually received only prophylactic-dose danaparoid. In contrast, HIT patients with thrombosis at baseline, and who were therefore treated with a therapeutic-dose regimen of danaparoid, had a similar outcome as patients receiving lepirudin ($P = 0.913$). However, the risk for major bleeding was lower in the danaparoid-treated group ($P = 0.012$) (Farner et al., 2001).

The major conclusions of these comparisons are (i) HIT patients seem to benefit from a longer treatment period with an alternative anticoagulant, with 10 days better than five days; and (ii) the prophylactic-dose regimen of danaparoid (750 U sc two or three times daily) approved in the European Union for HIT with isolated thrombocytopenia appears to be suboptimal. Thus, patients with acute HIT require anticoagulation generally in therapeutic doses (see also chap. 12).

More recently, fondaparinux has been used in case series for treatment of HIT (see chaps. 12 and 17). Two retrospective studies have compared outcomes between lepirudin and fondaparinux (Lobo et al., 2008; Al-Rossaies et al., 2011). Overall, the outcome of fondaparinux-treated HIT patients seems to be as least as good as the outcome of lepirudin-treated HIT patients. In particular, the rate of major bleeding seems to be less with fondaparinux (Greinacher, 2011). In a retrospective study on patients with suspected HIT (i.e., a confirmed fall in the platelet count to <100 × 10^9/L or a 50% reduction from baseline, four or more days after starting heparin therapy, with exclusion of other causes of thrombocytopenia) and a positive immunoassay test, five patients treated with fondaparinux had a similar time for platelets recovery as the lepirudin-treated patients (Al-Rossaies et al., 2011).

Antibody Formation

Because hirudin is a protein obtained from a nonhuman species, it can induce antibody formation in humans. Antibodies are induced by both iv therapeutic-dose and sc prophylactic-dose use (Greinacher et al., 2003a). Antihirudin antibodies have been detected in 44–74% of patients treated with lepirudin (Huhle et al., 1998; Song et al., 1999; Eichler et al., 2000). Of 196 HIT patients treated with lepirudin for five or more days, 44% developed antihirudin antibodies of the IgG class (Eichler et al., 2000). Reexposed patients developed antibodies in about 70% of cases (Lubenow et al., 2005). These antibodies were not associated with an increase in thrombin–antithrombin (TAT) complexes (Fig. 14.7). Antibody formation occurred as early as day 4 and peaked at days 8–9 (Eichler et al., 2000).

Antilepirudin antibodies can extend the half-life of lepirudin (Liebe et al., 2002; Linnemann et al., 2010), most likely by reduced renal filtration of

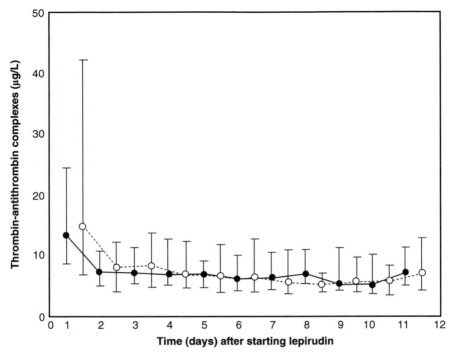

FIGURE 14.7 TAT complex concentrations in relation to antihirudin antibody formation. TAT complex concentrations did not differ between antihirudin antibody-positive (●, solid lines) and antihirudin antibody-negative (O, dotted lines) patients (median and 25% and 75% quartiles are given). *Abbreviation:* TAT, thrombin–antithrombin.

lepirudin–antilepirudin complexes (Fig. 14.8); in about 2–3% of patients with antilepirudin antibodies, an inhibitory effect is seen (Huhle et al., 2001; Fischer et al., 2003). The biologic effects of antilepirudin antibodies on anticoagulation can be easily compensated by changes in the lepirudin dose. Thus, ongoing daily aPTT measurements are recommended during lepirudin treatment, even when stable anticoagulation has been observed during the first five days.

Incidence of likelihood of antibody formation did not differ between lepirudin given in therapeutic dose and desirudin given in prophylactic dose (Greinacher et al., 2003a). Of 112 patients enrolled in a dose-finding study with sc desirudin following orthopedic hip surgery at 10 mg b.i.d. ($n = 17$), 15 mg b.i.d. ($n = 75$), and 20 mg b.i.d. ($n = 20$), 11 (9.8%) developed antihirudin antibodies independently of the dose. The rate of immunization did not differ from that observed in HIT patients treated with lepirudin ($P = 0.113$). Plasma concentrations of desirudin did not differ between antihirudin antibody-positive and -negative patients. Antihirudin antibodies had no impact on incidences of DVT and/or pulmonary embolism, allergic reactions, and hemorrhage. As the total number of immunized patients was low, adverse effects of antihirudin antibodies induced by desirudin cannot be excluded.

A subanalysis of the DESIRABLE trial found an antibody response rate to desirudin in 19/245 patients (7.7%) (Hamilton et al., 2012). However, the analysis

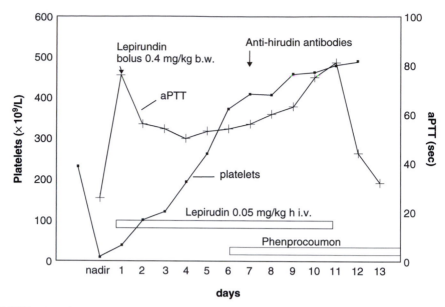

FIGURE 14.8 A 53-year-old woman was admitted to the hospital because of an ankle fracture. She received LMWH for 10 days, but was switched to unfractionated heparin because of a distal DVT. Ten days later she presented with proximal DVT, pulmonary embolism, and a rapid fall in platelet count from more than 200 to 12 × 10⁹/L. She was switched to iv lepirudin (schedule A1). After normalization of platelet counts, she received overlapping oral anticoagulation (phenprocoumon), with lepirudin stopped when the INR reached 2.0. Antihirudin antibodies were first detected on day 7; at the same time, the aPTT increased despite a stable hirudin dosage of 0.05 mg/kg b.w./hr. *Abbreviations*: aPTT, activated partial thromboplastin time; b.w., body weight; DVT, deep vein thrombosis; iv, intravenous; INR, international normalized ratio; LMWH, low molecular weight heparin.

was performed after five days of treatment, i.e., a time period during which antibody levels just start to rise.

Allergic Reactions

Lepirudin administration during prospective studies in patients with HIT was associated with a low incidence of allergic events, as well as during the much larger clinical trials in patients with ACS. Among the adverse events reported were eczema, rash, pruritus, hot flushes, fever, chills, urticaria, bronchospasm, cough, stridor, dyspnea, angioedema (face, tongue, larynx), and injection-site reactions. Any causal relationship of lepirudin to these adverse events is unclear.

Of 35,000–60,000 patients treated with lepirudin, nine patients were judged to have had severe anaphylaxis in close temporal association with lepirudin use (Greinacher et al., 2003b). All reactions occurred within minutes of iv bolus lepirudin administration, with four fatal outcomes (three acute cardiorespiratory arrests, one hypotension-induced MI). In these four cases, a previous uneventful treatment course with lepirudin was identified (1–12 weeks earlier). In an additional patient with nonfatal anaphylaxis (who did not receive a bolus), we found high-titer IgG antilepirudin antibodies. Since lepirudin had been used in approximately 35,000 patients, the risk of anaphylaxis was estimated at 0.015% (5/32,500) in first-exposure and 0.16% (4/2500) in reexposed patients (assuming 7.5% reexposure frequency). One other case has been reported with recurrent anaphylaxis during reexposure (Badger et al., 2004). We and others (Bircher et al., 1996) demonstrated high-titer antihirudin antibodies of the IgG class, but not of the IgE class in patients with hirudin-associated anaphylaxis. IgG-dependent anaphylaxis likely is Fc receptor-mediated and related to infusion dose. Thus, besides reducing bleeding risk, avoiding iv bolus administration of r-hirudin should also reduce the risk of severe anaphylactic reactions. There are two patients reported with delayed reactions to hirudin. One patient developed eczematous plaques accompanied by a positive lymphocyte transformation test (Zollner et al., 1996), the other had a granulomatous reaction (Smith et al., 2001). A third patient produced an Arthus-like reaction after intradermal application of lepirudin (Jappe et al., 2002). Approaches to test for these reactions are reviewed in Bircher et al. (2006).

R-HIRUDIN TREATMENT IN OTHER CLINICAL SETTINGS
ACS and Percutaneous Coronary Intervention
Due to their ability to inhibit clot-bound thrombin, DTIs have also been investigated as anticoagulants for ACS and percutaneous coronary intervention (PCI).

Desirudin
Angioplasty in Unstable Angina Patients
In the HELVETICA trial (Serruys et al., 1995), unfractionated heparin (UFH) was compared with desirudin in the prevention of restenosis after percutaneous transluminal coronary angioplasty in patients with unstable angina. A total of 1141 patients were randomly assigned to one of three treatment groups: (*i*) iv and sc desirudin (bolus of 40 mg followed by continuous infusion of 0.2 mg/kg/hr for 24 hours and 40 mg of desirudin sc b.i.d. for three consecutive days, $n = 378$); (*ii*) iv desirudin (bolus of 40 mg followed by continuous infusion of 0.2 mg/kg/hr for 24 hours, plus placebo sc b.i.d. for three consecutive days, $n = 381$); or (*iii*) iv UFH bolus of 10,000 IU followed by continuous infusion of 15 IU/kg for 24 hr plus placebo sc b.i.d. for three consecutive days, $n = 382$). After seven months of follow-up, no difference was observed among the treatment groups in the number of patients reaching the primary endpoint. However, desirudin therapy was associated with a significant reduction in early cardiac events at 96 hours (5.6% for iv and sc desirudin; 7.9% for iv desirudin; and 11.0% for UFH; combined desirudin *vs* UFH, $P = 0.023$). No differences in major or minor bleeding were observed among the three treatment groups.

ACS and ST-elevation MI
The Global Use of Strategies to Open Occluded Coronary Arteries (GUSTO-IIb) study (1996) enrolled 12,142 patients with ACS, who were stratified into two groups based on the presence ($n = 4131$) or absence ($n = 8011$) of ST-segment elevation at baseline. Study drugs were administered for three to five days: UFH, 5000 U bolus followed by 1000 U/hr ($n = 6073$) or desirudin, 0.1 mg bolus followed by 0.1 mg/kg/hr ($n = 6069$). There was no significant difference in the primary endpoint at 30 days in patients with or without ST-segment elevation

[9.8% of the UFH group *vs* 8.9% of the hirudin group; odds ratio (OR) 0.89, 95% confidence interval (CI) 0.79–1.00; $P = 0.06$], but also no increase in severe bleeding (1.2% *vs* 1.1%, $P = 0.49$) but an increase in moderate bleeding (8.8% *vs* 7.7%, $P = 0.03$).

Lepirudin
ACS and ST-elevation MI
Lepirudin was examined in large numbers of patients with unstable angina or suspected acute MI without ST segment elevation in the OASIS-1 (OASIS Investigators, 1997) ($n = 909$) and OASIS-2 ($n = 10,141$) trials (OASIS Investigators, 1999). These trials concluded that lepirudin is superior to heparin in preventing ischemic outcomes. A meta-analysis of 11 ACS trials involving over 35,000 patients revealed a 15% reduction in death or MI when bivalent DTIs (lepirudin or bivalirudin) were used to treat ACS patients, compared with heparin (Direct Thrombin Inhibitors Trialists' Collaborative Group, 2002). A retrospective subset analysis of the OASIS-2 trial examined the benefit of lepirudin in 117 ACS patients undergoing PCI within the first 72 hours (Mehta et al., 2002). Lepirudin was superior to heparin in reducing the risk of death or MI at 96 hours ($P = 0.036$) and 35 days ($P = 0.02$). Based on this evidence, lepirudin should be considered a treatment option in ACS patients with HIT.

Thrombosis Prophylaxis
Postorthopedic Surgery
The pivotal trials, which led to the approval of desirudin for thrombosis prophylaxis after major orthopedic joint replacement surgery, compared desirudin with UFH (5000 IU t.i.d.) (Eriksson et al., 1996; Eriksson et al., 1997a) or desirudin 15 mg b.i.d. with enoxaparin 40 mg once daily (Eriksson et al., 1997b). The duration of treatment was 8–12 days. In the first study, patients were randomly allocated to receive by sc injection either 10, 15, or 20 mg of desirudin b.i.d. or 5000 IU of UFH t.i.d. Thrombosis was reduced in desirudin-treated patients. It was 34.2% in the UFH group as compared with 23.9% ($P = 0.0113$), 18.4% ($P = 0.0003$), and 17.7% ($P = 0.0001$) in the 10, 15, and 20 mg desirudin groups, respectively. The frequency of proximal thrombosis was 19.6% in the UFH group as compared with 8.5% ($P < 0.001$), 3.1% ($P < 0.001$), and 2.4% ($P < 0.001$) in the 10, 15, and 20 mg desirudin groups, respectively.

In the second trial, 220 patients received heparin, and 225 desirudin. A per-protocol analysis of efficacy was performed for the 351 patients (79%). The prevalence of confirmed DVT was 13/174 (7%) desirudin-treated patients and 41/177 (23%) heparin treated patients ($P < 0.0001$). Also the prevalence of proximal DVT was reduced by desirudin (3% *vs* 16%; $P < 0.0001$) There was no significant difference between the treatment groups with respect to bleeding variables or bleeding complications.

In the third study (Eriksson et al., 1997b), 2079 eligible patients were randomly assigned to receive desirudin or enoxaparin. A total of 1587 patients were included in the primary analysis of efficacy. Desirudin-treated patients showed fewer proximal DVT compared with enoxaparin-treated patients (4.5% *vs* 7.5%, $P = 0.01$) and a lower overall rate of DVT (18.4 *vs* 25.5%, $P = 0.001$), with similar major bleedings in the two treatment groups.

In the desirudin postmarketing registry, Europe (DESIRE Registry) (Puente et al., 2011), 603 patients undergoing major orthopedic surgery were enrolled of whom 581 were analyzed. All patients received desirudin 15 mg b.i.d. Three hundred and three (52.2%) patients underwent hip replacement, 196 (33.7%) total knee replacement, 39 (6.7%) hip fracture repair, and 43 (7.4%) other types of surgery (e.g., spinal or trauma). Desirudin was given prior to surgery in 50.3% of the patients and after surgery in 48.8% of the patients. In this registry 14 patients had clinical HIT (six were confirmed with serology) and 37 a history of HIT. Of the patients with clinical HIT, none died or experienced a thrombotic event; there was one reported major bleeding event, but cessation of desirudin treatment was not required. Of the patients with a history of HIT, one patient developed DVT after receiving the first dose of desirudin, and six patients experienced major bleeding. Desirudin was not discontinued in any of these cases. The incidence of bleeding was low in the overall population and in the subgroup of patients with HIT. However, interpretation of the results is limited by the observational nature of the study.

Postcardiac Surgery

Twenty-eight patients undergoing elective coronary artery bypass graft (CABG) surgery who were positive for anti-PF4/heparin antibodies at baseline but had no clinical evidence of HIT, were treated with desirudin 15 mg b.i.d. preoperatively and/or postoperatively for thrombosis prophylaxis, while bivalirudin was used for anticoagulation during surgery. Eighteen patients received desirudin preoperatively and 24 patients were treated postoperatively (started within 12 hours after surgery in three patients, within 12–24 hours in eight patients, and longer than 24 hours after surgery in seven patients). One thrombotic event occurred about 30 days after the last dose of desirudin. No major bleeding events and no cases of clinical HIT were reported after surgery (Levy and Koster, 2011).

Intensive Care Unit Patients

In the DESIRABLE trial (Levy et al., 2011; Bergese et al., 2012), 516 critically ill patients received desirudin 15 mg sc b.i.d.. Patients with uncontrolled bleeding were excluded. The primary endpoint was major bleeding; secondary endpoints included new symptomatic thrombosis. Ninety-three patients had a platelet count $<150 \times 10^9$/L among whom 50 (54%) had a platelet count $<100 \times 10^9$/L. HIT was suspected in 27 (29%) of the thrombocytopenic patients but was not confirmed by platelet activation assay. No patient had clinical evidence of thrombosis at enrollment. The incidence of new VTE was 2 (2.2%) in patients with thrombocytopenia compared with six in the 423 non-thrombocytopenic patients (1.4%, P = NS). There were no bleeding events meeting criteria for the primary endpoint in either group. Serious adverse events occurred in 16 (17%) of the thrombocytopenic patients, all considered unrelated to the study drug. Serious adverse events were reported in 64 (15%) of the nonthrombocytopenic patients, five of which were considered "possibly related" to study drug. Thus the preliminary data of the DESIRABLE trial demonstrated the feasibility to use desirudin in a broad population of critically ill perioperative and medical patients. Thus desirudin may be a useful alternative for critically ill patients in whom HIT is suspected but who do not have an acute thrombosis. Additional randomized trials in thrombocytopenic patients are needed to confirm these findings (Levy et al., 2011; Bergese et al., 2012).

CPB and Vascular Surgery

Lepirudin was initially used to manage CPB patients in the HAT studies (Riess et al., 1995, 1996) and has also been used successfully by other investigators for CPB (Warkentin and Greinacher, 2003). It is now accepted that lepirudin is a suitable alternative for anticoagulation during CPB in patients with acute HIT, provided that ECT monitoring is performed (Koster et al., 1998, 2000a,b; Johnston et al., 1999; Follis and Schmidt, 2000; Latham et al., 2000; Longrois et al., 2000). Neither the activated clotting time (ACT) nor the aPTT is appropriate for monitoring r-hirudin plasma levels in such high-dose situations (see chap. 19).

Koster and colleagues (2000b) used lepirudin instead of heparin in 57 patients who had clinically diagnosed HIT and required CPB. The primary diagnoses included coronary artery disease ($n = 27$, including eight cases of MI), valvular heart disease ($n = 14$), combined coronary artery and valvular disease ($n = 9$), thoracic aortic aneurysms ($n = 4$), ventricular septal defect resulting from MI ($n = 2$), and atrial tumor ($n = 1$). In that study, anticoagulation was monitored with ECT, and lepirudin was maintained in the range of 3–4 µg/mL. The dose requirement for CPB was 0.016–0.035 mg/kg/min (1.0–2.1 mg/kg/hr), with concurrent 24-hr blood drainage of 50–2200 mL. Elimination of the drug at the conclusion of CPB was augmented through modified zero-balanced ultrafiltration and forced diuresis. However, drug removal was dependent on the prevailing renal function. Four patients with impaired renal function showed prolonged elimination and bleeding. Of the 57 patients, 54 achieved full recovery and showed no signs of thromboembolism over a 6-month follow-up. Three patient deaths were unrelated to perioperative management.

For patients undergoing vascular surgery, the dosage of lepirudin should be adjusted for the risk for reocclusion (Hach-Wunderle, 2001). In patients with a low risk of reocclusion (e.g., in the aortic, iliac, and carotid arteries), a bolus of 0.4 mg/kg (reduced in case of renal insufficiency) is given just before the vessel is clamped and is followed postoperatively by either an aPTT-adjusted infusion starting at 0.1 mg/kg/hr or 15 mg injected sc b.i.d. (assuming normal renal function). In patients with an increased risk for reocclusion (e.g., undergoing calf-vessel reconstruction or bypass), a preoperative bolus of lepirudin [0.4 mg/kg (less in case of renal impairment)] should be administered, followed by a postoperative infusion of 0.1 mg/kg/hr, aPTT-adjusted, for at least 3–4 days. For intraoperative flushing of the vessel during vascular surgery, up to 250 mL (0.1 mg/mL solution) of lepirudin can be used. As patients with acute HIT are at high risk for new TECs, therapeutic levels of anticoagulation should be achieved before surgery and maintained after surgery, at least until platelet counts are normalized.

Hemodialysis

Hirudin was the first anticoagulant to be used for hemodialysis, as performed by Haas (1924) in Germany. Because native hirudin preparations were crude and supply of leeches insufficient, hirudin was replaced by heparin to prevent clotting during dialysis.

Management of these patients requires careful dosing and frequent monitoring. HIT patients with transient renal failure are difficult to manage with lepirudin, because substantial dose adjustments are necessary, depending on the extent of renal failure. To reduce bleeding risk, we prefer administering a continuous iv infusion, starting at 0.005 mg/kg/hr, with adjustments made according to the aPTT, while others use intermittent iv boluses of 0.005–0.01 mg/kg (Fischer et al., 1999; Kern et al., 1999). Use of lepirudin in renal replacement therapy is reviewed in chapter 18.

r-Hirudins in Pregnancy

Data on the treatment of HIT during pregnancy are limited (Lindhoff-Last and Bauersachs, 2002). In general, the use of lepirudin during pregnancy is not recommended, as it crosses the placenta. Zebrafish experiments indicate that thrombin has an important role in early embryogenesis and that inhibition by lepirudin may cause cell regulation defects (Jagadeeswaran et al., 1997). Experiments in rabbits showed a fetal hirudin plasma concentration that was 1/60th that of the maternal concentration (Markwardt et al., 1988), and embryotoxic effects were seen in rabbits at high, but not low, doses (30 mg/kg/day *vs* 1–10 mg/kg/day, respectively) (Berlex Laboratories, Montville, NJ, USA, data on file).

A pregnant woman with systemic lupus erythematosus who was treated with dalteparin developed HIT at week 25. Her platelet count dropped from 230 to 59×10^9/L, after which she was treated with lepirudin (15 mg sc b.i.d.), with aPTT and ECT used to monitor her dosage. Following delivery by cesarean section, she experienced no postpartum bleeding complications, and treatment with lepirudin was continued for several weeks thereafter (Huhle et al., 2000a). Another pregnant woman with lupus anticoagulant and HIT was successfully treated for 36 weeks with lepirudin.

A case report described a breastfeeding woman diagnosed with HIT who was treated with sc lepirudin, 50 mg b.i.d. (Lindhoff-Last et al., 2000a). No lepirudin was detected in her breast milk, although plasma levels were within therapeutic range. Neither bleeding nor thrombosis occurred in mother or infant.

Lepirudin and danaparoid are each classified by the FDA as pregnancy category B, based on limited animal data. However, danaparoid does not cross the placenta, and it has been used for prophylaxis and therapy of HIT during pregnancy (Greinacher et al., 1993; Dager and White, 2002) (see chaps. 12 and 16).

Desirudin is classified as pregnancy category C. Teratology studies have been performed in rats at sc doses in a range of 1–15 mg/kg/day (about 0.3–4 times the recommended human dose based on BSA) and in rabbits at iv doses in a range of 0.6–6 mg/kg/day (about 0.3–3 times the recommended human dose based on BSA) and have revealed desirudin to be teratogenic. There are no adequate and well-controlled studies in pregnant women. Desirudin should be used during pregnancy only if the potential benefit justifies the potential risk to the fetus (Iprivask Product Insert [http://dailymed.nlm.nih.gov/dailymed/archives/fdaDrugInfo. cfm?archiveid=27742], Canyon Pharmaceuticals, 2010).

Lepirudin in Children

Although rare in children, HIT is important in the differential diagnosis of thrombocytopenia or unexplained thrombosis in the presence of heparin administration (Ranze et al., 1999; Klenner et al., 2004). Because of the rarity of HIT and its clinical heterogeneity in pediatric patients, it is difficult to design a standardized dosage protocol for lepirudin. Accordingly, current therapeutic recommendations are based on anecdotal experience. Given that children usually have normal renal function, the short half-life of lepirudin presents an advantage in the event of bleeding complications or the need for invasive procedures. However, the dose required may range between 0.05 and 0.22 mg/kg/hr, depending on comorbidity and renal function (Schiffmann et al., 1997; Deitcher et al., 2002; Nguyen et al., 2003) (see chap. 21).

CONCLUSION

The r-hirudins are DTIs that provide rapid and effective anticoagulation and lepirudin significantly reduces the risk of thrombosis in patients with HIT, including those with isolated thrombocytopenia. Less than 10% of all patient groups with HIT developed a new thrombosis after start of active treatment. Desirudin shows promising results but requires further study.

Lepirudin is given parenterally by iv infusion or sc injection. Recommended lepirudin dosage schedules have been established (Table 14.1). Desirudin is given by sc route at a dose of 15 mg b.i.d. (patients without thrombosis) or at a dose of 30 mg sc b.i.d. (patients with thrombosis), but has also been extensively assessed with iv aPTT-adjusted therapy in prospective randomized trials of patients with ACS.

r-Hirudins have a short half-life, which presents an advantage if invasive surgical procedures are indicated. However, their elimination strongly depends on renal function. The most important lessons learned after approval of lepirudin is that the approved dosage schedule is too high. The bolus should only be given in life- or limb-threatening thrombosis and also the starting maintenance dose should be greatly reduced (from 0.15 to 0.05–0.10 mg/kg/hr), especially in elderly patients. Lepirudin can be used safely and effectively in patients with renal impairment by appropriate dosing according to serum creatinine and regular monitoring. Lepirudin also allows for a safe and uncomplicated transition to warfarin, provided that warfarin is initiated after recovery of the platelet count.

After start of treatment, lepirudin should be monitored every 4 hours until a steady state is reached, then daily monitoring of aPTT is recommended with dosage adjustments made as needed to maintain the target aPTT value. Routine monitoring with ECT should be performed in high-dose situations, such as those required during CPB. All functional assays (aPTT, ECT) can give false high levels of anticoagulation in patients with prothrombin or fibrinogen deficiencies. In these patients a chromogenic assay (ECA) is more suitable to avoid underdosing.

The most common adverse event in the prospective clinical trials was bleeding. No antidote exists for the DTIs. Excess lepirudin can be removed by hemofiltration, and rFVIIa may also be used, but clinical data are limited.

Besides the 403 patients with HIT treated in prospective trials, an additional 1329 patients received lepirudin for HIT in a postmarketing surveillance study. Data on these patients, collected under routine clinical conditions, showed the lowest incidence of the clinical endpoints of death, new thrombosis, and amputations, with risk reductions exceeding those reported in the prospective clinical trials. Even more importantly, the incidence of major bleeding was low. These differences support the assumption that outcomes in patients with HIT can be substantially improved by immediately stopping heparin and starting lepirudin when HIT is strongly suspected on clinical grounds, without awaiting results of antibody testing, and that the bleeding risk has been reduced substantially as physicians have learned to handle this agent.

Postapproval observational studies also gave insights in the frequency of rare adverse effects associated with lepirudin treatment, such as anaphylaxis. The results of these trials and the DMP demonstrate that lepirudin is highly effective in reducing the risk of the potentially devastating complications of HIT.

Desirudin is given at a low dose by sc route. Monitoring might not be necessary at the dose of 15 mg b.i.d. but should be considered in patients receiving 30 mg b.i.d., especially in case of renal impairment. As desirudin has very similar characteristics as lepirudin, and extensive experience exists in giving desirudin iv, this drug might be used to substitute for lepirudin.

ACKNOWLEDGMENTS

The HAT studies were performed jointly by the combined clinical research team of Behring-Werke AG, Hoechst, and Aventis. The laboratory studies were supported by Deutsche Forschungsgemeinschaft GR 1096–2/2 and 2/3, and 2/4. Analysis of the HAT-3 data and the HAT-1, -2, -3 meta-analysis was supported by a grant from Berlex Laboratories (Montville, NJ, U.S.A.) and Pharmion (Cambridge, U.K.). The study on a comparison of danaparoid and lepirudin was supported by Organon NV (Oss, The Netherlands) and Thiemann/Celltech (Essen, Germany).

REFERENCES

AbuRahma AF, Boland JP, Witsberger T. Diagnostic and therapeutic strategies of white clot syndrome. Am J Surg 162: 175–179, 1991.

Al-Rossaies A, Alkharfy KM, Al-Ayoubi F, Al-Momen A. Heparin-induced thrombocytopenia: comparison between response to fondaparinux and lepirudin. Int J Clin Pharm 33: 997–1001, 2011.

Antman EM. Hirudin in acute myocardial infarction: safety report from the Thrombolysis and Thrombin Inhibition in Myocardial Infarction (TIMI) 9A trial. Circulation 90: 1624–1630, 1994.

Badger NO, Butler K, Hallman LC. Excessive anticoagulation and anaphylactic reaction after rechallenge with lepirudin in a patient with heparin-induced thrombocytopenia. Pharmacotherapy 24: 1800–1803, 2004.

Begelman SM, Deitcher SR. Outpatient management of venous thromboembolic disease with subcutaneous lepirudin: a case report. J Thromb Thrombolysis 13: 183–185, 2002.

Bergese SD, Minkowitz HS, Arpino PA, Sane DC, Levy JH. Multi-center trial of desirudin for the prophylaxis of thrombosis: an alternative to heparin-based anticoagulation – results from the DESIRABLE trial. Clin Appl Thromb Hemost 2012; in press.

Bircher AJ, Czendlik CH, Messmer SL, Muller P, Howard H. Acute urticaria caused by subcutaneous recombinant hirudin: evidence for an IgG-mediated hypersensitivity reaction. J Allergy Clin Immunol 98: 994–996, 1996.

Bircher AJ, Harr T, Hohenstein L, Tsakiris DA. Hypersensitivity reactions to anticoagulant drugs: diagnosis and management options. Allergy 61: 1432–1440, 2006.

Bove CM, Casey B, Marder VJ. DDAVP reduces bleeding during continued hirudin administration in the rabbit. Thromb Haemost 75: 471–475, 1996.

Boyce SW, Bandyk DF, Bartholomew JR, Frame JN, Rice L. A randomized, open-label pilot study comparing desirudin and argatroban in patients with suspected heparin-induced thrombocytopenia with or without thrombosis: PREVENT-HIT study. Am J Ther 18: 14–22, 2011.

Bucha E, Nowak G, Czerwinski R, Thieler H. r-Hirudin as anticoagulant in regular hemodialysis therapy: finding of therapeutic r-hirudin blood/plasma concentrations and respective dosages. Clin Appl Thromb Hemost 5: 164–170, 1999.

Butler KD, Dolan SL, Talbot MD, Wallis RB. Factor VIII and DDAVP reverse the effect of recombinant desulphatohirudin (CGB 39393) on bleeding in the rat. Blood Coagul Fibrinolysis 4: 459–464, 1993.

Callas DD, Hoppensteadt DA, Iqbal O, Rubsamen K, Fareed J. Ecarin clotting time (ECT) is a reliable method for the monitoring of hirudins, argatroban, efegatran and related drugs in therapeutic and cardiovascular indications [abstr]. Blood 86(10 Suppl 1): 866a, 1995.

Clore GM, Sukumaran DK, Nilges M, Zarbock J, Gronenborn AM. The conformation of hirudin in solution. A study using nuclear magnetic resonance, distance geometry and restrained molecular dynamics. EMBO J 6: 529–553, 1987.

Dager WE, White RH. Use of lepirudin in patients with heparin-induced thrombocytopenia and renal failure requiring hemodialysis. Ann Pharmacother 35: 885–890, 2001.

Dager WE, White RH. Treatment of heparin-induced thrombocytopenia. Ann Pharmacother 36: 489–503, 2002.

de Denus S, Spinier SA. Clinical monitoring of direct thrombin inhibitors using the ecarin clotting time. Pharmacotherapy 22: 433–435, 2002.

Deitcher SR, Topoulos AP, Bartholomew JR, Kichuk-Chrisant MR. Lepirudin anticoagulation for heparin-induced thrombocytopenia. J Pediatr 140: 264–266, 2002.

Dickneite G, Friesen HJ, Kumpe G, Reers M. Reduction of r-hirudin induced bleeding in pigs by the administration of von Willebrand factor. Platelets 7: 283–290, 1996.

Dickneite G, Nicolay U, Friesen HJ, Reers M. Development of an anti-bleeding agent for recombinant hirudin induced skin bleeding in the pig. Thromb Haemost 80: 192–198, 1998.

Diehl KH, Romisch J, Hein B, Jessel A, Ronneberger H, Paques EP. Investigation of activated prothrombin complex concentrate as potential hirudin antidote in animal models. Haemostasis 25: 182–192, 1995.

Direct Thrombin Inhibitors Trialists' Collaborative Group. Direct thrombin inhibitors in acute coronary syndrome: principal results of a meta-analysis based on individual patients' data. Lancet 359: 294–302, 2002.

Eichler P, Budde U, Haas S, Kroll H, Loreth RM, Meyer O, Pachmann U, Pötzsch B, Schabel A, Albrecht D, Greinacher A. First workshop for detection of heparin-induced antibodies: validation of the heparin-induced platelet activation test (HIPA) in comparison with a PF4/heparin ELISA. Thromb Haemost 81: 625–629, 1999.

Eichler P, Friesen HJ, Lubenow N, Jaeger B, Greinacher A. Antihirudin antibodies in patients with heparin-induced thrombocytopenia treated with lepirudin: incidence, effects on aPTT, and clinical relevance. Blood 96: 2373–2378, 2000.

Eriksson BI, Ekman S, Kalebo P, Zachrisson B, Bach D, Close P. Prevention of deep-vein thrombosis after total hip replacement: direct thrombin inhibition with recombinant hirudin, CGP 39393. Lancet 347: 635–639, 1996.

Eriksson BI, Ekman S, Lindbratt S, Baur M, Bach D, Torholm C, Kälebo P, Close P. Prevention of thromboembolism with use of recombinant hirudin. Results of a double-blind, multicenter trial comparing the efficacy of desirudin (Revasc) with that of unfractionated heparin in patients having a total hip replacement. J Bone Joint Surg Am 79: 326–333, 1997a.

Eriksson BI, Wille-Jorgensen P, Kalebo P, Mouret P, Rosencher N, Bosch P, Baur M, Ekman S, Bach D, Lindbratt S, Close P. A comparison of recombinant hirudin with a low molecular weight heparin to prevent thromboembolic complications after total hip replacement. N Engl J Med 337: 1329–1335, 1997b.

Fabrizio MC. Use of ecarin clotting time (ECT) with lepirudin therapy in heparin-induced thrombocytopenia and cardiopulmonary bypass. J Extra Corpor Technol 33: 117–125, 2001.

Farner B, Eichler P, Kroll H, Greinacher A. A comparison of danaparoid and lepirudin in heparin-induced thrombocytopenia. Thromb Haemost 85: 950–957, 2001.

Fischer KG. Hirudin in renal insufficiency. Semin Thromb Hemost 28: 467–482, 2002.

Fischer KG, van de Loo A, Böhler J. Recombinant hirudin (lepirudin) as anticoagulant in intensive care patients treated with continuous hemodialysis. Kidney Int 72(Suppl): S46–S50, 1999.

Fischer KG, Liebe V, Hudek R, Piazolo L, Haase KK, Borggrefe M, Huhle G. Anti-hirudin antibodies alter pharmacokinetics and pharmacodynamics of recombinant hirudin. Thromb Haemost 89: 973–982, 2003.

Follis F, Schmidt CA. Cardiopulmonary bypass in patients with heparin-induced thrombocytopenia. Ann Thorac Surg 70: 2173–2181, 2000.

Frame JN, Rice L, Bartholomew J, Whelton A. Rationale and design of the PREVENT-HIT Study: A randomized, open-label, pilot study to compare desirudin and argatroban in patients with suspected heparin-induced thrombocytopenia with or without thrombosis. Clin Ther 32: 626–636, 2010.

Frank RD, Farber H, Stefanidis I, Lanzmich R, Kierdorf HP. Hirudin elimination by hemofiltration: a comparative in vitro study of different membranes. Kidney Int 72(Suppl): S41–S45, 1999.

Glusa E. Pharmacology and therapeutic applications of hirudin, a new anticoagulant. Kidney Int 64(Suppl): S54–S56, 1998.

Glusa E, Markwardt F. Platelet functions in recombinant hirudin-anticoagulated blood. Haemostasis 20: 112–118, 1990.

Gosselin RC, King JH, Janatpour KA, Dager WE, Larkin EC, Owings JT. Comparing direct thrombin inhibitors using aPTT, ecarin clotting times, and thrombin inhibitor management testing. Ann Pharmacother 38: 1383–1388, 2004.

Graetz TJ, Tellor BR, Smith JR, Avidan MS. Desirudin: a review of the pharmacology and clinical application for the prevention of deep vein thrombosis. Expert Rev Cardiovasc Ther 9: 1101–1109, 2011.

Gray E, Harenberg J; ISTH Control of Anticoagulation SSC Working Group on Thrombin Inhibitors. Collaborative study on monitoring methods to determine direct thrombin inhibitors lepirudin and argatroban. Thromb Haemost 3: 2096–2097, 2005.

Greinacher A, Michels I, Kiefel V, Mueller-Eckhardt C. A rapid and sensitive test for diagnosing heparin-associated thrombocytopenia. Thromb Haemost 66: 734–736, 1991.

Greinacher A, Eckhardt T, Mubmann J, Mueller-Eckhardt C. Pregnancy complicated by heparin associated thrombocytopenia: management by a prospectively in vitro selected heparinoid (Org 10172). Thromb Res 71: 123–127, 1993.

Greinacher A, Völpel H, Janssens U, Hach-Wunderle V, Kemkes-Matthes B, Eichler P, Mueller-Velten HG, Pötzsch B. Recombinant hirudin (lepirudin) provides safe and effective anticoagulation in patients with heparin-induced thrombocytopenia: a prospective study. Circulation 99: 73–80, 1999a.

Greinacher A, Janssens U, Berg G, Böck M, Kwasny H, Kemkes-Matthes B, Eichler P, Völpel H, Pötzsch B, Luz M; For the Heparin-Associated Thrombocytopenia Study (HAT) investigators. Lepirudin (recombinant hirudin) for parenteral anticoagulation in patients with heparin-induced thrombocytopenia. Circulation 100: 587–593, 1999b.

Greinacher A, Eichler P, Lubenow N, Kwasny H, Luz M. Heparin-induced thrombocytopenia with thromboembolic complications: meta-analysis of 2 prospective trials to assess the value of parenteral treatment with lepirudin and its therapeutic APTT range. Blood 96: 846–851, 2000.

Greinacher A, Eichler P, Albrecht D, Strobel U, Pötzsch B, Eriksson BI. Antihirudin antibodies following low-dose subcutaneous treatment with desirudin for thrombosis prophylaxis after hip-replacement surgery: incidence and clinical relevance. Blood 101: 2617–2619, 2003a.

Greinacher A, Eichler P, Lubenow N. Anaphylactic reactions associated with lepirudin in patients with heparin-induced thrombocytopenia (HIT). Circulation 108: 2062–2065, 2003b.

Greinacher A, Warkentin TE. Recognition, treatment, and prevention of heparin-induced thrombocytopenia: review and update. Thromb Res 118: 165–176, 2006.

Greinacher A. Immunogenic but effective: the HIT-fondaparinux brain puzzler. J Thromb Haemost 9: 2386–2388, 2011.

Haas G. Über Versuche der Blutauswaschung am Lebenden mit Hilfe der Dialyse. Klin Wochenschr 4: 13–14, 1924. [in German]

Hach-Wunderle V. Hirudin in der Gefaesschirurgie. In: Greinacher A, ed. Hirudin in der vaskulaeren Medizin. Bremen: Uni-Med Verlag, 76–77, 2001.

Hacquard M, de Maistre E, Lecompte T. Lepirudin: is the approved dosing schedule too high? J Thromb Haemost 3: 2593–2596, 2005.

Hafner G, Roser M, Nauck M. Methods for the monitoring of direct thrombin inhibitors. Semin Thromb Hemost 28: 425–430, 2002.

Hamilton RG, Levy JH, Marder VJ, Sane DC. Interference of thrombin in immunological assays for hirudin specific antibodies. J Immunol Methods 381: 50–8, 2012.

Hermann JPR, Kutryk MJV, Serruys PW. Clinical trials of direct thrombin inhibitors during invasive procedures. Thromb Haemost 78: 367–376, 1997.

Hogg PJ, Jackson CM. Fibrin monomer protects thrombin from inactivation by heparin-antithrombin III: implications for heparin efficacy. Proc Natl Acad Sci USA 86: 3619–3623, 1989.

Huhle G, Song X, Wang LC, Hoffman U, Harenberg J. Generation and disappearance of anti-hirudin antibodies during treatment with r-hirudin. Fibrinol Proteol 12(Suppl 2): 91–113, 1998.

Huhle G, Geberth M, Hoffmann U, Heene DL, Harenberg J. Management of heparin-associated thrombocytopenia in pregnancy with subcutaneous r-hirudin. Gynecol Obstet Invest 49: 67–69, 2000a.

Huhle G, Hoffmann U, Hoffmann I, Liebe V, Harenberg JF, Heene DL. A new therapeutic option by subcutaneous recombinant hirudin in patients with heparin-induced thrombo-cytopenia type II: a pilot study. Thromb Res 99: 325–334, 2000b.

Huhle G, Liebe V, Hudek R, Heene DL. Anti-r-hirudin antibodies reveal clinical relevance through direct functional inactivation of r-hirudin or prolongation of r-hirudin's plasma halflife. Thromb Haemost 85: 936–938, 2001.

Ibbotson SH, Grant PJ, Kerry R, Findlay VS, Prentice CRM. The influence of infusions of l-desamino-8-D-arginine vasopressin (DDAVP) in vivo on the anticoagulant effect of recombinant hirudin (CGP 39393) in vitro. Thromb Haemost 65: 64–66, 1991.

Irami MS, White HJ Jr, Sexon RG. Reversal of hirudin-induced bleeding diathesis by pro-thrombin complex concentrate. Am J Cardiol 75: 422–423, 1995.

Jagadeeswaran P, Liu YC, Eddy CA. Effects of hirudin (thrombin specific inhibitor) in zebra-fish embryos: a developmental role for thrombin. Blood Cells Mol Dis 23: 410–414, 1997.

Jappe U, Reinhold D, Bonnekoh B. Arthus reaction to lepirudin, a new recombinant hirudin, and delayed-type hypersensitivity to several heparins and heparinoids, with tolerance to its intravenous administration. Contact Dermat 46: 29–32, 2002.

Johnston N, Jessen ME, DiMaio M, Douglass DS. The emergency use of recombinant hirudin in cardiopulmonary bypass. J Extra Corpor Technol 31: 211–215, 1999.

Kaiser B, Markwardt F. Antithrombotic and haemorrhagic effects of synthetic and naturally occurring thrombin inhibitors. Thromb Res 43: 613–620, 1986.

Kern H, Ziemer S, Kox WJ. Bleeding after intermittent or continuous r-hirudin during CVVH. Intensive Care Med 25: 1311–1314, 1999.

King DJ, Kelton JG. Heparin-associated thrombocytopenia. Ann Intern Med 100: 535–540, 1984.

Klenner AF, Lubenow N, Raschke R, Greinacher A. Heparin-induced thrombocytopenia in children: 12 new cases and review of the literature. Thromb Haemost 91: 719–724, 2004.

Kornalik F, Blomback B. Prothrombin activation induced by ecarin—a prothrombin convert-ing enzyme from Echis carinatus venom. Thromb Res 6: 57–63, 1975.

Koster A, Kuppe H, Hetzer R, Sodian R, Crystal GJ, Mertzlufft F. Emergent cardiopulmonary bypass in five patients with heparin-induced thrombocytopenia type II employing recom-binant hirudin. Anesthesiology 89: 777–780, 1998.

Koster A, Hansen R, Grauhan O, Hausmann H, Bauer M, Hetzer R, Kuppe H, Mertzlufft F. Hirudin monitoring using the TAS ecarin clotting time in patients with heparin-induced thrombocytopenia type II. J Cardiothorac Vasc Anesth 14: 249–252, 2000a.

Koster A, Hansen R, Kuppe H, Hetzer R, Crystal GJ, Mertzlufft F. Recombinant hirudin as an alternative for anticoagulation during cardiopulmonary bypass in patients with heparin-induced thrombocytopenia type II: a 1–year experience in 57 patients. J Cardiothorac Vasc Anesth 14: 243–248, 2000b.

Lange U, Nowak G, Bucha E. Ecarin chromogenic assay-a new method for quantitative determination of direct thrombin inhibitors like hirudin. Pathophysiol Haemost Thromb 33: 184–191, 2003.

Lange U, Olschewski A, Nowak G, Bucha E. [Ecarin chromogenic assay: an innovative test for quantitative determination of direct thrombin inhibitors in plasma]. Hamostaseologie 25: 293–300, 2005. [In German]

Latham P, Revelis AF, Joshi GP, DiMaio JM, Jessen ME. Use of recombinant hirudin in patients with heparin-induced thrombocytopenia with thrombosis requiring cardiopulmonary bypass. Anesthesiology 92: 263–266, 2000.

Levy J, Koster A. Safety of perioperative bridging with desirudin and intraoperative bivalirudin in patients with heparin antibodies undergoing coronary artery bypass surgery (CABG). Presented at the 33rd Annual Meeting and Workshops of the Society of Cardiovascular Anesthesiologists Savannah, GA; April 30–May 4, 2011.

Levy J, Kurz M, Whelton A. Lack of clinically significant interactions between the subcutaneously administered direct thrombin inhibitor desirudin and orally administered warfarin upon the international normalized ratio [abstr]. Blood 114: Abstr 3131, 2009.

Levy JH, Kurz MA, Koster A. Perioperative venous thromboembolism prophylaxis in patients with heparin-induced thrombocytopenia (HIT): the desirudin experience [abstr]. J Thromb Haemost 9: 332, 2011.

Liebe V, Bruckmann M, Fischer KG, Haase KK, Borggrefe M, Huhle G. Biological relevance of anti-recombinant hirudin antibodies-results from in vitro and in vivo studies. Semin Thromb Hemost 28: 483–489, 2002.

Lindhoff-Last E, Bauersachs R. Heparin-induced thrombocytopenia-alternative anticoagulation in pregnancy and lactation. Semin Thromb Haemost 28: 439–445, 2002.

Lindhoff-Last E, Willeke A, Thalhammer C, Nowak G, Bauersachs R. Hirudin treatment in a breastfeeding woman. Lancet 355: 467–468, 2000a.

Lindhoff-Last E, Piechottka GP, Rabe F, Bauersachs R. Hirudin determination in plasma can be strongly influenced by the prothrombin level. Thromb Res 100: 55–60, 2000b.

Linnemann B, Greinacher A, Lindhoff-Last E. Alteration of pharmacokinetics of lepirudin caused by anti-lepirudin antibodies occurring after long-term subcutaneous treatment in a patient with recurrent VTE due to Behcets disease. Vasa 39: 103–107, 2010.

Liu H, Fleming NW, Moore PG. Anticoagulation for patients with heparin-induced thrombocytopenia using recombinant hirudin during cardiopulmonary bypass. J Clin Anesth 14: 452–455, 2002.

Lobo B, Finch C, Howard A, Minhas S. Fondaparinux for the treatment of patients with acute heparin-induced thrombocytopenia. Thromb Haemost 99: 208–214, 2008.

Longrois D, de Maistre E, Bischoff N, Dopff C, Meistelman C, Angioi M, Lecompte T. Recombinant hirudin anticoagulation for aortic valve replacement in heparin-induced thrombocytopenia. Can J Anaesth 47: 255–260, 2000.

Lubenow N, Greinacher A. Hirudin in heparin-induced thrombocytopenia. Semin Thromb Hemost 28: 431–438, 2002.

Lubenow N, Eichler P, Greinacher A. Results of a large drug monitoring program confirms the safety and efficacy of Refludan (lepirudin) in patients with immune-mediated heparin-induced thrombocytopenia (HIT) [abstr]. Blood 100(Suppl l): 502a, 2002.

Lubenow N, Eichler P, Lietz T, Farner B, Greinacher A. Lepirudin for prophylaxis of thrombosis in patients with acute isolated heparin-induced thrombocytopenia: an analysis of 3 prospective studies. Blood 104: 3072–3077, 2004.

Lubenow N, Eichler P, Lietz T, Greinacher A; And the HIT Investigators Group. Lepirudin in patients with heparin-induced thrombocytopenia – results of the third prospective study (HAT-3) and a combined analysis of HAT-1, HAT-2, and HAT-3. J Thromb Haemost 3: 2428–2436, 2005.

Markwardt F. Development of hirudin as an antithrombotic agent. Semin Thromb Hemost 15: 269–282, 1989.

Markwardt F. Hirudin: the promising antithrombotic. Cardiovasc Drug Rev 10: 211–232, 1992.

Markwardt F, Fink G, Kaiser B, Klocking HP, Nowak G, Richter M, Sturzebecher J. Pharmacological survey of recombinant hirudin. Pharmazie 43: 202–207, 1988.

Mehta SR, Eikelboom JW, Rupprecht H-.J, Lewis BS, Natarajan MK, Yi C, Pogue J, Yusuf S. Efficacy of hirudin in reducing cardiovascular events in patients with acute coronary syndrome undergoing early percutaneous coronary intervention. Eur Heart J 23: 117–123, 2002.

Metz BK, White HD, Granger CB, Simes RJ, Armstrong PW, Hirsh J, Fuster V, MacAulay CM, Califf RM, Topol EJ. Randomized comparison of direct thrombin inhibition versus heparin in conjunction with fibrinolytic therapy for acute myocardial infarction: results from the GUSTO-IIb trial. J Am Coll Cardiol 31: 1493–1498, 1998.

Meyer BJ, Badimon JJ, Chesebro JH, Fallon JT, Fuster V, Badimon L. Dissolution of mural thrombus by specific thrombin inhibition with r-hirudin: comparison with heparin and aspirin. Circulation 97: 681–685, 1998.

Nafziger AN, Bertino JS Jr. Desirudin dosing and monitoring in moderate renal impairment. J Clin Pharmacol 50: 614–622, 2010.

Nand S, Wong W, Yuen B, Yetter A, Schmulbach E, Gross Fisher S. Heparin-induced thrombocytopenia with thrombosis: incidence, analysis of risk factors, and clinical outcomes in 108 consecutive patients treated at a single institution. Am J Hematol 56: 12–16, 1997.

Neuhaus KL, von Essen R, Tebbe U, Jessel A, Heinrichs H, Mäurer W, Doring W, Harnjanz D, Kötter V, Kalhammer E, et al. Safety observations from the pilot phase of the randomized r-Hirudin for Improvement of Thrombolysis (HIT-III) study: a study of the Arbeitsgemeinschaft Leitender Kardiologischer Krankenhausarzte (ALKK). Circulation 90: 1638–1642, 1994.

Neuhaus KL, Molhoek GP, Zeymer U, Tebbe U, Wegschieder K, Schroder R, Camez A, Laarman GJ, Grollier GM, Lok DJ, Kuckuck H, Lazarus P. Recombinant hirudin (lepirudin) for the improvement of thrombolysis with streptokinase in patients with acute myocardial infarction: results of the HIT-4 trial. J Am Coll Cardiol 34: 966–973, 1999.

Nguyen TN, Gal P, Ransom JL, Carlos R. Lepirudin use in a neonate with heparin-induced thrombocytopenia. Ann Pharmacother 37: 229–233, 2003.

Nishida S, Fujita T, Kohno N, Atoda H, Morita T, Takeya H, Kido I, Paine MJ, Kawabata S, Iwanaga S. cDNA cloning and deduced amino acid sequence of prothrombin activator (ecarin) from Kenyan Echis carinatus venom. Biochemistry 34: 1771–1778, 1995.

Novoa E, Seegers WH. Mechanisms of alpha-thrombin and beta-thrombin-E formation: use of ecarin for isolation of meizothrombin 1. Thromb Res 18: 657–668, 1980.

Nowak G. Clinical monitoring of hirudin and direct thrombin inhibitors. Semin Thromb Hemost 27: 537–541, 2001.

Nowak G, Bucha E. Prothrombin conversion intermediate effectively neutralizes toxic levels of hirudin. Thromb Res 80: 317–325, 1995.

Nowak G, Bucha E. Quantitative determination of hirudin in blood and body fluids. Semin Thromb Haemost 22: 197–202, 1996.

Nowak G, Bucha E, Goock T, Prasa D, Thieler H. Pharmakokinetik von Hirudin bei gestorter Nierenfunktion. Haemostaseologie 11: 152–157, 1991. [in German]

Nowak G, Bucha E, Goock T, Thieler H, Markwardt F. Pharmacology of r-hirudin in renal impairment. Thromb Res 66: 707–715, 1992.

Nowak G, Bucha E, Brauns I, Czerwinski R. Anticoagulation with r-hirudin in regular haemodialysis with heparin-induced thrombocytopenia (HIT II). The first long term application of r-hirudin in a haemodialysis patient. Wien Klin Wochenschr 109: 354–358, 1997.

Oh JJ, Akers WS, Lewis D, Ramaiah C, Flynn JD. Recombinant factor VIIa for refractory bleeding after cardiac surgery secondary to anticoagulation with the direct thrombin inhibitor lepirudin. Pharmacotherapy 26: 569–577, 2006.

Organization to Assess Strategies for Ischemic Syndromes (OASIS) Investigators. Comparison of the effects of two doses of recombinant hirudin compared with heparin in patients with acute myocardial ischemia without ST elevation: a pilot study. Circulation 96: 769–777, 1997.

Organization to Assess Strategies for Ischemic Syndromes (OASIS-2) Investigators. Effects of recombinant hirudin (lepirudin) compared with heparin on death, myocardial infarction, refractory angina, and revascularisation procedures in patients with acute myocardial ischemia without ST elevation: a randomised trial. Lancet 353: 429–438, 1999.

Parent F, Bridey F, Dreyfus M, Musset D, Grimon G, Duroux P, Meyer D, Simon-neau G. Treatment of severe thromboembolism with intravenous hirudin (HBW 023): an open pilot study. Thromb Haemost 70: 386–388, 1993.

Pieters J, Lindhout T, Hemker HC. In situ-generated thrombin is the only enzyme that effectively activates factor VIII and factor V in thromboplastin-activated plasma. Blood 74: 1021–1024, 1989.

Pötzsch B, Hund S, Madlener K, Unkrig C, Muller-Berghaus G. Monitoring of recombinant hirudin: assessment of a plasma-based ecarin clotting time assay. Thromb Res 86: 373–383, 1997a.

Pötzsch B, Madlener K, Seelig C, Riess CF, Greinacher A, Muller-Berghaus G. Monitoring of r-hirudin anticoagulation during cardiopulmonary bypass—assessment of the whole blood ecarin clotting time. Thromb Haemost 77: 920–925, 1997b.

Puente EG, Kurz M, Antor MA, Uribe AA, Erminy N, Bergese SD. Safety report from the desirudin post-marketing registry–Europe in patients undergoing major orthopedic surgery (DESIRE). Anesth Analg 112: S24, 2011.

Ranze O, Ranze P, Magnani HN, Greinacher A. Heparin-induced thrombocytopenia in paediatric patients—a review of the literature and a new case treated with danaparoid sodium. Eur J Pediatr 158(Suppl 3): S130–S133, 1999.

Refludan Package Insert. Monville, NJ: Berlex Laboratories, 2002.

Riess FC, Lower C, Seelig C, Bleese N, Kormann J, Muller-Berghaus G, Pötzsch B. Recombinant hirudin as a new anticoagulant during cardiac operations instead of heparin: successful for aortic valve replacement in man. J Thorac Cardiovasc Surg 110: 265–267, 1995.

Riess FC, Pötzsch B, Bader R, Bleese N, Greinacher A, Lower C, Madlener K, Muller-Berghaus G. A case report on the use of recombinant hirudin as an anticoagulant for cardiopulmonary bypass in open heart surgery. Eur J Cardiothorac Surg 10: 386–388, 1996.

Rupprecht HJ, Terres W, ozbek C, Luz M, Jessel A, Hafner G, vom Dahl J, Kromer EP, Prellwitz W, Meyer J. Recombinant hirudin (HBW 023) prevents troponin T release after coronary angioplasty in patients with unstable angina. J Am Coll Cardiol 26: 1637–1642, 1995.

Salmela B, Joutsi-Korhonen L, Saarela E, Lassila R. Comparison of monitoring methods for lepirudin: impact of warfarin and lupus anticoagulant. Thromb Res 1256: 538–544, 2010.

Schiele F, Vuillemenot A, Kramarz P, Kieffer Y, Soria J, Soria C, Camez A, Mirshahi MC, Bassand JP. A pilot study of subcutaneous recombinant hirudin (HBW 023) in the treatment of deep vein thrombosis. Thromb Haemost 71: 558–562, 1994.

Schiele F, Lindgaerde F, Eriksson H, Bassand JP, Wallmark A, Hansson PO, Grollier G, Sjo M, Moia M, Camez A, Smyth V, Walker M; For the International Multicenter Hirudin Study Group. Subcutaneous recombinant hirudin (HBW 023) *versus* intravenous sodium heparin in treatment of established acute deep vein thrombosis of the legs: a multicentre prospective dose-ranging randomized trial. Thromb Haemost 77: 834–838, 1997.

Schiffmann H, Unterhalt M, Harms K, Figulla HR, Völpel H, Greinacher A. Erfolgreiche behandlung einer heparin-induzierten thrombozytopenie typ II im kindesalter mit rekombinantem hirudin. Monatsschr Kinderheildk 145: 606–612, 1997. [in German]

Serruys PW, Herrman JP, Simon R, Rutsch W, Bode C, Laarman GJ, van Dijk R, van den Bos AA, Umans VA, Fox KA, et al. Helvetica Investigators. A comparison of hirudin with heparin in the prevention of restenosis after coronary angioplasty. N Engl J Med 333: 757–763, 1995.

Shepherd MF. Dosage of lepirudin in renal failure. Am J Health Syst Pharm 59: 77–78, 2002.

Shorr A, Eriksson BI, Jaffer A, Smith J. Impact of stage 3B chronic kidney disease on thrombosis and bleeding outcomes after orthopedic surgery in patients treated with desirudin or enoxaparin : insights from a randomized trial. J Thromb Haemost 4 Jun 2012. [Epub ahead of print]

Smith KJ, Rosario-Collazo J, Skelton H. Delayed cutaneous hypersensitivity reactions to hirudin. Arch Pathol Lab Med 125: 1585–1587, 2001.

Smythe MA, Stephens JL, Koerber JM, Mattson JC. A comparison of lepirudin and argatroban outcomes. Clin Appl Thromb Hemost 11: 371–374, 2005.

Song X, Huhle G, Wang L, Hoffmann U, Harenberg J. Generation of anti-hirudin antibodies in heparin-induced thrombocytopenic patients treated with r-hirudin. Circulation 100: 1528–1532, 1999.

Stephens JL, Koerber JM, Mattson JC, Smythe MA. Effect of lepirudin on the international normalized ratio. Ann Pharmacother 39: 28–31, 2005.

Stone S, Hofsteenge J. The kinetics of the inhibition of thrombin by hirudin. Biochemistry 25: 4622–4628, 1986.

Sukumaran DK, Clare GM, Presus A, Zarbock J, Gronenborn AM. Proton nuclear magnetic resonance study of hirudin: resonance assignment and secondary structure. Biochemistry 26: 333–338, 1987.

Tardy B, Lecompte T, Boelhen F, Tardy-Poncet B, Elalamy I, Morange P, Gruel Y, Wolf M, Francois D, Racadot E, Camarasa P, Blouch MT, Nguyen F, Doubine S, Dutrillaux F, Alhenc-Gelas M, Martin-Toutain I, Bauters A, Ffrench P, de Maistre E, Grunebaum L, Mouton C, Huisse MG, Gouault-Heilmann M, Lucke V, the GEHT-HIT Study Group. Predictive factors for thrombosis and major bleeding in an observational study in 181 patients with heparin-induced thrombocytopenia treated with lepirudin. Blood 108: 1492–1496, 2006.

The Global Use of Strategies to Open Occluded Coronary Arteries (GUSTO) IIb Investigators. A comparison of recombinant hirudin with heparin for the treatment of acute coronary syndromes. N Engl J Med 335: 775–782, 1996.

Vanholder RC, Camez AA, Veys N, Soria J, Mirshahi M, Soria C, Ringoir S. Recombinant hirudin: a specific thrombin inhibiting anticoagulant for hemodialysis. Kidney Int 45: 1754–1759, 1994.

Vanholder R, Camez A, Veys N, Van Loo A, Dhondt AM, Ringoir S. Pharmacokinetics of recombinant hirudin in hemodialyzed end-stage renal failure patients. Thromb Haemost 77: 650–655, 1997.

Warkentin TE. Should vitamin K be administered when HIT is diagnosed after administration of coumarin? J Thromb Haemost 4: 894–896, 2006.

Warkentin TE, Greinacher A, Craven S, Dewar L, Sheppard JI, Ofosu FA. Differences in the clinically effective molar concentrations of four direct thrombin inhibitors explain their variable prothrombin time prolongation. Thromb Haemost 94: 958–964, 2005.

Warkentin TE, Greinacher A. Heparin-induced thrombocytopenia and cardiac surgery. Ann Thorac Surg 76: 2121–2131, 2003.

Warkentin TE, Greinacher A. Heparin-induced thrombocytopenia: recognition, treatment, and prevention: the Seventh ACCP Conference on Antithrombotic and Thrombolytic Therapy. Chest 126(3 Suppl): 311S–337S, 2004.

Warkentin TE, Kelton JG. A 14–year study of heparin-induced thrombocytopenia. Am J Med 101: 502–507, 1996.

Weitz JI, Hudoba M, Massel D, Maraganore J, Hirsh J. Clot-bound thrombin is protected from inhibition by heparin-antithrombin III but is susceptible to inactivation by antithrombin III-independent inhibitors. J Clin Invest 86: 385–391, 1990.

Weitz JI, Leslie B, Hudoba M. Thrombin binds to soluble fibrin degradation products where it is protected from inhibition by heparin-antithrombin but susceptible to inactivation by antithrombin-independent inhibitors. Circulation 97: 544–552, 1998.

Wittkowsky AK, Kondo LM. Lepirudin dosing in dialysis-dependent renal failure. Pharmacotherapy 20: 1123–1128, 2000.

Zollner TM, Gall H, Völpel H, Kaufmann R. Type IV allergy to natural hirudin confirmed by in vitro stimulation with recombinant hirudin. Contact Dermatitis 35: 59–60, 1996.

15 Bivalirudin for the treatment of heparin-induced thrombocytopenia

John R. Bartholomew and Jayne Prats

INTRODUCTION

Bivalirudin (Angiomax), a direct thrombin inhibitor (DTI), has been approved in 42 countries worldwide. In the United States, Argentina, and Peru it is approved for use in heparin-induced thrombocytopenia (HIT), but only for those patients undergoing percutaneous transluminal coronary angioplasty (PTCA) or percutaneous coronary intervention (PCI). In Canada, it is approved for use in HIT patients undergoing PCI or cardiac surgery (Warkentin et al., 2008a). Bivalirudin is also approved in the United States, Canada, Australia, New Zealand, Israel, Argentina, Peru, Chile, Venezuela, India, Russia, Ukraine, Norway, Iceland, Switzerland, and the 27 members of the European Union (EU) for use as an anticoagulant in patients undergoing PCI (and in some countries with provisional use of glycoprotein (GP) IIb/IIIa inhibitor), and with concomitant aspirin. In some jurisdictions (e.g., the EU, Canada, Australia), the label also includes treatment of patients with moderate- to high-risk acute coronary syndrome (ACS)/unstable angina (UA)/non-ST segment elevation myocardial infarction (NSTEMI) who are undergoing early invasive management. In the EU it is marketed under the trade name Angiox (Warkentin and Koster, 2005).

Bivalirudin has seen increased use in cardiovascular medicine over the past decade through its primary indication as an anticoagulant used during PCIs; bivalirudin has also been further investigated and used as an "off-label" anticoagulation strategy in the setting of cardiac surgery and endovascular procedures (van De Car et al., 2010), particularly in the setting of HIT (either acute or previous). It has also been used as "off-label" for medical patients with HIT, especially those with renal and/or hepatic dysfunction including critically ill patients.

Bivalirudin is a hirulog, that is, one of a group of drugs designed from the structure of hirudin (analogue of hirudin). It was developed in the early 1990s by the Biogen Corporation (Cambridge, Massachusetts, U.S.A.), and was originally known as BG8967 or Hirulog. The U.S. Food and Drug Administration (FDA) mandated a name change to avoid confusion with Humalog (recombinant human insulin) when The Medicines Company (Parsippany, New Jersey, U.S.A.) acquired licensure for bivalirudin in 1997. The name was then changed to Angiomax. Currently, bivalirudin's major indications in the United States are for use in patients with UA undergoing PTCA or with provisional GP IIb/IIIa receptor inhibitor in patients undergoing PCI. For these latter indications, bivalirudin is to be used only in patients receiving concomitant aspirin (Angiomax (bivalirudin) Prescribing Information, The Medicines Company, Parsippany, NJ, U.S.A., 2010).

Bivalirudin has also been used with favorable results in both "on-pump" and "off-pump" cardiac surgery cases in patients with and without HIT. A clinical trial completed by Merry and colleagues (2004) in New Zealand compared bivalirudin with unfractionated heparin (UFH) (with protamine reversal) in non-HIT patients requiring off-pump coronary artery bypass (OPCAB) surgery. Favorable results, including improved graft patency and comparable hemorrhage and transfusion requirements, led to two subsequent multicenter trials. The CABG HIT/TS On- and Off-Pump Safety and Efficacy (CHOOSE-ON and CHOOSE-OFF) studies for patients with HIT, and the EValuation of Patients during coronary artery bypass graft Operations: Linking UTilization of bivalirudin to Improved Outcomes and New anticoagulation strategies (EVOLUTION-OFF and EVOLUTION-ON) trials, were conducted to evaluate the safety and efficacy of bivalirudin as an alternative to UFH (and protamine reversal) in the HIT and non-HIT settings, respectively. Results of these studies (Dyke et al., 2006, 2007; Smedira et al., 2006; Koster et al., 2007a) have revealed comparable safety and efficacy outcomes. As a result of these and other studies, bivalirudin is approved for on-pump surgery in Canada (for patients with or at risk for HIT) and in the EU its label gives recommendations for off-pump surgery.

BIVALIRUDIN
Chemistry
Bivalirudin is a small synthetic 20-amino acid peptide that is a specific and reversible inhibitor of thrombin (Parry et al., 1994) (Fig. 15.1). Although it is an analogue of hirudin, its amino acid sequence is considerably shorter. Bivalirudin unites a carboxy-terminal segment of 12 amino acids (dodecapeptide) derived from native hirudin (residues 53–64), plus a sulfated tyrosine at position 63, to an active site-binding tetrapeptide sequence (D-Phe-Pro-Arg-Pro) at its amino terminal (Maraganore et al., 1990; Nawarskas and Anderson, 2001; White and Chew, 2002). Four glycine residues bridge these two segments together. The amino-terminal segment has a high affinity and specificity for binding to the active site of thrombin (Fareed et al., 1999; Sciulli and Mauro, 2002), whereas the carboxy terminal binds to the fibrinogen recognition site of thrombin at exosite 1 (Thiagarajan and Wu, 1999; Reed and Bell, 2002). One difference between bivalirudin and hirudin is that the binding of bivalirudin to the active site of thrombin is transient, whereas with lepirudin, irreversible thrombin–hirudin complexes are formed (Weitz and Hirsh, 1998; Nawarskas and Anderson, 2001).

The manufacturing process of bivalirudin has evolved over time from a solid phase method to a liquid phase process (Maraganore et al., 1990) that was subsequently scaled up and further optimized. Its molecular mass is 2180 Da. Bivalirudin has no structural similarity to heparin.

Pharmacology
Bivalirudin is a bivalent DTI, that is, it binds two distinct regions of thrombin: the active (catalytic) site and the fibrinogen-binding (substrate-recognition) site. Moreover, like lepirudin and argatroban, bivalirudin binds to both free (soluble) and clot-bound (fibrin-bound) thrombin. It forms a 1:1 stoichiometric complex that neutralizes thrombin during coagulation and thrombus formation (Maraganore and Adelman, 1996). Thus, bivalirudin inhibits proteolytic cleavage of fibrinogen,

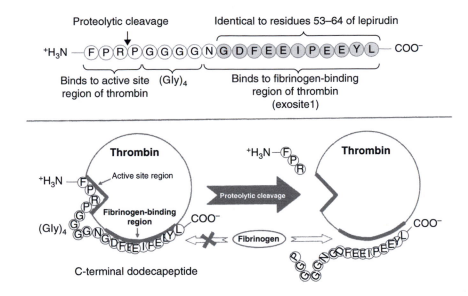

Bivalirudin binds _reversibly_ to thrombin

FIGURE 15.1 The structure of bivalirudin. (*Top*) Bivalirudin comprises 20 amino acids, with an N-(amino-) terminal D-Phe-Pro-Arg-Pro (F-P-R-P) region that binds with high affinity to the active site region of thrombin; a (gly)$_4$ (G4) "spacer" region; and a C-(carboxy-) terminal Asn-Gly-Asp-Phe-Glu-Glu-Ile-Pro-Glu-Glu-Tyr-Leu dodecapeptide (N-G-D-F-E-E-I-P-E-E-Y-L) that binds to the fibrinogen-binding region (exosite 1) of thrombin. The 11 C-terminal amino acids (shaded circles) correspond exactly to the 53- to 64-amino acid sequence of lepirudin. Highly specific, noncompetitive binding between bivalirudin and thrombin results. [Not shown is the heparin-binding region (exosite 2) of thrombin.] However, proteases [including other thrombin molecules (not shown)] can cleave the Arg$_3$-Pro$_4$ of bivalirudin, leading to loss of antithrombin activity. (*Bottom*) Initially, there is bivalent binding of bivalirudin to thrombin, as shown. Following cleavage at Arg$_3$-Pro$_4$, the N-terminal sequence of bivalirudin no longer binds to thrombin, leaving the residual C-terminal dodecapeptide with greatly reduced binding affinity for exosite 1 of thrombin. Thus, the bivalirudin remnant transforms to a competitive inhibitor of thrombin. Other substrates, e.g., fibrinogen, can compete with, and displace, bivalirudin, thus allowing thrombin to resume its prohemostatic functions. *Abbreviations*: Arg (R), arginine; Asn (N), asparagine; Asp (D), aspartic acid; Glu (E), glutamic acid; Gly (G), glycine; Ile (I), isoleucine; Leu (L), leucine; Phe (F), phenylalanine; Pro (P), proline; Tyr (Y), tyrosine.

thrombin-mediated activation of factors V, VIII, and XIII, and thrombin-induced platelet activation.

Bivalirudin (unlike lepirudin) is a *reversible* inhibitor of thrombin (Fig. 15.1). It acts initially as a noncompetitive inhibitor, rendering thrombin inactive. Circulating proteases (including other thrombin molecules) slowly cleave bivalirudin near the amino-terminal end (between Arg$_3$–Pro$_4$), thus eventually releasing the amino-terminal segment from the active site region of thrombin (Bates and Weitz, 1998; Carswell and Plosker, 2002; Reed and Bell, 2002; Sciulli and Mauro, 2002). This allows thrombin to resume catalytic function.

As mentioned, bivalirudin also inhibits thrombin by the binding of its carboxy-terminal segment to the fibrinogen-binding site on thrombin. This occurs at the same time that the amino-terminal segment attaches to the active site, thus resulting in dual blockage with complete inhibition of thrombin's multiple activities (Sciulli and Mauro, 2002). Once the ammo-terminal moiety of bivalirudin is cleaved, however, the carboxy-terminal region acquires low-affinity, weakly competitive binding properties. Fibrinogen can now displace the bivalirudin remnant from thrombin and align itself over the active site to be converted to fibrin (Parry et al., 1994).

Bivalirudin is not inactivated by platelet factor 4 (PF4), nor does it require any cofactor for its activity. It does not bind to red blood cells or proteins other than thrombin.

Pharmacokinetics

Bivalirudin has predictable pharmacokinetics and exhibits a linear dose–response relationship when given by the intravenous (iv) route to healthy volunteers. Its half-life is approximately 25 minutes in patients with normal renal function (Fox et al., 1993; Robson, 2000; Robson et al., 2002; Angiomax Prescribing Information, The Medicines Company, 2010). Peak bivalirudin plasma concentrations after a 15-minute iv infusion are related to dose (Fig. 15.2) and the anticoagulant effect is immediate, occurring within 2 minutes (earliest time tested) of drug bolus administration.

Bivalirudin has a volume of distribution of 0.24 L/kg and a clearance rate of approximately 3.4 mL/min/kg (Fox et al., 1993). It is cleared from plasma by both renal mechanisms and cleavage by plasma proteases. Bivalirudin undergoes glomerular filtration, secretion in the proximal convoluted tubule, and reabsorption in the distal convoluted tubule. The peptides are then further degraded within the

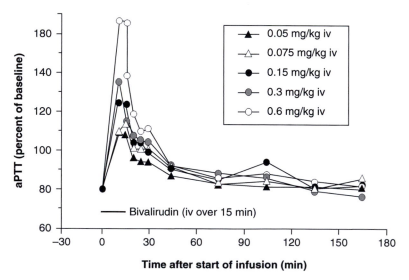

FIGURE 15.2 Prolongation of the aPTT by increasing doses of bivalirudin. Bivalirudin was given by iv infusion over 15 min to five groups (four subjects each) in doses ranging from 0.05 mg/kg per 15 min up to 0.6 mg/kg per 15 min. Each series of data points represents the mean of four study subjects. *Abbreviation*: aPTT, activated partial thromboplastin time. *Source*: From Fox et al. (1993).

intracellular lysosomes (Robson, 2000; Robson et al., 2002). In a study by Fox and colleagues (1993), only 20% of bivalirudin was recovered unchanged in the urine.

Clearance of bivalirudin is accomplished predominantly by proteolytic cleavage within plasma and elsewhere and accounts for approximately 80% of the drug's metabolism (Fox et al., 1993; Scatena, 2000; Robson et al., 2002; Warkentin and Greinacher, 2003). Indeed, proteolysis of bivalirudin appears to result mainly from thrombin, thus providing a mechanism of degradation that is independent of specific organ function (Bates and Weitz, 2000). This results in degradation to individual amino acids and small, inactive peptide fragments (Carswell and Plosker, 2002).

Patients with renal insufficiency may need dose adjustments for bivalirudin, according to their degree of impairment (Table 15.1). In a study of 45 patients with normal to severe renal disease, Robson (2000) found that patients with normal kidneys [glomerular filtration rate (GFR) >90 mL/min] and mildly impaired renal function (GFR = 60–89 mL/min) had similar renal clearance levels and required no dose adjustments. The clearance rate was reduced by 45% in individuals with moderate renal impairment (GFR = 30–59 mL/min) and by 68% in persons with severe renal impairment (GFR <30 mL/min). In dialysis-dependent patients, the clearance rate was reduced by 77% (Robson, 2000; Robson et al., 2002). The half-life of bivalirudin in patients with severe renal impairment is prolonged (about 1 hr) and in dialysis patients the half-life is approximately 3.5 hours (Nawarskas and Anderson, 2001).

Some investigators have suggested that dose reductions might be considered in patients with moderate or severe kidney dysfunction, including those on dialysis (Irvin et al., 1999; Robson, 2000; Robson et al., 2002). However, in the setting of PTCA/PCI, the current package insert states that no dose reduction in the bolus is required, and that only in those individuals on hemodialysis should the infusion dose be reduced; in those with a creatinine clearance (CrCl) <30 mL/min a reduction in the infusion dose should be considered (Angiomax Prescribing Information, The Medicines Company, 2010) (Table 15.1).

Pharmacodynamics

Bivalirudin produces an immediate effect after iv administration. It causes prolongation of the prothrombin time (PT)/international normalized ratio (INR), activated clotting time (ACT), the activated partial thromboplastin time (aPTT), and the

TABLE 15.1 Bivalirudin Pharmacokinetic Parameters in Patients with Renal Impairment

Renal function (Glomerular filtration rate, mL/min)	Bivalirudin clearance (mL/min/kg)	Half-life (min)
Normal renal function (>90 mL/min)	3.4	25
Mild renal impairment (60–89 mL/min)	3.4	22
Moderate renal impairment (30–59 mL/min)	2.7	34
Severe renal impairment (10–29 mL/min)[a]	2.8	57
Dialysis-dependent (while off dialysis) patients[b]	1.0	210

[a]For percutaneous coronary intervention, consider reduction in bivalirudin infusion rate to 1.0 mg/kg/hr (initial bolus unchanged).
[b]For percutaneous coronary intervention, reduce bivalirudin infusion rate to 0.25 mg/kg/hr (initial bolus unchanged).
Source: From Robson (2000); Robson et al. (2002); and Angiomax Prescribing Information, The Medicines Company (2010).

thrombin time (Fox et al., 1993; Lidon et al., 1993; Sharma et al., 1993; Topol et al., 1993). Although there is some interindividual variability, a dose of bivalirudin given as an infusion of 0.20 mg/kg/hr increased the aPTT from 27 to 62 seconds in one study, whereas an infusion rate of 1.0 mg/kg/hr resulted in an average aPTT of 98 seconds in another group of patients (Lidon et al., 1993).

The INR is also prolonged somewhat during bivalirudin infusion. In 54 healthy volunteers, a dose of 0.05–0.6 mg/kg of bivalirudin given over 15 minutes iv increased the INR to between 1.25 and 2.43 (Fox et al., 1993). In a study by Lidon and coworkers (1993), the PT was prolonged to between 12 and 16 seconds with a dose of 0.20 mg/kg/hr, whereas Francis and colleagues (2004) reported the mean INR on monotherapy to be 1.50 (range 1.23–2.18) in 52 patients with suspected HIT treated with bivalirudin. Although the increase in the INR is not as high as with the DTI argatroban, physicians need to be aware of DTI–coumarin interactions during overlapping therapy (see chap. 12).

Two studies have demonstrated differences among the DTIs with respect to their ability to prolong the PT (or INR). Gosselin et al. (2004) performed an *in vitro* study comparing bivalirudin, lepirudin, and argatroban using pooled normal plasma and 14 PT reagents commercially available in the United States, whereas Warkentin and colleagues (2005) used two reagents [of widely differing international sensitivity index (ISI) values] and compared four DTIs (lepirudin, bivalirudin, argatroban, and melagatran). Both groups reported that argatroban had the greatest effect on the INR, whereas lepirudin exhibited the least. Gosselin et al. (2004) also found that bivalirudin's effect on the INR was dependent on its concentration and the reagent used, with INR values ranging from 1.10 to 1.53. Warkentin and Koster found similar results, and noted that PT (INR) prolongation corresponded to the DTI molar concentrations required to prolong the aPTT, that is, if a higher molar concentration of the DTI is needed to prolong the aPTT, then its effect on PT (INR) prolongation will be relatively greater (Warkentin and Koster, 2005; Warkentin et al., 2005) (Fig. 15.3).

Bivalirudin decreases fibrinopeptide A levels (a marker of fibrinogen cleavage) in patients with coronary artery disease (Cannon et al., 1993; Ren et al., 1997). It may also increase the bleeding time in some patients (Topol et al., 1993).

Bivalirudin does not inhibit platelet activation or aggregation directly, but it has been shown to inhibit thrombin-mediated platelet aggregation without affecting adenosine 5′-diphosphate or collagen-mediated platelet activation (Weitz and Maraganore, 2001; Wiggins et al., 2002; Wittkowsky, 2002) (Fig. 15.4). Recently, Kimmelstiel and colleagues (2011) studied patients undergoing PCI, and found that bivalirudin did inhibit collagen-induced platelet activation. Bivalirudin has also been shown to be effective in blocking thrombin activation of both protease-activated receptor (PAR)1- and PAR4-dependent platelet aggregation (Leger et al., 2006; Kimmelstiel et al., 2011).

Schneider et al. (2006) demonstrated that bivalirudin inhibited thrombin-induced activation of platelets to a greater extent than heparin or heparin plus eptifibatide. Bivalirudin has also been shown to be effective (when used in combination with aspirin and clopidogrel) in suppressing thrombin generation and activity (Keating et al., 2005a). These antiplatelet effects, as well as bivalirudin's reported effects on inflammation (decreased concentration of high-sensitivity C-reactive protein seen 30 days after PCI), thrombin generation and activity (Keating et al., 2005a), decreased platelet reactivity and platelet–leukocyte aggregates, and leukocyte

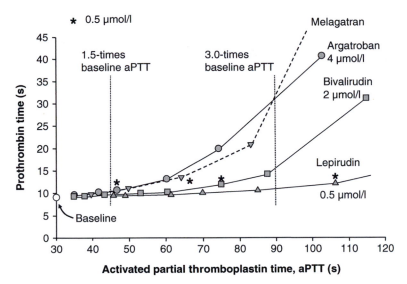

FIGURE 15.3 Effects of four DTIs on the INR–aPTT relationship. Pooled normal plasma was supplemented with serial twofold increases in the concentrations of each DTI. The asterisk (*) indicates the identical molar concentration (0.5 μmol/L) for each DTI. For a 1.5- to 3.0-fold increase in the aPTT (the range shown by the vertical dotted lines), the DTIs differ considerably in their ability to prolong the INR, as follows: argatroban > melagatran > bivalirudin > lepirudin. *Abbreviations*: aPTT, activated partial thromboplastin time; DTI, direct thrombin inhibitor; INR, international normalized ratio. *Source*: From Warkentin and Koster (2005), with modifications.

activation (Keating et al., 2005b) may make it more useful than heparin in the platelet-rich environment of active coronary lesions, where platelet activation and thrombin formation both play significant roles.

The anticoagulant effects of bivalirudin reverse rapidly, with coagulation times returning to baseline within 1–2 hours after stopping the infusion (Fox et al., 1993).

Dosage

Bivalirudin is approved for iv administration only and dosing regimens for patients undergoing PCI (including patients with HIT) are well established. There are no well-established dosing guidelines for other indications (Dager and White, 2002), although dosing regimens for certain indications have been reported. In three patients with venous and arterial thrombosis treated with bivalirudin for HIT, Chamberlin and associates (1994) used doses ranging from 0.05 to 0.20 mg/kg/hr. Their goal was to maintain a therapeutic aPTT greater than 50 seconds. Berilgen et al. (2003) initiated therapy at a mean dose of 0.16 mg/kg/hr in 15 suspected HIT patients maintaining a mean dose of 0.11 mg/kg/hr; all patients achieved a therapeutic aPTT within 24 hours.

Francis and colleagues (2004) have used bivalirudin in patients with both clinically suspected and confirmed HIT. Initial infusion rates ranged from 0.15 to 0.20 mg/kg/hr and their target aPTT was a 1.5- to 2.5-fold prolongation of the baseline aPTT value. Ramirez et al. (2005) reported doses ranging from 0.03 to 0.2 mg/kg/hr in 42 patients, many with multiorgan failure who were clinically

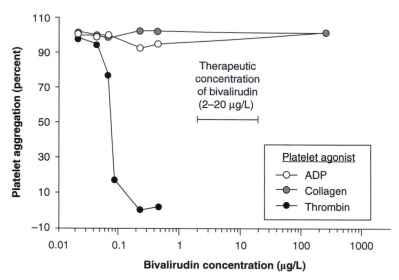

FIGURE 15.4   The effect of bivalirudin on thrombin-induced platelet aggregation. Bivalirudin completely inhibits thrombin-induced platelet aggregation at concentrations about 1/500 that of therapeutic doses achieved during percutaneous coronary intervention, without significant effect on platelet aggregation by collagen or ADP. *Abbreviation*: ADP, adenosine diphosphate. *Source*: From Wittkowsky (2002).

suspected of, or had a history of, HIT. Kiser and Fish (2006) reported mean bivalirudin doses for critically ill patients with hepatic and renal dysfunction, including 10 patients receiving continuous venovenous hemofiltration (CVVH) with or without dialysis. They recommended doses of 0.14 mg/kg/hr for patients with hepatic dysfunction, 0.03–0.05 mg/kg/hr in those with renal or combined renal/hepatic dysfunction, and 0.03–0.04 mg/kg/hr in patients receiving CVVH. Dang et al. (2006), reviewing their experience with 24 patients who received bivalirudin for confirmed or presumed HIT, used doses ranging from 0.10 to 0.17 mg/kg/hr.

   More recently, Skrupky and coworkers (2010) reported their dosing strategy for bivalirudin in 92 patients with known or suspected HIT. They recommended an initial bivalirudin dose of 0.06–0.1 mg/kg/hr for most of their patient population, with a lower dose range (0.02–0.06 mg/kg/hr) for those with renal dysfunction.

   Runyan et al. (2011) evaluated dosing requirement in 64 patients receiving bivalirudin for HIT-related disorders who were organized into five different groups of renal function based on their Cockcroft-Gault–estimated CrCl. The groups included patients with less than 30, 30–60, or >60 mL/min as well as individuals on intermittent hemodialysis or CVVH. In their retrospective medical record review, the authors reported that bivalirudin dosing requirements increased with increasing CrCl values with median bivalirudin dosing ranging from 0.15 mg/kg/hr for a CrCl of >60 mL/min to 0.04 mg/kg/hr for patients on hemodialysis.

   In the largest reported retrospective analysis to date, Tsu and Dager (2011) divided 135 patients treated with bivalirudin based on their renal function. The majority of their population consisted of intensive care unit (ICU) patients while one-third were obese. Patients not receiving dialysis and those on dialysis were

TABLE 15.2 Bivalirudin Initial Dosage Recommendations and Titration Nomogram (University of Colorado)

Estimated creatinine clearance (mL/min)	Initial bivalirudin dosage recommendation (mg/kg/hr)
>60	0.15
45–60	0.075
30–44	0.05
<30 or renal replacement therapy	0.025
Activated partial thromboplastin time (sec)	Bivalirudin dosage adjustment
<35	Increase dose by 50%
35–44	Increase dose by 25%
45–49	Increase dose by 10%
50–80	Target aPTT range, no change
81–90	Decrease dose by 10%
91–100	Hold infusion × 1 hr, decrease dose by 25%
>100	Hold infusion × 2 hr, decrease dose by 50%

aPTT monitoring schedule: baseline (prebivalirudin), then, 2 hr after initiation of bivalirudin, then every 4 hours; then every morning after 2 consecutive aPTTs in target range (50–80 seconds) on a stable DTI dose. Return to monitoring every 4 hours after any dose modification or aPTT result outside of goal range.
Note: the protocol would require modification if a target range other than 50–80 seconds was applicable.
Source: From Kiser et al. (2011), with modifications.

divided into three subgroups: the nondialysis categories were based on CrCl of >60, 30–60, and <30 mL/min, whereas the dialysis patients were grouped according to type of dialysis: intermittent hemodialysis, sustained low-efficiency daily diafiltration, or continuous renal replacement therapy. Tsu and Dager recommend dosage adjustments to 0.13, 0.08, and 0.05 mg/kg/hr in patients with CrCl of >60, 30–60, and <30 mL/min, respectively, and 0.07, 0.09, and 0.07 mg/kg/hr in patients on intermittent hemodialysis, sustained low-efficiency daily diafiltration or continuous renal replacement therapy, respectively.

Tsu and Dager (2012) also looked at total and ideal body weight as dosing strategies for initiating bivalirudin in obese patients. Forty-six patients were divided into two groups: a body mass index of between 30 and 40 kg/m² (33 patients) and >40 kg/m² (13 patients) and concluded that the total body weight was most accurate for achieving the target aPTT using bivalirudin in obese patients.

Kiser et al. (2011) recently reported their use of a DTI titration protocol with bivalirudin and argatroban to manage patients with suspected HIT. Twenty-one of the 46 patients utilizing the DTI protocol-driven dosage received bivalirudin and were found (vs non–protocol-driven adjustments) to have a shortened time to a therapeutic aPTT, as well as a decrease in the number of titrations required to achieve aPTT goals (Table 15.2).

Based on these studies, a reasonable regimen might be to start at 0.10–0.15 mg/kg/hr (no initial bolus) for non-interventional procedures in patients with normal renal function, with subsequent adjustments according to aPTT. However, in patients with renal (or hepatic dysfunction, or both), much lower doses are advised.

For HIT patients undergoing PCI, the dose initially recommended in the "Anticoagulant Therapy with Bivalirudin to Assist in the Performance of Percutaneous Coronary Intervention in Patients with Heparin-induced Thrombocytopenia"

(ATBAT) trial was a bolus of 1.0 mg/kg followed by an infusion of 2.5 mg/kg/hr for 4 hours. This dose was later changed to a bolus of 0.75 mg/kg followed by a 1.75 mg/kg/hr infusion for the duration of the procedure, based on data from the Comparison of Abciximab Complications with Hirulog Ischemic Events Trial (CACHET) and Randomized Evaluation in PCI Linking Angiomax to Reduced Clinical Events Trial (REPLACE-1) trials (Mahaffey, 2001; Lincoff et al., 2002a).

Bivalirudin is approved in the United States for PTCA in patients with UA and for patients undergoing PCI (with provisional GPIIb/IIIa). The current recommended dose for patients with (near) normal renal function is a bolus of 0.75 mg/kg followed immediately by a continuous infusion at 1.75 mg/kg/hr for the duration of the procedure (Sciulli and Mauro, 2002; Angiomax Prescribing Information, The Medicines Company, 2010). The bolus is given just prior to the procedure. Continuation of the infusion for up to 4 hours after the procedure is optional, at the discretion of the physician. After completing the 1.75 mg/kg/hr infusion period, additional bivalirudin may be given at a rate of 0.20 mg/kg/hr for up to 20 hours.

Bivalirudin infusion may need to be reduced in patients with moderate to severe renal impairment (estimated CrCl <30 mL/min) (Robson et al., 2002, Angiomax Prescribing Information, The Medicines Company, 2010), for example, to 1.0 mg/kg/hr (for CrCl <30 mL/min). In dialysis-dependent patients the dose is reduced to 0.25 mg/kg/hr and ideally should be given when the patient is off dialysis (Sciulli and Mauro, 2002; Angiomax Prescribing Information, The Medicines Company, 2010) (Table 15.1).

Allie et al. (2003) used doses similar to the modified ATBAT trial dose for percutaneous transluminal angioplasty (PTA) of the renal and iliac arteries. Following a 0.75 mg/kg iv bolus, bivalirudin was subsequently given by infusion (1.75 mg/kg/hr) until completion of the procedure. Similar bivalirudin doses were also used by Shammas and colleagues (2003) in a single-center experience, by Allie et al. (2004) in The Angiomax Peripheral Procedure Registry Of Vascular Events (APPROVE) Trial involving patients undergoing intervention for renal, iliac, and femoral vessels and by Katzen and colleagues (2005) in patients who underwent peripheral interventions of the lower extremities (iliac, femoropopliteal, or distal), and carotids, vertebrals, renal, aorta, and subclavian vessels. Of note, bivalirudin is not FDA approved for any of these indications.

For cardiac surgery using cardiopulmonary bypass (CPB), that is, on-pump surgery, about two- to threefold greater levels of anticoagulation are required, compared with OPCAB. [For details regarding these protocols, including important technical considerations for the cardiac surgeon and cardiac anesthesiologist, see chap. 19; see also Warkentin and Greinacher (2003); Warkentin and Koster (2005); Warkentin et al. (2008a,b).]

Administration

Bivalirudin is administered iv and produces a rapid anticoagulant effect (Fig. 15.2). In several small trials, however, it has also been given by subcutaneous (sc) injection. In contrast to its rapid clearance following iv injection, its anticoagulant effects are sustained for several hours after sc administration (Fox et al., 1993) (Fig. 15.5). The peak anticoagulant effect occurred between 1 and 2 hours after sc administration in a study of human volunteers, with detectable plasma levels measured up to 6 hours postinjection. Following sc injection of 0.3 mg/kg, the

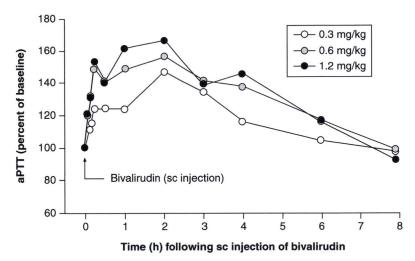

FIGURE 15.5 Prolongation of the aPTT by administration of sc bivalirudin. Three groups of study subjects containing four subjects each were given an increasing dose of sc bivalirudin. Each line represents the mean value of four study subjects. *Abbreviations*: aPTT, activated partial thromboplastin time; sc, subcutaneous. *Source*: From Fox et al. (1993).

aPTT was prolonged to $150 \pm 19.4\%$ of the baseline value, and after a $1\,mg/kg$ sc dose, to $176 \pm 19.4\%$ of the baseline value; the corresponding INR values increased to 1.18 ± 0.05 and to 1.48 ± 0.17 (Fox et al., 1993). Urinary excretion of the drug was complete by 8–12 hours. To date, there are no good efficacy data using the sc route of administration, and it is not approved for use in this manner.

A number of drugs commonly used in patients undergoing PCI have been tested for compatibility with bivalirudin when infused through the same line (Y-site compatibility). Testing was for short-term mixing, rather than longer-term interactions (4 hr). Drugs found to be compatible with bivalirudin included abciximab, dexamethasone, digoxin, diphenhydramine, dopamine, epinephrine, eptifibatide, esmolol, furosemide, heparin, lidocaine, morphine, nitroglycerin, potassium chloride, sodium bicarbonate, tirofiban, and verapamil (Reed and Bell, 2002; Angiomax Prescribing Information, The Medicines Company, 2010). Dobutamine was compatible at concentrations up to $4\,mg/mL$ but incompatible at a concentration of $12.5\,mg/mL$ (Trissel and Saenz, 2002; Hartman et al., 2004).

Trissel and Saenz (2002) looked at the compatibility of bivalirudin with 96 selected drugs including anti-infectives, analgesics, antihistamines, diuretics, steroids, and other supportive care agents by visual observation, turbidity measurement, and electronic particle content assessment. Eighty-seven were compatible with a bivalirudin dilution. Table 15.3 lists the nine drugs found by Reed and Bell (2002) and Trissel and Saenz to cause haze formation or gross precipitation, and which thus should not be administered in the same line as bivalirudin.

Drug–drug interaction studies have been performed with the thienopyridine derivative ticlopidine, the GPIIb/IIIa inhibitors abciximab, eptifibatide, and tirofiban, and low molecular weight heparin (LMWH) and UFH (Reed and Bell, 2002). No pharmacodynamic interactions occurred between bivalirudin and these agents.

TABLE 15.3   Drugs Incompatible with Bivalirudin

Alteplase
Amiodarone hydrochloride
Amphotericin B
Chlorpromazine hydrochloride
Diazepam
Prochlorperazine edisylate
Reteplase
Streptokinase
Vancomycin hydrochloride

Source: From Reed and Bell (2002); Angiomax Prescribing Information, The Medicines Company (2010).

In patients undergoing PTCA/PCI, coadministration of bivalirudin in conjunction with heparin, warfarin, thrombolytic therapy, or GPIIb/IIIa inhibitors has been associated with increased risk of bleeding compared with patients not receiving these concomitant medications (Angiomax Prescribing Information, The Medicines Company, 2010). Aspirin was associated with a mild increase in bleeding times in patients receiving bivalirudin infusions when compared with placebo. These changes were not felt to be clinically significant (Fox et al., 1993).

Monitoring

The PT (INR), ACT, aPTT, and thrombin time all rise linearly with increases in the dose of bivalirudin. The ACT can be used to monitor bivalirudin in patients undergoing PTCA, PCI, OPCAB, or PTA, whereas the aPTT has been used in patients treated for HIT and other noninterventional indications if desired. However, monitoring is optional for PTCA and PCI because of the linear pharmacokinetics of bivalirudin. Dosing in PCI generally results in ACTs above 300 or 350 seconds, although dosing is not adjusted based on the ACT, while at lower doses within the range of aPTT monitoring (used for certain nonapproved indications), the target range usually is a 1.5- to 2.5-fold increase in the baseline aPTT (Chew et al., 2001).

The ACT and aPTT have limitations, however, and questions regarding their adequacy for monitoring DTI therapy remain, particularly for anticoagulation during CPB (Pötzsch et al., 1997; Koster et al., 2000, 2003a; Despotis et al., 2001; de Denus and Spinier, 2002). As a result, other tests have been developed for monitoring these anticoagulants. One of these, the ecarin clotting time (ECT; see chap. 19) has been recommended for monitoring during on-pump cardiac surgery.

Koster et al. (2003a) found that an ECT ranging between 400 and 450 seconds provided acceptable anticoagulation during CPB, noting a close relationship between the ECT (but not the ACT) and bivalirudin concentrations. Nevertheless, a bivalirudin dosing protocol has now been developed that utilizes ACT (rather than ECT) monitoring, which has also provided acceptable monitoring during prospective evaluation for CPB anticoagulation (Dyke et al., 2006) (see chap. 19). The bivalirudin infusion rate in the EVOLUTION-ON cardiac surgery trial was usually not adjusted according to the ACT; rather, the ACT was used to assure that the protocol-specified dosing achieved an acceptable level of anticoagulation, although physicians could give extra bivalirudin boluses at their discretion (see chap. 19). More recently, Salemi et al. (2011) reported the use of a specific chromogenic antifactor IIa assay (Dade-Behring, Deerfield, Illinois, U.S.A.) in a patient with HIT to monitor bivalirudin concentrations during CPB.

As with other anticoagulants, monitoring may not be reliable if the patient has a lupus anticoagulant, hypofibrinogenemia, elevated fibrinogen–fibrin degradation products, or if the plasma contains heparin (Reid and Alving, 1993). Acquired coagulopathies are often seen in ICU patients (a patient group sometimes treated with bivalirudin), and associated low fibrinogen or prothrombin levels may lead to difficulties in judging appropriate drug levels. In these situations, other tests including high-performance liquid chromatography, immunoassays, and chromogenic assays may be superior. Although such assays have been used to measure levels of various DTIs (Griessbach et al., 1985; Bichler et al., 1991; Spannagl et al., 1991; Walenga et al., 1991), these assays are not widely available.

Reid and Alving (1993) developed a quantitative thrombin time in which bivalirudin (or hirudin) levels are measured using patient plasma (or whole blood) mixed with human fibrinogen solution, with the clotting time measured after adding human thrombin. The concentration of bivalirudin (or hirudin) is then determined by comparison with a standard curve that is generated by adding known concentrations of bivalirudin to pooled normal plasma.

Reversal

There is no specific antagonist to bivalirudin. If renal function is normal, bivalirudin is eliminated rapidly, and its anticoagulant effect clears within a few hours after discontinuing the infusion. Kaplan and Francis (2002) have suggested that recombinant factor VIIa (rFVIIa) may be of benefit if bleeding occurs. *Ex vivo* studies using thromboelastography support a possible role for rFVIIa for ameliorating bivalirudin-associated bleeding (Young et al., 2007b). Approximately 25% of bivalirudin can be removed by hemodialysis (Irvin et al., 1999; Angiomax Prescribing Information, The Medicines Company, 2010).

Koster and colleagues (2003b) demonstrated that large amounts of bivalirudin can be removed by hemofiltration and plasmapheresis. They utilized five different hemofilters in an *in vitro* study (conditions mimicking CPB) and observed a correlation between pore size and elimination rate. In their study, 65% of bivalirudin was removed using a hemofilter with a large pore size (65,000 Da) (Mintech Hemocor HPH 700, Minneapolis, Minnesota, U.S.A.), an amount comparable with that eliminated with a plasmapheresis filter system (69%). This represents a 50% improvement over the amount of lepirudin that can be removed through filtration (moreover, lepirudin filtration correlates poorly with pore size). These authors suggest that hemofiltration using appropriate filters may be useful for routine management of patients who receive bivalirudin for cardiac surgery.

Adverse Effects

Bleeding is the major adverse effect of bivalirudin and occurs more commonly in patients with renal impairment. Injection site pain has been reported in individuals who were given sc bivalirudin (Fox et al., 1993). Diarrhea and abdominal cramps have also been reported (Fox et al., 1993). The package insert includes two tables of treatment-related adverse events (other than bleeding) based on results from the Hirulog Angioplasty Study (HAS) [now known as the Bivalirudin Angioplasty Trial (BAT)], and the REPLACE-2 trial (Angiomax [bivalirudin] Prescribing Information, The Medicines Company, Parsippany, NJ, 2010). The most frequent adverse effects in the BAT trial (>10%) included nausea, back pain, hypotension, pain, and headache. Approximately 5–10% of patients reported insomnia, hypertension, bradycardia, vomiting, dyspepsia, urinary retention, anxiety, abdominal pain, fever, nervousness, pelvic pain, and pain at the injection site (Bittl et al., 1995; Sciulli and Mauro, 2002). In the REPLACE-2 trial, the most common adverse effects reported were thrombocytopenia, nausea, hypotension, angina pectoris, and headache (Lincoff et al., 2003). Of note, there was a difference in the dosage of bivalirudin used in these trials: in BAT, bivalirudin was dosed at 1.0 mg/kg iv followed by 2.5 mg/kg/hr compared with the 0.75 mg/kg iv and 1.75 mg/kg/hr used in the REPLACE-2 trial.

CLINICAL USE OF BIVALIRUDIN (NON-HIT PATIENTS)
Treatment of Deep Vein Thrombosis
Bivalirudin is not approved for the treatment of venous thromboembolism. However, it has been evaluated in animal models of venous and arterial thrombosis and in one study involving humans. In a rat model of venous thrombosis using injections of tissue thromboplastin combined with stasis, the administration of bivalirudin demonstrated a dose-dependent interruption of thrombus formation (Maraganore et al., 1991).

Ginsberg et al. (1994b) studied iv and sc injections of bivalirudin in 10 patients with calf-vein thrombosis to determine if single injections could inhibit thrombin generation in a sustained fashion. Prothrombin fragment (F1+2) levels were used as an index of thrombin generation. Significant reductions in F1+2 levels were noted at 6 hours postinjection, but by 24 hours, levels had increased significantly. These workers speculated that higher doses, more frequent sc injections, or prolonged infusions were required to achieve ongoing inhibition.

Prevention of Deep Vein Thrombosis
Bivalirudin (given as sc injection) has been evaluated for prevention of deep vein thrombosis (DVT) in patients undergoing hip or knee surgery. In a phase II, open-label, dose-optimization study of 222 patients, sc bivalirudin was given beginning 12–24 hours postoperatively for up to 14 days or until hospital discharge (Ginsberg et al., 1994a). Five dose regimens were used, ranging from 0.3 mg/kg twice a day to 1.0 mg/kg three times a day (Table 15.4). Patients were evaluated for the occurrence of symptomatic DVT or pulmonary embolism (PE) within 72 hours of discontinuing bivalirudin, and assessment of distal or proximal DVT by venography was performed on day 14 or just prior to discharge. Two patients suffered PE while three patients had major bleeding. The rate of DVT ranged from 59% in the lowest-dose regimen to only 17% in the highest-dose regimen (1.0 mg/kg three times a day). Proximal DVT occurred in only 2% of patients in the highest-dose regimen. Bleeding rates were low (<5%) with all regimens.

Percutaneous Coronary Intervention
Bivalirudin has been studied for several cardiology indications, including most prominently PCI, but also other nonintervention cardiac situations (Table 15.5). Bivalirudin has been approved by the FDA for use in patients undergoing PCI. To date, over 4,000,000 patients have been treated with bivalirudin (personal communication with The Medicines Company). Bivalirudin is a safe and effective alternative to heparin in this patient population.

TABLE 15.4 Efficacy and Safety of Bivalirudin in Preventing Deep Vein Thrombosis After Major Hip or Knee Surgery

Efficacy or safety endpoint	Bivalirudin dosing regimen				
	0.3 mg/kg every 12 hr	0.6 mg/kg every 12 hr	1.0 mg/kg every 12 hr for 3 days, then 0.6 mg/kg	1.0 mg/kg every 12 hr	1.0 mg/kg every 8 hr
n	17	54	40	20	46
Overall DVT rate	10 (59%)	23 (43%)	16 (40%)	7 (35%)	8 (17%)[a]
Proximal DVT rate	7 (41%)	9 (17%)	6 (15%)	4 (20%)	1 (2%)[b]
PE	0	2 (4%)	0	0	0
Major bleeding	0	1 (2%)	1 (3%)	0	1 (2%)
Minor bleeding	0	2 (4%)	0	1 (5%)	0

Note: Venous thrombosis was documented by bilateral venography or by the occurrence of PE. Of the 222 patients enrolled in the study, 177 patients had technically adequate bilateral venography or clinically documented PE and were considered in the analysis of efficacy. Major bleeding was defined as a fall in hemoglobin level of >2 g/dL or transfusion of >2 U of blood. All other clinically overt bleeding was classified as minor.
[a]Significantly lower overall DVT rate compared with the first four regimens combined: 8/46 (17%) *vs* 56/131 (43%); $P < 0.05$.
[b]Significantly lower proximal DVT rate compared with the first regimens combined: 1/46 (2%) *vs* 26/131 (20%); $P < 0.01$.
Source: From Ginsberg et al. (1994a).
Abbreviation: DVT, deep vein thrombosis; PE, pulmonary embolism.

The first clinical study using bivalirudin for coronary angioplasty was reported by Topol and coworkers (1993) in a multicenter, open-label, dose-finding trial of 291 patients. The encouraging results led to larger studies of patients requiring urgent angioplasty because of UA or postinfarction angina, the Hirulog (bivalirudin) Angioplasty Study [for review, see Nawarskas and Anderson (2001)]. The primary endpoint was in-hospital death, myocardial infarction (MI), or abrupt vessel closure within 24 hours of initiating PCI, or rapid clinical deterioration of cardiac origin. In the original publication, no statistically significant difference in the primary endpoint was noted between bivalirudin and heparin (Bittl et al., 1995); this, along with economic and other business considerations, caused the sponsor (Biogen) to abandon further drug development.

Subsequently, The Medicines Company reanalyzed the trial data (including an additional 214 patients analyzed by intention-to-treat principle who were not included in the per-protocol analysis initially reported). In this study, renamed as BAT, the frequency of endpoints (including death, revascularization or MI, and major hemorrhage) were found to be significantly reduced with bivalirudin. Bivalirudin was at least as effective as heparin in preventing ischemic complications in patients who underwent angioplasty for UA and included fewer episodes of major hemorrhage, retroperitoneal bleeding, and need for blood transfusion (Topol et al., 1993; Bittl et al., 1995, 2001; Campbell et al., 2000a; Antman and Braunwald, 2001).

CACHET (phases A, B, and C) evaluated the combination of bivalirudin plus the provisional use of a GPIIb/IIIa inhibitor (abciximab) in comparison with heparin and abciximab in patients undergoing balloon angioplasty and stenting.

TABLE 15.5 Major Clinical Studies Using Bivalirudin In Cardiac Patients (PCI and Non-PCI Indications)

Study acronym or description	Trial (Ref.)
PCI indications	
Dose-finding study	Multicenter, open-label study (Topol et al., 1993)
HAS	*H*irulog (Bivalirudin) *A*ngioplasty *S*tudy (Bittl, 1995; Bittl et al., 1995)
BAT	*B*ivalirudin *A*ngioplasty *T*rial (Bittl et al., 2001)[a]
CACHET	*C*omparison of *A*bciximab *C*omplications with *H*irulog Ischemic *E*vents *T*rial (Lincoff et al., 2002b)
REPLACE-1	*R*andomized *E*valuation in *P*CI *L*inking *A*ngiomax to Reduced *C*linical *E*vents (REPLACE)-1 Trial (Mahaffey 2001, Lincoff et al., 2002a)
REPLACE-2	*R*andomized *E*valuation in *P*CI *L*inking *A*ngiomax to Reduced *C*linical *E*vents (REPLACE)-2 Trial (Lincoff et al., 2003)
Angiomax in Practice Registry	Cho et al. (2003)
NAPLES	The *N*ovel *A*pproaches for *P*reventing or *L*imiting *E*vents *S*tudy (Tavano et al., 2009)
ARNO	The *A*ntithrombotic *R*egimens a*N*d *O*utcome trial (Parodi et al., 2010)
ACS Studies[b]	
TIMI-7	*T*hrombin *I*nhibition in *M*yocardial *I*schemia-7 (Fuchs and Cannon, 1995)
TIMI-8	*T*hrombolysis in *I*nhibition in *M*yocardial *I*schemia-8 (Antman et al., 2002)
HERO-1	*H*irulog *E*arly *R*eperfusion/*O*cclusion-1 (White et al., 1997)
HERO-2	*H*irulog *E*arly *R*eperfusion/*O*cclusion-2 (White, 2001)
ACUITY[c]	*A*cute *C*atheterization and *U*rgent *I*ntervention *T*riage Strateg*Y* Trial (Stone et al., 2004, 2006, 2007)
ISAR-REACT-3	*I*ntracoronary *S*tenting and *A*ntithrombotic *R*egimen-*R*apid *E*arly *A*ction for *C*oronary *T*reatment-3 Trial (Kastrati et al., 2008)
ISAR-REACT-4	*I*ntracoronary *S*tenting and *A*ntithrombotic *R*egimen-*R*apid *E*arly *A*ction for *C*oronary *T*reatment-4 Trial (Kastrati et al., 2011)
HORIZONS-AMI	*H*armonizing *O*utcomes with *R*evascular*IZ*ati*ON* and *S*tents in *A*cute *M*yocardial *I*nfarction trial (Mehran et al., 2009)
PROBI VIRI	*PRO*longed *B*ivalirudin *I*nfusion *V*ersus *I*ntraprocedural only *R*andom*I*zed trial (Cortese et al., 2009a,b)
PROBI VIRI-2	*PRO*longed *B*ivalirudin *I*nfusion *V*ersus *I*ntraprocedural only *R*andom*I*zed trial (Cortese et al., 2011)

[a]Bittl et al. (1995) reported the first study (combining two randomized, controlled trials) comparing bivalirudin against heparin for PCI; this study, subsequently called the *B*ivalirudin *A*ngioplasty *T*rial (BAT), was later reanalyzed (including data from an additional 214 patients) (Bittl et al., 2001).
[b]There is some overlap in the classification above (PCI, ACS) as many of the patients in the ACS trials also underwent PCI.
[c]Approximately 56% of patients in ACUITY underwent PCI, about 11% were triaged to CABG, and the rest were medically managed.
Abbreviations: ACS, acute coronary syndromes; PCI, percutaneous coronary intervention.

Bivalirudin was found to be safe and effective with stents and was associated with a lower combined incidence of death, MI, revascularization, or major hemorrhage at seven days (Nawarskas and Anderson, 2001; Lincoff et al., 2002b; Sciulli and Mauro, 2002).

In the REPLACE-1 trial, heparin was compared with bivalirudin in patients undergoing coronary stenting with any one of the GPIIb/IIIa inhibitors (at the discretion of the physician) in 1056 patients. The combined endpoint of death, MI, or revascularization showed a trend toward a reduction in bivalirudin-treated patients at 48 hours (Lincoff et al., 2002a).

The REPLACE-2 trial was a randomized, double-blind, active-controlled trial of 6010 patients who received bivalirudin with provisional use of GPIIb/IIIa blockage or heparin with planned GPIIb/IIIa inhibition. Bivalirudin was found to be superior to heparin alone and as effective as heparin plus GPIIb/IIIa inhibition for ischemic protection (Lincoff et al., 2003). A significant reduction in the incidence of bleeding and thrombocytopenia were also noted.

An Italian study, NAPLES, randomized 335 diabetic patients undergoing elective PCI to monotherapy with bivalirudin *versus* heparin and tirofiban. The endpoints included the 30-day composite incidence of death, urgent repeat revascularization, MI, and bleeding. The authors found the frequency of bleeding was lower in the bivalirudin group (mainly ascribed to the lower rate of minor bleeding) but concluded it to be safe and feasible with a significant reduction of in-hospital bleeding (Tavano et al., 2009).

In the ARNO trial, Parodi and coworkers (2010) compared bivalirudin and heparin plus protamine in patients undergoing elective PCI who were pretreated with aspirin and clopidogrel. A total of 850 patients with stable or unstable coronary artery disease were randomized to receive bivalirudin or UFH followed by protamine at the end of PCI. Bivalirudin was associated with less major bleeding and fewer ischemic complications compared with heparin.

Cortese et al. (2009a) retrospectively compared 109 patients with ACS undergoing complex PCI to UFH plus a GPIIb/IIIa inhibitor to periprocedural and post-PCI bivalirudin. They demonstrated that a prolonged infusion of bivalirudin (after PCI) was safe and effective with no significant difference in the rates of periprocedural MI or 30-day adverse cardiac events compared with heparin plus a GPIIb/IIIa inhibitor. In a single-center, randomized, single-blinded trial involving 178 consecutive patients with stable or UA and complex coronary anatomy, Cortese et al. (2009b) also demonstrated that a prolonged infusion of bivalirudin after PCI significantly decreased the incidence of periprocedural myocardial damage (PROBI VIRI). In the PROBI VIRI 2 study, Cortese et al. (2011) compared three different study populations; bivalirudin given only peri-PCI, or bivalirudin given additionally by a 4-hour prolonged infusion, and patients treated with standard care (UFH plus abciximab). Of the 264 patients undergoing PCI who were pretreated with aspirin and clopidogrel, the authors found that a prolonged infusion of bivalirudin after primary PCI was equivalent to heparin plus abciximab, with an improvement in early tissue reperfusion in the bivalirudin group.

Bivalirudin was compared directly with heparin in 4750 patients undergoing PCI for stable or UA who were pretreated with 600 mg of clopidogrel. Major bleeding occurred less often in the bivalirudin arm in the ISAR-REACT 3 trial; however, there was no major difference between the two anticoagulants in the primary end point of death, MI, or urgent target vessel revascularization (Kastrati et al., 2008). In ISAR-REACT 4, abciximab and UFH were compared with bivalirudin among 1721 patients with NSTEMI who were undergoing PCI. Compared with bivalirudin, abciximab and heparin failed to reduce the rate of the primary endpoint (death, large recurrent MI, urgent target-vessel revascularization, or major bleeding within 30 days) (Kastrati et al., 2011).

Bivalirudin may be a suitable substitute for heparin in patients with chronic renal disease who require PCI (Chew et al., 2003), because its clearance is primarily determined by proteolysis and not by renal excretion (Robson et al., 2002). ACT monitoring is recommended in patients with chronic renal disease. The dose of bivalirudin may need to be reduced in accordance with the degree of renal impairment, as discussed earlier. If the CrCl is 30mL/min or less, reduction of the infusion rate to 1.0mg/kg/hr should be considered, whereas if the patient is on hemodialysis, the infusion should be reduced to 0.25mg/kg/hr (Robson, 2000; Robson et al., 2002; Angiomax Prescribing Information, The Medicines Company, 2010) (Table 15.1).

Unstable Angina and Acute MI

One of the major experiences with bivalirudin is with patients who have had an acute MI or UA. Two open-label, uncontrolled trials were performed to evaluate the efficacy and tolerability of bivalirudin in patients with UA. Sharma et al. (1993) utilized a 5-day infusion of bivalirudin in patients with UA. Their primary endpoints included death, development of an MI, or the need for coronary intervention. Lidon and coworkers (1993) studied 55 patients with UA in a dose-ranging study. As a result of favorable findings in these two trials, the Thrombin Inhibition in MI (TIMI) 7 trial comparing four different doses of bivalirudin in combination with aspirin was performed in over 400 patients (Fuchs and Cannon, 1995). The TIMI-8 study compared bivalirudin in a single dose with heparin in patients with UA. This study was prematurely discontinued when Biogen suspended product development. Among the 133 patients enrolled, the primary endpoint (all-cause mortality and nonfatal MI at 14 days) was lower, and no major bleeding occurred in the bivalirudin group (Antman et al., 2002). These trials suggested that there is a role for bivalirudin in the management of UA.

A number of trials have evaluated the concomitant use of bivalirudin in patients who received streptokinase and aspirin for an acute MI. Lidon et al. (1994) compared bivalirudin with heparin in 45 patients who suffered an acute MI, whereas Theroux and colleagues (1995) utilized this same strategy in 68 patients. Higher early patency rates and a lower incidence of serious hemorrhage were noted (Nawarskas and Anderson, 2001).

The Hirulog Early Reperfusion/Occlusion (HERO) trial randomized 412 patients with acute MI to receive low-dose bivalirudin, high-dose bivalirudin, or heparin (White et al., 1997). Bivalirudin was found to be more effective than heparin in producing early patency rates at a reduced risk for bleeding.

The HERO-2 trial randomized 17,073 patients who received streptokinase to heparin or bivalirudin for 48 hours in patients who presented with an acute STEMI. Bivalirudin did not reduce mortality compared with heparin, but was associated with a 30% reduction in repeat MI, without significant increase in severe or life-threatening bleeding (White, 2001).

A meta-analysis by the Direct Thrombin Inhibitor Trialists' Collaborative Group (2002) based on individual patients' data reported on 11 studies (35,970 patients) receiving either heparin or DTI therapy (relative number of patients treated: hirudin > bivalirudin > argatroban > inogatran > efegatran). Overall, DTI therapy appeared to be superior over heparin for the prevention of MI in patients with ACS (although the larger number of patients treated with hirudin meant that this DTI contributed most to the overall result reported). Bivalirudin was associated with a 56% reduction in major bleeding risk.

The *A*cute *C*atheterization and *U*rgent *I*ntervention *T*riage Strateg*Y* (ACUITY) trial prospectively randomized 13,819 patients with NSTEMI/ACS to one of three antithrombotic regiments; UFH or LMWH (enoxaparin) plus IIb/IIIa inhibition; bivalirudin plus GPIIb/IIIa inhibition; or bivalirudin alone. Following coronary angiography, patients were randomized again at the discretion of the physician to PCI, CABG, or medical management. Primary endpoints were a composite ischemia endpoint (death, MI, or unplanned revascularization for ischemia), major bleeding, and the net clinical outcome, defined as the combination of composite ischemia or major bleeding. Coronary angiography was performed in 99% of patients. In this trial, bivalirudin plus GPIIb/IIIa inhibition was associated with rates of ischemia and bleeding that were similar to those of heparin plus GPIIb/IIIa inhibitor. Bivalirudin given without GPIIb/IIIa inhibition was also associated with similar rates of ischemia compared with the heparin plus GPIIb/IIIa inhibitor study arm, but with a significantly lower major bleeding rate (3.0% *vs* 5.7%; $P < 0.001$) (Stone et al., 2004, 2006, 2007).

In a substudy of the ACUITY trial involving 392 (4.2%) patients, Kumar et al. (2010) demonstrated that bivalirudin was an effective anticoagulant in the PCI of saphenous vein grafts. The primary endpoints of death, MI, or unplanned target vessel revascularization and major bleeding were similar with bivalirudin alone, bivalirudin plus a GPIIb/IIIa inhibitor, and heparin plus a GPIIb/IIIa inhibitor.

The HORIZONS-AMI trial randomized patients to bivalirudin *versus* heparin plus a GPIIb/IIIa inhibitor in 3602 patients presenting with an acute STEMI undergoing primary PCI (Stone et al., 2008). In a second randomization, patients undergoing PCI were randomly assigned to a paclitaxel-eluting stent or bare-metal stent. Primary endpoints for the first (pharmacology) randomization were major bleeding and the combination of death, reinfarction, urgent revascularization for ischemia or stroke, plus major bleeding (net adverse clinical events), at 30 days. Bivalirudin use resulted in significantly lower major bleeding, net adverse events, and mortality (all-cause and cardiac). The reduction in mortality was sustained at one-year follow-up (Mehran et al., 2009). Although the 24-hour rates of stent thrombosis were higher in the bivalirudin arm, the rates of stent thrombosis at 30 days and at one year were similar. Stone et al. (2011) assessed the three-year outcomes of the HORIZON-AMI trial and found that patients with STEMI treated with bivalirudin alone had a significant reduction in major bleeding, reinfarction, cardiac mortality, and all-cause mortality compared with heparin and a GPII/IIIa inhibitor.

Percutaneous Transluminal Angioplasty

There is limited experience using bivalirudin in the performance of PTA involving the renal or other peripheral arteries. Allie et al. (2003) performed 180 renal and 75 iliac artery PTAs for patients with severe arterial disease using bivalirudin as the only anticoagulant. Procedural success was achieved in 100% of patients, and no adverse thrombotic events were reported. The authors did note a decrease in sheath removal time, time to ambulation, and length of hospital stay. A decrease in vascular access complications was also seen. Shammas et al. (2003) performed PTA on 48 consecutive patients for lower extremity claudication or ulceration. Although there were two serious in-hospital procedural complications, no patient needed emergent revascularization, nor suffered death or limb loss. Allie and colleagues (2004) also assessed the safety and efficacy of bivalirudin in 505 patients undergoing percutaneous peripheral intervention (PPI) for renal, iliac, or femoral disease at 26 centers. Procedural success was achieved in 95% of patients and ischemic events and major hemorrhage rates were low.

Bivalirudin has also been used in carotid artery stenting (Lee et al., 2005; Lin et al., 2005; Finks, 2006). Lee et al. compared bivalirudin to heparin in 46 consecutive patients undergoing carotid artery stenting. Procedural success was 100% in the 24 patients receiving bivalirudin and there were no episodes of major bleeding, vascular complications, strokes, or death. Lin and colleagues performed 200 carotid artery stent procedures on 182 patients, the first 54 receiving heparin anticoagulation. Their protocol was changed, based on results from the REPLACE-2 trial for the next 128 consecutive individuals, resulting in a significant decrease in hemorrhagic complications (Lin et al., 2005). Although none of the series listed above were randomized or double-blind, the authors concluded that bivalirudin was safe, effective, and a reasonable alternative to heparin in peripheral interventions. In addition, the data appear favorable showing lower major bleeding rates and adverse events compared with heparin.

OPCAB Surgery

Merry et al. (2004) compared bivalirudin with UFH for OPCAB surgery in a semiopen label (surgeon-blinded), prospective study of 100 patients (half receiving bivalirudin). The primary endpoint was 12-hour blood loss, and secondary endpoints were ischemic complications and coronary artery patency at 12 weeks. No deaths were reported. The ACT took longer to return to normal after stopping bivalirudin, when compared with the UFH group (which received protamine reversal). Total blood loss was similar in both groups, however. An intriguing (and potentially important) finding was that graft patency was improved in the patients receiving bivalirudin.

Smedira et al. (2006) reported on 105 patients randomized to receive bivalirudin and 52 patients who were given UFH. Procedural success rates at 30 days and mortality were identical in both groups, whereas stroke rates were numerically more frequent in the UFH group (5.5% *vs* 0%), and repeat revascularization occurred more often in the bivalirudin group (3% *vs* 2%). The authors concluded that while data interpretation should be cautious given the small numbers, this study provides further evidence that bivalirudin is a safe and effective alternative to UFH plus protamine for OPCAB surgery. Recently, the American College of Chest Physicians Evidence-Based Clinical Practice Guidelines recommended bivalirudin over other anticoagulants for patients with acute or subacute HIT who required urgent cardiac surgery, either OPCAB or on-pump (discussed subsequently) (Linkins et al., 2012).

On-Pump (CPB) Cardiac Surgery

The EVOLUTION-ON study compared bivalirudin with UFH with protamine reversal in patients undergoing cardiac surgery with CPB (Dyke et al., 2006). Bivalirudin was used in 98 patients *versus* UFH and protamine in 52 individuals. There was no significant difference in procedural success (absence of death, non–Q-wave MI, stroke, repeat revascularization) in the two groups, although early postoperative blood loss and a numerically higher rate of reoperation for bleeding (5.1% *vs* 1.9%) were reported in the bivalirudin group (Warkentin, 2006). Secondary endpoints, including 24-hour blood loss and overall incidence of transfusions, were similar between the two study arms (Dyke et al., 2006).

Temporary Total Heart Implantation

Bivalirudin has also been used successfully in patients as an alternative to heparin following temporary total artificial heart implantation (Crouch et al., 2008). None of the five patients studied had HIT and the drug was tolerated without bleeding complications. One patient was found to have bilateral DVT during therapy but it could not be determined if these were new or pre-existing. The authors concluded that low-dose bivalirudin could be used as an alternative to heparin following temporary total artificial heart implantation.

Vascular Surgery

Kashyap et al. (2010) performed a single-arm, open-label, pilot prospective trial of bivalirudin in patients undergoing lower extremity bypass surgery to assess perioperative safety and efficacy. Eighteen patients with severe symptomatic peripheral arterial disease underwent a femoral–popliteal or femoral–tibial bypass procedure. There were no deaths, MI, or amputations at the 30-day postoperative period. Patency of the bypass was 100% at 30-day follow-up and only one patient had major bleeding requiring transfusion. The authors concluded that bivalirudin is a safe and effective anticoagulant for lower extremity bypass surgery and recommended a comparative trial to heparin be performed.

Pregnancy and Nursing Mothers

There are few data regarding bivalirudin use in pregnancy and nursing mothers. The Medicines Company reported no evidence for impaired fertility or harm to the fetus in rats and rabbits given bivalirudin in teratogenicity studies performed using higher doses than recommended for human use. There are no well-controlled studies in pregnant women, however. Given the potential for adverse effects on the neonate and the potential for increased maternal bleeding, bivalirudin and aspirin (normally used together in cardiac procedures) should be used only if clearly needed. Caution is also advised when giving bivalirudin to nursing women, as it is not known whether bivalirudin crosses the placenta or whether it is excreted in breast milk (Carswell and Plosker, 2002).

Pediatrics

There are limited data on the use of bivalirudin in children. Young et al. (2007a) performed a pilot (open-label, dose-finding) study to assess the safety and efficacy of bivalirudin in 16 younger than six months infants with thrombosis. Their patients received one of three bolus doses and one of two initial infusion doses while safety was assessed by bleeding endpoints. Based on their results, the authors recommended a bolus of 0.125 mg/kg and initial infusion rate of 0.125 mg/kg/hr for this patient population. Two patients experienced major bleeding (gross hematuria) that resolved with dose adjustments, whereas six had either complete or partial resolution of their thrombus burden.

Rayapudi et al. (2008) reported their experience with 16 children varying in age from a few days to 168 months of age. Bivalirudin was used in three patients with HIT and seven with a perceived heparin resistance, whereas the remainder were given bivalirudin for their thrombotic events because the attending physicians felt it had a better efficacy and safety profile. The thrombotic events included the following: seven DVTs, one superficial vein thrombosis, two arterial thrombosis, one right atrial thrombus, one tricuspid valve thrombus, and three patients (two with HIT) on extracorporeal membrane oxygenation (ECMO). Nine of the 16 received a bolus dose ranging from 0.15 to 0.25 mg/kg, whereas the infusion rate varied between 0.05 and 0.31 mg/kg/hr. Ultrasound evidence for clot regression was found in the 10 patients who had follow up imaging and the authors concluded that bivalirudin may be an effective alternative anticoagulant in pediatric patients unable to receive heparin therapy.

Forbes and coworkers (2011) reported pharmacologic data and clinical outcomes in 110 children (ranging from neonates to older children) receiving bivalirudin (0.75 mg/kg bolus; 1.75 mg/kg/hr) for percutaneous interventional procedures in the setting of congenital heart disease. They found predictable drug effects that resembled responses observed in adults.

Other Potential Uses

Bivalirudin has also been studied in animal models for its potential role in both surgical and interventional fields. Its antithrombotic effects were first studied in a baboon carotid endarterectomy model (Kelly et al., 1992). In later studies using end-arterectomized rats, significant decreases in platelet deposition with bivalirudin were shown using [111]Indium-labeled platelets (Hamelink et al., 1995) and scanning electron microscopy (Jackson et al., 1996).

Bivalirudin has also been studied for prevention of vascular restenosis in a rat carotid artery injury model. Xue and associates (2000, 2001) found that bivalirudin reduced platelet deposition on denuded intima. Platelet-derived growth factor levels were also decreased after bivalirudin infusion. The authors suggested that balloon catheter injury-induced neointima formation might be suppressed by bivalirudin.

Bivalirudin has been administered to rabbits after balloon injury and reduces vascular restenosis in the femoral artery of angioplasty-injured, diet-induced atherosclerotic rabbits (Sarembock et al., 1996). These studies support the possible role of thrombin in restenosis.

In contrast to the above study, Kranzhofer et al. (1999) administered bivalirudin to rabbits over three days immediately after balloon injury to the abdominal aorta and right iliac artery. Markers of inflammation, including intercellular adhesion molecule-1, macrophage colony-stimulating factor, tumor necrosis factor, and interleukin-1β, were examined by immunohistochemistry. These workers found that bivalirudin did not acutely reduce vascular smooth muscle cell proliferation or inflammation postangioplasty. They did not rule out other mechanisms by which thrombin inhibition could prevent restenosis.

Bivalirudin has also been shown to reduce thrombin-generated increase in levels of plasminogen activator inhibitor-1 (PAI-1) in cultured baboon aortic smooth muscle cells (Ren et al., 1997). Elevated levels of PAI-1 have been found in patients with coronary artery disease (Hamsten et al., 1985; Francis et al., 1988; Sakata et al., 1990), and numerous authors have suggested their role in the development of atherosclerosis and thrombosis (Ren et al., 1997). Bivalirudin may potentially prevent intravascular thrombogenesis through inhibition of thrombin-induced PAI-1 production (Ren et al., 1997; Shen et al., 1998).

Bivalirudin has also been studied in a rat model of endotoxemia and found to increase survival rate in one (but not the other) study (Cicala et al., 1995; Itoh et al.,

1996). Bivalirudin reduced endotoxin-induced thrombocytopenia, leukopenia, and fibrinogen consumption, suggesting a possible future therapeutic role in sepsis (Cicala et al., 1995).

BIVALIRUDIN FOR THE TREATMENT OF HIT
Miscellaneous Studies

Data on the use of bivalirudin in the treatment of HIT continues to accumulate. Chamberlin et al. (1994) reported three patients who received bivalirudin for HIT. One patient was treated for eight days due to bilateral lower extremity DVTs and recurrent PE with a positive heparin-induced platelet aggregation test, whereas the other two patients received bivalirudin for arterial ischemia due to HIT. One patient required an above-the-knee amputation and was given bivalirudin (for 12 days) to prevent loss of the other limb, whereas the other patient had worsening peripheral arterial disease and underwent angioplasty of his right superficial femoral artery using bivalirudin anticoagulation.

In another study, 39 patients with HIT were treated with bivalirudin (Berkowitz, 1999a; Campbell et al., 2000a; Gladwell, 2002). Seventeen patients had acute HIT, whereas 22 had previous HIT. Patients were treated for a variety of indications, including PCI, DVT, and PE. There were four deaths (10%), all due to complications from HIT. Bleeding complications were usually minor.

Francis and colleagues (2004) presented their experience using bivalirudin to treat 52 patients with a clinical suspicion of, or at an increased risk for, HIT. Forty-three tested positive for anti-PF4/polyanion antibodies, and 16 had thrombosis preceding bivalirudin treatment. Bivalirudin was given for an average of eight days, with transition to warfarin (median overlap four days) performed in 44 of 52 patients. The authors noted minimal increase in the INR on bivalirudin alone (mean increase 0.33). Minor bleeding was seen in only a few patients and there were no amputations or deaths attributable to HIT.

Berilgen et al. (2003) treated 15 patients with multiorgan failure and suspicion for HIT with bivalirudin. Thirteen of the patients had renal and liver dysfunction, 10 were on dialysis, and eight required mechanical ventilation. Fourteen of the 15 had a positive PF4-dependent enzyme immunoassay. One new catheter-related superficial thrombophlebitis developed and one patient with previous ischemic extremities required an amputation. Despite six deaths (not related to therapy), the authors concluded that bivalirudin can be safely and effectively administered in HIT patients with both renal and hepatic dysfunction. Dang et al. (2006) used bivalirudin, argatroban, or lepirudin in 42 confirmed or presumed HIT patients. A composite of clinical outcomes (DVT, nonfatal MI, nonfatal stroke, limb amputation, and all-cause mortality) were similar in all three groups. The authors concluded that bivalirudin was a viable treatment alternative for the management of HIT.

There are several additional series of critically ill patients with acute HIT (or a history of HIT) with multiorgan failure who received bivalirudin. Ramirez et al. (2005) reported their experience with 42 patients, of whom 78.6% required an ICU stay and 14 who had renal or liver dysfunction or both. Nine of their patients with a history of HIT underwent an interventional procedure or surgery requiring bivalirudin administration. Transfusion was required in 28.6% of the patients, five died from multiorgan failure, and three suffered a new thrombotic event during therapy, including a cephalic vein thrombosis, left ventricular thrombus, and an ischemic stroke (the latter occurred while the patient was on subtherapeutic doses of bivali-rudin). There were no amputations and bivalirudin was thought to be safe and efficacious in the ICU setting.

Similarly, Kiser and Fish (2006) evaluated the safety, effectiveness, and dosing of bivalirudin in 18 ICU patients with hepatic and/or renal dysfunction (12 had both). The mean duration of bivalirudin therapy was 15 ± 17 days. The authors reported no clinically significant bleeding episodes, there were no amputations or deaths associated with a thrombotic event, and there was only one reported new thrombosis (a lower extremity DVT). Of note, however, three patients had blood clots form on the filters used for CVVH during treatment, and hepatic dysfunction had only a minimal effect on bivalirudin dosing.

Skrupky et al. (2010) compared bivalirudin and argatroban for the treatment of HIT in 138 patients in a single-center, retrospective analysis. New thromboem-bolic events were reported in seven of the 92 (8%) patients who received bivalirudin while bleeding events occurred in 9%. The authors reported that bivalirudin and argatroban were similar in maintaining therapeutic target aPTTs, as well as clinical outcomes and safety.

In a retrospective review of 64 patients receiving bivalirudin for HIT with a wide range of renal function, Runyan and colleagues (2011) reported clinically sig-nificant bleeding leading to stopping therapy in only four (6%) patients; one of the bleeds was intracerebral. Two (3%) patients developed thrombotic strokes, one before bivalirudin therapy was initiated; both patients died.

In the largest published series to date, Tsu and Dager (2011) reported in a ret-rospective review the outcome of 135 patients with and without renal dysfunction. Only one patient developed a new thrombotic event. However, major bleeding occurred in 39%, which the authors attributed to the critically ill patient population, who frequently required blood transfusions related to surgery and other invasive procedures. They also noted that their all-cause mortality rate (24%) was similar to other reported rates of 17–22% (Dang et al., 2006; Kiser and Fish, 2006; Kiser et al., 2008; Skrupky et al., 2010).

A number of case reports describing bivalirudin use for patients with HIT have been published. Finks (2006) reported the successful use of bivalirudin as a primary anticoagulant during carotid endarterectomy; Robison et al. (2006) used it to maintain anticoagulation during femoral and tibial thromboembolectomy, whereas Alekshun et al. (2006) used bivalirudin in a patient with idiopathic giant-cell myocarditis requiring emergent biventricular assist device placement who had developed propagating clots in the chamber despite therapeutic heparin anticoagu-lation; both patients tested positive for anti-PF4/heparin antibodies. There is one report of long-term (two months) use of bivalirudin to treat serologically confirmed HIT complicated by recurrent left leg ischemia and arterial thrombosis while on LMWH (Bufton et al., 2002); this patient received a continuous infusion of bivaliru-din [22 mg/hr (0.27 mg/kg/hr)] using a continuous ambulatory drug delivery (CADD) pump. Bivalirudin has also been used in the prevention of thrombosis fol-lowing orthotopic liver transplantation in a patient with Budd–Chiari syndrome and a history of HIT (Anderegg, et al., 2008), for perioperative management of a partial face transplantation in a heparin antibody-positive donor (Edrich et al., 2011), and in two patients during radiofrequency catheter ablation procedures with a history of HIT (Baetz et al., 2010).

A few case reports have described patients with HIT where bivalirudin anti-coagulation was employed in a (noncardiac surgery) closed system, such as ECMO.

TABLE 15.6 Theoretical Advantages of Bivalirudin for Treatment of HIT

Features of bivalirudin	Comment
Short half-life (25 min)	Avoids need for initial iv bolus; rapid reversal of anticoagulation (useful if patient develops bleeding or if used for intraoperative anticoagulation)[a]
Predominant enzymic metabolism	Minor renal excretion (20%) means that risk of overdosing in renal failure less than with lepirudin; less risk of postoperative bleeding (compared with lepirudin) if used for intraoperative anticoagulation (in case of postoperative renal insufficiency)[b]
Minimal effect on PT/INR	Simplifies transition to oral anticoagulation (compared with argatroban)
Low immunogenicity	Reduced risk of allergy and anaphylaxis (compared with lepirudin)

[a]Possible disadvantages of a short half-life include need for frequent sc administration (e.g., three or four times daily) and rapid loss of anticoagulation (with risk of rebound thrombosis) if prematurely discontinued in patients with acute HIT.

[b]Possible disadvantage of enzymic metabolism includes loss of anticoagulant action in stagnant blood (implications for cardiac anesthesiology) (see chap. 19).

Abbreviations: HIT, heparin-induced thrombocytopenia; INR, international normalized ratio; iv, intravenous; PT, prothrombin time.

Koster et al. (2007b) reported successful use of bivalirudin for ECMO utilizing an initial bolus dose of 0.5 mg/kg followed by constant infusion of 0.5 mg/kg/hr. Pappalardo et al. (2009) employed a similar dosing strategy in managing a patient with HIT complicating a Bioline® heparin-coated ECMO circuit. Pollak et al. (2011) reported a case of HIT in a five-day-old newborn that developed cutaneous ischemia of the abdomen, hands, and feet, while receiving ECMO with heparin for a congenital diaphragmatic hernia. They used bivalirudin at a loading dose of 0.4 mg/kg followed by infusion of 0.15 mg/kg/hr, maintaining the ACT between 180 and 200 seconds. Although they reported gradual improvement in the thromboembolic cutaneous manifestations, the infant died following surgical repair of the hernia due to multiorgan failure.

Table 15.6 summarizes theoretic advantages of bivalirudin as a treatment for HIT.

Bivalirudin for PCI in HIT

The ATBAT trial was a prospective, open-label study to evaluate the safety and efficacy of bivalirudin in patients with acute HIT or a past history of HIT undergoing PCI (Campbell et al., 2000b; Mahaffey et al., 2003). The primary endpoint was major bleeding within 48 hours after completion of the bivalirudin infusion (1.0 mg/kg/hr iv bolus followed by 2.5 mg/kg/hr by iv infusion for 4 hr). This dose was later changed to a 0.75 mg/kg/hr iv bolus followed by a 1.75 mg/kg/hr infusion for up to 4 hours. Secondary endpoints included event rates for components of the primary endpoint and the ACT, aPTT, and platelet counts (at baseline, pre-PCI/post-PCI, and prior to discharge). Clinical success was defined as procedural success without death, emergency bypass surgery, or Q-wave MI. Only one of the 52 patients required a blood transfusion (1 U), and procedural and clinical success were achieved in 98% and 96% of the patients, respectively. There were no abrupt closures, nor was thrombus formation reported during or after PCI. One patient died of cardiac arrest about 46 hours after successful PCI.

Bivalirudin for Cardiac Surgery in HIT

Bivalirudin has been used off-label for cardiac surgery in a number of patients with acute or previous history of HIT, with both "on-pump" and "off-pump" experience reported, primarily as case reports (Spiess et al., 2002; Vasquez et al., 2002; Davis et al., 2003; Bott et al., 2003; Gordon et al., 2003; Koster et al., 2003a; Baker et al., 2004; Clayton et al., 2004; Jabr et al., 2004; Dyke et al., 2005; Veale et al., 2005; Wasowicz et al., 2005)—including two instances in which bivalirudin was used during heart transplantation (Mann et al., 2005; Almond et al., 2006).

Cardiac surgery experience with bivalirudin in the setting of HIT had been anecdotal until completion of the CHOOSE trials; these prospective studies employed bivalirudin for anticoagulation in HIT patients undergoing either CPB (CHOOSE-ON) or OPCAB surgery (CHOOSE-OFF). Results of these studies have revealed comparable safety and efficacy endpoints (Dyke et al., 2007; Koster et al., 2007a) (see chap. 19).

More recently, Koster et al. (2009) have reported their single-center experience using bivalirudin in "on-pump" and "off-pump" cardiac surgery in patients with and without antibodies (see chap. 19). Of the 141 patients treated with bivalirudin, 40 had heparin antibodies. The authors reported procedural success rates of 99.4% after 30 days and only two patients needing re-exploration owing to bleeding.

The rationale for using bivalirudin in these settings included its direct thrombin inhibition without the requirement of a cofactor, its rapid, dose-dependent prolongation of the ACT, its short half-life, lack of structural similarity to heparin (thus, no cross-reactivity with anti-PF4/heparin antibodies), avoidance of protamine use (and its potentially severe adverse reactions), no need for dose reduction in mild renal impairment, and an ability to "reverse" its anticoagulant effect through hemofiltration. Furthermore, there is the potential to avoid HIT antibody formation and, consequently, postoperative HIT. In addition, recent problems associated with heparin production have emphasized the need for alternative anticoagulant options for cardiac surgery (Koster et al., 2009).

ANTI-BIVALIRUDIN ANTIBODIES

Bivalirudin is a relatively small polypeptide and thus is expected to lack significant antigenicity (Fenton et al., 1998). In a study of plasma samples from seven patients, no evidence for antibody formation (IgG, IgM, or IgE) was found (Fox et al., 1993) with plasma samples obtained at seven and 14 days after iv administration. There was also no evidence for changes in the pharmacokinetics or pharmacodynamics of bivalirudin in their study. One patient exhibited antibody titers of greater than 1:2000 in the assay prior to administration of bivalirudin, although no explanation was given.

In another review of 494 bivalirudin-treated patients from nine different studies, 11 subjects initially tested positive for antibivalirudin antibodies (Berkowitz, 1999b). However, nine of these were found to be false positives on repeat testing. The remaining two (who could not be retested) did not develop any allergic or anaphylactic reactions. In clinical trials of bivalirudin performed from 1993 to 1995, only one of 3639 patients (0.03%) experienced an allergic reaction considered by the investigator to be related to study drug. In a study of 222 patients receiving bivalirudin subcutaneously two to three times daily for up to 14 days, no antibody formation occurred up to six weeks (Ginsburg et al., 1994a; Eichler et al., 2004).

Since bivalirudin shares a 11-amino acid sequence with hirudin, it is at least theoretically possible that patients with antilepirudin antibodies resulting from treatment with lepirudin could cross-react with bivalirudin. Eichler and colleagues (2004) found that 22 of 43 (51%) sera containing antilepirudin antibodies showed reactivity *in vitro* against bivalirudin. This suggests that if bivalirudin is used in patients previously treated with lepirudin, extra caution should be used, for example, careful anticoagulant monitoring, as antilepirudin antibodies sometimes influence pharmacokinetics.

COST ANALYSIS WITH BIVALIRUDIN

Bivalirudin is the only anticoagulant associated with lower rates of both ischemic and bleeding complications compared with heparin in studies of PCI. These complications are associated with increased morbidity and mortality, as well as higher costs and—as reported by Lauer (2000) and Compton (2002)—have a substantial impact on the cost of PCI, making bivalirudin financially more attractive. Bivalirudin may also be associated with a shorter hospital stay, use of fewer closure devices, lower incidence of hematoma formation, earlier sheath removal, and more selective use of the GPIIb/IIIa inhibitors.

An economic evaluation of bivalirudin was reported on the 4651 PCI patients enrolled in the REPLACE-2 trial. In-hospital and 30-day costs were reduced in the bivalirudin group. In addition, regression modeling demonstrated that the hospital savings were not only due to the cost savings of the anticoagulants themselves, but primarily due to the reduction in bleeding and thrombocytopenia that resulted from the use of bivalirudin (Cohen et al., 2004). A subsequent prospective economic analysis in the ACUITY trial involving 7851 patients found a shorter overall length of stay and a significant reduction in overall hospital costs (Pinto et al., 2008). Cost savings have also been observed in a budget model for the HORIZONS trial (Olchanski et al., 2010), as well as in an observational database (Pinto et al., 2012).

Dang and colleagues (2006) reviewed data on 42 hospitalized patients who were treated with bivalirudin, argatroban, or lepirudin for HIT or presumed HIT. Based on average treatment and wholesale price, bivalirudin cost less per day than the other two agents. Buckley and coworkers (2007) found bivalirudin to be more cost-effective than argatroban or lepirudin in the treatment of HIT using a decision-tree analysis to estimate the mean cost per patient employing average wholesale prices and a mean patient weight of 80 kg and 10.7 days treatment duration.

However, these analyses were all based on the cost structures in the U.S. healthcare system. In European health care systems, the use of bivalirudin is much less frequent, primarily due to economic considerations.

CONCLUSION

Bivalirudin is a unique anticoagulant with a number of already approved and several new potential applications. There is extensive experience in patients with UA undergoing PTCA, and it has received approval by the FDA for PCI in patients with HIT. Data are also accumulating on using bivalirudin for HIT, especially in the critically ill patient with multiorgan failure. It is also being used as an alternative anticoagulant in patients undergoing PTA in the peripheral arteries, including the carotid and renal and in the lower extremities.

Bivalirudin has emerged as the favored alternative anticoagulant to heparin in the setting of cardiac surgery, in patients both with and without HIT (Warkentin and Greinacher, 2003; Dyke et al., 2006; Smedira et al., 2006; Warkentin et al., 2008b; Linkins et al., 2012). Its short half-life, unique metabolism, and means of elimination (enzymic) and low immunogenicity provide it with certain advantages over heparin and the other DTIs. In addition, its reversible thrombin inhibition may be associated with decreased bleeding risk. Finally, although there are no antidotes available, the potential for reversibility with hemofiltration (which can be used routinely in the postcardiac surgery setting) adds to its attractiveness.

REFERENCES

Alekshun TJ, Lundbye J, Sokol L, Dailey ME. Use of bivalirudin to treat heparin-induced thrombocytopenia in a patient with idiopathic giant cell myocarditis. Conn Med 70: 69–71, 2006.

Allie DE, Lirtzman MD, Wyatt CH, Keller VA, Khan MH, Khan MA, Fail PS, Hebert CJ, Ellis SD, Mitran E, Chaisson G, Stagg S Jr, Allie AA, Walker CM. Bivalirudin as a foundation anticoagulant in peripheral vascular disease: a safe and feasible alternative for renal and iliac interventions. J Invasive Cardiol 15: 334–342, 2003.

Allie DE, Hall P, Shammas NW, Safian R, Laird JR, Young JJ, Virmani A. The Angiomax Peripheral Procedure Registry of Vascular Events Trial (APPROVE): in hospital and 30 day results. J Invasive Cardiol 16: 651–656, 2004.

Almond CSD, Harrington J, Thiagarajan R, Duncan CN, LaPierre R, Halwick D, Blume ED, del Nido PJ, Neufeld EJ, McGown FX. Successful use of bivalirudin for cardiac transplantation in a child with heparin-induced thrombocytopenia. J Heart Lung Transplant 25: 1376–1379, 2006.

Anderegg BA, Baillie GM, Uber WE, Chavin KD, Lin A, Baliga PK, Lazarchick J. Use of bivalirudin to prevent thrombosis following orthotopic liver transplant in a patient with Budd-Chiari syndrome and a history of heparin-induced thrombocytopenia. Ann Clin Lab Sci 38: 277–282, 2008.

Angiomax® Prescribing Information. The Medicines Company, updated, June 2010.

Antman EM, Braunwald E. A second look at bivalirudin. Am Heart J 142: 929–931, 2001.

Antman EM, McCabe CH, Braunwald E. Bivalirudin as a replacement for unfractionated heparin in unstable angina/non ST-elevation myocardial infarction: observations from the TIMI 8 trial. Am Heart J 143: 229–234, 2002.

Baetz BE, Gerstenfeld EP, Kolansky DM, Spinler SA. Bivalirudin use during radiofrequency catheter ablation procedures in two patients with a history of heparin-induced thrombocytopenia. Pharmacotherapy 30: 952, 2010.

Baker T, Chan R, Hill F. Anticoagulant monitoring techniques in a heparin-induced thrombocytopenia patient undergoing cardiopulmonary bypass using bivalirudin anticoagulant. J Extra Corpor Technol 36: 371–374, 2004.

Bates SM, Weitz JI. Direct thrombin inhibitors for treatment of arterial thrombosis: potential differences between bivalirudin and hirudin. Am J Cardiol 82: 12P-18P, 1998.

Bates SM, Weitz JI. The mechanism of action of thrombin inhibitors. J Invasive Cardiol 12(Suppl F): 27F-32F, 2000.

Berilgen JE, Nguyen PH, Baker KR, Rice L. Bivalirudin treatment of heparin-induced thrombocytopenia [abstr]. Blood 102: 537a, 2003.

Berkowitz SD. Bivalirudin in heparin-induced thrombocytopenia (HIT) or heparin induced thrombocytopenia and thrombosis syndrome (HITTS) patients [abstr]. Blood 94(Suppl 1): 101b, 1999a.

Berkowitz SD. Antigenic potential of bivalirudin [abstr]. Blood 94(Suppl 1): 102b, 1999b.

Bichler J, Siebeck M, Maschler R, Pelzer H, Fritz H. Determination of thrombin-hirudin complex in plasma with an enzyme-linked immunoabsorbent assay. Blood Coagul Fibrinolysis 2: 129–133, 1991.

Bittl JA. Comparative safety profiles of hirulog and heparin in patients undergoing coronary angioplasty. The Hirulog Angioplasty Study Investigators. Am Heart J 130: 658–665, 1995.

Bittl JA, Strony J, Brinker JA, Ahmed WH, Meckel CR, Chaitman BR, Maraganore J, Deutsch E, Adelman B. Treatment with bivalirudin (Hirulog) as compared with heparin during coronary angioplasty for unstable or postinfarction angina. Hirulog Angioplasty Study Investigators. N Engl J Med 333: 764–769, 1995.

Bittl JA, Chaitman BR, Feit F, Kimball W, Topol EJ. Bivalirudin versus heparin during coronary angioplasty for unstable or postinfarction angina: final report reanalysis of the Bivalirudin Angioplasty Study. Am Heart J 142: 952–959, 2001.

Bott JN, Reddy K, Krick S. Bivalirudin use in off-pump myocardial infarction revascularization in patients with heparin-induced thrombocytopenia. Ann Thorac Surg 76: 273–275, 2003.

Buckley M, Kane-Gill S, Seybert A, Dager W, Pathak D. Cost-effectiveness of direct thrombin inhibitors in heparin-induced thrombocytopenia [abstr]. Crit Care Med 35 (12 Suppl): A120, 439, 2007.

Bufton MG, Rubin WD, Springhorn ME, Miller CL, Senuty EJ, Gannon MK. Bivalirudin effect on the INR and experience with prolonged inpatient and outpatient anticoagulation with bivalirudin for treatment of leg ischemia and arterial thrombosis due to HIT-TS [abstr]. Blood 100: 124b, 2002.

Campbell KR, Mahaffey KW, Lewis BE, Weitz JI, Berkowitz SD, Ohman EM, Califf RM. Bivalirudin in patients with heparin-induced thrombocytopenia undergoing percutaneous coronary intervention. J Invasive Cardiol 12(Suppl F): 14F–19F, 2000a.

Campbell KR, Wildermann N, Janning C, Lewis B, Kelton J, Green D, Kottke-Marchant K, Berkowitz SD, Mahaffey KW. Bivalirudin during percutaneous coronary intervention in patients with heparin-induced thrombocytopenia: interim results of the ATBAT Trial [abstr]. Am J Cardiol 86(Suppl 1): 73i–74i, 2000b.

Cannon CP, Maraganore JM, Loscalzo J, McAllister A, Eddings K, George D, Selwyn AP, Adelman B, Fox I, Braunwald E, Ganz P. Anticoagulant effects of hirulog, a novel thrombin inhibitor, in patients with coronary artery disease. Am J Cardiol 71: 778–782, 1993.

Carswell CI, Plosker GL. Bivalirudin: a review of its potential place in the management of acute coronary syndromes. Drugs 62: 841–870, 2002.

Chamberlin JR, Lewis B, Leya F, Wallis D, Messmore H, Hoppensteadt D, Walenga JM, Moran S, Fareed J, McKiernan T. Successful treatment of heparin-associated thrombocytopenia and thrombosis using Hirulog. Can J Cardiol 11: 511–514, 1994.

Chew DP, Bhatt DL, Lincoff AM, Moliterno DJ, Brener SJ, Wolski KE, Topol EJ. Defining the optimal activated clotting time during percutaneous coronary intervention: aggregate results from 6 randomized, controlled trials. Circulation 103: 961–966, 2001.

Chew DP, Bhatt DL, Kimball W, Henry TD, Berger P, McCullough PA, Feit F, Bittl JA, Lincoff AM. Bivalirudin provides increasing benefit with decreasing renal function: a meta-analysis of randomized trials. Am J Cardiol 92: 919–923, 2003.

Cho L, Chew DP, Moliterno DJ, Roffi M, Ellis SG, Franco I, Bajzer C, Bhatt DL, Dorosti K, Simpfendorfer C, Yadav JS, Brener S, Raymond R, Whitlow P, Topol EJ, Lincoff AM. Safe and efficacious use of bivalirudin for percutaneous coronary intervention with adjunctive platelet glycoprotein IIb/IIIa receptor inhibition. Am J Cardiol 91: 742–743, 2003.

Cicala C, Bucci MR, Maraganore JM, Cirino G. Hirulog effect in rat endotoxin shock. Life Sci 57: 307–313, 1995.

Clayton SB, Acsell JR, Crumbley AJ, Uber WE. Cardiopulmonary bypass with bivalirudin in type II heparin-induced thrombocytopenia. Ann Thorac Surg 78: 2167–2169, 2004.

Cohen DJ, Lincoff AM, Lavelle TA, Chen HL, Bakhai A, Berezin RH, Jackman D, Sarembock IJ, Topol EJ. Economic evaluation of bivalirudin with provisional glycoprotein IIb/IIIa inhibition versus heparin with routine glycoprotein IIb/IIIa inhibition for percutaneous coronary intervention: Results from the REPLACE-2 Trial. J Am Coll Cardiol 44: 1792–1800, 2004.

Compton A. A practical cost analysis of bivalirudin. Pharmacotherapy 22: 119S–127S, 2002.

Cortese B, Cortese B, Micheli A, Picchi A, Bandinelli L, Brizi MG, Severi S, Limbruno U. Safety and efficacy of a prolonged bivalirudin infusion after urgent and complex percutaneous coronary interventions: a descriptive study. Coron Artery Dis 20: 348–353, 2009a.

Cortese B, Picchi A, Micheli A, Ebert AG, Parri F, Severi S, Limbruno U. Comparison of pro-longed bivalirudin infusion versus intraprocedural in preventing myocardial damage after percutaneous coronary intervention in patients with angina pectoris. Am J Cardiol 104: 1063–1068, 2009b.

Cortese B, Limbruno U, Severi S, De Matteis S, Diehl L, Pitì A. Effect of prolonged bivalirudin infusion on ST-segment resolution following primary percutaneous coronary interven-tion (from the PROBI VIRI 2 study). Am J Cardiol 108: 1220–1224, 2011.

Crouch MA, Kasirajan V, Cahoon W, Katlaps GJ, Gunnerson KJ. Successful use and dosing of bivalirudin after temporary total artificial heart implantation: A case series. Pharmaco-therapy 28: 1413–1420, 2008.

Dager WE, White RH. Treatment of heparin-induced thrombocytopenia. Ann Pharmacother 36: 489–503, 2002.

Dang CH, Durkalski VL, Nappi JM. Evaluation of treatment with direct thrombin inhibitors in patients with heparin-induced thrombocytopenia. Pharmacotherapy 26: 461–468, 2006.

Davis Z, Anderson R, Short D, Garber D, Valgiusti A. Favorable outcome with bivalirudin anticoagulation during cardiopulmonary bypass. Ann Thorac Surg 75: 264–265, 2003.

de Denus S, Spinier SA. Clinical monitoring of direct thrombin inhibitors using the ecarin clotting time. Pharmacotherapy 22: 433–435, 2002.

Despotis GJ, Hogue CW, Saleem R, Bigham M, Skubas N, Apostolidou I, Qayam A, Joist JH. The relationship between hirudin and activated clotting time: implications for patients with heparin-induced thrombocytopenia undergoing cardiac surgery. Anesth Analg 93: 28–32, 2001.

Dyke CM, Koster A, Veale JJ, Maier GW, McNiff T, Levy JH. Preemptive use of bivalirudin for urgent on-pump coronary artery bypass grafting in patients with potential heparin-induced thrombocytopenia. Ann Thorac Surg 80: 299–303, 2005.

Dyke CM, Smedira NG, Koster A, Aronson S, McCarthy HL, Kirshner R, Lincoff AM, Spiess BD. A comparison of bivalirudin to heparin with protamine reversal in patients undergoing cardiac surgery with cardiopulmonary bypass. The EVOLUTION-ON study. J Thorac Cardiovasc Surg 131: 533–539, 2006.

Dyke CM, Aldea G, Koster A, Smedira N, Avery E, Aronson S, Spiess BD, Lincoff AM. Off-pump coronary artery bypass with bivalirudin for patients with heparin-induced throm-bocytopenia or antiplatelet factor four/heparin antibodies. Ann Thorac Surg 84: 836–840, 2007.

Direct Thrombin Inhibitor Trialists' Collaborative Group. Direct thrombin inhibitors in acute coronary syndromes: principal results of a meta-analysis based on individual patients' data. Lancet 359: 294–302, 2002.

Edrich T, Pomahac B, Lu JT, Couper GS, Gerner P. Perioperative management of partial face transplantation involving a heparin antibody-positive donor. J Clin Anesth 23: 318–321, 2011.

Eichler P, Lubenow N, Strobel U, Greinacher A. Antibodies against lepirudin are polyspecific and recognize epitopes on bivalirudin. Blood 103: 613–616, 2004.

Fareed J, Lewis BE, Callas DD, Hoppensteadt DA, Walenga JM, Bick RL. Anti-thrombin agents: the new class of anticoagulant and antithrombotic drugs. Clin Appl Thromb Hemost 5(Suppl 1): S45–S55, 1999.

Fenton JW II, Ofosu FA, Brezniak DV, Hassouna HI. Thrombin and antithrombotics. Semin Thromb Hemost 24: 87–91, 1998.

Finks S. Bivalirudin use in carotid endarterectomy in a patient with heparin-induced throm-bocytopenia. Ann Pharmacother 40: 340–343, 2006.

Forbes TJ, Hijazi ZM, Young G, Ringewald JM, Aquino PM, Vincent RN, Qureshi AM, Rome JJ, Rhodes JF Jr, Jones TK, Moskowitz WB, Holzer RJ, Zamora R. Pediatric catheterization laboratory anticoagulation with bivalirudin. Catheter Cardiovasc Interv 77: 671–679, 2011.

Fox I, Dawson A, Loynds P, Eisner J, Findlen K, Levin E, Hanson D, Mant T, Wagner J, Maraganore J. Anticoagulant activity of Hirulog™, a direct thrombin inhibitor, in humans. Thromb Haemost 69: 157–163, 1993.

Francis RB Jr, Kawanishi D, Baruch T, Mahrer P, Rahimtoola S, Feinstein DL. Impaired fibrinolysis in coronary artery disease. Am Heart J 115: 776–780, 1988.

Francis JL, Drexler A, Gwyn G. Successful use of bivalirudin in the treatment of patients suspected, or at risk of, heparin-induced thrombocytopenia [abstr]. Blood 104(Suppl): 105b, 2004.

Fuchs J, Cannon CP. Hirulog in the treatment of unstable angina. Results of the Thrombin Inhibition in Myocardial Ischemia (TIMI) 7 trial. Circulation 92: 727–733, 1995.

Ginsberg JS, Nurmohamed MT, Gent M, MacKinnon B, Sicurella J, Brill-Edwards P, Levine MN, Panju AA, Powers P, Stevens P, Turpie AGG, Weitz J, Buller HR, ten Cate JW, Neemeh J, Adelman B, Fox I, Maraganore J, Hirsh J. Use of Hirulog in the prevention of venous thrombosis after major hip or knee surgery. Circulation 90: 2385–2389, 1994a.

Ginsberg JS, Nurmohamed MT, Gent M, MacKinnon B, Stevens P, Weitz J, Maraganore J, Hirsh J. Effects on thrombin generation of single injections of Hirulog in patients with calf vein thrombosis. Thromb Haemost 72: 523–525, 1994b.

Gladwell TD. Bivalirudin: a direct thrombin inhibitor. Clin Ther 24: 38–58, 2002.

Gordon G, Rastegar H, Schumann R, Deiss-Shrem J, Denman W. Successful use of bivalirudin for cardiopulmonary bypass in a patient with heparin-induced thrombocytopenia. J Cardiothorac Vasc Anesthesiol 17: 632–635, 2003.

Gosselin RC, Dager WE, King JH, Janatpour K, Mahackian K, Larkin EC, Owings JT. Effect of direct thrombin inhibitors, bivalirudin, lepirudin and argatroban, on prothrombin time and INR values. Am J Clin Pathol 121: 593–599, 2004.

Griessbach U, Sturzebecher J, Markwardt F. Assay of hirudin in plasma using a chromogenic thrombin substrate. Thromb Res 37: 347–350, 1985.

Hamelink JK, Tang DB, Barr CF, Jackson MR, Reid TJ, Gomez ER, Alving BM. Inhibition of platelet deposition by combined hirulog and aspirin in a rat carotid endarterectomy model. J Vasc Surg 21: 492–498, 1995.

Hamsten A, Wiman B, de Faire U, Blomback M. Increased plasma levels of a rapid inhibitor of tissue plasminogen activator in young survivors of myocardial infarction. N Engl J Med 313: 1557–1563, 1985.

Hartman CA, Faria CE, Mago K. Visual compatibility of bivalirudin with selected drugs. Am J Health Syst Pharm 61: 1774, 1776, 2004.

Irvin W, Sica D, Gehr T, McAllister A, Rogge M, Charenkavanich S, Adelman B. Pharmacodynamics (PD) and kinetics (PK) of bivalirudin (BIV) in renal failure (RF) and hemodialysis (HD) [abstr]. Clin Pharmacol Ther 65: 202, 1999.

Itoh H, Cicala C, Douglas GJ, Page CP. Platelet accumulation induced by bacterial endotoxin in rats. Thromb Res 83: 405–419, 1996.

Jabr K, Johnson JH, McDonald MH, Walsh DL, Martin WD, Johnson AC, Pickett JM. Plasma-modified ACT can be used to monitor bivalirudin (Angiomax®) anticoagulation for on-pump cardiopulmonary bypass surgery in a patient with heparin-induced thrombocytopenia. J Extra Corpor Technol 36: 174–177, 2004.

Jackson MR, Reid TJ, Tang DB, O'Donnell SD, Gomez ER, Alving BM. Anti-thrombotic effects of hirulog in a rat carotid endarterectomy model. J Surg Res 60: 15–22, 1996.

Kaplan KL, Francis CW. Direct thrombin inhibitors. Semin Hematol 39: 187–196, 2002.

Kashyap VS, Bishop PD, Bena JF, Rosa K, Sarac TP, Ouriel K. A pilot, prospective evaluation of a direct thrombin inhibitor, bivalirudin (Angiomax), in patients undergoing lower extremity bypass. J Vasc Surg 52: 369–374, 2010.

Kastrati A, Neumann FJ, Schulz S, Massberg S, Byrne RA, Ferenc M, Laugwitz KL, Pache J, Ott I, Hausleiter J, Seyfarth M, Gick M, Antoniucci D, Schömig A, Berger PB, Mehilli J; ISAR-REACT 4 Trial Investigators. Abciximab and heparin versus bivalirudin for non-ST-elevation myocardial infarction. N Engl J Med 365: 1980–1989, 2011.

Kastrati A, Neumann FJ, Mehilli J, Byrne RA, Iijima R, Büttner HJ, Khattab AA, Schulz S, Blankenship JC, Pache J, Minners J, Seyfarth M, Graf I, Skelding KA, Dirschinger J, Richardt G, Berger PB, Schörnig A; For the ISAR-REACT 3 Trial Investigators. Bivalirudin versus unfractionated heparin during percutaneous coronary intervention. N Engl J Med 359: 688–696, 2008. [Erratum in N Engl J Med 359: 983, 2008]

Katzen BT, Ardid MI, MacLean AA, Kovacs MF, Zemel G, Benenati JF, Powell A, Samuels S. Bivalirudin as an anticoagulation agent: safety and efficacy in peripheral interventions. J Vasc Interv Radiol 16: 1183–1187, 2005.

Keating FK, Dauerman HL, Whitaker DA, Sobel BE, Schneider DJ. The effects of bivalirudin compared with those of unfractionated heparin plus eptifibatide on inflammation and thrombin generation and activity during coronary intervention. Coron Artery Dis 16: 401–405, 2005a.

Keating FK, Dauerman HL, Whitaker DA, Sobel BE, Schneider DJ. Increased expression of platelet P-selectin and formation of platelet-leukocyte aggregates in blood from patients treated with unfractionated heparin plus eptifibatide compared with bivalirudin. Thromb Res 118: 361–369, 2005b.

Kelly AB, Maraganore JM, Bourdon P, Hanson SR, Harker LA. Antithrombotic effects of synthetic peptides targeting various functional domains of thrombin. Proc Natl Acad Sci USA 89: 6040–6044, 1992.

Kimmelstiel C, Zhang P, Kapur NK, Weintraub A, Krishnamurthy B, Castaneda V, Covic L, Kuliopulos A. Bivalirudin is a dual inhibitor of thrombin and collagen-dependent platelet activation in patients undergoing percutaneous coronary intervention. Circ Cardiovasc Interv 4: 171–179, 2011.

Kiser TH, Fish DN. Evaluation of bivalirudin treatment for heparin-induced thrombocytopenia in critically ill patients with hepatic and/or renal dysfunction. Pharmacotherapy 26: 452–460, 2006.

Kiser TH, Burch JC, Klem PM, Hassell KL. Safety, efficacy, and dosing requirements of bivalirudin in patients with heparin-induced thrombocytopenia. Pharmacotherapy 28: 1115–1124, 2008.

Kiser TH, Mann AM, Trujillo TC, Hassell KL. Evaluation of empiric versus nomogram-based direct thrombin inhibitor management in patients with suspected heparin-induced thrombocytopenia. Am J Hematol 86: 267–272, 2011.

Koster A, Hansen R, Grauhan O, Hausmann H, Bauer M, Hetzer R, Kuppe H, Mertzlufft F. Hirudin monitoring using TAS ecarin clotting time in patients with heparin-induced thrombocytopenia type II. J Cardiothorac Vasc Anesth 14: 249–252, 2000.

Koster A, Chew D, Grundel M, Bauer M, Kuppe H, Spiess BD. Bivalirudin monitored with the ecarin clotting time for anticoagulation during cardiopulmonary bypass. Anesth Analg 96: 383–386, 2003a.

Koster A, Chew D, Grundel M, Hausmann H, Grauhan O, Kuppe H, Spiess BD. An assessment of different filter systems for extracorporeal elimination of bivalirudin: an in vitro study. Anesth Analg 96: 1316–1319, 2003b.

Koster A, Dyke CM, Aldea G, Smedira NG, McCarthy HL II, Aronson S, Hetzer R, Avery E, Spiess BD, Lincoff AM. Bivalirudin during cardiopulmonary bypass in patients with previous or acute heparin-induced thrombocytopenia and heparin antibodies: results of the CHOOSE-ON trial. Ann Thorac Surg 83: 572–577, 2007a.

Koster A, Weng Y, Bottcher W, Gromann T, Kuppe H, Hetzer R. Successful use of bivalirudin as anticoagulant for ECMO in a patient with acute HIT. Ann Thorac Surg 83: 1865–1867, 2007b.

Koster A, Buz S, Krabatsch T, Yeter R, Hetzer R. Bivalirudin anticoagulation during cardiac surgery: a single-center experience in 141 patients. Perfusion 24: 7–11, 2009.

Kranzhofer R, Maraganore JM, Baciu R, Libby P. Systemic thrombin inhibition by Hirulog does not alter medial smooth muscle cell proliferation and inflammatory activation after vascular injury in the rabbit. Cardiovasc Drugs Ther 13: 429–434, 1999.

Kumar D, Dangas G, Mehran R, Kirtane A, Bertrand M, Ebrahimi R, Guagliumi G, Brar S, Fahy M, Heller E, Moses J, Stone G. Comparison of bivalirudin versus bivalirudin plus glycoprotein IIb/IIIa inhibitor versus heparin plus glycoprotein IIb/IIIa inhibitor in patients with acute coronary syndrome having percutaneous intervention for narrowed saphenous vein aorto-coronary grafts (the ACUITY trial investigators). Am J Cardiol 106: 941–945, 2010.

Lauer MA. Cost analysis of bivalirudin in percutaneous coronary intervention. J Invasive Cardiol 12(Suppl F): 37F–40F, 2000.

Lee A, Freeman J, Green SJ, Ong LY, Marchant D. Routine use of bivalirudin is safe and efficacious in carotid artery stenting [abstr]. Catheter Cardiovasc Interv 65: 112, 2005.

Leger AJ, Jacques SL, Badar J, Kaneider NC, Derian CK, Andrade-Gordon P, Covic L, Kuliopulos A. Blocking the protease-activated receptor 1–4 heterodimer in platelet mediated thrombosis. Circulation 113: 1244–1254, 2006.

Lidon RM, Theroux P, Juneau M, Adelman B, Maraganore J. Initial experience with a direct antithrombin, Hirulog, in unstable angina. anticoagulant, antithrombotic, and clinical effects. Circulation 88: 1495–1501, 1993.

Lidon RM, Theroux P, Lesperance J, Adelman B, Bonan R, Duval D, Levesque J. A pilot, early angiographic patency study using a direct thrombin inhibitor as adjunctive therapy to streptokinase in acute myocardial infarction. Circulation 89: 1567–1572, 1994.

Lin PH, Bush RL, Peden EK, Zhou W, Guerrero M, Henao EA, Kougias P, Mohiuddin I, Lumsden AB. Carotid artery stenting with neuroprotection: assessing the learning curve and treatment outcome. Am J Surg 190: 850–857, 2005.

Lincoff AM, Bittl JA, Kleiman NS, Kereiakes DJ, Harrington RA, Sarembook IJ, Jackman JD, Mehta S, Maierson EF, Chew DP, Topol EJ. The REPLACE 1 Trial: a pilot study of bivalirudin versus heparin during percutaneous coronary intervention with stenting and GP IIb/IIIa blockade [abstr]. J Am Coll Cardiol 39(Suppl A): 16A, 2002a.

Lincoff AM, Kleiman NS, Kottke-Marchant K, Maierson ES, Maresh K, Wolski KE, Topol EJ. Bivalirudin with planned or provisional abciximab versus low-dose heparin and abciximab during percutaneous coronary revascularization: results of the comparison of abciximab complications with hirulog for ischemic events trial (CACHET). Am Heart J 143: 847–853, 2002b.

Lincoff AM, Bittl JA, Harrington RA, Feit F, Kleiman NS, Jackman JD, Sarembock IJ, Cohen DJ, Spriggs D, Ebrahimi R, Keren G, Carr J, Cohen EA, Betriu A, Desmet W, Kereiakes DJ, Rutsch W, Wilcox RG, deFeyter PJ, Vahanian A, Topol EJ. Bivalirudin and provisional glycoprotein IIb/IIIa blockade compared with heparin and planned glycoprotein IIb/IIIa blockade during percutaneous coronary intervention: REPLACE-2 randomized trial. JAMA 289: 853–863, 2003.

Linkins LA, Dans AL, Moores LK, Bona R, Davidson BL, Schulman S, Crowther M. Treatment and prevention of heparin-induced thrombocytopenia: antithrombotic therapy and prevention of thrombosis, 9th ed. American College of Chest Physicians Evidence-Based Clinical Practice Guidelines. Chest 141: e495S–e530S, 2012.

Mahaffey KW. Anticoagulation for acute coronary syndromes and percutaneous coronary intervention in patients with heparin-induced thrombocytopenia. Curr Cardiol Rep 3: 362–370, 2001.

Mahaffey KW, Lewis BE, Wildermann NM, Berkowitz SD, Oliverio RM, Turco MA, Shalev Y, Lee PV, Traverse JH, Rodriguez AR, Ohman EM, Harrington RA, Califf RM, ATBAT Investigators. the anticoagulant therapy with bivalirudin to assist in the performance of percutaneous coronary intervention in patients with heparin-induced thrombocytopenia (ATBAT) study: main results. J Invasive Cardiol 15: 611–616, 2003.

Mann MJ, Tseng E, Ratcliffe M, Strattman G, De Silva A, DeMarco T, Achorn N, Moskalik W, Hoopes C. Use of bivalirudin, a direct thrombin inhibitor, and its reversal with modified ultrafiltration during heart transplantation in a patient with heparin-induced thrombocytopenia. J Heart Lung Transplant 24: 222–225, 2005.

Maraganore JM, Adelman BA. Hirulog: a direct thrombin inhibitor for management of acute coronary syndromes. Coron Artery Dis 7: 438–448, 1996.

Maraganore JM, Bourdon P, Jablonski J, Ramachandran KL, Fenton JW II. Design and characterization of hirulogs: a novel class of bivalent peptide inhibitors of thrombin. Biochemistry 29: 7095–7101, 1990.

Maraganore T, Oshima FA, Sugitachi A. Comparison of anticoagulant and anti-thrombotic activities of hirulog-1 and argatroban (MD-805) [abstr]. Thromb Haemost 65: 651, 1991.

Mehran R, Lansky AJ, Witzenbichler B, Guaqliumi G, Peruqa JZ, Brodie BR, Dudek D, Kornowski R, Hartmann F, Gersh BJ, Pocock SJ, Wong SC, Nikolsky E, Gambone L, Vandertie L, Parise H, Dangas GD, Stone GW. Bivalirudin in patients undergoing primary angioplasty for acute myocardial infarction (HORIZONS-AMI): 1-year results of a randomized controlled trial. Lancet 374: 1149–1159, 2009.

Merry AF, Raudkivi P, Middleton NG, McDougall JM, Nand P, Mills BP, Webber BJ, Frampton CM. Bivalirudin versus heparin and protamine in off pump coronary artery bypass surgery. Ann Thorac Surg 77: 925–931, 2004.

Nawarskas JJ, Anderson JR. Bivalirudin: a new approach to anticoagulation. Heart 3: 131–137, 2001.

Olchanski N, Slawsky KA, Plent S, Kado C, Cyr PL. Economic impact of switching to bivalirudin for a primary percutaneous coronary intervention in a US hospital. Hosp Pract (Minneap). 38: 138–146, 2010.

Pappalardo F, Scandroglio A, Sampietro F, Zangrillo A, Koster A. Bioline® heparin-coated ECMO with bivalirudin anticoagulation in a patient with acute heparin-induced thrombocytopenia: the immune reaction appeared to continue unabated. Perfusion 24: 135–137, 2009.

Parodi G, Migliorini A, Valenti R, Bellandi B, Signorini U, Moschi G, Buonamici P, Cerisano G, Antonuiucci D. Comparison of bivalirudin and unfractionated heparin plus protamine in patients with coronary heart disease undergoing percutaneous coronary intervention (from the antithrombotic regiments and outcome (ARNO) trial. Am J Cardiol 105: 1053–1059, 2010.

Parry MA, Maraganore JM, Stone SR. Kinetic mechanism for the interaction of Hirulog with thrombin. Biochemistry 33: 14807–14814, 1994.

Pinto DS, Stone GW, Shi C, Dunn ES, Reynolds MR, York M, Walczak J, Berezin RH, Mehran R, McLaurin BT, Cox DA, Ohman EM, Lincoff AM, Cohen DJ, ACUITY Investigators. Economic evaluation of bivalirudin with or without glycoprotein IIb/IIIa inhibition versus heparin with routine glycoprotein IIb/IIIa inhibition for early invasive management of acute coronary syndromes. J Am Coll Cardiol 52: 1758–1768, 2008.

Pinto DS, Ogbonnaya A, Sherman SA, Tung P, Normand SL. Bivalirudin therapy is associated with improved clinical and economic outcomes in ST-elevation myocardial infarction patients undergoing percutaneous coronary intervention: results from an observational database. Circ Cardiovasc Qual Outcomes 5: 52–61, 2012.

Pollak U, Yacobobich J, Tamary H, Dagan O, Manor-Shulman O. Heparin-induced thrombocytopenia and extracorporeal membrane oxygenation: A case report and review of the literature. J Extra Corpor Technol 43: 5–12, 2011.

Pötzsch B, Hund S, Madlener K, Unkrig C, Müller-Berhaus G. Monitoring of recombinant hirudin: assessment of a plasma-based ecarin clotting time assay. Thromb Res 86: 373–383, 1997.

Ramirez LM, Carman TL, Begelman SM, AlMahameed A, Joseph D, Kashyap V, White DA, Andersen-Harris K, Bartholomew JR. Bivalirudin in patients with clinically suspected HIT or history of HIT [abstr]. Blood 106: 269a, 2005.

Rayapudi S, Torres A Jr, Deshpande GG, Ross MP, Wohrley JD, Young G, Tarantino MD. Bivalirudin for anticoagulation in children. Pedatr Blood Cancer 51: 798–801, 2008.

Reed MD, Bell D. Clinical pharmacology of bivalirudin. Pharmacotherapy 22: 105S–111S, 2002.

Reid TJ III, Alving BM. A quantitative thrombin time for determining levels of hirudin and Hirulog. Thromb Haemost 70: 608–616, 1993.

Ren S, Fenton JWII, Maraganore JM, Angel A, Shen GX. Inhibition by Hirulog-1 of generation of plasminogen activator inhibitor-1 from vascular smooth-muscle cells induced by thrombin. J Cardiovasc Pharmacol 29: 337–342, 1997.

Robison JG, Crawford F Jr, Uber W. Use of bivalirudin for suspected heparin-induced thrombocytopenia during lower extremity revascularization. Vasc Dis Manag 3: 359–363, 2006.

Robson R. The use of bivalirudin in patients with renal impairment. J Invasive Cardiol 12(Suppl F): 33F–36F, 2000.

Robson R, White H, Aylward P, Frampton C. Bivalirudin pharmacokinetics and pharmacodynamics: effect of renal function, dose, and gender. Clin Pharmacol Ther 71: 433–439, 2002.

Runyan CL, Cabral KP, Riker RR, Redding D, May T, Seder DB, Savic M, Hedlund J, Abramson S, Fraser GL. Correlation of bivalirudin dose with creatinine clearance during treatment of heparin-induced thrombocytopenia. Pharmacotherapy 31: 850–856, 2011.

Sakata K, Kurata C, Taguchi T, Suzuki S, Kobayashi A, Yamazaki N, Rydzewski A, Takada Y, Takada A. Clinical significance of plasminogen activator inhibitor in patients with exercise-induced ischemia. Am Heart J 120: 831–838, 1990.

Salemi A, Agrawal YP, Fontes MA. An assay to monitor bivalirudin levels on cardiopulmonary bypass. Ann Thorac Surg 92: 332–334, 2011.

Sarembock IJ, Gertz SD, Thome LM, McCoy KW, Ragosta M, Powers ER, Maraganore JM, Gimple LW. Effectiveness of hirulog in reducing restenosis after balloon angioplasty of atherosclerotic femoral arteries in rabbits. J Vasc Res 33: 308–314, 1996.

Scatena R. Bivalirudin: a new generation antithrombotic drug. Exp Opin Invest Drugs 9: 1119–1127, 2000.

Schneider DJ, Keating F, Sobel BE. Greater inhibitory effects of bivalirudin compared with unfractionated heparin plus eptifibatide on thrombin-induced platelet activation. Coron Artery Dis 17: 471–476, 2006.

Sciulli TM, Mauro VF. Pharmacology and clinical use of bivalirudin. Ann Pharmacother 36: 1028–1041, 2002.

Sharma GVRK, Lapsley D, Vita JA, Sharma S, Coccio E, Adelman B, Loscalzo J. Usefulness and tolerability of hirulog, a direct thrombin-inhibitor, in unstable angina pectoris. Am J Cardiol 72: 1357–1360, 1993.

Shammas N, Lemke JH, Dippel EJ, McKinney DE, Takes VS, Youngblut M, Harris M. Bivalirudin in peripheral vascular interventions: a single center experience. J Invasive Cardiol 15: 401–404, 2003.

Shen GX, Ren S, Fenton JW II. Transcellular signaling and pharmacological modulation of thrombin-induced production of plasminogen activator inhibitor-1 in vascular smooth muscle cells. Semin Thromb Hemost 24: 151–156, 1998.

Skrupky LP, Smith JR, Deal EN, Arnold H, Hollands JM, Martinez EJ, Micek ST. Comparison of bivalirudin and argatroban for the management of heparin-induced thrombocytopenia. Pharmacotherapy 30; 1229–1238, 2010.

Smedira NG, Dyke CM, Koster A, Jurmann M, Bhatia DS, Hu T, McCarthy HL, Lincoff AM, Spiess BD, Aronson S. Anticoagulation with bivalirudin for off-pump coronary artery bypass grafting: The results of EVOLUTION-OFF study. J Thorac Cardiovasc 131: 686–692, 2006.

Spannagl M, Bichler J, Birg A, Lill H, Schramm W. Development of a chromogenic substrate assay for the determination of hirudin in plasma. Blood Coagul Fibrinolysis 2: 121–127, 1991.

Spiess BD, DeAnda A, McCarthy A, Yeatman D, Harness HL, Katlaps G. Off pump CABG in a patient with HITT anticoagulated with bivalirudin: a case report [abstr]. Anesth Analg 93: SCA70, 2002.

Stone GW, Bertrand M, Colombo A, Dangas G, Farkouh ME, Feit F, Lansky AJ, Lincoff AM, Mehran R, Moses JW, Ohman M, White HD. Acute catheterization and urgent intervention triage strategy (ACUITY) trial: Study design and rationale. Am Heart J 148: 764–775, 2004.

Stone GW, McLaurin BT, Cox DA, Bertrand ME, Lincoff AM, Moses JW, White HD, Pocock SJ, Ware JH, Feit F, Colombo A, Aylward PE, Cequier AR, Darius H, Desmet W, Ebrahimi R, Hamon M, Rasmussen LH, Rupprecht HJ, Hoeksktra J, Mehran R, Ohman EM. Bivalirudin for patients with acute coronary syndromes. N Engl J Med 355: 2203–2216, 2006.

Stone GW, White HD, Ohman EM, Bertrand ME, Lincoff AM, McLaurin BT, Cox DA, Pocock SJ, Ware JH, Feit F, Colombo A, Manoukian SV, Lansky AJ, Mehran R, Moses JW, Acute Catheterization and Urgent Intervention Triage strategy (ACUITY) trial investigators. Lancet 369: 907–919, 2007.

Stone GW, Witzenbichler B, Guagliumi G, Peruga JZ, Brodie BR, Dudek D, Kornowski R, Hartmann F, Gersh BJ, Pocock SJ, Dangas G, Wong SC, Kirtane AJ, Parise H, Mehran R for the HORIZONS-AMI Trial Investigators. Bivalirudin during primary PCI in acute myocardial infarction. N Engl J Med 358: 2218-2230, 2008.

Stone GW, Witzenbichler B, Guagliumi G, Peruga JZ, Brodie BR, Dudek D, Kornowski R, Hartmann F, Gersh BJ, Pocock SJ, Dangas G, Wong S C, Fahy M, Parise H, Mehran R.

Heparin plus a glycoprotein IIb/IIIa inhibitor versus bivalirudin monotherapy and paclitaxel-eluting stents versus bare-metal stents in acute myocardial infarction (HORIZONS-AMI): final 3-year results from a mulitcentre, randomised controlled trial. Lancet 377: 2193–2204, 2011.

Tavano D, Visconti G, D'Andrea D. Focaccio A, Golia B, Librera M, Caccavale M, Ricciarelli B, Briquori C. Comparison of bivalirudin monotherapy versus unfractionated heparin plus tirofiban in patients with diabetes mellitus undergoing elective percutaneous coronary intervention. Am J Cardiol 104: 1222–1228, 2009.

Theroux P, Perez-Villa F, Waters D, Lesperance J, Shabani F, Bonan R. Randomized double-blind comparison of two doses of Hirulog with heparin as adjunctive therapy to strepto-kinase to promote early patency of the infarct-related artery in acute myocardial infarction. Circulation 91: 2132–2139, 1995.

Thiagarajan P, Wu KK. Mechanisms of antithrombotic drugs. Adv Pharmacol 46: 297–324, 1999.

Topol EJ, Bonan R, Jewitt D, Sigwart U, Kakkar W, Rothman M, de Bono D, Ferguson J, Willerson JT, Strony J, Ganz P, Cohen MD, Raymond R, Fox I, Maraganore J, Adelman B. Use of a direct antithrombin, hirulog, in place of heparin during coronary angioplasty. Circulation 87: 1622–1629, 1993.

Trissel LA, Saenz CA. Compatibility screening of bivalirudin during simulated Y-site admin-istration with other drugs. Int J Pharm Compounding 6: 311–315, 2002.

Tsu LV, Dager WE. Bivalirudin dosing adjustments for reduced renal function with or without hemodialysis in the management of heparin-induced thrombocytopenia. Ann Pharmaco-ther 45: 1185–1192, 2011.

Tsu LV, Dager WE. Comparison of bivalirudin dosing strategies using total, adjusted, and ideal body weights in obese patients with heparin-induced thrombocytopenia. Pharmaco-therapy 32: 20–26, 2012.

Van de Car DA, Rao SV, Ohman EM. Bivalirudin: a review of the pharmacology and clinical application. Expert Rev Cardiovasc 8: 1673–1681, 2010.

Vasquez JC, Vichiendilokkul A, Mahmood S, Baciewicz FA Jr. Anticoagulation with bivaliru-din during cardiopulmonary bypass in cardiac surgery. Ann Thorac Surg 74: 2177–2179, 2002.

Veale JJ, McCarthy HLM, Palmer G, Dyke CM. Use of bivalirudin as an anticoagulant during cardiopulmonary bypass. J Am Soc Extra-Corporeal Technol 37: 296–302, 2005.

Walenga JM, Hoppensteadt D, Koza M, Pifarre R, Fareed J. Comparative studies on various assays for the laboratory evaluation of r-hirudin. Semin Thromb Hemost 17: 103–112, 1991.

Warkentin TE. Anticoagulation for cardiopulmonary bypass: Is a replacement for heparin on the horizon? J Thorac Cardiovasc Surg 131: 515–516, 2006.

Warkentin TE, Greinacher A. Heparin-induced thrombocytopenia and cardiac surgery. Ann Thorac Surg 76: 2121–2131, 2003.

Warkentin TE, Koster A. Bivalirudin: a review. Expert Opin Pharmacother 6: 1349–1371, 2005.

Warkentin TE, Greinacher A, Craven S, Dewar L, Sheppard JI, Ofosu FA. Differences in the clinically effective molar concentrations of four direct thrombin inhibitors explain their variable prothrombin time prolongation. Thromb Haemost 94: 958–964, 2005.

Warkentin TE, Greinacher A, Koster A. Bivalirudin. Thromb Haemost 99: 830–839, 2008a.

Warkentin TE, Greinacher A, Koster A, Lincoff AM. Treatment and prevention of heparin-induced thrombocytopenia. American College of Chest Physicians evidence-based clini-cal practice guidelines (8th edition). Chest 133(6 Suppl): 340S–380S, 2008b. [Erratum in Chest 139: 1261, 2011. Dosage error in article text]

Wasowicz M, Vegas A, Borger MA, Harwood S. Bivalirudin anticoagulation for cardiopulmo-nary bypass in a patient with heparin-induced thrombocytopenia. Can J Anesth 52: 1093–1098, 2005.

Weitz JI, Hirsh J. New antithrombotic agents. Chest 114(Suppl): 715S–727S, 1998.

Weitz J, Maraganore JM. The thrombin-specific anticoagulant, bivalirudin, completely inhib-its thrombin-mediated platelet aggregation [abstr]. Am J Cardiol 88(Suppl 5A): 83G, 2001.

White HD. Thrombin-specific anticoagulation with bivalirudin versus heparin in patients receiving fibrinolytic therapy for acute myocardial infarction: the HERO-2 randomised trial. Lancet 358: 1855–1863, 2001.

White HD, Chew DP. Bivalirudin: an anticoagulant for acute coronary syndromes and coronary interventions. Expert Opin Pharmacother 3: 777–788, 2002.

White HD, Aylward PE, Frey MJ, Adgey AAJ, Nair R, Hillis WS, Shalev Y, Brown MA, French JK, Collins R, Maraganore J, Adelman B. Randomized, double-blind comparison of hirulog versus heparin in patients receiving streptokinase and aspirin for acute myocardial infarction (HERO). Circulation 96: 2155–2161, 1997.

Wiggins BS, Spinier S, Wittkowsky AK, Stringer KA. Bivalirudin: a direct thrombin inhibitor for percutaneous transluminal coronary angioplasty. Pharmacotherapy 22: 1007–1018, 2002.

Wittkowsky AK. The role of thrombin inhibition during percutaneous coronary intervention. Pharmacotherapy 22: 97S–104S, 2002.

Xue M, Fenton JW II, Shen GX. Hirulog-1 reduces expression of platelet-derived growth factor in neointima of rat carotid artery induced by balloon catheter injury. J Vasc Res 37: 82–92, 2000.

Xue M, Ren S, Welch S, Shen GX. Hirulog-like peptide reduces balloon catheter injury induced neointima formation in rat carotid artery without increase in bleeding tendency. J Vasc Res 38: 144–152, 2001.

Young G, Tarantino MD, Wohrley J, Weber LC, Belvedere M, Nugent DJ. Pilot dose-finding and safety study of bivalirudin in infants <6 months of age with thrombosis. J Thromb Haemost 5: 1654–1659, 2007a.

Young G, Yonekawa KE, Nakagawa PA, Blain RC, Lovejoy AE, Nugent DJ. Recombinant activated factor VII effectively reverses the anticoagulant effects of heparin, enoxaparin, fondaparinux, argatroban, and bivalirudin ex vivo as measured using thromboelastography. Blood Coagul Fibrinolysis 18: 547–553, 2007b.

16 Danaparoid for the treatment of heparin-induced thrombocytopenia

Beng Hock Chong and Harry N. Magnani

INTRODUCTION

When a diagnosis of heparin-induced thrombocytopenia (HIT) is made, cessation of heparin is mandatory. Thereafter, an alternative anticoagulant is usually needed for the treatment of HIT-associated venous or arterial thrombosis, for the prevention of thrombosis in isolated HIT, or for other indications (Chong, 1995; Warkentin et al., 2008) (see chap. 12). Danaparoid (Orgaran), now manufactured by MSD (also known as Merck & Co. Inc; Oss, The Netherlands), is still widely used as an alternative antithrombotic drug for treatment of HIT outside of the United States (where it is not marketed). Worldwide, over 500,000 patients with HIT have been treated with danaparoid.

Chemistry, Pharmacology, Pharmacodynamics, and Pharmacokinetics
Chemistry
Although danaparoid is often referred to as a low molecular weight (LMW) "heparinoid," it differs chemically, pharmacologically, and pharmacokinetically from unfractionated heparin (UFH) and the LMW heparins (LMWHs) (Meuleman, 1992).

Danaparoid consists of a mixture of LMW glycosaminoglycans: heparan sulfate (84%), dermatan sulfate (12%), and chondroitin sulfate (4%). A small proportion of the heparan sulfate molecules (5%) have high affinity for antithrombin (AT) (Meuleman, 1992; Ofosu, 1992). Danaparoid has an average molecular mass of approximately 6000 Da. It does not contain heparin or heparin fragments. The repeating disaccharide subunits in heparan sulfate, its principal constituent, are predominantly glucuronic acid and N-acetyl-glucosamine, whereas in heparin and the LMWHs they are mostly iduronic acid and glucosamine-N-sulfate (Gordon et al., 1990) (Fig. 16.1). These chemical differences lower its degree of sulfation and overall charge density and probably account for the lack of danaparoid binding to plasma proteins and platelets (Casu, 1991).

Pharmacology
The antithrombotic activity of danaparoid is partly mediated by AT inhibition of factor Xa, partly by a small, heparin cofactor II-mediated anti-factor IIa (antithrombin) activity and partly by inhibition of factor IX activation by IIa, thereby dampening a major feedback loop for thrombin generation (Ofosu, 1992). The predominant anticoagulant effect of danaparoid is therefore thrombin generation inhibition.

Danaparoid does not interfere directly with platelet function (Meuleman et al., 1982; Mikhailidis et al., 1984, 1987; Meuleman, 1987) and unlike UFH has

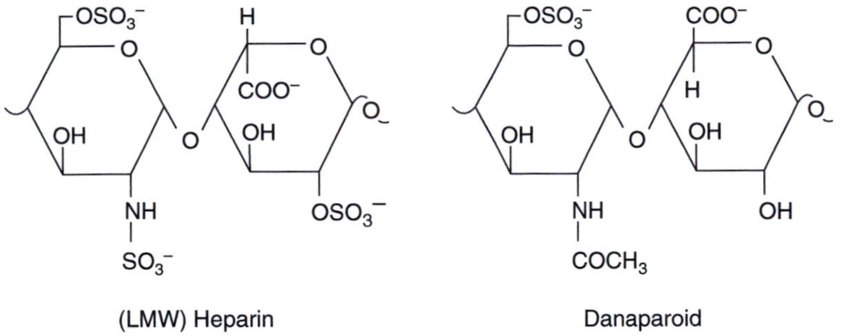

FIGURE 16.1 Comparison of predominant disaccharide structure of heparin with danaparoid. The LMW heparin disaccharide is mostly (*left*) glucosamine-*N*-sulfate and (*right*) iduronic acid, whereas danaparoid's principal constituent, heparan sulfate, is predominantly (*left*) *N*-acetyl-glucosamine and (*right*) glucuronic acid. The degrees of sulfation (sulfate groups per disaccharide unit) for heparin and danaparoid are approximately 2.0–2.5 and 1.0–1.5, respectively (see chap. 7). *Abbreviation*: LMW, low molecular weight.

minimal effect on formation of the platelet-dependent hemostatic plug (Meuleman, 1992). These characteristics of danaparoid contribute to its favorable benefit/risk ratio.

Danaparoid shows no or little overall binding to PF4 because the small fraction of heparan sulfate with high affinity to AT that can bind to PF4 is blocked by the overwhelming presence of the remaining heparan sulfate with low affinity to AT (Greinacher et al., 1992). This effect may also be responsible for its interference with the interactions between HIT antibodies and platelets (Chong et al., 1989) and subsequent prevention of platelet activation by HIT antibodies (Krauel et al., 2008).

Pharmacokinetics
Danaparoid has a pharmacokinetic profile different from that of UFH or LMWH. After subcutaneous (sc) or intravenous (iv) administration, its bioavailability approaches 100% (Stiekema et al., 1989; Danhof et al., 1992), compared with 87–92% for the LMWHs and 15–20% for UFH (Skoutakis, 1997). Danaparoid-induced plasma anti-Xa levels peak 4–5 hours following sc injection (Danhof et al., 1992). Unlike heparins, danaparoid is not neutralized by plasma proteins, such as PF4 and histidine-rich glycoprotein, accounting for its high bioavailability. Danaparoid exhibits linear pharmacokinetics and has relatively predictable plasma levels.

Danaparoid is eliminated mainly by the kidneys. Its biologic plasma half-life $(t_{1/2})$—which is best represented by its effect on thrombin generation inhibition activity—is approximately 7 hours (Bradbrook et al., 1987; Stiekema et al., 1989; Danhof et al., 1992). However, anti-factor Xa activity (measured using conventional chromogenic assays) has a $t_{1/2}$ of approximately 25 hours. In patients with moderate to severe renal impairment the drug tends to accumulate, but with suitable dose reduction, overdosing risk can be minimized.

Danaparoid's metabolism is not affected by hepatic cytochrome P-450, nor does it affect hepatic or renal handling of other drugs. It has no significant effect on the pharmacodynamics and pharmacokinetics of coumarins. Its pharmacokinetics are not modified by age or body weight (Stiekema et al., 1989; Danhof et al., 1992).

There is no antidote for danaparoid (Stiekema et al., 1989). Protamine sulfate only minimally neutralizes its anticoagulant activity. If severe bleeding occurs, the drug should be stopped and blood product replacement given, as indicated clinically. There is limited evidence that plasmapheresis can accelerate drug elimination (Schmahl et al., 1997), but this option is seldom practical.

CLINICAL USE OF DANAPAROID
Clinical Use of Danaparoid in Disorders Other than HIT
In eight prospective, randomized, controlled, and assessor-blind studies, danaparoid was more effective than other currently approved antithrombotics in preventing deep vein thrombosis (DVT) after total hip replacement (Hoek et al., 1992; Leyvraz et al., 1992; Org 10172 Report, 1994; Gent et al., 1996; Comp et al., 1998) or hip fracture surgery (Bergqvist et al., 1991; Gerhart et al., 1991), or ischemic stroke (Turpie et al., 1987, 1992). Danaparoid also compared favorably with LMWH in patients undergoing fractured hip surgery (TIFDED Study Group, 1999). These results led to worldwide approvals for one or more of these indications. In addition, prospective controlled studies have demonstrated the efficacy of danaparoid for DVT thromboprophylaxis after major thoracic and abdominal surgery for cancer (Cade et al., 1987; Gallus et al., 1993) and after spinal cord injury (Merli et al., 1991). Danaparoid (2000 U initial dose iv, then 2000 U twice daily by sc injection) was more effective than UFH in the treatment of DVT (de Valk et al., 1995). Case series also suggest efficacy in patients with disseminated intravascular coagulation (DIC) complicating promyelocytic leukemia (Nieuwenhuis and Sixma, 1986) (danaparoid is approved for treatment of DIC in Japan), as well as in the prevention of fibrinopeptide A release or fibrin deposition on the dialysis membrane during hemodialysis (Henny et al., 1983; Ireland et al., 1986; von Bonsdorff et al., 1990).

Clinical Use of Danaparoid in Patients with HIT
Danaparoid has been used extensively to treat patients with HIT (Chong and Magnani, 1992; Magnani, 1993, 1997; Magnani and Gallus, 2006). After the diagnosis of HIT and discontinuation of heparin administration, patients often require an alternative anticoagulant for any one of the following indications: (i) treatment of a recent or new thrombosis; (ii) prophylaxis of venous thromboembolism (VTE); (iii) anticoagulation for cardiopulmonary bypass (CPB) surgery or peripheral arterial surgery; (iv) anticoagulation for intermittent or continuous hemodialysis or continuous renal replacement therapy (CRRT); (v) cardiac catheterization or percutaneous coronary intervention (PCI); or (vi) maintenance of intravascular catheter patency. The rationale for the use of danaparoid in these various situations includes its nonheparin structure, its low degree of cross-reactivity with HIT antibodies compared with LMWH (Makhoul et al., 1986; Chong et al., 1989; Greinacher et al., 1992; Kikta et al., 1993; Vun et al., 1996), its ability to block ongoing platelet activation (Chong et al., 1989; Greinacher et al., 1992; Krauel et al., 2008), and its overall favorable efficacy and safety profile.

The largest clinical experience with the use of danaparoid in the treatment of patients with HIT is in the compassionate-use (named patient) program organized by the manufacturer (Magnani, 1993, 1997). From 1981 to 1997, more than 750 patients were treated under this program for the various indications listed earlier (Ortel and Chong, 1998). The duration of treatment ranged from 1 day to 3.5 years, and the post-treatment follow-up was a median 60 days (range, 2 days to 11 years). The overall success rate, defined as platelet count recovery without new, progressive, or recurrent thrombosis during the danaparoid treatment period, or thrombotic death during 3 months follow-up, and the absence of any adverse effect necessitating treatment cessation, has been over 90%, as judged by the local physician-investigators. However, as this definition does not include nonthrombotic death, the overall mortality observed in the program was 18%, including deaths during the post-treatment follow-up. Most patients in this program received danaparoid for the treatment of acute thromboembolism, often in the setting of severe illness, such as renal or multisystem organ failure.

Besides this compassionate-use program, other studies supporting the efficacy of danaparoid therapy for acute HIT include a randomized controlled trial comparing danaparoid with dextran (Chong et al., 2001), a retrospective analysis comparing danaparoid with lepirudin (Farner et al., 2001) and a historically controlled retrospective cohort study that compared danaparoid with ancrod (Lubenow et al., 2006).

Treatment of Venous and Arterial Thromboembolism

Patients with HIT frequently have one or more acute thromboses, which may have occurred before the development of HIT, as a complication of HIT itself, or both (Warkentin and Kelton, 1996). Venous thrombosis complicates HIT more often than does arterial occlusion. Indeed, in the compassionate-use program, the ratio of venous to arterial thrombosis was 2:1 (Ortel and Chong, 1998). Even without thrombosis, HIT patients require continuation of antithrombotic therapy after heparin cessation to prevent thromboembolism because without anticoagulant treatment approximately 50% of patients will develop thrombosis (Warkentin and Kelton, 1996).

As a result of the large clinical experience with the compassionate use program and the other clinical studies, the following guiding principles should be considered when using danaparoid in the treatment of HIT (Warkentin et al., 2008):

(i) to initiate danaparoid treatment at therapeutic doses in all HIT patients, even if no overt thrombosis is evident, by either the sc or preferably the iv route.

(ii) to attain therapeutic levels (0.5–0.8 U/mL) of plasma anti-Xa activity as soon as possible (unless contraindicated by bleeding risk) by using a loading iv bolus.

(iii) not to exceed a plasma level of 0.8 U/mL in patients with severe/complete renal failure [except to overcome severe initial extracorporeal circuit (ECC) clotting].

Table 16.1 describes the current protocol that takes into account the amount of danaparoid per marketed ampule (750 anti-factor Xa U/ampule), as well as certain initial bolus dose adjustments based on body weight. Danaparoid is also effective when administered sc so that 2250 U (three ampules) every 12 hours by sc injection is approximately equal to 190 U/hr by iv infusion given over 24 hours. In the compassionate-use program, 464 patients with acute thromboembolism were treated with danaparoid, with efficacy judged to be over 90% (Ortel and Chong, 1998).

Danaparoid also proved efficacious for HIT-associated thrombosis in a prospective, randomized, controlled study (Chong et al., 2001) in which HIT patients with an acute thrombosis (venous, arterial, or both) were randomized to receive either danaparoid plus warfarin or dextran 70 plus warfarin. Dextran 70—a weak

TABLE 16.1   Danaparoid Dosing Schedules in HIT Patients

Clinical indication	Danaparoid dosing schedule
Prophylaxis of VTE	750 U sc b.i.d. or t.i.d. for patients with history of HIT or who have low suspicion for HIT. For patients with (confirmed or strongly suspected) acute HIT with or without thrombosis, use treatment doses (see below)
Treatment of VTE or arterial thromboembolism	2250 U iv bolus[a] followed by 400 U/hr for 4 hr, 300 U/hr for 4 hr, then 150–200 U/hr for >5 days, aiming for a plasma anti-Xa level of 0.5–0.8 U/mL; or sc[b] administration: 1500–2250 U sc b.i.d.
Embolectomy or other peripheral vascular surgery	Preoperative: 2250 U iv bolus[a]; intraoperative flushes: 750 U in 250 mL saline, using up to 50 mL; postoperative: 750 U sc t.i.d. (low-risk patients) or 150–200 U/hr (high-risk patients) beginning at least 6 hr after surgery
Intermittent hemodialysis (on alternate days)	3750 U iv before first and second dialyses; 3000 U for third dialysis; then 2250 U for subsequent dialyses, aiming for plasma anti-Xa level of <0.3 U/mL predialysis, and 0.5–0.8 U/mL during dialysis
CRRT	2250 U iv bolus, followed by 400–600 U/hr for 4 hr, then 300 U/hr for 4 hr, then 150–400[c] U/hr aiming for a plasma anti-Xa level of 0.5–0.8 U/mL (or higher if more danaparoid is initially needed to overcome ECC clotting)
CPB	125 U/kg iv bolus after thoracotomy; 3 U/mL in priming fluid of apparatus; 7 U/kg/hr iv infusion commencing after CPB hookup, and continued until 45 min before expectation of stopping CPB
Cardiac catheterization	Preprocedure: 2250 U iv bolus (3000 U if 75–90 kg and 3750 U if >90 kg)
PCI or intra-aortic balloon pump	Preprocedure: bolus as per foregoing Postprocedure: 150–200 U/hr for 1–2 days post-PCI (or until removal of balloon pump)
Catheter patency	750 U in 50 mL saline, then 5–10 mL per port, or as required
Pediatric dosage considerations	Refer to Bidlingmaier et al., 2006; see also chap. 21

Note: Compatibility with intravenous solutions: Danaparoid is compatible for dilution with the following solutions: saline, dextrose, dextrose—saline, Ringer's, lactated Ringer's, 10% mannitol. Preparation of solution for infusion: One option is to add four ampules containing 3000 U (i.e., 750 anti-Xa U/0.6 mL ampule) of danaparoid to 300 mL of intravenous solution, i.e., a solution that comprises 10 U danaparoid per milliliter of intravenous solution: thus, an infusion rate of 40 mL/hr corresponds to a dose of 400 U/hr: 20 mL/hr to a dose of 200 U/hr, and so on.
[a]Adjust iv danaparoid bolus for body weight: <60 kg, 1500 U; 60–75 kg, 2250 U; 75–90 kg, 3000 U; >90 kg, 3750 U.
[b]Danaparoid should ideally be given iv during the acute (thrombocytopenic) phase of HIT (see above).
[c]Initially up to 600 U/hr may be required if the filter has recently shown excessive clotting. Once filter life is restored to normal, the rate can be lowered.
Abbreviations: b.i.d., twice daily; b.w., body weight; CPB, cardiopulmonary bypass surgery; CRRT, continuous renal replacement therapy; ECC, extracorporeal circuit; HIT, heparin-induced thrombocytopenia; iv, intravenous; PCI, percutaneous coronary intervention; sc, subcutaneous; t.i.d., three times daily; VTE, venous thromboembolism.

antithrombotic agent formerly used for DVT thromboprophylaxis (Aberg and Rausing, 1978; Bergqvist, 1980)—was the only other rapid-acting nonheparin anti-thrombotic drug available in Australia at study commencement in 1988.

Danaparoid was given as an iv bolus of 2400 U, followed by an infusion of 400 U/hr for 2 hours, 300 U/hr for 2 hours, and then 200 U/hr for 5 days. In the dextran 70 arm, patients received dextran, 1 L on day 1, and then 500 mL/day from days 2 to 5. The patients in both the treatment arms also received warfarin from day 1 for 3 months at doses adjusted to maintain an international normalized ratio (INR) of 2–4. Patients were also stratified at randomization, depending on the severity of their thrombosis, using predefined criteria.

Resolution of thrombocytopenia showed a nonsignificant trend in favor of danaparoid over dextran 70. Among the patients stratified as having "mild" thrombosis, a slightly higher percentage of patients treated with danaparoid (83%) improved compared with those who received dextran 70 (73%). By contrast, a substantial and significant difference in treatment outcome occurred in patients with "serious" thrombosis: 88% of danaparoid-treated thromboembolic events recovered, compared with only 44% of those treated with dextran 70. No serious bleeding events were observed. These data show the safety of danaparoid even when given concomitantly with therapeutic dose warfarin and suggest that the use of an effective anticoagulant to treat HIT-associated thromboembolism is particularly important in those with more severe disease.

In another study, patients treated prospectively with lepirudin were compared with patients treated over the same time period in the same institution with danaparoid (Farner et al., 2001). Although not a randomized trial, this study had important strengths. First, all patients had serologically confirmed HIT. Second, all patients met identical inclusion and exclusion criteria, had similar baseline characteristics (~70% had thrombosis at study entry, although danaparoid-treated patients were older by a mean of 6 yr), and were treated during the same time period (25 months ending April 1996). Third, many patients were studied (danaparoid, $n = 126$; lepirudin, $n = 175$). Furthermore, patients were subdivided into those treated with prophylactic or therapeutic doses. The results of this study suggest that both danaparoid and lepirudin have similar efficacy for treatment of HIT-associated thrombosis when given in *therapeutic* doses: the day 42 success rate was about 80% for either agent, when failure was defined as having a composite endpoint of new thrombosis, death, and/or limb loss (Fig. 16.2A). When evaluating the single endpoint of new thrombosis in patients who received therapeutic doses of study drug, danaparoid and lepirudin also showed similar efficacy (90.6% vs 92.1%; $P = 0.74$). Moreover, safety analysis of all patients (regardless of dose received) showed significantly fewer major bleeds with danaparoid (2.5% vs 10.4%; $P = 0.009$) (Fig. 16.2B). These data suggest that the favorable therapeutic index of danaparoid extends also to HIT complicated by thrombosis.

More recently, a retrospective evaluation of treatment outcomes was made between a period when HIT patients were often treated with the defibrinogenating snake venom, ancrod (usually with coumarin) or coumarin alone, and a later period when treatment of new HIT patients was mainly performed using danaparoid (usually with overlapping coumarin) (Lubenow et al., 2006). This historical "switch" in choice of HIT treatment (which occurred in Canada) was associated with a highly significant reduction in the composite endpoint of new/progressive/recurrent thrombosis, thrombotic death, and limb amputation among patients treated with danaparoid (day 7

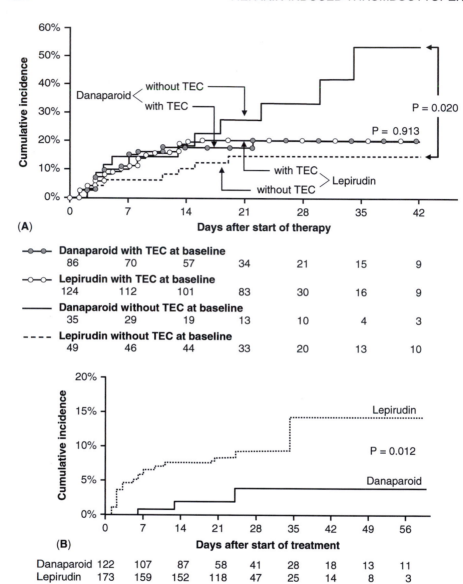

FIGURE 16.2   Efficacy and safety outcomes of HIT patients with and without TEC: comparison of danaparoid with lepirudin, showing the number of patients at risk on the starting day and at subsequent 7-day intervals (up to day 42). (**A**) Efficacy: time-to-event analysis of the incidences of a combined endpoint (new TECs, limb amputation, death; maximum, one endpoint per patient) up to day 42. Among patients without TEC at baseline (most of whom were treated with a *prophylactic-dose* regimen), there was a significantly higher incidence of the combined endpoint among patients treated with danaparoid, compared with lepirudin ($P = 0.02$, log-rank test). This suggests that a prophylactic-dose regimen for danaparoid (750 U b.i.d. or t.i.d. by sc injection, without anticoagulant monitoring) may be relatively less effective for managing patients with isolated HIT compared with a "prophylactic" regimen of lepirudin in which aPTT-adjusted monitoring occurs (Warkentin, 2001). In marked contrast, the combined endpoint did not differ significantly between danaparoid and lepirudin for patients with TEC at baseline (most of whom received *therapeutic-dose* danaparoid), (*Continued*)

FIGURE 16.2 (*Continued*) suggesting that therapeutic (treatment) doses of danaparoid (Table 16.1) results in efficacy similar to therapeutic-dose lepirudin. (**B**) Safety: Time-to-event analysis of the incidences of major bleeding. Major bleeding was defined as overt bleeding requiring transfusion of two or more red blood cell concentrates or intracerebral bleeding. The bleeding rate was significantly lower in patients treated with danaparoid (*P* = 0.012, log-rank test). This indicates that the therapeutic window of lepirudin is rather narrow. *Abbreviations*: aPTT, activated partial thromboplastin time; HIT, heparin-induced thrombocytopenia; TEC, thromboembolic complications. *Source*: From Farner et al. (2001).

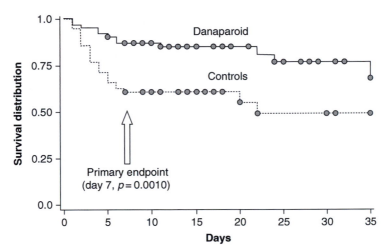

FIGURE 16.3 Efficacy outcomes: comparison of danaparoid (with or without coumarin) with ancrod (with or without coumarin) or coumarin alone. Time-to-event analysis of composite endpoint (new thrombosis, thrombotic death, amputation; maximum, one event per patient). The primary efficacy endpoint (at day 7) was reduced in the danaparoid-treated patients (*P* < 0.001, log-rank test); at day 35 (secondary endpoint), the composite endpoint remained reduced (*P* = 0.0022, log-rank test). When a different composite endpoint that included all-cause mortality was analyzed (i.e., new thrombosis, all-cause mortality, amputation; maximum, one event per patient), the differences remained significant (day 35; *P* = 0.0013 by log-rank test; data not shown). *Source*: From Lubenow et al. (2006).

outcomes: 12.9% *vs* 39.3%; *P* = 0.0014) (Fig. 16.3). In addition, significantly less major bleeding was observed with danaparoid (11.3% *vs* 28.6%; *P* = 0.0211). These investigators further compared the efficacy and safety outcomes using danaparoid treatment against those of published trials of lepirudin and argatroban (Table 16.2). The results suggest that the efficacy–safety relationship of danaparoid is more favorable, although the lack of head-to-head randomized comparisons between danaparoid and either direct thrombin inhibitors prevents any definitive conclusions.

A general review of 1478 danaparoid-treated patients available from the company files (i.e., the compassionate-use program and spontaneous adverse event reports) and independent published literature (Magnani and Gallus 2006) is also available. A wide variety of clinical scenarios in HIT were described, ranging from prophylaxis or treatment of thromboembolism in routine medical patients to intensive care unit (ICU) patients with sepsis and multiple organ failure and from major general and cardiovascular surgery to extracorporeal support for renal

TABLE 16.2 Comparison of Efficacy and Major Bleeding Endpoints of Danaparoid, Lepirudin, and Argatroban vs Control

Study	Drug studied	Composite endpoint[a]		Major bleeding[a]	
		Study drug	Control	Study drug	Control
Lubenow et al., 2006	Danaparoid	24.2%[b]	50.0%	12.9%[b]	33.9%
HAT-1 and HAT-2	Lepirudin	22.1%[b]	40.0%	19.5%	12.0%
Arg-911	Argatroban	43.8%	56.5%	11.1%	2.2%
Arg-915	Argatroban	41.5%	56.5%	6.1%	2.2%

[a]All deaths, amputations, and new thromboses up to day 35 for danaparoid and lepirudin: day 37 for argatroban.
[b]Statistically significant ($P < 0.01$) compared with control (by categoric analysis).
Abbreviation: HAT, heparin-associated thrombocytopenia. *Source*: From Lubenow et al. (2006).

failure. The frequency of a composite of adverse outcomes (new/extended thrombosis, new/persistent platelet count reduction, unplanned amputation) during the treatment period (range, 1 day to 3.5 years), plus a follow-up period (up to three months), was 16.4%. Thrombotic events occurred in 11.0% of the patients, whereas major bleeding was reported in 8.1%. This and specific reviews of its use for pediatric patients (Saxon et al., 1999; Bidlingmaier et al., 2006), pregnancy (Magnani, 2010a), and renal failure (Magnani and Wester, 2007; Magnani, 2010b) show that in all these settings, danaparoid appears to be safe and effective in treating HIT and associated thromboses.

Overlapping Oral Anticoagulants with Danaparoid

Some danaparoid-treated HIT patients received concurrent, and many received overlapping, warfarin treatment, since oral anticoagulation is usually indicated for longer-term control of thrombotic risk. However, as it generally takes at least five days for coumarin to achieve a therapeutic effect (Harrison et al., 1997), it is prudent to delay starting coumarin until the thrombotic process is controlled and substantial resolution of the thrombocytopenia has occurred (usually, to a platelet count $>150 \times 10^9/L$). This caveat is based on the observation that coumarin can aggravate the thrombotic process during the first few days of its administration by reducing levels of the natural anticoagulants protein C and protein S, particularly when thrombin generation is high (Pötzsch et al., 1996; Warkentin, 1996a; Warkentin et al., 1997) (see chaps. 2 and 12). Warfarin does not neutralize activated coagulation factors (which are increased in acute HIT), and even when sufficient time has passed for its antithrombotic effects to be achieved through reduction in the vitamin K-dependent procoagulant factors (particularly prothrombin), premature discontinuation of danaparoid prior to resolution of HIT has resulted in new thromboembolism and coumarin-induced microthrombosis. Once overlapping danaparoid–coumarin therapy is initiated, danaparoid should not be discontinued before at least five days of overlap have occurred and at least two INR measurements (at least 24 hours apart) are within the target therapeutic range (2.0–3.0).

Unlike lepirudin and argatroban, danaparoid does not interfere with INR or activated partial thromboplastin time (aPTT) measurements during oral anticoagulant therapy; thus, the potential for underdosing of direct thrombin inhibitor therapy due to aPTT confounding resulting from concomitant coumarin therapy (Warkentin, 2006) does not apply to danaparoid.

Prophylaxis During Acute HIT

In contrast to the comparable efficacy of danaparoid and lepirudin when used at therapeutic doses to treat HIT-associated thrombosis (discussed previously), lepirudin appeared somewhat more effective than danaparoid when prophylactic-dose regimens were compared for preventing the single endpoint of new thrombosis (91.4% vs 81.4%; $P = 0.138$); this difference was larger, and reached statistical significance, when the composite endpoint (new thrombosis, limb amputation, or death) was examined (Fig. 16.2A). However, superior efficacy of lepirudin came at a price: for patients without thrombosis at baseline (most of whom thus received prophylactic-dose therapy), lepirudin was associated with a trend to more major bleeding events than danaparoid (16.3% vs 2.9%; $P = 0.075$) (Farner et al., 2001).

Kodityal and colleagues (2003) also reported five patients who developed new thromboses while receiving relatively low doses of danaparoid (usually, 1250 U every 12 hours by sc injection). These data, the frequent delays in initiating danaparoid treatment (during which HIT progression occurred due to ineffective or no alternative antithrombotic being administered), and other observations describing early new thrombotic events in patients on prophylactic-dose danaparoid that responded favorably to increases in danaparoid dosing intensity (Lindhoff-Last et al., 2005; Magnani and Gallus, 2006), support the current recommendation that danaparoid treatment should be initiated at *therapeutic* doses for patients with acute HIT, even if they only have isolated HIT (Warkentin, 2001; Warkentin et al., 2008) (see chaps. 1 and 12). Furthermore, higher initial danaparoid dosing inhibits platelet activation in HIT more effectively (Ortel and Chong, 1998; Krauel et al., 2008) and may lead to faster platelet count recovery (Erdlenbruch et al., 2001). Delay in commencing danaparoid, and underdosing of danaparoid, were identified as risk factors for unfavorable clinical outcomes in a case–control report by Elalamy and coworkers (2009).

Prophylaxis of Venous Thromboembolism

Patients with a previous history of HIT may require an alternative anticoagulant to prevent VTE if they require prolonged bed rest and/or surgery or become pregnant. UFH should not be used, particularly when HIT antibodies are still present. Thereafter, although HIT antibodies are usually undetectable, and the risk of recurrent HIT is possibly relatively low (Warkentin and Kelton, 2001), most physicians are understandably reluctant to re-administer heparin.

Danaparoid is an effective and convenient drug for the prevention of VTE in patients with a history of prior HIT. In the compassionate-use program, 390 patients received danaparoid, 750 U by sc injection, usually twice daily for DVT prophylaxis for many postoperative nonacute HIT settings, including general, gynecologic, neurologic, cancer, and organ transplant surgeries. A high rate of success was observed (Magnani, 1997; Ortel and Chong, 1998).

Prophylaxis of Arterial Thromboembolism

Danaparoid has been used to prevent arterial thromboembolism in patients undergoing various vascular operations, including peripheral artery bypass graft surgery, embolectomy, and endarterectomy. In these patients, it was given as a preoperative iv bolus of 2500 or 2250 U, and in some it was also administered postoperatively. Given as an iv bolus of 2500 or 2250 U immediately before the procedure, danaparoid has also been used to provide antithrombotic cover during PCI, with or without stenting, and for insertion of intra-aortic balloon devices.

Anticoagulation for Cardiac Surgery

Patients with acute HIT, or recent previous HIT with persisting HIT antibodies, may need to undergo cardiac surgery. UFH is contraindicated during acute HIT, necessitating an alternative anticoagulant for use during CPB. After successful experiments in dogs (Henny et al., 1985a), danaparoid underwent use for CPB anticoagulation in such situations (Magnani, 1993; Wilhelm et al., 1996; Westphal et al., 1997; Christiansen et al., 1998; Fernandes et al., 2000; Olin et al., 2000) with some success. However, serious, mainly postoperative, bleeding occurred in 22% of the first 47 patients (Magnani et al., 1997) and remained as frequent after revision of the perioperative danaparoid dose schedule (Table 16.1) (Fernandes et al., 2000; Olin et al., 2000). Consequently, danaparoid is not recommended for CPB (Buys et al., 2003; Magnani and Gallus, 2006; see also chap. 19), unless no other suitable alternative is available.

The off-pump ("beating heart") technique for cardiac surgery that does not utilize CPB appears to require less antithrombotic cover, and thus a far lower dose of danaparoid may be feasible for intraoperative anticoagulation. This approach was used successfully to perform multiple coronary artery bypass grafting in a patient with acute HIT and unstable angina (Warkentin et al., 2001). A relatively low target plasma anti-factor Xa level (0.6 U/mL) was used, rather than the levels (>1.5 U/mL) sought during CPB (see chap. 19).

A randomized, double-blind comparison of danaparoid ($n = 34$) with UFH ($n = 37$) for off-pump coronary artery bypass grafting in non-HIT patients showed a nonsignificant trend to greater postoperative blood loss (mean, 264 mL) but a significant increase in patients exposed to homologous blood (53% vs 27%) with danaparoid (Carrier et al., 2003). Clinical outcomes appeared similar, and the authors concluded that danaparoid could be a valuable option in patients undergoing off-pump surgery when UFH is contraindicated.

Hemodialysis, Hemofiltration, and Intensive Care Use

Danaparoid was first used to anticoagulate non-HIT patients requiring intermittent hemodialysis in one of several clinical settings: stable chronic renal failure (Henny et al., 1983, 1985b; ten Cate et al., 1985; Ireland et al., 1986; von Bonsdorff et al., 1990) or ICU patients who developed postoperative acute renal failure (Henny et al., 1983, Wester et al., 2000; Statius van Eps et al., 2001). Danaparoid was then used to treat very ill patients in ICU settings who developed HIT during CRRT (Statius van Eps et al., 2000; Wester et al., 2000; Lindhoff-Last et al., 2001). The review by Magnani and Wester (2007) of 94 patients undergoing CRRT in critically ill patients suggests that clinical monitoring for bleeding and circuit clotting is better for controlling the danaparoid infusion rate than monitoring plasma anti-factor Xa levels. Switching from UFH to danaparoid prevents increases in fibrinopeptide A formation (Lane et al., 1989) and deposition of fibrin on the hemodialysis/filtration membranes, thus restoring the lifespan of the filters (Burgess and Chong, 1997; Lindhoff-Last et al., 2001; Statius van Eps et al., 2001; Magnani, 2010b). Such fibrin deposition may also be secondary to UFH-induced platelet aggregation and microthrombus formation and, because HIT antibodies are often absent, this may be a manifestation of nonimmune heparin-associated thrombocytopenia because significant thrombocytopenia usually does not occur (Burgess and Chong, 1997).

Danaparoid may accumulate in the blood of patients with moderate to severe renal dysfunction (creatinine clearance <30 mL/min) because it is cleared renally. During hemodialysis or hemofiltration, it is not cleared by the artificial kidney, but accumulation and the potential risk for bleeding can be minimized by suitable monitoring and danaparoid dose reduction (Table 16.1):

1. For intermittent hemodialysis, the aim is to maintain the plasma anti-factor Xa level between 0.5 and 0.8 U/mL during dialysis. Usually by hemodialysis number 4 or 5, a "steady-state" predialysis bolus dose has been found, which will allow effective anticoagulation during subsequent dialyses. Following this regimen, danaparoid has been used for up to 4 years for intermittent hemodialysis (three times per week).
2. For CRRT, the dosing regimen is similar to the iv infusion regimen used for the treatment of venous thrombosis (Table 16.1). However, if severe hemofilter clotting had occurred with UFH or LMWH, then an initial higher maintenance infusion rate (up to 600 U/hr if bleeding is not observed) may be needed until filter life has been restored to a reasonable duration. Danaparoid has been used for up to 39 days for continuous hemofiltration or hemodialysis in ICU patients.

Two recent reviews (Magnani and Wester, 2007; Magnani, 2010b;) described mainly seriously ill patients with HIT and chronic or acute renal failure (complicating sepsis, DIC, or multiple organ dysfunction syndrome). The above publications describe patients undergoing hemodialysis ($n = 122$) or CRRT ($n = 94$), respectively, and clinical outcome analyses showed major bleeding in 4.9% (none fatal) and 19.1% (eight fatal) respectively; thrombotic events (mainly circuit clotting) in 5.7% (four fatal systemic thrombotic events) and 12.8% (four fatal), respectively; and nonthrombotic/nonbleeding mortality rates were 11.5% and 24.4%, respectively. Most bleeding events and circuit clotting occurred during the danaparoid dose-adjustment phase and ceased after dose optimization (Lindhoff-Last et al., 2001). Most deaths appeared to be due to sepsis and/or multiple organ failure. A generally favorable experience in the use of danaparoid in 42 consecutive ICU patients with HIT was also reported by Tardy-Poncet and colleagues (1999), but the combination of renal failure and HIT is usually complicated by further adverse events.

Use in Children and Pregnant Women

A summary of danaparoid use in case reports of children (Bidlingmaier et al., 2006) (see chap. 21) reported 33 children aged between 2 weeks and 17 years who had suspected or confirmed HIT. The children required danaparoid for various indications, including maintenance of catheter patency, ECC use for renal failure, cardiac surgery, and thrombosis. In general, it was noted that children, particularly infants, often required higher doses of danaparoid than adults on a weight-adjusted basis. Twenty-six children survived (78.8%), five died, and for two, no outcome information was available. The causes of death were thrombotic (one of three patients with a thrombotic event), bleeding (two of four patients with a major bleeding event), treatment withdrawn (one), and septicemia-associated multiple organ failure (one).

Overall, danaparoid appeared safe and effective in children, except in cases requiring CPB, because this was associated with three of the four major bleeds.

Danaparoid is reported to have been used in 91 pregnancies of which 30 were complicated by acute HIT and 17 had past HIT (Magnani, 2010a). Patients with HIT (current or past) compared with non-HIT patients had more previous or current thromboses (89.4% *vs* 43.2%), more frequent serious underlying disorders (21.3% *vs* 11.4%) but the same frequency of coagulopathy (55.3% *vs* 61.4%). Danaparoid therapy for HIT was initiated in the first trimester in 60.2% and continued for up to 36 weeks overall (median 14 weeks). Treatment regimens for both HIT and non-HIT pregnancies were the same as those in nonpregnant women for the same indications. More non-HIT pregnancies ended at term with a live normal infant (94.9% *vs* 86.4%) of which 27.3% and 28.2%, respectively, were delivered by cesarian section. In eight pregnancies, danaparoid was stopped prematurely because of six early fetal deaths (three of which occurred in consecutive pregnancies in one woman who then had two successful pregnancies on danaparoid) and two maternal adverse events (both major bleeds, one due to placental abruption—fatal bleeding following cesarian section in a Jehovah's Witness—after 24 weeks of problem-free danaparoid use, and one due to placenta previa with fatal cardiopulmonary complications after cesarian section). One woman with a history of lupus developed hemolysis, elevated liver enzymes, low platelets (HELLP) syndrome after 6 weeks of danaparoid treatment; the danaparoid was replaced by warfarin and aspirin, but 2 weeks later an emergency cesarian was needed because of impaired fetal growth, and the premature, 24-week-old neonate died two days later of pulmonary hemorrhage.

In six cord plasmas no anti-factor Xa activity could be detected, and five breast milk samples obtained from nursing mothers receiving postpartum danaparoid had virtually undetectable anti-factor Xa activity. Thus, at least the main antithrombotic subfraction of danaparoid does not cross the placenta, and the tiny amounts measured in breast milk would probably be hydrolyzed in the infant's stomach (Lindhoff-Last and Bauersachs, 2002). One postpartum bleed was reported in a woman who was switched to dextran for delivery (Magnani, 2010a).

Postcesarean section danaparoid use has also been compared in 162 women (Nohira et al., 2004; Tani et al., 2005) with no therapy ($n = 124$) or a heparin ($n = 25$). A clinical thromboembolic event occurred in 0, 2, and 2 patients, respectively, and a major bleeding event in 1, 0, and 3 patients, respectively.

Laboratory Monitoring

Since danaparoid, unlike UFH and the LMWHs, does not significantly prolong the aPTT, prothrombin time/INR, or activated clotting time, except at very high doses, these assays cannot be used for its monitoring. However the dose-related effect on plasma anti-factor Xa activity measured in an amidolytic assay (Teien and Lie, 1977; Laposata et al., 1998) is suitable for monitoring. The method requires a standard calibration curve constructed using various dilutions of danaparoid diluted in pooled normal platelet-poor plasma. Control plasma samples, for example, 0.2, 0.7, and 1.25 U/mL, corresponding to low-, mid-, and high-control danaparoid levels, should be included in each assay run. Standard UFH and LMWH controls must not be used (Laposata et al., 1998); otherwise, danaparoid-induced plasma anti-factor Xa levels will be overestimated. Nevertheless, monitoring is not required for routine use of danaparoid for thrombosis prophylaxis or treatment, but it is recommended in patients with clinically significant renal impairment, adults with unusually low or high body weight, children, and clinically unstable patients to check for accumulation or underdosing. However, to avoid accumulation, at least in patients requiring an ECC to treat renal failure, control and adjustment of danaparoid dosing is best performed by careful clinical monitoring of the patient for signs of bleeding and thrombosis/circuit clotting (Magnani and Wester, 2007).

The 100% bioavailability of danaparoid allows predictable plasma levels after both sc or iv injection, but in some clinical treatment settings, it might be advisable to aim for a lower anti-Xa level (e.g., ~0.3 U/mL) for a patient judged to have a high risk of bleeding; sometimes, a higher target anti-Xa level should be sought (e.g., ~1.0 U/mL for a patient with life- or limb-threatening venous or arterial thrombosis or ECC clotting during CRRT, provided that bleeding is not a problem).

Cross-Reactivity of HIT Antibodies with Danaparoid

The mean overall frequency of *in vitro* danaparoid cross-reactivity rate in a large number of HIT patients was 7.6% (Magnani and Gallus, 2006). It is mediated by the 5% subfraction of heparan sulfate with high affinity for AT and in most patients is neutralized by the remaining subfractions of danaparoid with low/no affinity for AT (Greinacher et al., 1992). Nevertheless, this frequency depends on the sensitivity of the assay method, being lowest (~7%) for methods employing highly reactive donor platelets in platelet-rich plasma under standardized conditions (Makhoul et al., 1986; Kikta et al., 1993; Ramakrishna et al., 1995; Vun et al., 1996), higher with more sensitive assays using washed platelets (Warkentin, 1996b; Koster et al., 2000), with the greatest sensitivity and hence highest danaparoid cross-reactivity rate (~50%, Fig. 16.4) observed with an ultrasensitive fluid-phase enzyme immunoassay (Newman et al., 1998, Fig. 16.4). By comparison, all these types of assay showed a LMWH cross reactivity of 80–90%. Importantly, *in vitro* cross-reactivity with danaparoid is generally weak, and quantitatively much less than seen with LMWH (Fig. 16.4).

Newman et al. (1998) investigated the clinical significance of *in vitro* cross-reactivity in 21 patients treated with danaparoid. The eight patients who tested positive for cross-reactivity by the fluid-phase enzyme immunoassay, but negative by the [^{14}C]serotonin-release washed platelet assay, recovered with resolution of their thrombocytopenia and thrombosis, in a fashion similar to the 11 patients who did not manifest *in vitro* danaparoid cross-reactivity in either assay. Two patients tested positive in both assays: in one patient, both thrombocytopenia and pulmonary embolism resolved during danaparoid treatment. However, in the other patient, thrombocytopenia and extensive thrombosis persisted despite danaparoid therapy, although it was unclear whether this unusual patient course represented a specific danaparoid treatment failure (the patient's subsequent clinical course was characterized by consistent failure of all antithrombotic therapies used) (Fig. 16.5).

Warkentin (1996b) also evaluated the clinical significance of *in vitro* cross-reactivity with danaparoid in 29 HIT patients treated with danaparoid. This investigator found no difference in clinical outcomes, or in the time to platelet count recovery, between the two patient groups.

Some anecdotal reports of unfavorable clinical outcomes in HIT patients treated with danaparoid exist (Tardy-Poncet et al., 1995, 2009; Insler et al., 1997; Muhm et al., 1997). Cross-reactive antibodies were not always investigated, and their potential role in relation to other clinical factors remains uncertain.

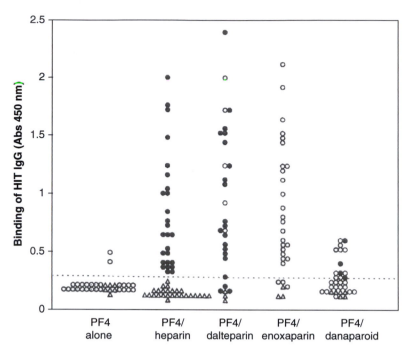

FIGURE 16.4 Cross-reactivity of HIT-IgG antibodies with PF4 complexed to heparin-like antico-agulants: The fluid-phase EIA was used to assess the degree to which IgG present in HIT sera or plasma bound to PF4 alone, PF4/heparin, PF4/dalteparin, PF4/enoxaparin, or PF4/danaparoid. The positive cutoff (dashed line) is three standard deviations above the mean (log transformed) absor-bance of the normal samples (triangles) using PF4/heparin. The binding of normal antibodies is indicated by triangles. Circles indicate HIT samples that have been positive (closed circle), negative (open circle), or not tested (speckled circle) in a functional assay with the corresponding drug. *Abbreviations*: EIA, enzyme immunoassay; HIT-IgG, heparin-induced thrombocytopenia-immunoglobulin G; PF4, platelet factor 4. *Source*: From Newman et al. (1998).

Magnani and Gallus (2006) found in a review of 1418 HIT patients treated with danaparoid that among 36 patients with apparent pretreatment danaparoid cross-reactivity, 23 had clinical events (platelet count fall, thrombotic event) possi-bly indicating *in vivo* cross-reactivity. The remaining 13 patients were treated for a median of 11 days without a problem. A more recent update (Magnani, unpub-lished), which includes patients reported by Warkentin (1996b) and Newman et al. (1998), shows that of 58 patients treated with danaparoid despite a positive danapa-roid pretreatment cross-reactivity test, 31 (53%) were treated for up to 42 days with full recovery of platelet counts and there were no further thromboembolic events. In 14 (24.2%) of the remaining patients, the platelet count did not recover (half of these developed a thromboembolic event).

A further 22 patients developed apparent cross-reactivity seroconversion (i.e., negative predanaparoid cross-reactivity test became positive 2–14 days after initiat-ing danaparoid treatment); a thromboembolic event occurred in seven (two fatal). Thus, in total, 3.2% of the 1418 patients reviewed by Magnani and Gallus (2006) were reported to have had serologically confirmed clinical cross-reactivity with

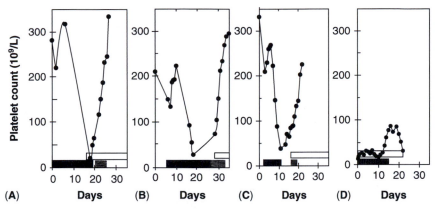

FIGURE 16.5 Serial platelet counts of representative HIT patients treated with danaparoid: Solid black bar shows duration of heparin administration, striped bar indicates danaparoid therapy, open bar shows warfarin therapy: (**A**) Typical profile of the 11 patients who were negative in both fluid phase EIA and functional assay. (**B**) Typical profile of the eight patients who were positive in the fluid-phase, but negative in a functional assay. (**C**) Profile of patient A, one of the two patients who were positive in both types of assay. She recovered during a short course of danaparoid. (**D**) Profile of patient B, the other patient positive in both assays. The profile indicates the course of HIT following transfer to a major hospital. Despite treatment with many antithrombotic agents, he eventually died after major thrombosis. *Abbreviations*: HIT, heparin-induced thrombocytopenia; EIA, enzyme immunoassay. *Source*: From Newman et al. (1998).

danaparoid (23 associated with pretreatment cross-reactivity, 22 associated with cross-reactivity seroconversion). However, the development of platelet count reduction and/or a thromboembolic event during danaparoid treatment is not necessarily a marker of cross-reactivity, since 10 patients re-tested at the time of suspected clinical cross-reactivity remained seronegative (Magnani and Gallus, 2006).

There are several important considerations regarding danaparoid cross-reactivity. First, it is clear that a positive pre-treatment test for *in vitro* cross-reactivity does not necessarily mean that adverse effects related to danaparoid therapy will follow (at least half the patients will do well). Second, more severe HIT, with the potential for greater risk of complications irrespective of which anticoagulant is given, is often mistaken for clinical cross-reactivity with danaparoid, thereby confusing the distinction between clinical cross-reactivity and the natural course of a severe episode of HIT (Newman et al., 1998; Warkentin, 1998; Baumgartel et al., 2000). Third, no standardized, validated testing method for cross-reactivity exists. Indeed, apparent *in vitro* cross-reactivity reported in some studies could even reflect the phenomenon of heparin-independent platelet activation caused by some HIT patient serum (see chap. 11). Besides mimicking *in vitro* cross-reactivity (as some serum-induced platelet activation will occur whether or not danaparoid is added), this serologic feature itself could portend a poor prognosis. Fourth, there are several other possible reasons for either persistent/new thrombocytopenia and/or the occurrence of extension of/new thromboses, for example, delay in danaparoid treatment initiation (Chong et al., 2001; Farner et al., 2001; Lubenow et al., 2006; Elalamy et al., 2009); underdosing, even in patients with isolated HIT (Farner et al., 2001; Elalamy et al., 2009; Magnani, 2010a, 2010b); continued heparin/LMWH; alternative causes, for example, sepsis, DIC, or possibly transfusion of platelets, but these patients are often critically ill with multiple reasons for developing new platelet count reductions or thromboses. Prospective and retrospective studies showed favorable clinical outcomes when danaparoid was given without delay for performing *in vitro* cross-reactivity, especially if initiated at therapeutic dosing levels.

Despite the issue of *in vitro* cross-reactivity with danaparoid, it is noteworthy that danaparoid-induced immune-mediated thrombocytopenia has never been reported. Indeed, danaparoid has the unique property among marketed anticoagulants that at *therapeutic* concentrations it often inhibits HIT antibody-induced platelet activation *in vitro* (Krauel et al., 2008). Based on all of these considerations, *in vitro* cross-reactivity testing is not recommended prior to commencing therapy with danaparoid for suspected HIT (Warkentin et al., 2008). However, cross-reactivity testing may be appropriate in patients who develop new, progressive, or recurrent thrombocytopenia or thrombosis during treatment with danaparoid, or in whom platelet counts do not increase within three to five days after starting danaparoid (Tardy-Poncet et al., 2009).

Adverse Effects

Major bleeding, the most serious adverse effect of danaparoid, is uncommon except in some HIT patients undergoing surgery with very high doses of the drug, for example, cardiac surgery using CPB: 42.3% (Magnani and Gallus, 2006), or in patients with acute renal failure: 20.1% (Magnani and Wester, 2007), or chronic renal failure: 6.2% (Magnani, 2010b). By contrast, bleeding was not seen in the randomized trial in which HIT patients with venous or arterial thromboses received danaparoid plus therapeutic warfarin (Chong et al., 2001). When CPB and renal failure patients are excluded, major bleeding episodes in relation to danaparoid use for medical and surgical patients drop in frequency from 8.1% to 3.2%.

Both recurrence of delayed-type hypersensitivity (DTH) skin reactions in patients with reactions to UFH or LMWHs (Magnani and Gallus, 2006) and successful use of danaparoid in such patients (de Saint-Blanquat et al., 2000; Grassegger et al., 2001; Harrison et al., 2001; Taylor, 2001) have been reported. Pretreatment skin cross-reactivity testing for DTH often reveals positive results (Harenberg et al., 1999; Figarella et al., 2001; Grassegger et al., 2001), but this does not necessarily translate into clinical problems, since in some patients, initial reactions have been observed to diminish with each danaparoid injection and disappear after a few days. In addition, iv treatment with danaparoid of patients with positive DTH has also proved successful (Boehnke et al., 1996; Jappe et al., 2002; Bircher et al., 2006).

Osteoporosis (a significant complication of prolonged UFH treatment) was not reported in any danaparoid-treated patients in the compassionate-use program, including pregnant patients treated for more than six months.

Availability of Danaparoid

Table 16.3 lists the countries where danaparoid has been approved for the treatment of HIT, either with or without associated thrombosis. In countries in which danaparoid is approved (and available) for DVT prophylaxis, physicians generally have the legal option to prescribe danaparoid for HIT (i.e., for "off-label" use in a nonapproved indication). Danaparoid is no longer marketed in some countries [e.g., United States (since April 2002), Norway, and Denmark] and manufacturing problems since 2009 have intermittently limited its availability in others.

TABLE 16.3 Countries in Which Danaparoid Is Available (as of Dec 2011)

Australia
Austria
Belgium
Canada
Finland
Israel
France
Germany
Great Britain
Greece
Japan
Netherlands
Sweden
Switzerland

Information courtesy of the manufacturer (Mr. Curtis Jorgensen).

CONCLUSION

Antithrombotic treatment with danaparoid is safe and effective for patients with HIT that combines a unique ability to inhibit HIT antibody-induced platelet activation with a favorable benefit:risk ratio for the prevention or treatment of venous or arterial thrombosis. It can be administered by sc and iv injection in a wide variety of clinical scenarios. *In vivo* cross-reactivity of danaparoid for HIT antibodies is an infrequent complication.

ACKNOWLEDGMENTS

Some of the studies described in this chapter were supported by a program grant from the National Health and Medical Research Council of Australia.

REFERENCES

Aberg M, Rausing A. The effect of dextran 70 on the structure of ex vivo thrombi. Thromb Res 12: 1113–1122, 1978.

Baumgartel MW, Eichler P, Glockner WM, Ranze O, Greinacher A. Heparin-induced thrombocytopenia (HIT): in vitro and in vivo cross-reactivity to danaparoid sodium and successful treatment with recombinant hirudin (lepirudin). Eur J Haematol 65: 148–149, 2000.

Bergqvist D. Prevention of postoperative deep vein thrombosis in Sweden. results of a survey. World J Surg 4: 489–495, 1980.

Bergqvist D, Kettunen K, Fredin H, Fauno P, Suomalainen S, Karjalainen P, Cederholm C, Jensen LJ, Justesen T. Thromboprophylaxis in patients with hip fractures: a prospective, randomized, comparative study between Org 10172 and dextran 70. Surgery 109: 617–622, 1991.

Bidlingmaier C, Magnani HN, Girisch M, Kurnik K. Safety and efficacy of danaparoid (Organan®) use in children. Acta Haematol 115: 237–247, 2006.

Bircher AJ, Harr T, Hohenstein L, Tsakiris DA. Hypersensitivity reactions to anticoagulant drugs: diagnosis and management options. Allergy 61: 1432–1440, 2006.

Boehnke WH, Weber L, Gall H. Tolerance to intravenous administration of heparin and heparinoid in a patient with delayed-type hypersensitivity to heparins and heparinoids. Contact Dermatitis 35: 73–75, 1996.

Bradbrook ID, Magnani HN, Moelker HCT, Morrison PJ, Robinson J, Rogers HJ, Spector RG, Van Dinther T, Wijnand H. Org 10172: a low molecular weight heparinoid anticoagulant with a long half-life in man. Br J Clin Pharmacol 23: 667–675, 1987.

Burgess JK, Chong BH. The platelet proaggregating and potentiating effects of unfractionated heparin, low molecular weight heparin and heparinoid in intensive care patients and healthy controls. Eur J Haematol 58: 279–285, 1997.

Buys S, Duterque D, Rouge P, Charlet J, Samii K. The use of danaparoid sodium in patients with heparin-induced thrombocytopenia requiring cardiac surgery with cardiopulmonary bypass is detrimental. Anesthesiol 99: A223, 2003.

Cade JF, Wood M, Magnani HN, Westlake GW. Early clinical experience of a new heparinoid, Org 10172, in prevention of deep venous thrombosis. Thromb Res 45: 497–503, 1987.

Carrier M, Robitaille D, Perrault LP, Pellerin M, Page P, Cartier R, Bouchard D. Heparin versus danaparoid in off-pump coronary bypass grafting: results of a prospective randomized clinical trial. J Thorac Cardiovasc Surg 125: 325–329, 2003.

Casu B. Structural features of chondroitin sulphate, dermatan sulphate and heparan sulphate. Semin Thromb Haemost 17(Suppl 1): 9–14, 1991.

ten Cate H, Henny ChP, ten Cate JW, Biiller HR, Mooy MC, Surachno S, Wilmink JM. Anticoagulant effects of a low molecular weight heparinoid (Org 10172) in human volunteers and haemodialysis patients. Thromb Res 38: 211–221, 1985.

Chong BH. Heparin-induced thrombocytopenia. Br J Haematol 89: 431–439, 1995.

Chong BH, Magnani HN. Orgaran in heparin-induced thrombocytopenia. Haemostasis 22: 85–91, 1992.

Chong BH, Ismail F, Cade J, Gallus AS, Gordon S, Chesterman CN. Heparin-induced thrombocytopenia: studies with a new molecular weight heparinoid, Org 10172. Blood 73: 1592–1596, 1989.

Chong BH, Gallus AS, Cade JF, Magnani H, Manoharan H, Oldmeadow M, Arthur C, Rickard K, Gallo J, Lloyd J, Seshadri P, Chesterman CN. Prospective randomised open-label comparison of danaparoid and dextran 70 in the treatment of heparin-induced thrombocytopenia and thrombosis. Thromb Haemost 86: 1170–1175, 2001.

Christiansen S, Geiger A, Splittgerber FH, Reidemeister JC. Coronary artery bypass grafting in a patient with type II heparin associated thrombopenia. Cardiovasc Surg 6: 90–93, 1998.

Comp PC, Voegeli T, McCutchen JW, Skoutakis VA, Trowbridge A, Overdyke WL, The Danaparoid Hip Arthroplasty Investigators Group. A comparison of danaparoid and warfarin for prophylaxis against deep vein thrombosis after total hip replacement. Orthopedics 21: 1123–1128, 1998.

Danhof M, de Boer A, Magnani HN, Stiekema JCJ. Pharmacokinetic considerations on Orgaran (Org 10172). Hemostasis 22: 73–84, 1992.

De Saint-Blanquat L, Simon L, Toubas MF, Hamza J. Treatment with danaparoid during pregnancy for a woman with a cutaneous allergy to low molecular weight heparin. Ann Fr Anesth Reanim 19: 751–754, 2000.

de Valk, HW, Banga JD, Wester JWJ, Brouwer CB, van Hessen MWJ, Meuwissen OJAT, Hart HC, Sixma JJ, Nieuwenhuis HK. Comparing subcutaneous danaparoid with intravenous unfractionated heparin for the treatment of venous thromboembolism. a randomized controlled trial. Ann Intern Med 123: 1–9, 1995.

Elalamy I, Tardy-Poncet B, Mulot A, de Maistre E, Pouplard C, Nguyen P, Cleret B, Gruel Y, Lecompte T, Tardy B, GEHT HIT Study Group. Risk factors for unfavorable clinical outcome in patients with documented heparin-induced thrombocytopenia. Thromb Res 124: 554–559, 2009.

Erdlenbruch W, Stephan B, Moersdorf S, Pindur G, Schenk JF. The dosage of danaparoid influences significantly the increase of platelet in patients with suspicious HIT II [abstr]. Ann Haematol 80(Suppl 1): 51, 2001.

Farner B, Eichler P, Kroll H, Greinacher A. A comparison of danaparoid and lepirudin in heparin-induced thrombocytopenia. Thromb Haemost 85: 950–957, 2001.

Fernandes P, Mayer R, MacDonald JL, Cleland A, Hay-McKay C. Use of danaparoid sodium (Orgaran) as an alternative to heparin sodium during cardiopulmonary bypass: a clinical evaluation of six cases. Perfusion 15: 531–539, 2000.

Figarella I, Barbaud A, Lecompte T, De Maistre E, Reichert-Penetrat S, Schmutz JL. Cutaneous delayed hypersensitivity reactions to heparins and heparinoids. Ann Dermatol Venereol 128: 25–30, 2001.

Gallus A, Cade J, Ockelford P, Hepburn S, Maas M, Magnani H, Bucknall T, Stevens J, Porteious F. Orgaran (Org 10172) or heparin for preventing venous thrombosis after elective surgery for malignant disease? a double-blind, randomised, multicentre comparison. Thromb Haemost 70: 562–567, 1993.

Gent M, Hirsh J, Ginsberg JS, Powers PJ, Levine MN, Geerts WH, Jay RM, Leclerc J, Neemeh JA, Turpie AG. Low molecular weight heparinoid Orgaran is more effective than aspirin in the prevention of venous thromboembolism after surgery for hip fracture. Circulation 93: 80–84, 1996.

Gerhart TN, Yett HS, Robertson LK, Lee MA, Smith M, Salzman EW. Low molecular weight heparinoid compared with warfarin for prophylaxis of deep-vein thrombosis in patients who are operated on for fracture of the hip. A prospective, randomized trial. J Bone Joint Surg 73A: 494–502, 1991.

Gordon DL, Linhardt R, Adams HP. Low molecular weight heparins and heparinoids and their use in acute or progressing ischaemic stroke. Clin Neuropharmacol 13: 522–543, 1990.

Grassegger A, Fritsch P, Reider N. Delayed-type hypersensitivity and cross-reactivity to heparins and heparinoids: a prospective study. Dermatol Surg 27: 47–52, 2001.

Greinacher A, Michels I, Muller-Eckhardt C. Heparin-associated thrombocytopenia: the antibody is not heparin specific. Thromb Haemost 67: 545–549, 1992.

Harenberg J, Huhle G, Wang L, Hoffman U, Bayerl Ch, Kerowgan M. Association of heparin-induced skin lesions, intracutaneous tests and heparin-induced IgG. Allergy 54: 473–477, 1999.

Harrison L, Johnston M, Massicotte MP, Crowther M, Moffat K, Hirsh J. Comparison of 5–mg and 10–mg loading doses in initiation of warfarin therapy. Ann Intern Med 126: 133–136, 1997.

Harrison SJ, Rafferty I, McColl MD. Management of heparin allergy during pregnancy with danaparoid. Blood Coagul Fibrinolysis 12: 157–159, 2001.

Henny CP, ten Cate H, ten Cate JW, Surachno S, van Bronswijk H, Wilmink JM, Ockelford PA. Use of a new heparinoid as anticoagulant during acute haemodialysis of patients with bleeding complications. Lancet 1: 890–893, 1983.

Henny CP, ten Cate H, ten Cate JW, Moulijn AC, Sie TH, Warren P, Buller HR. A randomized blind study comparing standard heparin and a new low molecular weight heparinoid in cardiopulmonary bypass surgery in dogs. J Lab Clin Med 106: 187–196, 1985a.

Henny CP, ten Cate H, Surachno S, Stevens P, Buller HR, den Hartog M, ten Cate JW. The effectiveness of a low molecular weight heparinoid in chronic intermittent haemodialysis. Thromb Haemost 54: 460–462, 1985b.

Hoek JA, Nurmohamed MT, Hamelynck KJ, Marti RK, Knipscheer HC, ten Cate H, Buller HR, Magnani HN, ten Cate JW. Prevention of deep vein thrombosis following total hip replacement by low molecular weight heparinoid. Thromb Haemost 67: 28–32, 1992.

Insler SR, Kraenzler EJ, Bartholomew JR, Kottke-Marchant K, Lytle B, Starr NJ. Thrombosis during the use of the heparinoid Organon 10172 in a patient with heparin-induced thrombocytopenia. Anesthesiology 86: 495–498, 1997.

Ireland H, Lane DA, Flynn A, Anastassiades E, Curtis JR. The anticoagulant effect of heparinoid Org 10172 during haemodialysis: an objective assessment. Thromb Haemost 55: 271–275, 1986.

Jappe U, Reinhold D, Bonnekoh B. Arthus reaction to lepirudin, a new recombinant hirudin, and delayed-type hypersensitivity to several heparins and heparinoids, with tolerance to its intravenous administration. Contact Dermatitis 46: 29–32, 2002.

Kikta MJ, Keller MP, Humphrey PW, Silver D. Can low molecular weight heparins and heparinoids be safely given to patients with heparin-induced thrombocytopenia syndrome? Surgery 114: 705–710, 1993.

Kodityal S, Manhas AH, Udden M, Rice L. Danaparoid for heparin-induced thrombocytopenia: an analysis of treatment failures. Eur J Haematol 71: 1–5, 2003.

Koster A, Meyer O, Hausmann H, Kuppe H, Hetzer R, Mertzlufft F. In vitro cross-reactivity of danaparoid sodium in patients with heparin-induced thrombocytopenia type II undergoing cardiovascular surgery. J Clin Anesth 12: 324–327, 2000.

Krauel K, Fürll B, Warkentin TE, Weitschies W, Kohlmann W, Sheppard JI, Greiniacher A. Heparin-induced thrombocytopenia—therapeutic concentrations of danaparoid, unlike fondaparinux and direct thrombin inhibitors, inhibit formation of PF4/heparin complexes. J Thromb Haemost 6: 2160–2167, 2008.

Lane DA, Tew C, Ireland H, Flynn A, Curtis JR. Heparin and low molecular weight heparin(oid)s as anticoagulants in haemodialysis for chronic renal failure. Ann NY Acad Sci 556: 456–458, 1989.

Laposata M, Green D, Van Cott EM, Barrowcliffe TW, Goodnight SH, Sosolik RC, College of American Pathologists Conference Therapy. The clinical use and laboratory monitoring of low molecular weight heparin, danaparoid, hirudin and related compounds, and argatroban. Arch Pathol Lab Med 122: 799–807, 1998.

Leyvraz P, Bachmann F, Bohnet J, Breyer HG, Estoppey D, Haas S, Hochreiter J, Jakubek H, Mair J, Sorensen R, et al. Thromboembolic prophylaxis in total hip replacement: a comparison between the low molecular weight heparinoid Lomoparan and heparin-dihydroergotamine. Br J Surg 79: 911–914, 1992.

Lindhoff-Last E, Bauersachs R. Heparin-induced thrombocytopenia—alternative anticoagulation in pregnancy and lactation. Semin Thromb Hemost 28: 439–445, 2002.

Lindhoff-Last E, Betz C, Bauersachs R. Use of a low molecular weight heparinoid (danaparoid sodium) for continuous renal replacement therapy in intensive care unit patients. Clin Appl Thromb/Hemost 7: 300–304, 2001.

Lindhoff-Last E, Magnani HN, Kreutzenbeck H-J. Treatment of 51 pregnancies with danaparoid because of heparin intolerance. Thromb Haemost 91/3: 63–69, 2005.

Lubenow N, Warkentin TE, Greinacher A, Wessel A, Sloane DA, Krahn EL, Magnani NH. A systematic evaluation of treatment outcomes for heparin-induced thrombocytopenia in patients receiving danaparoid, ancrod and/or coumarin explains the rapid shift in clinical practice during the 1990s. Thromb Haemost 117: 507–515, 2006.

Magnani HN. Heparin-induced thrombocytopenia (HIT): an overview of 230 patients treated with Orgaran (Org 10172). Thromb Haemost 70: 554–561, 1993.

Magnani HN. Orgaran (danaparoid sodium) use in the syndrome of heparin-induced thrombocytopenia. Platelets 8: 74–81, 1997.

Magnani HN. An analysis of clinical outcomes of 91 pregnancies in 83 women treated with danaparoid (Orgaran®). Thromb Res 125: 297–302, 2010a.

Magnani HN. A review of 122 published outcomes of danaparoid anticoagulation for intermittent haemodialysis. Thromb Res 125: 171–176, 2010b.

Magnani HN, Gallus A. Heparin-induced thrombocytopenia (HIT) a report of 1478 clinical outcomes of patients treated with danaparoid (Orgaran) from 1982 – mid-2004. Thromb Haemost 95: 967–981, 2006.

Magnani HN, Wester J. Orgaran® use in intensive care unit patients with heparin-induced thombocytopenia and renal failure. Critical Care 11(Suppl 2): P371, 2007.

Magnani HN, Beijering RJR, ten Gate JW, Chong BH. Orgaran anticoagulation for cardiopulmonary bypass in patients with heparin-induced thrombocytopenia. In: Pifarre R, ed. New Anticoagulants for the Cardiovascular Patient. Philadelphia: Hanley & Belfus, 487–500, 1997.

Makhoul RG, Greenberg CS, McCann RL. Heparin-induced thrombocytopenia and thrombosis: a serious clinical problem and potential solution. J Vasc Surg 4: 522–528, 1986.

Merli GJ, Doyle L, Crabbe S, Sciarra A, Herbison G, Ditunno J. Prophylaxis for deep vein thrombosis in acute spinal cord injury comparing two doses of low molecular weight heparinoid in combination with external pneumatic compression. J Rehabil Res Dev 28: 434–435, 1991.

Meuleman DG, Hobbelen PMJ, Van Dedem G, Moelker HCT. A novel anti-thrombotic heparinoid (Org 10172) devoid of bleeding inducing capacity: a survey of pharmacological properties in experimental animal models. Thromb Res 27: 353–363, 1982.

Meuleman DG. Synopsis of the anticoagulant and antithrombotic profile of the low molecular weight heparinoid Org 10172 in experimental models. Thromb Haemost 58: 376–380, 1987.

Meuleman DG. Orgaran (Org 10172): its pharmacological profile in experimental models. Haemostasis 22: 58–65, 1992.

Mikhailidis DP, Barradas MA, Mikhailidis AM, Magnani H, Dandona P. Comparison of the effect of a conventional heparin and a low molecular weight heparinoid on platelet function. Br J Clin Pharmacol 17: 43–48, 1984.

Mikhailidis DP, Fonseca VA, Barradas MA, Jeremy JY, Dandona P. Platelet activation following intravenous injection of a conventional heparin: absence of effect with a low molecular weight heparinoid (Org 10172). Br J Clin Pharmacol 24: 415–424, 1987.

Muhm M, Claeys L, Huk I, Koppensteiner R, Kyrle PA, Minar E, Stumpflen A, Ehringer H, Polterauer P. Thromboembolic complications in a patient with heparin-induced thrombocytopenia (HIT) showing cross-reactivity to a low molecular weight heparin-treatment with Org 10172 (Lomoparan). Wien Klin Wochenschr 109: 128–131, 1997.

Newman PM, Swanson RL, Chong BH. IgG binding to PF4-Heparin complexes in the fluid phase and cross-reactivity with low molecular weight heparin and heparinoid. Thromb Haemost 80: 292–297, 1998.

Nieuwenhuis HK, Sixma JJ. Treatment of disseminated intravascular coagulation in acute promyelocytic leukemia with low molecular weight heparinoid Org 10172. Cancer 58: 761–764, 1986.

Nohira T, Kim S, Nakai H, Okabe K. [Thromboembolic prophylaxis with danaparoid sodium for high thrombosis risk pregnant women after caesarean section]. Jap J Obstet Gynaecol Neonatal Haematol 13: 5–11, 2004. [In Japanese]

Ofosu FA. Anticoagulant mechanisms of Orgaran (Org 10172) and its fraction with high affinity to antithrombin III (Org 10849). Haemostasis 22: 66–72, 1992.

Olin DA, Urdaneta F, Lobato EB. Use of danaparoid during cardiopulmonary bypass in patients with heparin-induced thrombocytopenia. J Cardiothorac Vasc Anesth 14: 707–709, 2000.

Org 10172 hip joint replacement report. Research Protocol 004–023. West Orange, NJ: Organon Inc., 1994.

Ortel TL, Chong BH. New treatment options for heparin-induced thrombocytopenia. Semin Hematol 35(Suppl 5): 26–34, 1998.

Pötzsch B, Unrig C, Madlener K, Greinacher A, Müller-Berghaus G. APC resistance and early onset of oral anticoagulation are high thrombotic risk factors in patients with heparin-associated thrombocytopenia (HAT). Ann Hematol 72(Suppl 1): A6, 1996.

Ramakrishna R, Manoharan A, Kwan YL, Kyle PW. Heparin-induced thrombocytopenia: cross-reactivity between standard heparin, low molecular weight heparin, dalteparin (Fragmin) and heparinoid (Orgaran). Br J Haematol 91: 736–738, 1995.

Saxon BR, Black MD, Edgell D, Noel D, Leaker MT. Pediatric heparin-induced thrombocytopenia: management with danaparoid (Orgaran). Ann Thorac Surg 68: 1076–1078, 1999.

Schmahl TE, Ganjoo AK, Harloff MG. Orgaran (Org 10172) for cardiopulmonary bypass in heparin-induced thrombocytopenia: role of adjunctive plasmapheresis. J Cardiothorac Vasc Anesth 11: 262–263, 1997.

Skoutakis VA. Danaparoid in the prevention of thromboembolic complications. Ann Pharmacother 31: 876–887, 1997.

Statius van Eps R, Wester JPJ, de Ruiter FE, Girbes ARJ. Danaparoid sodium in continuous veno-venous hemofiltration in patients with multiple organ dysfunction syndrome [abstr]. Neth J Med 56: A40–A41, 2000.

Statius van Eps R, Wester JPJ, de Ruiter FE, Vervloet MG, Zweegman S, Thijs LG, Girbes ARJ. The incidence of heparin-induced thrombocytopenia in critically ill patients with the multiple organ dysfunction syndrome [abstr]. Thromb Haemost 86(Suppl): P2719, 2001.

Stiekema JC, Wijnand HP, van Dinther TG, Moelker HCT, Dawes J, Vinchenzo A, Toeberich H. Safety and pharmacokinetics of the low molecular weight heparinoid Org 10172 administered to healthy elderly volunteers. Br J Clin Pharmacol 27: 39–48, 1989.

Tani H, Itoh H, Kosaka K, Takemura M, Okada Y, Kawasaki K, Sagawa N, Fujii S. Prophylactic use of danaparoid sodium for deep-vein thromboembolism after cesarean section. Adv Obstet Gynaecol 57: 309–310, 2005.

Tardy-Poncet B, Mahul P, Beraud AM, Favre JP, Tardy B, Guyotat D. Failure of Orgaran therapy in a patient with a previous heparin-induced thrombocytopenia. Br J Haematol 90: 69–70, 1995.

Tardy-Poncet B, Tardy B, Reynaud J, Mahul P, Mismetti P, Mazet E, Guyotat D. Efficacy and safety of danaparoid sodium (ORG 10172) in critically ill patients with heparin-induced thrombocytopenia. Chest 115: 1616–1620, 1999.

Tardy-Poncet B, Wolf M, Lasne D, Bauters A, Ffrench P, Elalamy I, Tardy B. Danaparoid cross-reactivity with heparin-induced thrombocytopenia antibodies: report of 12 cases. Intensive Care Med 35: 1449–1453, 2009.

Taylor AA. Successful use of Heparinoids in a pregnancy complicated by allergy to heparin. Br J Obstet Gynaecol 108: 1011–1012, 2001.

Teien AN, Lie M. Evaluation of an amidolytic heparin assay method: increased sensitivity by adding purified antithrombin III. Thromb Res 10: 399–410, 1977.

The TIFDED Study Group. Thromboprophylaxis in fracture hip surgery: a pilot study comparing danaparoid, enoxaparin and dalteparin. Haemost 29: 310–317, 1999.

Turpie AGG, Hirsh J, Jay JM, Andrew M, Hull RD, Levine MN, Carter CJ, Powers PJ, Magnani HN, Gent M. Double-blind randomised trial of Org 10172 low molecular weight heparinoid in prevention of deep-vein thrombosis in thrombotic stroke. Lancet 1: 523–526, 1987.

Turpie AGG, Gent M, Cote R, Levine MN, Ginsbergt JS, Powers PJ, Leclerc J, Geerts W, Jay R, Neemeh J, Klimek M, Hirsh J. Low molecular weight heparinoid compared with unfractionated heparin in the prevention of deep vein thrombosis in patients with acute ischemic stroke. Ann Int Med 117: 353–375, 1992.

Von Bonsdorff M, Stiekema J, Harjanne A, Alapiessa U. A new low molecular weight heparinoid Org 10172 as anticoagulant in hemodialysis. Int J Artif Organs 13: 103–108, 1990.

Vun CH, Evans S, Chong BH. Cross-reactivity study of low molecular weight heparins and heparinoid in heparin-induced thrombocytopenia. Thromb Res 81: 525–532, 1996.

Warkentin TE. Heparin-induced thrombocytopenia: IgG-mediated platelet activation, platelet microparticle generation, and altered procoagulant/anticoagulant balance in the pathogenesis of thrombosis and venous limb gangrene complicating heparin-induced thrombocytopenia. Transfus Med Rev 10: 249–258, 1996a.

Warkentin TE. Danaparoid (Orgaran) for the treatment of heparin-induced thrombocytopenia (HIT) and thrombosis: effects on in vivo thrombin and cross-linked fibrin generation, and evaluation of the clinical significance of in vitro cross-reactivity of danaparoid for HIT-IgG. Blood 88: 626a, 1996b.

Warkentin TE. Limitation of conventional treatment options for heparin-induced thrombocytopenia. Semin Hematol 35(Suppl 5): 17–25, 1998.

Warkentin TE. Heparin-induced thrombocytopenia: yet another treatment paradox? Thromb Haemost 85: 947–949, 2001.

Warkentin TE. Should vitamin K be administered when HIT is diagnosed after administration of coumarin? J Thromb Haemost 4: 894–896, 2006.

Warkentin TE, Kelton JG. A 14–year study of heparin-induced thrombocytopenia. Am J Med 101: 502–507, 1996.

Warkentin TE, Kelton JG. Temporal aspects of heparin-induced thrombocytopenia. N Engl J Med 344: 1286–1292, 2001.

Warkentin TE, Elavathil LJ, Hayward CPM, Johnston MA, Russett JI, Kelton JG. The pathogenesis of venous limb gangrene associated with heparin-induced thrombocytopenia. Ann Intern Med 127: 804–812, 1997.

Warkentin TE, Dunn GL, Cybulsky IJ. Off-pump coronary artery bypass of grafting for acute heparin-induced thrombocytopenia. Ann Thorac Surg 72: 1730–1732, 2001.

Warkentin TE, Greinacher A, Koster A, Lincoff AM. Treatment and prevention of heparin-induced thrombocytopenia. American College of Chest Physicians Evidence-Based Clinical Practice guidelines, 8th edition. Chest 133(6 Suppl): 340S–380S, 2008.

Westphal K, Martens S, Strouhal U, Matheis G. Heparin-induced thrombocytopenia type II: perioperative management using danaparoid in a coronary artery bypass patient with renal failure. Thorac Cardiovasc Surg 45: 318–320, 1997.

Wester JPJ, Stolk M, Geers ABM, Vincent HH, Haas FJLM, Biesma DH, Veth G, Leusink JA, Wiltink HH. Danaparoid sodium in CAVHD in seriously ill patients with heparin-induced thrombocytopenia. Neth J Med 56: A44, 2000.

Wilhelm MJ, Schmid C, Kekecioglu D, Mollhoff T, Ostermann H, Scheld HH. Cardiopulmonary bypass in patients with heparin-induced thrombocytopenia using Org 10172. Ann Thorac Surg 61: 920–924, 1996.

Fondaparinux and other emerging anticoagulants to treat heparin-induced thrombocytopenia

Theodore E. Warkentin and John W. Eikelboom

INTRODUCTION
Progress in Drug Development

Historical approaches to anticoagulation have relied on partially purified or chemically derivatized natural products, such as heparin and warfarin (Hirsh et al., 2007). The utility of these agents, however, is limited by interpatient variability in pharmacologic effect, the requirement for routine coagulation monitoring, and, for warfarin, various food and drug interactions. The association of heparin and warfarin with prothrombotic complications—immune heparin-induced thrombocytopenia (HIT), and warfarin necrosis—is particularly troublesome. Low molecular weight heparin (LMWH) has replaced heparin for many indications because LMWH produces a more predictable anticoagulant effect and is associated with a lower risk of HIT. The parenterally administered selective factor Xa inhibitor, fondaparinux, represents a further advance over LMWH, and since the last edition of this book has emerged as a viable —albeit nonapproved ("off-label")— treatment for HIT. Several new orally administered anticoagulants that selectively target factor IIa (thrombin) or factor Xa have now been approved for (non-HIT) clinical use and in the future may also be attractive options for the treatment of HIT.

Rationale for Targeting Factor Xa and Thrombin

Table 17.1 lists anticoagulants, some established, some in development (names italicized), that inhibit factor Xa or thrombin (IIa) or both, either indirectly through antithrombin (AT; formerly, antithrombin III) or directly (AT-independent). The rationale for targeting these factors follows from their key roles in coagulation. Factor X is synthesized by the liver in a vitamin K-dependent manner. Positioned at the start of the final common pathway, factor X is activated by both the *extrinsic tenase complex* (VIIa/tissue factor [TF]) and the *intrinsic tenase complex* (IXa/VIIIa); the resulting factor Xa (a serine protease) then forms the prothrombinase complex with factor Va and ionic calcium on membranes, catalyzing the conversion of prothrombin to thrombin. Thrombin too is a serine protease with even more substrates within the coagulation cascade, notably soluble fibrinogen (converted to insoluble fibrin), and also factors XI, VIII, and V (Fig. 17.1).

There is debate surrounding the preferential targeting of factor Xa *versus* IIa, and the role of direct *versus* indirect (AT-mediated) inhibition (Ansell, 2007; Weitz, 2007). Direct inhibition of thrombin will likely suppress both procoagulant (fibrin, XIa, VIIIa, Va generation) and anticoagulant (protein C generation) functions (Fig. 17.1). However, the pharmacologic utility of commercially available direct

TABLE 17.1 Established and Emerging Parenteral and Oral Anticoagulants that Directly or Indirectly Block Thrombin or Factor Xa

	Indirect (AT-dependent unless indicated otherwise)	Direct (AT-independent)
Thrombin inhibitors		Argatroban Bivalirudin r-Hirudin (lepirudin, desirudin) Dabigatran etexilate (oral)
Combined thrombin and factor Xa inhibitors	Unfractionated heparin Low molecular weight heparins[a] (enoxaparin, dalteparin, nadroparin, reviparin, tinzaparin) Ultra-low molecular weight heparins (bemiparin, *semuloparin*)[b] Danaparoid[c]	
Factor Xa inhibitors	Fondaparinux *Idraparinux*[d] *Idrabiotaparinux*[d,e] *Otamixaban*	Apixaban (oral) Rivaroxaban (oral) Edoxaban (oral)[f]

Note: Agents are parenteral unless indicated otherwise. Agents mentioned in italics are not approved for clinical use. Several anti-factor Xa inhibitors in earlier phases of development are included in Table 17.3.
[a]Low molecular weight heparins have an anti-Xa:anti-IIa ratio of between 2:1 and 4:1.
[b]Bemiparin has an anti-Xa:anti-IIa ratio of about 8:1 and semuloparin has an anti-Xa:anti-IIa ratio of about 80:1.
[c]Danaparoid is a mixture of chondroitin sulfate, dermatan sulfate, and heparan sulfate (see chap. 16); it has an anti-Xa:anti-IIa ratio of >20:1.
[d]Idraparinux and idrabiotaparinux are no longer in clinical development.
[e]Biotinylated idraparinux.
[f]Approved only in Japan.
Abbreviations: AT, antithrombin; r-hirudin, recombinant hirudin.

thrombin inhibitors (DTIs) suggests that the dominant effect of targeting IIa is anti-coagulation. Additionally, thrombin has physiologic roles beyond coagulation that may be abrogated by DTI therapy, such as effects on platelets, wound-healing, and endothelium. By contrast, inhibition of factor Xa is expected to be associated with a purely anticoagulant pharmacodynamic effect, as factor Xa is not known to influence directly natural anticoagulant pathways.

Rationale for Exploring Treatment of HIT with New Anticoagulants
HIT is a markedly hypercoagulable state with a high risk of venous and arterial thrombosis (see chaps. 2 and 12). In most patients with suspected or proven HIT, there is a need for rapidly acting and effective anticoagulation with an alternative nonheparin anticoagulant (Warkentin, 2011). This chapter explores the potential role of emerging anticoagulants for the treatment of HIT with particular attention to the pentasaccharide anticoagulant, fondaparinux, for the treatment of patients with suspected and proven HIT. Indeed, with its low/absent cross-reactivity with HIT antibodies, relatively long half-life, and proven efficacy and safety in a variety of prophylactic and therapeutic anticoagulant settings, the success of fondaparinux for treating HIT suggests that other novel anticoagulants could have similar benefits

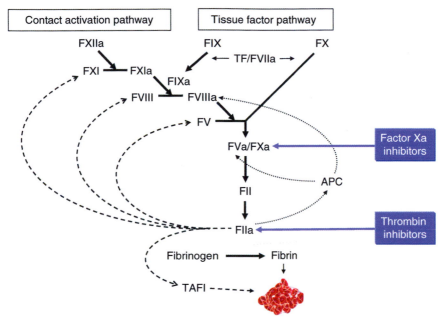

FIGURE 17.1 Blood coagulation is initiated when factor VII(a) is exposed to membrane-bound TF. The TF/VII(a) complexes activate factor IX (to IXa) and factor X (to Xa), leading ultimately to the formation of thrombin (IIa). Amplification of the process occurs when trace amounts of thrombin formed during the initiation of coagulation activate factor XI (to XIa), and the cofactors, VIII and V, to VIIIa and Va, respectively, in a series of positive feedback loops (denoted by dashed [- - - -] lines), resulting in the formation of the VIIIa/IXa ("tenase") and the Va/Xa ("prothrombinase") complexes, the generation of large amounts of thrombin, and the formation of a fibrin clot. Thrombin also exerts an inhibitory effect on coagulation by a negative feedback loop (denoted by dotted [. . . .] lines) that involves activation of the protein C anticoagulant pathway, resulting in degradation of factors Va and VIIIa. Anticoagulant drugs that inhibit factor Xa reduce the amount of thrombin formed. Anticoagulant drugs that inhibit IIa reduce thrombin activity and thus reduce (*i*) fibrin clot formation, (*ii*) positive feedback amplification of thrombin generation (including contact activation that occurs when blood is exposed to foreign surfaces), and (*iii*) negative feedback via the protein C pathway. *Abbreviations*: APC, activated protein C; TAFI, thrombin activatable fibrinolysis inhibitor; TF, tissue factor.

for treating HIT. If so, management of HIT could evolve in the coming years from the existing "niche" anticoagulants—particularly the parenteral DTIs—to these newer agents.

FONDAPARINUX
History
Unfractionated heparin (UFH) is comprised of a highly heterogeneous mixture of linear polysaccharide molecules of variable length (mean, 45–50 saccharide units). Seminal studies by Rosenberg in the 1970s and 1980s defined the structure–function relationship of heparin. The pharmacologic activity of UFH was ascribed to a subpopulation of polysaccharides capable of binding AT (Lam et al., 1976; Rosenberg et al., 1978). Anticoagulation resulted from the formation of an inhibitory ternary

complex among heparin, AT, and any of five clotting factors (factors IIa, Xa, IXa, XIa, and XIIa). Subsequent studies resolved the minimal chemical motif necessary for anticoagulation as a tetrasaccharide sequence (Rosenberg and Lam, 1979). Based on these findings, synthetic polysaccharides with potent anticoagulant activity were prepared (Choay et al., 1983; Grootenhuis et al., 1995; Petitou et al., 1999). One theoretical benefit of the small size of the synthetic heparin mimetics might be the potential not to cause HIT (Petitou et al., 1999).

Chemistry

Fondaparinux sodium (Arixtra, formerly Org31540/SR90107A), the first synthetic pentasaccharide anticoagulant, is prepared for injection as a decasodium salt. The chemical formula is $C_{31}H_{43}N_3Na_{10}O_{49}S_8$, and the molecular mass is 1728 Da (Arixtra Package Insert, 2006). The chemical structure is presented in Figure 7.8 of chapter 7.

Fondaparinux is a methyl glycoside analogue designed and optimized based on the AT-binding site of UFH. Binding to AT (1:1 stoichiometry) results in the allosteric induction of an irreversible conformational change in AT. This AT conformer exhibits high binding affinity for factor Xa, preventing thrombin generation (Arocas et al., 2001). After covalent binding of Xa to AT, fondaparinux is released without structural alteration, allowing subsequent binding once again to free AT. Unlike UFH and (longer fragments within) LMWH, binding of fondaparinux to AT does not facilitate inhibition of factor IIa, due to the structural absence of the heparin thrombin-binding domain.

Pharmacology

The pharmacodynamic impact of factor Xa inhibition is reduced thrombin generation. Studies performed *in vitro* with platelet-rich plasma have identified an inhibitory effect on both the initiation and propagation phases of thrombin generation, with reduction in the total amount of thrombin generated (Walenga et al., 1988; Gerotziafas et al., 2004b). Animal studies have demonstrated pronounced inhibition of thrombus extension (Amar et al., 1990).

The pharmacokinetics of fondaparinux were determined in young, healthy volunteers and in the elderly (Donat et al., 2002). Following subcutaneous (sc) injection, fondaparinux is absorbed completely, with peak plasma concentrations achieved within 1–3 hours. Maximal concentrations and area under the curve correlate linearly with dose, with the half-life being relatively constant in young volunteers (~17 hr). In the elderly, the half-life is mildly prolonged (~21 hr). The comparatively long elimination half-life permits a once-daily sc dosing schedule, with steady-state achieved following the fourth or fifth daily dose. Fondaparinux is excreted almost completely in the urine without metabolism.

The pharmacology of fondaparinux has not been well defined in special populations, such as pregnant women, children, or persons with severe renal impairment. Data from the orthopedic thromboprophylaxis trials provides insights into the impact of renal impairment on drug clearance (Turpie, 2002). With mild renal impairment (creatinine clearance, 50–80 mL/min), fondaparinux clearance is reduced by 25%; with moderate renal impairment (creatinine clearance, 30–50 mL/min), clearance is 40% reduced (Arixtra Package Insert, 2006). Thus, use of fondaparinux is not advised with severe renal impairment (creatinine clearance, <30 mL/min) (although two investigations investigating a total of 28 hemodialysis patients have provided parameters for its use to anticoagulate this patient population) (Kalicki et al., 2007; Sombolos et al., 2008). The safe, effective use of fondaparinux in pregnant patients has been reported in several case reports (Mazzolai et al., 2006; Wijesiriwardana et al., 2006; Gerhardt et al., 2007; Harenberg, 2007; Ciurzyński et al., 2011). Despite *in vitro* evidence to the contrary, transplacental passage of fondaparinux has been suggested by the detection of a low anti-factor Xa activity in umbilical cord blood, so caution in this context is warranted (Lagrange et al., 2002; Dempfle, 2004).

Dosage and Administration

Fondaparinux is supplied for use as a prefilled syringe with attached protective needle system. Individual syringes are available for the following doses: 2.5, 5.0, 7.5, and 10.0 mg. The drug is formulated in an isotonic solution of sodium chloride, with a pH varying between 5.0 and 8.0. The dose studied for thromboprophylaxis was determined by a wide dose-ranging phase II program in orthopedic surgery patients, which led to the selection of a 2.5 mg daily dose (Turpie et al., 2001).

The dose of fondaparinux selected for use in the treatment of venous thromboembolism (VTE) was also selected from a dose-ranging phase II study (Rembrandt Investigators, 2000). Guidance for dose selection was derived from a primary outcome measure of ultrasonographic change in thrombus mass balanced against tolerability data, with the data model supporting a 7.5 mg daily dose. The phase III VTE treatment program validated a simplified weight-based dosing scheme, where patients between 50 and 100 kg received 7.5 mg once-daily. Patients weighing in excess of 100 kg were administered 10.0 mg, whereas patients weighing less than 50 kg received 5.0 mg (Büller et al., 2003, 2004).

Dose selection for fondaparinux in the management of acute coronary syndrome (ACS) was based on the results of dose-ranging studies in patients with non–ST-segment elevation ACS (Simoons et al., 2004) and ST-segment elevation myocardial infarction (MI) (Coussement et al., 2001). In the absence of evidence of a dose response for efficacy, a 2.5 mg once-daily dose was selected for evaluation in the phase III trials.

Monitoring

Monitoring of fondaparinux drug level or pharmacodynamic effect was not routinely performed during the clinical studies establishing its efficacy. Consequently, monitoring has not been required by regulatory agencies. The pharmacodynamic effect of fondaparinux can be monitored using commercial assays for anti-factor Xa activity, although calibration to a standard curve derived from fondaparinux is required. However, the clinical utility of routine monitoring is uncertain (Klaeffling et al., 2006). Approximate plasma concentrations of fondaparinux attained during antithrombotic prophylaxis or therapy are approximately 0.3 and 1.4 µg/mL, respectively (Donat et al., 2002). Since 850 anti-factor Xa units of activity correspond to 1 mg of fondaparinux (Marilyn Johnston, personal communication), this indicates that the above-stated concentrations of 0.3 and 1.4 µg/mL correspond to anti-factor Xa activity concentrations of ~0.25 and ~1.2 U/mL (albeit with somewhat higher and lower levels corresponding to peak and trough drug levels).

Fondaparinux does not prolong the bleeding time (Boneu et al., 1995). Subtle prolongation of the prothrombin time (PT; 1 second) and partial thromboplastin time (PTT; 4 seconds), as well as a mild reduction in factor VIII have been reported (Smogorzewska et al., 2006).

Reversal

No specific antidote exists for fondaparinux. Studies performed *in vitro* have demonstrated the capacity of recombinant heparinase to depolymerize and inactivate fondaparinux (Daud et al., 2001). However, pharmaceutical preparations of this enzyme are not available. Notably, protamine sulfate does not neutralize the antifactor Xa effect of pentasaccharides (Bernat and Herbert, 1996). A clinical study of 16 healthy volunteers treated with fondaparinux suggests that recombinant factor VIIa (rFVIIa) may counteract its anticoagulant effects (Bijsterveld et al., 2002). A systematic review of the literature based mostly on *in vitro* studies (Lisman et al., 2003; Gerotziafas et al., 2004a; Young et al., 2007; Desmurs-Clavel et al., 2009) concluded that rFVIIa represented the preferred approach to manage fondaparinux-associated life-threatening bleeding situations, as compared with either activated or nonactivated prothrombin complex concentrates (Elmer and Wittels, 2012). A case report describes use of rFVIIa and tranexamic acid to help manage an orthopedic patient with hemorrhagic shock complicating fondaparinux use (Huvers et al., 2005), and another report described benefit of rFVIIa precardiocentesis in a patient with hemorrhagic pericarditis associated with therapeutic levels of fondaparinux (Ghanny et al., 2012). However, a recent case series suggests that rFVIIa may be less effective in bleeding patients with anti-factor Xa levels that exceed $1\,U/mL$ (Luporsi et al., 2011).

Adverse Effects

The most commonly reported adverse effect of fondaparinux is bleeding. In the large, prospective efficacy studies in VTE, the incidence of major bleeding among patients treated with (therapeutic-dose) fondaparinux was approximately 1% (Büller et al., 2003, 2004). In a registration study of patients undergoing elective total knee replacement, a statistically significant increase in bleeding, as defined by the bleeding index, was noted with fondaparinux, compared with enoxaparin, with no increase in fatal or clinically relevant bleeding (Bauer et al., 2001). A meta-analysis of the phase III registration program studies in VTE prevention identified a modest increase in major bleeding (compared with enoxaparin) but without an increase in bleeding leading to death, requiring surgical intervention, or bleeding in a critical site (Turpie et al., 2002a). When given at a dose of 2.5 mg once-daily in the ACS trials, fondaparinux was associated with reduced bleeding compared with enoxaparin or heparin (Yusuf et al., 2006a,b). Caution should be used in patients with cutaneous hypersensitivity to UFH, as the literature presents conflicting information regarding the tolerability of fondaparinux in this setting (Hirsch et al., 2004; Jappe et al., 2004; Utikal et al., 2005); however, a systematic review suggested that the risk of a cross-reaction with fondaparinux is relatively low (10%) (Weberschock et al., 2011).

CLINICAL USE OF FONDAPARINUX
Prevention of VTE After Orthopedic Surgery

The clinical utility of fondaparinux as a method of thromboprophylaxis following orthopedic surgery was established by four, large phase III studies in which patients were randomized to receive either fondaparinux or enoxaparin. Two studies (EPHESUS, PENTATHLON 2000) were performed in patients undergoing elective hip replacement (Lassen et al., 2002; Turpie et al., 2002b). With a primary outcome measure of venographically evident deep vein thrombosis (DVT) and symptomatic PE, fondaparinux demonstrated superior efficacy compared with once-daily dosing of enoxaparin (40 mg; EPHESUS) and comparable efficacy with twice-daily dosing (30 mg b.i.d.; PENTATHLON 2000). Major bleeding was not statistically different between the two groups. In a study of patients undergoing elective knee replacement surgery (PENTAMAKS), fondaparinux demonstrated superior efficacy (defined above) compared with enoxaparin (Bauer et al., 2001).

A fourth registration study (PENTHIFRA) enrolled patients undergoing hip fracture surgery (Eriksson et al., 2001). Here, fondaparinux demonstrated a marked reduction in VTE (postoperative DVT and PE) compared with enoxaparin (8.3% *vs* 19.1%; $P < 0.001$). Bleeding was not significantly different between the two treatment groups. To investigate the utility of extended prophylaxis following hip fracture surgery, a fifth orthopedic trial was undertaken (PENTHIFRA-Plus) (Eriksson and Lassen, 2003). Patients completing a standard course of therapy with 2.5 mg of fondaparinux given for 6–8 days were randomized to additional therapy *versus* placebo for 19–23 days. The primary efficacy outcome, symptomatic or venographically evident VTE, was markedly reduced by extended therapy (1.4% *vs* 35%; $P < 0.001$). Fondaparinux received approval from the U.S. Food and Drug Administration (FDA) for the prevention of VTE following major hip or knee surgery (Table 17.2).

Prevention of Venous Thrombosis in Other Clinical Settings

Additional clinical studies have examined the utility of fondaparinux in the prevention of VTE following general surgery and in the medical patient. In general surgery patients, the PEGASUS study compared the efficacy of 2.5 mg fondaparinux *versus* dalteparin administered preoperatively and then once-daily at a dose of 5000 IU (Agnelli et al., 2005). The primary endpoint was venographically evident DVT and symptomatic VTE to day 10. The objective of this noninferiority study was met, without a significant increase in major hemorrhage, prompting approval of fondaparinux by the FDA for the prevention of VTE following abdominal surgery.

In a population of medically ill patients, fondaparinux was compared with placebo in the prevention of venographically detected DVT and symptomatic VTE to day 15 of blinded therapy (Cohen et al., 2006). This international study of 849 patients, named ARTEMIS (ARixtra for ThromboEmbolism Prevention in a Medical Indications Study), illustrates the activity of fondaparinux in medical thromboprophylaxis, with a reduction in symptomatic and venographically evident VTE.

Treatment of VTE

The treatment of VTE was assessed in two large, international studies (Büller et al., 2003, 2004). The primary outcome measure for both noninferiority studies was the incidence of symptomatic VTE during a total treatment period of three months. In MATISSE-DVT, patients with acute DVT were randomized to receive either sc fondaparinux, given once-daily, or enoxaparin, given twice-daily at a dose of 1 mg/kg. Patients in both arms of the study were transitioned to vitamin K antagonist therapy for the remainder of the protocol. There was no significant difference in efficacy (fondaparinux 3.9%; enoxaparin 4.1%) or tolerability.

In MATISSE-PE, patients with symptomatic acute pulmonary embolism (PE) were randomized to once-daily sc fondaparinux *versus* standard therapy with UFH. Again, all patients were transitioned to oral therapy with a vitamin K antagonist.

TABLE 17.2 Indications for the Use of Fondaparinux in the United States

Indication	Dose and administration	U.S. approval
Venous thromboembolism prevention		
Hip fracture	2.5 mg/day sc o.d. for up to 32 days	Yes
Elective hip or knee replacement	2.5 mg/day sc o.d. for up to 11 days	Yes
Abdominal surgery	2.5 mg/day sc o.d. for up to 10 days	Yes
Venous thromboembolism treatment		
Acute treatment of deep vein thrombosis or pulmonary embolism	5 mg (<50 kg), 7.5 mg (50–100 kg), or 10 mg (>100 kg) sc o.d. in fixed weight adjusted dose for minimum of 5 days and until INR ≥ 2.0 on two occasions 24 hr apart[a]	Yes[a]

[a]Approved when administered in conjunction with warfarin; INR increase reflects overlapping treatment with warfarin (or another vitamin K antagonist).
Abbreviations: INR, international normalized ratio; iv, intravenous; MI, myocardial infarction; o.d., once-daily; sc, subcutaneous.

The incidence of recurrent VTE was not significantly reduced in patients treated with fondaparinux (3.8%) compared with UFH (5.0%). Notably, patients with a serum creatinine over 2.0 mg/dL were excluded from this study, which leaves some uncertainty regarding the tolerability of fondaparinux in patients with severe renal dysfunction. Based on the favorable results of the MATISSE studies, fondaparinux was approved for the treatment of VTE (Table 17.2).

Treatment of ACS
Recent clinical studies have explored the use of fondaparinux in the treatment of ACS, based on the rationale that antithrombotic therapy with UFH and LMWH is beneficial in this clinical context, as well as percutaneous coronary intervention (PCI). A pilot study was performed in patients undergoing elective or urgent PCI (Mehta et al., 2005). Fondaparinux was administered at either 2.5 or 5.0 mg, by intravenous (iv) infusion, and compared with iv UFH. Comparable efficacy was observed using a composite endpoint (all-cause mortality, infarction, revascularization, or need for glycoprotein IIb/IIIa antagonist therapy). However, a reduced incidence of hemorrhage in patients receiving 2.5 mg (3.4%) *versus* 5.0 mg (9.6%) provided further support for evaluation of the 2.5 mg dose of fondaparinux in registration studies.

The OASIS-5 study compared the efficacy of fondaparinux [2.5 mg once-daily] *versus* enoxaparin (1 mg/kg twice-daily) in patients with ACS (Yusuf et al., 2006a). In this large (*n* = 20,078) international study, patients were randomized and treated for 6–8 days. The primary endpoint of death, infarction, or ischemia was examined at day 9, without a significant difference noted between the groups. However, significant differences in mortality were noted at 30 days and at 180 days, favoring treatment with fondaparinux. Major bleeding was also markedly reduced by the use of fondaparinux (2.2% *vs* 4.1%; *P* < 0.001) and most of the excess deaths in the enoxaparin group occurred in patients who experienced bleeding.

With an interest in establishing the efficacy of fondaparinux in the treatment of ST-segment MI, fondaparinux was studied in another large (*n* = 12,092) randomized control trial (RCT) (Yusuf et al., 2006b). Patients were randomized to fondaparinux (2.5 mg once-daily) administered for an average of eight days or usual care, either UFH or no anticoagulation (placebo). The primary endpoint of this study, the composite of death or recurrent infarction at 30 days, was reduced by treatment with fondaparinux (9.7% *vs* 11.2%; $P = 0.008$). The benefit of therapy was durable through the study to final follow-up at 3–6 months, including a significant reduction in mortality. This large study allows for speculative examination of clinically meaningful subpopulations. Of note, there was no efficacy benefit among those patients undergoing primary therapy with PCI, whereas patients receiving thrombolytic therapy as well as those who received no reperfusion therapy derived a significant benefit from fondaparinux.

Prompted by the finding of a small but significant increase in the risk of catheter-related thrombotic complications among ACS patients randomized to receive fondaparinux in earlier ACS studies (Yusuf et al., 2006a,b), the OASIS-8 trial compared the safety of two doses of heparin during PCI in high-risk patients with non–ST-segment elevation ACS initially treated with fondaparinux (Steg et al., 2010). Catheter thrombosis rates were low with both doses of heparin but low-dose heparin did not reduce the risk of bleeding compared with standard doses, supporting the use of the standard dose at the time of PCI in ACS patients initially treated with fondaparinux.

Together, these studies have defined a striking activity and tolerability of fondaparinux in the cardiac patient. Fondaparinux is approved in many countries world wide (including Canada) for the management of patients with ACS but is not approved in the United States for this indication.

CLINICAL USE OF FONDAPARINUX IN THE TREATMENT OF HIT
Rationale
Fundamental to the development of HIT is the binding of (anionic) sulfated polysaccharides (UFH or LMWH) to (cationic) platelet factor 4 (PF4), resulting in an allosteric modulation of PF4 structure that presents neoantigens to the immune system. One motivation for the development of pentasaccharide anticoagulants was the inference that these comparatively small (~1700 Da) compounds might not associate significantly with PF4, potentially avoiding or minimizing risk of HIT (Petitou et al., 1999; see also chap. 7). However, there appear to be biologically relevant interactions between PF4 and fondaparinux, based on: (*i*) *in vitro* inhibition of HIT antibody-induced platelet activation at very high (supratherapeutic) concentrations of fondaparinux (Greinacher et al., 2006); (*ii*) sensitive studies of molecular interactions suggest PF4/fondaparinux binding occurs (Greinacher et al., 2006; discussed subsequently); (*iii*) formation of anti-PF4/heparin (anti-PF4/H) antibodies in patients treated with fondaparinux (Pouplard et al., 2005; Warkentin et al., 2005); (*iv*) rare cases implicating fondaparinux-dependent HIT antibodies that were triggered by preceding exposure to UFH (Warkentin and Lim, 2008); and (*v*) rare cases of HIT reported in patients who exclusively received fondaparinux for antithrombotic prophylaxis (discussed subsequently). At the same time, there is persuasive evidence that fondaparinux is an effective treatment for acute HIT (discussed subsequently). This points to an intriguing paradox: although fondaparinux is somewhat immunogenic and may rarely be associated with HIT, it can at the same time be an effective treatment for HIT (Warkentin, 2010; Greinacher, 2011). Indeed, a strong argument can be made supporting the use of fondaparinux as a frontline agent for the management of suspected or confirmed HIT (Warkentin, 2011).

An early hint to this fondaparinux paradox was the results of systematic studies of anti-PF4/H antibody formation in the orthopedic thromboprophylaxis trials that evaluated fondaparinux against the LMWH, enoxaparin. These studies showed that whereas both anticoagulants were associated with similar frequencies of anti-PF4/H antibody formation, only enoxaparin supported HIT antibody binding to PF4 (Warkentin et al., 2005). This dissociation between "immunogenicity" and "cross-reactivity" is illustrated in Figure 17.2, where both LMWH and fondaparinux are shown as equally sized icebergs (i.e., indicating similar immunogenicity), whereas LMWH exhibits much greater and more frequent cross-reactivity (shown as greater protrusion of the LMWH iceberg above the waterline); in comparison,

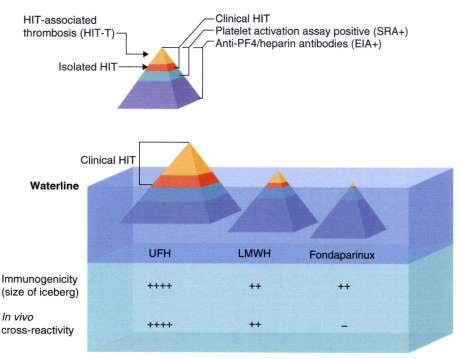

FIGURE 17.2 The relationship among the clinical expression of HIT (thrombocytopenia with or without thrombosis), the type of heparin used, and the antibodies that cause HIT. These concepts can be conceptualized as an "iceberg." The visible component of the iceberg (the portion above the waterline) represents clinically evident features of HIT, such as thrombocytopenia and/or thrombosis. The mass of the iceberg corresponds to the entire spectrum of anti-PF4/H antibodies generated. Some of these antibodies will be biologically active (platelet-activating), and other will be non–platelet-activating, which makes them unlikely to have clinical consequences. The type of heparin given to the patient determines the overall size of the iceberg, with UFH being the largest (most immunogenic) and LMWH and fondaparinux having lesser immunogenicity. Also illustrated in this figure is the *in vivo* cross-reactivity. UFH forms antigens which are readily recognized by HIT antibodies. By contrast, fondaparinux forms poorly recognized antigens, and LMWH is intermediate. *Abbreviations*: EIA: enzyme immunoassay; HIT, heparin-induced thrombocytopenia; HIT-T; HIT-associated thrombosis; LMWH, low molecular weight heparin; SRA, serotonin-release assay; UFH, unfractionated heparin. *Source*: From Kelton and Warkentin (2008).

UFH is both highly immunizing and highly cross-reactive, and so it is illustrated as the largest iceberg with the greatest degree of protrusion above the waterline (Kelton and Warkentin, 2008). All of these considerations support the differing frequencies of HIT with these three anticoagulants, as follows: UFH >> LMWH >> fondaparinux (see chap. 4).

Laboratory Cross-Reactivity Studies of Fondaparinux in HIT

Shortly after the identification of PF4/H as the major antigen in HIT (see chap. 6), various structural determinants for antigen formation were clarified by Greinacher and colleagues (1994, 1995; see chap. 7). Among these, increasing polysaccharide molecular weight and degree of sulfation increased the ability to form antigens with PF4 that were recognized by HIT antibodies. In addition, several studies described a lack of *in vitro* cross-reactivity when HIT antibodies were tested in the presence of fondaparinux. Elalamy et al. (1995) examined the ability of plasma (or purified IgG) from 25 patients with documented HIT to induce aggregation of platelets from healthy volunteers in the presence of UFH (100% of donor platelet samples aggregated), LMWH (76%), danaparoid (8%), or pentasaccharide (0%). Thus, platelet aggregation was induced in all samples in the presence of UFH but was not induced in the presence of fondaparinux.

These observations were confirmed shortly thereafter by another group in France using enzyme immunoassay (EIA) (Amiral et al., 1997). Plasmas from 49 patients with HIT (confirmed by platelet aggregometry) were compared with respect to their ability to induce the binding of antibodies to immobilized PF4 in the presence of increasing concentrations of fondaparinux or UFH. Although antibodies were fixed by a broad range of concentrations of UFH, no antibody binding was detected in the presence of fondaparinux.

A subsequent prospective study tested the cross-reactivity of fondaparinux with sera obtained from 39 patients with laboratory-confirmed HIT and 15 unaffected controls (Savi et al., 2005). Three functional (platelet activation) tests for cross-reactivity were performed by independent laboratories: the serotonin release assay (SRA), the heparin-induced platelet activation assay (both the aforementioned are washed platelet assays) and conventional platelet aggregometry (using platelet-rich plasma). Although cross-reactivity between HIT plasma and UFH was observed in 75 of 94 assays (79.8%), only three of 91 assays (3.3%) conducted in the presence of fondaparinux were reported as positive. The authors concluded that fondaparinux was essentially nonreactive with HIT sera.

Two subsequent studies investigated the potential for formation of PF4/fondaparinux complexes. Rauova et al. (2005) investigated the biophysical structure and polysaccharide determinants of ultra-large PF4 complexes (ULC). Using size exclusion high-performance liquid chromatography and electron microscopy, the authors observed that ULC formation was formed preferentially by UFH and less well by LMWH. By contrast, fondaparinux was incapable of forming ULC. However, using atomic force microscopy and photon correlation spectroscopy, Greinacher et al. (2006) provided evidence that fondaparinux can induce some formation of PF4 clusters, although this effect was much less marked than for UFH and LMWH.

These studies support the concept that fondaparinux usually exhibits no (or negligible) *in vitro* cross-reactivity with HIT antibodies, although the atomic force microscopy studies suggest that it might provoke an immune response against

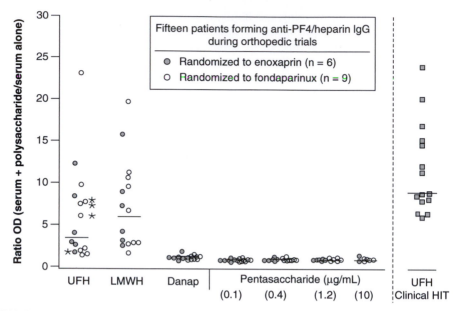

FIGURE 17.3 Ratio of antibody binding to PF4/polysaccharide complexes compared with PF4 alone by fluid-phase EIA. Results of fluid-phase EIA testing for sera from 15 patients who formed anti-PF4/H IgG antibodies (detected using solid-phase EIA) while receiving enoxaparin ($n = 6$, closed circles) or fondaparinux ($n = 9$, open circles). The data are expressed as ratios of binding to PF4 in the presence of polysaccharide (UFH, 0.6 IU/mL, LMWH 0.5 anti-Xa U/mL, danaparoid 0.1 anti-Xa U/mL, and fondaparinux, 0.1, 0.4, 1.2, and 10.0 µg/mL) over the baseline (buffer). Horizontal bars indicate medians. Asterisks indicate the four samples that tested positive (in the presence of UFH) in the platelet activation assay. For comparison, results are also shown for 15 patients with clinical HIT. Statistically significant increases in reactivity [null hypothesis, mean ratio of OD (presence of drug)/OD (presence of buffer) = 1] for the 15 sera obtained from patients in the orthopedic trials were observed for UFH ($P = 0.0032$), LMWH ($P = 0.0004$), danaparoid ($P = 0.0016$), but not with fondaparinux at any concentration ($P > 0.05$). Whereas 14 of 15 sera from patients in the orthopedic trials exhibited more than twofold greater reactivity than baseline against PF4/LMWH, none reacted similarly against PF4/fondaparinux ($P = 0.0002$ by McNemar's test, two tailed). *Abbreviations*: EIA, enzyme-linked immunoassay; HIT, heparin-induced thrombocytopenia; LMWH, low molecular weight heparin; UFH, unfractionated heparin. *Source*: From Warkentin et al. (2005).

PF4-dependent antigens. Indeed, in the four orthopedic thromboprophylaxis RCTs, anti-PF4/H antibodies were generated at similar frequencies in both the fondaparinux and enoxaparin study arms (Warkentin et al., 2005, 2010); although one patient [in the PENTHIFRA (hip fracture) study] who received fondaparinux developed HIT, this case was confounded by a 5000-U perioperative exposure to UFH, and the development of abrupt-onset HIT only occurred when fondaparinux was switched to LMWH for the treatment of DVT (Warkentin et al., 2010). Interestingly, the antibodies that were generated in these orthopedic surgery trials recognized PF4 in the presence of UFH and LMWH, but not in the presence of fondaparinux, even when the blood samples were obtained from patients who had formed antibodies while receiving fondaparinux (Fig. 17.3).

In a smaller study, Pouplard et al. (2005) also observed a low frequency of anti-PF4/H antibody formation among postorthopedic surgery patients undergoing fondaparinux thromboprophylaxis. One interpretation of these data is that anti-PF4/H antibodies formed in patients treated with fondaparinux likely would not cause clinical HIT even in the presence of fondaparinux, given the negligible degree of *in vitro* cross-reactivity. It should be further noted that neither of the above studies *proves* immunogenicity of fondaparinux, as a background frequency of "spontaneous" anti-PF4/H antibody formation (including development of clinical HIT) after orthopedic surgery has not been ruled out (Jay and Warkentin, 2008).

Clinical Cross-Reactivity Studies of Fondaparinux in HIT

A recent serologic substudy of the Matisse VTE trials provides direct evidence for a low risk of *in vivo* cross-reactivity of fondaparinux for HIT antibodies (Warkentin et al., 2011a). Baseline (prestudy) sera obtained from almost 4000 participants in these trials identified 14 patients whose blood harbored unrecognized platelet-activating HIT antibodies, that is, their sera tested positive in the platelet SRA. Four of these VTE patients received either UFH (PE trial) or LMWH (DVT trial), whereas the remaining 10 patients were randomized to the corresponding fondaparinux arms of the two Matisse trials, and accordingly received this novel study anticoagulant. Whereas all four UFH/LMWH-treated patients developed an abrupt >50% platelet count fall (indicating rapid-onset HIT), none of the 10 patients who received therapeutic-dose fondaparinux developed a similar platelet count fall (Fig. 17.4). This difference between UFH/LMWH and fondaparinux in risk of precipitating acute HIT was highly significant: 4/4 (100%) *versus* 0/10 (0%); $P < 0.001$. Although HIT was an exclusion criterion in the Matisse trials, in retrospect, it appears that three of the SRA-positive fondaparinux-treated patients likely had HIT at study entry (Fig. 17.4A–C); all three patients exhibited platelet count recovery, without developing new, progressive, or recurrent thrombosis.

Before evaluating the clinical experience using fondaparinux to treat HIT, we will examine an interesting question: does fondaparinux cause HIT?

Does Fondaparinux Cause HIT?

As of April 2012, there are six well-documented reports in the medical literature describing the HIT syndrome in patients receiving thromboprophylaxis with fondaparinux (Warkentin et al., 2007, 2012a; Rota et al., 2008; Salem et al., 2010; Burch and Cooper, 2012) (Table 17.3). In addition, Modi and coworkers (2009) reported an additional patient case consistent with fondaparinux-associated HIT but in which testing for HIT antibodies was not performed. Interestingly, two of the cases occurred in patients who were receiving fondaparinux because of a previous history of HIT (caused by LMWH or UFH) one to three years earlier (Rota et al., 2008; Modi et al., 2009). Other putative cases of fondaparinux-associated HIT (Ratuapli et al., 2010; Re and Legnani 2010) do not, in our opinion, likely represent "true" HIT.

All six cases listed in Table 17.3 occurred in the setting of antithrombotic prophylaxis (five surgical, one medical); four patients developed thrombotic events highly characteristic of HIT (e.g., adrenal hemorrhagic infarction, bilateral DVT, arterial thrombosis). The EIAs gave uniformly strong results [mean, ~3.00 optical density (OD) units]. For both patients who were studied in the SRA, strong heparin-*in*dependent platelet activation was observed, with only a small degree

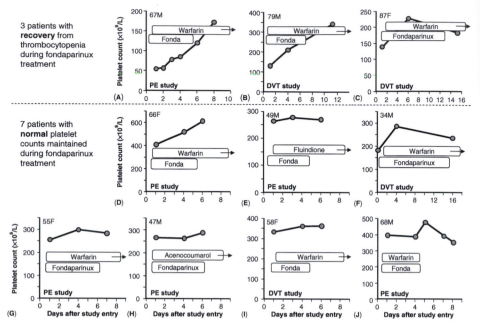

FIGURE 17.4 Ten patients with heparin-dependent, platelet-activating antibodies who were treated with fondaparinux. The boxes indicate start and stop dates for anticoagulant therapy (in relation to the day of study), except where arrows indicate continuation of anticoagulant beyond the period indicated. (A–C) Patients were thrombocytopenic at study entry and, thus, likely had unrecognized HIT. (D–J) Patients had normal platelet counts at study entry. None of the 10 patients developed thrombocytopenia (≥50% platelet count fall) during treatment with fondaparinux, and the three patients with thrombocytopenia at study entry developed platelet count recovery. *Abbreviations*: DVT, deep vein thrombosis; F, female; Fonda, fondaparinux; M, male; PE, pulmonary embolism. *Source*: From Warkentin et al. (2011a).

of fondaparinux-dependent platelet activation (Fig. 17.5). Taken together, these data raise the possibility that fondaparinux is a rare cause of the HIT syndrome; however, a definitive conclusion cannot be reached because—as pointed out by Salem and coworkers (2010)—HIT has also been reported in postorthopedic surgery patients exclusively prophylaxed with warfarin (see chap. 2) and thus epidemiologic studies would be required to determine whether fondaparinux is associated with a frequency of HIT greater than the "background" rate observed with warfarin. Intriguingly, given the minor degree of fondaparinux-dependent platelet activation induced by these unusual patient sera, it seems plausible that fondaparinux might even be an effective treatment of fondaparinux-associated HIT, that is, by increasing fondaparinux dosing from prophylactic to therapeutic, control of HIT-associated hypercoagulability could be achieved.

Treatment of Acute HIT with Fondaparinux
First Experience
The first published cases of fondaparinux use in patients with putative HIT were from Brazil and Spain. D'Amico et al. (2003) reported a patient with paroxysmal

TABLE 17.3   Reported Patients with Fondaparinux-Associated HIT

Reference	Age/Sex	Clinical setting	Platelet count nadir ($\times 10^9$/L)	Complications	Tests for HIT antibodies
Warkentin et al., 2007	48F	Bil TKR	39	Adr; DVT; DIC; nRBCs	EIA = 1.871; SRA = 90%–96%–0%
Rota et al., 2008	74F	THR[a]	50	Nil	EIA = 3.999; SRA ND
Salem et al., 2010	67M	TKR	35	Bil DVT; arterial stroke	EIA = 2.803; SRA ND
Burch and Cooper, 2012	47M	TKR	99; 50[b]	Bil Adr; DVT; PE	EIA = 2.807; SRA ND
Burch and Cooper, 2012	63M	TKR	240; 38[c]	Iliac artery thrombosis[d]	EIA = 3.081; SRA ND
Warkentin et al., 2012a	74F	ICU medical	51	Nil	EIA = 3.000; SRA = 90%–90%–0%

When two platelet count nadirs are shown, the first represents the lowest platelet count after receiving fondaparinux, but before receiving UFH or LMWH; the second nadir represents the lowest platelet count after receiving either UFH or LMWH (after HIT was already present). For the EIAs, results are expressed in OD units. For the SRA, the three test results shown sequentially are (**A**) percent serotonin release in the absence of heparin (buffer control); (**B**) peak percent serotonin release at 0.1–0.3 U/mL heparin; and (**C**) percent serotonin release at 100 U/mL heparin. The table excludes a patient case strongly suggestive of fondaparinux-associated HIT (Modi et al., 2009) but where tests for HIT antibodies were not performed.
[a]This patient had a history of HIT associated with nadroparin three years earlier.
[b]The platelet count abruptly fell to 50×10^9/L after starting UFH.
[c]The platelet count abruptly fell to 38×10^9/L after starting the LMWH, enoxaparin.
[d]The patient underwent urgent thromboembolectomy (with initial UFH anticoagulation, switched intraoperatively from UFH to argatroban), with successful limb salvage (personal communication from M. Burch).
Abbreviations: Adr, adrenal hemorrhagic necrosis (secondary to presumed adrenal vein thrombosis); Bil, bilateral; DIC, disseminated intravascular coagulation; DVT, deep vein thrombosis; EIA, enzyme immunoassay; F, female; Fonda, fondaparinux; HIT, heparin-induced thrombocytopenia; ICU, intensive care unit; LMWH, low molecular weight heparin; M, male; ND, not done; nRBCs, nucleated red blood cells (circulating normoblasts); OD, optical density; PE, pulmonary embolism; SRA, serotonin release assay; THR, total hip replacement; TKR, total knee replacement; UFH, unfractionated heparin.

nocturnal hemoglobinuria and Budd–Chiari syndrome who developed thrombo-cytopenia following administration of LMWH (dalteparin 5000 IU sc every 12 hours). The patient experienced spontaneous platelet count recovery, and received thrombolytic therapy. While receiving prophylactic doses of fondaparinux, the platelet count remained unchanged and the patient was transitioned uneventfully to oral anticoagulant therapy. Parody and coworkers (2003) reported a patient with lupus-associated thrombotic microangiopathy who developed apparent HIT as a consequence of receiving UFH for plasmapheresis. In neither case was a specific test for HIT antibodies performed. This experience highlights two issues: first, strong serologic support for "true" HIT in some of the reports is lacking (Warkentin, 2010), and second, the use of fondaparinux in medical settings with limited access to (expensive) DTIs. Subsequently, more than a dozen case reports describing fondaparinux to treat acute HIT have been published, with a high proportion

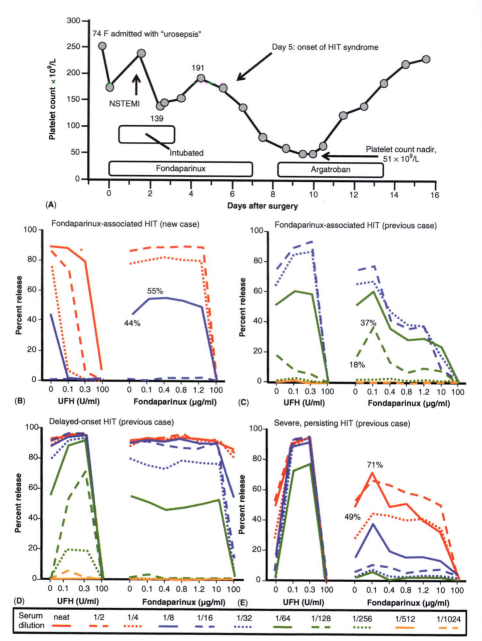

FIGURE 17.5   Serologic profile of fondaparinux-associated HIT (Patient No. 6 in Table 17.3). (**A**) Summary of clinical course of patient with fondaparinux-associated HIT syndrome. (**B–E**) Percent serotonin release is plotted against various concentrations of heparin (0.1, 0.3, 100 U/mL), fondaparinux (0.1, 0.4, 0.8, 1.2, 10, and 100 μg/mL), or buffer control. Results are shown using neat (undiluted) serum as well as serum diluted up to 1/1024 (represented by solid or dashed or dotted lines of different colors—see legend at bottom of figure). For the three patients with evidence of fondaparinux-dependent platelet activation (shown in panels B, C, and E), the actual percent serotonin release results are indicated in the graph. (*Continued*)

FIGURE 17.5 (*Continued*) **(B)** Platelet activation profile of the patient with fondaparinux-associated HIT shown in panel A. The asterisk (*) beside the solid red line indicates the results of the initial SRA performed using neat serum. Subsequent studies were performed using 1/2 to 1/16 serum dilutions. **(C)** Serologic profile of a previously reported case of fondaparinux-associated HIT (Warkentin et al., 2007). **(D)** Serologic profile of patient with delayed-onset HIT. **(E)** Serologic profile of patient with persisting HIT. *Abbreviations*: F, female; HIT, heparin-induced thrombocytopenia; NSTEMI, non–ST-segment elevation myocardial infarction. *Source*: From Warkentin et al. (2012a).

showing successful outcomes (for review: Warkentin, 2010). However, unsuccessful outcomes have also been reported (Jankowski et al., 2007; Miranda et al., 2012). Fondaparinux has also been used successfully to anticoagulate patients with suspected HIT who required hemodialysis (Haase et al., 2005; Montagnac et al., 2010; Wellborn-Kim et al., 2010).

Case Series

There are six case series (minimum, five patients per report) that in total describe 65 patients with HIT who were treated with fondaparinux (Table 17.4). It seems likely that most of these patients were "true" HIT cases, based on the reported serologic findings (particularly, the positive SRA results in the two Canadian studies) and the high overall frequency of HIT-associated thrombosis (65%). Most of the patients received therapeutic doses of fondaparinux (i.e., 7.5 mg daily for a patient weighing between 50 and 100 kg), although we adjusted fondaparinux dosing in some renally compromised patients based on anti-factor Xa levels (Warkentin et al., 2011b).

Remarkably, none of the 65 patients developed new, progressive, or recurrent thrombosis after initiation of fondaparinux (upper 95% CI, 5.5%). Moreover, the frequencies of major bleeding (3%) and limb amputation (5%) were relatively low. The authors of these six reports concluded that fondaparinux appeared to be an effective treatment of HIT.

Table 17.4 excludes a case series that reported on 11 critically ill post-cardiac surgery patients (Pappalardo et al., 2010), as in our view the low frequency of apparent HIT-associated thrombosis and the clinical setting suggests that most patients likely did not have HIT. None of the 11 patients developed thrombosis after starting fondaparinux, however, so the study is not inconsistent with fondaparinux being efficacious for HIT. Three (27%) of the patients, however, developed major bleeding.

Table 17.4 also excludes data from 38 EIA+ patients with possible HIT from the Massachusetts General Hospital reported in the previous edition of this book (Bradner and Eikelboom, 2007), since the low frequency of HIT-associated thrombosis suggested that most patients did not have true HIT. Moreover, 17 of the patients received a DTI during the acute phase of HIT, with subsequent transition to fondaparinux. Nevertheless, the Boston investigators noted that none of the 38 patients developed evidence of *in vivo* cross-reactivity with fondaparinux (i.e., platelet count recovery occurred in all), and they further remarked that "there was a low incidence of thromboses in the treated cohorts (2/38).

Table 17.4 also excludes a series of 20 patients (17 with thrombosis) reported in abstract form (Piovella et al., 2006); however, no patient developed thrombosis or required amputation, and only one (postsurgical) patient developed major bleeding. Persistent thrombocytopenia in one patient triggered switch to lepirudin, with eventual platelet recovery. Interestingly, serial EIAs in the seven patients so tested showed progressive declines in OD levels to near-normal while receiving therapeutic-dose fondaparinux for HIT-associated thrombosis.

TABLE 17.4 Case Series of Fondaparinux for Treatment of Acute HIT

Study	N	N with HIT-T[a]	Platelet count nadir, $\times 10^9$/L (mean)	Serology	Thrombosis rate[b]	Amputation rate[b]	Major bleeding[b]
Kuo and Kovacs, 2005	5	5 (100%)	43	EIA >1.0 SRA ND	0 (0%)	0 (0%)	0 (0%)
Lobo et al., 2008	7	6 (86%)	66	EIA 0.7 (median) SRA ND	0 (0%)	1 (14%)[c]	0 (0%)
Grouzi et al., 2010	24	14 (58%)	66[d]	EIA 1.4 (mean)[e] SRA ND	0 (0%)	1 (4%)[f]	0 (0%)
Al-Rossaies et al., 2011	5	2 (40%)	89	EIA >0.4 SRA ND	0 (0%)	0 (0%)	1 (5%)
Goldfarb and Blostein, 2011	8	6 (75%)	56	EIA >1.0 SRA+ 4/4[g]	0 (0%)	0 (0%)	0 (0%)
Warkentin et al., 2011b	16	9 (56%)	79	EIA 2.5 (mean) SRA+ (all 16)	0 (0%)	1 (6%)[h]	1 (6%)
Pooled data	65	42 (65%)	68	EIA+ 63/65[i]	0 (0%)	3 (5%)	2 (3%)

Most patients listed in the Table received 7.5 mg daily by sc injection (10.0 mg if >100 kg and 5.0 mg if <50 kg body weight, respectively), although a few received lower or higher doses, and in some patients doses were adjusted based on anti-factor Xa levels.

[a]HIT-T defined here as thrombosis that was present before beginning fondaparinux therapy; in most cases, the thrombosis occurred as a result of HIT.

[b]Indicates thrombosis and amputation that occurred within 30 days after starting fondaparinux, and bleeding that occurred while receiving fondaparinux.

[c]One patient with popliteal artery thrombosis and failed thrombectomy required amputation; however, the ischemic limb necrosis was judged to have been present before fondaparinux treatment.

[d]The mean platelet count nadir excludes two patients with myeloproliferative disease who had baseline thrombocytosis.

[e]The mean OD was significantly greater (2.0 units) in the subset of 14 patients with HIT-associated thrombosis.

[f]One patient had limb amputation before commencing fondaparinux.

[g]The SRA was strongly positive in four patients, and was not performed in the remaining four EIA+ patients because their EIAs were strongly positive (>2.00 OD units) and the patients had a high pretest probability score for HIT.

[h]One patient with upper-limb amputation due to brachial artery thrombosis was judged to have ischemic limb necrosis established before initiation of fondaparinux.

[i]The SRA was positive in one of the two EIA-negative patients.

Abbreviations: EIA, enzyme immunoassay; ND, not done; OD, optical density; SRA, serotonin release assay; +, positive.

Adjunct Therapy for HIT (e.g., "Bridging" to Warfarin)

Some authors have reported the use of a DTI for initial management of acute HIT, but then transitioning to fondaparinux following platelet count recovery. In some cases, fondaparinux was used for longer-term anticoagulation (e.g., because warfarin was contraindicated) (Patterson et al., 2006; Ekbatani et al., 2010), or "as a bridge to warfarin from a DTI," as reported by Baroletti and coworkers (2009) in eight patients. Experience was generally favorable, except for one patient who developed propogation of DVT during bridging to warfarin (Baroletti et al., 2009).

Fondaparinux Use in Patients with Previous HIT

Two reports describe a total of 25 patients who received fondaparinux—either for prophylactic or therapeutic indications—in which there was a history of "previous HIT" (Harenberg et al., 2004; Baroletti et al., 2009); only the six patients reported by Harenberg had well-documented previous HIT (positive platelet activation test). None of the 25 patients developed recurrent HIT as a result of administering fondaparinux, and only one of the 25 patients developed a thrombotic event (which occurred four days after stopping fondaparinux) (Baroletti et al., 2009). By contrast, two cases of putative fondaparinux-associated HIT occurred in patients who were receiving fondaparinux for thromboprophylaxis because of a previous history of LMWH-associated HIT three years earlier (Rota et al., 2008) and UFH-associated HIT one year earlier (Modi et al., 2009). Recently, the American College of Chest Physicians (ACCP) Evidence-based Clinical Practice Guidelines recommended fondaparinux in full therapeutic doses (pending transition to vitamin K antagonist) for a patient with a previous history of HIT who has acute thrombosis (not related to HIT) and who has normal renal function (Linkins et al., 2012).

Can Fondaparinux be Recommended for Treatment of Acute HIT?

The recent ACCP Clinical Practice Guidelines specifically recommended argatroban, lepirudin, or danaparoid over fondaparinux for the treatment of acute HIT, noting that further studies evaluating the role of fondaparinux and the new oral anticoagulants in the treatment of HIT are needed (Linkins et al., 2012). However, we believe that fondaparinux can already be regarded as a first-tier agent for treatment of HIT, particularly in a noncritically ill patient with "isolated" HIT or with HIT-associated VTE. Our recommendation is based on: (*i*) theoretical factors (low risk for *in vitro*/*in vivo* cross-reactivity or for triggering further immunization; (*ii*) favorable clinical experience—including patients with well-documented HIT (Table 17.4); (*iii*) its ease of use (including for both prophylactic- and therapeutic-dose settings) and infrequent requirement for monitoring; and (*iv*) comparatively low cost. Moreover, (*v*) fondaparinux has been shown to be safe and effective in a wide range of therapeutic and prophylactic clinical settings; since HIT is confirmed in only approximately 10% of patients who undergo laboratory investigations triggered by clinical suspicion, in most cases, the clinician will be treating a patient who (ultimately) is shown *not* to have HIT. In this regard, the different dosing options are advantageous: if the patient is strongly suspected (or confirmed) to have HIT, or has thrombosis, then therapeutic-dose fondaparinux is appropriate; in contrast, if the physician has only a low or intermediate suspicion for HIT, then low-dose fondaparinux is a reasonable option. Among the three anticoagulants recommended for treatment of acute HIT by the ACCP, only danaparoid has a similar profile of well-established prophylactic- and therapeutic-dosing regimes. Regarding the lower cost of fondaparinux—this includes not only the actual drug cost (<10% that of the approved DTIs or danaparoid), but also the prospect of avoiding one week of hospitalization (for DTI–warfarin overlap) because patients can be discharged to home on once-daily sc fondaparinux.

Table 17.5 describes the dosing and monitoring that we have used for fondaparinux treatment of acute HIT.

TABLE 17.5   Fondaparinux Dosing for Treatment of Acute HIT

A. Therapeutic-dose regimen for treatment of acute HIT, including HIT-T
First dose (afternoon[a]): 7.5 mg (or 10 mg[b]) by sc injection[c] for patient weighing 50–100 kg[d]
Second and subsequent doses (morning[e]): 7.5 mg by sc injection
Dosing adjustments for renal failure:
Do not reduce first dose or two; subsequently, reduce daily dose to 5 or 2.5 mg, depending on the
   extent of renal dysfunction, and results of anti-factor Xa levels (if available)
Monitoring of drug levels and efficacy
Anti-factor Xa monitoring (if available), especially if renal dysfunction is present[f]
Baseline and serial markers of hemostasis[g]: PT/INR, PTT, fibrinogen, fibrin D-dimer, fibrin
   monomer (or protamine sulfate paracoagulation test), LD
B. Prophylactic-dose regimen for fondaparinux[h]
2.5 mg by sc injection[i]

[a]HIT is often diagnosed by platelet count monitoring, and thus treatment is frequently started in the afternoon or evening.
[b]Ten milligrams, rather than 7.5 mg, may be appropriate even for a 50–100 kg patient if HIT is judged very severe (e.g., with overt DIC), or if the initial dose is given in the morning and therefore a 20–24 hr interval before the next (morning) dose is anticipated.
[c]Intravenous (iv) injection can be considered if immediate anticoagulation is desired. If given iv, flush the line afterwards, or administer the fondaparinux in 25–50 mL normal saline over 3–5 min.
[d]Five milligrams if body weight <50 kg and 10 mg if body weight >100 kg.
[e]The rationale for administering 2nd and subsequent doses in the morning (~0800 hr)—even if the first dose was given in the preceding afternoon or evening—is that it will help to achieve early therapeutic levels of anticoagulation (since there will usually be <20 hr interval between the first two doses); in addition, it will facilitate determining plasma anticoagulant levels (trough) by the morning blood draw (~0600 hr), using anti-factor Xa levels, if desired.
[f]A target drug (trough) level of 0.6–1.0 anti-factor Xa U/mL is currently being used by the Author.
[g]The Author frequently follows serial markers of hemostasis activation, especially in patients with severe HIT-associated DIC, where effective anticoagulation should result in increase in fibrinogen levels, and decrease in fibrin D-dimer, fibrin monomer levels, and LD levels (marker of intravascular hemolysis).
[h]Low-dose (prophylactic-dose) fondaparinux regimen may be appropriate if: (*i*) patient has low (or intermediate) probability for acute HIT and (*ii*) no thrombosis; or (*iii*) for various other typical settings of prophylactic-dose anticoagulation, e.g., patient with history of previous HIT who requires postoperative prophylaxis.
[i]Assumes normal renal function.
Abbreviations: DIC, disseminated intravascular coagulation; LD, lactate dehydrogenase; PT/INR, prothrombin time/international normalized ratio; PTT, (activated) partial thromboplastin time; sc, subcutaneous.
Source: From Warkentin (2010).

OTHER FACTOR Xa INHIBITORS
History
Historical antecedents for the development of direct factor Xa inhibitors and the rationale for targeting factor Xa are discussed above. The success of fondaparinux has fueled the development of a large number of new oral and parenteral factor Xa inhibitors that are currently in various stages of clinical development or have been approved for use (Table 17.6). Because the greatest clinical need for new anticoagulants is for a replacement for warfarin, the major focus of drug development has been on *oral* direct factor Xa inhibitors (Hirsh et al., 2007).

Pharmacology
Direct factor Xa inhibitors bind to the active site of factor Xa and block the interaction of factor Xa with its substrates (Hirsh et al., 2007). Unlike indirect factor Xa inhibitors, which are catalytic and result in AT-mediated irreversible inhibition of free factor Xa, the direct factor Xa inhibitors are reversible, and not only inhibit free

TABLE 17.6 Established and Emerging Parenteral and Oral Factor Xa Inhibitors

Agent	Company	Phase	Therapeutic applications evaluated to date
Oral			
Apixaban	BMS	Phase III/approved	ACS, AF, VTE prevention (medical, orthopedic surgery), VTE treatment
Edoxaban	Daiichi Sankyo	Phase III/approved[a]	AF, VTE prevention (orthopedic surgery), VTE treatment
Rivaroxaban	Bayer	Phase III/approved	ACS, AF, DVT treatment, PE treatment, VTE prevention (medical, orthopedic surgery)
Parenteral			
Fondaparinux	GSK	Phase III/approved	ACS, DVT treatment, PE treatment, VTE prevention (general surgery, medical, orthopedic surgery)
Idraparinux	Sanofi	Phase III[b]	AF, DVT treatment, PE treatment
Idrabiotaparinux	Sanofi	Phase III[b]	PE treatment
Otamixaban	Sanofi	Phase III	ACS

[a]Approved only in Japan.
[b]No longer in development.
Abbreviations: ACS, acute coronary syndrome; AF, atrial fibrillation; DVT, deep vein thrombosis; PE, pulmonary embolism; VTE, venous thromboembolism.

factor Xa, but also inactivate factor Xa bound to platelets within the prothrombinase complex (Table 17.7). This represents an important theoretical advantage of direct factor Xa inhibitors over the indirect inhibitors, because prothrombinase-bound factor Xa that is not inhibited can continue to generate thrombin and thereby promote thrombus formation. Because of the pharmacologic differences between direct and indirect factor Xa inhibitors, it cannot be assumed that direct factor Xa inhibitors will achieve the same success as indirect factor Xa inhibitors, such as fondaparinux.

Direct Factor Xa Inhibitors in Clinical Development or Approved for Use
Factor Xa inhibitors currently being evaluated in RCTs and those approved for use are listed in Table 17.6.

Oral Direct Factor Xa Inhibitors
Apixaban
Apixaban is a selective competitive active direct factor Xa inhibitor with a bioavailability of 60% (Raghavan et al., 2009). Maximum drug levels occur 3 hours after oral intake in healthy men, the drug is highly protein bound and the half life is 8–14 hours. Apixaban is cleared via multiple pathways; about 25% is cleared via the kidneys and the remainder undergoes oxidative metabolism and is cleared via the feces. Apixaban is partly metabolized via CYP3A4. Consequently, drugs that strongly inhibit CYP3A4 (e.g., ketoconazole, clarithromycin) elevate drug levels and are contraindicated in patients treated with apixaban. Apixaban is given twice-daily and causes dose-dependent prolongation of the PTT (although prolongation is minimal at therapeutic concentrations). Because of its high protein binding, apixaban is not expected to be cleared by hemodialysis. Apixaban does not have a specific antidote.

TABLE 17.7   Comparison of Indirect and Direct Factor Xa Inhibitors

Characteristic	Indirect	Direct
Inhibitory mechanism	AT dependent Catalytic	AT independent Stoichiometric
Binding	Irreversible (i.e., covalent AT-Xa complexes are formed)	Reversible
Drug target	Free Xa	Free and tissue-bound Xa

Abbreviation: AT, antithrombin.

Apixaban has been extensively evaluated in phase III RCTs for the prevention of VTE in medical patients and in those undergoing major orthopedic surgery, stroke prevention in patients with atrial fibrillation (AF), and the management of patients who have been stabilized after presenting with ACS (Weitz et al., 2012). Trials evaluating apixaban for the treatment of VTE are ongoing. Apixaban is being considered by regulatory authorities for the prevention of VTE after hip and knee surgery and for stroke prevention in AF. At the time of writing, it has been approved in Europe for the prevention of VTE after hip and knee surgery.

Edoxaban

Edoxaban is a selective competitive direct factor Xa inhibitor with a bioavailability of 50–60% (Ogata et al., 2010). Maximum plasma levels are achieved 1–2 hours after oral ingestion and the drug half-life is 9–11 hours. One-third of the drug is cleared via the kidneys and the remainder is eliminated via the feces. Edoxaban is approximately 50% protein bound, raising the possibility that it can be at least partially removed with hemodialysis. Like other oral direct factor Xa inhibitors, edoxaban lacks an antidote. It is being given once-daily in RCTs.

Edoxaban has been evaluated for the prevention of VTE in phase III RCTs in patients undergoing hip and knee arthroplasty and in patients undergoing hip fracture surgery and is approved for these indications in Japan (Weitz et al., 2012). Edoxaban is currently being evaluated in phase III trials for the treatment of VTE and for stroke prevention in patients with AF. It has not been approved in North America or Europe.

Rivaroxaban

Rivaroxaban is another selective competitive direct factor Xa inhibitor and has a bioavailability of 80% (Perzborn et al., 2011). Maximum plasma drug levels occur 2–3 hours after oral administration, and the half-life is 7–11 hours. One-third is cleared as unchanged drug via the kidneys, one-third is metabolized by the liver (in part via CYP3A4), and excreted in the feces and one-third is metabolized to inactive metabolites that are excreted in the feces. Drugs that inhibit both CYP3A4 and P-glycoprotein (e.g., ketoconazole, ritinovir) increase drug levels and are contraindicated in patients treated with rivaroxaban. Rivaroxaban is given once-daily or twice-daily. It causes dose-dependent prolongation of the PT and PTT (Kubitza and Haas, 2006), but the effect of rivaroxaban on these tests is short-lived, with prolongation only seen at peak drug levels. Rivaroxaban is not expected to be cleared by hemodialysis because it is highly protein bound. Rivaroxaban does not have an antidote.

Rivaroxaban has been extensively evaluated in phase III RCTs for the prevention of VTE in medical patients and in those undergoing major orthopedic surgery, the treatment of DVT and PE, stroke prevention in patients with AF, and the management of patients who have been stabilized after presenting with ACS (Weitz et al., 2012). It has been approved in the United States, Canada, and Europe for the prevention of VTE after hip or knee surgery and stroke prevention in AF, and in some countries for the treatment of VTE. It is also under consideration for use in the treatment of patients with ACS.

Parenteral Factor Xa Inhibitors
Idraparinux and Idrabiotaparinux
Idraparinux is a hypermethylated derivative of fondaparinux that inhibits factor Xa in an AT-dependent manner (Herbert et al., 1998). Idraparinux binds so tightly to AT that its plasma half-life is similar to that of AT (~80 hr), which enables it to be given by once-weekly sc injection. Idraparinux has been evaluated in phase III trials for the treatment of VTE and for stroke prevention in patients with AF but its development was halted because of an excess of bleeding, including intracranial bleeding.

Idrabiotaparinux is a biotinylated form of idraparinux that has the same pharmacokinetic and pharmacodynamic properties. The presence of biotin enables reversal of the anticoagulant effect of idrabiotaparinux with an iv infusion of avidin. Idrabiotaparinux has been evaluated for the treatment of PE and for stroke prevention in patients with AF but has not been approved for clinical use (Weitz et al., 2012).

Otamixaban
Otamixaban is a parenteral direct factor Xa inhibitor with a short half-life that is less than 25% renally cleared (Hinder et al., 2006). Otamixaban is currently being evaluated as an alternative to heparin for the management of patients presenting with ACS. It is not approved for clinical use.

Role of Factor Xa Inhibitors in the Treatment of HIT
Orally active direct factor Xa inhibitors have not been evaluated for the treatment of patients with suspected or proven HIT but are attractive for this indication because they do not interact with PF4 or cross-react with anti-PF4/H antibodies (Walenga et al., 2008; Krauel et al., 2012). Oral direct factor Xa inhibitors are also not expected to cause a syndrome analogous to coumarin-induced microthrombosis (for which HIT is a risk factor) and are therefore potentially suitable for use during the acute or subacute phase of HIT.

ORAL DIRECT THROMBIN (FACTOR IIA) INHIBITORS
History
DTIs were developed to overcome the limitations of the heparin/AT complex to inactivate tissue-bound thrombin (Weitz and Buller, 2002). The prototype DTI is hirudin, a naturally occurring 65-amino acid polypeptide first isolated from the salivary gland of medicinal leeches but now manufactured using recombinant DNA technology. Argatroban and lepirudin are approved for the treatment of HIT (see chaps. 13 and 14); argatroban is also approved for use in patients with or at risk of HIT undergoing PCI (see chap. 13), and bivalirudin is licensed as an alternative to heparin in patients with or without HIT undergoing PCI (see chap. 15). Although

widely used for the treatment of suspected or proven HIT in the United States, where danaparoid is not available, parenteral DTIs have important limitations. Lepirudin and argatroban are "niche" agents that did not gain wide approvals for non-HIT indications, require frequent coagulation monitoring, cause serious bleeding and are expensive and inconvenient because of the need for continuous iv infusion (Warkentin, 2011, 2012). Furthermore, the parenteral DTIs do not address the unmet need for an oral anticoagulant to replace warfarin for the treatment of HIT. Several oral DTIs have been developed; ximelagatran was the first orally available DTI but was withdrawn because of hepatotoxicity. Dabigatran etexilate has completed evaluation in phase III RCTs and is approved for several indications world wide.

Pharmacology

Thrombin bound to fibrin or fibrin degradation products is protected from being inhibited by AT-heparin but is susceptible to inactivation by DTIs (Weitz and Buller, 2002). Thus, DTIs block both free and fibrin-bound thrombin, which is an important theoretical advantage over heparin because fibrin-bound thrombin can continue to promote thrombus formation. Because DTIs do not bind nonspecifically plasma proteins and cells, they also produce a more predictable anticoagulant response than heparin (Weitz and Buller, 2002).

Oral DTIs in Clinical Development

Ximelagatran

Ximelagatran is a prodrug of melagatran, a dipeptide mimetic of the portion of fibrinopeptide A that interacts with the active site of thrombin and blocks the enzyme's interaction with its substrate (Linkins and Weitz, 2005). After oral ingestion, ximelagatran undergoes rapid biotransformation to melagatran. Melagatran is eliminated via the kidneys and has a half-life in the plasma of 4–5 hours. It has no known interactions with food, drugs, or alcohol and is administered twice-daily.

Ximelagatran has been evaluated in phase III RCTs for the prevention and treatment of VTE, for the prevention of stroke or systemic embolism in patients with AF, and for the management of patients who have been stabilized after presenting with ACS. Despite favorable efficacy and bleeding results, ximelagatran was not approved for use in North America because 5–10% of patients developed abnormal liver function tests, typically between six weeks and 6 months of treatment, and several deaths possibly related to hepatotoxicity occurred. The drug was initially approved but subsequently withdrawn from other markets (Bauer, 2006).

Dabigatran Etexilate

Dabigatran etexilate is a prodrug of dabigatran, a specific, competitive, and reversible inhibitor of thrombin with a bioavailability of 5–7% (Stangier, 2008). For an account of dabigatran development, see Hauel and coworkers (2002). The drug is rapidly absorbed after oral administration and is converted to the active moiety, dabigatran, by esterases in the blood and liver. The plasma half-life is 12–17 hours. Dabigatran is 80% renally cleared. Because it is only one-third protein bound, dabigatran can be substantially cleared by hemodialysis (Warkentin et al., 2012b), but it lacks a specific antidote.

On the basis of positive results in phase III RCTs, dabigatran has been approved in many countries worldwide for the prevention of VTE in patients undergoing major orthopedic surgery and for prevention of stroke and systemic embolism in patients with AF (Ageno et al., 2012). Dabigatran has also been evaluated for the treatment of VTE but has not yet been approved for this indication.

Role of Oral DTIs in the Treatment of HIT

Oral DTIs have not been evaluated for the treatment of patients with suspected or proven HIT, but may have several important advantages over parenteral DTIs for this indication. (Although dabigatran was used in a patient who had anti-PF4/H antibodies, clinical HIT was not diagnosed; Fieland and Taylor, 2012). Unlike parenteral DTIs, orally administered dabigatran etexilate is approved worldwide as an alternative to warfarin, does not require routine coagulation monitoring, and is easy to use. The availability of dabigatran etexilate as an alternative to warfarin may reduce the potential for HIT-associated microthrombosis, as has been reported during warfarin administration during the acute or subacute phase of HIT (see chaps. 2 and 12).

SUMMARY

New anticoagulants that selectively target factor Xa or thrombin have begun replacing heparin and warfarin for several indications. As a consequence of this evolution in anticoagulant practice, the use of UFH is likely to decline, resulting in a reduction in the incidence of HIT, and there is likely to be an expansion of the treatment options for HIT. Fondaparinux has an extensive track record as a highly effective and safe parenteral anticoagulant, and is replacing UFH and LMWH across a broad spectrum of clinical indications. Fondaparinux only rarely cross-reacts with anti-PF4/H antibodies and there are persuasive observational data supporting its effectiveness and safety for the treatment of HIT. New oral factor Xa inhibitors and oral DTIs are theoretically attractive for the treatment of HIT, but further evaluation is needed for all of these agents.

REFERENCES

Ageno W, Gallus AS, Wittkowsky A, Crowther M, Hylek EM, Palareti G. Oral anticoagulant therapy: antithrombotic therapy and prevention of thrombosis, 9th ed: American College of Chest Physicians Evidence-Based Clinical Practice guidelines. Chest 141(Suppl): e44S–e88S, 2012.

Agnelli G, Bergqvist D, Cohen AT, Gallus AS, Gent M. Randomized clinical trial of postoperative fondaparinux versus perioperative dalteparin for prevention of venous thromboembolism in high-risk abdominal surgery. Br J Surg 92: 1212–1220, 2005.

Al-Rossaies A, Alkharfy KM, Al-Ayoubi F, Al-Momen A. Heparin-induced thrombocytopenia: comparison between response to fondaparinux and lepirudin. Int J Clin Pharm 33: 997–1001, 2011.

Amar J, Caranobe C, Sie P, Boneu B. Antithrombotic potencies of heparins in relation to their antifactor Xa and antithrombin activities: an experimental study in two models of thrombosis in the rabbit. Br J Haematol 76: 94–100, 1990.

Amiral J, Lormeau JC, Marfaing-Koka A, Vissac AM, Wolf M, Boyer-Neumann C, Tardy B, Herbert JM, Meyer D. Absence of cross-reactivity of SR90107A/ORG31540 pentasaccharide with antibodies to heparin-PF4 complexes developed in heparin-induced thrombocytopenia. Blood Coagul Fibrinolysis 8: 114–117, 1997.

Ansell J. Factor Xa or thrombin: is factor Xa a better target? J Thromb Haemost 5(Suppl 1): 60–64, 2007.

Arixtra Package Insert, Philadelphia, Pennsylvania. GlaxoSmithKline, 2006.

Arocas V, Bock SC, Raja S, Olson ST, Bjork I. Lysine 114 of antithrombin is of crucial importance for the affinity and kinetics of heparin pentasaccharide binding. J Biol Chem 276: 43809–43817, 2001.

Baroletti S, Labreche M, Niles M, Fanikos J, Goldhaber SZ. Prescription of fondaparinux in hospitalised patients. Thromb Haemost 101: 1091–1094, 2009.

Bauer KA. New anticoagulants. Hematology Am Soc Hematol Educ Program: 450–456, 2006.

Bauer KA, Eriksson BI, Lassen MR, Turpie AGG. Fondaparinux compared with enoxaparin for the prevention of venous thromboembolism after elective major knee surgery. N Engl J Med 345: 1305–1310, 2001.

Bernat A, Herbert JM. Protamine sulphate inhibits pentasaccharide (SR80027)-induced bleeding without affecting its antithrombotic and anti-factor Xa activity in the rat. Haemostasis 26: 195–202, 1996.

Bijsterveld NR, Moons AH, Boekholdt SM, van Aken BE, Fennema H, Peters RJ, Meijers JC, Buller HR, Levi M. Ability of recombinant factor VIIa to reverse the anticoagulant effect of the pentasaccharide fondaparinux in healthy volunteers. Circulation 106: 2550–2554, 2002.

Boneu B, Necciari J, Cariou R, Sie P, Gabaig AM, Kieffer G, Dickinson J, Lamond G, Moelker H, Mant T, et al. Pharmacokinetics and tolerance of the natural pentasaccharide (SR90107/Org31540) with high affinity to antithrombin III in man. Thromb Haemost 74: 1468–1473, 1995.

Bradner JE, Eikelboom JW. Emerging anticoagulants and heparin-induced thrombocytopenia: indirect and direct factor Xa inhibitors and oral thrombin inhibitors. In: Warkentin TE, Greinacher A, eds. Heparin-Induced Thrombocytopenia, 4th edn. New York: Informa, 441–461, 2007.

Büller HR, Davidson BL, Decousus H, Gallus A, Gent M, Piovella F, Prins MH, Raskob G, Van den Berg-Segers AE, Cariou R, Leewenkamp O, Lensing AW. Subcutaneous fondaparinux versus intravenous unfractionated heparin in the initial treatment of pulmonary embolism. N Engl J Med 349: 1695–1702, 2003.

Büller HR, Davidson BL, Decousus H, Gallus A, Gent M, Piovella F, Prins MH, Raskob G, Segers AE, Cariou R, Leeuwenkamp O, Lensing AW. Fondaparinux or enoxaparin for the initial treatment of symptomatic deep venous thrombosis: a randomized trial. Ann Intern Med 140: 867–873, 2004.

Burch M, Cooper B. Fondaparinux-associated heparin-induced thrombocytopenia. Proc (Bayl Univ Med Center) 25: 13–15, 2012.

Choay J, Petitou M, Lormeau JC, Sinay P, Casu B, Gatti G. Structure-activity relationship in heparin: a synthetic pentasaccharide with high affinity for antithrombin III and eliciting high anti-factor Xa activity. Biochem Biophys Res Commun 116: 492–499, 1983.

Ciurzyński M, Jankowski K, Pietrzak B, Mazanowska N, Rzewuska E, Kowalik R, Pruszczyk P. Use of fondaparinux in a pregnant woman with pulmonary embolism and heparin-induced thrombocytopenia. Med Sci Monit 17: 56–59, 2011.

Cohen AT, Davidson BL, Gallus AS, Lassen MR, Prins MH, Tomkowski W, Turpie AGG, Egberts JF, Lensing AW. Efficacy and safety of fondaparinux for the prevention of venous thromboembolism in older acute medical patients: randomized placebo controlled trial. BMJ 332: 325–329, 2006.

Coussement PK, Bassand JP, Convens C, Vrolix M, Boland J, Grollier G, Michels R, Vahanian A, Vanderheyden M, Rupprecht HJ, Van de Werf F. A synthetic factor-Xa inhibitor (ORG31540/SR9017A) as an adjunct to fibrinolysis in acute myocardial infarction: the PENTALYSE study. Eur Heart J 22: 1716–1724, 2001.

D'Amico EA, Villaca PR, Gualandro SF, Bassitt RP, Chamone DA. Successful use of Arixtra in a patient with paroxysmal nocturnal hemoglobinuria, Budd-Chiari syndrome and heparin-induced thrombocytopenia. J Thromb Haemost 1: 2452–2453, 2003.

Daud AN, Ahsan A, Iqbal O, Walenga JM, Silver PJ, Ahmad S, Fareed J. Synthetic heparin pentasaccharide depolymerization by heparinase I: molecular and biological implications. Clin Appl Thromb Hemost 7: 58–64, 2001.

Dempfle CE. Minor transplacental passage of fondaparinux in vivo. N Engl J Med 350: 1914–1915, 2004.

Desmurs-Clavel H, Huchon C, Chatard B, Negrier C, Dargaud Y. Reversal of the inhibitory effect of fondaparinux on thrombin generation by rFVIIa, aPCC and PCC. Thromb Res 123: 796–798, 2009.

Donat F, Duret JP, Santoni A, Cariou R, Necciari J, Magnani H, De Greef R. The pharmacokinetics of fondaparinux sodium in healthy volunteers. Clin Pharmacokinet 41(Suppl 2): 1–9, 2002.

Ekbatani A, Asaro LR, Malinow AM. Anticoagulation with argatroban in a parturient with heparin-induced thrombocytopenia. Int J Obstet Anesth 19: 82–87, 2010.

Elalamy I, Lecrubier C, Potevin F, Abdelouahed M, Bara L, Marie JP, Samama M. Absence of in vitro cross-reaction of pentasaccharide with the plasma heparin-dependent factor of twenty-five patients with heparin-associated thrombocytopenia. Thromb Haemost 74: 1384–1385, 1995.

Elmer J, Wittels KA. Emergency reversal of pentasaccharide anticoagulants: a systematic review of the literature. Transfus Med 22: 108–115, 2012.

Eriksson BI, Lassen MR. Duration of prophylaxis against venous thromboembolism with fondaparinux after hip fracture surgery: a multicenter, randomized, placebo controlled, double-blind study. Arch Intern Med 163: 1337–1342, 2003.

Eriksson BI, Bauer KA, Lassen MR, Turpie AGG. Fondaparinux compared with enoxaparin for the prevention of venous thromboembolism after hip-fracture surgery. N Engl J Med 345: 1298–1304, 2001.

Fieland D, Taylor M. Dabigatran use in a postoperative coronary artery bypass surgery with nonvalvular atrial fibrillation and heparin-PF4 antibodies. Ann Pharmacother 46: e1, 2012.

Gerhardt A, Zotz RB, Stockschlaeder M, Scharf RE. Fondaparinux is an effective alternative anticoagulant in pregnant women with high risk of venous thromboembolism and intolerance to low molecular weight heparins and heparinoids. Thromb Haemost 97: 496–497, 2007.

Gerotziafas GT, Depasse F, Chakroun T, Samama MM, Elalamy I. Recombinant factor VIIa partially reverses the inhibitory effect of fondaparinux on thrombin generation after tissue factor activation in platelet rich plasma and whole blood. Thromb Haemost 91: 531–537, 2004a.

Gerotziafas GT, Depasse F, Chakroun T, Van Dreden P, Samama MM, Elalamy I. Comparison of the effect of fondaparinux and enoxaparin on thrombin generation during in-vitro clotting of whole blood and platelet-rich plasma. Blood Coagul Fibrinolysis 15: 149–156, 2004b.

Ghanny S, Warkentin TE, Crowther MA. Reversing anticoagulant therapy. Curr Drug Discov Technol 9: 143–149, 2012.

Goldfarb MJ, Blostein MD. Fondaparinux in acute heparin-induced thrombocytopenia: a case-series. J Thromb Haemost 9: 2501–2503, 2011.

Greinacher A. Immunogenic but effective: the HIT-fondaparinux brain puzzler. J Thromb Haemost 9: 2386–2388, 2011.

Greinacher A, Pötzsch B, Amiral J, Dummel V, Eichner A, Mueller-Eckhardt C. Heparin-associated thrombocytopenia: isolation of the antibody and characterization of a multimolecular PF4-Heparin complex as the major antigen. Thromb Haemost 71: 247–251, 1994.

Greinacher A, Alban S, Dummel V, Franz G, Mueller-Eckhardt C. Characterization of the structural requirements for a carbohydrate based anticoagulant with a reduced risk of inducing the immunological type of heparin-associated thrombocytopenia. Thromb Haemost 74: 886–892, 1995.

Greinacher A, Gopinadhan M, Günther JU, Omer-Adam MA, Strobel U, Warkentin TE, Papastavrou G, Weitschies W, Helm CA. Close approximation of two platelet factor 4 tetramers by charge neutralization forms the antigens recognized by HIT antibodies. Arterioscler Thromb Vasc Biol 26: 2386–2393, 2006.

Grootenhuis PD, Westerduin P, Meuleman D, Petitou M, van Boeckel CA. Rational design of synthetic heparin analogues with tailor-made coagulation factor inhibitory activity. Nat Struct Biol 2: 736–739, 1995.

Grouzi E, Kyriakou E, Panagou I, Spiliotopoulou I. Fondaparinux for the treatment of acute heparin-induced thrombocytopenia: a single-center experience. Clin Appl Thromb Hemost 16: 663–667, 2010.

Haase M, Bellomo R, Rocktaeschel J, Ziemer S, Kiesewetter H, Morgera S, Neumayer HH. Use of fondaparinux (ARIXTRA) in a dialysis patients with symptomatic heparin-induced thrombocytopenia type II. Nephrol Dial Transplant 20: 444–446, 2005.

Harenberg J. Treatment of a woman with lupus and thromboembolism and cutaneous intolerance to heparins using fondaparinux during pregnancy. Thromb Res 119: 385–388, 2007.

Harenberg J, Jorg I, Fenyvesi T. Treatment of heparin-induced thrombocytopenia with fondaparinux. Haematologica 89: 1017–1018, 2004.

Hauel NH, Nar H, Priepke H, Ries U, Stassen JM, Wienen W. Structure-based design of novel potent nonpeptide thrombin inhibitors. J Med Chem 45: 1757–1766, 2002.

Herbert JM, Hérault JP, Bernat A, van Amsterdam RG, Lormeau JC, Petitou M, van Boeckel C, Hoffmann P, Meuleman DG. Biochemical and pharmacological properties of SANORG 34006, a potent and long-acting synthetic pentasaccharide. Blood 91: 4197–4205, 1998.

Hinder M, Frick A, Jordaan P, Hesse G, Gebauer A, Maas J, Paccaly A. Direct and rapid inhibition of factor Xa by otamixaban: a pharmacokinetic and pharmacodynamic investigation in patients with coronary artery disease. Clin Pharmacol Ther 80: 691–702, 2006.

Hirsch K, Ludwig RJ, Lindhoff-Last E, Kaufmann R, Boehncke WH. Intolerance of fondaparinux in a patient allergic to heparin. Contact Dermatitis 50: 383–384, 2004.

Hirsh J, O'Donnell M, Eikelboom JW. Beyond unfractionated heparin and warfarin. Circulation 116: 552–560, 2007.

Huvers F, Slappendel R, Benraad B, van Hellemondt G, van Kraaij M. Treatment of postoperative bleeding after fondaparinux with rFVIIa and tranexamic acid. Neth J Med 63: 184–186, 2005.

Jankowski K, Ozdzenska-Milke E, Lichodziejewska B, Huba M, Ciurzyński M, Pruszczyk P. [Recurrent pulmonary embolism in a patient with heparin-induced thrombocytopenia. Article in Polish]. Pol Arch Med Wewn 117: 524–526, 2007.

Jappe U, Juschka U, Kuner N, Hausen BM, Krohn K. Fondaparinux: a suitable alternative in cases of delayed-type allergy to heparins and semisynthetic heparinoids? a study of 7 cases. Contact Dermatitis 51: 67–72, 2004.

Jay RM, Warkentin TE. Fatal heparin-induced thrombocytopenia (HIT) during warfarin thromboprophylaxis following orthopedic surgery: another example of 'spontaneous' HIT? J Thromb Haemost 6: 1598–1600, 2008.

Kalicki RM, Aregger F, Alberio L, Lämmle B, Frey FJ, Uehlinger DE. Use of the pentasaccharide fondaparinux as an anticoagulant during hemodialysis. Thromb Haemost 98: 1200–1207, 2007.

Kelton JG, Warkentin TE. Heparin-induced thrombocytopenia: a historical perspective. Blood 112: 2607–2616, 2008.

Klaeffling C, Piechottka G, Daemgen-von Brevern G, Mosch G, Mani H, Luxembourg B, Lindhoff-Last E. Development and clinical evaluation of two chromogenic substrate methods for monitoring fondaparinux sodium. Ther Drug Monit 28: 375–381, 2006.

Krauel K, Hackbarth C, Fürll B, Greinacher A. Heparin-induced thrombocytopenia: in vitro studies on the interaction of dabigatran, rivaroxaban, and low-sulfated heparin, with platelet factor 4 and anti-PF4/heparin antibodies. Blood 119: 1248–1255, 2012.

Kubitza D, Haas S. Novel factor Xa inhibitors for prevention and treatment of thromboembolic diseases. Expert Opin Investig Drugs 99: 999–1000, 2006.

Kuo KHM, Kovacs MJ. Successful treatment of heparin induced thrombocytopenia (HIT) with fondaparinux. Thromb Haemost 93: 999–1000, 2005.

Lagrange F, Vergnes C, Brun JL, Paolucci F, Nadal T, Leng JJ, Saux MC, Banwarth B. Absence of placental transfer of pentasaccharide (Fondaparinux, Arixtra) in the dually perfused human cotyledon in vitro. Thromb Haemost 87: 831–835, 2002.

Lam LH, Silbert JE, Rosenberg RD. The separation of active and inactive forms of heparin. Biochem Biophys Res Commun 69: 570–577, 1976.

Lassen MR, Bauer KA, Eriksson MI, Turpie AGG. Postoperative fondaparinux versus preoperative enoxaparin for prevention of venous thromboembolism in elective hip-replacement surgery: a randomised double-blind comparison. Lancet 359: 1715–1720, 2002.

Linkins LA, Weitz JI. New anticoagulant therapy. Annu Rev Med 56: 63–77, 2005.

Linkins LA, Dans LA, Moores LK, Bona R, Davidson BL, Schulman S, Crowther M. Treatment and prevention of heparin-induced thrombocytopenia: antithrombotic therapy and prevention of thrombosis, 9th ed: american college of chest physicians evidence-based clinical practice guidelines. Chest 141(Suppl): e495–e530, 2012.

Lisman T, Bijsterveld NR, Adelmeijer J, Meijers JC, Levi M, Nieuwenhuis HK, De Groot PG. Recombinant factor VIIa reverses the in vitro and ex vivo anticoagulant and profibrinolytic effects of fondaparinux. J Thromb Haemost 1: 2368–2373, 2003.

Lobo B, Finch C, Howard A, Minhas S. Fondaparinux for the treatment of patients with acute heparin-induced thrombocytopenia. 99: 208–214, 2008.

Luporsi P, Chopard R, Janin S, Racadot E, Bernard Y, Ecarnot F, Séronde MF, Briand F, Guignier A, Descotes-Genon V, Meneveau N, Schiele F. Use of recombinant factor VIIa (NovoSeven®) in 8 patients with ongoing life-threatening bleeding treated with fondaparinux. Acute Card Care 13: 93–98, 2011.

Mazzolai L, Hohlfeld P, Spertini F, Hayoz D, Schapira M, Duchosal MA. Fondaparinux is a safe alternative in case of heparin intolerance during pregnancy. Blood 108: 1569–1570, 2006.

Mehta SR, Steg PG, Granger CB, Bassand JP, Faxon DP, Weitz JI, Afzal R, Rush B, Peters RJ, Natarajan MK, Velianou JL, Goodhart DM, Labinaz M, Tanguay JF, Fox KA, Yusuf S. Randomized, blinded trial comparing fondaparinux with unfractionated heparin in patients undergoing contemporary percutaneous coronary intervention: Arixtra study in percutaneous coronary intervention: a randomized evaluation (ASPIRE) pilot trial. Circulation 111: 1390–1397, 2005.

Miranda AC, Donovan JL, Tran MT, Gore JM. A case of unsuccessful treatment of heparin-induced thrombocytopenia (HIT) with fondaparinux. J Thromb Thrombolysis 33: 133–135, 2012.

Modi C, Satani D, Cervellione KL, Cervantes J, Gintautas J. Delayed-onset heparin-induced thrombocytopenia type-2 during fondaparinux (Arixtra®) therapy. Proc West Pharmacol 52: 5–7, 2009.

Montagnac R, Brahimi S, Janian P, Melin JP, Bertocchio JP, Wynckel A. [Use of fondaparinux during hemodialysis in heparin-induced thrombocytopenia. About a new observation.] Article in French. Nephrol Ther 6: 581–584, 2010.

Ogata K, Mendell-Harary J, Tachibana M, Masumoto H, Oguma T, Kojima M, Kunitada S. Clinical safety, tolerability, pharmacokinetics, and pharmacodynamics of the novel factor Xa inhibitor edoxaban in healthy volunteers. J Clin Pharmacol 50: 743–753, 2010.

Pappalardo F, Scandroglio A, Maj G, Zangrillo A, D'Angelo A. Treatment of heparin-induced thrombocytopenia after cardiac surgery: preliminary experience with fondaparinux. J Thorac Cardiovasc Surg 139: 790–792, 2010.

Parody R, Oliver A, Souto JC, Fontcuberta J. Fondaparinux (ARIXTRA) as an alternative antithrombotic prophylaxis when there is hypersensitivity to low molecular weight and unfractionated heparins. Haematologica 88: ECR32, 2003.

Patterson SL, LaMonte MP, Mikdashi JA, Haines ST, Hursting MJ. Anticoagulation strategies for treatment of ischemic stroke and antiphospholipid syndrome: case report and review of the literature. Pharmacotherapy 26: 1518–1525, 2006.

Perzborn E, Roehrig S, Straub A, Kubitza D, Misselwitz F. The discovery and development of rivaroxaban, an oral direct factor Xa inhibitor. Nat Rev Drug Discov 10: 61–75, 2011.

Petitou M, Herault JP, Bernat A, Driguez PA, Duchaussoy P, Lormeau JC, Herbert JM. Synthesis of thrombin-inhibiting heparin mimetics without side effects. Nature 398: 417–422, 1999.

Piovella F, Barone M, Beltrametti C, Piovella C, D'Armini AM, Marzani FC, Arici V, De Amici M, Barco SL, Castellani G, Langer M. Efficacy of fondaparinux in the treatment of heparin-induced thrombocytopenia with venous thromboembolism: reduction of thromboembolic burden, normalization of platelet count and disappearance of anti-platelet factor 4/heparin antibodies. Blood 108(Suppl 1): 173a, 2006.

Pouplard C, Couvret C, Regina S, Gruel Y. Development of antibodies specific to polyanion-modified platelet factor 4 during treatment with fondaparinux. J Thromb Haemost 3: 2813–2815, 2005.

Raghavan N, Frost CE, Yu Z, He K, Zhang H, Humphreys WG, Pinto D, Chen S, Bonacorsi S, Wong PC, Zhang D. Apixaban metabolism and pharmacokinetics after oral administration to humans. Drug Metab Dispos 37: 74–81, 2009.

Ratuapli SK, Bobba B, Zafar H. Heparin-induced thrombocytopenia in a patient treated with fondaparinux. Clin Adv Hematol Oncol 8: 61–62, 2010.

Rauova L, Poncz M, McKenzie SE, Reilly MP, Arepally G, Weisel JM, Nagaswami C, Cines DB, Sachais BS. Ultralarge complexes of PF4 and heparin are central to the pathogenesis of heparin-induced thrombocytopenia. Blood 105: 131–138, 2005.

Re G, Legnani C. Thrombocytopenia during fondaparinux prophylaxis: HIT or something different? Intern Emerg Med 5: 361–363, 2010.

Rembrandt Investigators. Treatment of proximal deep vein thrombosis with a novel synthetic compound (SR90107A/ORG31540) with pure anti-factor Xa activity: a phase II evaluation. Circulation 102: 2726–2731, 2000.

Rosenberg RD, Lam L. Correlation between structure and function of heparin. Proc Natl Acad Sci USA 76: 1218–1222, 1979.

Rosenberg RD, Armand G, Lam L. Structure-function relationships of heparin species. Proc Natl Acad Sci USA 75: 3065–3069, 1978.

Rota E, Bazzan M, Fantino G. Fondaparinux-related thrombocytopenia in a previous low molecular weight heparin (LMWH)-induced heparin-induced thrombocytopenia. Thromb Haemost 99: 779–781, 2008.

Salem M, Elrefai S, Shrit MA, Warkentin TE. Fondaparinux thromboprophylaxis-associated heparin-induced thrombocytopenia syndrome complicated by arterial thrombotic stroke. Thromb Haemost 104: 1071–1072, 2010.

Savi P, Chong BH, Greinacher A, Gruel Y, Kelton JG, Warkentin TE, Eichler P, Meuleman D, Petitou M, Herault JP, Cariou R, Herbert JM. Effect of fondaparinux on platelet activation in the presence of heparin-dependent antibodies: a blinded comparative multicenter study with unfractionated heparin. Blood 105: 139–144, 2005.

Simoons ML, Bobbink IWG, Boland J, Gardien M, Klootwijk P, Lensing AWA, Ruzyllo W, Umans VAWM, Vahanian A, Van De Werf F, Zeymer U; PENTUA Investigators. A dose-finding study of fondaparinux in patients with non-ST-segment elevation acute coronary syndromes: the pentasaccharide in unstable angina (PENTUA) Study. J Am Coll Cardiol 43: 2183–2190, 2004.

Smogorzewska A, Brandt JT, Chandler WL, Cunningham MT, Hayes TE, Olson JD, Kottke-Marchant K, Van Cott EM. Effect of fondaparinux on coagulation assays: results of college of american pathologists proficiency testing. Arch Pathol Lab Med 130: 1605–1611, 2006.

Sombolos KI, Fragia TK, Gionanlis LC, Veneti PE, Bamichas GI, Fragidis SK, Georgoulis IE, Natse TA. Use of fondaparinux as an anticoagulant during hemodialysis: a preliminary study. Int J Clin Pharmacol Ther 46: 198–203, 2008.

Stangier J. Clinical pharmacokinetics and pharmacodynamics of the oral direct thrombin inhibitor dabigatran etexilate. Clin Pharmacokinet 47: 285–295, 2008.

Steg PG, Jolly SS, Mehta SR, Afzal R, Xavier D, Rupprecht HJ, López-Sendón JL, Budaj A, Diaz R, Avezum A, Widimsky P, Rao SV, Chrolavicius S, Meeks B, Joyner C, Pogue J, Yusuf S. Low-dose vs standard-dose unfractionated heparin for percutaneous coronary intervention in acute coronary syndromes treated with fondaparinux: the FUTURA/OASIS-8 randomized trial. JAMA 304: 1339–1349, 2010.

Turpie AGG. Use of selective factor Xa inhibitors in special populations. Am J Orthop 31: 11–15, 2002.

Turpie AGG, Gallus AS, Hoek JA. A synthetic pentasaccharide for the prevention of deep-vein thrombosis after total hip replacement. N Engl J Med 344: 619–625, 2001.

Turpie AGG, Bauer KA, Eriksson BI, Lassen MR. Fondaparinux vs enoxaparin for the prevention of venous thromboembolism in major orthopedic surgery: a meta-analysis of 4 randomized double-blind studies. Arch Intern Med 162: 1833–1840, 2002a.

Turpie AGG, Bauer KA, Eriksson BI, Lassen MR. Postoperative fondaparinux versus postoperative enoxaparin for prevention of venous thromboembolism after elective hip-replacement surgery: a randomized double-blind trial. Lancet 359: 1721–1726, 2002b.

Utikal J, Peitsch WK, Booken D, Velten F, Dempfle CE, Goerdt S, Bayerl C. Hypersensitivity to the pentasaccharide fondaparinux in patients with delayed-type heparin allergy. Thromb Haemost 94: 895–896, 2005.

Walenga JM, Bara L, Petitou M, Samama M, Fareed J, Choay J. The inhibition of the generation of thrombin and the antithrombotic effect of a pentasaccharide with sole anti-factor Xa activity. Thromb Res 51: 23–33, 1988.

Walenga JM, Prechel M, Jeske WP, Hoppensteadt D, Maddineni J, Iqbal O, Messmore HL, Bakhos M. Rivaroxaban—an oral, direct Factor Xa inhibitor—has potential for the management of patients with heparin-induced thrombocytopenia. Br J Haematol 143: 92–99, 2008.

Warkentin TE. Fondaparinux: does it cause HIT? can it treat HIT? Exp Rev Hematol 3: 567–581, 2010.

Warkentin TE. How I diagnose and manage HIT. Hematology Am Soc Hematol Educ Program 2011: 143–149, 2011.

Warkentin TE. HIT: treatment easier, prevention harder. Blood 119: 1099–1100, 2012.

Warkentin TE, Lim W. Can heparin-induced thrombocytopenia be associated with fondaparinux use? reply to a rebuttal. J Thromb Haemost 6: 1243–1246, 2008.

Warkentin TE, Cook RJ, Marder VJ, Sheppard JI, Moore JC, Eriksson BI, Greinacher A, Kelton JG. Anti-platelet factor 4/heparin antibodies in orthopedic surgery patients receiving antithrombotic therapy with fondaparinux or enoxaparin. Blood 106: 3791–3796, 2005.

Warkentin TE, Maurer BT, Aster RH. Heparin-induced thrombocytopenia associated with fondaparinux. N Engl J Med 356. 2653–2655, 2007.

Warkentin TE, Cook RJ, Marder VJ, Greinacher A. Anti-PF4/heparin antibody formation post-orthopedic surgery thromboprophylaxis: the role of non-drug risk factors and evidence for a stoichiometry-based model of immunization. J Thromb Haemost 8: 504–512, 2010.

Warkentin TE, Davidson BL, Büller HR, Gallus A, Gent M, Lensing AWA, Piovella F, Prins MH, Segers AEM, Kelton JG. Prevalence and risk of preexisting heparin-induced thrombocytopenia antibodies in patients with acute VTE. Chest 140: 366–373, 2011a.

Warkentin TE, Pai M, Sheppard JI, Schulman S, Spyropoulos AC, Eikelboom JW. Fondaparinux treatment of acute heparin-induced thrombocytopenia confirmed by the serotonin-release assay: a 30-month, 16-patient case series. J Thromb Haemost 9: 2389–2396, 2011b.

Warkentin TE, Chakraborty AK, Sheppard JI, Griffin DK. The serological profile of fondaparinux-associated heparin-induced thrombocytopenia syndrome. Thromb Haemost 108: 394–396, 2012a.

Warkentin TE, Margetts P, Connolly SJ, Lamy A, Ricci C, Eikelboom JW. Recombinant factor VIIa (rFVIIa) and hemodialysis to manage massive dabigatran-associated postcardiac surgery bleeding. Blood 119: 2172–2174, 2012b.

Weberschock T, Meisster AC, Bohrt K, Scmitt J, Boehncke WH, Ludwig RJ. The risk for cross-reactions after a cutaneous delayed-type hypersensitivity reaction to heparin preparations is independent of their molecular weight: a systematic review. Contact Dermatitis 65: 187–194, 2011.

Weitz JI. Factor Xa or thrombin: is thrombin a better target? J Thromb Haemost 5 Suppl 1: 65–67, 2007.

Weitz JI, Buller HR. Direct thrombin inhibitors in acute coronary syndromes: present and future. Circulation 105: 1004–1011, 2002.

Weitz JI, Eikelboom JW, Samama MM. American College of Chest Physicians Therapy and Prevention of Thrombosis, 9th New Antithrombotic Drugs : Antithrombotic Evidence-Based Clinical Practice Guidelines. Chest 141(Suppl): e120S–e151S, 2012.

Wellborn-Kim JJ, Mitchell GA, Terneus WF Jr, Stowe CL, Malias MA, Sparkman GM, Hanson GW. Fondaparinux therapy in a hemodialysis patient with heparin-induced thrombocytopenia type II. Am J Health Syst Pharm 67: 1075–1079, 2010.

Wijesiriwardana A, Lees DA, Lush C. Fondaparinux as anticoagulant in a pregnant woman with heparin allergy. Blood Coagul Fibrinolysis 17: 147–149, 2006.

Young G, Yonekawa KE, Nakagawa PA, Blain RC, Lovejoy AE, Nugent DJ. Recombinant activated factor VII effectively reverses the anticoagulant effects of heparin, enoxaparan, fondaparinux, argatroban, and bivalirudin ex vivo as measured using thromboelastography. Blood Coagul Fibrinolysis 18: 547–553, 2007.

Yusuf S, Mehta SR, Chrolavicius S, Afzal R, Pogue J, Granger CB, Budaj A, Peters RJ, Bassand JP, Wallentin L, Joyner C, Fox KA; Fifth Organization to Assess Strategies in Acute Ischemic Syndromes Investigators. Comparison of fondaparinux and enoxaparin in acute coronary syndromes. N Engl J Med 354: 1464–1476, 2006a.

Yusuf S, Mehta SR, Chrolavicius S, Afzal R, Pogue J, Granger CB, Budaj A, Peters RJ, Bassand JP, Wallentin L, Joyner C, Fox KA. Effects of fondaparinux on mortality and reinfarction in patients with acute ST-segment elevation myocardial infarction: the OASIS-6 randomized trial. JAMA 295: 1519–1530, 2006b.

18 Hemodialysis in heparin-induced thrombocytopenia

Karl-Georg Fischer

HEPARIN-INDUCED THROMBOCYTOPENIA IN HEMODIALYSIS PATIENTS
Given the major role of unfractionated heparin (UFH) for anticoagulation in hemodialysis (HD), it is important to define the potential impact of immune heparin-induced thrombocytopenia (HIT) in contributing to morbidity and mortality in patients with dialysis-dependent renal failure.

Within the prospective cohort study Choices for Healthy Outcomes in Caring for End-Stage Renal Disease (CHOICE), sera from 740 incident kidney failure patients starting outpatient dialysis (HD, $n = 596$; peritoneal dialysis, $n = 144$) were tested for anti-PF4/heparin (anti-PF4/H) antibodies approximately six months after enrolment (Asmis et al., 2008). Early after treatment initiation, antibodies were detected in almost 20% of the patients. At six months, 76/740 (10.3%) of patients had a positive polyspecific enzyme immunoassay (EIA) based on an absorbance ≥ 0.4 optical density (OD) units. Mean platelet counts were not significantly different between antibody-positive and -negative patients. The presence of anti-PF4/H antibodies did not predict subsequent thrombocytopenia at three, six, or nine months postmeasurement. Over a mean follow-up of 3.6 years, antibody positivity did not predict development of arterial cardiovascular events, venous thromboembolism, vascular access occlusion, or mortality. Nine of 740 patients (1.2%, all on HD) presented with clinical features possibly compatible with HIT [positive test result and thrombocytopenia (mean platelet count nadir, 124×10^9/L; range, 106–147)] with one patient having a venous thromboembolic event (1/740, 0.13%); However, neutralization of a positive EIA by the high heparin step was seen in only six of these nine patients.

One further study reported on the incidence of HIT in new HD patients. Six of 154 patients (3.9%) were clinically suspected of having developed HIT because of a fall in the platelet count accompanied by clotting of the dialyzer and extracorporeal circuit (Yamamoto et al., 1996). The clinical diagnosis was confirmed by the detection of HIT antibodies in all but one patient. Only one patient developed organ damage from thrombosis (myocardial infarction and stroke).

In cross-sectional studies involving more than 3000 patients, antibody positivity (by EIA) ranged from 0% to 17.9% (Table 18.1). Anti-PF4/H antibodies were detected by EIA in 117 of 1450 patients (8.1%) on UFH and in four of 218 patients (1.8%) on low molecular weight heparin (LMWH) (Syed and Reilly, 2009). Functional assays were positive in 3.7% of 730 patients exposed to UFH. Interestingly, in some patients antibodies were not detected by EIA, whereas functional assays were positive. Only in a few patients did antibodies appear to be associated with thrombocytopenia or thromboembolic events.

TABLE 18.1 Frequency of Anti-PF4/Heparin Antibodies and Clinical HIT in Hemodialysis Patients

Reference	N[a]	Frequency of HIT antibodies		Frequency of HIT	
		Antigen test	Functional test	Thrombocytopenia	Thrombosis
De Sancho et al., 1996	45	0% (0/45)	NA	NA	NA
Yamamoto et al., 1996	154	6.8% (5/73)	NA	3.8% (6/154)[b]	3.8% (6/154)[c]
Greinacher et al., 1996	165	NA	4.2% (7/165)	0% (0/165)	0% (0/165)
Boon et al., 1996	261	1.9% (5/261)	NA	0% (2/261)	0% (0/261)
Sitter et al., 1998	70	2.8% (2/70)	NA	0% (0/70)	0% (0/70)
Luzzato et al., 1998	50	12% (6/50)	NA	0% (0/50)	0% (0/50)
O'Shea et al., 2002	88	1.1% (1/88)	NA	0% (0/88)	0% (0/88)
Peña de la Vega et al., 2005	57	3.5% (2/57)	NA	1.7% (1/57)	0% (0/57)
Palomo et al., 2005	207	17.9% (37/207)	5.8% (12/207)	18.5% (29/156)	12.4% (21/207)
Carrier et al., 2007	419	12.9% (54/419)	0% (0/419)	NA	—[d]

[a]All patients are chronic hemodialysis patients except Yamamoto et al. (acute HD patients, $n = 50$; chronic HD patients, $n = 104$).
[b]Defined as a greater than 20% reduction in platelet counts.
[c]Dialyzer clotting defined as a consequence of HIT (other forms of thrombosis observed only in one patient).
[d]Of 419 patients, 107 patients had access thrombosis. However, no significant correlation was observed between presence of HIT antibodies and access thrombosis.
Abbreviations: HIT, heparin-induced thrombocytopenia; NA, not available.

In a UK survey covering 10,564 end-stage renal disease (ESRD) patients on maintenance HD, renal units were asked to report on HIT cases, being defined as patients who developed thrombocytopenia with heparin in the absence of other causes, and where HIT antibodies were detected. Based on returned questionnaires, incidence and prevalence of HIT were given as 0.32% and 0.26%, respectively (Hutchison and Dasgupta, 2007). Seventeen percent of the 28 HIT patients were reported to have suffered from complications, most often deep vein thrombosis (8%).

Taken together, mainly focusing on ESRD patients—the population studied by Yamamoto et al. (1996) also included 50 patients with acute kidney injury—these studies suggest that only a few patients who form anti-PF4/H antibodies in association with chronic intermittent HD develop related clinical events.

The risk of clinical HIT may be higher in patients starting HD (the aforementioned study of Yamamoto and colleagues) than in patients in the long-term phase of HD (as per the remaining studies). Anecdotal case reports of HIT complicating HD also seem frequently to include patients undergoing short-term HD (Matsuo et al., 1989; Hall et al., 1992; Nowak et al., 1997; Gupta et al., 1998), or HD given in a postoperative setting (Hartman et al., 2006).

In HD patients, anti-PF4/H antibody positivity appears to diminish over time: Early after HD initiation in the CHOICE study, nearly 20% of incident HD outpatients were antibody positive, whereas at six months this percentage decreased to 10.3% (Asmis et al., 2008). In a series of 305 prevalent HD patients in Japan, three of seven antibody-positive patients had been on HD for less than one year; by contrast, none of the 62 patients on HD for more than 10 years was antibody positive (Matsuo et al., 2006; Syed and Reilly, 2009).

Clinical conditions requiring hospital admission may increase the risk of developing HIT: In a recent study evaluating data of 25,653 medical inpatients, 55 of which were HIT cases, HD patients had a relative risk (RR) of 9.68 (95% CI, 4.90–19.1; $P < 0.0001$ in multivariate analysis) of developing HIT (Kato et al., 2011). The risk of developing HIT was also increased upon full anticoagulation dose and prolonged duration of UFH treatment [RR, 7.66 (95% CI, 3.31–17.8; $P < 0.0001$) and RR, 3.66 (95% CI, 1.98–6.75; $P < 0.0001$)]. Therefore, these circumstances may require an increased surveillance for HIT by repeated platelet counts.

At present, it is unclear if HIT antibody positivity of HD patients is associated with increased mortality. In 419 patients on chronic HD with a median follow-up of 2.5 years, Carrier et al. (2007) showed IgG-specific anti-PF4/H antibodies to constitute an independent predictor of mortality (adjusted hazard ratio, 2.68; 95% CI, 1.08–6.63). Of 1203 chronic HD patients followed over a 5-year period, 45 patients (3.7%) tested positive for antibodies in a functional assay (Mureebe et al., 2004). Not only were thrombotic and hemorrhagic complications significantly more frequent in antibody-positive *versus* antibody-negative patients (60% *vs* 8.7%, respectively), but the mortality rate also was significantly higher (28.6% *vs* 4.35%, respectively). By contrast, studying 596 incident HD patients over a mean follow-up of 3.6 years, Asmis et al. (2008) did not find an association between anti-PF4/H antibody positivity at baseline and the various clinical outcomes (e.g., hazard ratio for mortality, 1.18; 95% CI, 0.85–1.64). Whether the test used to detect heparin-dependent antibodies (functional assay in the first two studies and EIA in the last study) can explain these differences—as suggested by Syed and Reilly (2009)—remains to be elucidated. Another study adds to difficulties in interpreting a potential association of anti-PF4/H antibody positivity and mortality: Peña de la Vega et al. (2005) reported data concerning the impact of elevated absorbance (by EIA) below the threshold permitting serologic diagnosis of HIT on cardiovascular outcome in HD patients. Absorbance values in the EIA of 57 patients were ranked in tertiles and patients were then followed for a median of 798 days. After risk adjustment, patients in the highest tertile (still below the threshold of EIA positivity) had a 2.47-fold greater risk ($P = 0.03$) of all-cause mortality and a 4.14-fold greater risk of cardiovascular mortality ($P = 0.02$) compared with the lower tertiles.

Additional studies are needed to clarify if anti-PF4/H antibody-positive patients are at increased mortality risk. In my view, testing the antibody status of nonthrombocytopenic HD patients on a regular basis, as proposed by others (Chang and Parikh, 2006), is not recommended. Furthermore, switching antibody-positive HD patients to alternative anticoagulants in the absence of thrombocytopenia appears justified only if clinical symptoms or signs of HIT occur (Greinacher et al., 1996).

CLINICAL PRESENTATION OF HIT IN HEMODIALYSIS PATIENTS

The diagnosis of HIT and respective management decisions should be primarily based on clinical criteria supported by a confirmatory laboratory test for HIT antibodies (Lewis et al., 1997; Davenport, 2009).

Concerning clinical criteria, it should be underlined that HIT in HD patients may present with a nontypical course of platelet count with regard to timing and absolute platelet numbers: Typically, acute HIT presents with a drop in platelet count to $<150 \times 10^9$/L or by 30–50% that begins 5–10 days after the onset of heparin therapy ("typical-onset HIT") (Linkins et al., 2012). In HD patients, acute HIT may occur beyond this typical time frame: In the UK survey, only 20% of patients were diagnosed with HIT between day 5 and day 10 after commencement of hemodialysis; the mean time between starting HD and HIT was 61 (range, 5–390) days with 20% of patients having developed HIT after 90 days (Hutchison and Dasgupta, 2007). Acute HIT may rarely occur even after years of uneventful HD with UFH (Tholl et al., 1997; see below). The fall in platelet count in HD patients developing HIT may be only moderate (Matsuo et al., 1997; Asmis et al., 2008).

Intensive care unit (ICU) patients constitute a subpopulation in which both diagnosis and treatment of HIT face several difficulties. According to an excellent review summarizing the respective data, HIT is uncommon in ICU patients (0.3–0.5%), whereas thrombocytopenia from other causes is frequent (30–50%) (Selleng et al., 2007). Given the complexity of multiorgan failure, multiple interventions, a broad range of differential diagnoses for thrombocytopenia, the timely identification of HIT in the ICU is particularly challenging.

In HD patients, some additional aspects must be considered: The HD procedure itself is associated with a relative decrease in platelet count, even when so-called biocompatible dialyzer membranes are used (Schmitt et al., 1987; Beijering et al., 1997). UFH can exert a platelet proaggregatory effect in the absence of anti-PF4/H antibodies, particularly in critically ill patients undergoing continuous venovenous HD (Burgess and Chong, 1997); this heparin-induced platelet proaggregatory effect is less marked with LMWH, and absent or negligible with the heparinoid, danaparoid sodium. Apart from this proaggregatory effect of UFH, continuous renal replacement therapy (CRRT) alone causes a drop in platelet count, which may also influence the evaluation of HIT pretest probability applying the "4Ts" score (Holmes et al., 2009).

The occurrence of fibrin formation, or even frank clotting of the extracorporeal circuit despite apparent sufficient anticoagulation, should lead to suspicion of possible HIT (Koide et al., 1995; Yamamoto et al., 1996; Gregorini et al., 2002; Lasocki et al., 2008). The study of Yamamoto and coworkers (1996) found an association between heparin-dependent antibody positivity and extracorporeal circuit clotting. In a study on unexpected filter clotting during continuous veno-venous hemofiltration (CVVH) being ascribed to acute HIT, CVVH duration was significantly shorter (5 *vs* 12 hours) and urea reduction ratio was significantly lower (17% *vs* 44%) in antibody-positive *versus* antibody-negative patients (Lasocki et al., 2008). Given these data, it is tempting to speculate that in the setting of acute HIT—with activation of platelets and the clotting cascade—the additional contact of blood to artificial surfaces may potentiate thrombotic events within the extracorporeal circuit.

One of the most serious complications, occlusion of vascular access (the "Achilles' heel" of HD), may also indicate HIT, and has been described both for native fistulae as well as prosthetic grafts (Laster et al., 1989; Hall et al., 1992). However, whereas vascular access thrombosis frequently occurs in HD patients, it appears questionable whether HIT increases the risk of this complication (O'Shea et al., 2002; Nakamoto et al., 2005; Palomo et al., 2005; Chang and Parikh, 2006; Carrier et al., 2007; Asmis et al., 2008; Davenport, 2009).

The occurrence of an anaphylactoid reaction, sometimes termed an "acute systemic reaction," upon initiating HD with UFH or LMWH, is a sign of possible acute HIT (Davenport, 2006; Hartman et al., 2006; Matsuo et al., 2012; Warkentin, 2012), and represents systemic manifestations of rapid platelet activation (see chap. 2). Symptoms and signs include fever, chills, tachycardia, and dyspnea, sometimes mimicking pulmonary embolism ("pseudopulmonary embolism"). Here, air embolism, reactions to the dialyzer (in cases aggravated by angiotensin-converting enzyme inhibitors) or sterilization agents may constitute differential causes for anaphylactoid reactions (Davenport, 2009).

Severe skin necrosis, even in the presence of normal platelet count, has been reported in association with the presence of HIT antibodies in patients after both short- and long-term HD (Leblanc et al., 1994; Bredlich et al., 1997).

Rarely, patients can develop HIT after years of regular long-term maintenance HD. Tholl et al. (1997) reported a patient who developed HIT following surgery after 9 years of long-term intermittent HD performed with UFH. In this patient, an anaphylactic reaction to heparin, accompanied by a platelet count fall, led to the diagnosis of HIT. It is possible that the surgery itself contributed to HIT antibody formation, as the highest reported rates of HIT are in postoperative patients receiving UFH (see chap. 4).

Unfortunately, HD complications associated with HIT are nonspecific. Thus, the clinician must consider other factors that could compromise patency of the extracorporeal circuit (e.g., low blood flow, high ultrafiltration rate, excess turbulence within the circuit, or foam formation with blood–air interfaces in the drip chambers). The quality of the vascular access plays a crucial role in this. Other patient-related factors include low arterial blood pressure, high hematocrit, and the need for intradialytic blood transfusion or lipid infusion (Hertel et al., 2001). In addition to insufficient anticoagulation, these factors should be ruled out first as the underlying causes of clotting within the extracorporeal circuit. Given the long-term implications of labeling HD patients as having HIT, laboratory testing for HIT antibodies should be performed when HIT is clinically suspected (O'Shea et al., 2003).

MANAGEMENT OF HEMODIALYSIS IN HIT PATIENTS
Discontinuation of Heparin Treatment and Start of Suitable Alternative Systemic Anticoagulation

As HIT is frequently associated with potentially life-threatening thrombotic events (Warkentin et al., 1995; Warkentin and Kelton, 1996), discontinuation of heparin treatment and initiation of adequate alternative anticoagulation is generally considered mandatory (Linkins et al., 2012). This critical first treatment decision most often is required before the result of HIT antibody testing is available. Given the high rate of thrombosis in the first days of acute HIT without anticoagulation (combined patient event rate 6.1% per day; Greinacher et al., 2000), stopping heparin alone appears insufficient to prevent further thromboembolism.

In HD patients, especially in the ICU, critical assessment is required as to the risk of thrombosis *versus* the risk of bleeding upon use of alternative anticoagulants, as drug clearance may depend on renal function. In this regard, treatment decisions are influenced by the patient's renal function: In a retrospective study analyzing data of 97 anti-PF4/H antibody-positive patients, 62 of whom were primarily suspected of having acute HIT, the percentage of patients being treated with alternative anticoagulants was lowest in the patient group with a glomerular filtration rate (GFR) <30 mL/min/1.73 m^2, as estimated by the Modification of

Diet in Renal Disease (MDRD) GFR calculation formula, even if they had a thromboembolic event (Perry et al., 2009). In patients on intermittent or continuous renal replacement therapy (RRT), GFR is not necessarily nil. Especially in acute kidney injury recovery of renal function may occur. Repetitive estimation of renal function should rely not only on serum creatinine-based GFR calculation, but also on urinary output. In patients with renal insufficiency, choice of a specific suitable alternative anticoagulant constitutes a second, and finally its dosing a third, critical treatment decision.

HIT is an acute systemic drug-induced disease, which therefore requires systemic alternative (= nonheparin) anticoagulation. Provided the patient is not at significantly elevated risk of bleeding or is overtly bleeding, exclusive regional anticoagulation for RRT in acute HIT without systemic anticoagulation often is not adequate.

With regard to strict heparin avoidance, heparin must not be added to any flushing solution, and no heparin-coated systems can be used. Indeed, heparin flushes and heparin-coated devices can both initiate and sustain HIT (Moberg et al., 1990; Kadidal et al., 1999).

Unsuitable Approaches
Low Molecular Weight Heparin
LMWH is not recommended as an alternative anticoagulant for managing acute HIT. *In vitro* tests for HIT antibodies show a high degree of cross-reactivity between UFH and LMWH (Greinacher et al., 1992b; Vun et al., 1996). Furthermore, *in vivo* cross-reactivity manifesting as persistent or recurrent thrombocytopenia or thrombosis during LMWH treatment of HIT appears to be common (Horellou et al., 1984; Roussi et al., 1984; Greinacher et al., 1992a). Because nonheparin anticoagulants are available, LMWH should not be used even if *in vitro* cross-reactivity is reported to be negative.

Regional Heparinization
Regional heparinization is defined as application of heparin at the inlet of the extracorporeal circuit and its neutralization by protamine at the outlet of the circuit. However, its use in HIT is problematic because of the potential for heparin "contamination" of the patient, as well as for heparin "rebound anticoagulation" (recurrence of heparin anticoagulation owing to shorter half-life of protamine compared with heparin) (Blaufox et al., 1966). Moreover, direct injurious effects of protamine on the clotting cascade can occur. Consequently, this regimen is not recommended for HD of patients with HIT.

Aspirin
Acetylsalicylic acid has been used as an antiplatelet agent together with continued anticoagulation with UFH for HD of patients with HIT (Janson et al., 1983; Matsuo et al., 1989; Hall et al., 1992). This approach is not recommended for at least two reasons: (*i*) protection against heparin-induced platelet activation may be incomplete or absent, as aspirin's effects on blocking the thromboxane-dependent pathway of platelet activation does not reliably inhibit platelet activation by HIT antibodies (Kappa et al., 1987; Polgár et al., 1998; Selleng et al., 2005); and (*ii*) the bleeding risk of uremic patients is increased.

Hemodialysis Without Anticoagulant

HD without an anticoagulant (Romao et al., 1997) is not ideal for maintenance HD. Without anticoagulation, the artificial surfaces become coated, first by plasma proteins, followed by adhesion and activation of platelets, with accompanying activation of the coagulation cascade (Basmadjian et al., 1997). This will markedly reduce dialysis quality in removal of fluid and solutes long before clotting of the circuit is visible. Moreover, this approach may aggravate HIT-associated thrombosis. However, in patients at high risk of bleeding (e.g., owing to hepatic disorders or multiorgan failure, or those requiring surgery), temporary HD without anticoagulant may be appropriate.

Adequate Anticoagulants for Hemodialysis in HIT Patients

Patients with renal failure show plasma hypercoagulability as well as uremic platelet defects, both of which can be worsened by HD (Sreedhara et al., 1995; Ambühl et al., 1997; Vecino et al., 1998). Clearance of several alternative anticoagulants is significantly influenced by renal function. Therefore, selection of an appropriate anticoagulant in HD patients who also suffer from HIT is difficult. However, as probably most strikingly exemplified in patients acutely suffering from pseudopulmonary embolism, once acute HIT is suspected, stopping heparin and starting a suitable systemic alternative anticoagulant must not be delayed.

Reports on specific anticoagulant strategies for HD in HIT patients most often are anecdotal. Large studies, especially those comparing different anticoagulant regimens, are lacking. Therefore, no treatment recommendations based on level A or B evidence (i.e., randomized trials) can be provided. Furthermore, because UFH is the routine anticoagulant for HD, considerable additional time, effort, and costs are usually required to manage a new anticoagulant, especially during initial use. Ideally, therefore, a center should try to gain experience with a single appropriate alternative anticoagulant for management of these difficult patients. Fear of inducing bleeding should not lead to under-anticoagulation, with the potential risk of thrombotic complications.

Choice of the alternative anticoagulant is influenced by numerous nonclinical factors, such as approval status of the specific drug, availability, cost, clinician experience, and so on. The overall clinical condition of the given patient, however, should be the main determinant for which alternative anticoagulation is tailored.

Fortunately, HIT is a relatively rare disease. Unfortunately, this often implies relevant nonexperience of the treating physician in detecting and moreover in treating this life-threatening disease. This specifically holds true for alternative anticoagulation in renal insufficiency. As dosing of alternative anticoagulants given in the manufacturer's package insert often is too high for patients with renal insufficiency, the recommendations given therein should not be uncritically followed. If not experienced in this area, the treating physician is advised to consult an appropriate expert.

In addition to the information given below, the reader is also referred to two excellent reviews covering the complex field of HIT in HD patients (Davenport, 2009; Syed and Reilly, 2009). Furthermore, the most recently published 9th edition of the American College of Chest Physicians (ACCP) guidelines on treatment and prevention of HIT (Linkins et al., 2012) contains recommendations as to choice and dosing of different alternative anticoagulants in renal insufficiency and RRT.

Danaparoid Sodium

Danaparoid sodium (Orgaran, formerly known as Org 10172) is an alternative anti-coagulant that has been widely used for management of HD in patients with HIT (Henny et al., 1983; Chong and Magnani, 1992; Greinacher et al., 1992a, 1993; Ortel et al., 1992; Magnani, 1993, 2010; Tholl et al., 1997; Wilde and Markham, 1997; Roe et al., 1998; Neuhaus et al., 2000; Magnani and Gallus, 2006; see chap. 16). In 2002, danaparoid was withdrawn from the U.S. market by the manufacturer, but still is available in numerous other countries. Some of its characteristics require specific attention:

1. The anticoagulant activity of danaparoid can be monitored only by measurement of anti-factor Xa (anti-Xa) levels based on a danaparoid calibration curve; however, many laboratories do not routinely perform these assays. Except for an emergency situation, such as when HIT is strongly suspected and danaparoid is the only available alternative, HD should not be performed without monitoring the anti-Xa activity to evaluate the dose required for adequate anticoagulation. Once the optimal dose is identified, it can often be used without alteration for several subsequent HD sessions, provided no bleeding or inappropriate clotting occurs and no surgical intervention is scheduled. Periodic measurement of anti-Xa activity thereafter to validate the dosing of danaparoid is recommended. For maintenance HD without complications, single determination of pre-HD anti-Xa activity probably suffices. If there are concerns about adequate or excess anticoagulation, then monitoring of levels at three time points is appropriate (e.g., 30–60 minutes pre-HD, 30 minutes after beginning HD, and just before completion).

2. Regarding the pharmacokinetics of danaparoid, renal excretion accounts for approximately 40–50% of total plasma clearance; accordingly, diminished clearance of anti-Xa activity occurs in HD patients (Danhof et al., 1992). Elimination half-life of the anti-Xa activity has been determined as 30.8 hours in HD patients compared to 18.4 hours in healthy individuals (Henny et al., 1985). Significant anti-Xa levels can be detected in patients undergoing HD with danaparoid even during the interdialytic interval: In a pharmacokinetic study in 21 stable chronic HD patients, seven HD patients received the same single predialysis danaparoid dose of 34 U/kg for four weeks. Compared with dalteparin and enoxaparin, after one week patients who were administered danaparoid still had significant anticoagulation 24 hours postdose (anti-Xa activity: 1 hour peak, 0.67 ± 0.051, 24 hours postdose, 0.22 ± 0.021). After four weeks, anti-Xa activity 24 hours postdose had even further increased (anti-Xa activity: 1 hour peak, 0.74 ± 0.059; 24 hours postdose, 0.31 ± 0.039), indicating that a steady state had not been reached after one week (Polkinghorne et al., 2002). An increase in interdialytic bleeding episodes was not reported. The authors concluded that danaparoid dose can be safely reduced without loss of efficacy. If pharmacokinetic modeling aims at full patency of the extracorporeal circuit during the HD session and a reduction of interdialytic bleeding risk in non-HIT patients, this conclusion appears reasonable. With regard to sufficient systemic anticoagulation in acute HIT, however, a single predialysis danaparoid bolus may lead to danaparoid "underdosing," even if HD is performed on a daily schedule (Magnani, 2010). In this analysis of 122 published outcomes of danaparoid anticoagulation for intermittent HD, none of the HIT patients who developed new

thromboses received the therapeutic intravenous (iv) danaparoid infusion regimen. Based on these data, the therapeutic regimen (continuous iv application) was recommended for all HD-dependent HIT patients including those with isolated HIT only (Magnani, 2010). When the patient is on continuous danaparoid anticoagulation, the initial iv bolus prior to HD should be adapted, starting no higher than 2250 U. Non-HIT and past HIT patients without thrombosis appear to be adequately anticoagulated by predialysis danaparoid bolus only (Magnani, 2010), which normally is sufficient to prevent clotting within the extracorporeal circuit during the procedure.

3. Danaparoid anticoagulation may also be useful in critically ill patients on CRRT. In 13 consecutive ICU patients clinically suspected to have HIT, danaparoid was administered by initial bolus (750 U) followed by continuous infusion (Lindhoff-Last et al., 2001). This regimen was sufficient to prevent clotting within the extracorporeal circuit both in CVVH (eight patients) and in continuous venovenous HD (CVVHD, five patients), respectively (Lindhoff-Last et al., 2001). Thromboembolic complications did not occur. Despite a mean danaparoid infusion rate of approximately 140 U/hr (CVVH: 140 ± 86 U/hr; CVVHD: 138 ± 122 U/hr), which is markedly reduced compared with the recommendation of the manufacturer, major bleeding was observed in six of 13 patients (which could be explained by disseminated intravascular coagulation in five patients). Here, HIT was confirmed by antibody detection in only two patients. In seven of 13 patients, even a low mean infusion rate of 88 ± 35 U/hr was efficient to prevent clotting of the extracorporeal circuit. Mean anti-Xa levels were 0.4 ± 0.2 U/mL (Lindhoff-Last et al., 2001).

    Another study designed a dosing scheme for danaparoid aiming at anti-Xa levels of 0.5–0.7 U/mL (de Pont et al., 2007), which was investigated in five ICU patients with acute renal failure (ARF) and suspicion of HIT. Following a loading dose of 3500 U, danaparoid was given as continuous infusion at a rate of 100 U/hr. After 15 minutes, median anti-Xa activity reached a maximum of 1.02 (0.66–1.31) anti-Xa U/mL and gradually declined to 0.40 (0.15–0.58) anti-Xa U/mL over the next 24 hours. Bleeding or thromboembolic events were not observed (de Pont et al., 2007).

    In the second study, the high initial loading dose led to comparably high anti-Xa levels over hours, which may increase the risk of bleeding. Furthermore, with regard to invasive procedures, the long half-life of danaparoid should be considered.

4. No antidote to danaparoid exists. Accordingly, we evaluated hemofiltration as a potential means to rapidly reduce danaparoid plasma concentration. Whereas five different high-flux hemodialyzer membranes did not allow for danaparoid filtration, a plasmapheresis membrane was capable of removing danaparoid from the blood compartment (Schneider et al., 2004). Hence, plasmapheresis may be a way to reduce danaparoid levels in situations of overdosing or bleeding. Again, careful dosing of danaparoid is important to avoid bleeding.

5. HIT antibodies potentially cross-react with danaparoid. Although the respective clinical risk has been claimed to be less than 5% (Warkentin et al., 1998), individual patients, nevertheless, may be threatened if this condition occurs. As positive *in vitro* cross-reactivity is of uncertain clinical significance (Warkentin, 1996; Wilde and Markham, 1997; Newman et al., 1998), attention should focus

on platelet count monitoring. A further fall in platelet count, or new fibrin deposits and clot formation within the extracorporeal circuit after application of danaparoid, may indicate clinically relevant cross-reactivity. To differentiate *in vivo* cross-reactivity from "under-anticoagulation" owing to insufficient dosage, determination of anti-Xa levels and HIT antibody cross-reactivity studies are needed.

6. Recently, new data have been reported highlighting a unique property of danaparoid, which had already been reported decades ago (Chong et al., 1989): At therapeutic concentration (e.g., 0.6 anti-Xa U/mL) danaparoid inhibits formation of the pathogenic complexes of PF4 and heparin, blocks binding of PF4 and PF4/H complexes to cell surfaces, and removes PF4/H complexes from cell surfaces (Krauel et al., 2008). Most interestingly, neither the direct thrombin inhibitors (DTIs)—lepirudin, argatroban, dabigatran, and rivaroxaban—nor the pentasaccharide, fondaparinux, exhibited similar effects (Krauel et al., 2008, 2012). These data further underline that in acute HIT danaparoid should be used in therapeutic concentration. Again, danaparoid dosing is a critical task.

Table 18.2 lists dosing examples of danaparoid for RRT (cf. also Keeling et al., 2006; Davenport, 2009; Syed and Reilly, 2009; Magnani, 2010; Linkins et al., 2012). These dosing examples should not be followed uncritically in any individual patient. If not experienced in this area, the treating physician is advised to consult an appropriate expert.

If applied with appropriate care, danaparoid provides adequate anticoagulation for HD of HIT patients with a favorable benefit/risk ratio, even during long-term use.

Recombinant Hirudin (Lepirudin)

Native hirudin was the first anticoagulant used for HD over 75 years ago (Haas, 1925). In recent years, interest in its use for HD has redeveloped because of the availability of recombinant preparations, as well as the clinical need for managing patients with HIT. A preparation of r-hirudin, lepirudin (Refludan or HBW023), has been used successfully in humans for anticoagulation of both intermittent (Nowak et al., 1992, 1997; Vanholder et al., 1994; Van Wyk et al., 1995; Bucha et al., 1999b; Steuer et al., 1999) and continuous HD (Fischer et al., 1999; Schneider et al., 2000; Saner et al., 2001; Vargas Hein et al., 2001; Gajra et al., 2007).

For use of lepirudin anticoagulation in HD, some aspects should be specifically addressed (see also Fischer, 2002):

1. There remains debate as to which laboratory parameter is best suited for monitoring lepirudin treatment. Initial studies addressing this in HD patients yielded conflicting results (Vanholder et al., 1994, 1997; van Wyk et al., 1995). However, it appears that the ecarin clotting time (ECT) (Nowak and Bucha, 1996) and chromogenic substrate assays (Griessbach et al., 1985) measure the lepirudin plasma concentration with adequate precision over a wide concentration range and correlate well with each other (Hafner et al., 2000, 2002). However, as these tests are often not available, monitoring of lepirudin anticoagulation is usually performed with the (activated) partial thromboplastin time (aPTT). A meta-analysis of two lepirudin treatment trials for HIT revealed a suitable aPTT ratio for reducing clinical thromboembolic complications to be between 1.5 and 2.5, which was associated with only a moderately increased

TABLE 18.2 Anticoagulation in Hemodialysis of HIT Patients—Dosage Examples of Suitable Alternative Anticoagulants

Agent	Dialysis procedure		Bolus	Continuous infusion	Monitoring parameter[a]	Target range
Danaparoid sodium[1] (Org10172, Orgaran®)	Intermittent HD (every 2nd day)	Before first two HDs	3750 (2500)[b,c]	—	Anti-Xa activity	0.5–0.8[d,e]
		Subsequent HD	*Predialytic anti-Xa activity*[d,f]			
		<0.3	3000 (2000)	—		
		0.3–0.35	2500 (1500)	—		
		0.35–0.4	2000 (1500)	—		
		>0.4	0[g]	—		
	Intermittent HD (daily)	1st HD	3750 (2500)[b,c]	—	Anti-Xa activity	0.5–0.8[d,e]
		2nd HD	2500 (2000)	—		
		Subsequent HD	See above	—		
	Continuous HD/HF	Initial bolus	2500 (2000)[b,c]	—	Anti-Xa activity	0.5–1.0[d,j]
		First 4 hr	—	600 (600)[c,h]		
		Next 4 hr	—	400 (400)[c,h]		
		Subsequently	—	200–600[g,h,j] (150–400)[c,g,h,j]		
Lepirudin[2] (HBW023, Refludan®)	Intermittent HD (every 2nd day)		0.08–0.15 mg/kg bw[k,l,m]	—	aPTT ratio[n,o,p] Hirudin conc.[r]	2–3[e,q] 0.5–1.2[e,s]
	Continuous HD	Initial bolus	0.01 mg/kg bw[k,l,m,t]	—	aPTT ratio[n,o,p]	1.5–2.0[u,v]
		Subsequent boluses	0.005–0.01 mg/kg bw[k,l,m,t]	—		
		Alternatively	—	0.005–0.01 mg/kg bw/hr[t,w]		
Argatroban[3] (MD-805, Novastan®)	Intermittent HD (every 2nd day)	Initial bolus	250 µg/kg bw	2.0 µg/kg bw/min	aPTT ratio[n,o]	1.5–3.0[q]
	Continuous HD	Initial bolus	100 µg/kg bw	0.5 (–2.0) µg/kg bw/min[x]	aPTT ratio[n,o]	1.5–2.0[u,v]

Many of the approaches discussed in this chapter have not been formally studied, none has been approved. Treatment examples are given based on a limited number of cases successfully treated with the respective regimen. The different anticoagulants thus cannot be uncritically applied in the dosage given here. The choice of anticoagulant should depend on the experience of the center and the anticoagulant monitoring available. Dosing of each alternative anticoagulant must primarily be based on a critical on-site evaluation of the risk of thrombosis *vs* the risk of bleeding. In case of acute HIT with its predominant risk of thrombosis, levels of alternative anticoagulants must be sufficiently high.

[1]Dosing on danaparoid mainly follows the recommendations of the manufacturer. For intermittent procedures, they appear adequate in clinical practice. For continuous procedures, markedly lower doses (i.e., both of the initial bolus and the continuous infusion) proved successful in ICU patients (cf. text).

[2]Compared with danaparoid, lepirudin is extremely potent in thrombin inhibition, the binding to which is irreversible, leading to an increased and prolonged bleeding risk (cf. text). To this end and provided the patient is not suffering from or at high risk of thrombotic events, lepirudin dosing should be very cautious and monitoring is to be performed sufficiently frequent. Dosage examples given herein do not reflect the SmPC; the recommended lepirudin doses given therein are generally regarded too high.

[3]In many centers, argatroban has become the alternative anticoagulant of choice in patients with renal insufficiency. Dosing for intermittent procedures follows the recommendations of the manufacturer. For continuous procedures, dosing is to be cautious, especially if performed in critically ill patients (cf. text).

[a]Monitoring the condition of the dialyzer after a HD session as well as the time required for termination of bleeding of the fistula should be included as well.

[b]Dosage given in anti-Xa units (bolus).

[c]Dosage given in parentheses for patients with body weight <55 kg.

[d]Data given in U/mL.

[e]Peak activity determined after approximately 30 min of HD; this level is not required throughout the whole HD session.

[f]Determination 30–60 min before start of the respective HD session.

[g]If fibrin deposition in the dialyzer or clots in the extracorporeal circuit occur, addition of 1500 anti-Xa units as a single bolus.

[h]Dosage given in anti-Xa units/hr (infusion).

[i]To achieve the same anti-Xa activity, smaller doses may be required in *hemodialysis* as compared with *hemofiltration*.

[j]Maintenance dosage dependent on actual anti-Xa activity; determination every 12 hr (provided that no bleeding or clotting occurs).

[k]Dosage given in mg/kg body weight for hemodialysis performed with polysulfone high-flux hemodialyzers.

[l]The dosage required to reach the target range may vary, e.g., due to residual renal function or the type of dialyzer used (cf. text).

[m]If larger doses are needed to achieve the target range or to avoid clotting of the extracorporeal circuit, changing to another type of dialyzer may be helpful.

[n]In our center aPTT is determined with the BCS coagulometer and Pathromtin SL as aPTT reagent (both Dade-Behring, Liederbach, Germany).

[o]According to the literature, alternative tests such as ECT or ACT also appear suitable for monitoring.

[p]It is unclear which test is best suited to monitor anticoagulation with r-hirudin, as no test has been prospectively evaluated in HD patients so far.

[q]A peak aPTT of 100 sec should not be exceeded.

[r]Determination in plasma by chromogenic assays.

[s]Data given in µg/mL.

[t]Dosage given for anuric patients; in case of polyuria a higher dosage may be required; the required daily dosage may vary significantly between patients.

[u]As patients requiring continuous procedures often are at an increased risk of bleeding, a lower aPTT is to be preferred (50–70 sec).

[v]To be initially controlled every 4–6 hr to avoid overdosage especially in patients at bleeding risk.

[w]In our experience a continuous infusion is more often associated with bleeding events; however, this aspect has not been prospectively studied yet.

[x]Adequate argatroban dosing in intensive care patients appears facilitated using nomograms based on actual critical illness severity score.

Abbreviations: ACT, activated clotting time; aPTT, activated partial thromboplastin time; conc., concentration; ECT, ecarin clotting time; HD, hemodialysis; HF, hemofiltration; Xa, clotting factor Xa.

bleeding risk (Greinacher et al., 2000). Control of lepirudin treatment by the aPTT is problematic: there is considerable assay variability among patients and different aPTT reagents (Nurmohamed et al., 1994; Hafner et al., 2000; Lubenow and Greinacher, 2000). In contrast to the foregoing tests, correlation between aPTT and plasma lepirudin concentration is not linear over a broad concentration range. Instead, linear correlation is observed only with lepirudin concentrations up to $0.5\,\mu g/mL$ (Nowak and Bucha, 1996), a concentration often insufficient for HD. Above this concentration, the correlation between aPTT and lepirudin concentration is poor (Nowak and Bucha, 1996; Hafner et al., 2000), especially for aPTT values >70 seconds (Lubenow and Greinacher, 2000). Nevertheless, because of its wide availability, aPTT monitoring of lepirudin treatment is likely to remain common. If available, ECT or chromogenic assays are preferred. A frequent problem in ICU patients with HIT and renal failure are low prothrombin levels, which can cause falsely high values in the aPTT and ECT during therapy with lepirudin or argatroban (risk of underdosing).

2. The elimination of lepirudin is markedly prolonged in renal impairment. Nowak and colleagues (1992) reported elimination half-lives of up to 316 hours in HD patients. Vanholder and coworkers (1997) found a prolongation of lepirudin half-life by a factor of 31 in HD patients compared with healthy controls. Both studies showed a correlation between the residual creatinine clearance (CrCl) and the lepirudin clearance, in that a minor improvement in CrCl resulted in a shorter elimination half-life of lepirudin. This was confirmed in a study of HD patients repeatedly anticoagulated with lepirudin (Bucha et al., 1999b). As with HD patients treated with danaparoid, lepirudin-treated patients remain anticoagulated during the interdialytic interval (Nowak et al., 1997).

It should be emphasized that the approved lepirudin dose as given in the manufacturer's package insert is too high and frequently leads to over-anticoagulation (Hacquard et al., 2005; Tschudi et al., 2009; Linkins et al., 2012). Whereas this already holds true for patients with normal renal function (Hacquard et al., 2005; Tschudi et al., 2009), lepirudin dosing is a particularly critical aspect in renal insufficiency. Application of a "normal" (i.e., approved) lepirudin dose in a patient with severe renal dysfunction will cause greatly increased bleeding risk lasting for a prolonged period of time. Safety analysis of the HAT trials showed a significant increase of major bleeding in patients with reduced renal function, occurring already at comparably mildly elevated serum creatinine (Lubenow et al., 2005).

Lepirudin dosing has been markedly reduced in clinical practice without significant impact on efficacy (Tschudi et al., 2009; Linkins et al., 2012). Actual guidelines for HIT patients with renal insufficiency recommend the initial lepirudin bolus either to be completely omitted (or in case of life-threatening thrombosis to be applied at a reduced dose, 0.2 mg/kg) (Linkins et al., 2012). Furthermore, lepirudin doses required to reach the aPTT target range (1.5–2.5 times baseline aPTT) appear minimal: Based on a retrospective analysis of lepirudin dose requirements in 53 patients, Tschudi and coworkers prospectively investigated markedly reduced lepirudin doses (Tschudi et al., 2009). Initial lepirudin bolus was omitted. Instead, lepirudin was administered at hourly rates of 0.08 mg/kg (CrCl >60 mL/min), 0.04 mg/kg (CrCl 30–60 mL/min), and 0.01–0.02 mg/kg (CrCl <30 mL/min), respectively. In 15 patients, this lepirudin dosing appeared both efficacious and safe (Tschudi et al., 2009). Significantly reduced lepirudin infusion rates depending on actual serum creatinine have also been recommended in the current ACCP guideline (Linkins et al., 2012). Recent case reports also underline the need to markedly reduce lepirudin dose in severe renal insufficiency (Tardy-Poncet et al., 2009; Desconclois et al., 2011).

3. In patients suffering from ARF, further deterioration or partial recovery of renal function frequently occurs (Fischer et al., 1999; Tardy-Poncet et al., 2009). Hence, lepirudin anticoagulation should be closely monitored in these patients for timely dose adjustments. Preferably, lepirudin should be given in repeated small boluses, rather than administered continuously, to minimize bleeding risk (Fischer et al., 1999; Kern et al., 1999). For the same reason, use of lepirudin permeable high-flux hemodialyzers for patients with HD-dependent ARF is recommended, especially as the patients often need vessel punctures, biopsies, or surgical interventions.

4. Pharmacokinetics of lepirudin are also influenced by the type of dialyzer used. The pharmacology of lepirudin (molecular mass ~7 kDa; volume of distribution 0.20–0.25 L/kg b.w.; low protein binding) should favor its elimination by high-flux hemodialyzers with a nominal cutoff point of approximately 60 kDa. Indeed, most high-flux hemodialyzers are permeable to lepirudin, whereas most of the low-flux hemodialyzers tested appear to be lepirudin impermeable (Bucha et al., 1999a; Frank et al., 1999, 2002; Koster et al., 2000; Benz et al., 2007). However, high-flux hemodialyzers vary considerably in their capacity to filter lepirudin (Fischer, 2002; Willey et al., 2002). Furthermore, a specific type of hemophan low-flux dialyzer has been reported to show high permeability for lepirudin (Nowak et al., 1997), whereas a specific type of polysulfone high-flux dialyzer, with a cutoff point of approximately 50 kDa, did not eliminate lepirudin from the circulation (Vanholder et al., 1997). Thus, knowledge of the actual filtration characteristics for lepirudin of a specific type of hemodialyzer improves safety of treatment with lepirudin in HD.

Given the prolonged half-life of lepirudin in renal impairment, use of polyethylene glycol–hirudin (molecular mass 17 kDa), which has an even greater elimination half-life compared with uncoupled lepirudin (Pöschel et al., 2000), does not seem appropriate for HD, as bleeding risk likely would be increased.

5. As there is repetitive exposure to lepirudin when used for regular, intermittent HD, immunogenicity of lepirudin is of particular interest. Initially, lepirudin appeared to be a weak immunogen (Bichler et al., 1991). However, recent studies revealed frequent development of antihirudin antibodies (aHAb) in patients receiving lepirudin for more than five days (Huhle et al., 1999, 2001; Song et al., 1999; Eichler et al., 2000; Lubenow et al., 2005). In addition, allergic reactions (including fatal anaphylaxis) to lepirudin have been reported (Huhle et al., 1998; Eichler et al., 2000; Greinacher et al., 2003).

Studies of HIT patients treated with lepirudin suggest that aHAb reduce renal lepirudin clearance (Huhle et al., 1999; Eichler et al., 2000). Indeed, marked reduction of renal lepirudin clearance due to monoclonal aHAb has been demonstrated in rats with normal renal function (Fischer et al., 2003). This was accompanied by a significant increase of both maximal plasma concentration and area under the curve of the alternative anticoagulant when compared with non–aHAb-treated animals. Accumulation of lepirudin by aHAb at normal renal function has also been reported in humans, requiring repetitive reduction of lepirudin dose (Linnemann et al., 2010). In chronic renal failure patients undergoing HD this may not be an issue. However, even small reductions in residual renal function have been shown to account for relevant prolongation of lepirudin decay in plasma (Vanholder et al., 1997; Bucha et al., 1999b). Further reduction of renal lepirudin clearance due to aHAb thus may influence lepirudin dosing in these patients.

In ARF requiring HD treatment for a prolonged period, reduction of renal lepirudin clearance attributable to aHAb may be more relevant. Here, in patients suffering from multiorgan failure, the lepirudin dosage required for sufficient anticoagulation is to be reduced significantly compared with the dosage needed in patients with normal renal function. In addition, lepirudin dosage varied markedly depending on the residual renal function (Fischer et al., 1999). aHAb are likely to further reduce the amount of lepirudin required, and thus may complicate anticoagulation in this challenging patient population.

The animal study also showed a significant decrease in the volume of distribution of lepirudin at steady state in the presence of aHAb (Fischer et al., 2003). Hence, even if further reduction of renal lepirudin clearance owing to aHAb was negligible, major alterations in lepirudin plasma concentration could still occur.

Given the risk of anaphylactic reactions and the impairment of pharmacokinetics by aHAb, re-application of lepirudin should be carefully considered, even if a first treatment period was uneventful. In this regard, risk–benefit considerations for repetitive lepirudin application in HD patients remain uncertain. As to pharmacokinetics and immunogenicity, argatroban appears a more suitable long-term treatment option.

6. Lepirudin overdosing or unexpected drug accumulation can lead to severe bleeding (Kern et al., 1999; Müller et al., 1999; Fischer et al., 2000). In this situation, lepirudin can be removed from the circulation using hemofiltration (Bauersachs, 1999; Fischer et al., 2000; Mon et al., 2006). However, several hours may be needed to lower lepirudin plasma levels by 50%, even at high ultrafiltration rates. Thus, careful lepirudin dosing is of utmost importance. Recent case reports have shown application of recombinant factor VIIa to be of additional value in patients suffering from renal insufficiency and postoperative bleeding upon lepirudin anticoagulation (Hein et al., 2005; Oh et al., 2006). In the presence of aHAb, hemofiltration may no longer suffice to eliminate lepirudin (Fischer et al., 2003). Here, plasmapheresis may be the only means to clear lepirudin from the circulation. Preliminary studies in animals suggest that a theoretic treatment might be use of certain aHAb with lepirudin-neutralizing capacity (Liebe et al., 2001).

Table 18.2 lists dosing examples of lepirudin for RRT (cf. also Keeling et al., 2006; Davenport, 2009; Syed and Reilly, 2009; Linkins et al., 2012). These dosing examples should not be followed uncritically in any individual patient. If not experienced in this area, the treating physician is advised to consult an appropriate expert.

In summary, lepirudin is a valid alternative anticoagulant for HD procedures in HIT patients, but it should be used with caution and careful monitoring.

Argatroban
Argatroban (Novastan; MD-805) is a potent arginine-derived, synthetic, catalytic site-directed thrombin inhibitor lacking antiplatelet and antifibrinolytic activities (Matsuo et al., 1992; Koide et al., 1995). This agent is approved as an alternative anticoagulant for HIT in the United States, Canada, and a number of European countries. It does not cross-react with HIT antibodies. Apart from an even better relative ability to inhibit fibrin-bound *versus* soluble thrombin (Berry et al., 1996; Lunven et al., 1996), the principal advantages of argatroban over heparin are similar to lepirudin (Markwardt, 1991; Matsuo et al., 1992). Some of the characteristics of argatroban should be specifically addressed:

1. In contrast to (renally eliminated) lepirudin, argatroban is excreted primarily by the liver. Argatroban half-life is only moderately extended in patients with renal insufficiency: In patients with CrCl of 0–29 mL/min, argatroban half-life is 64 ± 35 minutes compared with 47 ± 22 minutes in patients with CrCl > 80 mL/min ($P = 0.58$) (Swan and Hursting, 2000). Although a correlation of CrCl and aPTT-adjusted argatroban dose has been described (Arpino and Hallisey, 2004; Guzzi et al., 2006), a recent retrospective analysis of multicenter trial data suggests this correlation is not of clinical significance (Guzzi et al., 2006), as argatroban dose adjustments were found not to be necessary in patients with renal impairment (Tang et al., 2005; Guzzi et al., 2006).

   In a retrospective analysis of 269 patients with clinically diagnosed HIT treated with argatroban, renal impairment was found not to constitute a risk factor for major bleeding (Hursting and Verme-Gibboney, 2008). An evaluation of argatroban anticoagulation during percutaneous coronary intervention (PCI) in 219 patients with or at risk of HIT did not reveal an association between CrCl (as estimated with the Cockcroft–Gault equation) and initial activated clotting time (ACT) or mean argatroban infusion dose (Hursting and Jang, 2010). Whether renal dysfunction prolongs decay of argatroban effect in this patient population remains to be discussed: Although significant, the approximately 17 minutes slower ACT effect decay after argatroban cessation per 30 mL/min CrCl decrease was influenced by two extreme values and not detected in the HIT group. Argatroban was well tolerated in PCI patients with renal impairment (Hursting and Jang, 2010). One may conclude from these published data that argatroban dosing as given by the manufacturer's package insert (i.e., continuous iv argatroban infusion at a rate of 2 µg/kg/min) is adequate in patients with stable renal dysfunction. However, current consensus guidelines favor reduced infusion rates (Alatri et al., 2012; Linkins et al., 2012).

2. After argatroban proved to be a valuable anticoagulant in HD (Matsuo et al., 1986), it was applied successfully to HIT patients undergoing this procedure (Matsuo et al., 1992; Koide et al., 1995). Concerning intermittent HD, a prospective crossover study of 13 maintenance HD patients compared three different argatroban dosing regimens (250 µg/kg bolus alone, with an additional 250 µg/kg bolus allowed; 250 µg/kg bolus followed by 2 µg/kg/min infusion, or 2 µg/kg/min infusion at steady state with initiation of argatroban infusion 4 hours before dialysis) to be safe and well tolerated (Murray et al., 2004). In a retrospective analysis of 47 patients with HIT and renal failure requiring RRT (with at least 11 patients receiving CVVHD or

arteriovenous HD), argatroban provided effective anticoagulation with an acceptable safety profile (Reddy et al., 2005). Initially, argatroban was given according to current dosing recommendations used for the prophylaxis or treatment of thrombosis in HIT, that is, $2\,\mu g/kg/min$ (or $0.5\,\mu g/kg/min$ if hepatically impaired), adjusted to target aPTT range 1.5- to 3-times baseline. To reach this target aPTT range, argatroban dosing had to be more frequently adjusted downward than upward. To successfully run a HD session in patients on continuous argatroban anticoagulation with sufficient aPTT prolongation, usually no additional argatroban bolus and no increase of argatroban dose is required.

3. Alternative anticoagulation with argatroban in critically ill patients requires specific attention. In ICU patients, to reach the intended aPTT target range, significantly smaller argatroban doses may be required depending on the specific clinical situation (Koster et al., 2007a; Alatri et al., 2012). Apart from the known influence of hepatic impairment, heart failure leading to hepatic congestion, severe anasarca, the postoperative period, and/or multiple organ failure may additionally play a significant role in this setting (de Denus and Spinler, 2003; Reichert et al., 2003; Guzzi et al., 2006). Especially in multiple organ failure and after cardiac surgery, argatroban dosing to reach the aPTT target range may be small (Reichert et al., 2003; Beiderlinden et al., 2007; Saugel et al., 2010). Argatroban dose nomograms—based on the respective critical illness severity scores (APACHE II, SAPS II, SOFA)—have been developed from recent study data, which may help to individually adjust argatroban anticoagulation (Link et al., 2009a,b; Alatri et al., 2012).

   Recently, data have been published regarding RRT in the ICU: In critically ill patients with ARF at high risk of bleeding, intermittent HD procedures can successfully be performed at reduced argatroban dose (Sun et al., 2011). For CRRT in ICU patients, likewise, argatroban dose requirements are significantly reduced (Koster et al., 2007b; Link et al., 2009a,b). To control argatroban anticoagulation and especially to avoid over-anticoagulation with increased bleeding risk, aPTT should frequently be measured in ICU patients. Again, dosing of the alternative anticoagulant primarily depends on the individual clinical situation. If, for example, ICU patients suffer from life-threatening thrombotic events, initial argatroban anticoagulation nonetheless may be required at full dose.

4. Dialytic argatroban clearance by high-flux hemodialyzer membranes is regarded as clinically insignificant (Murray et al., 2004; Tang et al., 2005). However, as both low-flux and high-flux membranes show significant argatroban sieving (Krieger et al., 2007), hemofiltration appears to be a suitable rescue measure if rapid removal of argatroban is required, for example, in the case of bleeding or accidental overdose.

5. Argatroban has also proved safe and effective in HD patients with antithrombin deficiency (Ota et al., 2003). Whether anticoagulation with argatroban alone is always sufficient to prevent clotting in the extracorporeal circuit is unclear: In one HD patient treated with argatroban, marked spontaneous platelet aggregation occurred, perhaps due to HIT together with additional platelet activation known to occur in HD (Koide et al., 1995). Because platelet aggregation could not be suppressed by argatroban alone in this patient, aspirin was added to achieve patency of the extracorporeal circuit.

6. Periodic monitoring of the anticoagulant activity of argatroban is recommended (Matsuo et al., 1992), for example, using the aPTT (Matsuo et al., 1992; Koide et al., 1995), the ECT (Berry et al., 1998), or the ACT (Murray et al., 2004; Tang et al., 2005). Frequent aPTT measurements especially are recommended in ICU patients.

Table 18.2 lists dosing of argatroban for RRT (cf. also Davenport, 2009; Syed and Reilly, 2009; Linkins et al., 2012). These dosing suggestions should not be followed uncritically in any individual patient. If not experienced in this area, the treating physician is advised to consult an appropriate expert.

In summary, argatroban appears to be well suited for anticoagulation of HIT patients requiring HD. Its predominant hepatic elimination favors argatroban for alternative anticoagulation in chronic renal failure. With regard to the complicated clinical setting of ICU patients suffering from ARF requiring intermittent or CRRT, alternative anticoagulation with argatroban is feasible. However, careful argatroban dosing, close monitoring, and respective clinical expertise is needed.

Vitamin K Antagonists

For HIT patients requiring long-term anticoagulation, vitamin K antagonists (coumarins) are usually given (after recovery of the platelet count). Although coumarins decrease hemostasis and thrombosis, fibrin formation within the extracorporeal circuit is not always sufficiently blocked. In these cases, additional low-dose iv anticoagulation with UFH is usually given for regular maintenance HD. However, in HIT patients requiring HD, alternative low-dose anticoagulation has not been formally studied. The need for additional iv anticoagulation depends on the increase of the INR, which should be checked regularly before HD. Priming of the extracorporeal circuit by addition of a compatible anticoagulant to the filling solution with subsequent washout before start of the respective HD session may be of value in diminishing the risk of "over-anticoagulation." An alternative option is regional citrate anticoagulation.

Other Approaches

Bivalirudin

Bivalirudin constitutes a synthetic DTI with a molecular mass of 2.18 kDa (Warkentin et al., 2008), being licensed for PCI and treatment of unstable angina/non-ST elevation myocardial infarction planned for urgent or early intervention in the United States and the European countries. The half-life of bivalirudin is approximately 25 minutes, which is the shortest half-life of the marketed DTIs. In contrast to lepirudin and argatroban, elimination of bivalirudin is predominantly by proteolysis, and only 20% is renally excreted. Despite this, a correlation of bivalirudin dose with CrCl has been established (Runyan et al., 2011). Reduction of bivalirudin dosing is required depending on the degree of renal insufficiency (Tsu et al., 2011; Wisler et al., 2012). Bivalirudin anticoagulation has also been evaluated in intermittent hemodialysis (IHD, $n = 24$), sustained low-efficiency daily diafiltration (SLEDD, $n = 12$), and CRRT ($n = 5$). Compared with patients with normal renal function, dose reduction was required in all three modalities (IHD, 0.07; SLEDD, 0.09; CRRT, 0.07 mg/kg/hr) (Tsu et al., 2011). To achieve systemic anticoagulation in HD patients, bivalirudin dosing has been given as a 1 mg/kg bolus followed by an infusion starting at 0.25 mg/kg/hr, further being adjusted to achieve an aPTT ratio of 1.5–2.5 (Davenport, 2009). It should be noted, however, that bivalirudin has not been licensed for HD procedures. Moreover, in Europe, bivalirudin is contraindicated in patients with severe renal insufficiency (CrCl < 30 mL/min) and in dialysis-dependent patients. In addition, sharing 12 amino acid residues with lepirudin, cross-reactivity with aHAb may constitute an additional risk. In summary, bivalirudin anticoagulation is feasible in patients with renal insufficiency. However, given the availability of other alternative anticoagulants, its use currently cannot be advocated.

Fondaparinux

Fondaparinux constitutes a synthetic pentasaccharide, which binds to antithrombin, thereby enhancing the inactivation of factor Xa. An elimination half-life of 17–21 hours enables once-daily dosing (Nagler et al., 2012). As fondaparinux is predominantly eliminated by the kidneys in unchanged form (Donat et al., 2002), this drug accumulates with declining renal function: In patients with a GFR <60 mL/min and <30 mL/min (estimated by the MDRD GFR equation) fondaparinux clearance was decreased by 25% and 43%, respectively (Turpie et al., 2009). In patients with moderate renal impairment (GFR 30–60 mL/min), fondaparinux at a dose of 1.5 mg resulted in a drug exposure being comparable to 2.5 mg in patients with normal renal function (Turpie et al., 2009).

Successful fondaparinux anticoagulation in HD patients has been described in several case reports, each demonstrating that fondaparinux dose reduction is required (Haase et al., 2005; Sharathkumar et al., 2007; Wellborn-Kim et al., 2010). A recent study on fondaparinux use in 12 stable maintenance HD patients showed a predialysis fondaparinux dose of 0.05 mg/kg to result in peak anti-Xa activity of 0.61 ± 0.14 µg/L after the first dose to 0.89 ± 0.24 µg/L after a ninth dose. In parallel, predialysis anti-Xa activity continuously increased to 0.32 ± 0.09 µg/L (Kalicki et al., 2007). In six of the 12 patients minor bleeding problems occurred during the interdialytic interval. Therefore, although fondaparinux was applied only before dialysis (i.e., on an alternate day basis), patients were systemically anticoagulated on the days off dialysis. Comparable data have been reported in a study on 16 chronic HD patients having received 2.5 mg fondaparinux prior to start of the HD session. Again, increased anti-Xa levels were observed before the next HD session (Sombolos et al., 2008). As postdialysis anti-Xa levels were significantly higher after HD sessions with low-flux as compared with high-flux hemodialyzers, high-flux dialyzers appeared to be capable of sieving fondaparinux (Sombolos et al., 2008).

Despite high anti-Xa levels, fondaparinux appeared inferior to UFH in achieving sufficient anticoagulation within the extracorporeal circuit (Kalicki et al., 2007). As all but one HD session could be finished without changing dialyzer and/or tubing, this may be no significant issue in non-HIT patients. Given the marked prothrombotic state in HIT, however, one may question whether fondaparinux would sufficiently prevent clotting within the extracorporeal circuit when dialyzing a patient with acute HIT.

In summary, intermittent HD with fondaparinux anticoagulation is feasible. However, as suitable alternative anticoagulants are available, currently it is premature to recommend this agent for use in RRT. It should be underlined that patients on pre-dialysis bolus fondaparinux are systemically anticoagulated into the interdialytic interval, thereby increasing the risk of bleeding. Conversely, this theoretically may constitute an approach comparable to chronic oral anticoagulation, which may be of interest in HD patients with recent HIT.

Dermatan Sulfate
Dermatan sulfate is a natural glycosaminoglycan that selectively inhibits both solu-ble and fibrin-bound thrombin through potentiation of endogenous heparin cofac-tor II. It does not interfere with platelet function. Dermatan sulfate has been used successfully to anticoagulate patients with HIT (Agnelli et al., 1994), and has also been applied successfully as an anticoagulant for HD (Boccardo et al., 1997).

Nafamostat Mesilate
Nafamostat mesilate (FUT-175), a synthetic nonspecific serine protease inhibitor with a short half-life, has been evaluated for regional HD in patients at risk of bleed-ing (Akizawa et al., 1993). It has also been applied occasionally to HIT patients on HD (Koide et al., 1995). However, owing to significant clot formation at the dialyzer outlet, despite a twofold prolongation of aPTT, reported both in HIT and non-HIT patients (Matsuo et al., 1993; Koide et al., 1995; Takahashi et al., 2003), this anti-coagulant cannot currently be recommended for HD of HIT patients.

Prostacyclin
Prostacyclin (PGI_2, epoprostenol), a potent antiplatelet agent with a short half-life, has been evaluated both as a substitute for, and as an adjunct to, UFH for HD of patients with acute or chronic renal insufficiency (Turney et al., 1980; Smith et al., 1982; Samuelsson et al., 1995). Adverse effects, such as nausea, vomiting, and hypo-tension, can be avoided by dose reduction, use of bicarbonate- instead of acetate-containing dialysate, or infusion of the drug at the inlet of the extracorporeal circuit. Because of its mode of action, prostacyclin cannot inhibit activation of coagulation during HD (Rylance et al., 1985; Novacek et al., 1997). Moreover, in a HIT patient receiving CVVHD, prostacyclin was unable to suppress platelet consumption effec-tively after heparin had been reinstituted, owing to a false-negative platelet aggre-gation assay (Samuelsson et al., 1995). Prostacyclin thus does not seem to be a suitable antithrombotic agent for HD in HIT. Whether it may be a useful adjunct in selected cases remains to be clarified.

Regional Citrate Anticoagulation
Anticoagulation by regional citrate is based on the concept of inhibition of clotting by chelation of ionized calcium, and it was first developed as an alternative antico-agulant regimen in HD patients at risk of bleeding (Pinnick et al., 1983). Metabolic alkalosis, hypernatremia, alterations in calcium homeostasis, and hyperalbumin-emia are reported side effects that are generally manageable (Ward and Mehta, 1993; Flanigan et al., 1996; Janssen et al., 1996). Regional citrate anticoagulation is a valuable approach in experienced centers. Efficient and safe long-term citrate anti-coagulation in a HIT patient over a period of nine months was reported (Unver et al., 2002). Regional citrate anticoagulation is a treatment option only in patients with a history of HIT as it does not suppress the prothrombotic state in acute HIT.

RESUMPTION OF HEPARIN ANTICOAGULATION FOR HEMODIALYSIS IN A PATIENT WITH PREVIOUS HIT

HIT antibodies are surprisingly transient, and usually become undetectable within a few weeks or months following an episode of HIT (Davenport, 2009; Wanaka et al., 2010; Warkentin and Kelton, 2001). Moreover, after their disappearance, the antibodies do not usually recur (or are regenerated in low levels) if a deliberate rechallenge with heparin is administered, such as for cardiac or vascular surgery (Pötzsch et al., 2000; Warkentin and Kelton, 2001). This experience at least suggests the possibility that resumption of heparin for HD may be feasible too following an episode of HIT. In contrast, however, in some patients HIT antibodies persist for years (Hartman et al., 2006), which could result in life-threatening complications upon heparin rechallenge (Davenport, 2009). Different centers have reported strategies to re-institute heparin (Hartman et al., 2006; Davenport, 2009; Wanaka et al., 2010). After confirmation of HIT antibody seronegativity, heparin was resumed [either UFH (Wanaka et al., 2010) or LMWH (Hartman et al., 2006; Davenport, 2009)]. In all three small cohorts, this approach was successful, with none of the patients developing recurrent HIT. However, before rechallenge with LMWH and, possibly, UFH for HD anticoagulation can be recommended, carefully designed studies are necessary, balancing the costs and risks of indefinite anticoagulation with nonheparin agents against the potential risk of recurrent HIT.

SUMMARY

An alternative anticoagulant is required for HD in patients with HIT. Available agents are danaparoid sodium and the DTIs lepirudin and argatroban. Dosing of these agents is an ongoing critical task, especially in critically ill patients. As experience with these agents has been gained with a limited number of patients, larger prospective trials are desirable to define the best treatment options in this setting. Bivalirudin and fondaparinux constitute additional agents, the role of which has to be further defined in the future. Even today, though, HIT should no longer be a life-threatening problem for patients requiring dialysis.

REFERENCES

Agnelli G, Iorio A, De Angelis V, Nenci GG. Dermatan sulphate in heparin-induced thrombocytopenia. Lancet 344: 1295–1296, 1994.

Akizawa T, Koshikawa S, Ota K, Kazama M, Mimura N, Hirasawa Y. Nafamostat mesilate: a regional anticoagulant for hemodialysis in patients at high risk for bleeding. Nephron 64: 376–381, 1993.

Alatri A, Armstrong AE, Greinacher A, Koster A, Kozek-Langenecker SA, Lancé MD, Link A, Nielsen JD, Sandset PM, Spanjersberg AJ, Spannagl M. Results of a consensus meeting on the use of argatroban in patients with heparin-induced thrombocytopenia requiring antithrombotic therapy – a European Perspective. Thromb Res 129: 426–433, 2012.

Ambühl PM, Wüthrich RP, Korte W, Schmid L, Krapf R. Plasma hypercoagulability in haemodialysis patients: impact of dialysis and anticoagulation. Nephrol Dial Transplant 12: 2355–2364, 1997.

Arpino PA, Hallisey RK. Effect of renal function on the pharmacodynamics of argatroban. Ann Pharmacother 38: 25–29, 2004.

Asmis LM, Segal JB, Plantinga LC, Fink NE, Kerman JS, Kickler TS, Coresh J, Gardner LB. Heparin-induced antibodies and cardiovascular risk in patients on dialysis. Thromb Haemost 100: 498–504, 2008.

Basmadjian D, Sefton MV, Baldwin SA. Coagulation on biomaterials in flowing blood: some theoretical considerations. Biomaterials 18: 1511–1522, 1997.

Bauersachs RM, Lindhoff-Last E, Ehrly AM, Betz C, Geiger H, Hauser IA. Treatment of hirudin overdosage in a patient with chronic renal failure. Thromb Haemost 81: 323–324, 1999.

Beiderlinden M, Treschan TA, Görlinger K, Peters J. Argatroban anticoagulation in critically ill patients. Ann Pharmacother 41: 749–754, 2007.

Beijering RJR, ten Gate H, Nurmohamed MT, ten Cate JW. Anticoagulants and extracorporeal circuits. Semin Thromb Hemost 23: 225–233, 1997.

Benz K, Nauck MA, Böhler J, Fischer KG. Hemofiltration of recombinant hirudin by different hemodialyzer membranes: implications for clinical use. Clin J Am Soc Nephrol 2: 470–476, 2007.

Berry CN, Girardot C, Lecoffre C, Lunven C. Effects of the synthetic thrombin inhibitor argatroban on fibrin- or clot-incorporated thrombin: comparison with heparin and recombinant hirudin. Thromb Haemost 72: 381–386, 1996.

Berry CN, Lunven C, Girardot C, Lechaire I, Girard D, Charles MC, Ferrari P, O'Brien DP. Ecarin clotting time: a predictive coagulation assay for the anti-thrombotic activity of argatroban in the rat. Thromb Haemost 79: 228–233, 1998.

Bichler J, Gemmerli R, Fritz H. Studies for revealing a possible sensitization to hirudin after repeated intravenous injections in baboons. Thromb Res 61: 39–51, 1991.

Blaufox MD, Hampers CL, Merrill JP. Rebound anticoagulation occurring after regional heparinization for hemodialysis. Trans Am Soc Artif Intern Organs 12: 207–209, 1966.

Boccardo P, Melacini D, Rota S, Mecca G, Boletta A, Casiraghi F, Gianese F. Individualized anticoagulation with dermatan sulphate for haemodialysis in chronic renal failure. Nephrol Dial Transplant 12: 2349–2354, 1997.

Boon DMS, van Vliet HHDM, Zietse R, Kappers-Klunne MC. The presence of antibodies against a PF4-heparin complex in patients on haemodialysis. Thromb Haemost 76: 480, 1996.

Bredlich RO, Stracke S, Gall H, Proebstle TM. Heparin-associated platelet aggregation syndrome with skin necrosis during haemodialysis. Dtsch Med Wochenschr 122: 328–332, 1997.

Bucha E, Kreml R, Nowak G. In vitro study of r-hirudin permeability through membranes of different haemodialyzers. Nephrol Dial Transplant 14: 2922–2926, 1999a.

Bucha E, Nowak G, Czerwinski R, Thieler H. r-Hirudin as anticoagulant in regular hemodialysis therapy: finding of therapeutic r-hirudin blood/plasma concentrations and respective dosages. Clin Appl Thromb Hemost 5: 164–170, 1999b.

Burgess JK, Chong BH. The platelet proaggregating and potentiating effects of unfractionated heparin, low molecular weight heparin and heparinoid in intensive care patients and healthy controls. Eur J Haematol 58: 279–285, 1997.

Carrier M, Knoll GA, Kovacs MJ, Moore JC, Fergusson D, Rodger MA. The prevalence of antibodies to the platelet factor 4-heparin complex and association with access thrombosis in patients on chronic hemodialysis. Thromb Res 120: 215–220, 2007.

Carrier M, Rodger MA, Fergusson D, Doucette S, Kovacs MJ, Moore J, Kelton JG, Knoll GA. Increased mortality in hemodialysis patients having specific antibodies to the platelet factor 4-heparin complex. Kidney Int 73: 213–219, 2007.

Chang JJ, Parikh CR. When heparin causes thrombosis: significance, recognition, and management of heparin-induced thrombocytopenia in dialysis patients. Semin Dial 19: 297–304, 2006.

Chong BH, Magnani HN. Orgaran in heparin-induced thrombocytopenia. Haemostasis 22: 85–91, 1992.

Chong BH, Ismail F, Cade J, Gallus AS, Gordon S, Chesterman CN. Heparin-induced thrombocytopenia: studies with a new low molecular weight heparinoid, Org 10172. Blood 73: 1592–1596, 1989.

Danhof M, De Boer A, Magnani HN, Stiekema JC. Pharmacokinetic considerations of Orgaran (Org 10172) therapy. Haemostasis 22: 73–84, 1992.

Davenport A. Sudden collapse during haemodialysis due to immune-mediated heparin-induced thrombocytopaenia. Nephrol Dial Transplant 21: 1721–1724, 2006.

Davenport A. Antibodies to heparin-platelet factor 4 complex: pathogenesis, epidemiology, and management of heparin-induced thrombocytopenia in hemodialysis. Am J Kidney Dis 54: 361–374, 2009.

De Denus S, Spinler SA. Decreased argatroban clearance unaffected by hemodialysis in anasarca. Ann Pharmacother 37: 1237–1240, 2003.

De Pont AC, Hofstra JJ, Pik DR, Meijers JC, Schultz MJ. Pharmacokinetics and pharmacodynamics of danaparoid during continuous venovenous hemofiltration: a pilot study. Crit Care 11: R102, 2007.

De Sancho M, Lema MG, Amiral J, Rand J. Frequency of antibodies directed against heparinplatelet factor 4 in patients exposed to heparin through chronic hemodialysis. Thromb Haemost 75: 695–696, 1996.

Desconclois C, Ract C, Boutekedjiret T, Alhenc-Gelas M, Duranteau J, Dreyfus M, Proulle V. Heparin-induced thrombocytopenia: successful biological and clinical management with lepirudin despite severe renal impairment. Thromb Haemost 105: 568–569, 2011.

Donat F, Duret JP, Santoni A, Cariou R, Necciari J, Magnani H, de Greef R. The pharmacokinetics of fondaparinux sodium in healthy volunteers. Clin Pharmacokinet 41(Suppl 2): 1–9, 2002.

Eichler P, Friesen HJ, Lubenow N, Jaeger B, Greinacher A. Antihirudin antibodies in patients with heparin-induced thrombocytopenia treated with lepirudin: incidence, effects on aPTT, and clinical relevance. Blood 96: 2373–2378, 2000.

Fischer KG. Hirudin in renal insufficiency. Semin Thromb Hemost 28: 4674–4682, 2002.

Fischer KG, van de Loo A, Böhler J. Recombinant hirudin (lepirudin) as anticoagulant in intensive care patients treated with continuous hemodialysis. Kidney Int 56(Suppl 72): S46–S50, 1999.

Fischer KG, Weiner SM, Benz K, Nauck M, Böhler J. Treatment of hirudin overdose with hemofiltration [abstr]. Blood Purif 18: 80–81, 2000.

Fischer KG, Liebe V, Hudek R, Piazolo L, Haase KK, Borggrefe M, Huhle G. Anti-hirudin antibodies alter pharmacokinetics and pharmacodynamics of recombinant hirudin. Thromb Haemost 89: 973–982, 2003.

Flanigan MJ, Pillsbury L, Sadewasser G, Lim VS. Regional hemodialysis anticoagulation: hypertonic trisodium citrate or anticoagulant citrate dextrose-A. Am J Kidney Dis 27: 519–524, 1996.

Frank RD, Farber H, Stefanidis I, Lanzmich R, Kierdorf HP. Hirudin elimination by hemofiltration: a comparative in vitro study of different membranes. Kidney Int 56(Suppl 72): S41–S45, 1999.

Frank RD, Farber H, Lazmich R, Floege J, Kierdorf HP. In vitro studies on hirudin elimination by haemofiltration: comparison of three high-flux membranes. Nephrol Dial Transplant 17: 1957–1963, 2002.

Gajra A, Vajpayee N, Smith A, Poiesz BJ, Narsipur S. Lepirudin for anticoagulation in patients with heparin-induced thrombocytopenia treated with continuous renal replacement therapy. Am J Hematol 82: 391–393, 2007.

Gregorini G, Bellandi D, Martini G, Volpi R. Heparin-induced thrombocytopenia syndrome and thrombosis in patients undergoing periodic haemodialysis. G Ital Nefrol 19: 672–692, 2002.

Greinacher A, Drost W, Michels I, Leitl J, Gottsmann M, Kohl HJ, Glaser M, Mueller-Eckhardt C. Heparin-associated thrombocytopenia: successful therapy with the heparinoid Org 10172 in a patient showing cross-reaction to LMW heparins. Ann Hematol 64: 40–42, 1992a.

Greinacher A, Michels I, Mueller-Eckhardt C. Heparin-associated thrombocytopenia: the antibody is not heparin specific. Thromb Haemost 67: 545–549, 1992b.

Greinacher A, Philippen KH, Kemkes-Matthes B, Möckl M, Mueller-Eckhardt C, Schaefer K. Heparin-associated thrombocytopenia type II in a patient with end-stage renal disease: successful anticoagulation with the low molecular weight heparinoid Org 10172 during haemodialysis. Nephrol Dial Transplant 8: 1176–1177, 1993.

Greinacher A, Zinn S, Wizemann U, Birk W. Heparin-induced antibodies as a risk factor for thromboembolism and haemorrhage in patients undergoing chronic haemodialysis. Lancet 348: 764, 1996.

Greinacher A, Eichler P, Lubenow N, Kwasny H, Luz M. Heparin-induced thrombocytopenia with thromboembolic complications: meta-analysis of 2 prospective trials to assess the value of parenteral treatment with lepirudin and its therapeutic aPTT range. Blood 96: 846–851, 2000.

Greinacher A, Lubenow N, Eichler P. Anaphylactic and anaphylactoid reactions associated with lepirudin in patients with heparin-induced thrombocytopenia. Circulation 108: 2062–2065, 2003.

Griessbach U, Stürzebecher J, Markwardt F. Assay of hirudin in plasma using a chromogenic thrombin substrate. Thromb Res 37: 347–350, 1985.

Gupta AK, Kovacs MJ, Sauder DN. Heparin-induced thrombocytopenia. Ann Pharmacother 32: 55–59, 1998.

Guzzi LM, McCollum DA, Hursting MJ. Effect of renal function on argatroban therapy in heparin-induced thrombocytopenia. J Thromb Thrombolysis 22: 169–176, 2006.

Haas G. Versuche der Blutauswaschung am Lebenden mit Hilfe der Dialyse. Klin Wochen-schr 4: 13–14, 1925.

Haase M, Bellomo R, Rocktaeschel J, Ziemer S, Kiesewetter H, Morgera S, Neumayer HH. Use of fondaparinux (ARIXTRA) in a dialysis patient with symptomatic heparin-induced thrombocytopaenia type II. Nephrol Dial Transplant 20: 444–446, 2005.

Hacquard M, de Maistre E, Lecompte T. Lepirudin: is the approved dosing schedule too high? J Thromb Haemost 3: 2593–2596, 2005.

Hafner G, Peetz D, Klingel R, Prellwitz W. Methods for hirudin determination in plasma. J Lab Med 24: 172–178, 2000.

Hafner G, Roser M, Nauck M. Methods for the monitoring of direct thrombin inhibitors. Semin Thromb Hemost 28: 425–430, 2002.

Hall AV, Clark WF, Parbtani A. Heparin-induced thrombocytopenia in renal failure. Clin Nephrol 38: 86–89, 1992.

Hartman V, Malbrain M, Daelemans R, Meersman P, Zachee P. Pseudo-pulmonary embolism as a sign of acute heparin-induced thrombocytopenia in hemodialysis patients: safety of resuming heparin after disappearance of HIT antibodies. Nephron Clin Pract 104: c143–c148, 2006.

Hein OV, von Heymann C, Morgera S, Konertz W, Ziemer S, Spies C. Protracted bleeding after hirudin anticoagulation for cardiac surgery in a patient with HIT II and chronic renal failure. Artif Organs 29: 507–510, 2005.

Henny CP, ten Cate H, ten Cate JW, Surachno S, Van Bronswijk H, Wilmink JM, Ockelford PA. Use of a new heparinoid as anticoagulant during acute haemodialysis of patients with bleeding complications. Lancet 1: 890–893, 1983.

Henny CP, ten Cate H, Surachno S, Stevens P, Büller HR, den Hartog M, ten Cate JW. The effectiveness of a low molecular weight heparinoid in chronic intermittent haemodialysis. Thromb Haemost 54: 460–462, 1985.

Hertel J, Keep DM, Caruana RJ. Anticoagulation. In: Daugirdas JT, Blake PG, Ing TS, eds. Handbook of Dialysis, 3rd edn. Boston: Little, Brown, 182–198, 2001.

Holmes CE, Huang JC, Cartelli C, Howard A, Rimmer J, Cushman M. The clinical diagnosis of heparin-induced thrombocytopenia in patients receiving continuous renal replacement therapy. J Thromb Thrombolysis 27: 406–412, 2009.

Horellou MH, Conard I, Lecrubier C, Samama M, Roque-D'Orbcastel O, de Fenoyl O, Di Maria G, Bernadou A. Persistent heparin induced thrombocytopenia despite therapy with low molecular weight heparin. Thromb Haemost 51: 134, 1984.

Huhle G, Hoffmann U, Wang L, Bayerl C, Harenberg J. Allergy and positive IgG in a patient reexposed to r-hirudin [abstr]. Ann Hematol 76(Suppl 1): A97, 1998.

Huhle G, Hoffmann U, Song X, Wang LC, Heene DL, Harenberg J. Immunologic response to recombinant hirudin in HIT type II patients during long-term treatment. Br J Haematol 106: 195–201, 1999.

Huhle G, Liebe V, Hudek R, Heene DL. Anti-r-hirudin antibodies reveal clinical relevance through direct functional inactivation of r-hirudin or prolongation of r-hirudin's plasma halflife. Thromb Haemost 85: 936–938, 2001.

Hursting MJ, Verme-Gibboney CN. Risk factors for major bleeding in patients with heparin-induced thrombocytopenia treated with argatroban: a retrospective study. J Cardiovasc Pharmacol 52: 561–566, 2008.

Hursting MJ, Jang IK. Impact of renal function on argatroban therapy during percutaneous coronary intervention. J Thromb Thrombolysis 29: 1–7, 2010.

Hutchison CA, Dasgupta I. National survey of heparin-induced thrombocytopenia in the haemodialysis population of the UK population. Nephrol Dial Transplant 22: 1680–1684, 2007.

Janson PA, Moake JL, Carpinito G. Aspirin prevents heparin-induced platelet aggregation in vivo. Br J Haematol 53: 166–168, 1983.

Janssen MJFM, Deegens JK, Kapinga TH, Beukhof JR, Huijgens PC, Van Loenen AC, Van der Meulen J. Citrate compared to low molecular weight heparin anticoagulation in chronic hemodialysis patients. Kidney Int 49: 806–813, 1996.

Kadidal VV, Mayo DJ, Home MK. Heparin-induced thrombocytopenia (HIT) due to heparin flushes: a report of three cases. J Intern Med 246: 325–329, 1999.

Kalicki RM, Aregger F, Alberio L, Lämmle B, Frey FJ, Uehlinger DE. Use of the pentasaccharide fondaparinux as an anticoagulant during haemodialysis. Thromb Haemost 98: 1200–1207, 2007.

Kappa JR, Fisher CA, Berkowitz HD, Cottrel ED, Addonizio VP. Heparin-induced platelet activation in sixteen surgical patients: diagnosis and management. J Vasc Surg 5: 101–109, 1987.

Kato S, Takahashi K, Ayabe K, Samad R, Fukaya E, Friedmann P, Varma M, Bergmann SR. Heparin-induced thrombocytopenia: analysis of risk factors in medical inpatients. Br J Haematol 154: 373–377, 2011.

Keeling D, Davidson S, Watson H. Haemostasis and Thrombosis Task Force of the British committee for standards in haematology. Br J Haematol 133: 259–269, 2006.

Kern H, Ziemer S, Kox WJ. Bleeding after intermittent or continuous r-hirudin during CVVH. Intensive Care Med 25: 1311–1314, 1999.

Koide M, Yamamoto S, Matsuo M, Suzuki S, Arima N, Matsuo T. Anticoagulation for heparin-induced thrombocytopenia with spontaneous platelet aggregation in a patient requiring haemodialysis. Nephrol Dial Transplant 10: 2137–2140, 1995.

Koster A, Merkle F, Hansen R, Loebe M, Kuppe H, Hetzer R, Crystal GJ, Mertzlufft F. Elimination of recombinant hirudin by modified ultrafiltration during simulated cardiopulmonary bypass: assessment of different filter systems. Anesth Analg 91: 265–269, 2000.

Koster A, Fischer KG, Harder S, Mertzlufft F. The direct thrombin inhibitor argatroban: a review of its use in patients with and without HIT. Biologics 1: 105–112, 2007a.

Koster A, Hentschel T, Groman T, Kuppe H, Hetzer R, Harder S, Fischer KG. Argatroban anticoagulation for renal replacement therapy in patients with heparin-induced thrombocytopenia after cardiovascular surgery. J Thorac Cardiovasc Surg 133: 1376–1377, 2007b.

Krauel K, Fürll B, Warkentin TE, Weitschies W, Kohlmann T, Sheppard JI, Greinacher A. Heparin-induced thrombocytopenia—therapeutic concentrations of danaparoid, unlike fondaparinux and direct thrombin inhibitors, inhibit formation of platelet factor 4-heparin complexes. J Thromb Haemost 6: 2160–2167, 2008.

Krauel K, Hackbarth C, Fürll B, Greinacher A. Heparin-induced thrombocytopenia: in vitro studies on the interaction of dabigatran, rivaroxaban, and low-sulfated heparin, with platelet factor 4 and anti-PF4/heparin antibodies. Blood 119: 1248–1255, 2012.

Krieger D, Geisen U, Is A, Fischer KG. Hemodialyzer membranes allow for removal of argatroban [abstr]. J Thromb Haemost 5(Suppl 2): P-S-669, 2007.

Lasocki S, Piednoir P, Ajzenberg N, Geffroy A, Benbara A, Montravers P. Anti-PF4/heparin antibodies associated with repeated hemofiltration-filter clotting: a retrospective study. Crit Care 12: R84, 2008.

Laster J, Elfrink R, Silver D. Reexposure to heparin of patients with heparin-associated antibodies. J Vasc Surg 9: 677–682, 1989.

Leblanc M, Roy LF, Legault L, Dufresne LR, Morin C, Thuot C. Severe skin necrosis associated with heparin in hemodialysis. Nephron 68: 133–137, 1994.

Lewis BE, Walenga JM, Wallis DE. Anticoagulation with Novastan (argatroban) in patients with heparin-induced thrombocytopenia and heparin-induced thrombocytopenia and thrombosis syndrome. Semin Thromb Hemost 23: 197–202, 1997.

Liebe V, Piazolo L, Fischer KG, Hudek R, Heene DL, Huhle G. A monoclonal mouse anti-r-hirudin antibody neutralizes r-hirudin in vivo—potential use as antidote [abstr]. Ann Hematol 80(Suppl 1): A42, 2001.

Lindhoff-Last E, Betz C, Bauersachs R. Use of a low molecular weight heparinoid (danaparoid sodium) for continuous renal replacement therapy in intensive care patients. Clin Appl Thromb Hemost 7: 300–304, 2001.

Link A, Girndt M, Selejan S, Mathes A, Böhm M, Rensing H. Argatroban for anticoagulation in continuous renal replacement therapy. Crit Care Med 37: 105–110, 2009a.

Link A, Selejan S, Mathes A, Böhm M, Rensing H. Argatroban for anticoagulation in continuous renal replacement therapy (the authors reply). Crit Care Med 37: 2139–2140, 2009b.

Linkins LA, Dans AL, Moores LK, Bona R, Davidson BL, Schulman S, Crowther M. Treatment and prevention of heparin-induced thrombocytopenia: Antithrombotic Therapy and Prevention of Thrombosis, 9th ed: American College of Chest Physicians Evidence-Based Clinical Practice Guidelines. Chest 141(2 Suppl): e495S–e530S, 2012.

Linnemann B, Greinacher A, Lindhoff-Last E. Alteration of pharmacokinetics of lepirudin caused by anti-lepirudin antibodies occurring after long-term subcutaneous treatment in a patient with recurrent VTE due to Behcets disease. Vasa 39: 103–107, 2010.

Lubenow N, Greinacher A. Heparin-induced thrombocytopenia. Recommendations for optimal use of recombinant hirudin. BioDrugs 14: 109–125, 2000.

Lubenow N, Eichler P, Lietz T, Greinacher A; Hit Investigators Group. Lepirudin in patients with heparin-induced thrombocytopenia - results of the third prospective study (HAT-3) and a combined analysis of HAT-1, HAT-2, and HAT-3. J Thromb Haemost 3: 2428–2436, 2005.

Lunven C, Gauffeny C, Lecoffre C, O'Brien DP, Roome NO, Berry CN. Inhibition by argatroban, a specific thrombin inhibitor, of platelet activation by fibrin clot-associated thrombin. Thromb Haemost 75: 154–160, 1996.

Luzzatto G, Bertoli M, Cella G, Fabris F, Zaia B, Girolami A. Platelet count, anti-heparin/platelet factor 4 antibodies and tissue factor pathway inhibitor plasma antigen level in chronic dialysis. Thromb Res 89: 115–122, 1998.

Magnani HN. Heparin-induced thrombocytopenia (HIT): an overview of 230 patients treated with Orgaran (Org 10172). Thromb Haemost 70: 554–561, 1993.

Magnani HN. A review of 122 published outcomes of danaparoid anticoagulation for intermittent hemodialysis. Thromb Res 125: e171–e176, 2010.

Magnani HN, Gallus A. Heparin-induced thrombocytopenia (HIT). A report of 1,478 clinical outcomes of patients treated with danaparoid (Orgaran) from 1982 to mid-2004. Thromb Haemost 95: 967–981, 2006.

Markwardt F. Past, present and future of hirudin. Haemostasis 21: 11–26, 1991.

Matsuo T, Nakao K, Yamada T, Matsuo O. Effect of a new anticoagulant (MD 805) on platelet activation in the hemodialysis circuit. Thromb Res 41: 33–41, 1986.

Matsuo T, Yamada T, Chikahira Y, Kadowaki S. Effect of aspirin on heparin-induced thrombocytopenia (HIT) in a patient requiring hemodialysis. Blut 59: 393–395, 1989.

Matsuo T, Kario K, Kodama K, Okamoto S. Clinical application of the synthetic thrombin inhibitor, argatroban (MD-805). Semin Thromb Hemost 18: 155–160, 1992.

Matsuo T, Kario K, Nakao K, Yamada T, Matsuo M. Anticoagulation with nafamostat mesilate, a synthetic protease inhibitor, in hemodialysis patients with a bleeding risk. Haemostasis 23: 135–141, 1993.

Matsuo T, Koide M, Kario K. Application of argatroban, a direct thrombin inhibitor, in heparin-intolerant patients requiring extracorporeal circulation. Artif Organs 21: 1035–1038, 1997.

Matsuo T, Kobayashi H, Matsuo M, Wanaka K, Nakamoto H, Matsushima H, Sakai R. Frequency of anti-heparin-PF4 complex antibodies (HIT antibodies) in uremic patients on chronic intermittent hemodialysis. Pathophysiol Haemost Thromb 35: 445–450, 2006.

Matsuo T, Wanaka K, Miyasita K, Prechel M, Walenga JM. Clinical evaluation of acute systemic reaction and detection of IgG antibodies against PF4/heparin complexes in hemodialysis patients. Thromb Res 129: 474–478, 2012.

Moberg PQ, Geary VM, Sheikh FM. Heparin-induced thrombocytopenia: a possible complication of heparin-coated pulmonary artery catheters. J Cardiothorac Anesth 4: 226–228, 1990.

Mon C, Moreno G, Ortiz M, Diaz R, Herrero JC, Oliet A, Rodriguez I, Ortega O, Gallar P, Vigil A. Treatment of hirudin overdosage in a dialysis patient with heparin-induced thrombocytopenia with mixed hemodialysis and hemofiltration treatment. Clin Nephrol 66: 302–305, 2006.

Müller A, Huhle G, Nowack R, Birck R, Heene DL, van der Woude FJ. Serious bleeding in a haemodialysis patient treated with recombinant hirudin. Nephrol Dial Transplant 14: 2482–2483, 1999.

Mureebe L, Coats RD, Silliman WR, Shuster TA, Nichols WK, Silver D. Heparin-associated antiplatelet antibodies increase morbidity and mortality in hemodialysis patients. Surgery 136: 848–853, 2004.

Murray PT, Reddy BV, Grossman EJ, Hammes MS, Trevino S, Ferrell J, Tang I, Hursting MJ, Shamp TR, Swan SK. A prospective comparison of three argatroban treatment regimens during hemodialysis in end-stage renal disease. Kidney Int 66: 2446–2453, 2004.

Nagler M, Haslauer M, Wuillemin WA. Fondaparinux – data on efficacy and safety in special situations. Thromb Res 129: 407–417, 2012.

Nakamoto H, Shimada Y, Kanno T, Wanaka K, Matsuo T, Suzuki H. Role of platelet factor 4-heparin complex antibody (HIT antibody) in the pathogenesis of thrombotic episodes in patients on hemodialysis. Hemodial Int 9(Suppl 1): S2–S7, 2005.

Neuhaus TJ, Gotschel P, Schmugge M, Leumann E. Heparin-induced thrombocytopenia type II on hemodialysis: switch to danaparoid. Pediatr Nephrol 14: 713–716, 2000.

Newman PM, Swanson RL, Chong BH. IgG binding to PF4-heparin complexes in the fluid phase and cross-reactivity with low molecular weight heparin and heparinoid. Thromb Haemost 80: 292–297, 1998.

Novacek G, Kapiotis S, Jilma B, Quehenberger P, Michitsch A, Traindl O, Speiser W. Enhanced blood coagulation and enhanced fibrinolysis during hemodialysis with prostacyclin. Thromb Res 88: 283–290, 1997.

Nowak G, Bucha E. Quantitative determination of hirudin in blood and body fluids. Semin Thromb Hemost 22: 197–202, 1996.

Nowak G, Bucha E, Gööck T, Thieler H, Markwardt F. Pharmacology of r-hirudin in renal impairment. Thromb Res 66: 707–715, 1992.

Nowak G, Bucha E, Brauns I, Czerwinski R. Anticoagulation with r-hirudin in regular haemodialysis with heparin-induced thrombocytopenia (HIT II). The first long term application of r-hirudin in a haemodialysis patient. Wien Klin Wochenschr 109: 354–358, 1997.

Nurmohamed MT, Berckmans RJ, Morriën-Salomons WM, Berends F, Hommes DW, Rijnierse JJMM, Sturk A. Monitoring anticoagulant therapy by activated partial thromboplastin time: hirudin assessment. Thromb Haemost 72: 685–692, 1994.

Oh JJ, Akers WS, Lewis D, Ramaiah C, Flynn JD. Recombinant factor VIIa for refractory bleeding after cardiac surgery secondary to anticoagulation with the direct thrombin inhibitor lepirudin. Pharmacotherapy 26: 569–577, 2006.

Ortel TL, Gockermann JP, Califf RM, McCann RL, O'Connor CM, Metzler DM, Greenberg CS. Parenteral anticoagulation with the heparinoid Lomoparan (Org 10172) in patients with heparin-induced thrombocytopenia and thrombosis. Thromb Haemost 67: 292–296, 1992.

O'Shea SI, Sands JJ, Nudo SA, Ortel TL. Frequency of anti-heparin-platelet factor 4 antibodies in hemodialysis patients and correlation with recurrent vascular access thrombosis. Am J Hematol 69: 72–73, 2002.

O'Shea SI, Ortel TL, Kovalik EC. Alternative methods of anticoagulation for dialysis-dependent patients with heparin-induced thrombocytopenia. Semin Dial 16: 61–67, 2003.

Ota K, Akizawa T, Hirasawa Y, Agishi T, Matsui N. Effects of argatroban as an anticoagulant for haemodialysis in patients with antithrombin III deficiency. Nephrol Dial Transplant 18: 1623–1630, 2003.

Palomo I, Pereira J, Alarcon M, Diaz G, Hidalgo P, Pizarro I, Jara E, Rojas P, Quiroga G, Moore-Carrasco R. Prevalence of heparin-induced antibodies in patients with chronic renal failure undergoing hemodialysis. J Clin Lab Anal 19: 189–195, 2005.

Peña de la Vega L, Miller RS, Benda MM, Grill DE, Johnson MG, McCarthy JT, McBane RD 2nd. Association of heparin-dependent antibodies and adverse outcomes in hemodialysis patients: a population-based study. Mayo Clin Proc 80: 995–1000, 2005.

Perry SL, Whitlatch NL, Ortel TL. Heparin-dependent platelet factor 4 antibodies and the impact of renal function on clinical outcomes: a retrospective study in hospitalized patients. J Thromb Thrombolysis 28: 146–150, 2009.

Pinnick RV, Wiegmann TB, Diederich DA. Regional citrate anticoagulation for hemodialysis in the patient at high risk for bleeding. N Engl J Med 308: 258–261, 1983.

Polgár J, Eichler P, Greinacher A, Clemetson KJ. Adenosine diphosphate (ADP) and ADP receptor play a major role in platelet activation/aggregation induced by sera from heparin-induced thrombocytopenia patients. Blood 91: 549–554, 1998.

Polkinghorne KR, McMahon LP, Becker GJ. Pharmacokinetic studies of dalteparin (Fragmin), enoxaparin (Clexane), and danaparoid sodium (Orgaran) in stable chronic hemodialysis patients. Am J Kidney Dis 40: 990–995, 2002.

Pöschel KA, Bucha E, Esslinger HU, Nörtersheuser P, Jansa U, Schindler S, Nowak G, Stein G. Pharmacodynamics and pharmacokinetics of polyethylene glycol-hirudin in patients with chronic renal failure. Kidney Int 58: 2478–2484, 2000.

Pötzsch B, Klövekorn WP, Madlener K. Use of heparin during cardiopulmonary bypass in patients with a history of heparin-induced thrombocytopenia. N Engl J Med 343: 515, 2000.

Reddy BV, Grossman EJ, Trevino SA, Hursting MJ, Murray PT. Argatroban anticoagulation in patients with heparin-induced thrombocytopenia requiring renal replacement therapy. Ann Pharmacother 39: 1601–1605, 2005.

Reichert MG, MacGregor DA, Kincaid EH, Dolinski SY. Excessive argatroban anticoagulation for heparin-induced thrombocytopenia. Ann Pharmacother 37: 652–654, 2003.

Roe SD, Cassidy MJD, Haynes AP, Byrne JL. Heparin-induced thrombocytopenia (HIT) and thrombosis in a haemodialysis-dependent patient with systemic vasculitis. Nephrol Dial Transplant 13: 3226–3229, 1998.

Romao JE Jr, Fadil MA, Sabbaga E, Marcondes M. Haemodialysis without anticoagulant: haemostasis parameters, fibrinogen kinetic, and dialysis efficiency. Nephrol Dial Transplant 12: 106–110, 1997.

Roussi JH, Houbouyan LL, Goguel AF. Use of low molecular weight heparin in heparin-induced thrombocytopenia with thrombotic complications. Lancet 1: 1183, 1984.

Runyan CL, Cabral KP, Riker RR, Redding D, May T, Seder DB, Savic M, Hedlund J, Abramson S, Fraser GL. Correlation of bivalirudin dose with creatinine clearance during treatment of heparin-induced thrombocytopenia. Pharmacotherapy 31: 850–856, 2011.

Rylance PB, Gordge MP, Ireland H, Lane DA, Weston MJ. Haemodialysis with prostacyclin (epoprostenol) alone. Proc Eur Dial Transplant Assoc Eur Renal Assoc 21: 281–286, 1985.

Samuelsson O, Amiral J, Attman P-O, Bennegard K, Björck S, Larsson G, Tengborn L. Heparin-induced thrombocytopenia during continuous haemofiltration. Nephrol Dial Transplant 10: 1768–1771, 1995.

Saner F, Hertl M, Broelsch CE. Anticoagulation with hirudin for continuous veno-venous hemodialysis in liver transplantation. Acta Anaesthesiol Scand 45: 914–918, 2001.

Saugel B, Phillip V, Moessmer G, Schmid RM, Huber W. Argatroban therapy for heparin-induced thrombocytopenia in ICU patients with multiple organ dysfunction syndrome: a retrospective study. Crit Care 14: R90, 2010.

Schmitt GW, Moake JL, Rudy CK, Vicks SL, Hamburger RJ. Alterations in hemostatic parameters during hemodialysis with dialyzers of different membrane composition and flow design. Platelet activation and factor VII-related von Willebrand factor during hemodialysis. Am J Med 83: 411–418, 1987.

Schneider T, Heuer B, Deller A, Boesken WH. Continuous haemofiltration with r-hirudin (lepirudin) as anticoagulant in a patient with heparin induced thrombocytopenia (HIT II). Wien Klin Wochenschr 112: 552–555, 2000.

Schneider SA, Nauck MS, Nauck MA, Fischer KG. Only plasmapheresis allows for danaparoid elimination from blood [abstr]. Kidney Blood Press Res 27: a360, 2004.

Selleng K, Selleng S, Raschke R, Schmidt CO, Rosenblood GS, Greinacher A, Warkentin TE. Immune heparin-induced thrombocytopenia can occur in patients receiving clopidogrel and aspirin. Am J Hematol 78: 188–192, 2005.

Selleng K, Warkentin TE, Greinacher A. Heparin-induced thrombocytopenia in intensive care patients. Crit Care Med 35: 1165–1176, 2007.

Sharathkumar AA, Crandall C, Lin JJ, Pipe S. Treatment of thrombosis with fondaparinux (Arixtra) in a patient with end-stage renal disease receiving hemodialysis therapy. J Pediatr Hematol Oncol 29: 581–584, 2007.

Sitter T, Spannagl M, Banas B, Schiffl H. Prevalence of heparin-induced PF4-heparin antibodies in hemodialysis patients. Nephron 79: 245–246, 1998.

Smith MC, Danviriyasup K, Crow JW, Cato AE, Park GD, Hassid A, Dunn MJ. Prostacyclin substitution for heparin in long-term hemodialysis. Am J Med 73: 669–678, 1982.

Sombolos KI, Fragia TK, Gionanlis LC, Veneti PE, Bamichas GI, Fragidis SK, Georgoulis IE, Natse TA. Use of fondaparinux as an anticoagulant during hemodialysis: a preliminary study. Int J Clin Pharmacol Ther 46: 198–203, 2008.

Song X, Huhle G, Wang L, Hoffmann U, Harenberg J. Generation of anti-hirudin antibodies in heparin-induced thrombocytopenic patients treated with r-hirudin. Circulation 100: 1528–1532, 1999.

Sreedhara R, Itagaki I, Lynn B, Hakim RM. Defective platelet aggregation in uremia is transiently worsened by hemodialysis. Am J Kidney Dis 25: 555–563, 1995.

Steuer S, Boogen C, Plum J, Deppe C, Reinauer H, Grabensee B. Anticoagulation with r-hirudin in a patient with acute renal failure and heparin-induced thrombocytopenia. Nephrol Dial Transplant 14(Suppl 4): 45–47, 1999.

Sun X, Chen Y, Xiao Q, Wang Y, Zhou J, Ma Z, Xiang J, Chen X. Effects of argatroban as an anticoagulant for intermittent veno-venous hemofiltration (IVVH) in patients at high risk of bleeding. Nephrol Dial Transplant 26: 2954–2959, 2011.

Swan SK, Hursting MJ. The pharmacokinetics and pharmacodynamics of argatroban: effects of age, gender, and hepatic or renal dysfunction. Pharmacotherapy 20: 318–329, 2000.

Syed S Reilly RF. Heparin-induced thrombocytopenia: a renal perspective. Nat Rev Nephrol 5: 501–511, 2009.

Takahashi H, Muto S, Nakazawa E, Yanagiba S, Masunaga Y, Miyata Y, Tamba K, Kusano E, Matsuo M, Matsuo T, Asano Y. Combined treatment with nafamostat mesilate and aspirin prevents heparin-induced thrombocytopenia in a hemodialysis patient. Clin Nephrol 59: 458–462, 2003.

Tang IY, Cox DS, Patel K, Reddy BV, Nahlik L, Trevino S, Murray PT. Argatroban and renal replacement therapy in patients with heparin-induced thrombocytopenia. Ann Pharmacother 39: 231–236, 2005.

Tardy-Poncet B, Charier D, Diconne E, Zeni F, Garraud O, Tardy B, Campos L. Extremely low doses of lepirudin in a patient with heparin-induced thrombocytopenia, high bleeding risk and renal insufficiency. Br J Haematol 146: 456–457, 2009.

Tholl U, Greinacher A, Overdick K, Anlauf M. Life-threatening anaphylactic reaction following parathyroidectomy in a dialysis patient with heparin-induced thrombocytopenia. Nephrol Dial Transplant 12: 2750–2755, 1997.

Tschudi M, Lämmle B, Alberio L. Dosing lepirudin in patients with heparin-induced thrombocytopenia and normal or impaired renal function: a single-center experience with 68 patients. Blood 113: 2402–2409, 2009.

Tsu LV, Dager WE. Bivalirudin dosing adjustments for reduced renal function with or without hemodialysis in the management of heparin-induced thrombocytopenia. Ann Pharmacother 45: 1185–1192, 2011.

Turney JH, Williams LC, Fewell MR, Parsons V, Weston MJ. Platelet protection and heparin sparing with prostacyclin during regular dialysis therapy. Lancet 2: 219–222, 1980.

Turpie AG, Lensing AW, Fuji T, Boyle DA. Pharmacokinetic and clinical data supporting the use of fondaparinux 1.5 mg once daily in the prevention of venous thromboembolism in renally impaired patients. Blood Coagul Fibrinolysis 20: 114–121, 2009.

Unver B, Sunder-Plassmann G, Hörl WH, Apsner R. Long-term citrate anticoagulation for high-flux haemodialysis in a patient with heparin-induced thrombocytopenia type II. Acta Med Austriaca 29: 146–148, 2002.

Vanholder RC, Camez AA, Veys NM, Soria J, Mirshahi M, Soria C, Ringoir S. Recombinant hirudin: a specific thrombin inhibiting anticoagulant for hemodialysis. Kidney Int 45: 1754–1759, 1994.

Vanholder R, Camez A, Veys N, van Loo A, Dhondt AM, Ringoir S. Pharmacokinetics of recombinant hirudin in hemodialyzed end-stage renal failure patients. Thromb Haemost 77: 650–655, 1997.

Van Wyk V, Badenhorst PN, Luus HG, Kotze HF. A comparison between the use of recombinant hirudin and heparin during hemodialysis. Kidney Int 48: 1338–1343, 1995.

Vargas Hein O, von Heymann C, Lipps M, Ziemer S, Ronco C, Neumayer HH, Morgera S, Welte M, Kox WJ, Spies C. Hirudin versus heparin for anticoagulationin continuous renal replacement therapy. Intensive Care Med 27: 673–679, 2001.

Vecino A, Navarro-Antolin J, Teruel J, Navarro J, Cesar J. Lipid composition of platelets in patients with uremia. Nephron 78: 271–273, 1998.

Vun CM, Evans S, Chong BH. Cross-reactivity study of low molecular weight heparins and heparinoid in heparin-induced thrombocytopenia. Thromb Res 81: 525–532, 1996.

Wanaka K, Matsuo T, Matsuo M, Kaneko C, Miyashita K, Asada R, Matsushima H, Nakajima Y. Re-exposure to heparin in uremic patients requiring hemodialysis with heparin-induced thrombocytopenia. J Thromb Haemost 8: 616–618, 2010.

Ward DM, Mehta RL. Extracorporeal management of acute renal failure patients at high risk of bleeding. Kidney Int 43(Suppl): S237–S244, 1993.

Warkentin TE. Danaparoid (Orgaran) for the treatment of heparin-induced thrombocytopenia (HIT) and thrombosis: effects on in vivo thrombin and cross-linked fibrin generation, and evaluation of the clinical significance of in vitro cross-reactivity (XR) of danaparoid for HIT-IgG [abstr]. Blood 88: 626a, 1996.

Warkentin TE. Hemodialysis-associated acute systemic reactions and heparin-induced thrombocytopenia. Thromb Res 129: 405–406, 2012

Warkentin TE, Kelton JG. A 14-year study of heparin-induced thrombocytopenia. Am J Med 101: 502–507, 1996.

Warkentin TE, Kelton JG. Temporal aspects of heparin-induced thrombocytopenia. N Engl J Med 344: 1286–1292, 2001.

Warkentin TE, Chong BH, Greinacher A. Heparin-induced thrombocytopenia: towards consensus. Thromb Haemost 79: 1–7, 1998.

Warkentin TE, Levine MN, Hirsh J, Horsewood P, Roberts RS, Gent M, Kelton JG. Heparin-induced thrombocytopenia in patients treated with low molecular weight heparin or unfractionated heparin. N Engl J Med 332: 1330–1335, 1995.

Warkentin TE, Greinacher A, Koster A. Bivalirudin. Thromb Haemost 99: 830–839, 2008.

Wellborn-Kim JJ, Mitchell GA, Terneus WF Jr, Stowe CL, Malias MA, Sparkman GM, Hanson GW. Fondaparinux therapy in a hemodialysis patient with heparin-induced thrombocytopenia type II. Am J Health Syst Pharm 67: 1075–1079, 2010.

Wilde MI, Markham A. Danaparoid. A review of its pharmacology and clinical use in the management of heparin-induced thrombocytopenia. Drugs 54: 903–924, 1997.

Willey ML, de Denus S, Spinier SA. Removal of lepirudin, a recombinant hirudin, by hemodialysis, hemofiltration, or plasmapheresis. Pharmacotherapy 22: 492–499, 2002.

Wisler JW, Washam JB, Becker RC. Evaluation of dose requirements for prolonged bivalirudin administration in patients with renal insufficiency and suspected heparin-induced thrombocytopenia. J Thromb Thrombolysis 33: 287–295, 2012.

Yamamoto S, Koide M, Matsuo M, Suzuki S, Ohtaka M, Saika S, Matsuo T. Heparin-induced thrombocytopenia in hemodialysis patients. Am J Kidney Dis 28: 82–85, 1996.

19

Management of intraoperative anticoagulation in patients with heparin-induced thrombocytopenia undergoing cardiovascular surgery

Andreas Koster and Sixten Selleng

INTRODUCTION

Immediate cessation of, and avoidance of reexposure to, heparin are important principles underlying the management of patients with immune-mediated heparin-induced thrombocytopenia (HIT) (Chong and Berndt, 1989). Because further antithrombotic therapy is often necessary for these patients, several alternative anti-coagulant strategies have been developed (see chaps. 12–17). However, patients with HIT who require cardiac surgery present exceptional problems. Apart from the inherent disturbances of the hemostatic system in this patient population, considerable activation of the hemostatic system results from the surgical trauma itself. Furthermore, during cardiopulmonary bypass (CPB), there is exposure of blood to the large nonendothelial surfaces of the CPB circuit and reinfusion of tissue factor-activated blood aspirated from the operative field into the CPB system. This profound hemostatic activation requires potent high-dose anticoagulation to prevent thrombosis within both the CPB system and the patient (Edmunds, 1993; Slaughter et al., 1994). Anticoagulation with unfractionated heparin (UFH), point-of-care monitoring by activated clotting time (ACT) systems, and reversal via the antidote protamine comprise a long-standing and well-established strategy permitting cardiac surgery. This approach is so universally entrenched that there is very minor experience with all other forms of anticoagulation in this patient setting.

With regard to vascular surgery, dramatic changes in practice and technique have occurred in recent years. In particular, a large number of procedures, which classically were performed exclusively as "open" surgery, are now increasingly managed as percutaneous endovascular interventional (PEVI) procedures. Examples are the treatment of abdominal and thoracic aneurysms with endovascular stent-prostheses and stenting in peripheral vascular intervention. Due to the similarity of such procedures with percutaneous coronary intervention (PCI), where alternative anticoagulants and particularly the direct thrombin inhibitors (DTIs) have been assessed in large multicenter trials, dosing protocols have been translated into the world of PEVI procedures and from there into classic vascular surgery.

In this chapter, alternative anticoagulation strategies for cardiac surgery with and without CPB, and for PEVI and classic vascular surgery will be discussed. The underlying premise is that performing cardiac surgery with UFH in a patient who has acute HIT or who has platelet-activating antibodies at the time of cardiac surgery is dangerous. However, this might not be true. Thousands of patients undergo cardiac surgery each year and presumably many of them have clinically significant antibodies present at the time of cardiac surgery. Yet, to our knowledge, no one has reported intraoperative thrombotic events due to precipitating acute HIT in patients undergoing cardiac surgery. On the contrary, there is an intriguing report of a patient who was proved in retrospect to have been in the early phase of acute HIT at the time of cardiac surgery that was performed as per routine with UFH (Fig. 19.1). This patient suffered no intraoperative adverse events, and was diagnosed as having HIT when the platelet count continued to fall during the early postoperative period. It is possible that the very high doses of heparin given during cardiac surgery are somewhat protective against consequences of HIT, perhaps for

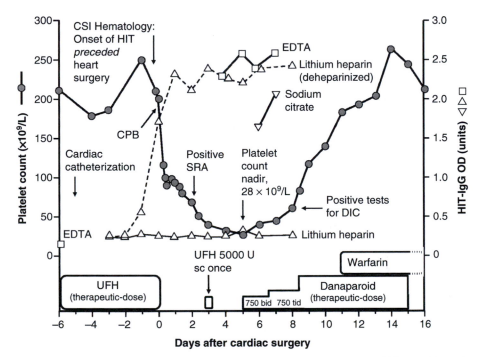

FIGURE 19.1 Clinical course of a 67-year-old female patient who developed HIT coincident with cardiac surgery. The patient presented with acute heart failure (severe mitral valve regurgitation). She received therapeutic-dose UFH for six days pre–cardiac surgery. Progressive thrombocytopenia led to testing for HIT antibodies on POD 2, with strong positive SRA reported on POD8. Testing for DIC on POD8 was positive; with danaparoid dosing increased to therapeutic, DIC markers improved/normalized. Serial HIT-IgG levels (by EIA) were performed using as-yet-undiscarded blood samples from different laboratories: hematology/transfusion medicine (EDTA), coagulation (sodium citrate), chemistry (lithium heparin). Ecteola cellulose was needed to remove heparin from the lithium heparin-anticoagulated plasma, giving interpretable EIA-IgG results. Elucidating the precise timeline of anti-PF4/H IgG seroconversion showed that acute HIT had commenced (with 20% platelet count fall) on the morning of surgery. *Abbreviations*: bid, twice daily; CPB, cardiopulmonary bypass; CSI, clinical sample investigation; DIC, disseminated intravascular coagulation; EDTA, ethylene diamine tetraacetic acid; HIT, heparin-induced thrombocytopenia; OD, optical density; POD, postoperative day; SRA, serotonin release assay; UFH, unfractionated heparin. *Source*: From Warkentin and Sheppard, 2006.

at least three reasons: (*i*) high heparin concentrations can inhibit HIT antibody-induced platelet activation; (*ii*) the high heparin concentrations control thrombin generation or the effects of thrombin; and (*iii*) acute platelet count declines of cardiac surgery result in fewer platelets to cause HIT-related complications.

Preoperative Anti-PF4/Heparin Antibodies and Adverse Prognosis

Five studies provide information on the prognostic significance of antiplatelet factor 4/heparin (anti-PF4/H) antibodies present prior to cardiac surgery (a situation where UFH is routinely given) (for review: Yusuf et al., 2012). While no correlation was found between the preoperative presence of antibodies and the rate of postoperative thromboembolic events, two studies reported an association between preoperative presence of antibodies and postoperative *nonthrombotic* adverse events (Kress et al., 2007; Selleng et al., 2010), and together with a third study (Bennett-Guerrero et al., 2005) also found increased length-of-stay. However, only one of these studies (Selleng et al., 2010) evaluated the different antibody classes, and this study found that the association with nonthrombotic adverse events and increased length-of-stay only held for the IgM class of anti-PF4/H antibodies. As IgM antibodies do not cause HIT, the explanation for an association between anti-PF4/H antibodies and postoperative adverse events remains uncertain. Gluckmann and coworkers (2009) used multidetector computed tomography coronary angiography to assess whether preoperative or postoperative antibodies predicted for saphenous vein graft occlusion, but no association was detected.

In our view, preoperative screening for anti-PF4/H antibodies on a routine basis cannot be recommended (Warkentin et al., 2008). First, the vast majority of anti-PF4/H antibodies detected would not be expected to cause clinical HIT. Second, a causal role of preoperative antibodies for postoperative adverse events has not been established. Third, there is no evidence that alternative nonheparin anticoagulation for heart surgery is safer than for UFH, either in general or in patients with anti-PF4/H antibodies.

ALTERNATIVE STRATEGIES FOR ANTICOAGULATION IN CARDIAC SURGERY FOR PATIENTS WITH HIT

Any alternative anticoagulant considered for HIT patients in cardiac surgery should ideally meet certain requirements. First, the agent should be effective in minimizing activation of coagulation during CPB and in preventing thrombus formation. Second, a rapid and simple method of monitoring its anticoagulant effects should be available, so as to avoid inappropriate under- or over-anticoagulation. Finally, rapid and complete reversibility of the anticoagulant effects is important to minimize postoperative bleeding complications. Unfortunately, no existing agent meets all of these requirements.

A variety of approaches to perform anticoagulation in HIT patients who require cardiac surgery with and without CPB has been reported, including the use of danaparoid, the thrombin inhibitors lepirudin and bivalirudin, the combination of UFH with short-acting antiplatelet agents, such as platelet glycoprotein (GP) IIb/IIIa antagonists or prostaglandins, and the combination of UFH with plasma exchange. Experience with a planned reexposure to UFH to permit CPB in patients with a previous history of HIT, but who no longer have detectable HIT antibodies at the time of subsequent UFH reexposure, will also be discussed.

Danaparoid Sodium

Danaparoid is a low molecular weight heparinoid, which achieves its anticoagulant effect predominately by inhibition of coagulation factor Xa (see chap. 16). The plasma anti-factor Xa activity half-life is approximately 20 hours and somewhat dependent on renal function. No antidote is available. Monitoring of its anticoagulant effect is performed by measuring plasma anti-factor Xa activity.

Danaparoid has been used in various protocols for CPB anticoagulation in HIT patients (Magnani, 1993; Magnani et al., 1997; Magnani and Gallus, 2006). However, due to its long plasma elimination half-life, lack of a reversal agent, and the fact that danaparoid cannot be monitored with current point-of-care tests, such as the ACT, its use during cardiovascular surgery with CPB is problematic, including a high major bleeding rate (42%), as well as potential for CPB thrombosis due to inadequate dosing (Magnani and Gallus, 2006).

By contrast, in a controlled prospective trial comparing danaparoid (bolus of 40 U/kg) and UFH in non-HIT patients undergoing coronary artery bypass grafting (CABG) without use of CPB [so-called off-pump coronary artery bypass (OPCAB) grafting surgery], danaparoid was effective and associated with bleeding rates comparable to that seen with UFH, with only a minor increase in transfusion requirements (Carrier et al., 2003). Favorable experience with danaparoid in the setting of OPCAB for a patient with acute HIT has also been reported (Warkentin et al., 2001).

Conclusion

Based on these results, we believe that danaparoid should not be used for anticoagulation during CPB. However, danaparoid is an option in HIT patients undergoing OPCAB surgery.

Recombinant Hirudin

Recombinant hirudin (r-hirudin), a DTI naturally produced by the salivary gland of the leech (*Hirudo medicinalis*), is now approved in most countries for clinical use by the iv route. Hirudin is a single-chain polypeptide of 65 amino acids (7000 Da) that forms a tight 1:1 stoichiometric complex with thrombin. Currently, three hirudins are approved (lepirudin, desirudin, RB-hirudin), although data on use in cardiac surgery are available only for lepirudin.

Because of its potent anticoagulant effect, r-hirudin has been studied as an anticoagulant for use in open heart surgery in both dogs (Walenga et al., 1991) and pigs (Riess et al., 1997). In both animal models, effective CPB anticoagulation could be achieved by administration of r-hirudin as a bolus injection [1 mg/kg body weight (b.w.)] followed by a continuous infusion of 1 mg/kg b.w./hr, started after initiation of CPB, and continuing until end of CPB. In humans, however, recovery of hirudin in the plasma following b.w.-adjusted dosing shows a high interindividual variability (Koza et al., 1993). Therefore, a fixed-dose protocol for r-hirudin in the CPB setting bears the risk of both inadequate anticoagulation and overdosing. Although the latter is complicated by excessive and potentially fatal postoperative bleeds, the former may result in the occurrence of thromboembolic complications while on pump, including catastrophic total pump occlusion.

To establish a treatment schedule that is adjusted to the individual's response to hirudin, different monitoring systems for hirudin plasma levels have been

TABLE 19.1   Whole Blood Ecarin Clotting Time

---

50 µL citrate-anticoagulated whole blood to be analyzed
+ 50 µL standard normal human plasma
Incubate for 1 min at 37°C
+ 50 µL ecarin solution (20 U/mL) containing 0.025 M calcium chloride
Determination of the clotting time

---

investigated. Several *in vitro* and *in vivo* experiments demonstrated that the ACT and activated partial thromboplastin time were not sufficiently sensitive to monitor hirudin plasma levels (Pötzsch et al., 1997). However, reliable results were obtained by using the whole blood ecarin clotting time (ECT) (Pötzsch et al., 1997; Koster et al., 2000a).

Ecarin is a prothrombin-activating enzyme, derived from the venom of the snake, *Echis carinatus*, which activates prothrombin to an intermediate product, meizothrombin (Nishida et al., 1995). Meizothrombin expresses only moderate clotting activity, but is fully reactive toward, and thus inhibited by, hirudin. As a result, in r-hirudin-containing plasma, meizothrombin forms stable 1:1 complexes with r-hirudin. Only when hirudin is neutralized does clotting become initiated, either by meizothrombin or by subsequently generated thrombin. Ecarin is available from commercial sources.

Table 19.1 outlines the whole blood ECT method, which can be performed using the KC10a coagulometer (Pötzsch et al., 1997). The method is easily adaptable to any other coagulometer. A calibration curve is constructed by using citrate-anticoagulated whole blood spiked with r-hirudin to achieve final concentrations of 0.5, 1.0, 1.5, 2.0, 3.0, and 4.0 µg/mL. A reliable ECT requires adequate prothrombin levels, which can be reduced in severely ill patients and/or by hemodilution after beginning CPB. This problem can be overcome by mixing patient blood with normal human plasma (1:1).

Critical levels of r-hirudin during CPB were established in an *in vitro* CPB setting and in a first series of HIT patients undergoing cardiac surgery (Pötzsch et al., 1993; Riess et al., 1995, 1996). Clot formation in the CPB apparatus was seen at levels of r-hirudin below 1.8 µg/mL, and increasing levels of fibrinopeptide A (an indicator of thrombin-mediated fibrinogen cleavage) occurred at r-hirudin plasma levels less than 2.0 µg/mL. Based on these results, the therapeutic level of r-hirudin during CPB was set between 3.5 and 4.5 µg/mL. Higher intraoperative levels of r-hirudin could be complicated by a higher postoperative bleeding risk, especially because no antidote is available.

A treatment protocol based on the ECT monitoring of hirudin levels is given in Table 19.2. The data obtained from 10 patients with HIT, treated with r-hirudin for heart surgery, demonstrated that stable r-hirudin plasma levels in the range from 3.5 to 5.0 µg/mL could be obtained using the ECT-adjusted treatment schedule. Because of the relatively short half-life of r-hirudin of approximately 1 hour, plasma levels of r-hirudin declined rapidly after stopping its infusion. However, in renally impaired patients, r-hirudin can accumulate, leading to postoperative bleeding (Koster et al., 2000b). In this situation, elimination can be augmented by the use of hemofilters, for example, as modified ultrafiltration after termination of CPB (Koster et al., 2000c).

TABLE 19.2 Treatment Protocol for r-Hirudin (Lepirudin) Anticoagulation During CPB

Initial lepirudin dosing (pre-CPB)	
Initial iv lepirudin bolus	0.25 mg/kg body weight
Initiate continuous iv infusion[a]	30 mL/h (0.5 mg/min)
Lepirudin added to priming solution	0.2 mg/kg body weight
Target lepirudin plasma levels[b]	>2.5 µg/mL before start of CPB
	If <2.5 µg/mL, give additional bolus (10 mg)
Lepirudin dosing and monitoring while on CPB	
Frequency of lepirudin level monitoring	Every 15 min using ECT
Intraoperative dose adjustments, based on ECT	
Lepirudin plasma level	Dosing modification
>4.5 µg/mL	Reduce infusion rate by 10 mL/hr
3.5–4.5 µg/mL	No change in infusion rate
<3.5 µg/mL	Increase infusion rate by 10 mL/hr
Special steps toward end of CPB	
Stop lepirudin infusion 15 min before anticipated end of CPB	
After disconnection of CPB, administer 5 mg hirudin to the heart–lung machine to avoid clot formation	

[a]50 mg of lepirudin are dissolved in 50 mL 0.9% sodium chloride.
[b]The target lepirudin level pre-CPB (>2.5 µg/mL) is lower than the ones sought during CPB (3.5–4.5 µg/mL) because of the addition of lepirudin to the pump circuit volume (0.2 mg/kg body weight).
Abbreviations: CPB, cardiopulmonary bypass; ECT, ecarin clotting time; iv, intravenous.

To date, the clinical data demonstrate that r-hirudin is a suitable alternative for anticoagulation of CPB in selected HIT patients. The ECT provides adequate monitoring and allows an adjusted treatment schedule with apparently minimal risk for thrombotic problems on pump. Because of the relatively short half-life, plasma levels of r-hirudin decline rapidly after stopping its infusion. However, there are two key aspects, which must be considered for safe management of CPB with r-hirudin. As no commercial point-of-care test for measurement of the ECT is available, care must be taken that reliable measurement of the ECT in the operating room can be provided. Moreover, due to the dramatic prolongation of the r-hirudin plasma half-life to >100 hours in case of renal failure and associated risk of severe hemorrhage, only patients at low risk for postoperative renal impairment should be selected for this strategy. Moreover, hirudin should be restricted to patients who may not be exposed to heparin because the bleeding risk is increased also in patients without renal impairment (Riess et al., 2007).

The experience with the use of lepirudin for OPCAB surgery is limited to a small number of case reports. The dosages used varied from 0.2 to 0.4 mg/kg bolus followed by a continuous infusion of 0.15 mg/kg/hr (Iqbal et al., 2005). Therefore, as no adequate dose finding study has been performed to date, this strategy should only be used if no other option is available.

Conclusion

Based on current data, we conclude that lepirudin can be safely used for anticoagulation during CPB in patients with unimpaired renal function, provided there is reliable ECT monitoring. For OPCAB surgery and vascular surgery, the limited available data suggest that lepirudin should only be used if no other option is available.

Bivalirudin

Bivalirudin is a short-acting, bivalent, reversible DTI (see chap. 15). Its pharmaco-kinetics are characterized by rapid onset of effect and a short half-life of approximately 25 minutes. The drug's elimination is predominantly achieved by proteolytic cleavage and to a minor extent by renal excretion. These pharmaco-logic features, particularly its rapid elimination essentially independent of spe-cific organ involvement, render bivalirudin a potentially valuable alternative to UFH/protamine for high-dose anticoagulation during cardiac surgery with and without CPB (Warkentin and Koster, 2005).

Bivalirudin has been assessed in large trials (>40,000 patients) in patients undergoing PCI, including formal evaluation in patients with or at risk for HIT. Bivalirudin is approved by the U.S. Food and Drug Administration for angioplasty in patients with or without HIT (see chap. 15).

Based on the favorable results in PCI, a large program was started for the assessment of safety and efficacy of bivalirudin use in cardiac surgery. The first of these investigations was performed in OPCAB surgery in non-HIT patients, and involved a comparison between bivalirudin (given in the PCI dose) and UFH/protamine. This investigation revealed comparable results with respect to safety parameters, such as perioperative hemorrhage and transfusion requirements. Inter-estingly, bivalirudin demonstrated improved efficacy, as shown by enhanced graft patency (Merry et al., 2004).

A second pilot investigation assessing the use of bivalirudin in cardiac sur-gery with CPB also demonstrated an acceptable safety and efficacy profile (Koster et al., 2003a). Based on these data, dosing schemes, perfusion strategies, and moni-toring recommendations were formulated (Koster et al., 2004a, 2005; Veale et al., 2005; Zucker et al., 2005) (Table 19.3). Due to the fact that in areas of stagnant blood bivalirudin is cleaved by thrombin, surgical and perfusion practice must be adjusted to the unique pharmacology of the drug. In particular, any area of stasis within the CPB circuit must be avoided and cardiotomy suction from the operating field mini-mized whenever possible (Table 19.3).

After defining dosing protocols, and monitoring guidelines and surgical/perfusion strategies, two multicenter investigations were begun with the goal of obtaining regulatory approval for cardiac surgery in HIT patients, either with CPB (CHOOSE-ON study) or OPCAB surgery (CHOOSE-OFF study). These investigations (The acronym CHOOSE, indicates *CABG HIT/TS On-* and *Off-*Pump *Safety and Efficacy*) were accompanied by "back-up safety studies" in non-HIT patients that compared bivalirudin with UFH/protamine in OPCAB surgery (EVOLUTION-OFF study) and in CPB (EVOLUTION-ON study) sur-gery. (The acronym, EVOLUTION, indicates *EV*aluation of Patients during coro-nary artery bypass graft *O*perations: *L*inking *UT*ilization of bivalirudin to *I*mproved *O*utcomes and *N*ew anticoagulant strategies.) The two EVOLUTION studies had comparable safety and efficacy endpoints (Dyke et al., 2006; Smedira et al., 2006). Results of the CHOOSE-ON study also demonstrated an acceptable safety and efficacy profile even in patients with impaired renal function (Koster et al., 2007a). The results of the CHOOSE-OFF study also showed good results in safety and efficacy data (Dyke et al., 2007). We have also reported very good results in our single-center experience with bivalirudin anticoagulation for car-diac surgery in 141 patients, 40 of whom had heparin-dependent antibodies (Koster et al., 2009).

TABLE 19.3   Treatment Protocol for Bivalirudin Anticoagulation During CPB and OPCAB Surgery

I. CPB

Dosing of bivalirudin

Initial iv bivalirudin bolus: 1.0 mg/kg body weight and initiate continuous iv infusion: 2.5 mg/kg/hr

Bivalirudin added to pump circuit volume: 50 mg

ACT: A prolongation of ≥2.5-fold baseline ACT level (varies between different commercially available assays) indicates adequate anticoagulation with bivalirudin

Bivalirudin dosing and monitoring while on CPB

Continue iv infusion: ≥2.5 mg/kg/hr

Frequency of bivalirudin level monitoring: Every 30 min by ACT

A prolongation of ≥2.5-fold baseline ACT level (varies between different commercially available assays) indicates adequate anticoagulation with bivalirudin. Keep bivalirudin infusion rate constant, and only increase bivalirudin infusion rate if the ACT levels decrease below target (alternatively, maintain the same infusion rate but give repeat fractionated boluses of 0.25 mg/kg to maintain ACT in therapeutic range); do not reduce infusion rate if ACT exceeds target

Performance of CPB

Due to the unique pharmacology of bivalirudin, stasis in the CPB circuit should be avoided/minimized. This can be achieved by the following strategies: the use of closed systems whenever possible; the creation of shunting lines from the arterial filter to the cardiotomy reservoir; intermittent compression of the collapse venous reservoir with flushing back in the hard shell cardiotomy reservoir to provide flow of systemic blood in the cardiotomy reservoir and to maintain bivalirudin levels; storage of excessive blood in citrated bags instead of the hard shell cardiotomy reservoir; or processing excessive blood with the use of cell savers. The use of cardiotomy suction should be minimized whenever possible and replaced by the use of a cell saver to avoid aspiration and systemic infusion of "activated" blood from the operative field. If "blood cardioplegia" is used, constant flow should be provided in the lines to avoid clot formation and danger of thromboembolism of coronary arteries

Temperature

Due to the enzymatic metabolism of bivalirudin, hypothermia may lead to drug accumulation. Therefore, in the absence of a specific test to monitor bivalirudin levels, periods of hypothermia should be brief, and if possible only mild hypothermia (30–34°C.) should be instituted

Extracorporeal elimination

Bivalirudin elimination can be enhanced *after* CPB by the use of modified ultrafiltration using standard commercially available hemofilters. However, due to the possibility of eliminating bivalirudin via hemofiltration, this procedure is discouraged *during* CPB (Koster et al., 2003b, 2004a)

Management of circuit after CPB

After cessation of CPB, the venous line should be infused into the patient, the system refilled with saline, the arterial and venous line reconnected, and circulation of the closed system started to avoid stasis and thrombosis of the system. With the beginning of recirculation, a bivalirudin bolus of 50 mg, followed by a continuous infusion of 50 mg/hr, should be added to provide adequate bivalirudin concentrations. When it is definitively determined that CPB will not need to be reestablished, this volume has to be processed with a cell saver before reinfusion to avoid overdosage with bivalirudin

Cell saver

A cell saver should be used with sodium citrate as anticoagulant for flushing line

II. OPCAB surgery

Dosing of bivalirudin

Bolus: 0.75 mg/kg followed by continuous infusion of 1.75 mg/kg/hr (stop infusion approx 20 min before end of grafting)

ACT: >300 sec when measured with the ACT+ device (Hemochrone Jr, New Jersey, U.S.A.)

Considerations of graft handling

Assessments of grafts for patency and leakage should be performed with saline or, if bivalirudin-containing blood is used, grafts should thereafter be flushed with saline and "bulldogged" while applying pressure on the saline syringe. If a left or right internal thoracic artery is used for grafting, the vessel should be transected shortly before grafting in order to avoid stasis and potential risk of thrombus formation in the graft

Abbreviations: ACT, activated clotting time; CPB, cardiopulmonary bypass; OPCAB, off-pump coronary artery bypass.

Conclusion

To date bivalirudin is the only alternative anticoagulant that has been assessed in prospective trials for intraoperative anticoagulation during cardiac surgery in HIT patients. Based on the currently available data, bivalirudin can be recommended as a firstline option in HIT patients undergoing OPCAB surgery. It also is the drug-of-choice in a large variety of procedures in cardiac surgery requiring CPB, at least where experience exists in adjusting surgical and perfusion techniques to reflect the unique pharmacology of the agent (Table 19.3).

Argatroban

Argatroban is a synthetic, small-molecule (532 Da) DTI derived from L-arginine that binds reversibly to thrombin. Its half-life is about 40–50 minutes. The potential of argatroban to be an effective anticoagulant in patients with HIT has been documented by the studies of Lewis et al. (1997a,b, 2001, 2003) (see chap. 13). Its feasibility for anticoagulation of HIT patients is *after* cardiac surgery, with dosing reduced to 0.5–1 µg/kg/min (Koster et al., 2006). However, only limited information (<30 patients) is available for use during cardiac surgery (Kawada et al., 2000; Furukawa et al., 2001; Edwards et al., 2003; Kieta et al., 2003; Ohno et al., 2003; Cannon et al., 2004; Gasparovic et al., 2004; Martin et al., 2007; Azuma et al., 2010; Genzen et al., 2010) and no standardized dosing/monitoring protocol exists. Moreover, several of these cases were complicated by intraoperative thrombosis or severe postprocedure bleeding. Therefore, argatroban cannot be recommended for these indications.

Platelet Inhibition as a Strategy to Permit Heparinization for CPB

Another approach for managing CPB in a patient with acute or previous HIT is to combine full heparinization with one or more antiplatelet agents. Following surgery, an alternative nonheparin anticoagulant (e.g., a DTI or danaparoid) is initiated as soon as deemed safe.

Several groups of investigators have used iloprost for this situation (Kappa et al., 1985; Long, 1985; Palmer Smith et al., 1985; Addonizio et al., 1987; Kraenzler and Starr, 1988), following the original observation by Olinger et al. (1984) that iloprost inhibited heparin-dependent platelet activation in the presence of HIT serum. Iloprost is a stable analogue of prostacyclin; thus, it stimulates adenylate cyclase, resulting in increased platelet cAMP levels, which prevents platelet activation by various platelet agonists, including HIT antibodies. In one larger case series Antoniou et al. (2002) preoperatively determined the individual concentrations of iloprost *in vitro* to inhibit the HIT-induced platelet activation and thereafter used these individual concentrations to attenuate the HIT reaction during CPB.

This approach experienced a resurgence with epoprostenol sodium (Flolan), a freeze-dried preparation of prostacyclin itself (Mertzlufft et al., 2000; Aouifi et al., 2001). Epoprostenol is approved for use in patients with primary pulmonary hypertension. Its very short half-life (6 minutes) means that continuous iv infusion is necessary. Complete inhibition of heparin-dependent platelet aggregation by HIT antibodies is generally achieved by doses ranging from 15 to 30 ng/kg/min. One protocol that does not require intraoperative monitoring of platelet aggregation gradually increases epoprostenol infusion (in 5 ng/kg/min increments made at 5-minute intervals) until the target rate (30 ng/kg/min) is reached, whereupon standard-dose UFH anticoagulation is commenced (Aouifi et al., 2001). The epoprostenol infusion is continued until 15 minutes following reversal of UFH with protamine. The major adverse effect is vasodilatation, leading to severe hypotension that requires intraoperative vasopressors.

Another strategy is the combination of the short-acting GPIIb/IIIa inhibitor, tirofiban, with UFH for anticoagulation during CPB (Koster et al., 2000e, 2001a,b). Tirofiban is predominantly eliminated by the kidneys, and has a plasma half-life of about 2 hours. However, in contrast to prostaglandins, tirofiban exhibits no effect on vascular tone. Tirofiban is given 10 minutes before standard-dose UFH as a 10 μg/kg bolus followed by 0.15 μg/kg/min continuous infusion. The tirofiban infusion is stopped 1 hour before the end of surgery. UFH is neutralized with protamine as per usual. Using this treatment protocol, no thromboses occurred. However, in patients with severe renal impairment, tirofiban persists in the circulation and can cause major bleeding refractory to platelet transfusions: three such cases led the manufacturer to discourage use of this off-label protocol (Warkentin and Greinacher, 2003). In such patients, extracorporeal elimination of tirofiban (e.g., ultrafiltration at the end of CPB or modified zero-balanced ultrafiltration after CPB) appears to be an appropriate strategy to augment tirofiban elimination and prevent excessive hemorrhage (Koster et al., 2004b).

However, although there are no reports about thromboembolic complications following these strategies, theoretically there is a danger that HIT-associated platelet activation or thromboembolism might occur when platelet function recovers and PF4/H/IgG complexes still circulate. Therefore, immediately postoperatively iv thrombosis prophylaxis should be started with argatroban, lepirudin, or danaparoid.

With regard to OPCAB surgery and vascular surgery no data are available. In theory, UFH plus antiplatelet therapy could be used during these procedures.

Conclusion

Based on the current available data, we believe that the strategy of UFH plus antiplatelet therapy, particularly during CPB, is easy to perform and is associated with a minimal risk of bleeding complications, even in extended, complex surgeries. Tirofiban might be preferred in hemodynamically unstable or hypotensive patients, whereas prostaglandins might be advisable for procedures that also require profound reduction of the pulmonary artery pressure, such as in heart transplantation or implantation of a left ventricular assist device (VAD). However, as HIT might be only attenuated, with the theoretical potential for a prothrombotic state during recovery of platelet function, these strategies are not the first choice in a patient with acute HIT.

Concerning OPCAB surgery and vascular surgery, it should be noted that it is difficult to establish hemofiltration for augmented elimination of tirofiban intraoperatively.

Plasmapheresis as a Strategy to Permit Heparinization for CPB

Based on the experience that patients with acute HIT have been treated successfully with plasmapheresis (see chap. 12), this procedure has also been used in patients with acute HIT who required urgent CPB surgery to permit standard heparinization on CPB (Kajitani et al., 2001; Voeller et al., 2010; Welsby et al., 2010; Jaben et al., 2011). The concept is to lower the level of HIT antibodies using plasma exchange and thereby to reduce the risk of thromboembolic events with subsequent heparin exposure; this is based on the observation that anti-PF4/H antibody titers [when estimated by enzyme immunoassay (EIA) optical density] directly correlate with their platelet-activating properties in functional assays [e.g., the serotonin release assay (SRA); see chap. 11]. In order to achieve this, different approaches have been used. Some performed a 1.0 plasma volume exchange immediately before CPB with albumin and fresh frozen plasma as replacement fluids (Jaben et al., 2011), whereas others performed a series of three (Kajitani et al., 2001) or seven plasmaphereses (Voeller et al., 2010) before CPB until the HIT antibody test was negative. The authors of an 11-patient case series described intraoperative 1.3 plasma volume exchange with fresh frozen plasma as replacement fluid and thereby reduced the anti-PF4/H antibody titers (estimated with EIA optical density) by 50–84%; in all reported patients, standard heparin was used for anticoagulation during CPB without any HIT-related complications or excessive bleeding (Welsby et al., 2010).

However, none of the available reports provide functional test results, the number of patients treated with plasmapheresis before or during CPB is still small and no controlled or randomized study exists that proves the clinical utility of this approach. Unresolved questions include the timing of plasmapheresis, the kind of replacement fluid, the type of monitoring, and target endpoint of HIT antibody assessment, and the necessity and kind of postoperative anticoagulation. Nevertheless, in patients with acute HIT requiring urgent or emergent CPB surgery, pre- or intraoperative plasmapheresis in combination with standard heparinization on CPB represents a therapeutic option.

Conclusion

Plasmapheresis, using plasma as replacement fluid, as a strategy to reduce HIT antibody levels, combined with standard heparinization during CPB and postoperative nonheparin anticoagulation, is a treatment option in patients with acute HIT who require urgent or emergent CPB surgery.

USE OF HEPARIN FOR CPB IN PATIENTS WITH A PREVIOUS HISTORY OF HIT

An intriguing option for patients with a history of HIT, but in whom HIT antibodies can no longer be detected, is to consider reexposure to UFH for CPB, and to avoid heparin completely both before surgery (e.g., at heart catheterization) and in the postoperative period. This approach has been used successfully (Makhoul et al., 1987; Pötzsch et al., 2000; Selleng et al., 2001; Warkentin and Kelton, 2001), and is based on the following rationale. First, HIT antibodies are transient, and are usually not detectable after several weeks or a few months following an episode of HIT (see chap. 2). Thus, no immediate problems would be expected in a patient without residual HIT antibodies. Second, it appears that a minimum of five days are required before clinically significant levels of HIT antibodies are generated after any episode of heparin treatment (Warkentin and Kelton, 2001). In the event that a recurrent immune response to PF4/H is induced by reexposure to heparin during CPB, it is unlikely that the newly generated antibodies will contact exogenously administered heparin. As a consequence, platelet activation by HIT antibodies should not occur, and thus the thrombotic risk should not be increased. Pötzsch et al. (2000) reported 10 patients with a documented history of HIT, but no detectable HIT antibodies at the time of the proposed surgery, who thus underwent CPB anticoagulation with heparin. In none of the 10 patients was a thromboembolic complication or prolonged thrombocytopenia observed. Furthermore, no increase in anti-PF4/H antibody concentrations occurred during 10-day follow-up. These data are consistent with the findings of Warkentin and Kelton (2001), who also observed no evidence for a rapid "anamnestic" type of immune response when heparin reexposure was used as a strategy for intraoperative anticoagulation for cardiac and vascular surgery in patients with previous HIT.

We recommend that HIT antibody-negative patients with a history of HIT who require CPB for heart surgery should be treated according to established heparin protocols (Fig. 19.2). The use of heparin should be restricted to the operative period itself; if necessary, postoperative anticoagulation should be achieved with an alternative anticoagulant (see chaps. 12–17).

Testing for HIT antibodies in patients with a history of HIT before anticipated heparin reexposure at heart surgery should be performed using one or more sensitive tests (see chap. 11). Particularly in cardiac surgical centers where there is limited experience with nonheparin anticoagulation for CPB, risk–benefit considerations strongly favor a brief use of heparin for these patients. For example, a patient who developed near-fatal CPB circuit thrombosis during danaparoid anticoagulation had had HIT 11 years earlier and had no detectable HIT antibodies at the time danaparoid was used (Grocott et al., 1997). It should also be noted that the recommendation to use heparin for cardiac surgery in patients with a previous history of HIT and in whom platelet-activating HIT antibodies are no longer detectable is a strong consensus conference recommendation (Warkentin et al., 2008; Linkins et al., 2012).

Studies using EIA show that the frequency of anti-PF4/H antibody formation following heart surgery (Visentin et al., 1996; Bauer et al., 1997; Warkentin and Sheppard, 2006) is as high as 70% (see chap. 4). Even with the SRA, platelet-activating antibodies are detected in 13–20% of patients (Bauer et al., 1997; Warkentin et al., 2000). However, despite this high seroconversion rate, only about 1–2% of patients

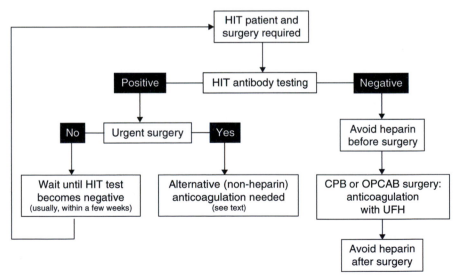

FIGURE 19.2 Algorithm for decision making for alternative anticoagulation in HIT patients. "Negative" testing for HIT antibodies includes a weak (gray zone) enzyme immunoassay result plus a negative functional test using washed platelets, such as the serotonin release assay or heparin-induced platelet activation assay (see chap. 11). *Abbreviations*: CPB, cardiopulmonary bypass; OPCAB, off-pump coronary artery bypass; UFH, unfractionated heparin.

who receive further postoperative anticoagulation with UFH develop HIT. Currently, there is no convincing evidence that patients who form anti-PF4/H antibodies in the absence of thrombocytopenia are at increased risk for thrombosis (Bauer et al., 1997; Trossaert et al., 1998; Warkentin et al., 2000). However, postoperative cardiac surgery patients who develop clinical HIT appear to be at increased risk for both venous and arterial thrombotic events (Walls et al., 1990; Van Dyck et al., 1996; Pouplard et al., 1999). Therefore, if HIT is clinically highly suspected or confirmed, an alternative nonheparin anticoagulant should be initiated (see chap. 12).

HEPARIN FOR CPB IN PATIENTS WITH *SUBACUTE* HIT

Subacute HIT is characterized by the condition after the acute phase of HIT where the platelet count has normalized but platelet-activating HIT antibodies in particular are still detectable. Schroder et al. (2007) reported the successful use of standard UFH as anticoagulant during CPB in patients who developed HIT after implantation of a left VAD (LVAD) and who underwent heart transplantation. While being on nonheparin anticoagulation before surgery, the average antibody titer (estimated with EIA optical density) decreased by >50% compared with the level when HIT was diagnosed, but was still positive in 12 patients at the time of heart transplantation. In an undefined number of these patients intraoperative plasmapheresis or the prostaglandin iloprost was employed, thus making it hard to evaluate in how many patients UFH anticoagulation was the sole strategy. Additionally, dosing and timing of stoppage of the DTIs is not described.

Selleng et al. (2008) presented three cases of patients who underwent heart transplantation with UFH during CPB. In these patients, the platelet count had already recovered after the start of nonheparin anticoagulation, the functional assay [i.e., the heparin-induced platelet activation assay (HIPA)] was negative, but patients were still positive for anti-PF4/H IgG by EIA. Transplantation was performed successfully in all patients without any thromboembolic complications.

Another case series reports 14 HIT patients who successfully underwent VAD implantation and/or heart transplantation using UFH on CPB, although anti-PF4/H antibodies were still detectable in the EIA (Zucker et al., 2010). Unfortunately, the diagnosis was not confirmed by a functional assay so that it is unknown how many of these patients had platelet-activating antibodies in their plasma.

These reports demonstrate that in patients with subacute HIT, anticoagulation during CPB may be performed with UFH. Interestingly, all these patients with subacute HIT in the context of cardiac surgery reported to date have been heart failure patients. This patient population presents frequently with thrombocytopenia as well as with a positive EIA for PF4/H antibodies (Schenk et al., 2006) bearing the risk of overdiagnosis of HIT. Our view is that the presence of platelet-activating antibodies using a functional assay, such as the SRA or the HIPA, has to be proved before a nonheparin therapy can be considered.

Conclusion

Reexposure to heparin, when restricted to time on CPB, seems to be possible in certain patients with subacute HIT, namely those patients with a recent history of HIT in whom platelet counts have normalized, who test negative for platelet-activating antibodies, but continue to test positive in the EIA. Although further studies in this regard are desirable, this strategy appears to be an important option particularly for the complex and high-risk surgery of VAD implantation and heart transplantation (particularly when performed after previous VAD implantation).

HIT IN PATIENTS WITH MECHANICAL CIRCULATORY SUPPORT

The incidence of HIT and its clinical impact varies among different patient populations. Patients who receive UFH during implantation and early anticoagulant management of mechanical circulatory support (MCS), that is, a VAD or total artificial heart (TAH), appear to be at very high risk for HIT and HIT-related complications. Schenk and coworkers (2006) assessed 115 patients on MCS. The incidence of HIT, as defined by an *in vitro* platelet activation test, was 10.6%. The risk of developing a thromboembolic event was more than doubled when compared with non-HIT patients, particularly in the first month of MCS.

Koster and colleagues (2007b) performed a retrospective investigation of 358 VAD patients. The incidence of HIT was 8.6%. The clinical outcome of patients who developed HIT after VAD implantation was detrimental, with a procedural success rate of only 31% compared with 50% in non-HIT patients. However, in patients who had HIT before surgery, and who therefore received nonheparin anticoagulation pre- and post-VAD implantation, together with UFH plus an antiplatelet agent for intraoperative anticoagulation, the procedural success rate was 67%.

Considering the high incidence and complication rate of HIT in this patient population, it could be appropriate for an alternative nonheparin anticoagulant to be used preemptively for postoperative anticoagulation (Warkentin et al., 2009). Samuels et al. (2008) reported the successful use of argatroban in 28 patients after implantation of a VAD. In this small group of patients, thromboembolic complication rates (15%) were comparable with the use of heparin (20%). Furthermore, the incidence of bleeding complication requiring re-exploration was very low (5% compared with 15% in heparin-treated patients) suggesting an adequate safety profile of argatroban (despite the lack of an antidote). Of note, preemptive bivalirudin anticoagulation was used successfully for managing extracorporeal membrane oxygenation post–cardiac surgery (Ranucci et al., 2011). Further studies will be needed to determine if the pre-emptive use of alternative anticoagulants, such as argatroban and bivalirudin, will improve outcomes of patients after MCS or whether the intended aim at reducing the incidence of HIT is counterbalanced by an increased risk of bleeding or other complications.

SUMMARY OF RECOMMENDATIONS FOR CARDIAC SURGERY

In patients with a history of HIT and a negative antibody test result at the time of surgery, anticoagulation during surgery should be performed with UFH (Fig. 19.2). Postoperatively, if further anticoagulation is needed, an alternative nonheparin anticoagulant should be given. In patients with detectable antibodies, the operation should be postponed whenever possible to allow for disappearance of the antibodies (usually within several weeks). Surgery is likely also safe if the antibodies are of the (nonplatelet-activating) IgA and/or IgM classes, or if the IgG antibodies are "weak" [i.e., negative testing in a functional assay (SRA, HIPA)]. It is reasonable to repeat testing for HIT antibodies at short intervals (e.g., every two or three weeks), as antibodies can disappear quickly in some patients. Thereafter, surgery is performed with UFH, as above.

In patients with a positive antibody test before surgery requiring urgent operation, an alternative approach should be used. Based on current data, bivalirudin appears to be the firstline strategy for OPCAB surgery, and for a large variety of standard CPB procedures (CABG, isolated valve surgery, combined CABG and valve procedures). However, consideration should be given to the modifications of CPB and surgical practice that are necessary due to the pharmacology of bivalirudin (Table 19.3). r-Hirudin should only be used in patients with normal renal function and a low probability of developing perioperative renal impairment. Moreover, point-of-care monitoring with the ECT is a further obligation for use of r-hirudin in this indication. Argatroban and danaparoid cannot be recommended for CPB procedures, although danaparoid might be an option in OPCAB surgery.

In complex procedures or institutions with minor experience in alternative anticoagulation strategies, risk reduction might be achieved best by combination of UFH with a short-acting potent antiplatelet agent in order to attenuate the HIT reaction. The safest class of agents appears to be prostaglandins as the elimination half-life is very short, and major bleeding complications appear to be uncommon. However, their potent hypotensive effect should be considered. The short-acting platelet GPIIb/IIIa antagonist tirofiban may also be used for this purpose, if there is a low probability that the patient will develop perioperative renal failure. Pre- and intraoperative plasmapheresis may also be used to reduce HIT antibody concentrations and reduce the risk of thromboembolic events, but needs further validation. The same applies for the use of UFH without any concomitant antiplatelet agent in patients with subacute HIT.

ANTICOAGULATION IN VASCULAR SURGERY AND PERCUTANEOUS ENDOVASCULAR VASCULAR INTERVENTIONS

As mentioned earlier, PEVI procedures increasingly are replacing conventional vascular surgery. It is conceivable that due to the similarity of PEVI and PCI, anticoagulation strategies that have been validated in large PCI studies can also be used during PEVI and may also be used in classic vascular surgery.

Bivalirudin

In contrast to the large pool of data describing the use of bivalirudin for anticoagulation of PCI and controlled studies in cardiac surgery, in PEVI procedures and vascular surgery much less data are available. Bivalirudin, using the PCI dose (bolus of 0.75 mg/kg followed by continuous infusion of 1.75 mg/kg/hr), has been studied in 98 non-HIT patients for endovascular abdominal aneurysm repair (Stamler et al., 2009). Major bleeding was observed in 10.2% and thrombosis in 4.8% of patients. These complication rates were comparable with the results observed with heparin anticoagulation at the same institution. In a registry report, data of 369 patients undergoing peripheral vascular interventions with bivalirudin, also given the aforementioned PCI dose, were published (Shammas et al., 2010). The procedural success rate was 97.3% with low complication rates.

With regard to vascular surgery, theoretically, use of bivalirudin could be problematic since clamping of the vessel results in ischemia (stimulating generation of thrombin) and stagnation (preventing influx of fresh nondegraded bivalirudin molecules) with the potential for bivalirudin concentrations to decrease to critically low levels, resulting in local thrombosis. However, in a series of 18 patients undergoing lower extremity bypass surgery, and employing the PCI dose, bivalirudin was successfully used without thrombotic events and with acceptable rates of major (one patient) and minor (three patients) bleeding complications (Kashyap et al., 2010). In this study, ACTs were simultaneously determined in the systemic circulation as well as from samples collected from the clamped vessel. No significant differences between the measured values were observed, indicating that the plasma concentrations of bivalirudin measured from blood obtained from the cross-clamped vessel were mostly within the target range. However, in one patient, the distal limb ACT value had decreased below the critical value of ≤ 200 seconds so that a further bolus of 0.075 mg/kg bivalirudin was directly administered into the clamped vessel. Due to the fact that the mean arterial cross clamp time was relatively lengthy (>30 minutes), it can be speculated that due to the mostly chronic condition of the disease, collateral arterial blood flow maintained adequate bivalirudin concentrations. Further studies will need to be performed to establish whether bivalirudin can also be safely used when more central vessels (abdominal aorta) are clamped or when surgery is performed in patients with aneurysmal disease (where usually less collateral flow occurs).

Argatroban
In contrast to bivalirudin, no fixed dosing protocol for argatroban during PCI has been established. The bolus varies between 250 and 350 µg/kg and continuous infusion rates between 15 and 25 µg/kg/min (Lewis et al., 2002; Rössig et al., 2011).

Argatroban has been used in 48 patients diagnosed with HIT undergoing PEVI for peripheral arterial disease (Baron et al., 2008). The mean dose used was a bolus of 174 ± 143 µg/kg followed by a continuous infusion of 10.7 ± 9.64 µg/kg/min. In 25% of these patients the composite endpoint of death (two patients), urgent revascularization (one patient), amputation (nine patients) was observed, and 6% of patients experienced major bleeding.

Intraoperative Anticoagulation for Thromboembolectomy in Acute HIT
Patients with acute HIT may need urgent thromboembolectomy, for example, for removal of "white clots" within large arteries. However, no data are available regarding the optimal anticoagulation for this procedure. Thromboembolectomy has features of both PCI and PEVI procedures; this suggests that bivalirudin could be the drug of choice. Arguments for bivalirudin include its parenteral administration, its short half-life, and its clearance which is largely independent of the function of a special organ system. Moreover, the validation of a fixed-dose protocol for PCI, PEVI procedures and OPCAB surgery is an important consideration. However, studies will be required to establish the safety and efficacy of bivalirudin for acute thromboembolectomy.

Warkentin et al. (2012) presented data of 13 patients with acute HIT-related arterial thrombosis requiring 14 urgent thrombectomies. In 10 of these procedures, UFH was used as an anticoagulant during the procedure, and in four procedures an alternate nonheparin strategy was used (lepirudin, danaparoid, argatroban, saline). In the UFH group, only two of 10 (20%) patients needed amputations, compared with three of four (75%) in the other group. This small study suggests that the use of UFH—unintended or otherwise—does not necessarily result in adverse

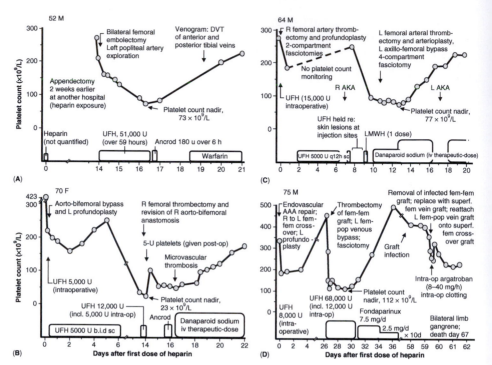

FIGURE 19.3 Four patients who underwent vascular surgery at a time when HIT antibodies were present: cases A and B were performed using UFH for intraoperative anticoagulation, whereas case C was performed using danaparoid. For case D, the first vascular surgery was performed using UFH, and the second procedure was performed using argatroban. *Abbreviations*: AAA, abdominal aortic aneurysm; AKA, above-knee amputation; DVT, deep-vein thrombosis; fem, femoral; iv, intravenous; LMWH, low molecular weight heparin; pop, popliteal; sc, subcutaneous; superf., superficial; UFH, unfractionated heparin. *Source*: From Warkentin et al. (2012).

consequences when used for intraoperative anticoagulation in the setting of acute HIT requiring urgent thromboembolectomy. Figure 19.3 shows representative patients from this study.

Conclusion

During PEVI procedures and vascular surgery, bivalirudin—used according to the PCI protocol—appears to be a safe and effective option. This, however, needs further assessment in large prospective trials, particularly in patients with central and aneurysmal disease.

Given the fact that a large number of vascular surgery patients also are diabetics suffering from renal impairment, this suggests that argatroban, due to its short half-life and hepatic elimination, is a theoretically attractive option for this indication. However, dosing protocols vary largely and safety and efficacy data for this special indication are limited.

The fact that UFH has been used successfully for thromboembolectomy in patients with acute HIT, similar to that seen in patients undergoing CPB (Fig. 19.1), is surprising and demonstrates that further investigation into the pathomechanism of HIT and HIT-associated thrombosis is necessary.

REFERENCES

Addonizio VP Jr, Fisher CA, Kappa JR, Ellison N. Prevention of heparin-induced thrombocytopenia during open heart surgery with iloprost (ZK36374). Surgery 102: 796–807, 1987.

Antoniou T, Kapetanakis EI, Theodoraki K, Rellia P, Thanapoulos A, Kotiou M, Zarkalis D, Alivizatos P. Cardiac surgery in patients with heparin-induced thrombocytopenia using preoperatively determined dosages of iloprost. Heart Surg Forum 5: 354–357, 2002.

Aouifi A, Blanc P, Piriou V, Bastien OH, Ffrench P, Hanss M, Lehot JJ. Cardiac surgery with cardiopulmonary bypass in patients with type II heparin-induced thrombocytopenia. Ann Thorac Surg 71: 678–683, 2001.

Azuma K, Maruyama K, Imanishi H, Nakagawa H, Kitamura A, Hayashida M. Difficult management of anticoagulation with argatroban in a patient undergoing on-pump cardiac surgery. J Cardiothorac Vasc Anesth 24: 831–833, 2010.

Baron SJ, Yeh RW, Cruz-Gonzales I, Healy JL, Pomerantsev E, Garasic J, Drachman D, Rosenfield K, Jang IK. Efficacy and safety of argatroban in patients with heparin induced thrombocytopenia undergoing endovascular intervention for peripheral arterial disease. Catheter Cardiovasc Interv 72: 116–120, 2008.

Bauer TL, Arepally G, Konkle BA, Mestichelli B, Shapiro SS, Cines DB, Poncz M, McNulty S, Amiral J, Hauck WW, Edie RN, Mannion JD. Prevalence of heparin-associated antibodies without thrombosis in patients undergoing cardiopulmonary bypass surgery. Circulation 95: 1242–1246, 1997.

Bennett-Guerrero E, Slaughter TF, White WD, Welsby IJ, Greenberg CS, El-Moalem H, Ortel TL. Preoperative anti-PF4/heparin antibody level predicts adverse outcome after cardiac surgery. J Thorac Cardiovasc Surg 130: 1567–1572, 2005.

Cannon MA, Butterworth J, Riley RD, Hyland JM. Failure of argatroban anticoagulation during off-pump coronary artery bypass surgery. Ann Thorac Surg 77: 711–713, 2004.

Carrier M, Robitaille D, Perrault LP, Pellerin M, Page P, Cartier R, Bouchard D. Heparin versus danaparoid in off-pump coronary bypass grafting: results of a prospective randomized clinical trial. J Thorac Cardiovasc Surg 125: 325–329, 2003.

Chong BH, Berndt MC. Heparin-induced thrombocytopenia. Blut 58: 53–57, 1989.

Dyke CM, Smedira N, Koster A, Aronson S, McCarthy HL 2nd, Kirshner R, Lincoff AM, Spiess BD. A comparison of bivalirudin to heparin with protamine reversal in patients undergoing cardiac surgery with cardiopulmonary bypass: the EVOLUTION-ON study. J Thorac Cardiovasc Surg 131: 533–539, 2006.

Dyke CM, Aldea G, Koster A, Smedira N, Avery E, Aronson S, Spiess BD, Lincoff AM. Off-pump coronary artery bypass with bivalirudin for patients with heparin-induced thrombocytopenia or antiplatelet factor 4/heparin antibodies. Ann Thorac Surg 84: 836–839, 2007.

Edmunds LH Jr. Blood-surface interactions during cardiopulmonary bypass. J Cardiovasc Surg 8: 404–410, 1993.

Edwards JT, Hamby JK, Worrall NK. Successful use of argatroban as a heparin substitute during cardiopulmonary bypass: heparin-induced thrombocytopenia in a high-risk cardiac surgical patient. Ann Thorac Surg 75: 1622–1624, 2003.

Furukawa K, Ohteki H, Hirahara K, Narita Y, Koga S. The use of argatroban as an anticoagulant for cardiopulmonary bypass in cardiac operations. J Thorac Cardiovasc Surg 122: 1255–1257, 2001.

Gasparovic H, Nathan NS, Fitzgerald D, Aranki SF. Severe argatroban-induced coagulopathy in a patient with a history of heparin-induced thrombocytopenia. Ann Thorac Surg 78: e89–e91, 2004.

Genzen JR, Farreed J, Hoppensteadt D, Kurup V, Barash P, Coady M, Wu YY. Prolonged elevation of plasma argartoban in a cardiac transplant patient with a suspected history of heparin-induced thrombocytopenia with thrombosis. Transfusion 50: 801–807, 2010.

Gluckman TJ, Segal JB, Schulman SP, Shapiro EP, Kickler TS, Prechel MM, Conte JV, Walenga JM, Shafique I, Rade JJ. Effect of anti-platelet factor-4/heparin antibody induction on early saphenous vein graft occlusion after coronary artery bypass surgery. Thromb Haemost 7: 1457–1464, 2009.

Grocott HP, Root J, Berkowitz SD, deBruijn N, Landolfo K. Coagulation complicating cardiopulmonary bypass in a patient with heparin-induced thrombocytopenia receiving the heparinoid, danaparoid sodium. J Cardiothorac Vasc Anesth 11: 875–877, 1997.

Iqbal O, Tobu M, Aziz S, Gerdisch M, DaValle M, Demir M, Hoppensteadt DA, Ahmad S, Walenga JM, Fareed J. Successful use of recombinant hirudin and its monitoring by ecarin clotting time in patients with heparin-induced thrombocytopenia undergoing off-pump coronary artery revascularization. J Card Surg 20: 42–51, 2005.

Jaben EA, Torloni AS, Pruthi RK, Winters JL. Use of plasma exchange in patients with heparin-induced thrombocytopenia: a report of two cases and a review of the literature. J Clin Apher 26: 219–224, 2011.

Kajitani M, Aguinaga M, Johnson CE, Scott MA, Antakli T. Use of plasma exchange and heparin during cardiopulmonary bypass for a patient with heparin induced thrombocytopenia: a case report. J Card Surg 16: 313–318, 2001.

Kappa JR, Horn D, McIntosh CL, Fisher CA, Ellison N, Addonizio VP. Iloprost (ZK36374), a new prostacyclin analogue, permits open cardiac surgery in patients with heparin-induced thrombocytopenia. Surg Forum 36: 285–286, 1985.

Kashyap VS, Bishop PD, Bensa JF, Rosa K, Sarac TP, Ouriel K. A pilot, prospective evaluation of a direct thrombin inhibitor, bivalirudin (Angiomax), in patients undergoing lower extremity bypass. J Vasc Surg 52: 369–374, 2010.

Kawada T, Kitagawa H, Hoson M, Okada Y, Shiomura J. Clinical application of argatroban as an alternative anticoagulant for extracorporeal circulation. Hematol Oncol Clin North Am 14: 445–457, 2000.

Kieta DR, McCammon AT, Holman WL, Nielsen VG. Hemostatic analysis of a patient undergoing off-pump coronary artery bypass surgery with argatroban anticoagulation. Anesth Analg 96: 956–958, 2003.

Koster A, Hansen R, Grauhan O, Hausmann H, Bauer M, Hetzer R, Kuppe H, Mertzlufft F. Hirudin monitoring using the TAS ecarin clotting time in patients with heparin-induced thrombocytopenia type II. J Cardiothorac Vasc Anesth 14: 249–252, 2000a.

Koster A, Pasic M, Bauer M, Kuppe H, Hetzer R. Hirudin as anticoagulant for cardiopulmonary bypass: importance of reoperative renal function. Ann Thorac Surg 69: 37–41, 2000b.

Koster A, Merkle F, Hansen R, Loebe M, Kuppe H, Hetzer R, Crystal GJ, Mertzlufft F. Elimination of recombinant hirudin by modified ultrafiltration during simulated cardiopulmonary bypass: assessment of different filter systems. Anesth Analg 91: 265–269, 2000c.

Koster A, Loebe M, Merztlufft F, Kuppe H, Hetzer R. Cardiopulmonary bypass in a patient with heparin induced thrombocytopenia II and impaired renal function using heparin and platelet GP IIb/IIIa inhibitor tirofiban as anticoagulant. Ann Thorac Surg 70: 2160–2161, 2000e.

Koster A, Kukucka M, Bach F, Meyer O, Fischer T, Mertzlufft F, Loebe M, Hetzer R, Kuppe H. Anticoagulation during cardiopulmonary bypass in patients with heparin-induced thrombocytopenia type II and renal impairment using heparin and the platelet glycoprotein IIb-IIIa antagonist tirofiban. Anesth 94: 245–251, 2001a.

Koster A, Meyer O, Fischer T, Kuschka M, Krabatsch T, Bauer M, Kuppe H, Hetzer R. One-year experience with the platelet glycoprotein IIb/IIIa antagonist tirofiban and heparin during cardiopulmonary bypass in patients with heparin-induced thrombocytopenia type II. J Thorac Cardiovasc Surg 122: 1254–1255, 2001b.

Koster A, Chew D, Grundel M, Bauer M, Kuppe H, Spiess BD. Bivalirudin monitored with the ecarin clotting time for anticoagulation during cardiopulmonary-bypass. Anesth Analg 96: 383–386, 2003a.

Koster A, Chew D, Gruendel M, Hausmann H, Grauhan O, Kuppe H, Spiess BD. An assessment of different filter systems for extracorporeal elimination of bivalirudin: an in vitro study. Anesth Analg 96: 1316–1319, 2003b.

Koster A, Spiess BD, Chew DP, Krabatsch T, Tambeur L, DeAnda A, Hetzer R, Kuppe H, Smedira NG, Lincoff AM. Effectiveness of bivalirudin as a replacement for heparin during cardiopulmonary bypass in patients undergoing coronary artery bypass grafting. Am J Cardiol 93: 356–359, 2004a.

Koster A, Chew D, Merkle F, Gruendel M, Jurmann M, Kuppe H, Oertel R. Extracorporeal elimination of large concentrations of tirofiban by zero-balanced ultrafiltration during cardiopulmonary bypass: an in vitro investigation. Anesth Analg 99: 989–92, 2004b.

Koster A, Yeter R, Buz S, Kuppe H, Hetzer R, Lincoff AM, Dyke CM, Smedira NG, Spiess BD. Assessment of hemostatic activation during cardiopulmonary bypass for coronary artery bypass grafting with bivalirudin: results of a pilot study. J Thorac Cardiovasc Surg 129: 1391–1394, 2005.

Koster A, Buz S, Hetzer R, Kuppe H, Breddin K, Harder S. Anticoagulation with argatroban in patients with heparin-induced thrombocytopenia antibodies after cardiac surgery with cardiopulmonary bypass: first results from the ARG-E03 trial. J Thorac Cardiovasc Surg 132: 699–700, 2006.

Koster A, Dyke CM, Aldea G, Smedira NG, McCarthy HL 2nd, Aronson S, Hetzer R, Avery E, Spiess BD, Lincoff M. Bivalirudin during cardiopulmonary bypass in patients with previous or acute heparin-induced thrombocytopenia and heparin antibodies: results of the CHOOSE-ON trial. Ann Thorac Surg 83: 572–577, 2007a.

Koster A, Huebler S, Potapov E, Meyer O, Jurmann M, Weng Y, Pasic M, Drews T, Kuppe H, Loebe M, Hetzer R. Impact of heparin-induced thrombocytopenia on outcome in patients with ventricular assist device support: single-institution experience in 358 consecutive patients. Ann Thorac Surg 83: 72–76, 2007b.

Koster A, Buz S, Krabatsch T, Yeter R, Hetzer R. Bivalirudin anticoagulation during cardiac surgery: a single-center experience in 141 patients. Perfusion 24: 7–11, 2009.

Koza MJ, Walenga JM, Fareed J, Pifarre R. A new approach in monitoring recombinant hirudin during cardiopulmonary bypass. Semin Thromb Hemost 19: 90–96, 1993.

Kraenzler EJ, Starr NJ. Heparin-associated thrombocytopenia: management of patients for open heart surgery. Case reports describing the use of iloprost. Anesthesiology 69: 964–967, 1988.

Kress DC, Aronson S, McDonald ML, Malik MI, Divgi AB, Tector AJ, Downey FX III, Anderson AJ, Stone M, Clancy C. Positive heparin-platelet factor 4 antibody complex and cardiac surgical outcomes. Ann Thorac Surg 83: 1737–1743, 2007.

Lewis BE, Johnson SA, Grassman ED, Wrona LL. Argatroban as an anticoagulant for coronary procedures in patients with HIT antibody. In: Pifarre R, ed. New Anticoagulants for the Cardiovascular Patient. Philadelphia: Hanley & Belfus, 301–308, 1997a.

Lewis BE, Walenga JM, Pifarre R, Fareed J. Argatroban in the management of patients with heparin-induced thrombocytopenia and heparin-induced thrombocytopenia and thrombosis syndrome. In: Pifarre R, ed. New Anticoagulants for the Cardiovascular Patient. Philadelphia: Hanley & Belfus, 223–229, 1997b.

Lewis BE, Wallis DE, Berkowitz SD, Matthai WH, Fareed J, Walenga JM, Bartholomew J, Sham R, Lerner RG, Zeigler ZR, Rustagi PK, Jang IK, Rifkin SD, Moran J, Hursting MJ, Kelton JG for the ARG-911 Study Investigators. Argatroban anticoagulant therapy in patients with heparin-induced thrombocytopenia. Circulation 103: 1838–1843, 2001.

Lewis BE, Matthai WH Jr, Cohen M, Moses JW, Hursting MJ, Leya F, ARG-216/310/311 Study Investigators. Argatroban anticoagulation during percutaneous coronary intervention in patients with heparin-induced thrombocytopenia. Catheter Cardiovas Interv 57: 177–184, 2002.

Lewis BE, Wallis DE, Leya F, Hursting MJ, Kelton JG, Argatroban-915 Investigators. Argatroban anticoagulation in patients with heparin-induced thrombocytopenia. Arch Intern Med 163: 1849–1856, 2003.

Long RW. Management of patients with heparin-induced thrombocytopenia requiring cardiopulmonary bypass. J Thorac Cardiovasc Surg 89: 950–951, 1985.

Magnani HN. Heparin-induced thrombocytopenia (HIT): an overview of 230 patients treated with Orgaran (Org 10172). Thromb Haemost 70: 554–561, 1993.

Magnani HN, Beijering RJR, ten Cate JW, Chong BH. Orgaran anticoagulation for cardiopulmonary bypass in patients with heparin-induced thrombocytopenia. In: Pifarre R, ed. New Anticoagulants for the Cardiovascular Patient. Philadelphia: Hanley & Belfus, 487–500, 1997.

Magnani HN, Gallus A. Heparin-induced thrombocytopenia (HIT). A report of 1,478 clinical outcomes of patients treated with danaparoid (Orgaran) from 1982 to mid 2004. Thromb Haemost 95: 967–981, 2006.

Makhoul RG, McCann RL, Austin EH, Greenberg CS, Lowe JE. Management of patients with heparin-associated thrombocytopenia and thrombosis requiring cardiac surgery. Ann Thorac Surg 43: 617–621, 1987.

Martin ME, Kloecker GH, Laber DA. Argatroban for anticoagulation during cardiac surgery. Eur J Haematol 78: 161–166, 2007.

Merry AF, Raudkivi PJ, Middleton NG, McDougall JM, Nand P, Mills BP, Webber BJ, Frampton CM, White HD. Bivalirudin versus heparin and protamine in off-pump coronary artery bypass surgery. Ann Thorac Surg 77: 925–931, 2004.

Mertzlufft F, Kuppe H, Koster A. Management of urgent high-risk cardiopulmonary bypass in patients with heparin-induced thrombocytopenia type II and coexisting disorders of renal function: use of heparin and epoprostenol combined with online monitoring of platelet function. J Cardiothorac Vasc Anesth 14: 304–308, 2000.

Nishida S, Fujita T, Kohno N, Atoda H, Morita T, Takeya H, Kido I, Paine MJI, Kawabata S, Iwanaga S. cDNA cloning and deduced amino acid sequence of prothrombin activator (ecarin) from Kenyan Echis carinatus venom. Biochemistry 34: 1771–1778, 1995.

Ohno H, Higashidate M, Yokosuka T. Argatroban as an alternative anticoagulant for patients with heparin allergy during coronary bypass surgery. Heart Vessels 18: 40–42, 2003.

Olinger GN, Hussey CV, Olive JA, Malik MI. Cardiopulmonary bypass for patients with previously documented heparin-induced platelet aggregation. J Thorac Cardiovasc Surg 87: 673–677, 1984.

Palmer Smith J, Walls JT, Muscato MS, Scott McCord E, Worth ER, Curtis JJ, Silver D. Extracorporeal circulation in a patient with heparin-induced thrombocytopenia. Anesthesiology 62: 363–365, 1985.

Pötzsch B, Iversen S, Riess FC, Tzanova N, Seelig C, Nowak G, Müller-Berghaus G. Recombinant hirudin as an anticoagulant in open-heart surgery: a case report [abstr]. Ann Hematol 68(Suppl 2): A46, 1993.

Pötzsch B, Madlener K, Seelig C, Riess CF, Greinacher A, Müller-Berghaus G. Monitoring of r-hirudin anticoagulation during cardiopulmonary bypass—assessment of the whole blood ecarin clotting time. Thromb Haemost 77: 920–925, 1997.

Pötzsch B, Klovekorn WP, Madlener K. Use of heparin during cardiopulmonary bypass in patients with a history of heparin-induced thrombocytopenia. N Engl J Med 343: 515, 2000.

Pouplard C, May MA, Iochmann S, Amiral J, Vissac AM, Marchand M, Gruel Y. Antibodies to platelet factor 4-Heparin after cardiopulmonary bypass in patients anticoagulated with unfractionated heparin or a low molecular weight heparin: clinical implications for heparin-induced thrombocytopenia. Circulation 99: 2530–2536, 1999.

Ranucci M, Ballotta A, Kandil H, Isgrò G, Carlucci C, Baryshnikova E, Pistuddi V. Bivalirudin-based versus conventional heparin anticoagulation for postcardiotomy extracorporeal membrane oxygenation. Crit Care 15: R275, 2011.

Riess FC, Löwer C, Seelig C, Bleese N, Kormann J, Müller-Berghaus G, Pötzsch B. Recombinant hirudin as a new anticoagulant during cardiac operations instead of heparin: successful for aortic valve replacement in man. Thorac Cardiovasc Surg 110: 265–267, 1995.

Riess FC, Pötzsch B, Bader R, Bleese N, Greinacher A, Löwer C, Madlener K, Müller-Berghaus G. A case report on the use of recombinant hirudin as an anticoagulant for cardiopulmonary bypass in open heart surgery. Eur J Cardiothorac Surg 10: 386–388, 1996.

Riess FC, Pötzsch B, Müller-Berghaus G. Recombinant hirudin as an anticoagulant during cardiac surgery. In: Pifarre R, ed. New Anticoagulants for the Cardiovascular Patient. Philadelphia: Hanley & Belfus, 197–222, 1997.

Riess FC, Pötzsch B, Madlener K, Cramer E, Doll KN, Doll S, Lorke DE, Kormann J, Müller-Berghaus. Recombinant hirudin for cardiopulmonary bypass anticoagulation: a randomized, prospective, and heparin-controlled pilot study. Thorac Cardiovasc Surg 55: 233–238, 2007.

Rössig L, Genth-Zotz S, Rau M, Heyndrickx GR, Schneider T, Gulba DC, Desaga M , Buerke M, Harder S, Zeiher AM, ARG-E04 study group. Argatroban for elective percutaneous coronary intervention: the ARG-E04 multi-center study. Int J Cardiol 148: 214–219, 2011.

Samuels LE, Kohout J, Casanova-Ghosh E, Hagan K, Garwood P, Ferdinand F, Goldmann SM. Aratroban as a primary or secondary postoperative anticoagulant in patients with ventricular assist devices. Ann Thorac Surg 85: 1651–1655, 2008.

Schroder JN, Daneshmand MA, Villamizar NR, Petersen RP, Blue LJ, Welsby IJ, Lodge AJ, Ortel TL, Rogers JG, Milano CA. Heparin-induced thrombocytopenia in left ventricular assist device bridge-to-transplant patients. Ann Thorac Surg 84: 841–845, 2007.

Schenk S, El-Banayosy A, Prohaska W, Arusoglu L, Morshuis M, Koester-Eiserfunke WS, Kizner L, Murray E, Eichler P, Koerfer R, Greinacher A. Heparin-induced thrombocytopenia in patients receiving mechanical circulatory support. J Thorac Cardiovasc Surg 131: 1373–1381, 2006

Selleng S, Lubenow N, Wollert HG, Müllejans B, Greinacher A. Emergency cardiopulmonary bypass in a bilaterally nephrectomized patient with a history of heparin-induced thrombocytopenia: successful reexposure to heparin. Ann Thorac Surg 71: 1041–1042, 2001.

Selleng S, Haneya A, Hirt S, Selleng K, Schmid C, Greinacher A. Management of anticoagulation in patients with subacute heparin-induced thrombocytopenia scheduled for heart transplantation. Blood 112: 4024–4027, 2008.

Selleng S, Malowsky B, Itterman T, Bagemühl J, Wessel A, Wollert HG, Warkentin TE, Greinacher A. Incidence and clinical relevance of anti-platelet factor 4/heparin antibodies before cardiac surgery. Am Heart J 160: 362–369, 2010.

Shammas NW, Shammas GA, Jerin M, Dippel EJ, Shammas AN. In-hospital safety and effectiveness of bivalirudin in percutaneous peripheral interventions: data from a real-world registry. J Endovasc Ther 17: 31–36, 2010.

Slaughter TF, LeBleu TH, Douglas JM Jr, Leslie JB, Parker JK, Greenberg CS. Characterization of prothrombin activation during cardiac surgery by hemostatic molecular markers. Anesthesiology 80: 520–526, 1994.

Smedira NG, Dyke CM, Koster A, Jurmann M, Bhatia DS, McCarthy HL 2nd, Lincoff AM, Spiess BD, Áraonson S. Anticoagulation with bivalirudin for off-pump coronary artery bypass grafting: results of the EVOLUTION-OFF study. J Thorac Cardiovasc Surg 131: 686–692, 2006.

Stamler S, Katzen BT, Tsoukas AI, Baum SZ, Diehm N. Clinical experience with the use of bivalirudin in a large population undergoing abdominal aortic aneurysm repair. J Vasc Interv Radiol 20: 17–21, 2009.

Trossaert M, Gaillard A, Commin PL, Amiral J, Vissac AM, Fressinaud E. High incidence of anti-heparin/platelet factor 4 antibodies after cardiopulmonary bypass surgery. Br J Haematol 101: 653–655, 1998.

Van Dyck MJ, Lavenne-Pardonge E, Azerad MA, Matta AG, Moriau M, Comunale ME. Thrombosis after the use of heparin-coated cardiopulmonary bypass circuit in a patient with heparin-induced thrombocytopenia. J Cardiothorac Vasc Anesth 10: 809–815, 1996.

Veale JJ, McCarthy HM, palmer G, Dyke CM. Use of bivalirudin as an anticoagulant during cardiopulmonary bypass. J Extra Corpor Technol 37: 296–302, 2005.

Visentin GP, Malik M, Cyganiak KA, Aster RH. Patients treated with unfractionated heparin during open heart surgery are at high risk to form antibodies reactive with heparin: platelet factor 4 complexes. J Lab Clin Med 128: 376–383, 1996.

Voeller RK, Melby SJ, Grizzell BE, Moazami N. Novel use of plasmapheresis in a patient with heparin-induced thrombocytopenia requiring urgent insertion of a left ventricular assist device under cardiopulmonary bypass. J Thorac Cardiovasc Surg 140: e56–e58, 2010.

Walenga JM, Bakhos M, Messmore HL, Koza M, Wallock M, Orfei E, Fareed J, Pifarre R. Comparison of recombinant hirudin and heparin as an anticoagulant in a cardiopulmonary bypass model. Blood Coagul Fibrinolysis 2: 105–111, 1991.

Walls JT, Curtis JJ, Silver D, Boley TM. Heparin-induced thrombocytopenia in patients who undergo open heart surgery. Surgery 108: 686–693, 1990.

Warkentin TE, Greinacher A. Heparin-induced thrombocytopenia and cardiac surgery. Ann Thorac Surg 76: 2121–2131, 2003.

Warkentin TE, Kelton JG. Temporal aspects of heparin-induced thrombocytopenia. N Engl J Med 344: 1286–1292, 2001.

Warkentin TE, Koster A. Bivalirudin: a review. Expert Opin Pharmacother 6: 1349–1371, 2005.

Warkentin TE, Sheppard JI. No significant improvement in diagnostic specificity of an anti-PF4/polyanion immunoassay with use of high heparin confirmatory procedure. J Thromb Haemost 4: 281–282, 2006.

Warkentin TE, Sheppard JI. Clinical sample investigation (CSI) hematology: pinpointing the precise onset of heparin-induced thrombocytopenia. J Thromb Haemost 5: 636–637, 2006.

Warkentin TE, Sheppard JI, Horsewood P, Simpson PJ, Moore JC, Kelton JG. Impact of the patient population on the risk of heparin-induced thrombocytopenia. Blood 96: 1703–1708, 2000.

Warkentin TE, Dunn GL, Cybulsky IJ. Off-pump coronary artery bypass grafting for acute heparin-induced thrombocytopenia. Ann Thorac Surg 72: 1730–1732, 2001.

Warkentin TE, Greinacher A, Koster A, Lincoff AM. Treatment and prevention of heparin-induced thrombocytopenia. American College of Chest Physicians evidence-based clinical practice guidelines, 8th edition. Chest 133(6 Suppl): 340S–380S, 2008.

Warkentin TE, Pai M, Cook RJ. Intraoperative anticoagulation and limb amputations in patients with immune heparin-induced thrombocytopenia who require vascular surgery. J Thromb Haemost 10: 148–150, 2012.

Warkentin TE, Greinacher A, Koster A. Heparin-induced thrombocytopenia in patients with ventricular assist devices: are new prevention strategies required? Ann Thorac Surg 87: 1633–1640, 2009.

Welsby IJ, Um J, Milano CA, Ortel TL, Arepally G. Plasmapheresis and heparin reexposure as a management strategy for cardiac surgical patients with heparin-induced thrombocytopenia. Anesth Analg 110: 30–35, 2010.

Yusuf AM, Warkentin TE, Arsenault KA, Whitlock R, Eikelboom JW. Prognostic importance of preoperative anti-PF4/heparin antibodies in patients undergoing cardiac surgery. A systematic review. Thromb Haemost 107: 8–14, 2012.

Zucker ML, Koster A, Prats J, Laduca FM. Sensitivity of a modified ACT test to levels of bivalirudin used during cardiac surgery. J Extra Corpor Technol 37: 364–368, 2005.

Zucker MJ, Sabnani I, Baran DA, Balasubramanian S, Camacho M. Cardiac transplantation and/or mechanical circulatory support device placement using heparin anticoagulation in the presence of heparin-induced thrombocytopenia. J Heart Lung Transplant 29: 53–60, 2010.

20

Heparin-coated intravascular devices and heparin-induced thrombocytopenia

Theodore E. Warkentin

INTRODUCTION

The clinical use of medical devices that make contact with blood has increased considerably in recent years. Exposure of blood to artificial materials, however, is associated with a number of adverse reactions, such as thrombus formation and associated device occlusion, embolization with distal ischemic events, as well as inflammatory responses. Coating of such artificial surfaces with heparin is one approach for improving compatibility with blood.

Previously, most commercially available products with a heparinized surface were central venous catheters and components for extracorporeal blood oxygenator systems. In more recent years, heparin-coated vascular and endovascular prostheses have achieved widespread use.

Although several different types of heparin-coated devices have been shown to reduce thrombogenicity, they rarely have also been implicated in heparin-induced thrombocytopenia (HIT). However, a causal relationship is difficult to establish, for two reasons. First, there invariably is confounding by exposure to unfractionated heparin (UFH) administered through more traditional intravenous (iv) and/or subcutaneous (sc) routes; and second, it is now well recognized that HIT can be caused by antibodies with prominent heparin-*independent* platelet activating properties. With such antibodies, HIT can occur without the need for any ongoing heparin exposure. Thus, the few instances of device-associated HIT might be related to coincidental formation of such highly pathogenic antibodies, rather than a process in which the heparin-coated device is maintaining HIT. *In other words, the disease course would be identical with or without the device being present.*

The purpose of this chapter is first to summarize different approaches to heparin coating, and to describe some of these devices (focusing on those approved for use and marketed in the United States and European Union). The second goal is to review the theoretical issues implicating—or absolving—these devices from HIT, and to review studies that have evaluated the immune response against platelet factor 4/heparin (PF4/H) complexes when heparin-coated devices are used. Finally, we will critically assess the available literature regarding reports of HIT associated with use of these devices.

COATING OF DEVICES

Heparin coating techniques can be broadly classified into those involving (*i*) covalently bound heparin (noneluting), and (*ii*) ionically bound heparin (these latter devices elute heparin over time). For covalently bound heparin, there are two main

TABLE 20.1 Partial List of Various Heparin Coating Techniques

Heparin coating	Company	Approach
Carmeda® Bioactive Surface (CBAS®)	Carmeda AB	Covalent, end-linked heparin, reduced molecular weight; well established
BioLine Coating	Maquet	Heparin bound covalently to albumin
INTERGARD Heparin	Maquet	Ionically bonded heparin
Polymaille Flow Plus Heparin®	Perouse Medical	Heparin bound covalently
FlowLine Bipore® Heparin	Jotec GmbH	Heparin covalently and ionically bonded
Astute™ Advanced Heparin Coating (marketed as Trillium® Biopassive Surface by Medtronic and Tal Palindrom™ Emerald™ by Covidien)	BioInteractions Ltd	Heparin bound covalently to immobilized polyethylene glycol (PEG)
GBS® (Gish Biocompatible Surface) heparin coating	Gish Biomedical (Sorin Group)	Hyaluronan (hyaluronic acid) based with covalently attached heparin
Corline® Heparin Surface (CHS™)	Corline Systems AB	Macromolecular water-soluble heparin conjugate (70 heparin molecules to one polyamine carrier chain) is preassembled; subsequently used to coat biomedical devices
Atrium HydraGlide™	Atrium Medical Corporation	Covalently bonded heparin in combination with passively released heparin (over 24–48 hr)
AMC Thromboshield® Treatment	Edwards Life Sciences Inc	Ionic (heparin–benzalkonium chloride complex)
Duraflo II®	Edwards Life Sciences Inc.	Ionic (heparin–benzalkonium chloride complex)

categories: endpoint-linked and multipoint-linked (crosslinked). Table 20.1 provides a selected list of various heparin coatings (Wendel et al., 1999; Larsson, 2004; Tanzi, 2005).

Types of Bonding and Terminology
Materials Commonly Used in Intravascular Devices

Before discussing heparin bonding, we will briefly discuss the substrates commonly used in the construction of coated devices, particularly intravascular grafts.

"PET" refers to "polyethyleneterephthalate," commercially known as "Dacron." The use of this material has been associated with high rates of restenosis (Ahmadi et al., 2002), and consequently heparin-bonded Dacron grafts are now available, for example, INTERGARD heparin grafts (Maquet), which are composed of Dacron impregnated with collagen and immobilized heparin.

"PTFE" refers to polytetrafluoroethylene, whereas "ePTFE" refers to "expanded" PTFE, and indicates a modified manufacturing process whereby the solid material is altered into a porous lattice. In essence, by rapidly stretching PTFE under appropriate conditions, a strong, microporous material is created. As with Dacron, PTFE and ePTFE grafts are now often coated with heparin.

Ionic bonding (noncovalent)

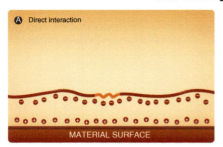

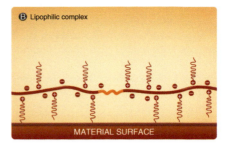

Covalent bonding

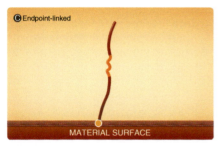

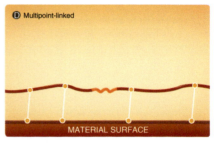

FIGURE 20.1 Four approaches for heparin bonding to device surfaces. (**A**) Ionic bonding (noncovalent) by direct surface interaction. (**B**) Ionic bonding between heparin and a positively charged lipophilic compound. The resulting complex is adsorbed to the device surface. (**C**) Covalent endpoint-linked heparin (CBAS®). The active site of heparin (depicted by the coiled central orange region) is not directly bound to the device surface and thus its anticoagulant function is preserved. (**D**) Covalent multipoint-linked heparin. *Source*: Courtesy of Carmeda AB, Upplands Väsby, Sweden.

Noncovalent or Ionic Heparin Bonding

Noncovalent or "ionic bonding" is a relatively simple way to immobilize heparin, and was the first approach to be developed (Gott et al., 1963). Here, direct interaction between the negative charge of the (heparin) molecule and the positively charged surface achieves surface heparin coating (Fig. 20.1A). Alternatively, heparin is allowed to form water-insoluble complexes with lipophilic quaternary ammonium compounds, such as tridodecyl methyl ammonium chloride (TDMAC); subsequently, the heparin bonds to a noncharged graft surface by hydrophobic interactions between the TDMAC and the polyester (Fig. 20.1B). A key feature of grafts that employ noncovalent bonding of heparin is that the heparin elutes off the graft over time.

Ionically bound heparin is sometimes used for central venous catheters, pulmonary artery (Swan Ganz) catheters, and other devices. As discussed later, some investigators have implicated these devices with HIT. The rationale includes the fact that heparin elutes off these catheters, and soluble heparin is a well-known trigger of HIT.

The time frame for leaching of heparin off the devices appears to be relatively rapid (hours to a few days). For example, for graphite–benzalkonium–heparin surfaces, dog studies using radioactive heparin found 70% of the heparin eluted off within 4 hours, and >90% after four days; moreover, this loss of heparin activity appeared to correlate with loss of thromboresistance (Kramer et al., 1967).

Covalent (Noneluting) Heparin Bonding

As previously noted, two broad types of *covalent* heparin bonding are available, endpoint-linked (Fig. 20.1C) and multipoint (or crosslinked) (Fig. 20.1D).

Endpoint-Linked Heparin

Endpoint-linked (or endpoint-immobilized) heparin is widely used for coating grafts and other devices (for review: Olsson et al., 2000). Most widely used is "CBAS®" ("Carmeda® Bioactive Surface"), which denotes a proprietary heparin bioactive surface comprised of heparin covalently attached via endpoint linkage. CBAS-heparin is a reduced molecular weight derivative of porcine heparin sodium that is produced by controlled chemical depolymerization; an aldehyde functional group is formed at the reducing terminus of the heparin chains, allowing the CBAS–heparin to become covalently bound at its terminus to synthetic materials that have been pretreated with a base polymeric matrix (Larm et al., 1983). This preserves the active site [antithrombin (AT)-binding pentasaccharide sequence] of heparin and, consequently, its anticoagulant function (Fig. 20.2). Heparin immobilized according to this technology remains bound to the surface, that is, is noneluting.

CBAS is used in a wide variety of intravascular devices (Table 20.2). For example, the Gore PROPATEN® Vascular Graft is an ePTFE vascular graft that has heparin bonded to its luminal surface via the CBAS proprietary endpoint covalent-bonded mechanism, thereby imparting thromboresistant properties. Another example is the Gore VIABAHN® Endoprosthesis with Heparin ("stent-graft"), which is constructed

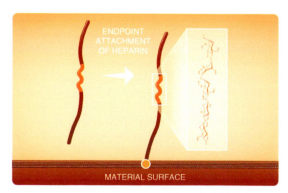

FIGURE 20.2 Covalent endpoint-linked heparin (CBAS®). CBAS-heparin is a reduced molecular weight derivative of porcine heparin sodium produced by controlled chemical depolymerization; an aldehyde functional group is formed at the reducing terminus of the heparin chains, allowing the CBAS-heparin to become covalently bound at its terminus to synthetic materials that have been pretreated with a base polymeric matrix. This preserves the active site of heparin (depicted by the coiled central orange region) and, consequently, its anticoagulant function. Heparin immobilized according to this technology remains bound to the surface, i.e., is noneluting. *Source*: Courtesy of Carmeda AB, Upplands Väsby, Sweden.

of a nitinol stent and an ePTFE graft, and which has CBAS on its surface (Kwa et al., 2010). This is currently the only stent-graft for femoral artery use approved by the U.S. Food and Drug Administration (FDA) (Kwa et al., 2010). (A "stent-graft" is a device that is placed permanently within an obstructed blood vessel so as to relieve an obstruction.)

Reported antithrombotic effects of CBAS (reviewed in Olsson et al., 2000) include the following: inhibition of coagulation factor Xa and thrombin (Elgue et al., 1993), prevention of thrombus formation in animal models (Begovac et al., 2003), inhibition of contact system activation (Sanchez et al., 1995, 1997, 1998), prevention of complement activation (Mollnes et al., 1995), and markedly reduced platelet attachment (Mollnes et al., 1999; Kocsis et al., 2000) and leukocyte activation (Lappegård et al., 2004). These antiplatelet and anticoagulant effects of CBAS, as well as its lack of activation of the contact system, are all crucially dependent on binding of AT to the immobilized heparin.

TABLE 20.2 Partial List of Medical Devices Utilizing Heparin Surface Coatings

Heparin coating	Device manufacturer[a]	Representative devices
Carmeda® Bioactive Surface (CBAS®)	W.L. Gore & Associates, Inc.	PROPATEN® vascular graft; VIABAHN® endoprosthesis with Heparin BioActive Surface; Hybrid Vascular Graft (combines graft and stent); ACUSEAL Vascular Graft (for dialysis access); TIGRIS Vascular Stent
	Berlin Heart	Ventricular assist devices (Excor® and Incor®)
	Spire	Decathlon Gold End Point Bonded Heparin Coated Catheter; Alta Gold End Point Bonded Heparin Coated Catheter (no longer marketed)
	Cordis	Bx Velocity™ coronary stent with Hepacoat™ (no longer marketed)
	Medtronic Inc.	Affinity NT® oxygenator, Minimax Plus® oxygenator, Affinity™ CP centrifugal blood pump, Affinity® arterial filter
Astute™ Advanced Heparin Coating	Medtronic Inc.	Cardiac Surgery (Trillium® Biopassive Surface)
	Covidien	Tal Palindrome™ Emerald™ (hemodialysis catheter)
BioLine Coating	Maquet	Cardiopulmonary bypass products; FUSION BioLine vascular graft
INTERGARD Heparin	Maquet	INTERGARD Heparin grafts
FlowLine Bipore®	Jotec	FlowLine Bipore® Heparin vascular graft
Polymaille Flow Plus Heparin®	Perouse	Polymaille Flow Plus Heparin® vascular graft
HydraGlide™	Atrium	HydraGlide™ thoracic drainage catheters
AMC Thromboshield® Treatment	American Edwards Laboratories	Multi-Med central venous infusion catheters, IntroFlex percutaneous sheath introducers, Swan-Ganz catheters, Vantex central venous catheters, AVA 3Xi device, AVA high-flow device

[a]The manufacturers listed in this Table are those who make the representative devices, who in some cases, may license the heparin coating technology from another manufacturer, e.g., W. L. Gore, Berlin Heart and Medtronic license CBAS® from Carmeda, and Medtronic and Covidien license Astute™ (Table 20.1).

Heparin-coated surfaces with high-affinity (i.e., AT-binding) heparin do not cause platelet activation as much as surfaces with low-affinity heparin, perhaps because of lower heparin–platelet interactions (Kocsis et al., 2000). Indeed, for low molecular weight heparin (LMWH), there is an inverse relationship between heparin activity (AT-binding capacity) and potentiation of platelet activation (Salzman et al., 1980). Cornelius and coworkers (2003) reported that low-activity immobilized heparin is thrombogenic, for the reason that it recruits factor XIIa to the surface but is not able to catalyze factor XIIa inhibition (i.e., it functions as a contact system activator through its high negative charge density but without offsetting AT-dependent XIIa inactivation). Although a recent study by Gao and collaborators (2011) found that both UFH or LMWH—whether in solution or immobilized onto glass tissue culture slides—potentiated activation of platelets to various platelet agonists, endpoint-linked heparin was not investigated.

In a human *ex vivo* model developed in Utrecht, non-anticoagulated blood drawn from healthy donors was aspirated directly and in parallel into heparin-bonded (endpoint-linked) and nonbonded ePTFE grafts at a constant flow and controlled shear rate (74/second), with measurement of various markers of coagulation activation (Heyligers et al., 2006). Significantly greater levels of fibrinopeptide A—a sensitive marker of fibrin formation—were seen in the non–heparin-bonded grafts; furthermore, platelet adhesion and fibrin deposition were observed by electron microscopy only on the surface of the standard grafts.

Although heparin is concentrated at the graft surface in CBAS, the absolute amount of heparin is relatively small, for example, less than 400 U for a PROPATEN vascular graft (W. L. Gore & Associates, 2009 Website). As noted, this heparin does not leach (elute) from the graft. In theory, even if all the heparin from a larger vascular graft suddenly entered the circulation, the concentration of heparin would be lower than 0.1 U/mL.

There is substantial long-term persistence of CBAS heparin activity (at least up to 12 weeks), based on a chronic canine model (Begovac et al., 2003). Analysis of an explanted PROPATEN vascular graft implanted eight months earlier showed residual heparin activity that was within the end-of-shelf-life specification for the product (information provided by Gore); and a Berlin Heart ventricular assist device (VAD) explanted after two years had 50% of estimated initial heparin activity (Riesenfeld et al., 2007).

The rationale for clinical use of heparin-coated vascular grafts is their good-to-excellent short-term and long-term patency (Kirkwood et al., 2011), including in high-risk infragenicular (below-the-knee) bypasses (Dorrucci et al., 2008). In a multicenter randomized trial, superior one-year patency was shown for the heparin-bonded ePTFE (PROPATEN) compared with non–heparin-bonded ePTFE grafts (Lindholt et al., 2011) (Fig. 20.3). It is unclear, however, whether all types of heparin-coated devices would necessarily show an advantage over the corresponding non–heparin-coated device, as specific properties of any given coating technology—for example, functional heparin activity and its persistence—may be crucial for their long-term clinical benefit.

Other Covalent Heparin-Bonding Technologies
Other devices utilize heparin that is covalently immobilized through proprietary techniques distinct from CBAS (Table 20.1). Relatively little technical information is available regarding these approaches used for heparin bonding. To the extent that

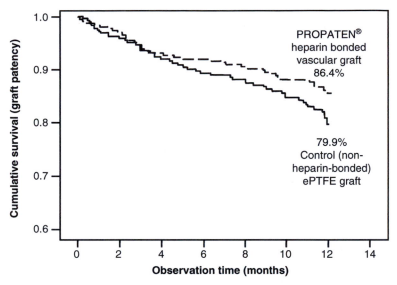

FIGURE 20.3   One-year primary patency of heparin-bonded ePTFE vascular grafts (PROPATEN®) and (nonheparin-bonded) ePTFE vascular grafts, including silent occlusions discovered after one year. The higher one-year primary graft patency rate for heparin-bonded (*vs* nonheparin-bonded) ePTFE grafts (86.4% *vs* 79.9%) was statistically significant (*P* = 0.043). *Abbreviation*: ePTFE, expanded polytetrafluoroethylene. *Source*: From Lindholt et al. (2011).

some techniques might achieve some proportion of multipoint-linked heparin, there could be a decrease in heparin bioactivity relative to endpoint-linked heparin.

THEORETICAL ISSUES

Suh and coworkers (1998) showed that HIT antibodies bind to PF4 that is bound to immobilized heparin, but only when the heparin is bound as endpoint linkage, rather than via multipoint linkages. For this reason, this section will focus on the theoretical issues of HIT involving endpoint linkage of heparin.

Given that standard enzyme immunoassay (EIA) technology to detect HIT antibodies uses heparin bound to a surface, it might seem obvious that HIT antibodies would bind to heparin immobilized through endpoint linkage. However, in commercial EIAs, PF4/H complexes are first formed in the fluid-phase at stoichiometrically optimal concentrations (and using purified PF4), and only then bound to the solid phase; moreover, subsequent incubations to detect HIT antibodies use diluted patient plasma or serum, and consequently the role of competing proteins in these various steps is not physiologic. Furthermore, the specific mechanism of heparin binding employed by Suh and coworkers—although similar to—is likely not identical to any of the commercial products. For these reasons, one cannot extrapolate to the clinic these *in vitro* studies of HIT antibody binding.

Approximately 50% of the protein eluted from a model CBAS surface in acute *in vitro* blood contact experiments is AT, with the remaining being well-known heparin-binding proteins, such as apolipoproteins, plasminogen, and serine protease inhibitors, for example, heparin cofactor II (Biran et al., 2011). Of note, PF4 was *not* identified in these studies as one of the eluted proteins.

Furthermore, following implantation of a CBAS-coated graft, a protein layer covers the CBAS surface, which presumably restricts platelets and other cells from making contact (Fisher et al., 2011).

IMMUNIZATION STUDIES

It is not possible to perform nonconfounded studies of anti-PF4/H immunization associated with the use of many heparin-coated devices. For example, heparin-coated arterial grafts devices will invariably be implanted with intraoperative UFH (and often additional prophylactic- or therapeutic-dose UFH or LMWH given pre- or postoperatively).

Koster and colleagues (2000, 2001) reported on the frequency of anti-PF4/H antibodies in patients who received heparin-coated *versus* non–heparin-coated VADs (Koster et al., 2000, 2001). Besides routine intraoperative UFH, these patients all received postoperative UFH for at least seven days (and for at least one month in one-third of the patients). In their first report (2000), they compared 30 patients who received the Berlin Heart (with CBAS-heparin) against 25 patients who received one of three non–heparin-coated VADs (Novacor, TCI, DeBakey). On day 14, 20 (67%) of 30 Berlin Heart recipients had positive anti-PF4/H antibodies (by polyspecific EIA), *versus* 20 (80%) of 25 controls. Confounding with systemic UFH was shown by the observation that all of the control patients were already seropositive prior to VAD implantation, and 15 of 20 Berlin Heart patients were seropositive preimplantation. At three months, five (25%) of the 20 Berlin Heart patients had become seronegative *versus* six (30%) of the 20 controls; in all seronegative patients, concomitant administration of systemic UFH had also been stopped. The authors concluded that "[c]oating the surfaces of the VADs with [CBAS] was not associated with an increased formation or persistence of positive [anti-PF4/H] antibody status."

Koster and colleagues (2001) extended these studies in a further 45 patients, reporting the entire 100-patient population (heparin-coated, $n = 57$; controls, $n = 43$). Overall, positive testing for anti-PF4/H antibodies was seen in 32 (56%) of 57 who received CBAS-coated VADs *versus* 31 (72%) of 43 who received a non–heparin-coated device. Importantly, 14 (44%) of 32 seropositive patients who had the Berlin Heart became seronegative [*vs* 18/31 (58%) controls], indicating that antibodies disappeared despite ongoing exposure to CBAS-heparin.

More recently, Heyligers et al. (2008) studied 20 patients who underwent implantation of a femoropopliteal bypass graft—10 with a CBAS-heparin ePTFE graft and 10 with an uncoated ePTFE graft—and found that none of the 20 patients developed anti-PF4/H antibodies (at six-week follow-up). However, besides small patient numbers, blood sampling was additionally performed only on postoperative days 1, 3, and 5, so a transient immune response peaking at postoperative days 10–14 and disappearing within a month would have been missed.

HIT REPORTS
Heparin-Eluting Devices and HIT

Historically, the first association between heparin-coated devices and HIT was reported for ionically bonded (heparin-eluting) catheters. These studies, which were performed under the aegis of the vascular surgeon, Don Silver, at the University of Columbia, combined clinical observations with *in vitro* studies using (ionically bound) heparin-coated catheters as the source of heparin for performing conventional platelet aggregometry. As reviewed in chapter 11, these investigations test for effects of HIT antibodies by assessing aggregation of platelets in platelet-rich plasma (PRP) obtained from normal blood donors in the presence of platelet-poor plasma (PPP) obtained from HIT patients or controls.

Laster and Silver (1988) reported 10 patients with putative HIT in whom the platelet counts did not recover until removal of the heparin-coated catheters; *in vitro* studies using catheter segments as a source of heparin for patient PPP and normal PRP observed that platelet aggregation only occurred with pretreatment using heparin-bonded segments and not with (control) non–heparin-bonded catheter segments. It is difficult to discern from the clinical descriptions whether or not the patients had HIT (some reports were suggestive of transient perioperative thrombocytopenia). Furthermore, PRP aggregation studies are not as diagnostically specific for HIT antibodies, given the nonspecific effects of UFH in aggregating platelets in PRP (see chaps. 5 and 11).

Subsequently, this group (Laster et al., 1989) reported on 12 patients with putative HIT associated with heparin-coated catheters (two new cases plus the previous 10). One of the newly reported cases had features that were atypical for HIT, including "white clot syndrome" that occurred unusually early (postoperative day 1) following abdominal aortic aneurysm surgery. The authors reported an abrupt decrease in the platelet count when a heparin-coated pulmonary artery catheter was placed four days later; however, the catheter was placed because "the patient's cardiovascular function was deteriorating," a clinical event that could also be associated with thrombocytopenia.

The research group extended their studies to experimental (nonmarketed) heparin-bonded vascular grafts, testing three types of grafts obtained from two manufacturers (Almeida et al., 1998). In preliminary experiments, they identified the length of graft segment that would leach an equivalent of $1\,U/mL$ of UFH, and then performed platelet aggregation experiments using known HIT plasmas that had been exposed to the grafts for 30 minutes, prior to removal of the grafts and addition of PRP for studies of platelet aggregation. They found that the heparin-bonded (but not control non–heparin-bonded) grafts supported platelet aggregation by HIT plasmas. The authors argued that industry should avoid development of heparin-bonded grafts. However, given that graft implantation at the time of vascular surgery would invariably require heparin administration, the role of additional small amounts of heparin on immunogenicity and HIT pathogenicity would seem unlikely, particularly since most of the ionically bound UFH would be expected to have leached off the grafts prior to the formation of HIT antibodies (at least five days later). Moreover, the relatively high concentrations of UFH achieved under their experimental conditions are unlikely to be reached when the heparin elutes into a patient's whole blood volume over a period of hours to days.

Mureebe et al. (2007) repeated these studies several years later with a marketed heparin-bonded Dacron graft (INTERGARD heparin-knitted polyester graft). In these experiments, 1 cm sections of graft were incubated in 5 mL of PPP—the resulting UFH concentrations measured at $1.82\,U/mL$ (mean) if the PPP was incubated with heparin-coated graft, and $0\,U/mL$ when incubated with control (non–heparin-coated) graft. As before, platelet aggregation was caused by HIT patient PPP when incubated with UFH that had "leached" from these grafts to which heparin had been ionically bonded using TDMAC.

A Japanese group (Nasuno et al., 2003) reported a case of HIT in which a large thrombus had formed around the heparin-coated central venous catheter. However, it is known that (non–heparin-coated) central venous lines are strongly associated with thrombus formation [upperlimb deep vein thrombosis (DVT)] at the site of the central line in patients with HIT (Hong et al., 2003).

Given that UFH can rapidly elute within several hours to a few days after catheter insertion, it is at least theoretically conceivable that insertion of a catheter with ionically bonded UFH might exacerbate HIT. Potentially, there could be locally increased UFH concentrations and associated formation of HIT-related thrombus at the site of the catheter releasing UFH. However, as noted above, the concentrations of systemic UFH that would arise from catheter use would likely be substantially lower than the concentrations achieved *in vitro* when the catheter segments were placed in relatively small volumes of PPP. Also, with insertion of permanent grafts ionically coated with heparin, it seems likely that only minor amounts of residual UFH would continue to be leached after several days, that is, at the time that pathogenic HIT antibodies could arise because of UFH administered during the preceding graft implantation surgery. However, contemporary techniques of ionic heparin-bonding employ slower release profiles (extended over days) compared with direct ionic interaction (Hsu et al., 1991).

Non-Heparin Eluting Devices and HIT
Difficulties in Attributing Causation: Persisting HIT after Implantation of a Non–Heparin-Coated Graft
Bürger et al. (2001) reported a case of HIT that occurred following implantation of a Dacron vascular graft. Surgery was performed with perioperative and intraoperative administration of UFH. However, the HIT-associated period of thrombocytopenia persisted for approximately 50 days, despite anticoagulation with sc desirudin 15 mg twice-daily and transient platelet count increase with high-dose iv immunoglobulin G (iv IgG). The authors concluded that the Dacron graft—despite the manufacturer's insistence that there was no heparin coating—must have played a role in the HIT. However, arguing against the role of the graft is the recognition that for approximately 1% of patients with HIT there is delay in recovery of the platelet count for more than one month (Warkentin and Kelton, 2001a) (see chap. 2).

Delayed-Onset and Persisting HIT
Approximately 3–5% of patients develop HIT several days after their last exposure to heparin, a phenomenon that has been called "delayed-onset HIT" (Rice et al., 2001; Warkentin and Kelton, 2001a). Perhaps even more common are patients who develop HIT while receiving heparin, but in whom the thrombocytopenia and hypercoagulability state worsen for several days despite discontinuing all heparin (Warkentin, 2010; Linkins and Warkentin, 2011). Usually, the platelet count nadir is reached approximately 14 days after the immunizing heparin exposure (e.g., intraoperative UFH), although in a small number of patients the platelet count may take several weeks or even months to recover to normal levels ("persisting HIT"). The key observation is that numerous cases of delayed-onset HIT have occurred in patients who have no ongoing systemic or device-associated heparin exposure whatsoever, indicating that this phenomenon can simply represent the natural history of HIT. The fact that such cases exist calls into question the common assumption that in a patient who develops postoperative HIT and whose only ongoing

heparin exposure is a heparin-coated graft or other device, that the graft must be the explanation for development of and/or the persistence of HIT.

Patients exhibiting the phenomenon of delayed-onset HIT have certain characteristic serologic findings. First, they usually have very strong positive results in PF4-dependent EIAs [>2.0 units of optical density (OD)]. Second, their serum exhibits strong heparin-independent platelet-activating properties, that is, the serum often triggers substantial platelet activation with buffer control [>80% serotonin release in the platelet serotonin release assay (SRA)], with a further increase in platelet activation in the presence of pharmacologic heparin concentrations (as with conventional HIT antibodies, there is also inhibition of platelet activation at very high heparin concentrations). Third, these patients appear to have a high frequency of HIT-associated disseminated intravascular coagulation (DIC) and thrombotic events.

Reports of HIT with CBAS-Coated Vascular Grafts

Thakur and coworkers (2009) reported a 79-year-old man who received a PRO-PATEN graft from superficial femoral artery to tibioperoneal trunk; 6000-U intraoperative UFH were given, as well as postoperative LMWH (enoxaparin) 70 mg every 12 hours by sc injection. On day 9 the platelet count was 11×10^9/L, and LMWH was replaced by argatroban. The platelet count further declined to 8×10^9/L after four days of argatroban. Although no limb ischemia was reported, the severe persisting thrombocytopenia prompted explantation of the graft, which was replaced with a standard graft. Rapid platelet count recovery ensued (likely aided by a platelet transfusion). The explanted graft contained "friable, nonocclusive clots." The EIA showed a strong positive test for HIT antibodies (3.58 OD units). The authors concluded that "If HIT is confirmed, the entire heparin-bonded graft should be explanted and an alternative prosthesis inserted."

Gabrielli et al. (2011) described a 67-year-old woman who received a heparin-coated PTFE (PROPATEN) left femoropopliteal bypass graft to the popliteal artery (above the knee), with 5000-U intraoperative UFH given and postoperative antiplatelet therapy (ASA, clopidogrel); no postoperative heparin was given. The platelet count nadir was 29×10^9/L on day 9, and the patient had symptomatic left lower limb ischemia attributed to combined thrombosis of the bypass graft and DVT. A PF4-dependent EIA was positive. The patient was anticoagulated with argatroban, and an emergency graft explant—with replacement by non–heparin-coated ePTFE graft—was performed while continuing argatroban. The platelet count recovered to 189×10^9/L one week postexplant. The authors concluded that "[h]eparin-coated PTFE graft-induced HIT requires an entire graft explant and an alternative prosthesis placement."

Wheatcroft et al. (2011) reported a 92-year-old woman who received a profunda to tibioperoneal trunk bypass using a heparin-bonded ePTFE graft (PRO-PATEN), with intraoperative UFH anticoagulation and postoperative enoxaparin prophylaxis. On day 8, after the platelet count declined by >50% to approximately 140×10^9/L, the patient was switched from enoxaparin to argatroban. A diagnosis of HIT was supported by the EIA-IgG measuring 1.95, and the SRA showing heparin-independent platelet activation (94% serotonin release at 0 U/mL heparin, 100% release at 0.2 U/mL heparin, and 0% at 100 U/mL). The platelet count continued to decline to a nadir of 42×10^9/L despite five days of argatroban (Fig. 20.4A). Moreover, the distal foot (at the site of a recently amputated toe) developed progressive

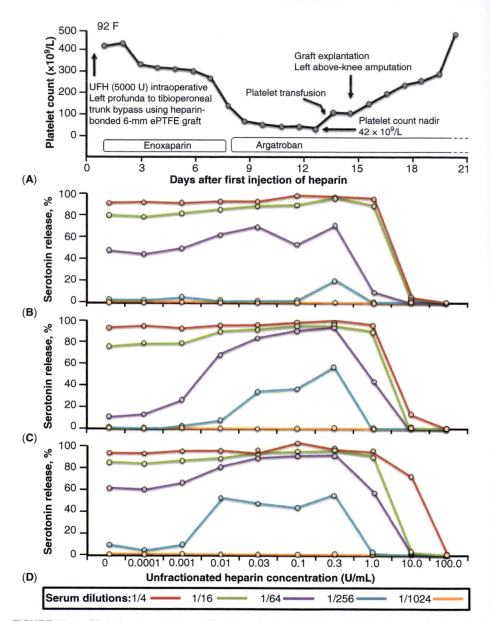

FIGURE 20.4 Clinical and serologic profile of a patient with HIT associated with use of a heparin-coated vascular graft: comparison with serologic profiles of two patients with delayed-onset HIT phenotype. (**A**) Serial platelet counts and clinical course of patient reported by Wheatcroft and colleagues (2011). (**B**) For the patient depicted in panel A, serum-induced percent serotonin release in the presence of buffer control (0 U/mL heparin) and various concentrations of heparin (ranging from 0.0001 to 100 U/mL) are shown, performed with serial four-fold serum dilutions ranging from 1/4 to 1/1024. The patient's serum induced "strong" (approximately 80% serotonin release or greater) platelet activation in the absence of heparin (at 1/4 and 1/16 serum dilutions). As is characteristic of HIT sera, high concentrations of UFH (10 and 100 U/mL) inhibited platelet activation. (*Continued*)

FIGURE 20.4 (*Continued*) (**C**) and (**D**) Similar serologic profiles of strong serum-induced heparin-independent platelet activation (i.e., substantial serotonin release at buffer control at 1/4 and 1/16 dilutions) were also observed in two patients with delayed-onset HIT phenotype. Panel C corresponds to patient 1 from Warkentin and Kelton (2001a), i.e., a patient with "classic" delayed-onset HIT [68-year-old woman who developed transient global amnesia, venous thrombosis, and DIC eight days following the first of three perioperative injections of UFH for thromboprophylaxis (platelet count nadir, 14×10^9/L)]. Panel D corresponds to a 78-year-old woman with colon cancer who developed HIT postcolectomy while receiving sc UFH and whose platelet count continued to fall from 53 to 19×10^9/L after stopping UFH. The serologic studies shown in panel B (and appropriate controls shown in panels C and D) were performed after discussions with the patient's attending surgeon (Dr. Graham Roche-Nagle, Department of Surgery, University of Toronto) and with the approval of the McMaster Research Ethics Board. *Abbreviations*: DTI, direct thrombin inhibitor; HIT, heparin-induced thrombocytopenia; iv IgG, intravenous (high-dose) gammaglobulin; PF4/H, platelet factor 4/heparin; PTT, partial thromboplastin time; DIC, disseminated intravascular coagulation; ePTFE, expanded polytetrafluoroethylene; F, female; sc, subcutaneous; U, units; UFH, unfractionated heparin.

ischemic changes. Although there was no evidence of graft occlusion by duplex, the graft was explanted and an above-the-knee amputation was performed. The authors remarked: "if symptoms persist or the health of the patient appears compromised, strong consideration must be given to the removal of the heparin-bonded graft if the thrombocytopenia is to be reversed and complications avoided."

Because the case reported by Wheatcroft and colleagues occurred in Toronto, the blood had been referred for serologic investigations for HIT in our nearby laboratory in Hamilton (at McMaster University). To test the hypothesis that the serologic features were consistent with delayed-onset HIT, we performed the SRA at various concentrations of heparin, and with various dilutions of patient's serum: 1/4, 1/16, 1/64, and 1/256 (Fig. 20.4B). We compared the reactivity against two other sera we had previously shown to have strong heparin-independent platelet-activating properties, and whose clinical features were consistent with HIT that either began after stopping heparin (Fig. 20.4C), or that substantially worsened after stopping heparin (Fig. 20.4D). As predicted, the serologic profile of strong heparin-independent platelet activation consistent with a "delayed-onset HIT" phenotype was observed in the Toronto patient, thus calling into question any role for the heparin-bonded graft in the patient's clinical course.

Kasirajan et al. (2012) performed a retrospective analysis of suspected cases of HIT following implant of PROPATEN vascular grafts. The investigator analyzed published reports, as well as cases reported to the manufacturer (W. L. Gore & Associates). As of June 2011, there have been 27 patients (30 vascular grafts) with suspected HIT post–graft implant. At least one positive test for HIT antibodies was obtained in 17 of 18 patients tested (in five patients, discrepant negative and positive results were obtained with two different assays). A mean of 4850 U of UFH was given at operation; the mean platelet count at HIT diagnosis was 53×10^9/L (mean preoperative platelet count, 227×10^9/L). Argatroban was the most frequent alternative anticoagulant used for management. Of the 26 patients with known outcomes, 16 had grafts remain implanted and in circulation, eight were explanted, and two were ligated *in situ*. Among the 16 patients with grafts remaining in circulation, four grafts required thrombectomy for occlusion, two patients died, and one other patient had a remote thrombotic event; the remaining patients had no reported adverse events. Among the 10 patients with graft removal or ligation, six patients had a graft occlusion (four patients required amputation, and two died). Among the cases in which platelet count recovery was reported after systemic heparin was discontinued, the majority were cases in which the grafts were left in circulation. The author concluded that systemic heparin seemed to be the likely trigger of HIT, and that the platelet counts typically normalized even when the grafts remained *in situ*.

Reports of HIT with CBAS-Coated Stents or Stent-Grafts

Cruz and coworkers (2003) reported a case of HIT associated with the use of a heparin-coated stent. The 66-year-old man with acute inferior myocardial infarction received a heparin-coated stent (Bx Velocity™ coronary stent with Hepacoat™, Cordis) and was discharged to home on clopidogrel and aspirin (discharge platelet count, $413 \times 10^9/L$). He was readmitted 15 days post–stent placement with a thrombotic stroke and bilateral DVT; a patent foramen ovale was detected. The platelet count was only $130 \times 10^9/L$ at the time of readmission, and fell to 51 within three days of administering UFH. HIT antibodies were reported "positive." Heparin was changed to argatroban, and the platelet count "returned to baseline." Thirty-four days post–stent placement, and three days after stopping clopidogrel (but while receiving warfarin), the patient developed complete occlusion of the right coronary artery, and reestablishment of flow was made with balloon angioplasty. As noted by Bittl (2003) in an editorial, this case might well fit within the spectrum of "delayed-onset HIT."

SUMMARY AND INTERPRETATION OF DATA

In my view, these aforementioned reports of HIT cases suggesting a pathogenic role of covalently bound heparin-coated grafts have not considered the important confounding role of strong HIT antibodies with heparin-independent platelet-activating effects. Delayed-onset (or "autoimmune-like") HIT is an increasingly recognized complication of UFH (and sometimes LMWH) given intra-/perioperatively, and occurs in 3–5% of HIT patients. The frequency is probably higher when one additionally considers patients in whom the HIT worsens or persists despite stopping heparin (Linkins and Warkentin, 2011). The relative paucity of cases of HIT in the setting of heparin-coated grafts suggests that these cases may represent delayed-onset HIT with the presence of the heparin-coated device being merely coincidental. Indeed, direct evidence for the presence of such antibodies was observed in the patient case reported by Wheatcroft and colleagues (2011) (Fig. 20.4B).

Also, most physicians are not aware of the remarkable transience of HIT antibodies (Warkentin and Kelton, 2001b)—including even when systemic heparin continues to be given (Greinacher et al., 2009). Kasirajan's finding (2012) that resolution of thrombocytopenia occurred even when the grafts remained *in situ* and in circulation is in keeping with HIT antibody transience. Thus, thrombocytopenia that has resolved upon explantation of the heparin-coated device likely is coincidental with the natural history of HIT.

Most explanted grafts to date have not exhibited occlusion by platelet-rich thrombi. Although some adherence of platelet-rich thrombi might be expected (as even with non–heparin-coated grafts it is relatively common for HIT to involve thrombotic occlusion of newly implanted grafts), this has only been observed in a minority of cases (Kasirajan et al., 2012). If noneluting heparin-bonded grafts were directly activating platelets and thereby maintaining clinically evident HIT, one might expect that the most prominent clinical feature would be graft thrombosis or associated thromboembolism.

Management Plan in Case of HIT Occurring in Patients with Implanted Heparin-Bonded Devices

Explantation of a new vascular graft is not an inconsequential procedure; there will be loss of vascular integrity, possible interruption of anticoagulation (e.g., for postoperative hemostasis), and intraoperative platelet transfusions might also be given. Table 20.3 lists a therapeutic approach that avoids preemptive graft explantation, and which emphasizes: (*i*) optimal anticoagulation with an alternative nonheparin

TABLE 20.3 Suggested Management for a Patient with Acute HIT Occurring One to Two Weeks After Implantation of a Heparin-Coated Graft or Stent-Graft

Anticoagulation
1. Therapeutic-dose anticoagulation with an alternative, nonheparin anticoagulant, aiming for high-therapeutic levels, either:
   a. Indirect factor Xa inhibitor (e.g., danaparoid[a], fondaparinux) with antifactor Xa monitoring (if available); or
   b. DTI (e.g., bivalirudin, argatroban, hirudin)—caution: beware "PTT confounding" due to HIT-associated consumptive coagulopathy or recent use of warfarin; ideally, patients should be monitored by direct DTI levels, if available.
2. Use ancillary coagulation parameters to assess response to therapy (e.g., measure daily D-dimer and fibrinogen levels).[b]
3. Avoid warfarin until thrombocytopenia has resolved (give vitamin K by iv route if HIT is diagnosed only after a vitamin K antagonist has already been given).[c]

Antiplatelet therapy
1. Adjunctive therapy with aspirin and/or clopidogrel.
2. High-dose iv IgG (1 g/kg given twice [one or two days apart]) to interrupt HIT antibody-induced platelet activation.
3. Avoid platelet transfusions.

Surgical considerations
1. Recommend "watchful waiting" *without* graft explantation.
2. Thromboembolectomy in case of partial or complete obstruction of the heparin-coated vascular graft.

Laboratory investigations for HIT antibodies
1. Refer blood to laboratory that can assess heparin-independent platelet activation by functional (platelet activation) assay (e.g., McMaster Platelet Immunology, Hamilton, Canada; or Ernst-Moritz-Arndt University, Greifswald, Germany).
2. Repeat testing every 5–10 days to document waning of anti-PF4/H immune response (including decrease in heparin-independent platelet-activating properties).

The above treatment recommendations are based on the rationale that the HIT is related to "delayed-onset" (autoimmune) HIT mechanisms and that the heparin-coated graft is likely an "innocent bystander" (see text). Moreover, the natural history is for the HIT intensity to peak approximately two weeks after the immunizing heparin exposure (i.e., heparin given during the preceding surgery wherein the device was implanted), and to diminish either rapidly (most often) or gradually thereafter.

[a]Danaparoid has theoretical advantages in this clinical situation: (a) rapid anticoagulation can be achieved with iv bolus administration; (b) antifactor Xa levels can be measured; (c) high-therapeutic concentrations of danaparoid inhibit HIT antibody-induced platelet activation (Krauel et al., 2008).

[b]D-dimer levels should decrease, and fibrinogen levels should increase, if satisfactory anticoagulation is being achieved.

[c]Vitamin K antagonists (e.g., warfarin) are contraindicated during the acute phase of HIT treatment because of the risk of precipitating microthrombosis (e.g., venous limb gangrene).

Abbreviations: DTI, direct thrombin inhibitor; HIT, heparin-induced thrombocytopenia; iv IgG, intravenous (high-dose) gammaglobulin; PF4/H, platelet factor 4/heparin; PTT, partial thromboplastin time.

agent; (ii) antiplatelet therapy (including high-dose iv IgG); (iii) thromboembolectomy (if indicated) with "watchful waiting" rather than graft explantation; and
(iv) laboratory testing to document presence of heparin-independent platelet-
activating properties, and to follow the expected diminution of antibody levels and
associated platelet-activating properties over days to a few weeks.

REFERENCES

Ahmadi R, Schillinger M, Maca T, Minar E. Femoropopliteal arteries: immediate and long-
    term results with a Dacron-covered stent-graft. Radiology 223: 345–350, 2002.
Almeida JI, Liem TK, Silver D. Heparin-bonded grafts induce platelet aggregation in the pres-
    ence of heparin-associated antiplatelet antibodies. J Vasc Surg 27: 896–901, 1998.
Begovac PC, Thomson RC, Fisher JL, Hughson A, Gällhagen A. Improvements in GORE-TEX®
    vascular graft performance by Carmeda® BioActive surface heparin immobilization. Eur J
    Vasc Endovasc Surg 25: 432–437, 2003.
Biran R, Gore S, Pond D, Andersson J, Sundin G, Riesenfeld J. Analysis of proteins associated
    with the Carmeda Bioactive Surface (CVAS) after acute blood contact [abstr]. Presented at
    the 12th Biennial Meeting of the International Society for Applied Cardiovascular Biology
    (ISACB), Boston, MA, Sep 22–25, 2010. Cardiovascular Pathology 20: e122, 2011.
Bittl JA. Heparin-coated stent and heparin-induced thrombocytopenia: true, true, and con-
    ceivably related. Catheter Cardiovasc Intervent 58: 84–85, 2003.
Bürger T, Tautenhahn J, Böck M, Fahlke J, Halloul Z, Lippert H. Can a coated Dacron vascular
    graft maintain a heparin-induced thrombocytopenia type II? Langenbecks Arch Surg 386:
    267–271, 2001.
Cornelius RM, Sanchez J, Olsson P, Brash JL. Interactions of antithrombin and proteins in the
    plasma contact activation system with immobilized functional heparin. J Biomed Mater
    Res A 67: 475–483, 2003.
Cruz D, Karlsberg R, Takano Y, Vora D, Tobis J. Subacute stent thrombosis associated with a
    heparin-coated stent and heparin-induced thrombocytopenia. Catheter Cardiovasc Inter-
    vent 58: 80–83, 2003.
Dorrucci V, Griselli F, Petralia G, Spinamano L, Adornetto R. Heparin-bonded expanded
    polytetrafluoroethylene grafts for infragenicular bypass in patients with critical limb isch-
    emia: 2-year results. J Cardiovasc Surg (Torino) 49: 145–149, 2008.
Elgue G, Blombäck M, Olsson P, Riesenfeld J. On the mechanism of coagulation inhibition on
    surfaces with end point immobilized heparin. Thromb Haemost 70: 289–293, 1993.
Fisher JL, Riesenfeld J, Begovac PC. Reduced protein deposition on heparinized CBAS-ePTFE
    vascular grafts: a mechanism for in vivo persistence of heparin bioactivity. Cardiovasc
    Pathol 20: e118, 2011. [Presented at the 12th Biennial Meeting of the International Society
    for Applied Cardiovascular Biology (ISACV), Boston, MA, 22–25, Sep 2010.]
Gabrielli R, Siani A, Rosati MS, Antonelli R, Accrocca F, Giordano GA, Marcucci G. Heparin-
    induced thrombocytopenia type II because of heparin-coated polytetrafluoroethylene
    graft used to bypass. Ann Vasc Surg 25: 840.e9–e12, 2011.
Gore WL, Associates Inc. Frequently asked questions, Gore PROPATEN vascular
    graft, October, 2009 [Available from: www.goremedical.com/resources/dam/assets/
    AK0409EN3.PVG.FAQ.BRO.FNL.mr.pdf] (Accessed Jan 28, 2012).
Gao C, Boylan B, Fang J, Wilcox DA, Newman DK, Newman PJ. Heparin promotes platelet
    responsiveness by potentiating αIIbβ3-mediated outside-in signaling. Blood 117: 4946–4952,
    2011.
Gott VL, Whiffen JD, Dutton RC. Heparin bonding on colloidal graphite surfaces. Science 142:
    1297–1298, 1963.
Greinacher A, Kohlmann T, Strobel U, Sheppard JI, Warkentin TE. The temporal profile of the
    anti-PF4/heparin immune response. Blood 113: 4970–4976, 2009.
Heyligers JMM, Verhagen HJM, Rotmans JI, Weeterings C, de Groot PG, Moll FL, Lisman T.
    Heparin immobilization reduces thrombogenicity of small-caliber expanded polytetra-
    fluoroethylene grafts. J Vasc Surg 43: 587–591, 2006.

Heyligers JMM, Lisman T, Verhagen HJM, Weeterings C, de Groot PG, Moll FL. A heparin-bonded vascular graft generates no systemic effect on markers of hemostasis activation or detectable heparin-induced thrombocytopenia-associated antibodies in humans. J Vasc Surg 47: 324–329, 2008.

Hong AP, Cook DJ, Sigouin CS, Warkentin TE. Central venous catheters and upper-extremity deep-vein thrombosis complicating immune heparin-induced thrombocytopenia. Blood 101: 3049–3051, 2003.

Hsu LC. Principles of heparin-coating techniques. Perfusion 6: 209–219, 1991.

Kasirajan K. Outcomes after heparin-induced thrombocytopenia in Patients with Propaten vascular grafts. Ann Vasc Surg 26: 802–808, 2012.

Kirkwood ML, Wang GJ, Jackson BM, Golden MA, Fairman RM, Woo EY. Lower limb revascularization for PAD using a heparin-coated PTFE conduit. Vasc Endovascular Surg 45: 329–334, 2011.

Kocsis JF, Llanos G, Holmer E. Heparin-coated stents. J Long Term Eff Med Implants 10: 19–45, 2000.

Koster A, Sänger S, Hansen R, Sodian R, Mertzlufft F, Harke C, Kuppe H, Hetzer R, Loebe M. Prevalence and persistence of heparin/platelet factor 4 antibodies in patients with heparin coated and noncoated ventricular assist devices. ASAIO J 46: 319–322, 2000.

Koster A, Loebe M, Sodian R, Potapov EV, Hansen R, Müller J, Mertzlufft F, Crystal GJ, Kuppe H, Hetzer R. Heparin antibodies and thromboembolism in heparin-coated and noncoated ventricular assist devices. J Thorac Cardiovasc Surg 121: 331–335, 2001.

Kramer RS, Vasko JS, Morrow AG. Stability of graphite-benzalkonium-heparin surfaces. J Thorac Cardiovasc Surg 53: 130–137, 1967.

Krauel K, Fürll B, Warkentin TE, Weitschies W, Kohlmann T, Sheppard JI, Greinacher A. Heparin-induced thrombocytopenia—therapeutic concentrations of danaparoid, unlike fondaparinux and direct thrombin inhibitors, inhibit formation of PF4/heparin complexes. J Thromb Haemost 6: 2160–2167, 2008.

Kwa AT, Yeo KK, Laird JR. The role of stent-grafts for prevention and treatment of restenosis. J Cardiovasc Surg (Torino) 51: 579–589, 2010.

Lappegård KT, Fung M, Bergseth G, Riesenfeld J, Lambris JD, Videm V, Mollnes TE. Effect of complement inhibition and heparin coating on artificial surface-induced leukocyte and platelet activation. Ann Thorac Surg 77: 932–941, 2004.

Larm O, Larsson R, Olsson P. A new non-thrombogenic surface prepared by selective covalent binding of heparin via a modified reducing terminal residue. Biomater Med Devices Artif Organs 11: 161–173, 1983.

Larsson R. Heparin-binding to improve biocompatibility. In: Bowlin GL, Wnek G, eds. Encyclopedia of Biomaterials and Biomedical Engineering. Informa Healthcare, USA 753–761, 2004.

Laster J, Silver D. Heparin-coated catheters and heparin-induced thrombocytopenia. J Vasc Surg 7: 667–672, 1988.

Laster J, Nichols WK, Silver D. Thrombocytopenia associated with heparin-coated catheters in patients with heparin-associated antiplatelet antibodies. Arch Intern Med 149: 2285–2287, 1989.

Lindholt JS, Gottschalksen B, Johannesen N, Dueholm D, Ravn H, Christensen ED, Viddal B, Flørenes T, Pedersen G, Rasmussen M, Carstensen M, Grøndal N, Fasting H. The Scandinavian Propaten® trial—1-year patency of PTFE vascular prostheses with heparin-bonded luminal surfaces compared to ordinary pure PTFE vascular prostheses—a randomized clinical controlled multi-centre trial. Eur J Vasc Endovasc Surg 41: 668–673, 2011.

Linkins LA, Warkentin TE. Heparin-induced thrombocytopenia: real world issues. Semin Thromb Hemost 37: 653–663, 2011.

Mollnes TE, Riesenfeld J, Garred P, Nordström E, Høgåsen K, Fosse E, Götze O, Harboe M. A new model for evaluation of biocompatibility: combined determination of neoepitopes in blood and on artificial surfaces demonstrates reduced complement activation by immobilization of heparin. Artif Organs 19: 909–917, 1995.

Mollnes TE, Videm V, Christiansen D, Bergseth G, Riesenfeld J, Hovig T. Platelet compatibility of an artificial surface modified with functionally active heparin. Thromb Haemost 82: 1132–1136, 1999.

Mureebe L, Graham JA, Bush RL, Silver D. Risk of heparin-induced thrombocytopenia from heparin-bonded vascular prostheses. Ann Vasc Surg 21: 719–722, 2007.

Nasuno A, Matsubara T, Hori T, Higuchi K, Tsuchida K, Mezaki T, Tanaka T, Hanzawa K, Moro H, Hayashi J, Tanaka K, Fuse I, Aizawa Y. Acute pulmonary thromboembolism induced by prophylactic heparin use and a heparin-coated catheter—a case of heparin-induced thrombocytopenia and thrombosis syndrome. Circ J 67: 96–98, 2003.

Olsson P, Sanchez J, Mollnes TE, Riesenfeld J. On the blood compatibility of end-point immo-bilized heparin. J Biomater Sci Polym Ed 11: 1261–1273, 2000.

Rice L, Attisha WK, Drexler A, Francis JL. Delayed-onset heparin-induced thrombocytopenia. Ann Intern Med 136: 210–215, 2001.

Riesenfeld J, Ries D, Hetzer R. Analysis of the heparin coating of an EXCOR® ventricular assist device after 855 days in a patient. Presented at the 32nd Society for Biomaterials Annual Meeting, Chicago, IL, 18–21 Apr 2007. Abstract 180.

Salzman EW, Rosenberg RD, Smith MH, Lindon JN, Favreau L. Effect of heparin and heparin fractions on platelet aggregation. J Clin Invest 65: 64–73, 1980.

Sanchez J, Elgue G, Riesenfeld J, Olsson P. Control of contact activation on end-point immo-bilized heparin: the role of antithrombin and the specific antithrombin-binding sequence. J Biomed Mater Res 29: 655–661, 1995.

Sanchez J, Elgue G, Riesenfeld J, Olsson P. Inhibition of the plasma contact activation system of immobilized heparin: relation to surface density of functional antithrombin binding sites. J Biomed Mater Res 37: 37–42, 1997.

Sanchez J, Elgue G, Riesenfeld J, Olsson P. Studies of absorption, activation, and inhibition of factor XII on immobilized heparin. Thromb Res 89: 41–50, 1998.

Suh JS, Aster H, Visentin GP. Antibodies from patients with heparin-induced thrombocyto-penia/thrombosis recognize different epitopes on heparin: platelet factor 4. Blood 91: 916–922, 1998.

Tanzi MC. Bioactive technologies for hemocompatibility. Expert Rev Med Devices 2: 473–492, 2005.

Thakur S, Pigott JP, Comerota AJ. Heparin-induced thrombocytopenia after implantation of a heparin-bonded polytetrafluoroethylene lower extremity bypass graft: a case report and plan for management. J Vasc Surg 49: 1037–1040, 2009.

Warkentin TE. Agents for the treatment of heparin-induced thrombocytopenia. Hematol/Oncol Clin N Am 24: 755–775, 2010.

Warkentin TE, Kelton JG. Delayed-onset heparin-induced thrombocytopenia and thrombosis. Ann Intern Med 135: 502–506, 2001a.

Warkentin TE, Kelton JG. Temporal features of immune heparin-induced thrombocytopenia. N Engl J Med 344: 1286–1292, 2001b.

Wendel HP, Ziemer G. Coating-techniques to improve the hemocompatibility of artificial devices used for extracorporeal circulation. Eur J Cardiothorac Surg 16: 342–350, 1999.

Wheatcroft MD, Greco E, Tse L, Roche-Nagle G. Heparin-induced thrombocytopenia in the presence of a heparin-bonded bypass graft. Vascular 19: 338–341, 2011.

21 Heparin-induced thrombocytopenia in children

Anne F. Klenner and Andreas Greinacher

INTRODUCTION

Heparin-induced thrombocytopenia (HIT) can occur in children, with the potential for severe venous and arterial thrombotic complications (Table 21.1). Unlike in adults, few data exist regarding pediatric HIT. Only 116 children have been reported with HIT between 1990 and 2011 (Oriot et al., 1990; Potter et al., 1992; Murdoch et al., 1993; Boon et al., 1994; Klement et al., 1996; Wilhelm et al., 1996; Butler et al., 1997; Schiffmann et al., 1997; Barth, 1998; Sauer et al., 1998; Scurr et al., 1998; Bocquet et al., 1999; Saxon et al., 1999; Weigel et al., 1999; Neuhaus et al., 2000; Ranze et al., 1999, 2001; Girisch et al., 2001, 2002; Severin and Sutor, 2001; Zöhrer et al., 2001; Deitcher et al., 2002; Schmugge et al., 2002; Severin et al., 2002a; Boshkov et al., 2002, 2003a,b, 2004; Gatti et al., 2003; Schlegel and Hurtaud-Roux, 2003; Klenner et al., 2003b, 2004; Newall et al., 2003; Nguyen et al., 2003; Porcelli et al., 2003; Alsoufi et al., 2004; Dager and White, 2004; Lischetzki et al., 2004; Malherbe et al., 2004; Mejak et al., 2004; Rischewski et al., 2004; Tcheng and Wong, 2004; Verso et al., 2004; Frost et al., 2005; Grabowski et al., 2005; Iannoli et al., 2005; John and Hallisey, 2005; Martchenke and Boshkov, 2005; Bidlingmaier et al., 2006; Knoderer et al., 2006; Schreiber et al., 2006; Scott et al., 2006; von Heymann et al., 2006; Potter et al., 2007; Breinholt et al., 2008; Ciccolo et al., 2008; Hanke et al., 2009; Maurer et al., 2009; Dragomer et al., 2011; Pollak et al., 2011).

PATHOPHYSIOLOGY

Studies of the pathophysiology of HIT have been performed using adult blood. In our laboratory, pediatric and adult HIT sera react similarly in various *in vitro* assays. Therefore, it seems reasonable to infer that the pathophysiology of HIT in children resembles that in adults (see chaps. 5–10).

FREQUENCY

Thirteen studies have addressed the frequency of HIT in children.

Pediatric Intensive Care Unit Patients

Spadone and coworkers (1992) collected cases of suspected HIT in a neonatal intensive care unit (ICU) between 1988 and 1990. Of 1329 newborns enrolled, about 70% received unfractionated heparin (UFH), either 0.5–1.0 IU/mL added to central venous or peripheral/umbilical artery catheters or via flushing of peripheral venous catheters (10 IU/mL UFH/saline every 4 hours). In 34 (3.7%) newborns, HIT was

TABLE 21.1   Clinical Complications of HIT in Children ($n = 116$)

Complication	Absolute	Percentage
Venous thrombosis		
Iliac vein	11	9.5
Femoral vein	10	8.6
Inferior vena cava	10	8.6
Pulmonary embolism	8	6.9
Progression of venous thrombosis	9	7.7
Superior vena cava	5	4.3
Calf vein	5	4.3
Subclavian vein	4	3.3
Jugular vein	3	2.6
Rare: Innominate vein, pulmonary vein, arm veins, renal vein, dural sinus veins	9	7.7
Arterial thrombosis		
Femoral artery	4	3.3
Iliac artery	2	1.6
Foot arteries	3	2.6
Rare: renal artery, arterial embolism	4	3.3
Others		
Clotted lines (ECMO, hemodialyzer, catheters)	9	7.7
Bleeding	7	6.0
Intracardiac thrombi	7	6.0
Neurological deficits	4	3.3
Clotted shunt	6	5.2
Decreased ventricular function	5	4.3
Reoperation	2	1.6
Skin necrosis	4	3.3

Note: Patients may have had more than one complication.
Abbreviation: ECMO, extracorporeal membrane oxygenation.

suspected because the platelet count fell to $<70 \times 10^9/L$ or because of new thrombo-embolic events. In 14 of these 34 infants, HIT antibodies were detected by platelet aggregation assay (incidence $14/930 = 1.5\%$). However, this study has several limitations. It is an observational study without a defined protocol. As differentiation of HIT from other causes of thrombocytopenia or thrombosis is difficult and the specificity of the applied platelet aggregation test for HIT antibodies may be low in ICU patients (see chap. 11), the incidence of HIT might have been overestimated.

In a retrospective cohort study in a pediatric ICU, 57 patients developed arterial and/or venous thrombosis among 612 children treated with UFH for more than five days (Schmugge et al., 2002). In 14 children (2.3%), HIT was suspected based on thrombosis and a platelet count below $150 \times 10^9/L$ (or platelet fall exceeding 50%) occurring after five or more days of UFH use. In six patients (1.0%), HIT antibodies were demonstrated by platelet factor 4 (PF4)-dependent enzyme immunoassay (EIA), using adult cutoff values in determining a positive assay result. The eight other patients with clinically suspected HIT had antibody levels below adult cutoff. Eleven of the 14 patients had received UFH following cardiac surgery. Four were newborns and five others were also younger than one year (mean age, 6.5 months).

Newall et al. (2003) retrospectively collected cases of HIT in a tertiary pediatric hospital. During the 2-year study, 116 patients received UFH over a seven-day period (25 re-exposures). HIT was suspected in four patients who received therapeutic-dose UFH and developed a platelet count fall of >85% of the preheparin value. Three of the patients were tested for HIT antibodies, with one positive result (incidence $1/116 = 0.9\%$).

Etches et al. (2003) conducted a prospective pilot study to determine the incidence of HIT in a pediatric ICU population. Patients received UFH during cardiopulmonary bypass (CPB), continuous intravenous (iv), and/or intra-arterial infusion and/or subcutaneous (sc) injection. During a 41-month study period, 233 patients with a median age of 2.3 years were enrolled. Three of 233 study patients had a positive HIT assay (by platelet lumiaggregometry), giving a seroconversion incidence of 1.3%. All the three patients had undergone cardiovascular surgery. None of the HIT assay-positive patients showed a ≥50% decrease in platelet count, and none had clinically evident thrombosis.

In a randomized, double-blind, placebo-controlled trial in neonatal ICU patients receiving either iv UFH or saline to prolong patency of peripheral venous catheters (Klenner et al., 2003a), of 108 neonates receiving UFH (0.5 IU/mL) and 105 receiving saline for at least five days, none developed HIT or anti-PF4/heparin (anti-PF4/H) antibodies (assessed by EIA). This suggests that the incidence of HIT is lower in neonatal ICU patients than previously reported. However, no neonates following cardiac surgery were enrolled. The results of this study were confirmed by a smaller trial (Kumar et al., 2004). None of the 42 newborns receiving UFH for prolonging patency of a central venous access line developed heparin-dependent antibodies, either in the anti-PF4/H EIA or in a functional (platelet activation) assay. Although 57% of the newborns developed thrombocytopenia, none had clinical suspicion of thrombosis.

Pediatric Cardiac Surgery Patients

Boshkov et al. (2003a) reported a retrospective case series in pediatric cardiac surgery patients. HIT antibodies were demonstrated by positive functional assay in five of 433 children following open heart surgery (incidence, 1.2%). Martchenke and colleagues (2004) found an incidence of HIT with thrombotic complications of 2.5% in pediatric patients after congenital heart surgery. Boning et al. (2005) performed a retrospective analysis to identify the incidences of HIT and of anti-PF4/H antibodies in pediatric patients undergoing cardiac surgery. There were 559 cardiac procedures with extracorporeal circulation using UFH in 415 patients with congenital heart defects performed over a 2-year period. The 144 patients undergoing a scheduled second procedure on extracorporeal circulation were screened preoperatively. Of these 144 patients, 41 underwent a third procedure and were screened before each procedure for the presence of anti-PF4/H antibodies and clinical signs of HIT. The incidence of anti-PF4/H antibodies was 1.4% (2/144). In none of the patients did clinical HIT occur.

Punzalan and colleagues (2005) performed a prospective study in children receiving heparin during CPB. Of 30 children between two days and 50 months of age, one patient had a borderline positive result and another a positive anti-PF4/H EIA; both tested negative by a functional test (serotonin release assay). Neither patient developed thrombosis.

Hanson and colleagues (2007) performed a prospective, observational study in a tertiary care pediatric ICU in children requiring heparin for more than five days after CPB surgery. In 30 patients screened by anti-PF4/H EIA, there were no confirmed cases of heparin-dependent platelet antibodies.

Mullen et al. (2008) screened 135 patients undergoing cardiac surgery in a prospective study using the anti-PF4/H EIA. On postoperative day 10, antibodies were present in 1.7% of the 60 neonates after primary cardiac surgery and in 52% of the 75 children undergoing reoperation with a history of UFH exposure. HIT was not diagnosed in any neonatal patient; one reoperated patient (1.3%) seroconverted and developed HIT without thrombosis or skin lesions.

Pediatric Dialysis Patients

Skouri et al. (2006) performed a prospective study in the pediatric hemodialysis unit, evaluating 38 children between one and 16 years of age (mean, 10.5 years) undergoing chronic hemodialysis thrice weekly. Patients received iv UFH as a single bolus (70 IU/kg body weight). Plasma samples were tested for antibodies by anti-PF4/H EIA and by a washed platelet functional assay, the heparin-induced platelet activation assay (HIPA). Of 38 patients, nine patients (21%) tested positive by EIA and/or HIPA, but none had thrombocytopenia or clinical thrombosis. Sequential EIAs performed every three months in seven of the eight patients with antibodies detected by EIA showed gradual reductions in antibody levels in six children, with a persistently positive EIA seen in only one patient at one-year follow-up.

CLINICAL PRESENTATION

Between 1990 and 2011, 116 children have been reported with HIT: 19 (16.4%) were newborns, 47 (40.5%) were children aged one month to 3 years, 23 (19.8%) were between 4 and 11 years of age, and 27 (23.3%) ranged in age from 12 to 18 years (Fig. 21.1). In most newborns and young children (under four years of age), HIT occurred after cardiac surgery (46/66 = 69.7%). In contrast, among 27 children aged 12 years or older, HIT complicated the use of UFH given because of preceding thrombosis in 13 (48.1%) patients, and following use of antithrombotic prophylaxis in eight (29.6%); only two of the older children had undergone cardiac surgery.

Five patients developed HIT during low-dose UFH given for catheter patency (4.3%). Hemodialysis or hemofiltration accounted for UFH use in eight (6.9%) patients. In 23 of the 116 patients, the laboratory test for HIT was negative or not performed (19.8%).

The most frequent manifestation of HIT in children was a decrease in platelet count (90/116, 77.6%). HIT was associated with thromboembolic complications in about two thirds of the patients, most commonly involving iliac and femoral veins, the inferior vena cava, and pulmonary embolism (PE) (Table 21.1). Less commonly, intracardiac thrombi or neurologic events occurred, or clotting of the dialyzer. Only about 11% (13/116) of patients developed arterial thrombosis. Thus, there is a strong preponderance of venous thrombosis in pediatric HIT.

Fifteen (12.8%) of the 116 children died (Butler et al., 1997; Weigel at al., 1999; Deitcher et al., 2002; Boshkov et al., 2003a; Klenner et al., 2003b; Newall et al., 2003; Porcelli et al., 2003; Alsoufi et al., 2004; Mejak et al., 2004; Martchenke and Boshkov 2005; Bidlingmaier et al., 2006; Potter et al., 2007), and three required amputations. In four children, only partial recanalization of thrombosed veins occurred.

This summary does not include the 14 newborns reported by Spadone and colleagues (1992). These workers primarily observed arterial thrombosis, with at

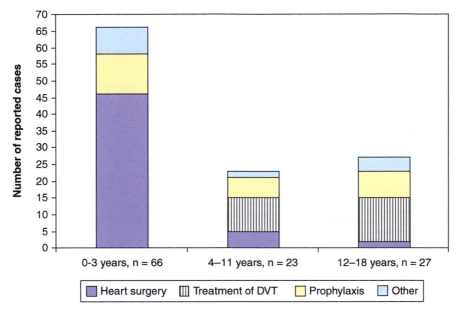

FIGURE 21.1 Reasons for preceding heparin therapy in children with HIT. Among the various age groups, the reasons for heparin therapy that led to HIT varied considerably: newborns and infants usually developed HIT after cardiac surgery, whereas among teenagers, HIT more often complicated the use of heparin during treatment of thrombosis. *Abbreviations*: DVT, deep vein thrombosis; HIT, heparin-induced thrombocytopenia.

least 11 (78.6%) developing aortic thrombosis (one infant died without imaging studies). Two newborns with thrombosis had normal platelet counts. Eleven (78.6%) survived, the remaining three developing mesenteric ischemia. Arterial thrombosis likely was related to umbilical artery catheters (used in all but one of the 14 neonates). In adults, intravascular catheters are a risk factor for HIT-associated thrombosis (Hong et al., 2003), but whether the arterial thrombi observed by Spadone et al. (1992) indeed were HIT-related is unclear.

LABORATORY TESTING

As in adults, no data exist to justify routine screening for HIT antibodies during heparin use in children. Testing for HIT antibodies should be used to exclude or confirm clinically suspected HIT. During UFH therapy, platelet counts should be monitored regularly, particularly between days 5 and 14 of heparin use (when >90% of HIT begins; see chap. 2).

For laboratory testing, functional and antigen tests are available (see chap. 11). Commercial antigen assays (EIAs) are often used and are especially appropriate for neonates and infants because small blood volumes are needed (<100 μL *vs* >1 mL for most platelet activation assays). However, the appropriate cutoff level that defines a positive EIA result suitable for children is debated. In a retrospective study, Schmugge and coworkers (2002) investigated cutoff levels for children using a commercial EIA (Asserachrom, Stago , Asnieres sur Seine, France). Among 612 children,

HIT was suspected in 14 because of thrombocytopenia and thrombosis. Positive test results (using the adult cutoff) were seen in six of the 14 patients. In the remaining eight children with suspected HIT, test results ranged from 26% to 80% of the adult cutoff level, that is, levels that were higher than among controls (with wide overlap).

A retrospective analysis performed by Risch and colleagues (2003) of the same 612 pediatric ICU patients initially reported by Schmugge et al. (2002) addressed whether there was an association between anti-PF4/H antibody levels and thrombosis. Ten patients who developed thrombosis without thrombocytopenia constituted the study group and were compared with 19 matched controls with neither thrombosis nor thrombocytopenia. All 29 subjects had lower antibody levels than the adult cutoff level. However, median assay results were significantly higher in the thrombosis patients than in controls (51% vs 23% of the manufacturer's cutoff; $P = 0.004$). The authors concluded that there might be an association between anti-PF4/H antibody levels and thrombosis, even in the absence of thrombocytopenia or a positive test result (by conventional criteria).

However, in our randomized, double-blind trial (Klenner et al., 2003a), none of the infants developed anti-PF4/H antibodies using the adult cutoff [UFH group: mean optical density (OD), 0.020; maximum, 0.328; saline group: mean OD, 0.019, maximum, 0.239; anti-PF4/polyvinyl sulfonate EIA (Gen-Probe GTI Diagnostics, Wausheka, Wisconsin, U.S.A.)]. Minor increase in OD (>0.100) occurred in six patients (three in each group) (Fig. 21.2). Therefore, these minor increases in OD are unlikely to be related to UFH use and could represent a nonspecific increase in antibody levels in ill patients (acute phase reaction). Among the subjects receiving placebo, all OD values were below 0.400 (the accepted adult cutoff value), suggesting that this level is also appropriate for neonates.

The limitations of antigen assays observed in adults likely also apply to children. In some cases, the antigen assay could be false-negative if HIT antibodies recognize a non–PF4-dependent antigen (Greinacher et al., 1994) (see chaps. 5 and 11). Thus, a functional test for HIT antibodies should be performed when HIT remains strongly suspected despite a negative EIA. However, when the pretest probability of HIT is low, a negative antigen test usually excludes HIT.

THERAPY OF PEDIATRIC HIT

Numerous case reports describe the occurrence of new or recurrent thromboembolic events during continued or repeated use of heparin in adult patients with acute HIT. Thus, all heparin should be discontinued in patients strongly suspected of having HIT, including heparin "flushes," heparin-coated catheters, and heparin-containing blood products (Severin et al., 2002b) (see chap. 12). As in adults, low molecular weight heparin (LMWH) should not be used to treat acute HIT in children (see chap. 12).

Because HIT is a prothrombotic ("hypercoagulability") state with high risk of thromboembolic complications, alternative anticoagulation is usually required after stopping heparin. In adults, there are prospective studies of anticoagulation for HIT patients using danaparoid, lepirudin, or argatroban. However, in children, experience with these agents is anecdotal and heterogenous. Expert opinions are available in reviews (Young, 2004; Balasa, 2005; Bidlingmaier et al., 2006; Hursting et al., 2006; Risch et al., 2006; Takemoto and Streiff, 2011).

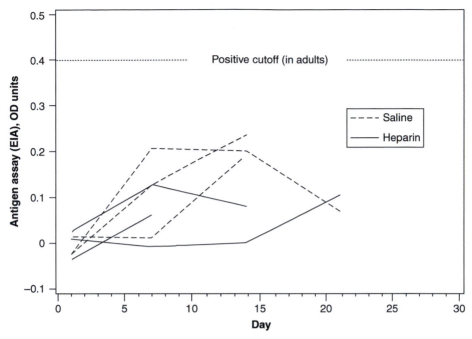

FIGURE 21.2 Six neonates with rising absorbance levels in platelet factor 4 (PF4)-dependent EIA. Six of 213 neonates participating in a randomized, double-blind trial comparing heparin with normal saline for maintenance of peripheral venous catheter patency developed a rise in absorbance of more than 0.100 OD units by anti-PF4/polyvinyl sulfonate EIA (Gen-Probe GTI Diagnostics, Waukesha, Wisconsin, U.S.A.). All OD values were less than the positive adult cutoff (0.400 OD units). No differences were observed between patients receiving heparin (solid lines) compared with patients receiving saline (dotted lines). As the maximum OD in saline controls was 0.239, the 0.400 cutoff seems appropriate also for pediatric patients. *Abbreviations*: EIA, enzyme immunoassay; OD, optical density. *Source*: From Klenner et al. (2003b).

Danaparoid use has been reported in 39 patients (with additional aspirin, thrombolysis, or lepirudin given in some cases). In two children, danaparoid was stopped because of apparent cross-reactivity, with further anticoagulation with lepirudin. Sixteen patients received lepirudin (one combined with aspirin). Eight children were treated with LMWH. Three infants received aspirin, three were given argatroban plus aspirin, one argatroban and fondaparinux, and 21 were treated with argatroban alone. Two children received bivalirudin, one child was anticoagulated primarily with bivalirudin and warfarin and was switched to fondaparinux and argatroban later. Nineteen children received oral anticoagulants, six received thrombolytics. (Note, however, that oral anticoagulants should not be given during acute HIT; see chaps. 2 and 12.) In five children, no anticoagulant was given. In fifteen cases, alternative anticoagulation was not mentioned.

Danaparoid
Danaparoid (see chap. 16) is a mixture of low molecular weight glycosaminoglycans that catalyze the inactivation of factor Xa (FXa) by antithrombin (formerly,

antithrombin III). It has relatively minor anti-factor IIa (anti-thrombin) activity. Dosing schedules for adults (appropriately weight-adjusted for the child) can be used for guidance. For antithrombotic prophylaxis, 10 IU/kg body weight given twice daily by sc injection is recommended. For therapeutic anticoagulation in pediatric HIT patients, an initial iv bolus of 30 IU/kg is followed by continuous infusion of 1.2–2.0 IU/kg/hr (Monagle et al., 2004, 2012). The anti-FXa level should be measured during treatment for optimal dosing. Target levels of anti-FXa activity are 0.4–0.6 IU/mL for standard and 0.5–0.8 IU/mL for higher danaparoid doses (Severin et al., 2002b). Danaparoid is not available in the United States and the manufacturer has increasing supply problems.

Fondaparinux

Fondaparinux is a selective but indirect inhibitor of FXa by catalyzing antithrombin. It is approved for thromboprophylaxis in adults undergoing orthopedic surgery and abdominal surgery, and for treatment of adults with deep vein thrombosis (DVT) and PE (see chap. 17). The agent does not usually cross-react with HIT antibodies. There are few reports of fondaparinux use in children (Boshkov et al., 2004; Young and Nugent, 2004). In both cases, therapeutic levels could be achieved with a dose of 0.15 mg/kg given once daily. No adverse effects were noted during a period of several months. Maurer et al. (2009) reported a case of an 11-year-old girl with putative HIT during therapy for DVT and PE (however, HIT antibodies tested negative). Transition from bivalirudin to warfarin resulted in extensive re-thrombosis, and fondaparinux therapy similarly failed, so the patient was treated with argatroban.

Young et al. (2011b) performed an open-label, single-arm, dose-finding, pharmacokinetic, and safety study of fondaparinux as primary treatment for DVT or HIT in children between one and 18 years of age. In 24 patients enrolled into the study (only one of whom had HIT), a dose of 0.1 mg/kg administered once daily was safe and effectively achieved concentrations approximately equal to those achieved in adults known to provide therapeutic dose anticoagulation.

Clinical trials with fondaparinux are warranted before any further recommendations of its use in children can be made, especially in children younger than one year. Expert opinions are available in reviews (Streif and Ageno, 2011; Young, 2011a,b).

Hirudins

Lepirudin (see chap. 14) is a direct inhibitor of free and clot-bound thrombin through noncovalent, irreversible binding. In adults with HIT, lepirudin is given as continuous iv infusion (0.1 mg/kg/hr; greatly reduced in case of renal impairment) adjusted by (activated) partial thromboplastin time (aPTT). The usual target aPTT ratio should be 1.5–2.5 times the normal laboratory mean aPTT. Dosing in children is based on anecdotal experience. Schiffmann et al. (1997) gave a bolus of lepirudin (0.2 mg/kg) and a continuous infusion (ranging between 0.1 and 0.7 mg/kg/hr) adjusted by aPTT. Severin et al. (2002b) achieved therapeutic anticoagulation with a continuous infusion of 0.1 mg/kg/hr in a 15-year-old boy, and with an infusion rate of about 0.15 mg/kg/hr in an eight-year-old girl. In an 11-year-old girl, 0.15–0.22 mg/kg/hr was given. In a premature infant, Nguyen and coworkers (2003) gave a 0.2 mg/kg bolus followed initially by 0.1 mg/kg/hr infusion rate; the dose was adjusted daily based on the aPTT, and 0.03–0.05 mg/kg/hr provided adequate anticoagulation. Hanke et al. (2009) started anticoagulation with an initial dose of

5.5 µg/kg/hr in a 6-year-old boy with HIT and renal failure, lepirudin dosage was increased later, the maximum dose being 46 µg/kg/hr after renal improvement and discontinuation of continuous renal replacement therapy. Because pharmacokinetics depend largely on renal function, we recommend starting lepirudin in children with an iv infusion of 0.10 mg/kg/hr (if renal function is normal) and to adjust the dose according to aPTT 4 hr later, without initial bolus (see chap. 14).

Argatroban

Argatroban (see chap. 13) is a synthetic direct thrombin inhibitor that binds reversibly to the active site of thrombin. In adults, the recommended initial dose of argatroban is 2 µg/kg/min given by continuous iv infusion and adjusted by aPTT (target range, 1.5–3.0 times the baseline aPTT). Argatroban also prolongs the international normalized ratio (INR), which makes subsequent transition to vitamin K antagonist therapy, if required, more difficult.

Safety and efficacy of argatroban in pediatric patients have not been established. However, there are several case reports and a chart review (Liedel et al., 2003). Hursting et al. (2006) conducted a comprehensive search and critical analysis of the literature on argatroban use in 34 children. Overall, the patients were between one week and 16 years of age. All patients received a continuous iv infusion of argatroban, titrated to achieve a target aPTT. The aPTT-adjusted doses ranged from 0.1 to 12 µg/kg/min. Four patients also received an initial argatroban bolus of 75 to 200 µg/kg. Bleeding occurred in three patients while on argatroban.

Young et al. (2011a) performed an open-label, safety, efficacy, and pharmacokinetic study in 18 patients between 1.6 week and 16 years of age. The authors concluded that for continuous anticoagulation, argatroban 0.75 µg/kg/min, adjusted by aPTT, should be used in children (in case of hepatic impairment, 0.2 µg/kg/min).

In neonates (Kawada et al., 2000; Okada et al., 2000; Boshkov et al., 2003a,b), an argatroban bolus of 200–250 µg/kg has been described, followed by a continuous infusion rate of 7.5–10 µg/kg/min. Of note, this dose is much higher than the 1–2 µg/kg/min recommended in adults. In a newborn, argatroban was used for anticoagulation during extracorporeal membrane oxygenation (ECMO). After an initial bolus of 200 µg/kg, a continuous infusion at a rate of 3.0–7.5 µg/kg/min was started. During use of a ventricular assist device (VAD), safe anticoagulation with argatroban could be achieved in this infant with an infusion rate of 0.005–1.8 µg/kg/min. Scott et al. (2006) achieved the target aPTT using 1–2 µg/kg/min in a 17-month-old boy requiring ECMO and hemofiltration, while Potter et al. (2007) used 0.1–1 mg/kg/min in two term infants and a 1-year-old girl, who required extracorporeal life support.

The literature reviewed by Hursting et al. (2006) provides information regarding argatroban dosing during CPB, ECMO, VAD use, hemodialysis, and cardiac catheterization. In general, although generally safe anticoagulation with argatroban was reported, further evaluation of the efficacy and safety of argatroban in pediatric patients is needed to make further recommendations.

Bivalirudin

Bivalirudin (see chap. 15) is a direct inhibitor of free and clot-bound thrombin. Data on the use of bivalirudin in pediatric patients are available from two studies, each including 16 children (Young et al., 2007; Rayapudi et al., 2008). After an initial bolus of 0.25 mg/kg, a continuous infusion at a dose of 0.03–0.55 mg/kg/hr was used to achieve a target aPTT. Streif and Ageno (2011) found an initial bolus of either 0.125 or 0.25 or 0.75 mg/kg followed by continuous infusion of 0.125–0.195 mg/kg/hr to be effective for providing sufficient anticoagulation. Young (2011a,b) suggested a bolus of 0.125 mg/kg followed by a continuous infusion of 0.125 mg/kg/hr. Breinholt et al. (2008) presented a case of a two-year-old boy with HIT who underwent recanalization of an occluded superior vena cava and stent placement using bivalirudin for anticoagulation (bolus 0.75 mg/kg followed by infusion at 1.75 mg/kg/hr).

Coumarin

Oral anticoagulants of the coumarin class (warfarin, phenprocoumon) are not appropriate for therapy of acute HIT (see chap. 12). HIT patients are at relatively high risk of developing coumarin-induced microthrombosis (venous limb gangrene and skin necrosis syndromes (see chap. 2)). Therefore, coumarin should be delayed until the patient is adequately anticoagulated with danaparoid, lepirudin, or argatroban, and the platelet counts have substantially recovered (usually $>150 \times 10^9$/L).

Cardiac Interventions in Children with HIT

Recommendations concerning anticoagulation in children with HIT undergoing cardiac surgery have been published in several reviews (Alsoufi et al., 2004; Greinacher and Klenner, 2005; Boshkov et al., 2006). In patients with a history of HIT who need repeat cardiac surgery, the intraoperative use of UFH is recommended for anticoagulation during CPB, if a sensitive assay excludes the presence of HIT antibodies (Warkentin et al., 2008). This is because rapid recurrence of HIT antibodies (before postoperative day 5) will not occur. Furthermore, whereas UFH is the standard anticoagulant for CPB, and its effects can be readily antagonized (protamine), there is minimal experience with newer anticoagulants for CPB (particularly in children) and no antidotes exist. However, for pre- and postoperative anticoagulation, a nonheparin anticoagulant should be given.

For patients with acute HIT or patients with persistently circulating antibodies, this approach cannot be used. Therefore, these patients require alternative anticoagulation during cardiac surgery. The most practical approach (when feasible) is to postpone surgery until the antibodies disappear or reach very low levels (usually, within four to 10 weeks). After their disappearance, heparin can be used (discussed above). If surgery cannot be delayed, alternative nonheparin regimen can be used (see chap. 19). In children, Boshkov and coworkers (2002) started argatroban (250 μg/kg bolus followed by continuous infusion of 10 μg/kg/min) in a 6-month-old child with HIT for anticoagulation during CPB.

For patients with subacute or previous HIT who require cardiac catheterization, the use of an alternative anticoagulant, such as argatroban, lepirudin, bivalirudin, or danaparoid, is recommended over the use of heparin (as heparin use might boost antibody levels, complicating use of heparin for subsequent surgery). Porcelli and coworkers (2003) gave 150 μg/kg of argatroban iv over 10 minutes at the start of cardiac catheterization in a six-year-old boy with HIT with congenital heart disease. No continuous infusion of argatroban was given due to the relatively brief procedure. In a 14-month-old boy with tetralogy of Fallot and HIT after cardiac surgery, danaparoid was used for cardiac catheterization (Girisch et al., 2001), with a loading dose (30 U/kg) followed by an iv infusion (2 U/kg/hr).

Boning et al. (2005) reported four children with anti-PF4/H antibodies without clinically manifest HIT requiring cardiac surgery with CPB. In these four patients, surgery was performed using lepirudin. Three of the four children had an uneventful procedure and postoperative course. In one patient, after total cavopulmonary connection, re-operation was necessary on postoperative day 7 because of partial thrombosis of the lateral tunnel.

There are several case reports on bivalirudin for CPB in children with HIT (Almond et al., 2006; Gates et al., 2010; Dragomer et al., 2011). In a five-month-old child with HIT (Gates et al., 2010), effective anticoagulation was achieved by the following regimen: an initial bolus of 1 mg/kg bivalirudin followed by a second bolus of 0.5 mg/kg given 5 minutes later; the CPB circuit was primed with 50 mg/kg bivalirudin/400 cc volume; and with the initiation of CPB, a continuous infusion of 2.5 mg/kg/min was started. Activated clotting time (ACT) was monitored every 15 minutes. Dragomer et al. (2011) used repetitive bolus application (1.0, 0.5, 0.5, 0.5 mg/kg) prior to CPB followed by continuous infusion with 2.5 mg/kg/hr in a 17-month-old child with HIT.

PREVENTION OF HIT IN CHILDREN

Since the pivotal trial in adult orthopedic patients (Warkentin et al., 1995), it is known that LMWH induces HIT less frequently than does UFH. In children, HIT appears to occur most often among the very young following cardiac surgery, and among adolescents given UFH to treat spontaneous thrombosis. Data from Pouplard and colleagues (1999) suggest that HIT might also occur less with LMWH than with UFH thromboprophylaxis after cardiac surgery. This approach should be investigated in children.

Similarly, in the second group of at-risk pediatric patients (adolescents with thrombosis), it is possible that the frequency of HIT would be reduced if LMWH is given instead of UFH. Pharmacokinetic studies of LMWH in infants and children have been conducted for several LMWH preparations. The safety and efficacy of prophylactic and therapeutic doses of LMWH in children have been evaluated in clinical trials for a variety of conditions. LMWH is safe and effective for anticoagulation of infants and children of varying age (Albisetti and Andrew, 2002; Massicotte et al., 2003a,b,c; Monagle et al., 2004, 2012; Sutor et al., 2004; Merkel et al., 2006; Tousovska et al., 2009). Increased dosing seems to be required for obese children and neonates (Lewis et al., 2011; Malowany et al., 2008).

SUMMARY

HIT appears to be rare in children. The incidence depends somewhat on patient age and indication for heparin. Two major pediatric at-risk groups are apparent: newborns/infants after cardiac surgery (incidence ~1%), and adolescents treated with UFH for spontaneous thrombosis. HIT can be life-threatening in children (~12% mortality). Venous thrombosis is the most frequent HIT-associated complication. For laboratory support for a diagnosis of HIT, antigen assays are most appropriate (small blood volumes required), although whenever possible a functional assay should be used for confirmation if the EIA is positive. Although there are conflicting data on the optimal laboratory cutoff for antigen assays, a randomized, double-blind clinical trial suggests that the cutoff level established in adults is also appropriate for children. There are no prospective studies of alternative anticoagulants in children with HIT. Most available data are for lepirudin, danaparoid, and argatroban, and (for cardiac surgery) also for bivalirudin. Greater use of LMWH in children may lead to a reduced risk for HIT, as is seen in adults.

REFERENCES

Albisetti M, Andrew M. Low molecular weight heparin in children. Eur J Pediatr 161: 71–77, 2002.

Almond CS, Harrington J, Thiagarajan R, Duncan CN, LaPierre R, Halwick D, Blume ED, del Nido PJ, Neufeld EJ, McGowan FX. Successful use of bivalirudin for cardiac transplantation in a child with heparin-induced thrombocytopenia. J Heart Lung Transplant 25: 1376–1379, 2006.

Alsoufi B, Boshkov LK, Kirby A, Ibsen L, Dower N, Shen I, Ungerleider R. Heparin-induced thrombocytopenia (HIT) in pediatric cardiac surgery: an emerging cause of morbidity and mortality. Semin Thorac Cardiovasc Surg Pediatr Card Surg Annu 7: 155–171, 2004.

Balasa VV. New anticoagulants: a pediatric perspective. Pediatr Blood Cancer 45: 741–752, 2005.

Barth KSA. [Incidence of heparin-induced thrombocytopenia at the Justus Liebig University Hospital (MD thesis)]. Gießen, Germany: Justus Liebig University, 1998. [in German]

Bidlingmaier C, Magnani HN, Girisch M, Kurnik K. Safety and efficacy of Danaparoid (Orgaran) use in children. Acta Haematol 115: 237–247, 2006.

Bocquet R, Blanot S, Dautzenberg MD, Pierre-Kahn A, Carli P. [Antiphospholipid antibody syndrome in pediatric neurosurgery: a hemostasis problem]. Ann Fr Anesth Reanim 18: 991–995, 1999. [in French]

Boning A, Morschheuser T, Blase U, Scheewe J, von der Breie M, Grabitz R, Cremer JT. Incidence of heparin-induced thrombocytopenia and therapeutic strategies in pediatric cardiac surgery. Ann Thorac Surg 79: 62–65, 2005.

Boon DM, Michiels JJ, Stibbe J, van Vliet HH, Kappers-Klunne MC. Heparin-induced thrombocytopenia and antithrombotic therapy. Lancet 344: 1296, 1994.

Boshkov LK, Thomas G, Kirby A, Shen I, Swanson V, Burch G, Ungerleider R. Pharmacokinetics of argatroban infusion in a 6 month old congenital cardiac patient with previously diagnosed heparin-induced thrombocytopenia (HIT) [abstr]. Blood 100: 269a, 2002.

Boshkov LK, Ibsen L, Kirby A, Ungerleider R, Shen I. Heparin-induced thrombocytopenia (HIT) in neonates and very young children undergoing congenital cardiac surgery: a likely under-recognized complication with significant morbidity and mortality: report of 4 sequential cases [abstr]. J Thromb Haemost 1(Suppl 1): P1494, 2003a.

Boshkov LK, Ibsen L, Kirby A, Ungerleider R, Shen I. Report of argatroban infusions for heparin-induced thrombocytopenia (HIT) diagnosed by functional assay in 2 congenital cardiac surgery patients, a neonate and a 5 month old [abstr]. J Thromb Haemost 1(Suppl 1): P1495, 2003b.

Boshkov LK, Kirby A, Heuschkel M. Pharmacokinetics of Fondaparinux by anti-Xa levels and clinical response to anticoagulation in a 4-month old congenital cardiac patient with heparin-induced thrombocytopenia (HIT) and established venous thrombosis transitioned from argatroban to fondaparinux [abstr]. Blood 104: 104b, 2004.

Boshkov LK, Kirby A, Shen I, Ungerleider RM. Recognition and management of heparin-induced thrombocytopenia in pediatric cardiopulmonary bypass patients. Ann Thorac Surg 81: S2355–S2359, 2006.

Breinholt JP, Moffett BS, Texter KM, Ing FF. Successful use of bivalirudin for superior vena cava recanalization and stent placement in a child with heparin-induced thrombocytopenia. Pediatr Cardiol 29: 804–807, 2008.

Butler TJ, Sodoma LJ, Doski JJ, Cheu HW, Berg ST, Stokes GN, Lancaster KJ. Heparin-associated thrombocytopenia and thrombosis as the cause of a fatal thrombus on extracorporeal membrane oxygenation. J Pediatr Surg 32: 768–771, 1997.

Ciccolo ML, Bernstein J, Collazos JC, Acherman RJ, Restrepo H, Winters JM, Krueger J, Evans WN. Argatroban anticoagulation for cardiac surgery with cardiopulmonary bypass in an infant with double outlet right ventricle and a history of heparin-induced thrombocytopenia. Congenit Heart Dis 3: 299–302, 2008.

Dager WE, White RH. Low molecular weight heparin-induced thrombocytopenia in a child. Ann Pharmacother 38: 247–250, 2004.

Deitcher SR, Topoulos AP, Bartholomew JR, Kichuk-Chrisant MR. Lepirudin anticoagulation for heparin-induced thrombocytopenia. J Pediatr 140: 264–266, 2002.

Dragomer D, Chalfant A, Biniwale R, Reemtsen B, Federman M. Novel techniques in the use of bivalirudin for cardiopulmonary bypass anticoagulation in a child with heparin-induced thrombocytopenia. Perfusion 26: 516–518, 2011.

Etches WS, Stang LJ, Conradi AG. Incidence of heparin-induced thrombocytopenia in a pediatric intensive care population [abstr]. Blood 102: 536a, 2003.

Frost J, Mureebe L, Russo P, Russo J, Tobias J. Heparin-induced thrombocytopenia in the pediatric intensive care unit population. Pediatr Crit Care Med 6: 216–219, 2005.

Gates R, Yost P, Parker B. The use of bivalirudin for cardiopulmonary bypass anticoagulation in pediatric heparin-induced thrombocytopenia patients. Artif Organs 34: 667–669, 2010.

Gatti L, Carnelli V, Rusconi R, Moia M. Heparin-induced thrombocytopenia and warfarin-induced skin necrosis in a child with severe protein C deficiency: successful treatment with dermatan sulfate and protein C concentrate. J Thromb Haemost 1: 387–388, 2003.

Girisch M, Buheitel G, Ries M, Klinge J. Safe and effective use of Danaparoid during cardiac catheterization in a 14 month old boy with tetralogy of fallot and heparin-induced thrombocytopenia [abstr]. Ann Hematol 80(Suppl 1): A68, 2001.

Girisch M, Klinge J, Lischetzki G, Buheitel G. In neonates higher doses orgaran may be needed to achieve effective doses [abstr]. Ann Hematol 81(Suppl 1), A22, 2002.

Grabowski EF, Buonanno FS, Doody D, Van Cott EM, Grant PE, Jones RM, Whalen M, Nowski N. Two cases of pediatric HIT requiring unusually high doses of direct thrombin inhibitors: does a subset of such patients exist? [abstr] Blood 106: A4161, 2005.

Greinacher A, Klenner AF. Heparin-induced thrombocytopenia with a focus on children undergoing cardiac surgery. Prog Pediatr Cardiol 21: 71–79, 2005.

Greinacher A, Amiral J, Dummel V, Vissac A, Kiefel V, Mueller-Eckhardt C. Laboratory diagnosis of heparin-associated thrombocytopenia and comparison of platelet aggregation test, heparin-induced platelet activation test, and platelet factor 4/heparin enzyme-linked immunosorbent assay. Transfusion 34: 381–385, 1994.

Hanke CA, Barth K, Nakamura L, Budde U, Arnold R, Zieger B, Stiller B. Lepirudin treatment in a boy with suspected HIT II after surgery because of tetralogy of Fallot. Hamostaseologie 2: 168–170, 2009.

Hanson SJ, Punzalan RC, Ghanayem N, Havens P. Prevalence of heparin-dependent platelet antibodies in children after cardiopulmonary bypass. Pediatr Crit Care Med 8: 358–361, 2007.

Hong AP, Cook DJ, Sigouin CS, Warkentin TE. Central venous catheters and upper-extremity deep-vein thrombosis complicating immune heparin-induced thrombocytopenia. Blood 101: 3049–3051, 2003.

Hursting MJ, Dubb J, Verme-Gibboney CN. Argatroban anticoagulation in pediatric patients. J Pediatr Hematol Oncol 28: 4–10, 2006.

Iannoli ED, Eaton MP, Shapiro JR. Bidirectional Glenn shunt surgery using lepirudin anticoagulation in an infant with heparin-induced thrombocytopenia with thrombosis. Anesth Analg 101: 74–76, 2005.

John TE, Hallisey RK. Argatroban and lepirudin requirements in a 6-year-old patient with heparin-induced thrombocytopenia. Pharmacotherapy 25: 1383–1388, 2005.

Kawada T, Kitagawa H, Hoson M, Okada Y, Shiomura J. Clinical application of argatroban as an alternative anticoagulant for extracorporeal circulation. Hematol Oncol Clin North Am 14: 445–457, 2000.

Klement D, Rammos S, Kries R, Kirschke W, Kniemeyer HW, Greinacher A. Heparin as a cause of thrombus progression. Heparin-associated thrombocytopenia is an important differential diagnosis in paediatric patients even with normal platelet counts. Eur J Pediatr 155: 11–14, 1996.

Klenner AF, Fusch C, Rakow A, Kadow I, Beyersdorff E, Eichler P, Wander K, Lietz T, Greinacher A. Benefit and risk of heparin for maintaining peripheral venous catheters in neonates: a placebo-controlled trial. J Pediatr 143: 741–745, 2003a.

Klenner AF, Fusch C, Varnholt V, Ringe H, Meyer O, Stiller B, Greinacher A. Heparin-induced thrombocytopenia in pediatrics and its therapy – case-report review of the literature. Monatsschr Kinderheilkd 151: 1180–1187, 2003b.

Klenner AF, Lubenow N, Raschke R, Greinacher A. Heparin-induced thrombocytopenia in children: 12 new cases and review of the literature. Thromb Haemost 91: 719–724, 2004.

Knoderer CA, Knoderer HM, Turrentine MW, Kumar M. Lepirudin anticoagulation for heparin-induced thrombocytopenia after cardiac surgery in a pediatric patient. Pharmacotherapy 26: 709–712, 2006.

Kumar P, Hoppensteadt DA, Prechel MM, Deddish RB, Walenga JM. Prevalence of heparin-dependent platelet-activating antibodies in preterm newborns after exposure to unfractionated heparin. Clin Appl Thromb Hemost 10: 335–339, 2004.

Lewis TV, Johnson PN, Nebbia AM, Dunlap M. Increased enoxaparin dosing is required for obese children. Pediatrics 127: e787–e790, 2011.

Liedel JL, Panicker N, Kahana MD. Argatroban for anticoagulation in children with heparin-induced platelet antibodies [abstr]. Crit Care Med 31: A132, 2003.

Lischetzki G, Dittrich S, Klinge J. Pediatric heparin-induced thrombocytopenia type II on hemodialysis [abstr]. Ann Hematol 24: P38, 2004.

Malherbe S, Tsui BCH, Stobart K, Koller J. Argatroban as an anticoagulant in cardiopulmonary bypass in an infant and attempted reversal with recombinant activated factor VII. Anesthesiology 100: 443–445, 2004.

Malowany JI, Monagle P, Knoppert DC, Lee DSC, Wu J, McCusker P, Massicotte MP, Williams S, Chan AKC. Enoxaparin for neonatal thrombosis: a call for a higher dose for neonates. Thromb Res 122: 826–830, 2008.

Martchenke J, Boshkov L. Heparin-induced thrombocytopenia in neonates. Neonatal Netw 24: 33–37, 2005.

Martchenke J, Pate MF, Cruz M, Phromsivarak S. What is the incidence of heparin-induced thrombocytopenia (HIT) in children? Crit Care Nurse 24: 66–67, 2004.

Massicotte P, Julian JA, Gent M, Shields K, Marzinotto V, Szechtman B, Andrew M; REVIVE Study Group. An open-label randomized controlled trial of low molecular weight heparin compared to heparin and coumarin for the treatment of venous thromboembolic events in children: the REVIVE trial. Thromb Res 109: 85–92, 2003a.

Massicotte P, Julian JA, Gent M, Shields K, Marzinotto V, Szechtman B, Chan AK, Andrew M; PROTEKT Study Group. An open-label randomized controlled trial of low molecular weight heparin for the prevention of central venous line-related thrombotic complications in children: the PROTEKT trial. Thromb Res 109: 101–108, 2003b.

Massicotte P, Julian JA, Marzinotto V, Gent M, Shields K, Chan AK, Szechtman B, Kohne S, Shepherd S, Bacher P, Andrew M. Dose-finding and pharmacokinetic profiles of prophylactic doses of a low molecular weight heparin (reviparin-sodium) in pediatric patients. Thromb Res 109: 93–99, 2003c.

Maurer SH, Wilimas JA, Wang WC, Reiss UM. Heparin induced thrombocytopenia and re-thrombosis associated with warfarin and fondaparinux in a child. Pediatr Blood Cancer 53: 468–471, 2009.

Mejak B, Giacomuzzi C, Heller E, You X, Ungerleider R, Shen I, Boshkov L. Argatroban usage for anticoagulation for ECMO on a post-cardiac patient with heparin-induced thrombocytopenia. J Extra Corpor Technol 36: 178–181, 2004.

Merkel N, Gunther G, Schobess R. Long-term treatment of thrombosis with enoxaparin in pediatric and adolescent patients. Acta Haematol 115: 230–236, 2006.

Monagle P, Chan A, Massicotte P, Chalmers E, Michelson AD. Antithrombotic therapy in children: the Seventh ACCP Conference on Antithrombotic and Thrombolytic Therapy. Chest 126(Suppl): 645S–687S, 2004.

Monagle P, Chan A, Goldenberg NA, Ichord RN, Journeycake JM, Nowak-Göttl U, Vesely SK. Antithrombotic therapy in neonates and children: Antithrombotic Therapy and Prevention of Thrombosis, 9th ed: American College of Chest Physicians Evidence-Based Clinical Practice Guidelines. Chest 141(2 Suppl): e737S–e801S, 2012.

Mullen MP, Wessel DL, Thomas KC, Gauvreau K, Neufeld EJ, McGowan FX Jr, Dinardo JA. The incidence and implications of anti-heparin-platelet factor 4 antibody formation in a pediatric cardiac surgical population. Anesth Anal 107: 371–378, 2008.

Murdoch IA, Beattie RM, Silver DM. Heparin-induced thrombocytopenia in children. Acta Paediatr 82: 495–497, 1993.

Neuhaus TJ, Goetschel P, Schmugge M, Leumann E. Heparin-induced thrombocytopenia type II on hemodialysis: switch to danaparoid. Pediatr Nephrol 14: 713–716, 2000.

Newall F, Barnes C, Ignjatovic V, Monagle P. Heparin-induced thrombocytopenia in children. J Paediatr Child Health 39: 289–292, 2003.

Nguyen TN, Gal P, Ransom JL, Carlos R. Lepirudin use in a neonate with heparin-induced thrombocytopenia. Ann Pharmacother 37: 229–233, 2003.

Okada Y, Kawada T, Hoson M. Use of an antithrombotic agent, argatroban, in two patients with ECMO after pediatric open heart surgery. Jpn J Thromb Hemost 11: 201–204, 2000.

Oriot D, Wolf M, Wood C, Brun P, Sidi D, Devictor D, Tchernia G, Hualt G. [Severe thrombocytopenia induced by heparin in an infant with acute myocarditis]. Arch Fr Pediatr 47: 357–359, 1990. [in French]

Pollak U, Yacobobich J, Tamary H, Dagan O, Manor-Shulman O. Heparin-induced thrombocytopenia and extracorporal membrane oxygenation: a case-report and review of the literature. J Extra Corpor Technol 43: 5–12, 2011.

Porcelli R, Moskowitz BC, Cetta F, Graham LC, Godwin JE, Eidem BW, Prechel MM, Walenga JM. Heparin-induced thrombocytopenia with associated thrombosis in children after the Fontan operation: report of two cases. Tex Heart Inst J 30: 58–61, 2003.

Potter C, Gill JC, Scott JP, McFarland JG. Heparin-induced thrombocytopenia in a child [see comments]. J Pediatr 121: 135–138, 1992.

Potter KE, Raj A, Sullivan JE. Argatroban for anticoagulation in pediatric patients with heparin-induced thrombocytopenia requiring extracorporeal life support. J Pediatr Hematol Oncol 29: 265–268, 2007.

Pouplard C, May MA, Iochmann S, Amiral J, Vissac AM, Marchand M, Gruel Y. Antibodies to platelet factor 4-heparin after cardiopulmonary bypass in patients anticoagulated with unfractionated heparin or a low molecular weight heparin: clinical implications for heparin-induced thrombocytopenia. Circulation 99: 2530–2536, 1999.

Punzalan RC, Hanson SJ, Ghanayem N, Curtis BR, Murkowski K, Havens PL, McFarland JG. Prevalence of heparin-dependent platelet antibodies in children after cardiopulmonary bypass surgery [abstr]. Blood 106: 845a, 2005.

Ranze O, Ranze P, Magnani HN, Greinacher A. Heparin-induced thrombocytopenia in paediatric patients–a review of the literature and a new case treated with danaparoid sodium. Eur J Pediatr 158: S130–S133, 1999.

Ranze O, Rakow A, Ranze P, Eichler P, Greinacher A, Fusch C. Low-dose danaparoid sodium catheter flushes in an intensive care infant suffering from heparin-induced thrombocytopenia. Pediatr Crit Care Med 2: 175–177, 2001.

Rayapudi S, Torres Jr A, Deshpanade GG, Ross MP, Wohrley JD, Young G, Tarantino MD. Bivalirudin for anticoagulation in children. Pediatr Blood Cancer 51: 798–801, 2008.

Risch L, Fischer JE, Schmugge M, Huber AR. Association of anti-heparin platelet factor 4 antibody levels and thrombosis in pediatric intensive care patients without thrombocytopenia. Blood Coagul Fibrinolysis 14: 113–116, 2003.

Risch L, Huber AR, Schmugge M. Diagnosis and treatment of heparin-induced thrombocytopenia in neonates and children. Thromb Res 118: 123–135, 2006.

Rischewski J, Eifrig B, Müller-Wiefel D, Neu A, Schneppenheim R, Ganschow R. Heparin-induced thrombocytopenia type 2 (HIT 2) in a 3 year old child after 2nd liver transplantation [abstr]. Ann Hematol 24: P40, 2004.

Sauer M, Gruhn B, Fuchs D, Altermann W, Zintl F. [Heparin-induced type II thrombocytopenia within the scope of high dose chemotherapy with subsequent stem cell rescue]. Klin Padiatr 210: 102–105, 1998. [in German]

Saxon BR, Black MD, Edgell D, Noel D, Leaker MT. Pediatric heparin-induced thrombocytopenia: management with danaparoid (Orgaran). Ann Thorac Surg 68: 1076–1078, 1999.

Schiffmann H, Unterhalt M, Harms K, Figulla HR, Völpel H, Greinacher A. Successful treatment of heparin-induced thrombocytopenia type II in childhood with recombinant hirudin. Monatsschr Kinderheilk 145: 606–612, 1997.

Schlegel N, Hurtaud-Roux MF. TIH en pediatrie. Presented at the HIT-School Paris 28.03.2003. [in French]

Schmugge M, Risch L, Huber AR, Benn A, Fischer JE. Heparin-induced thrombocytopenia-associated thrombosis in pediatric intensive care patients. Pediatrics 109: E10, 2002.

Schreiber C, Dietrich W, Braun S, Kostolny M, Eicken A, Lange R. Use of heparin upon reoperation in a pediatric patient with heparin-induced thrombocytopenia after disappearance of antibodies. Clin Res Cardiol 95: 379–382, 2006.

Scott LK, Grier LR, Conrad SA. Heparin-induced thrombocytopenia in a pediatric patient receiving extracorporeal membrane oxygenation managed with argatroban. Pediatr Crit Care Med 7: 473–475, 2006.

Scurr J, Baglin T, Burns H, Clements RV, Cooke T, de Swiet M, Paxton Dewar E, Forbes C, Frostick S, Greer I, Hobbs R, Jenkins T, Klein L, Lanigan D, Lowe G, Warwick D, Wilson J. Risk of and prophylaxis for venous thromboembolism in hospital patients. Phlebology 13: 87–97, 1998.

Severin T, Sutor AH. Heparin-induced thrombocytopenia in pediatrics. Semin Thromb Hemost 27: 293–299, 2001.

Severin T, Dittrich S, Zieger B, Kampermann J, Kececioglu D, Sutor AH. HIT II after Fontan procedure—treatment with lepirudin [abstr]. Ann Hematol 81: A77, 2002a.

Severin T, Zieger B, Sutor AH. Anticoagulation with recombinant hirudin and danaparoid sodium in pediatric patients. Semin Thromb Hemost 28: 447–454, 2002b.

Skouri H, Gandouz R, Abroug S, Kraiem I, Euch H, Gargouri J, Harbi A. A prospective study of the prevalence of heparin-induced antibodies and other associated thromboembolic risk factors in pediatric patients undergoing hemodialysis. Am J Hematol 81: 328–334, 2006.

Spadone D, Clark F, James E, Laster J, Hoch J, Silver D. Heparin-induced thrombocytopenia in the newborn. J Vasc Surg 15: 306–311, 1992.

Streif W, Ageno W. Direct thrombin and factor Xa inhibitors in children: a quest for new anticoagulants for children. Wien Med Wochenschr 161: 73–79, 2011.

Sutor AH, Chan AKC, Massicotte M. Low molecular weight heparin in pediatric patients. Semin Thromb Hemost 30(Suppl 1): 31–39, 2004.

Takemoto CM, Streiff MB. Heparin-induced thrombocytopenia screening and management in pediatric patients. Hematology Am Soc Hematol Educ Program 2011: 162–169, 2011.

Tcheng WY, Wong W-Y. Successful use of argatroban in pediatric patients requiring anticoagulant alternatives to heparin [abstr]. Blood 104: 107b, 2004.

Tousovska K, Zapletal O, Skotakova J, Bukac J, Sterba J. Treatment of deep venous thrombosis with low molecular weight heparin in pediatric cancer patients: safety and efficacy. Blood Coagul Fibrinolysis 20: 583–589, 2009.

Verso M, Mazzarino I, Agnelli G, Stefanelli M, Ceppi S, Paoletti F. Dermatan sulphate for heparin-induced thrombocytopenia and central venous catheter-related deep vein thrombosis in a child with acute lymphoblastic leukemia. Haematologica 89: ECR06, 2004.

von Heymann C, Hagemeyer E, Kastrup M, Ziemer S, Proqitte H, Konertz WF, Spies C. Heparin-induced thrombocytopenia type II in an infant with congenital heart defect- anticoagulation during cardiopulmonary bypass with epoprostenol sodium and heparin. Pediatr Crit Care Med 7: 383–385, 2006.

Warkentin TE, Levine MN, Hirsh J, Horsewood P, Roberts RS, Gent M, Kelton JG. Heparin-induced thrombocytopenia in patients treated with low molecular weight heparin or unfractionated heparin. N Engl J Med 332: 1330–1335, 1995.

Warkentin TE, Greinacher A, Koster A, Lincoff AM. Treatment and prevention of heparin-induced thrombocytopenia. American College of Chest Physicians evidence-based clinical practice guidelines, 8th edition. Chest 133(6 Suppl): 340S–380S, 2008.

Weigel B, Laky A, Krishnamurti L. Danaparoid (Organan) anticoagulation of pediatric patients with heparin-induced thrombocytopenia (HIT) [abstr]. J Pediatr Hematol Oncol 21: 327, 1999.

Wilhelm MJ, Schmid C, Kececioglu D, Mollhoff T, Ostermann H, Scheld HH. Cardiopulmonary bypass in patients with heparin-induced thrombocytopenia using Org 10172. Ann Thorac Surg 61: 920–924, 1996.

Young G. Current and future antithrombotic agents in children. Expert Rev Cardiovasc Ther 2: 523–534, 2004.

Young G. New anticoagulants in children: a review of recent studies and a look to the future. Thromb Res 127: 70–74, 2011a.

Young G. Old and new antithrombotic drugs in neonates and infants. Semin Fetal Neonatal Med 16: 349–354, 2011b.

Young G, Nugent DJ. Use of argatroban and fondaparinux in a child with heparin-induced thrombocytopenia. Pediatr Blood Cancer 42: 507, 2004.

Young G, Tarantino MMD, Wohrley J, Weber LC, Belvedere M, Nugent DJ. Pilot dose-finding and safety study of bivalirudin in infants <6 months of age with thrombosis. J Thromb Hemost 5: 1654–1659, 2007.

Young G, Boshkov LK, Sullivan JE, Raffini LJ, Cox DS, Boyle DA, Kallender H, Tarka EA, Soffer J, Hursting MJ. Argatroban therapy in pediatric patients requiring nonheparin anticoagulation: an open-label, safety, efficacy, and pharmacokinetic study. Pediatr Blood Cancer 56: 1103–1109, 2011a.

Young G, Yee DL, O'Brien SH, Khanna R, Barbour A, Nugent DJ. FondaKIDS: a prospective pharmacokinetic and safety study of fondaparinux in children between 1 and 18 years of age. Pediatr Blood Cancer 57: 1049–1054, 2011b.

Zöhrer B, Zenz W, Rettenbacher A, Covi P, Kurnik K, Kroll H, Grubbauer HM, Muntean W. Danaparoid sodium (Orgaran) in four children with heparin-induced thrombocytopenia type II. Acta Paediatr 90: 765–771, 2001.

A clinician's perspective on heparin-induced thrombocytopenia: Paradoxes, myths, and continuing challenges

Lawrence Rice

INTRODUCTION

I was never given a choice but to develop an interest in heparin-induced thrombo-cytopenia (HIT). As a medical resident in 1976, I had just read articles in the *New England Journal of Medicine* and *Annals of Internal Medicine* (Babcock et al., 1976; Bell et al., 1976) championing different mechanisms of this phenomenon, when a 50-year-old man came under my care at the Veterans Administration Hospital with deep vein thrombosis (DVT) after back surgery. After intravenous (iv) heparin was infused for 1 week, he experienced worsening leg signs, new pulmonary emboli (PE), and a fall in platelet count from 441 to 83 × 10⁹/L. Proud of my astuteness, I immediately stopped the heparin, gave a "loading dose" of warfarin (10 mg), pro-tected his lungs with an inferior vena cava (IVC) filter, and confirmed the diagnosis by observing that heparin produced *in vitro* aggregation of normal platelets in the presence of the patient's platelet-poor plasma. Within days, a necrotic thigh lesion emerged; sepsis and death ensued, leaving me to marvel at the incredibly bad luck that could deal a person with both HIT and warfarin-induced skin necrosis. Today we understand that these two drug reactions are not coincidental and that the war-farin therapy likely contributed to the catastrophic outcome. We published this case 27 years later, including it within a case series illustrating the dangers of warfarin use during acute HIT (Srinivasan et al., 2004).

Sealing a personal abiding clinical interest in HIT were five more cases I encountered during my first three months of Hematology Fellowship. As impres-sionable as my first case was, each of these proved more dramatic and more chal-lenging than the last, such that I can still recount many details. One patient was a middle-aged man admitted for leg pain and swelling, administered heparin while awaiting a contrast venogram. The procedure was postponed over the weekend when he was mistakenly served breakfast. All signs and symptoms resolved in the interim, and the venogram proved negative, but on discharge, walking to the door, he collapsed. Brought back to life by electric countershock, he was found to have suffered a massive anterior myocardial infarction (MI); also discovered was a pre-cipitous fall in the platelet count on a blood sample drawn that morning but not checked until postarrest (Rice and Jackson, 1981). Another of the patients received heparin for MI only to develop thrombocytopenia and fatal bowel necrosis 1 week later. By that time, a case series from Missouri had delineated clinical features of the HIT syndrome and highlighted the occurrence of thromboembolic complications (Rhodes et al., 1977; see chap. 1).

I first presented Grand Rounds on HIT more than 30 years ago, and sought speaking opportunities at state, national, and international society meetings. I joined a small cadre of "HITophiles" who naively believed that just getting the word out would greatly diminish the amputations, strokes, PE, and deaths we were seeing in afflicted patients. When I lectured, questioners frequently protested that this syndrome had to be incredibly rare or downright imaginary. One venerated practitioner at my hospital assured the audience that he had never seen a case despite using heparin for decades; I restrained myself from pointing out that his resident had just shared with me hospital records indicating that one of his patients had developed low platelets and recurrent multiple arterial and venous clots while receiving more and more heparin. Perhaps I should have realized back then that as awareness increased, case numbers would escalate—my colleagues and I collected 50 cases with thrombotic complications at our institution from the mid-1970s to the mid-1980s (which we felt represented an enormous problem), but by the late-1990s we were seeing 100 cases every year.

My interest in HIT opened vistas that could never be gleaned from lecture halls or textbooks, covering issues of what is important in medical education, medical orthodoxies and their evolution, medical economics, medicolegal challenges, and relationships between academic medicine, clinical medicine, and industry. It was long very troubling that appreciation and recognition of HIT lagged far behind, even as new anticoagulant strategies in cardiology quickly become standard practice, sometimes despite marginal benefit. Textbooks (in critical care medicine, vascular medicine, and others) provided scant attention to this problem for the longest time, and only recently have begun to catch up. Did HIT find a crack, some manner of "perfect storm," as Hematology/Oncology training shifted emphasis to solid tumors and thought-leaders in thrombosis left the intensive care unit for the laboratory? Whatever the other factors, I believe that a major impediment to the widespread recognition and treatment for this problem continues to be the numerous paradoxes and myths that surround HIT. Awareness of the paradoxes and myths may allow physicians to advance past these obstacles (Rice, 2004).

HIT PARADOXES

1. Heparin, the most powerful anticoagulant of the twentieth century, has saved countless lives and limbs, yet may *also precipitate the most extreme hypercoagulable state, costing thousands yearly their lives and limbs.*
2. Despite the fall in platelet count during use of heparin, patients rarely develop bleeding; rather, attempts to correct the platelet count with platelet transfusions could worsen the prothrombotic problem.
3. This is a humoral immune reaction, yet it usually does not recur with future heparin exposure, and classic anamnestic responses do not appear to occur.
4. This drug reaction continues for a time even after the drug has been stopped, and even asymptomatic patients who have already recovered from their only initial manifestation of the reaction (thrombocytopenia) may develop a thrombotic event following platelet count recovery.
5. One would think that medical professionals (doctors, nurses, pharmacists) would be especially attuned to this problem, given that it is common, serious, treatable, preventable, a major source of malpractice litigation, and iatrogenic, *but many are not, and scant attention has been paid in textbooks and in medical school curricula.*

HIT MYTHS
HIT is Rare
Traditionally, this has been one of the most detrimental myths, leading health professionals not to learn about the problem and not to be vigilant for it. In fact, HIT occurs in up to 3–5% of patients receiving 1 week or more of prophylactic-dose unfractionated heparin (UFH) for postoperative thromboprophylaxis, as well as in about 1% of patients receiving iv UFH for treatment of DVT, PE, or unstable angina (see chap. 4). Any heparin exposure can cause HIT, with documented cases following single or brief exposures to heparin (Warkentin and Bernstein, 2003). Relatively recent data from the CATCH registry suggests that there is still much to be done to increase HIT awareness among medical personnel. Data were collected from 48 U.S. hospitals on 4000 patients who were exposed to heparin for more than four days or who became thrombocytopenic while in the Coronary Care Unit (Crespo et al., 2009). Thrombocytopenia was common and was the strongest independent predictor of complications (including thromboemboli) and death, yet shockingly few patients had HIT considered, testing ordered, alternative anticoagulation given, or a hematologist consulted.

Heparin Flushes are Needed to Maintain Catheter Patency and are Benign
We observed decades ago that the small amounts of heparin used in catheter flush solutions can sometimes cause the full-blown HIT syndrome or more often promulgate new complications in affected patients (Rice and Jackson, 1981; Rice et al., 1986, 1988), observations which have been verified by others (Doty et al., 1986). Even small amounts of heparin that leach from heparin-bonded central venous or pulmonary artery catheters may have caused HIT (Laster and Silver, 1988). It is clear from a meta-analysis of randomized trials that there is no advantage to heparin flush over saline in maintaining patency of traditional "hep lock" peripheral venous catheters (Randolph et al., 1998). The data are scant with regard to other types of catheters (e.g., intra-arterial catheters, percutaneously inserted central catheters), but exploration of risks/benefits are warranted. Clearly, it is prudent to eliminate exposures to heparin that are unnecessary and to eliminate all heparin exposures completely when HIT is suspected.

We can Just Use Low Molecular Weight Heparin and Forget about HIT
Low molecular weight heparin (LMWH) preparations cause HIT about one-tenth as often as does UFH (Martel et al., 2005). Nevertheless, given that there are millions of patients exposed to LMWH each year, it should not be surprising that I regularly encounter some patients with HIT who have been exposed exclusively to LMWH. Indeed, as LMWH use increases, it can become a more common trigger of HIT than UFH (Linkins and Warkentin, 2011). Importantly, once a patient has HIT, LMWH is contraindicated, as the antibodies usually cross-react with LMWH, leading to more complications (see chap. 12).

This cannot be HIT Because it is Too Early, Too Late, or the Platelets are Not Low Enough, or They are Too Low
"Classic" HIT ensues 5–10 days (occasionally, a few days later) after beginning a course of heparin, but rapid-onset HIT may occur within minutes of heparin administration if the patient has had prior sensitization to heparin within the preceding three months (Warkentin and Kelton, 2001a; Mims et al., 2004). Although

the degree of thrombocytopenia with HIT is often moderate (median platelet count, $60 \times 10^9/L$), 10% of patients may experience severe thrombocytopenia (platelet count $<20 \times 10^9/L$) (Warkentin, 2003, 2007); remarkably such patients rarely bleed, although many are fully anticoagulated, and in fact those patients with the lowest platelet counts have the highest risk for thromboembolic complications and thus the most dire need for alternative anticoagulation. Another 10% of HIT patients may have nadir platelet counts that fall within the normal range, but usually these are patients who had substantially elevated platelet counts a few days earlier (Warkentin et al., 2003). Thus, one should not completely dismiss the possibility of HIT when temporal features or the magnitudes of the platelet count decline are somewhat atypical.

This cannot be HIT Because the Patient is not on Heparin Now

The syndrome of "delayed-onset HIT" was elucidated a decade ago, and is now widely recognized (Warkentin and Kelton, 2001b; Rice et al., 2002). The patients are often recuperating at home from a hospitalization that included heparin exposure, having received no heparin for a few days or more. They return to hospital with an arterial or venous thrombotic event. Upon return, the platelet count is often (although not necessarily) low. These people are often given heparin for their presenting thrombosis, which invariably leads to an abrupt fall in platelet count, frequently clinical deterioration, and substantial mortality. Invariably, their serum contains high-titer antibodies against platelet factor 4/heparin (PF4/H) complexes. The message to emergency room doctors, intensivists, and hospitalists is to consider the possibility of delayed-onset HIT—and not to initiate heparin reflexively—when a recently hospitalized patient returns with thrombosis. The U.S. Food and Drug Administration mandated a special warning section on delayed-onset HIT in the prescribing information for heparin (December 8, 2006).

We can Wait for the Test to Come Back

The time immediately after heparin is stopped may be the most dangerous for the emergence of thromboemboli, because heparin may exert some protective anticoagulant effect at the same time it is feeding a prothrombotic maelstrom. The protocol for the lepirudin registration trials in Europe called for heparin to be stopped when HIT was suspected, but lepirudin was initiated only after obtaining positive serologic results; a 6% per day thrombosis event rate was observed while physicians awaited the test results (Greinacher et al., 2000). The initial suspicion for HIT depends on clinical features, such as the 4Ts (Thrombocytopenia, Timing, Thrombosis, oTher causes of thrombocytopenia unlikely) (Lo et al., 2006); when HIT is reasonably suspected, an alternative anticoagulant should be initiated, and the results of serologic tests considered later.

If the Test is Positive, the Patient has HIT

Serologic tests are crucial for diagnosis confirmation and should be ordered whenever HIT is reasonably suspected. Nevertheless, clinicians must appreciate the practical limitations of currently available PF4-dependent immunoassays and that test results alone cannot tell you if your patient has HIT or not (it only aids your clinical decision making). No assay is highly satisfactory in terms of sensitivity–specificity tradeoffs, reproducibility, and availability in "real time." Commercially available enzyme(-linked) immuno(sorbent) assays (EIAs or ELISAs) are most widely used and have advantages of standardization, ease of performance, wide availability, and high sensitivity, but the major problem is their very high rate of "false positives" for diagnosing clinical HIT. The question of where appropriate cutoff values should be between "positive" and "negative" may be misplaced, if one recognizes that all results need to be interpreted in the context of the clinical situation, the pretest probability, and the optical density (OD) measurement. For example, one to two weeks after heart surgery, 25–70% of patients will have a "positive" EIA test (OD > 0.4 U), but only 2–5% of these will actually have clinical HIT. The interpretation of the EIA result must take into account the OD reading (a proxy for antibody titer). Warkentin and colleagues (2008b) found that "positive" EIAs with ODs of 0.4–1.0 had only a 2–5% rate of platelet-activating antibodies in a functional serotonin release assay (SRA); when the OD was >2.0, approximately 90% had platelet-activating antibodies detected. Functional (platelet activation) assays, such as the platelet SRA, may aid clinical interpretation in the few cases where diagnosis remains equivocal. An unfortunate fact of life is that interpreting HIT serologic tests is much like interpreting many other tests obtained in clinical medicine: one has to understand the disease process, its likelihood, and the limitations of testing (see chap. 11). As always, the interpretation of the test begins with clinical judgment and assessment of pretest probability. Accordingly, information on the temporal course of platelet counts in relation to heparin exposure, or a scoring system, such as the 4Ts, can be invaluable (Lo et al., 2006; see chap. 3).

Overdiagnosis Creates no Big Problem

Although there still remains a need to increase awareness of HIT, "overdiagnosis" has emerged as a substantial problem at many institutions (Lo et al., 2007; Berry et al., 2011; Cuker and Cines, 2012). Overdiagnosis has deleterious consequences (Smythe et al., 2011). Anticoagulant drugs in general have narrow therapeutic ratios, and when treating HIT, physicians often institute expensive agents with which they are unfamiliar with the nuances of use. Needed procedures may be postponed, we have seen transplant lists culled, and patients can become permanently "branded." Undoubtedly, the use of overly sensitive EIA assays by those not skilled in their interpretation has contributed to the overdiagnosis problem. However, even before this, we and others have found that the test is frequently ordered "willy–nilly" in patients with low platelet counts whose course is not at all compatible with HIT—the fact that only 10% of ordered specimens are positive at even low titer speaks toward this (Trehel-Tursis et al., 2012; Wanat et al., 2012). Thus, physicians must learn about the disease process, know when to suspect it and when it is clearly not a reasonable possibility. They must further understand that ordering an unwarranted test may have harmful repercussions. In recent years, when my colleagues and I are consulted on cases of suspected HIT, more often than not we find that the patient does not have the problem.

We can Just Stop the Heparin

As awareness and recognition of HIT have increased, the myth that one can simply stop heparin is generating proportionally more harm. When Warkentin and Kelton (1996) followed up 62 patients with serologically confirmed "isolated HIT" (HIT with no thrombosis) whose UFH had been stopped, and in whom either no anticoagulant was given or warfarin was initiated or continued, 53% developed new clots, usually in the first two weeks; in three (5%), the new clot was manifest as sudden death. Other case series have confirmed the high risk for new thromboemboli after heparin is stopped (Wallis et al., 1999; Lewis et al., 2001). Indeed, it seems wise to investigate systematically the lower limbs for DVT when isolated HIT is diagnosed (Warkentin et al., 2008a). In getting physicians thinking beyond paradox 4 (p. 609) that stopping the drug will end the danger, one will also confront the "minor paradox" that prophylactic doses of anticoagulation will not suffice in isolated HIT (Farner et al., 2001; Warkentin, 2001; Kodityal et al., 2003) and the myth that HIT with thrombosis is somehow a different disorder than HIT without thrombosis—the only real difference is that clots have not (yet) appeared in the latter. Continuing to promulgate type I and type II HIT terminology (see chap. 1) further confuses physicians into believing that some cases of true HIT are benign and do not require intervention (Rice, 2004). My colleagues and I see many cases where new devastating thromboses appear after doctors have recognized HIT and stopped the heparin, but failed to institute an alternative anticoagulant. Among untreated patients we have also seen many clots emerge after the platelet count has recovered to normal.

We can Just Give Warfarin

Unlike most anticoagulants, warfarin does not inhibit any activated coagulation factors, and thus will not inhibit the hypercoagulable state that characterizes acute HIT. Worse, warfarin will produce an early and rapid decrease of the short-lived vitamin K-dependent natural anticoagulant factor, protein C. Thus, in the extreme prothrombotic milieu of HIT, warfarin's earliest effects can precipitate or exacerbate thromboembolic phenomena, including microvascular thrombosis. The syndrome of venous limb gangrene first came to light as a complication of warfarin use in the setting of HIT, and may be a more common cause of limb loss in HIT than arterial thrombosis (Warkentin et al., 1997). Examples of "classic" warfarin-induced central skin necrosis are also recognized as complications of HIT (Warkentin et al., 1999; Srinivasan et al., 2004). Observations made in HIT patients have taught us about warfarin's significant risks when used in any active procoagulant process, especially when it is used unopposed, early and/or in excessive doses (ironically, supra-therapeutic levels of anticoagulation—as judged by the international normalized ratio (INR)—are a surrogate marker for very low protein C levels, and correlate with increased risk of microvascular thrombosis). The magnitude of warfarin danger during acute HIT is such that current treatment guidelines recommend reversal with vitamin K if a patient with HIT has already begun warfarin therapy: this not only prevents the exacerbation of thrombotic complications *per se*, but also prevents underdosing of alternative anticoagulants due to warfarin's contribution to the prolongation of global coagulation tests used for monitoring (Warkentin and Greinacher, 2004; Warkentin, 2006; Warkentin et al., 2008a) (see chap. 12).

We can Protect the Patient with an Inferior Vena Cava Filter

The scant available evidence for the efficacy and safety of IVC filters best support use when anticoagulation is contraindicated in a patient at high risk for PE or when adequate anticoagulation therapy has failed. With HIT, anticoagulation with an alternative agent is strongly indicated, not contraindicated. In the extreme hypercoagulable milieu of HIT, the foreign-body filter is likely to exacerbate thrombotic tendencies. A retrospective eight-year chart review at our hospital revealed 18 HIT patients who had IVC filters placed, and 15 of these developed new thromboses, some catastrophic (Jung et al., 2011).

Alternative Anticoagulants are Expensive and do not Improve Outcomes with HIT

A small, randomized controlled trial of HIT therapies (danaparoid *vs* dextran-70) experienced very slow patient recruitment, probably because of the widely perceived (and ultimately demonstrable) superiority of danaparoid (Chong et al., 2001) (see chap. 16). In the pivotal studies of the direct thrombin inhibitors lepirudin and argatroban, it was deemed unethical to have placebo controls, and so historical controls were used (see chaps. 13 and 14). Nevertheless, benefit has been demonstrated consistently, not only for the designated primary composite endpoints (all-cause mortality, limb amputation, new thromboemboli) but particularly for the endpoint in which an effective antithrombotic agent would be expected to show the most impact, namely, new thromboemboli (Lewis et al., 2006). (This is because most deaths in HIT patient series are due to nonthrombotic events, such as multiorgan failure, cancer, and other non-HIT comorbidities, and amputations are often performed on limbs already doomed by the time of initiation of alternative anticoagulation, and perhaps too because these prospective cohort studies were done before warfarin's adverse effect profile was appreciated.) Newer therapies (generic fondaparinux, bivalirudin, desirudin, generic argatroban) and those on the horizon (dabigatran, rivoraxoban) may simplify therapy and reduce expense. There is no question of efficacy of alternative anticoagulants among those with experience managing HIT, who have often witnessed dramatic reversals of the thrombotic "storm" with therapy.

HIT and its Complications are Inevitable, Unpredictable, and cannot be Prevented

LMWHs have a number of advantages over UFH, one being the lower risk of inducing HIT by one order of magnitude (Martel et al., 2005). Fondaparinux (like LMWH) also has a low risk of causing significant antibody formation, and in addition (unlike LMWH) does not usually cross-react with pathogenic HIT antibodies: thus, fondaparinux almost certainly has an even lower risk of causing HIT (Warkentin et al., 2005; Salem et al., 2010). In my opinion, either LMWH or fondaparinux should be preferred to UFH in the great majority of situations where anticoagulation is indicated. (Exceptions to this would be in the cardiovascular operating room, hemodialysis unit, and, perhaps in the cardiac catheterization laboratory, or in renally impaired or high bleeding risk critical care patients.) Furthermore, effective and safe new oral anticoagulants, such as dabigatran and rivoroxaban, will further diminish exposures to heparin. Such a change in practice has the potential to diminish greatly both HIT incidence and sequelae. Short-sighted administrators cannot be allowed to "save money" by divorcing pharmacy acquisition costs for UFH from the institution's costs of monitoring for, treating, and defending lawsuits arising from HIT. The last bastion of UFH use is likely to be cardiac surgery using extracorporeal circulation, because of the established experience with heparin, including reliable intraoperative monitoring and its rapid reversibility with protamine, although even here potentially safer alternative anticoagulants have been studied (see chap. 19). Furthermore, appropriate monitoring of platelet counts in patients at risk for HIT, followed by appropriate action when thrombocytopenia occurs, is likely to reduce the thromboembolic catastrophes that might otherwise occur (Warkentin et al., 2008a); this is likely to be advanced by "systems-based" approaches.

HIT REALITIES

Medical professionals have to be highly knowledgeable about HIT, a relatively common and serious clinical problem. It can be prevented by avoiding unnecessary heparin exposures (e.g., heparin flushes), by increasing, where appropriate, the use of LMWH or fondaparinux rather than UFH, and through appropriate platelet count monitoring. In addition to the lack of attention traditionally devoted to HIT in medical curricula and textbooks, obstacles to addressing the problem include promoting greater awareness of the paradoxes and myths surrounding it. HIT produces the most extreme prothrombotic diathesis, so upon reasonable clinical suspicion, an alternative anticoagulant must be initiated. Key to preventing catastrophes is knowledge, vigilance, and maintenance of a high degree of suspicion: HIT must be a prime consideration whenever a patient in the hospital (or recently hospitalized) suffers a fall in platelet count or a new venous or arterial thrombotic event. The temporal relationship of such events to heparin exposure has to be analyzed. Physician thinking must get past the notion that this drug reaction can be reversed simply by stopping the drug. By appreciating the paradoxes and exposing the myths, we can move forward, particularly now that effective agents and strategies are available for prevention and treatment.

REFERENCES

Babcock RB, Dumper CW, Scharfman WB. Heparin-induced thrombocytopenia. N Engl J Med 295: 237–241,1976.

Bell WR, Tomasulo PA, Alving BM, Duffy TP. Thrombocytopenia occurring during the administration of heparin: a prospective study in 52 patients. Ann Intern Med 85: 155–160, 1976.

Berry C, Tcherniantchouk O, Ley EJ, Salim A, Mirocha J, Martin-Stone S, Stolpner D, Margulies DR. Overdiagnosis of heparin-induced thrombocytopenia in surgical ICU patients. J Am Coll Surg 213: 10–17, 2011.

Chong BH, Gallus AS, Cade JF, Magnani H, Manoharan A, Oldmeadow M, Arthur C, Rickard K, Gallo J, Seshadri P, Chesterman CN, Australian HIT Study Group. Prospective randomized open-label comparison of danaparoid with dextran 70 in the treatment of heparin-induced thrombocytopenia with thrombosis: a clinical outcome study. Thromb Haemost 86: 1170–1175, 2001.

Crespo EM, Oliveira GB, Honeycutt EF, Becker RC, Berger PB, Moliterno DJ, Anstrom KJ, Abrams CS, Kleiman NS, Moll S, Rice L, Rodgers JE, Steinhubl SR, Tapson VF, Granger CB, Ohman EM, CATCH Registry Investigators. Evaluation and management of thrombocytopenia and suspected heparin-induced thrombocytopenia in hospitalized patients: The Complications After Thrombocytopenia Caused by Heparin (CATCH) registry. Am Heart J 157: 651–657, 2009.

Cuker A, Cines DB. How I treat heparin-induced thrombocytopenia. Blood 119: 2209–2218, 2012.

Doty JR, Alving BM, McDonnell DE, Ondra SL. Heparin-associated thrombocytopenia in the neurosurgical patient. Neurosurgery 19: 69–72, 1986.

Farner B, Eichler P, Kroll H, Greinacher A. A comparison of danaparoid and lepirudin in heparin-induced thrombocytopenia. Thromb Haemost 85: 950–957, 2001.

Greinacher A, Eichler P, Lubenow N, Kwasny H, Luz M. Heparin-induced thrombocytopenia with thromboembolic complications: meta-analysis of 2 prospective trials to assess the value of parenteral treatment with lepirudin and its therapeutic aPTT range. Blood 96: 846–851, 2000.

Jung M, McCarthy JJ, Baker KR, Rice L. Safety of IVC filters with heparin-induced thrombocytopenia: a retrospective study. Blood (ASH Annual Meeting Abstract) 118: Abstract 2225, 2011.

Kodityal S, Manhas AH, Udden M, Rice L. Danaparoid for heparin-induced thrombocytopenia: an analysis of treatment failures. Eur J Haematol 7: 109–113, 2003.

Laster J, Silver D. Heparin-coated catheters and heparin-induced thrombocytopenia. J Vasc Surg 7: 667–672, 1988.

Lewis BE, Wallis DE, Berkowitz SD, Matthai WH, Fareed J, Walenga JM, Bartholomew J, Sham R, Lerner RG, Zeigler ZR, Rustagi PK, Jang IK, Rifkin SD, Moran J, Hursting MJ, Kelton JG, ARG-911 Investigators. Argatroban anticoagulant therapy in patients with heparin-induced thrombocytopenia. Circulation 103: 1838–1843, 2001.

Lewis BE, Wallis DE, Hursting MJ, Levine RL, Leya F. Effects of argatroban therapy, demographic variables, and platelet count on thrombotic risks in heparin-induced thrombocytopenia. Chest 129: 1407–1416, 2006.

Linkins LA, Warkentin TE. Heparin-induced thrombocytopenia: real world issues. Semin Thromb Hemost 37: 653–663, 2011.

Lo GK, Juhl D, Warkentin TE, Sigouin CS, Eichler P, Greinacher A. Evaluation of pretest clinical score (4 T's) for the diagnosis of heparin-induced thrombocytopenia in two clinical settings. J Thromb Haemost 4: 759–765, 2006.

Lo GK, Sigouin CS, Warkentin TE. What is the potential for overdiagnosis of heparin-induced thrombocytopenia? Am J Hematol 82: 1037–1043, 2007.

Martel N, Lee J, Wells PS. Risk for heparin-induced thrombocytopenia with unfractionated heparin and low molecular weight heparin thromboprophylaxis: a metaanalysis. Blood 106: 2710–2715, 2005.

Mims MP, Manian P, Rice L. Acute cardiorespiratory collapse from heparin: a consequence of heparin-induced thrombocytopenia. Eur J Haematol 72: 366–369, 2004.

Randolph AG, Cook DJ, Gonzales CA, Andrew M. Benefit of heparin in peripheral venous and arterial catheters: systematic review and meta-analysis of randomized controlled trials. BMJ 316: 969–975, 1998.

Rhodes GR, Dixon RH, Silver D. Heparin induced thrombocytopenia: eight cases with thrombotic-hemorrhagic complications. Ann Surg 186: 752–758, 1977.

Rice L. Heparin-induced thrombocytopenia: myths and misconceptions (that will cause trouble for you and your patient). Arch Intern Med 164: 1961–1964, 2004.

Rice L, Jackson D. Can heparin cause clotting? Heart Lung 10: 331–335, 1981.

Rice L, Huffman DM, Levine ML, Udden MM, Waddell CC, Luper WE. Heparin-induced thrombocytopenia/thrombosis syndrome: clinical manifestation and insights [abstr]. Blood 68(Suppl 1): 339a, 1986.

Rice L, Huffman DM, Waddell CC, Luper WE, Udden MM, Levine ML. Therapy of thromboembolic disease: the heparin thrombocytopenia/thrombosis syndrome. In: Thrombosis, Anticoagulants and Antiplatelet Agents in Clinical Practice. New York: Park Row Publishers, 31–36, 1988.

Rice L, Attisha W, Francis JL, Drexler AJ. Delayed onset heparin-induced thrombocytopenia. Ann Intern Med 136: 210–215, 2002.

Salem M, Elrefai S, Shrit MA, Warkentin TE. Fondaparinux thromboprophylaxis-associated heparin-induced thrombocytopenia syndrome complicated by arterial thrombotic stroke. Thromb Haemost 104: 1071–1072, 2010.

Smythe MA, Warkentin TE, Woodhouse AL, Zakalik D. Venous limb gangrene and fatal hemorrhage: adverse consequences of HIT "overdiagnosis" in a patient with antiphospholipid syndrome. Am J Hematol 86: 188–191, 2011.

Srinivasan AF, Rice L, Bartholomew JR, Rangaswamy C, La Perna L, Thompson JE, Murphy S, Baker KR. Warfarin-induced skin necrosis and venous limb gangrene with heparin-induced thrombocytopenia. Arch Intern Med 164: 66–70, 2004.

Trehel-Tursis V, Louvain-Quintard V, Zarrouki Y, Imbert A, Doubine S, Stéphan F. Clinical and biological features of patients suspected or confirmed to have heparin-induced thrombocytopenia in a cardiothoracic surgical ICU. Chest 8 Mar 2012. [Epub ahead of print]

Wallis DE, Workman DL, Lewis BE, Steen L, Pifarre R, Moran JF. Failure of early heparin cessation as treatment for heparin-induced thrombocytopenia. Am J Med 106: 629–635, 1999.

Wanat M, Fitousis K, Hall J, Rice L. PF4/heparin antibody testing and treatment of heparin-induced thrombocytopenia in the intensive care unit. Clin Appl Thromb Haemost 2 Mar 2012. [Epub ahead of print]

Warkentin TE. Heparin-induced thrombocytopenia: yet another treatment paradox? Thromb Haemost 85: 947–949, 2001.

Warkentin TE. Heparin-induced thrombocytopenia: pathogenesis and management. Br J Haematol 121: 535–555, 2003.

Warkentin TE. Should vitamin K be administered when HIT is diagnosed after administration of coumarin? J Thromb Haemost 4: 894–896, 2006.

Warkentin TE. Drug-induced immune-mediated thrombocytopenia—from purpura to thrombosis. N Engl J Med 356: 891–893, 2007.

Warkentin TE, Bernstein RA. Delayed-onset heparin-induced thrombocytopenia and cerebral thrombosis after a single administration of unfractionated heparin. N Engl J Med 348: 1067–1069, 2003.

Warkentin TE, Greinacher A. Heparin-induced thrombocytopenia: recognition, treatment, and prevention: the Seventh ACCP Conference on antithrombotic and thrombolytic therapy. Chest 126(3 Suppl): 311S–337S, 2004.

Warkentin TE, Kelton JG. A 14-year study of heparin-induced thrombocytopenia. Am J Med 101: 502–507, 1996.

Warkentin TE, Kelton JG. Temporal aspects of heparin-induced thrombocytopenia. N Engl J Med 344: 1286–1292, 2001a.

Warkentin TE, Kelton JG. Delayed-onset heparin-induced thrombocytopenia and thrombosis. Ann Intern Med 135: 502–506, 2001b.

Warkentin TE, Elavathil LJ, Hayward CPM, Johnston MA, Russett JI, Kelton JG. The pathogenesis of venous limb gangrene associated with heparin-induced thrombocytopenia. Ann Intern Med 127: 804–812, 1997.

Warkentin TE, Sikov WM, Lillicrap DP. Multicentric warfarin-induced skin necrosis complicating heparin-induced thrombocytopenia. Am J Hematol 62: 44–48, 1999.

Warkentin TE, Roberts RS, Hirsh J, Kelton JG. An improved definition of immune heparin-induced thrombocytopenia. Arch Intern Med 163: 2518–2524, 2003.

Warkentin TE, Cook RJ, Marder VJ, Sheppard JI, Moore JC, Eriksson BI, Greinacher A, Kelton JG. Anti-platelet factor 4/heparin antibodies in orthopedic surgery patients receiving antithrombotic prophylaxis with fondaparinux or enoxaparin. Blood 106: 3791–3796, 2005.

Warkentin TE, Greinacher A, Koster A, Lincoff AM. Treatment and prevention of heparin-induced thrombocytopenia. American College of Chest Physicians evidence-based clinical practice guidelines, 8th edition. Chest 133(6 Suppl): 340S–380S, 2008a.

Warkentin TE, Sheppard JI, Moore JC, Sigouin CS, Kelton JG. Quantitative interpretation of optical density measurements using PF4-dependent enzyme-immunoassays. J Thromb Haemost 6: 1304–1312, 2008b.

Appendices

APPENDIX 1: TEN CLINICAL "RULES" FOR DIAGNOSING HIT

Rule 1
A thrombocytopenic patient whose platelet count fall began between days 5 and 10 of heparin treatment (inclusive) should be considered to have heparin-induced thrombocytopenia (HIT) unless proved otherwise (first day of heparin use is considered "day 0").

Rule 2
A rapid fall in the platelet count that began soon after starting heparin therapy is unlikely to represent HIT unless the patient has received heparin in the recent past, usually within the past 30, and latest, 100 days.

Rule 3
A platelet count fall of more than 50% from the postoperative peak between days 5 and 14 after surgery associated with heparin treatment can indicate HIT even if the platelet count remains higher than 150×10^9/L.

Rule 4
Petechiae, mucosal hemorrhages, and other signs of spontaneous bleeding are not clinical features of HIT, even in patients with very severe thrombocytopenia.

Rule 5
HIT is associated with a high frequency of thrombosis despite discontinuation of heparin therapy with or without substitution by coumarin: the initial rate of thrombosis is about 5–10% per day over the first 1–2 days; the 30–day cumulative risk is about 50%.

Rule 6
Localization of thrombosis in patients with HIT is strongly influenced by independent acute and chronic clinical factors, such as the postoperative state, arteriosclerosis, or the location of intravascular catheters in central veins or arteries.

Rule 7
In patients receiving heparin, the more unusual or severe a subsequent thrombotic event, the more likely the thrombosis is caused by HIT.

Rule 8
Venous limb gangrene is characterized by (*i*) *in vivo* thrombin generation associated with acute HIT; (*ii*) active deep vein thrombosis (DVT) in the limb(s) affected by venous gangrene; and (*iii*) a supratherapeutic INR during coumarin anticoagulation. This syndrome can be prevented by (*i*) delaying initiation of coumarin

anticoagulation during acute HIT until there has been substantial recovery of the platelet count (to at least $150 \times 10^9/L$) while receiving an alternative parenteral anticoagulant (e.g., lepirudin, argatroban, danaparoid, fondaparinux), and only if the thrombosis has clinically improved; (*ii*) initiating coumarin in low maintenance doses (e.g., 2–5 mg warfarin); (*iii*) ensuring that both parenteral and oral anticoagulant overlap for at least five days, with at least the last two days in the target therapeutic range; and (*iv*) if applicable, physicians should reverse coumarin anticoagulation with iv vitamin K in a patient recognized with acute HIT after coumarin therapy has been commenced.

Rule 9

Erythematous or (especially) necrotizing skin lesions at heparin injection sites should be considered dermal manifestations of the HIT syndrome, irrespective of the platelet count, unless proved otherwise. Patients who develop thrombocytopenia in association with heparin-induced skin lesions are at an increased risk for venous and, especially, arterial thrombosis.

Rule 10

Any inflammatory, cardiopulmonary, or other unexpected acute event that begins 5–30 minutes after an iv heparin bolus, or within 60 minutes of an sc low–molecular weight heparin (LMWH) injection, should be considered acute HIT unless proved otherwise. The postreaction platelet count should be measured promptly and compared with prereaction levels, because the platelet count fall is abrupt and often transient.

APPENDIX 2: RECOMMENDATIONS FOR THE TREATMENT OF HIT

THERAPY OF (IMMUNE) HIT
Discontinuation of Heparin for Clinically Suspected HIT

Recommendation. All heparin administration should be discontinued in patients clinically suspected of having (immune) HIT.

The routine use of heparin (e.g., line flushing) is pervasive in hospitals. Thus, based on our experience, it can be helpful to institute methods to reduce the risk for inadvertent heparin use in hospitalized patients with HIT.

Recommendation. A clearly visible note should be placed above the patient's bed stating "NO HEPARIN: HIT."

Recommendation. Heparin can be restarted in patients proved not to have HIT antibodies by a sensitive platelet activation assay or a PF4-dependent antigen assay.

Anticoagulation of the HIT Patient with Thrombosis
Anticoagulants Evaluated for Treatment of HIT: Indirect Factor Xa Inhibitors and Direct Thrombin Inhibitors

Recommendation. Therapeutic-dose anticoagulation with a rapidly acting alternative, nonheparin anticoagulant should be given to a patient with thrombosis complicating acute HIT. Treatment should not be delayed pending laboratory confirmation in a patient strongly suspected to have HIT. The specific choice of anticoagulant depends on many factors, including drug availability, physician experience with any particular agent, and pharmacologic considerations (especially regarding renal and hepatic function).

PTT Confounding

Recommendation. In patients with underlying coagulopathy (e.g., disseminated intravascular coagulation or warfarin-related), DTI monitoring should be performed by an assay that is independent of prothrombin concentrations (more widely available in Europe), especially when early posttreatment PTT values seem higher than expected for the DTI dose given.

Danaparoid Cross-Reactivity

Recommendation. *In vitro* cross-reactivity testing for danaparoid using HIT patient serum or plasma is not recommended prior to danaparoid administration.

Anticoagulation of the HIT Patient Without Thrombosis

Recommendation. Patients suspected to have acute HIT should undergo imaging studies for lower limb DVT, especially those at highest risk for venous thromboembolism, such as postoperative patients.

Recommendation. Therapeutic-dose anticoagulation with a rapidly acting alternative, nonheparin anticoagulant should be considered in patients strongly suspected (or confirmed) to have HIT even in the absence of symptomatic thrombosis. Anticoagulation should be continued at least until recovery of the platelet counts to a stable plateau.

Longer-Term Anticoagulant Management of the HIT Patient with Thrombosis
Transition to Vitamin K Antagonist (Coumarin) Therapy
Recommendation. To minimize the risk of coumarin necrosis in a patient with acute HIT, vitamin K antagonist (coumarin) therapy should be delayed until the patient is adequately anticoagulated with a rapidly acting parenteral anticoagulant, and not until there has been substantial platelet count recovery (at least $>150 \times 10^9/L$). The vitamin K antagonist should be started in low maintenance doses (e.g., ≤ 5 mg warfarin), with at least five days of overlap with the parenteral anticoagulant (including at least two days in the target-therapeutic range), and the parenteral anticoagulant should not be stopped until the platelet count has reached a stable plateau.
Recommendation. Oral or iv vitamin K should be given to reverse coumarin anticoagulation in a patient recognized as having acute HIT after coumarin has been commenced.
Recommendation. Prothrombin complex concentrates should not be used to reverse coumarin anticoagulation in a patient with acute or recent HIT unless bleeding is otherwise unmanageable.

Management of the Patient with a Low or Intermediate Probability of HIT (Pending Results of HIT Antibody Testing)
Recommendation. In a patient with a low probability for HIT (e.g., 4Ts score ≤ 3) pending the results of laboratory testing for HIT antibodies, we suggest either continuing the use of heparin or using alternative, nonheparin anticoagulation in prophylactic, rather than in therapeutic, doses (assuming there is no other reason for therapeutic-dose anticoagulation).
Recommendation. In a patient with an intermediate probability for HIT (e.g., 4Ts score of 4 or 5), who has an alternative explanation for thrombocytopenia and who does not require therapeutic-dose anticoagulation for other reasons, we suggest alternative anticoagulation in prophylactic, rather than in therapeutic, doses.

Reexposure of the HIT Patient to Heparin
Heparin Reexposure of the Patient with Acute or Recent HIT
Recommendation. Deliberate reexposure to heparin of a patient with acute or recent HIT for diagnostic purposes is not recommended. Rather, the diagnosis should first be excluded or confirmed in most situations by testing acute patient serum or plasma for HIT antibodies using a sensitive activation or antigen assay.

Heparin Reexposure of the Patient with a History of Remote HIT
Recommendation. Heparin should not be used for antithrombotic prophylaxis or therapy in a patient with a previous history of HIT, except under special circumstances (e.g., cardiac or vascular surgery, or hemodialysis).

HIT IN SPECIAL CLINICAL SITUATIONS
Cardiac or Vascular Surgery
Management of the Patient with Acute or Recent HIT
Recommendation. Alternative anticoagulation should be used for heart or vascular surgery in a patient with acute or recent HIT with detectable heparin-dependent,

platelet-activating antibodies. Bivalirudin is an appropriate alternative for intraoperative anticoagulation.

Management of the Patient Following Disappearance of HIT Antibodies

Recommendation. In a patient with a previous history of HIT, heart or vascular surgery can be performed using heparin, provided that (platelet-activating) HIT antibodies are absent (by sensitive functional assay) and heparin use is restricted to the surgical procedure itself.

HIT During Pregnancy

Recommendation. If available, danaparoid (and possibly fondaparinux) is preferred for parenteral anticoagulation of pregnant patients with HIT, or in those who have a previous history of HIT.

ADJUNCTIVE THERAPIES

Medical Thrombolysis

Recommendation. Regional or systemic pharmacologic thrombolysis should be considered as a treatment adjunct in selected patients with limb-threatening thrombosis or pulmonary embolism with severe cardiovascular compromise.

Surgical Thromboembolectomy and Fasciotomies

Recommendation. Surgical thromboembolectomy is an appropriate adjunctive treatment for selected patients with limb-threatening large-vessel arterial thromboembolism. Thrombocytopenia is not a contraindication to surgery. An alternative anticoagulant to heparin should preferably be used for intraoperative anticoagulation, although choice of anticoagulant and dosing remain unknown.

Intravenous Gammaglobulin

Recommendation. Intravenous gammaglobulin is a possible adjunctive treatment in selected patients requiring rapid blockade of the Fc receptor-dependent platelet-activating effects of HIT antibodies (e.g., management of patients with cerebral venous thrombosis, severe limb ischemia, or severe and/or persisting thrombocytopenia).

Plasmapheresis

Recommendation. Plasmapheresis, using plasma as replacement fluid, may be a useful adjunctive therapy in selected patients with acute HIT and life- or limb-threatening thrombosis who are suspected or proved to have acquired deficiency of one or more natural anticoagulant proteins, as well as for pre- or intraoperative removal of HIT antibodies when unfractionated heparin is planned for intraoperative anticoagulation.

Antiplatelet Agents

Dextran

Recommendation. Dextran should not be used as primary therapy for acute HIT complicated by thrombosis.

Acetylsalicylic Acid, Dipyridamole, and Clopidogrel
Recommendation. Antiplatelet agents, such as aspirin or clopidogrel, may be used as adjuncts to anticoagulant therapy of HIT, particularly in selected (arteriopathic) patients at high risk for arterial thromboembolism. The possible benefit in preventing arterial thrombosis should be weighed against the potential for increased bleeding.

Platelet Glycoprotein IIb/IIIa Inhibitors
Recommendation. GPIIb/IIIa inhibitors should be considered as experimental treatment in HIT and used with caution if combined with anticoagulant drugs.

CAVEATS FOR THE TREATMENT OF HIT
Low–Molecular Weight Heparin
Recommendation. LMWH should not be used to treat patients with acute HIT.

Vitamin K Antagonists
Recommendation. Vitamin K antagonist (coumarin) therapy is *contraindicated* during the acute (thrombocytopenic) phase of HIT. In patients who have already received coumarin when HIT is diagnosed, reversal with vitamin K is recommended. (See pp 334–335 for specific details of managing coumarin therapy in HIT.)

Platelet Transfusions
Recommendation. Prophylactic platelet transfusions are relatively contraindicated in patients with acute HIT, but may be appropriate with very severe thrombocytopenia, bleeding, major invasive procedure, or in the context of diagnostic uncertainty.

APPENDIX 3: TIMELINES OF AN EPISODE OF HIT

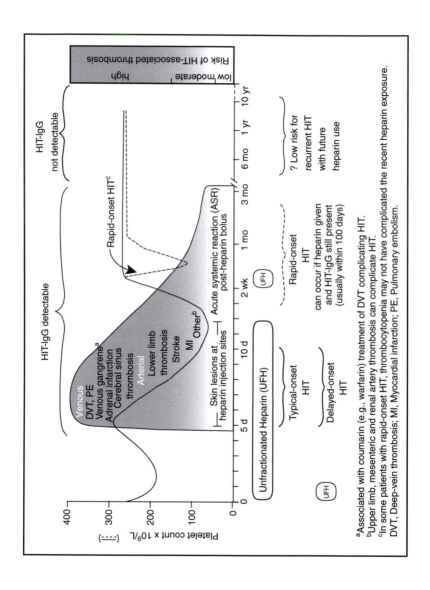

[a] Associated with coumarin (e.g., warfarin) treatment of DVT complicating HIT.
[b] Upper limb, mesenteric and renal artery thrombosis can complicate HIT.
[c] In some patients with rapid-onset HIT, thrombocytopenia may not have complicated the recent heparin exposure.
DVT, Deep-vein thrombosis; MI, Myocardial infarction; PE, Pulmonary embolism.

APPENDIX 4. SIX TREATMENT PRINCIPLES OF HIT[a]

TWO DO'S
Do stop all heparin (including heparin flushes, low molecular weight heparin, etc.)[b]
Do start an alternative, non-heparin anticoagulant[c] (usually in therapeutic doses[d,e])

TWO DON'TS
Don't administer coumarin (warfarin) during the acute thrombocytopenic phase of HIT[f] (give vitamin K if coumarin has already been given when HIT is diagnosed)
Don't give prophylactic platelet transfusions[g]

TWO DIAGNOSTICS
Test for HIT antibodies[h]
Investigate for lower-limb deep-vein thrombosis (e.g., duplex ultrasound)[i]

---

[a]These principles apply when HIT is strongly-suspected or confirmed.
[b]Sometimes HIT begins after all heparin has been stopped ("delayed-onset HIT").
[c]Danaparoid (Chapter 16), recombinant hirudin (Chapter 14), and argatroban (Chapter 13) are three alternative, non-heparin anticoagulants that are approved for treatment of HIT, although approval status and drug availability varies in different jurisdictions. Other nonapproved treatment options include fondaparinux (Chapter 17) and bivalirudin (Chapter 16).
[d]Therapeutic-dose regimens include aPTT-adjusted iv dosing schedules for lepirudin and argatroban; for danaparoid, there is evidence that a therapeutic-dose regimen (e.g., initial iv bolus, then 400 U/h iv × 4 h, followed by 300 U/h iv × 4 h, followed by 200 U/h iv (with subsequent dose adjustments made using anti-factor Xa levels, if available) is more effective than low-dose danaparoid (e.g., 750 U b.i.d. or t.i.d. by subcutaneous injection).
[e]There is evidence that therapeutic-dose anticoagulation of "isolated HIT," i.e., HIT recognized because of thrombocytopenia and in the absence of clinically-apparent thrombosis, reduces risk of subsequent thrombosis.
[f]Coumarin is a risk factor for microvascular thrombosis, e.g., venous limb gangrene; further, aPTT prolongation by coumarin can lead to underdosing of lepirudin or argatroban therapy ("aPTT confounding").
[g]Petechiae and other signs of thrombocytopenic bleeding are not characteristic of HIT.
[h]PF4-dependent enzyme-immunoassays have high sensitivity (>99%) for clinical HIT; however, their diagnostic specificity is lower than washed platelet activation assays. In experienced laboratories, the latter "functional" (platelet activation) assays also have high sensitivity for diagnosis of clinical HIT (see Chapter 11).
[i]Up to 50% of patients with isolated HIT have deep vein thrombosis.
Abbreviations: aPTT, activated partial thromboplastin time; b.i.d., twice daily; HIT, heparin-induced thrombocytopenia; iv, intravenous; PF4, platelet factor 4; t.i.d., three times daily.

Index